The Immunopathology of Lymphoreticular Neoplasms

Comprehensive Immunology

Series Editors: ROBERT A. GOOD and STACEY B. DAY

Sloan-Kettering Institute for Cancer Research
New York, New York

The Immunopathology of Lymphoreticular Neoplasms

Edited by

J. J. TWOMEY, M. B. (N. U. I.), F. A. C. P.
Veterans Administration Hospital
Houston, Texas

and

ROBERT A. GOOD, Ph. D., M. D.
Sloan-Kettering Institute for Cancer Research
New York, New York

PLENUM MEDICAL BOOK COMPANY
New York and London

Library of Congress Cataloging in Publication Data

Main entry under title:

The Immunopathology of lymphoreticular neoplasms.

   (Comprehensive immunology; v. 4)
   Includes bibliographies and index.
   1. Lymphoma—Immunological aspects. 2. Reticuloendothelial system—Tumors—Immunological aspects. 3. Immunopathology. I. Twomey, Jeremiah John, 1934-   II. Good, Robert A., 1922-   III. Series. [DNLM: 1. Lymphoma—Immunology. 2. Lymphoma—Pathology. W1 CO4523 v. 4/QZ350 I33]
RC280.L9I45   616.9'94'42   77-27315
ISBN-13: 978-1-4613-4017-1   e-ISBN-13: 978-1-4613-4015-7
DOI: 10.1007/978-1-4613-4015-7

©1978 Plenum Publishing Corporation
227 West 17th Street, New York, N. Y. 10011
Softcover reprint of hardcover 1st edition 1978

Plenum Medical Book Company is an imprint of
Plenum Publishing Corporation

Contributors

Joel Buxbaum   Research Service, Department of Medicine, Manhattan Veterans Administration, New York, New York

Delvyn C. Case, Jr.   Portland, Maine

Max D. Cooper   The Cellular Immunobiology Unit of the Tumor Institute, Departments of Pediatrics and Microbiology, and The Comprehensive Cancer Center, University of Alabama in Birmingham, Birmingham, Alabama

Maria de Sousa   Memorial Sloan-Kettering Cancer Center, New York, New York

Mehdi Farhangi   Department of Medicine, University of Missouri–Columbia, Columbia, Missouri

G. Fernandes   Memorial Sloan-Kettering Cancer Center, New York, New York

Edward C. Franklin   Irvington House Institute, Rheumatic Diseases Study Group, Department of Medicine, New York University Medical Center, New York, New York

Richard K. Gershon   Laboratory of Cellular Immunology, Howard Hughes Medical Institute, and Department of Pathology, Yale University Medical School, New Haven, Connecticut

Robert A. Good   Memorial Sloan-Kettering Cancer Center, New York, New York

Sudhir Gupta   Memorial Sloan-Kettering Cancer Center, New York, New York

William D. Hardy, Jr.   Laboratory of Veterinary Oncology, Memorial Sloan-Kettering Cancer Center, New York, New York

John H. Kersey   Departments of Pediatrics, and Laboratory Medicine and Pathology, University of Minnesota, Minneapolis, Minnesota

Benjamin Koziner   Memorial Sloan-Kettering Cancer Center, New York, New York

Alexander R. Lawton   The Cellular Immunobiology Unit of the Tumor Institute, Departments of Pediatrics and Microbiology, and The Comprehensive Cancer Center, University of Alabama in Birmingham, Birmingham, Alabama

Arthur E. Lindner   New York University School of Medicine, New York, New York

Robert J. Lukes   Department of Pathology, University of Southern California School of Medicine, Los Angeles, California, and Los Angeles County–University of Southern California Medical Center

Daniel Maklansky   The Mount Sinai School of Medicine, New York, New York

Richard H. Marshak   The Mount Sinai School of Medicine, New York, New York

Charles M. Metzler   Laboratory of Cellular Immunology, Howard Hughes Medical Institute, and Department of Pathology, Yale University Medical School, New Haven, Connecticut

Mark E. Nesbit   Department of Pediatrics, University of Minnesota, Minneapolis, Minnesota

Elliott F. Osserman   Department of Medicine, College of Physicians and Surgeons, Columbia University, New York, New York

John W. Parker   Department of Pathology, University of Southern California School of Medicine, Los Angeles, California, and Los Angeles County–University of Southern California Medical Center

Israel Penn   Department of Surgery, University of Colorado School of Medicine, and Veterans Administration Hospital, Denver, Colorado

Guy S. Perry III   Department of Laboratory Medicine and Pathology, University of Minnesota, Minneapolis, Minnesota

Raymond D. A. Peterson   Department of Pediatrics, University of South Alabama College of Medicine, Mobile, Alabama

Jean-Claude Rambaud   Department of Gastroenterology and Research Unit on Physiopathology of Digestion, Hôpital Saint-Lazare, Paris, France

Saul A. Rosenberg   Division of Oncology, Stanford University School of Medicine, Stanford, California

Bijan Safai   Memorial Sloan-Kettering Cancer Center, New York, New York

Maxime Seligmann   Laboratory of Immunochemistry and Immunopathology, Research Institute on Blood Diseases, Hôpital Saint-Louis, Paris, France

Frederick P. Siegal   Memorial Sloan-Kettering Cancer Center, New York, New York

Beatrice D. Spector   Department of Laboratory Medicine and Pathology, University of Minnesota, Minneapolis, Minnesota

Jeremiah J. Twomey   Baylor College of Medicine and Veterans Administration Hospital, Houston, Texas

Nicholas J. Vianna   Cancer Control Bureau, New York State Department of Health, Albany, New York

Norma Wollner   Memorial Sloan-Kettering Cancer Center, New York, New York

Dennis H. Wright   University of Southampton Medical School, Southampton, England

E. J. Yunis   Sidney Farber Cancer Institute, Harvard Medical School, Boston, Massachusetts

Preface

Until recently, understanding of the lymphomas was limited and largely descriptive. Attention has been focused, for the most part, upon morphological issues and clinical matters. Although useful, this approach has many shortcomings. The true cytoidentity of primary neoplastic cells was not established by these methods, nor could their clonal nature be recognized. The more overt changes in immunological function, such as monoclonal gammopathies and immunodeficiencies, were appreciated as important components of these diseases. However, subtle immunological perturbations were not recognized. Furthermore, associations were not established between the lymphoreticular neoplasms on the one hand and both primary and secondary immunological abnormalities on the other. There has been considerable recent progress in the fields of immunobiology, cytology, and immunochemistry. These new approaches have proved readily applicable to studies on the lymphomas.

The term "lymphoma" has been applied to a heterogeneous group of neoplasms that involve lymphoid tissues. This term is not altogether satisfactory, since it implies that cells of primarily the lymphoid series are involved in the neoplastic process. Some neoplasms, heretofore classified as "lymphomas," now appear, from the results of penetrating analysis using newer methodology, to be malignancies of the macrophage series, rather than of the lymphocytic series. These neoplasms include Hodgkin's disease and a minority of neoplasms previously referred to as "histiocytic" lymphomas. The majority of these "histiocytic" lymphomas are now known to be lymphoid malignancies involving the B-cell series. We suggest that *primary neoplasms of lymphoid tissues* is a more accurate descriptive term than "lymphomas" for this group of diseases. In this volume, the knowledge that now exists regarding the two arms of the immune system and their digits has been assembled and used to analyze the nature, pathogenesis, and immunopathology of primary tumors of lymphoid tissues from a modern perspective.

Infection, hemorrhage, and anemia remain cardinal clinical problems with these neoplasms. It has therefore become vitally important to understand the immunological and hematological changes that, in a sense, are consequences of these malignancies. When considering immunological changes, it is important that both positive and negative aspects of immunological controls be brought into account. Clearly, effector, helper, and suppressor cells cooperate to maintain immunological homeostasis. It now appears that these subsets of immune reactive cells are also the primary malignant cells of different neoplasms of lymphoid tissues. These cells and their activities undergo maturation and involution, which are dynamic concomitants of age. They are, in turn, affected by age, virus infections, tissue transplantation, immunosuppressive drugs, and genetic factors. These factors interrelate in special ways to permit the occurrence of neoplasms of this class.

These complex interacting factors are most easily studied from experimental models. There now exists a variety of experimental models of lymphoid and histiocytic neoplasms. These models permit epidemiological studies on vertical and horizontal transmission and on genetic susceptibility to primary neoplasms of lymphoid tissues. Study of these experimental neoplasms suggests new bases for understanding relationships among malignancies of the lymphoreticular system and viral infections, immunological breakdown, autoimmunity, and the major histocompatibility system. These experimental models are highly relevant to their human counterparts, as is exemplified by the combined viral infection and promotor influence(s) that participate in the pathogenesis of Burkitt's lymphoma. There occur in the animal world outbreaks of lymphoma that may reflect underlying infectious processes. These outbreaks in animals may be paralleled in man, as evidenced by contact and familial spread in the epidemiology of Hodgkin's disease. Familial clusters suggest that genetic predisposition, perhaps to oncogenic infection, exists with human as well as with experimental tumors of lymphoid tissues. Furthermore, autoimmune perturbations are coincident to lymphoid tumors in man as well as in certain inbred mice. The infectious basis of many experimental tumors raises the possibility that vaccines will be introduced for experimental systems, and may ultimately be anticipated for some of these diseases in man.

Experimental primary tumors of lymphoid tissues opened the door to the new classifications of the "lymphomas." These experimental models include the lymphoid leukemia in AKR mice and RPLI2-virus-induced visceral lymphomatosis in chickens. These experimental neoplasms made it possible to show that lymphoreticular neoplasms originate focally in central lymphoid organs. These organs include the thymus of AKR mice and the bursa of Fabricius of chickens. These malignancies, like solid tumors, only later spread throughout the lymphoid system and other parts of the body. Prevention of these murine and fowl lymphoid malignancies can be accomplished by surgical removal of the appropriate central lymphoid organ. The nature and other details of these model systems are defined and described in several chapters in this volume.

Of great importance is the high frequency of malignancies in patients with primary, genetically determined immunodeficiency. This relationship was predicted by Lewis Thomas in his initial statement on the modern concept of immunosurveillance. The very special relationship between immunity and the lymphomas is reviewed in this volume. The results of an international effort to collect data on malignancies that occur in patients with primary immunodeficiencies are presented. Although the observations fulfill the predictions that there is a high frequency of cancer in children suffering from primary immunodeficiencies, the data do not support a general concept of faulty immunosurveillance. This survey points out that the malignancies that occur in immunodeficient patients are predominently "lymphomas," "lymphosarcomas," "reticulum-cell sarcomas," gastrointestinal cancers, and brain tumors, but few among the many other kinds of cancer.

Most neoplasms that occur in patients receiving immunosuppressive chemotherapy for organ transplantation are also predominantly lymphoreticular, skin, and brain tumors. These findings are targets for considerable further investigation, which should shed additional light on the etiopathology of these malignancies. Specifically, understanding of the role played by infection, potentially carcinogenic chemicals, antigenic stimulation, and interactions between graft and host in the pathogenesis of these predominantly lymphoreticular tumors could be of great importance. From analysis of experience with malignancy occurring in organ transplant recipients comes the encouraging information that disseminated epithelial cancers with trillions of malignant cells, which occur when malignant cells are inadvertently transplanted along with desired organs, can be eradicated by permitting reemergence of vigorous immune function. This portends much from an immunological approach to the treatment of cancer.

New marker techniques have been introduced that permit the identification of normal polyclonal and neoplastic monoclonal cells. Chapters are devoted to these new techniques and the relationship between data obtained through the use of these techniques and observations made from classic morphological analysis. It is apparent that these advances offer new ways to classify and analyze primary tumors of lymphoid tissues. These new approaches should form the basis for ultimately understanding these malignancies in terms that permit improved treatment and prevention. An important development now possible through technical advances is the ability, in some instances, to identify the cell of origin of lymphomas. Furthermore, it is now realized that with respect to normal cells, the morphology of stimulated lymphocytes differs considerably from that of resting lymphocytes. This new look at morphology, in terms of surface markers, gives additional meaning to follicular arrangements, hairy cell morphology, and nuclear and cytoplasmic features.

Hodgkin's disease receives much attention in this volume. There are observations of fluctuations in immune reactivity from activation to severe immunodeficiency that follow a complex and changing sequence. The immunodeficiency of Hodgkin's disease is placed in focus in terms of its lymphocyte-depleting and recently described suppressor components. This disease is very complex, but its pathophysiology is now becoming understood and its clinical prognosis is rapidly being improved.

A chapter is devoted to dynamic lymphoid cell movement through blood, lymph, and solid lymphoid tissue compartments. The principles of ecotaxis and its perturbations are detailed by one of the founders of this new field.

Important lessons have been learned in the field of molecular biology and, in particular, antibody synthesis, structure, and function, through studies on the lymphoreticular neoplasms. These neoplasms include multiple myeloma, macroglobulinemia, and other lymphoid tumors. A chapter is devoted to the excesses, aberrations, and deficiencies of antibody synthesis with these malignancies. The interference with blood circulation, through hyperviscosity, by excessive amounts of macroglobulins and the correction and treatment of this complication by plasmaphoresis are the results of modern clinical investigation.

Burkitt's lymphoma and its relationship to infectious mononucleosis through the Epstein–Barr virus receives attention. The fascinating clustering of Burkitt's lymphoma and its geographical distribution and epidemiological associations are presented. It is now known that B lymphocytes have receptors for the Epstein–Barr virus. Presumably, B lymphocytes thus infected undergo morphological transformation. This in turn leads to a T-lymphocyte response that includes blast transformation of T lymphocytes. This sequence is the probable explanation for the morphologically bizarre lymphocytes that are characteristic of infectious mononucleosis.

Alpha-chain disease is given special attention because of evidence that interactions between infection and a defective immune system, which probably has a genetic basis, ultimately lead to malignant adaptation. The complete understanding of this model may prove valuable in clarifying the etiopathology of lymphoreticular neoplasms.

The gut is a major lymphoid organ. A chapter is therefore devoted to the characteristic radiological changes observed in the gastrointestinal tract with primary and secondary immunodeficiencies and with the lymphoreticular malignancies. This presentation should prove useful to the physician.

There has been tremendous recent progress in the treatment of primary tumors of lymphoid tissues. A series of chapters is devoted to this subject. The nature and consequences of the immunodeficiencies secondary to these neoplasms are discussed. New approaches to understanding controls over the immune system have been applied to this subject and are greatly enhancing our understanding of these immunodeficiencies.

We hope that this new comprehensive look at the immunopathology of lymphoreticular neoplasms presented in the context of the rapidly expanding new knowledge of the immunological apparatus will contribute to better understanding of these important diseases. It is to be hoped (and we certainly anticipate that it will come about) that new studies from this point of departure will further improve our classifications of these diseases and our understanding of their pathology and pathogenesis and thereby lead to better approaches toward therapy and ultimately provide means of preventing this class of malignancy in man.

Jeremiah J. Twomey, M.D.
Robert A. Good, M.D.

Contents

Chapter 7

Immunodeficiency Diseases and Malignancy   203

*Beatrice D. Spector, Guy S. Perry III, Robert A. Good, and
John H. Kersey*

Chapter 8

Immunosuppression and Malignant Disease   223

Israel Penn

Chapter 9

The Pathology of Lymphoreticular Neoplasms   239

Robert J. Lukes and John W. Parker

Chapter 16
Proliferative Disorders of the T-Cell Series   493
Bijan Safai

Chapter 17
Lymphoreticular Malignancies in Childhood   533
John H. Kersey and Mark E. Nesbit

Chapter 18
Immunodeficiency States Associated with Acute Leukemias, Multiple Myeloma, and Waldenström's Macroglobulinemia   543
Benjamin Koziner and Robert A. Good

1

Development of Lymphoid Tissues

MAX D. COOPER and ALEXANDER R. LAWTON

1. Introduction

Knowledge of the pathways of differentiation of immunocompetent cells holds promise of providing a unique perspective on the biology of cancer. Many lymphoid malignancies of man and animals can now be classified not only as to cell of origin, but also in terms of a precise stage of differentiation of that cell type. Moreover, the oncogenic potential of several animal viruses is restricted both to a particular lymphoid cell type and to a discrete stage in the life history of that cell. Accumulation of more information on the regulation of normal lymphoid differentiation will have an important impact on the diagnosis and treatment of lymphoreticular malignancy.

In this chapter, the development, migratory characteristics, and function of T and B cells will be outlined. Although the emphasis will be on development of the human lymphoid system, we will draw freely on ideas derived from study of a variety of animals under the assumption that the biological principals are likely to be generally valid. Our purpose is to present a selective overview of this area, rather than a comprehensive review, for which the reader is referred to Greaves *et al.* (1973); more detailed information will be provided in subsequent chapters.

2. The T-Cell System

2.1. General Remarks

Lymphoid cells beginning their development within the thymus before migrating to populate the rest of the body play a fundamental role in body defense. All lymphoid cells developing along this axis will be called *T cells* in this discussion,

MAX D. COOPER and ALEXANDER R. LAWTON • The Cellular Immunobiology Unit of the Tumor Institute, Departments of Pediatrics and Microbiology, and The Comprehensive Cancer Center, University of Alabama in Birmingham, Birmingham, Alabama 35294.

although the term T cell was originally used to denote thymus-derived cells; many authorities reserve the term for cells in the periphery and refer to all lymphoid cells within the thymus as *thymocytes*. On recognition of antigens, T cells initiate immunological reactions collectively referred to as *cell-mediated immunity* (CMI). The term CMI originated with observations that this type of immunity could be transferred from one individual to another by lymphoid cells, but not by immune serum. The immunological phenomena that have CMI as their basis include delayed hypersensitivity reactions to protein, bacterial, fungal, and viral antigens; graft-versus-host reactions; and, to a large extent, rejection of histoincompatible grafts and transplanted tumor cells. T cells elicit the cooperation of other cell types, especially macrophages, in these reactions. CMI is essential for host protection in most viral and fungal infections. In addition to their primary responsibility for CMI, T cells play an important role as regulators of B-cell function. For most antigens, specific T-cell recognition is required for triggering B-cell maturation (Katz and Benacerraf, 1972). Besides this helper function, T cells also act as suppressors of humoral and cellular immune responses (see Chapter 2).

2.2. Early Thymus Development

The thymus begins its development by specialized differentiation of endodermal cells lining the 3rd and 4th pharyngeal pouches. Formation of the epithelial thymus begins around the 7th week in human gestation with formation of paired lobes that migrate caudally into the thoracic mediastinal area overlying the base of the heart and great vessels (Norris, 1938). Lymphopoiesis is a secondary development, and after it begins, some of the epithelial cells form whorls called Hassall's corpuscles. Keratin formation accompanies other features of the more differentiated epithelial cells in these distinct thymic structures. The frequent occurrence of cellular debris in Hassall's corpuscles and the tendency for injected particulate substances to be localized here has led to the idea that Hassall's corpuscles perform a cleanup function for the thymus (Blau *et al.,* 1968). The absence of Hassall's corpuscles in the thymus of patients who fail to achieve thymic lymphopoiesis contrasts with their prominence in the "stress-involuted" thymus and is helpful in distinguishing the two conditions.

Although the thymic framework is composed chiefly of epithelial cells, the fully developed thymus also contains reticular stromal cells, mainly in the inner medulla (Pereira and Clermont, 1971), and a few scattered myoid cells that contain striations typical of muscle (Bockman, 1968). These, and the blood vessels of the thymus, are of mesenchymal origin.

2.3. Stem-Cell Migration to the Thymus

This migration has been studied mainly in rodents and chickens. The stem cells that populate the embryonic thymus appear to be relatively large mononuclear cells having an undifferentiated nuclear appearance and cytoplasmic basophilia (Moore and Owen, 1967). Circulating stem cells are attracted by the epithelial thymus at a precise time in its development (Le Douarin and Jotereau, 1975). The nature of the thymic signal and the stem cell's reception of it are still unknown, but the result is stem-cell migration from the circulation through the perithymic connective tissue and thence into the epithelial thymus. The initial inflow of stem cells into the thymus is followed by successive waves of migrant stem cells later in life. Although the extent of this continued traffic is imprecisely defined, it appears to slow with advancing age.

2.4. T-Cell Differentiation within the Thymus

Within the first few days after stem cells arrive in the thymus, they are influenced to begin lymphoid differentiation, a process that involves extensive cell replication and results in compartmentalization of thymic lobules into distinct cortical and medullary zones (Metcalf, 1964; Matsuyama *et al.,* 1966). The youngest thymocytes are located in the cortical areas. Because of their rapid replication rate (mean generation time of approximately 8 hr), large numbers of immature T cells accumulate in the thymic cortex. With maturation, some of these T cells migrate into the thymic medulla and there exhibit a slower rate of cell division. In human fetuses, thymic lymphopoiesis is well under way by the 8th week (Norris, 1938).

Immature cortical thymocytes differ in several ways from the more mature T cells of the medulla (for a review, see Greaves *et al.,* 1973). For example, the latter can recognize and respond to histoincompatible cells and more conventional antigens, and they are responsive to the polyclonal T-cell mitogen, phytohemagglutinin (PHA), while the more numerous cortical thymocytes lack these capabilities. Although medullary T cells are relatively resistant to the cytolytic effects of corticosteroids, cortical thymocytes are very susceptible. The human thymus can therefore be drastically reduced in size by increased levels of corticosteroids of either intrinsic or extrinsic origin (Caffey, 1961).

The growth rate of the thymus is determined primarily by the production rate of thymocytes, since thymocytes are by far the predominant cell type in the thymus of young individuals. In humans, the thymus reaches its peak size near puberty or earlier, when it may weigh as much as 50 g (Boyd, 1932). Thereafter, the rate of T-cell production slowly declines to the point that the thymus of an old person may contain relatively few lymphoid cells and weigh as little as 3 g. As would be expected, the size of the thymus is also influenced by the rate of T-cell destruction and exodus. In young guinea pigs, for example, approximately one quarter of the millions of thymocytes produced each day are exported via the blood (Ernström and Sandberg, 1970). This phenomenon suggests that many emigrant T cells are relatively immature; indeed, evidence obtained in mice indicates the existence in spleen of immature postthymic cells that have a relatively limited life span in the absence of thymic humoral factors (Cantor, 1972) (see also Section 2.9).

2.5. Routes of T-Cell Migration

On leaving the thymus, T cells migrate via the circulation into all the lymphoid tissues of the body, including the spleen, lymph nodes, Peyer's patches, appendix, tonsils, and, to a lesser extent, the bone marrow (Weissmann, 1967) (Table 1). The

TABLE 1. Distribution of T Cells in
Adults[a]

Lymphoid tissue[b]	T-cell content (% ± S.D.)[c]
Thymus (7)	96 ± 3
Lymph node (7)	56 ± 6
Spleen (17)	40 ± 8
Bone marrow (10)	12 ± 8
Blood lymphocytes (16)	75 ± 6

[a]The data were obtained by Dr. C. M. Balch.
[b]The number of specimens examined is given in parentheses.
[c]Determined by enumeration of cells stained by a fluoresceinated antiserum specific for T cells.

mode of exit from the bloodstream has been best studied in lymph nodes (Gowans and Knight, 1964), where it has been shown that lymphocytes slip out between the cuboidal endothelial cells lining postcapillary venules of the paracortex. In all the organized lymphoid tissues, the T cells have special zones of residence that are distinct from those occupied by B cells (Figure 1); T cells accumulate in the paracortical areas of lymph nodes, in cuffs surrounding the penicillary arteries of the spleen, and in the interfollicular areas of the gut-associated lymphoid tissues (Parrott *et al.,* 1966; Howard *et al.,* 1972). Lymphoid cells leave the bloodstream in nonlymphoid tissues as well, but this traffic is usually less heavy except under special circumstances such as localized infections or invasions by other foreign materials.

Most T cells do not remain long in the lymphoid tissues, but migrate through the T-cell zones, enter the efferent lymphatics, and eventually pass through the thoracic duct or other lymphaticovenous communications to reenter the blood (Figure 2). In rodents, lymphocytes that shuttle in this way between blood and lymph may make the entire circuit twice or more in a day. Interruption of this circuit by thoracic duct drainage leads to a drastic depletion of T cells; within a few days, and T-cell zones in lymph nodes may appear virtually vacant (Fish *et al.,* 1970).

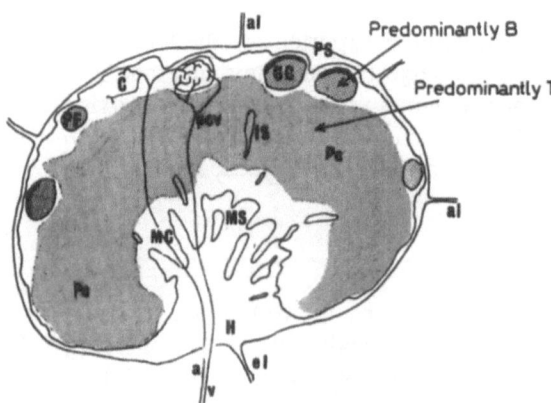

Figure 1. Anatomy of lymph node. (C) Cortex; (Pc) paracortex; (MS) medullary sinuses; (MC) medullary cords; (GC) germinal center; (PF) primary follicle; (H) hilum; (a) artery; (v) vein; (pcv) postcapillary venule; (el) efferent lymphatic; (al) afferent lymphatic; (IS) intermediary sinus; (PS) peripheral sinus. Reproduced from Greaves *et al.* (1973) with permission of the authors and publisher.

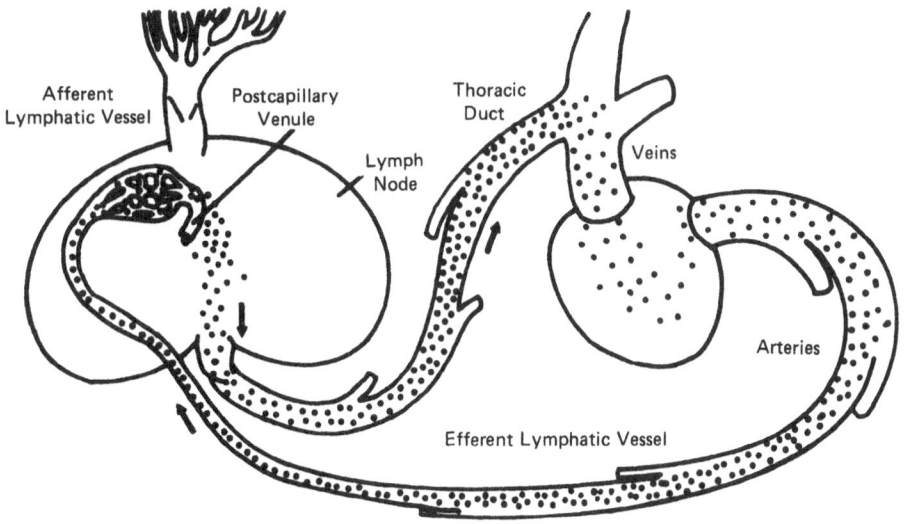

Figure 2. Recirculation of small lymphocytes. Redrawn with permission of the author and publisher from Gowans (1971).

2.6. Life Span of T Cells

T cells are highly variable in their longevity. Some T cells may die even before leaving the thymus (Matsuyama *et al.*, 1966). Others migrate into the intestinal epithelium and may be lost into the gut lumen together with epithelial cells (Lemmel and Fichtelius, 1971). The life span of a T cell can also be shortened by encounter with an antigen for which it has receptors or by exposure to noxious agents such as irradiation or immunosuppressive drugs. Despite all this, many T cells are relatively long-lived. In women given X-irradiation therapy for breast cancer, lymphocytes carrying a radiation-induced, morphologically distinct chromosomal abnormality that could not be passed on to daughter lymphocytes disappeared from the blood with a half-life of 2 years (Ottesen, 1954). From other evidence, life spans of over 10 years have been estimated for human lymphocytes (Buckton and Pike, 1964). Although these studies were done before T and B cells were defined, T cells are generally thought to live longer than B cells. One other point deserves mention. Lymphocyte life spans are usually calculated from the intermitotic period (Everett *et al.*, 1964). Since cell division generally gives rise to identical daughter cells, a short life span does not imply disappearance of the antigen specificity carried by a particular cell.

From this fragmentary picture, it can be deduced that even were the thymic source of T cells obliterated, the T-cell lineage might sustain itself in the body for years. Clinical and laboratory evidence in a few thymectomized patients suggests that this is so, but evidence from mice indicates that some subpopulations of T cells do not survive and function well for long after thymus removal and that the overall functional integrity of the T-cell system eventually diminishes (Taylor, 1965). It therefore seems reasonable to expect that some continuation of lymphopoietic activity in the thymus is needed throughout life. This might be especially important if peripheral T cells were destroyed at an unusually rapid rate.

MAX D. COOPER AND
ALEXANDER R.
LAWTON

2.7. Differentiation Antigens of T Cells

In inbred strains of mice, alloantisera have been produced that recognize antigens that are characteristically present on the surface of T cells but are not detectable on B cells or other types of blood cells (Boyse *et al.,* 1971; Greaves *et al.,* 1973). Some of these, e.g., the Thy-1 antigens, may be shared by other cell types such as brain and skin cells, while others, like the thymus leukemia (TL) antigens, appear to be unique to thymocytes. The stage of differentiation of T cells can be discerned by the variable expression of these antigens at different points in their life history. Stem cells lack these differentiation antigens when they enter the thymus, but are induced to express surface Thy-1 and TL antigens as soon as they begin lymphoid differentiation (Owen and Raff, 1970). By the time of migration from the thymus, T cells no longer express TL antigens, but continue to display Thy-1 antigens, although in reduced amounts.

Alloantisera for human T-cell antigens have not been defined as yet, but antisera against human T cells have been raised in other species. After appropriate absorption, these antisera react specifically with T cells from all locations within the body. The distribution of T cells can be determined using these antisera (Table 1) (see also Chapter 10).

Another practical marker for human T cells in tissues containing a mixture of cell types is the presence of a surface binding site for sheep erythrocytes (SRBC). Incubation of T cells with SRBC in the cold results in SRBC adherence in a rosette distribution around the T cell; these are called *E rosettes,* and virtually all human T cells can form them (see Chapter 10). Galactopeptides on erythrocyte membranes may participate in the formation of these rosettes (Boldt and Armstrong, 1976).

2.8. T-Cell Subpopulations

We have alluded to the existence of subpopulations of T cells that may have different functions, migratory habits, and life spans. One such subpopulation of T cells, defined in mice, home to the spleen and show little tendency to enter the recirculating pool. Another T-cell subpopulation has a homing predilection for lymph nodes and recirculates extensively. The former subpopulation is relatively short-lived and thus depends on continuous replenishment from the thymus to be maintained, whereas the latter subpopulation is more self-sustaining (Cantor, 1972; Stutman, 1975). T-cell subpopulations may exhibit different patterns of responsiveness to the T-cell mitogens, PHA and concanavalin A, and may have different functional capabilities as well. For example, there is increasing evidence in mice that helper T cells, those capable of helping B cells respond to antigen stimulation, and suppressor T cells (see Chapter 2) may belong to distinct T-cell subpopulations. Recent evidence suggests that T-cell subpopulations may express characteristic patterns of differentiation antigens. Alloantigens designated Ly (for lymphocyte) are products of three genetic loci, *Ly1, Ly2,* and *Ly3,* each of which has two alleles. *Ly2* and *3* are closely linked. Approximately half of adult mouse T cells in the periphery express all three antigens, while a third express *Ly1* and approximately 7% *Ly23* exclusively. The *Ly1* and *Ly23* subpopulations have different functions; *Ly1* T cells have helper activity and mediate delayed hypersensitivity reactions, while *Ly23* cells suppress antibody responses and are the source of killer T cells (Cantor and Boyse, 1975a,b).

Recently, subpopulations of human T cells have been defined on the basis of having cell-surface receptors for either IgM or IgG. Approximately 40–70% of circulating T cells have receptors for IgM, and another distinct subpopulation of T cells (3–20%) bears surface receptors for IgG (Moretta *et al.*, 1975, 1976). The functional capabilities of the two subpopulations have yet to be characterized fully, but early results suggest that T cells with IgM receptors can help B cells respond to pokeweed mitogen, whereas T cells with IgG receptors do not help B cells in this experimental system.

2.9. Thymic Humoral Factors

Convincing evidence for a humoral function of the thymus stemmed largely from studies showing that immunological competence of thymectomized mice could be enhanced by implantation of thymus grafts within cell-impermeable diffusion chambers or by injection of thymic extracts (reviewed by Bach *et al.*, 1975; Stutman, 1975). The active factors appear to be low-molecular-weight substances, for a discussion of which the reader is referred to a symposium on the subject (Friedman, 1975). Much of the *in vivo* evidence regarding activity of thymic hormones on T cells suggests that the function of postthymic cells is enhanced by hormonal exposure. Although thymic hormones probably exert most of their influence on T-cell differentiation within the thymus or on postthymic cells, evidence has now been brought forth suggesting that stem-cell commitment to T-cell differentiation may occur at a prethymic level, and that thymus hormones and other agents can induce such cells to begin T-cell development outside the thymic environment (Scheid *et al.*, 1975). This issue must still be regarded as unsettled in our view, since there is much evidence that must be discounted before it can be accepted that T-cell differentiation can normally begin anywhere else than in the thymus. It seems particularly germane to the subject of this book that T-cell lymphomagenesis in mice always appears to begin in the thymus (see Chapter 4).

The available evidence suggests that thymus hormone levels in the circulation are high in young mice, but decline dramatically during adult life (Bach *et al.*, 1975). An inbred strain of mice that appears deficient in thymic hormone production develops first deficiency and later excessive suppressor-T-cell activity and may have an unusually high incidence of lymphomas (Talal and Steinberg, 1974).

2.10. Antigen Receptors of T Cells

There is abundant evidence that T cells carry surface receptors that are complementary to particular antigenic configurations. Clonal distribution of T cells, whereby members of each clone bear receptors for only one or very few antigens, is suggested by the fact that depletion of T cells reactive to one antigen does not eliminate T cells capable of responding to other antigens (Basten *et al.*, 1971). The nature of the antigen receptors for T cells is not so clear. Prior to recognition that T and B lymphocytes were developmentally different populations, it was assumed that antigen-specific receptors for both humoral and CMI reactions would be similar in nature to circulating antibodies. This view was challenged with observations that only B cells were capable of secreting antibodies, and that chickens or humans lacking the B-cell line were still capable of manifesting normal CMI. Following a period of considerable controversy concerning whether or not T cells might synthesize small amounts of immunoglobulins (Ig's) expressed as cell-surface receptors, two major candidates for the role of the receptor have emerged. One possibility is that the receptors are as yet undefined products of the immune response (*Ir*) genes, which are closely associated with the major histocompatibility locus of mouse and man (Benacerraf and McDevitt, 1972). A second, and somewhat more likely, possibility is that T-cell receptors are either Ig's or molecules consisting of the variable portions of Ig's. The latter concept is supported by recent evidence that the receptors of T cells that recognize foreign histocompatibility antigens may be molecules of approximately 40,000 daltons in size that have combining sites very similar or identical to the Ig receptors of B lymphocytes with the same specificity (Binz and Wigzell, 1975). Since a proportion of T cells are capable of binding either IgG or IgM via an Fc receptor, it remains possible that Ig-like molecules found on the surface of T cells may be the products of B cells.

2.11. T-Cell Recognition of Viral Antigens

Virus-specific cytotoxic T cells, generated in infected mice, lyse infected target cells only when both cell types share major histocompatibility antigens (Doherty and Zinkernagel, 1975). The same phenomenon was also shown for other antigens (Shearer, 1974). The simplest explanation of this phenomenon is the "altered-self" concept, which proposes that T cells are sensitized not only against viral antigens, but also against structures coded by major histocompatibility genes that are modified by virus infection or chemical manipulation. While a molecular explanation for this is not yet available, the observations raise important questions, the answers to which should also provide new insight into the nature of T-cell antigen receptors.

2.12. Soluble Factors Produced by T Cells

A low-molecular-weight substance ($\leq$10,000 daltons) called *transfer factor* can be extracted from human lymphocytes. Transfer factor has the capacity to transfer specific CMI from a donor sensitized by previous antigen exposure to a nonimmune recipient (Lawrence, 1969). By inference, transfer factor seems likely to be a product of T cells, but exactly what this antigen-specific factor is or how it works is still unknown, and a counterpart in nonprimate experimental animals has not been verified.

Activated lymphocytes, including T cells, produce a wide variety of biologically active substances that are not antigen-specific; these substances are referred to collectively as *lymphokines* (Bloom and Glade, 1971). Lymphokines serve as biological amplifiers of CMI by attracting and promoting the activity of other cells, particularly macrophages. Most of the lymphokines have been defined by biological assays under *in vitro* conditions. Among them are migration-inhibition factor (MIF), a factor that both activates and inhibits migration of macrophages, and other factors that are chemotactic for a variety of cell types, or are cytotoxic, or can induce blastogenesis of lymphocytes. Interferon is also produced by activated T cells. The nature and activities of these factors are discussed in more detail in Chapter 2.

3.1. General Remarks

Many features of the B-cell line are remarkably similar to those of T cells. B cells come from the same ancestral stem cells, travel virtually the same routes (see Figure 2), albeit more slowly, have their own special zones of residence in lymphoid tissues (see Figure 1), have unique surface antigens, produce many of the lymphokines, and respond to a select group of mitogens. The most unique characteristic of B cells is their commitment to the synthesis of antibodies.

Because of the well-defined and diverse nature of its Ig products, the B-cell system is a favorite model of cell differentiation in higher vertebrates. This popularity has led to a relative wealth of information about this cell line. The ability to identify and accurately measure the various kinds of antibodies has enhanced recognition of both malignancies and deficiencies of members of the B-cell population.

We will emphasize in this discussion of B-cell development the generation of diversity at three different levels: (1) the life history of B cells in terms of stages in cellular differentiation; (2) the generation of diversity in expression of genes coding for the variable regions of heavy and light chains, which together determine antibody specificity; and (3) the generation of diversity in expression of genes coding for the different classes of Ig H chains. Although these are related issues, this division provides a relatively straightforward framework for consideration of abnormalities in B-cell differentiation.

3.2. Basic Structure of Immunoglobulin Molecules

Since B cells are identifiable primarily by Ig expression, we will begin with a brief consideration of Ig structure (Porter, 1967; Edelman, 1970). The basic unit of Ig molecules consists of two paired chains of amino acids (Figure 3). The larger pair are designated *heavy (H) chains;* the smaller are called *light (L) chains.* The four chains of the bi-symmetrical molecule are held together by disulfide bonds. The L chains may be either of two types, κ or λ, although both are always of the same type in any one molecule. Likewise, the paired H chains are always identical, but they may belong to any of five basic types (μ, γ, α, δ, and ϵ), which determine the Ig class of the antibody (IgM, IgG, IgA, IgD, and IgE). Some Ig molecules have additional polypeptide chains, and some form oligomeric associations of two to five paired units of L and H chains. The various combinations are shown in Table 2. Multiple subclasses have been identified within some of the classes. In addition, there are allelic variations in this polymorphic system.

The paired H and L chains of Ig molecules are divided into relatively homologous subunits called *domains,* each composed of around 110 amino acids and containing an intrachain disulfide bond. This type of structure suggests that genes for both chains evolved from a smaller subunit by gene duplication. In terms of amino acid sequence, the L and H chains can be further subdivided into constant regions (C_L and C_H), in which the amino acid sequences are invariant, and variable regions (V_L and V_H). Much of the variability of the V regions is found in small stretches of amino acids that are called *hypervariable;* there are three hypervariable

MAX D. COOPER AND
ALEXANDER R.
LAWTON

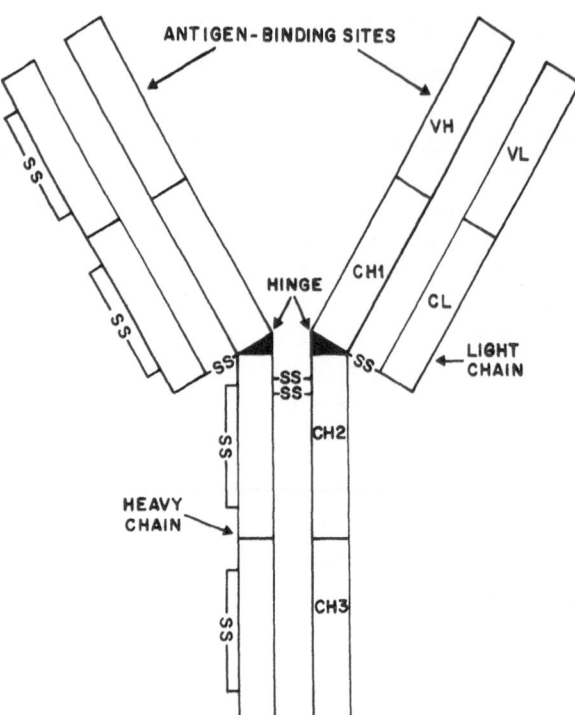

Figure 3. Bilaterally symmetrical basic subunit of the Ig molecule. The subunit consists of paired H and L chains linked by disulfide bonds. Each chain is divided into units called domains, approximately 110 amino acid molecules in length, each of which contains an internal disulfide loop. The amino-terminal V_H and V_L domains have amino acid sequences that vary from one molecule to the other. These variations are present largely in hypervariable regions that form the contact areas of the antigen-binding cleft of the native molecule. The remaining domains (C_L, C_H1, C_H2, and C_H3) have an invariant sequence for molecules of a given H-chain class and L-chain type.

regions in V_L and four in V_H (Capra and Kehoe, 1975). The polypeptide chains are folded so that most of the hypervariable regions form a part of the antigen-binding cleft, one for each V_H–V_L domain (Poljak *et al.*, 1973). The amino acid sequences of the H-chain C-region domains determine the Ig classes and their different biological roles, such as complement fixation and selective transport across membranes.

Antibodies can also serve as antigens; because of the variations in structure of Ig's, antibodies can be raised with specificity for different classes and subclasses of

TABLE 2. Classes of Immunoglobulins

Immunoglobulin	Light chains	Heavy chains	Other chains[a]	Formulas[b]
IgM	κ or λ	μ	J chain	$(\mu_2L_2)_5$ J (serum)
				μ_2L_2 (cell surface)
IgG	κ or λ	$\gamma 1$	None	γ_2L_2
		$\gamma 2$		
		$\gamma 3$		
		$\gamma 4$		
IgA	κ or λ	$\alpha 1$	SC	α_2L_2 (serum)
		$\alpha 2$	J chain	$(\alpha_2L_2)_2$ J SC
IgD	κ or λ	δ	None	δ_2L_2
IgE	κ or λ	ϵ	None	ϵ_2L_2

[a] J (joining) chain is the designation for a polypeptide found in association with polymeric Ig's which may facilitate polymer formation; SC (secretory component) is a polypeptide synthesized by epithelial cells that becomes linked to secretory IgA during transport of this molecule across mucosal surfaces.
[b] L in this column refers to either κ or λ L chains.

Ig H chains, κ and λ L chains, different Ig allotypes, and even the different antigen-combining regions. Such Ig-specific antibodies can be coupled to convenient markers, such as radioactive isotopes, fluorochromes, and large particulate substances, and used to identify the cellular origins of particular kinds of antibodies.

3.3. Genes That Code for Immunoglobulin Determinants

There are three families of Ig genes that are not closely linked and presumably are located on separate autosomes: κ, λ, and H (reviewed by Hood *et al.*, 1975). Each family consists of a group of V genes that are closely linked to a smaller number of C genes. At least four genetic decisions are required for a B cell to make an antibody. With certain exceptions, each B cell makes antibodies of a single class, subclass, L-chain type, allotype, and specificity. The phenomenon of *allelic exclusion*—the term refers to the fact that individual B cells from heterozygous persons express only one Ig allele—indicates that an early genetic decision involves selection of one of the chromosome pairs from each family for expression. Another primary decision is the selection of either the κ or the λ L-chain family. The remaining two decisions involve the pairing of a unique V_L gene with either $C\kappa$ or $C\lambda$, and the selection and pairing of a V_H gene with one of the C_H genes. The V_L and V_H genes to be expressed by the cell apparently are physically translocated to join with C_L and C_H genes, such that a single mRNA for the complete L chain and another for the complete H chain are transcribed (Milstein *et al.*, 1974). Ig molecules are assembled after the synthesis of L and H chains on cytoplasmic polyribosomes (Scharff and Laskov, 1970; Parkhouse, 1973).

3.4. Stages of B-Cell Differentiation

The stem-cell precursors of B cells are thought to be the same as for T cells. It has been postulated that some stem cells become committed solely for differentiation along T and B cell lines, but this concept of a lymphoid stem cell lacks a solid experimental basis. The stem-cell precursors in the yolk sac do not express Ig's at either cytoplasmic or surface levels, whereas this is the primary identifying feature of B cells at all stages of their life history (Figure 4).

3.5. Pre-B Cells

The earliest expression of Ig's in mammals occurs in lymphoid cells of fetal liver (Raff *et al.*, 1976). IgM molecules can be detected within the cytoplasm of large lymphoid cells in human fetal liver by the early part of the 7th week in gestation (Gathings *et al.*, 1976). These cells, which by present convention are called *pre-B cells*, do not have detectable amounts of surface IgM. Such cells are later located exclusively in the bone marrow. They appear to be rapidly dividing cells in humans (Okos and Gathings, 1977) and in mice (Osmond and Nossal, 1974; Ryser and Vassalli, 1974), but their precise kinetics, morphology, and metabolism need further definition.

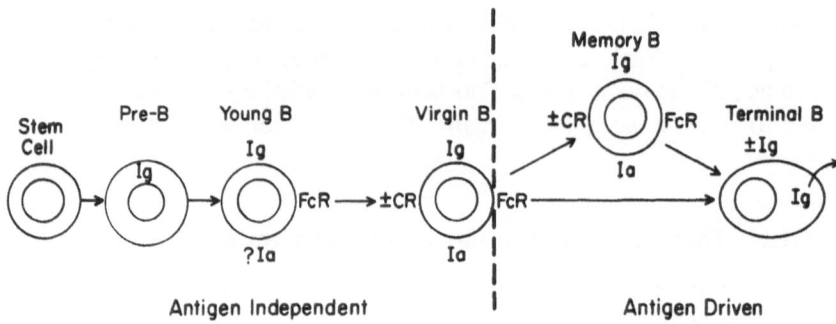

Figure 4. Scheme showing various stages in the development of B cells. The pre-B cell, identified by the presence of intracytoplasmic IgM in the absence of SIg, is thought to give rise to an immature B lymphocyte. Immature B lymphocytes are distinguished from more mature B lymphocytes by the ease with which they are inactivated by cross-linkage of SIg with multivalent antigens or anti-Ig. The acquisition of non-Ig membrane components such as the Fc receptor (FcR), Ia antigens (Ia), and complement receptor (CR) occurs subsequent to expression of cell-surface IgM. These components can be used to aid in estimation of the stage in B-cell maturation, but their roles in this process are still poorly understood.

3.6. Young B Lymphocytes

The expression of surface IgM (SIgM) marks the next stage in B-cell differentiation. The molecular form of SIgM expressed at this stage and also by more mature B lymphocytes is an 8 S monomer, rather than the 19 S pentamer that is secreted by IgM-producing plasma cells (Vitetta and Uhr, 1972). For want of a better term, we will call cells at this stage *young B lymphocytes*. The earliest B lymphocytes appear in human fetal liver during the 9th week of gestation (Lawton *et al.*, 1972); bone marrow later becomes the major site for their production. Young B lymphocytes are relatively small, do not express detectable amounts of IgD on their surface or in their cytoplasm (Gathings *et al.*, 1976), and lack C3 receptors (Gelfand *et al.*, 1974), but appear to have as much SIgM as do B lymphocytes from older subjects (Raff *et al.*, 1975).

With both young and mature B lymphocytes, cross-linkage of SIgM molecules by bivalent antibodies results in capping and subsequent endocytosis of the complex (Raff *et al.*, 1975). An important functional distinction between young and mature B lymphocytes has thus far been determined in mice: young B lymphocytes are very easily and persistently inhibited by cross-linkage of their surface antibodies either by anti-μ treatment or by exposure to the appropriate antigen (Nossal and Pike, 1975; Kearney *et al.*, 1976; Metcalf and Klinman, 1976). This phenomenon may explain the relative ease with which neonatal animals can be rendered tolerant, and seems indicative of an important mechanism for elimination of clones of B cells with antibody receptors directed against self antigens.

3.7. Virgin B Lymphocytes

Virgin B lymphocytes, untouched by antigen, circulate in blood, through lymphoid tissues, and in lymphatic channels. They appear to differ in a number of ways both from their immediate precursors and from memory cells to which they give rise following antigenic stimulation. These mature B lymphocytes lack detectable cytoplasmic Ig, but many bear other classes of SIg's in addition to SIgM. Most simultaneously bear SIgD (Rowe *et al.,* 1973), and a smaller number may also bear SIgG or even SIgA. These cells have roughly 10^5 SIg molecules/cell; these surface antibodies are continually replaced as approximately half are shed each day (Vitetta and Uhr, 1972; Melchers *et al.,* 1975).

In addition to surface antibodies, most virgin B lymphocytes have surface receptors for the Fc fragment of IgG, receptors for activated C3, and poorly defined antigen or antigens that are unique for B lymphocytes (reviewed by Warner, 1974). Most murine B lymphocytes carry alloantigens coded for by *I*-region genes that are located in the major histocompatibility gene complex (Klein, 1975). These Ia antigens may be involved in cooperative interactions between B and T cells (Pierce, S. K., and Klinman, 1975), and may also define different functional subsets of B lymphocytes (Press *et al.,* 1975). Similar alloantigens have now been found on human B lympocytes (Winchester *et al.,* 1975; Mann *et al.,* 1975).

To this point in the B lymphocyte's life history, its differentiation is influenced primarily by intrinsic signals, not by exogenous antigens and T cells. The latter influences or suitable substitutes are required for further B-cell differentiation.

3.8. Memory B Cells

Daughter memory cells are produced when virgin B lymphocytes are induced to divide following contact with an appropriate antigen. In this way, the clonal size is amplified. There is considerable evidence that suggests that memory cells differ in several ways from their immediate precursors (Klinman, 1972; Strober and Dilley, 1973). They appear to circulate more, are more easily triggerable by antigens, are usually smaller, and may have different generation times. Memory cells induced by antigens that elicit little or no T-cell help, or in the absence of T cells, bear SIgM primarily, whereas memory cells produced with T-cell help more often bear SIgG or SIgA (Davie and Paul, 1973).

3.9. Terminal B Cells or Plasma Cells

On contact with antigen, especially with T-cell help, some virgin B lymphocytes and memory B lymphocytes are induced to become plasma cells that synthesize and secrete approximately 1000 identical antibody molecules per second (Salmon and Smith, 1970). The antibodies produced may be of any one of the five Ig classes, depending on the genetic commitment of the individual plasma cells. Some, but not all, plasma cells bear detectable SIg. The SIg may be of a different class than that being produced in the cytoplasm for secretion. For example, plasma cells secreting IgG may express SIgM, reflecting the fact that a switch in expression of Ig H-chain genes has occurred during the life history of that cell or its immediate precursors (Pernis *et al.,* 1971). The class of SIg on IgM-secreting plasma cells always appears to be IgM, and the secreted IgM molecules are usually pentameric.

MAX D. COOPER AND
ALEXANDER R.
LAWTON

Plasma cells normally represent the terminal stage in B-cell differentiation; most apparently die within a few days. However, division of plasma cells or preplasma cells may be especially prominent among myeloma cells.

3.10. Generation of Clonal Diversity

Although immunologists agree that the number of different kinds of antibodies that an individual subject can produce is very large, actual estimates vary from 10^5 to 10^8. Since individual B cells at all stages in their life history make antibodies of identical specificity, or in other words express only one set of V_L and V_H genes, each different potential antibody is represented by at least one lymphocyte. Antibody specificity is determined by both the V_H and V_L regions. The existence of a mechanism allowing for all possible V_L and V_H regions to be paired would therefore reduce the number of V_L and V_H genes required to 1000 for each if the antibody repertoire is one million.

The foregoing considerations indicate that the problem of generation of clonal diversity can be divided into two separate but related issues. The first is the question of how the very large number of V-region genes is generated in the first place, and the second is the program for generating the even larger number of different B-cell clones, each of which expresses just one combination of V_L and V_H genes.

There are two competing types of theories for the mechanism of generating diversity of V-region genes. The germ-line theory holds that all the V-region genes have been generated during evolution, and that each fertilized egg contains virtually all the V genes that may be expressed during the lifetime of an individual subject. Somatic theories hold that the fertilized egg contains a smaller number of V genes, and that during the lifetime of the individual subject, these genes are diversified by mutational events. There are two subdivisions of somatic theories, one in which the mutations occur spontaneously before antigen contact and another in which contact with antigens exerts selective pressure for useful mutations. The evidence bearing on these theories and the arguments for and against each have been reviewed extensively elsewhere (Cohn *et al.*, 1974; Hood *et al.*, 1975) and will not be discussed in detail here.

A large body of evidence bearing on the generation of diversity of antibodies expressed by individual B cells during development places constraints on the various theories mentioned above. In the mouse, the clonal diversity of B cells generated during embryonic life is extensive. By a few weeks of age, generation of clonal diversity appears to be essentially complete (Klinman *et al.*, 1976; D'Eustachio and Edelman, 1975). This is true even for mice born and raised in a germ-free environment. This clearly suggests that exogenous antigens play no significant role in the generation of clonal diversity. An interesting question currently under study is whether or not antibody diversity is expressed by mammalian pre-B cells lacking surface antibodies. Antibody diversity expressed during this stage of B-cell development would almost surely be independent of the influence of either endogenous or exogenous antigens. Evidence obtained in mice and chickens also strongly implies that the generation of B-cell clonal diversity occurs by a pre-programmed sequence of expression. In the chicken, each stem cell appears to give rise to multiple clones of B cells (Lydyard *et al.*, 1976), and this phenomenon was also shown to occur in lethally irradiated mice (Trentin *et al.,* 1967). This has several interesting implications both for normal B-cell differentiation and for the means by which malignant clones of B cells are induced.

In summary, the available evidence favors the idea that clonal diversity of B lymphocytes is developed independently of antigen and in a programmed fashion. This concept is consistent with either the germ-line theory or a somatic mutational mechanism that successively modified a smaller number of germ-line genes. Antigens then selectively induce further B-cell differentiation by triggering precommitted B lymphocytes.

3.11. Generation of Immunoglobulin-Class Diversity

It is now generally accepted that the earliest class of Ig expressed during B-cell differentiation is IgM, and that expression of the other classes of Ig's occurs by a sequential switch mechanism occurring at a gene level. Important issues that remain unresolved are the precise order of the switch in Ig-class expression, the factors that regulate it, and the genetic mechanisms by which it occurs. Nevertheless, because of their importance in considering the mechanisms by which clones of B cells may become malignant, current ideas on these problems will be briefly discussed.

There is abundant evidence that a single V_H gene may become associated with any of the C-region genes for the H chain (Hood *et al.,* 1975). Thus, during development of a single clone, which begins with a progenitor cell expressing a V_H gene together with the μ H-chain gene, a switch may occur to expression of other C_H genes without any change in expression of V_H, V_L, or C_L. It is also known that during clonal development, members of an individual clone may simultaneously produce more than one Ig class as an expression of this switch. Largely on the basis of experiments in chickens, but with consideration of available relevant information in mammals, we originally proposed that this switch occurred (1) within special inductive microenvironments for B-cell differentiation, (2) at a B-lymphocyte level of differentiation, (3) independently of the influences of antigens and T cells, and (4) in the sequence IgM $\rightarrow$ IgG $\rightarrow$ IgA (Cooper *et al.,* 1972; Lawton *et al.,* 1975). In this view, the special need for T-cell help in antigen-triggering of B lymphocytes to mature into IgG- and IgA-producing plasma cells reflects differences in triggering requirements for the different subpopulations of B lymphocytes precommitted to these pathways of plasma-cell maturation. An alternative hypothesis is that T-cell modulation induces the derepression of $C\gamma$ and $C\alpha$ genes during the antigen-driven stage of B-cell differentiation (Pierce, C. W., *et al.,* 1973). There is little doubt that the virgin precursors of plasma cells synthesizing IgG are IgM-bearing cells. The fundamental issue that remains to be resolved is whether the genetic switch has occurred prior to antigen contact, in which case the influence of T cells and antigens is permissive, or whether the gene switch itself is regulated by antigen and T-cell modulation. Another important issue still in contention is the sequence of IgA expression. There is evidence both for the IgG $\rightarrow$ IgA switch, as we proposed, and for a direct IgM $\rightarrow$ IgA switch. It is also possible that both pathways are operative under various conditions.

Another fundamental problem was raised with the discovery that most B lymphocytes in peripheral tissues that bear SIgM also carry SIgD. Because IgD is quantitatively a major class of SIg but is present in extremely small amounts in

MAX D. COOPER AND
ALEXANDER R.
LAWTON

serum, it has been postulated that this Ig class has a unique role as a cell-surface receptor. The possibility that the IgD might precede IgM during primary B-cell development was excluded by ontogenetic studies in man (Gathings *et al.*, 1976) and mouse (Abney and Parkhouse, 1974; Vitetta and Uhr, 1975). Another suggestion is that B cells expressing both SIgD and SIgM are pivotal in the switch to SIgG and SIgA (Vitetta and Uhr, 1975). A likely alternative is that the pivotal cell in the switch to other classes is the early B cell expressing only SIgM (Cooper and Seligmann, 1976). By the time this book is published, this issue should be resolved. This is of obvious importance to a consideration of the means by which malignant accumulation of B cells may occur at different stages in differentiation.

Since the general phenomenon of a switch from IgM to other H-chain classes during B-cell differentiation is firmly established, it is worth considering why the precise details are important. One reason is that more complete understanding of the switch may shed considerable light on the genetic mechanisms involved in joining V and C genes. For example, the existence of a sequential switch from $C\mu$ to $C\gamma$ and then $C\alpha$ might imply a translocation mechanism by which a single copy of a V_H gene was integrated successively with $C\mu$, $C\gamma$, and $C\alpha$ genes linked in that order. On the other hand, the observation that single B cells simultaneously express two Ig classes implies the existence of two integrated V-gene copies. This suggests a mechanism through which mulitple copies of a single V_H gene become simultaneously inserted in front of each C_H gene.

4. Conclusion

An extremely fruitful relationship, unique in many ways, has existed between the basic science of immunology and clinical studies on patients with either immunodeficiency or lymphoid malignancy. The nature of multiple myeloma became apparent after the association of antibodies with the γ-globulin fraction of serum was recognized. Once myeloma proteins were identified as homogeneous products of a single clone of malignant plasma cells, it became possible to establish both the amino acid sequence and three-dimensional structure of antibody molecules. The current hypotheses for the genetic basis of antibody diversity, the concept that two genes are involved in the synthesis of a single Ig chain, and the discovery of hypervariable regions in V genes that determine antibody specificity were all derived from sequence studies of myeloma proteins. From the developmental approach, discovery of independent T- and B-cell lines of lymphoid differentiation made it possible to predict that lymphoid malignancies would belong to one or the other of these lines. This was quickly confirmed for several animal tumors. The discovery of markers for human T and B cells has made it possible to confirm this prediction for many human lymphoid malignancies. As is fully discussed in other chapters, most cases of Burkitt's lymphoma, chronic lymphocytic leukemia, and adult lymphocytic lymphoma represent monoclonal accumulations of B lymphocytes. Thus, the major identifiable stages of normal B-cell differentiation all have their malignant counterparts. (An exception so far is the malignant counterpart for the "pre-B" cell stage, but the search for this has just begun.) Lymphoid malignancies belonging to the T-cell line have also been identified, including the Sézary syndrome and some cases of childhood acute lymphoblastic leukemia.

It seems likely that the pure morphological classification of lymphoid malignancies will soon be replaced by a new system based primarily on relationships to normal pathways of lymphoid differentiation. This approach has already proved extremely valuable. For example, the absence of *monoclonal* lymphoid proliferation, as determined by study of cell-surface markers, often makes it possible to exclude a diagnosis of lymphoid malignancy in patients with primary immunodeficiency in whom clinical evaluation and routine morphological study of biopsy specimens may initially suggest the possibility of lymphoma.

The future holds great promise for parallel advances in both basic immunology and the study of lymphoid malignancy. The existence of monoclonal T-cell lymphomas may serve as the primary resource for unraveling the precise nature of the T-cell receptor for antigen, just as the myelomas made this possible for B-cell antibodies. On the other hand, one of the most fascinating aspects of the genesis of lymphoid malignancy is the tropism of oncogenic viruses in experimental animals not just for either T- or B-cell lines, but also for lymphocytes at a particular point in differentiation. More precise knowledge of the genetic events that regulate lymphoid differentiation should help us learn the ways in which viruses induce malignant transformation.

Note Added in Proof: Since this paper was completed in April of 1976, much new information has been gained with regard to the genetic constraints on functional interactions of cells of the immune system, subpopulations of human T cells, and genetic aspects of the generation of B-cell diversity. In addition, pre-B-cell malignancies have been identified among the acute lymphoblastic leukemias of childhood. Information on these recent developments can be found in Katz (1977), Lawton *et al.* (1978), Moretta *et al.* (1977, 1978), Paul and Benacerraf (1977), Parkhouse and Cooper (1977), and Vogler *et al.* (1978).

References

Abney, E. R., and Parkhouse, R. M. E., 1974, Candidate for immunoglobulin D present on murine B lymphocytes, *Nature (London)* **252**:600–602.

Bach, J.-F., Dardenne, M., Pleau, J.-M., and Bach, M.-A., 1975, Isolation, biochemical characteristics, and biological activity of a circulating thymic hormone in the mouse and in the human, *Ann. N.Y. Acad. Sci.* **249**:186–210.

Basten, A., Miller, J. F. A. P., Warner, N. L., and Pye, J., 1971, Specific inactivation of thymus-derived (T) and non-thymus (B) lymphocytes by ^{125}I-labelled antigens, *Nature (London) New Biol.* **231**:104–106.

Benacerraf, B., and McDevitt, H. O., 1972, Histocompatibility-linked immune response genes, *Science* **175**:273–279.

Binz, H., and Wigzell, H., 1975, Similar or identical idiotypes on IgG molecules and T cell receptors with specificity for the same alloantigens, in: *Membrane Receptors of Lymphocytes* (M. Seligmann, J. L. Preud'homme, and F. M. Kourilsky, eds.), pp. 101–116, North-Holland, Amsterdam—Oxford, and American Elsevier, New York.

Blau, J. N., Jones, R. N., and Kennedy, L. A., 1968, Hassall's corpuscles: A measure of activity in the thymus during involution and reconstitution, *Immunology* **15**:561–570.

Bloom, B. R., and Glade, P. (eds.), 1971, *In Vitro Methods in Cell-Mediated Immunity*, Academic Press, New York.

Bockman, D. E., 1968, Myoid cells in adult human thymus, *Nature (London)* **218**:286–287.

Boyd, E., 1932, The weight of the thymus gland in health and disease, *Am. J. Dis. Child.* **43**:1162–1214.

Boldt, D., and Armstrong, J., 1976, Rosette formation between human lymphocytes and sheep erythrocytes, *J. Clin. Invest.* **57**:1068–1078.

MAX D. COOPER AND
ALEXANDER R.
LAWTON

Boyse, E. A., Old, L. J., and Scheid, M., 1971, Selective gene action in the specification of cell surface structure, *Am. J. Pathol.* **65**:439–450.

Buckton, K. E., and Pike, M. C., 1964, Chromosome investigations on lymphocytes from irradiated patients: Effect of time in culture, *Nature (London)* **202**:714–715.

Caffey, J., 1961, *Pediatric X-Ray Diagnosis,* Year Book Medical Publishers, Chicago.

Cantor, H., 1972, T cells and the immune response, *Prog. Biophys. Mol. Biol.* **25**:73–82.

Cantor, H., and Boyse, E. A., 1975a, Functional subclasses of T lymphocytes bearing different Ly antigens. I. The generation of functionally distinct T-cell subclasses is a differentiative process independent of antigen, *J. Exp. Med.* **141**:1376–1389.

Cantor, H., and Boyse, E. A., 1975b, Functional subclasses of T lymphocytes bearing different Ly antigens. II. Cooperation between subclasses of Ly$^+$ cells in the generation of killer activity, *J. Exp. Med.* **141**:1390–1399.

Capra, J. D., and Kehoe, J. M., 1975, Hypervariable regions, idiotypy and the antibody combining site, *Adv. Immunol.* **20**:1–40.

Cohn, M., Blomberg, B., Geckeler, W., Raschke, W., Riblet, R., and Weigert, M., 1974, First order considerations in analyzing the generator of diversity, in: *The Immune System,* Third ICN–UCLA Symposium on Molecular Biology (E. E. Sercarz, A. R. Williamson, and C. F. Fox, eds.), p. 89, Academic Press, New York and London.

Cooper, M. D., and Seligmann, M., 1976, B and T lymphocytes in lymphoproliferative and immunodeficiency diseases, in: *B and T Cells in Immune Recognition* (F. Loor and G. E. Roelants, eds.), pp. 377–405, John Wiley & Sons, Great Britain.

Cooper, M. D., Lawton, A. R., and Kincade, P. W., 1972, A two-stage model for development of antibody-producing cells, *Clin. Exp. Immunol.* **11**:143–149.

Davie, J. M., and Paul, W. E., 1973, Antigen-binding receptors on lymphocytes, in: *Contemporary Topics in Immunobiology,* Vol. 3 (M. D. Cooper and N. L. Warner, eds.), pp. 171–192, Plenum Press, New York.

D'Eustachio, P., and Edelman, G. M., 1975, Frequency and avidity of specific antigen-binding cells in developing mice, *J. Exp. Med.* **142**:1078–1091.

Doherty, P. C., and Zinkernagel, R. M., 1975, H-2 compatibility is required for T-cell mediated lysis of target cells infected with lymphocytic choriomeningitis virus, *J. Exp. Med.* **141**:502–507.

Edelman, G. M., 1970, The structure and function of antibodies, *Sci. Am.* **223**:34–42.

Ernström, U., and Sandberg, G., 1970, Quantitative relationship between release and intrathymic death of lymphocytes, *Acta Pathol. Microbiol. Scand.* **78**:362–363.

Everett, N. B., Caffrey, R. W., and Rieke, W. O., 1964, Recirculation of lymphocytes, *Ann. N.Y. Acad. Sci.* **113**:887–897.

Fish, J. C., Beathard, G., Sarles, H. E., Remmers, A. R., and Ritzmann, S. E., 1970, Circulating lymphocyte depletion: Effect on lymphoid tissue, *Surgery* **67**:658–666.

Friedman, H. (ed.), 1975, Thymus factors in immunity, *Ann. N.Y. Acad. Sci.* **249**:1–547.

Gathings, W. E., Cooper, M. D., Lawton, A. R., and Alford, C. A., Jr., 1976, B cell ontogeny in humans, *Fed. Proc. Fed. Am. Soc. Exp. Biol.* **35**:393.

Gelfand, M. C., Elfenbein, G. J., Frank, M. M., and Paul, W. E., 1974, Ontogeny of B lymphocytes. II. Relative rates of appearance of lymphocytes bearing surface immunoglobulin and complement receptors, *J. Exp. Med.* **139**:1125–1141.

Gowans, J. L., 1971, Immunobiology of the small lymphocyte, in: *Immunobiology* (R. A. Good and D. W. Fisher, eds.), pp. 18–27, Sinauer Associates, Stanford, Connecticut.

Gowans, J. L., and Knight, E. J., 1964, The route of recirculation of lymphocytes in the rat, *Proc. R. Soc. London Ser. B* **159**:257–282.

Greaves, M. F., Owen, J. J. T., and Raff, M. C., 1973, *T and B Lymphocytes: Origins, Properties and Roles in Immune Responses,* Excerpta Medica, Amsterdam, and American Elsevier, New York.

Hood, L., Campbell, J. H., and Elgin, S. C. R., 1975, The organization, expression, and evolution of antibody genes and other multigene families, *Annu. Rev. Genet.* **9**:305–353.

Howard, J. C., Hunt, S. V., and Gowans, J. L., 1972, Identification of marrow-derived and thymus-derived small lymphocytes in the lymphoid tissue and thoracic duct lymph of normal rats, *J. Exp. Med.* **135**:200–219.

Katz, D. H., 1977, *Lymphocyte Differentiation, Recognition, and Regulation,* Academic Press, New York.

Katz, D. H., and Benacerraf, B., 1972, The regulatory influence of activated T cells on B cell responses to antigen, *Adv. Immunol.* **15**:1–94.

Kearney, J. F., Cooper, M. D., and Lawton, A. R., 1976, B lymphocyte differentiation induced by lipopolysaccharide. III. Suppression of B cell maturation by anti-mouse immunoglobulin antibodies, *J. Immunol.* **117**:1567–1572.

Klein, J., 1975, *Biology of the Mouse Histocompatibility-2 Complex,* Springer-Verlag, New York, Heidelberg, Berlin.

Klinman, N. R., 1972, The mechanism of antigenic stimulation of primary and secondary clonal precursor cells, *J. Exp. Med.* **136**:241–260.

Klinman, N. R., Press, J. L., Sigal, N. H., and Gearhart, P. J., 1976, The acquisition of the B cell specificity repertoire: The germ line theory of predetermined permutation of genetic information, in: *Generation of Diversity: A New Look* (A. J. Cunningham, ed.), p. 127, Academic Press, London.

Lawrence, H. S., 1969, Transfer factor, *Adv. Immunol.* **11**:195–266.

Lawton, A. R., Self, K. S., Royal, S. A., and Cooper, M. D., 1972, Ontogeny of B-lymphocytes in the human fetus, *Clin. Immunol. Immunopathol.* **1**:104–121.

Lawton, A. R., Kincade, P. W., and Cooper, M. D., 1975, Sequential expression of germ line genes in development of immunoglobulin class diversity, *Fed. Proc. Fed. Am. Soc. Exp. Biol.* **34**:33–39.

Lawton, A. R., Kearney, J. F., and Cooper, M. D., 1978, Control of expression of C region genes during development of B cells, in: *Progress in Immunology III,* pp. 171–182, Academic Press, New York.

Le Douarin, N. M., and Jotereau, F. V., 1975, Tracing of cells of the avian thymus through embryonic life in interspecific chimeras, *J. Exp. Med.* **142**:17–40.

Lemmel, E.-M., and Fichtelius, K. E., 1971, Life span of lymphocytes within intestinal epithelium, Peyer's patch epithelium, epidermis, and liver of mice, *Int. Arch. Allergy* **41**:716–728.

Lydyard, P. M., Grossi, C. E., and Cooper, M. D., 1976, Ontogeny of B cells in the chicken. I. Sequential development of clonal diversity in the bursa, *J. Exp. Med.* **144**:79–97.

Mann, D. L., Abelson, L., Harris, S., and Amos, D. B., 1975, Detection of antigens specific for B-lymphoid cultured cell lines with human alloantisera, *J. Exp. Med.* **142**:84–89.

Matsuyama, M., Wiadrowski, M. N., and Metcalf, D., 1966, Autoradiographic analysis of lymphocytopoiesis and lymphocyte migration in mice bearing multiple thymus grafts, *J. Exp. Med.* **123**:559–576.

Melchers, F., von Boehmer, H., and Phillips, R. A., 1975, B-lymphocyte subpopulations in the mouse, *Transplant. Rev.* **25**:26–58.

Metcalf, D., 1964, The thymus and lymphopoiesis, in: *The Thymus in Immunobiology* (R. A. Good and A. E. Gabrielsen, eds.), pp. 150–182, Harper and Row, New York.

Metcalf, E. S., and Klinman, N. R., 1976, *In vitro* tolerance induction of neonatal murine B cells, *J. Exp. Med.* **143**:1327–1340.

Milstein, C., Brownlee, G. G., Cartwright, E. M., Jarvis, J. M., and Proudfoot, N. J., 1974, Sequence analysis of immunoglobulin light chain messenger RNA, *Nature (London)* **252**:354–359.

Moore, M. A. S., and Owen, J. J. T., 1967, Experimental studies on the development of the thymus, *J. Exp. Med.* **126**:715–726.

Moretta, L., Ferrarini, M., Durante, M. L., and Mingari, M. C., 1975, Expression of a receptor for IgM by human T cells *in vitro, Eur. J. Immunol.* **5**:565–569.

Moretta, L., Webb, S. R., Grossi, C. E., Lydyard, P. M., and Cooper, M. D., 1976, Functional analysis of two subpopulations of human T cells and their distribution in immunodeficient patients, *Clin. Res.* **24**:448A.

Moretta, L., Webb, S. R., Grossi, C. E., Lydyard, P. M., and Cooper, M. D., 1977, Functional analysis of two human T-cell subpopulations: Help and suppression of B cell responses by T cells bearing receptors for IgM ($T_{,M}$) or IgG ($T_{,G}$), *J. Exp. Med.* **146**:184–200.

Moretta, L., Ferrarini, M. and Cooper, M. D., 1978, Characterization of human T cell subpopulations as defined by specific receptors for immunoglobulins, in: *Contemporary Topics in Immunobiology,* Vol. 8 (M. D. Cooper and N. L. Warner, eds.), Plenum Press, New York.

Norris, E. H., 1938, The morphogenesis and histogenesis of the thymus gland in man, *Contrib. Embryol.* **27**:193–207.

Nossal, G. J. V., and Pike, B. L., 1975, Evidence for the clonal abortion theory of B lymphocyte tolerance, *J. Exp. Med.* **141**:904–917.

Osmond, D. G., and Nossal, G. J. V., 1974, Differentiation of lymphocytes in mouse bone marrow. II. Kinetics of maturation and renewal of antiglobulin-binding cells studied by double labeling, *Cell. Immunol.* **13**:132–145.

Ottesen, J., 1954, On the age of human white cells in peripheral blood, *Acta Physiol. Scand.* **32**:75–93.

Owen, J. J. T., and Raff, M. C., 1970, Studies on the differentiation of thymus-derived lymphocytes, *J. Exp. Med.* **132**:1216–1232.

Parkhouse, R. M., 1973, Assembly and secretion of immunoglobulin M (IgM) by plasma cells and lymphocytes, *Transplant. Rev.* **14**:131–144.

Parkhouse, R. M. E., and Cooper, M. D., 1977, A model for the differentiation of B lymphocytes with implications for the biological role of IgD, in: *Immunological Reviews,* Vol. 37 (G. Möller, ed.), pp. 105–126, Munksgaard, Copenhagen.

Parrott, D. M. V., DeSousa, M. A. B., and East, J., 1966, Thymus-dependent areas in the lymphoid organs of neonatally thymectomized mice, *J. Exp. Med.* **123**:191–204.

Paul, W. E., and Benacerraf, B., 1977, Functional specificity of thymus-dependent lymphocytes, *Science* **195**:1293–1300.

Pereira, G., and Clermont, Y., 1971, Distribution of cell web-containing epithelial reticular cells in the rat thymus, *Anat. Rec.* **169**:613–626.

Pernis, B., Forni, L., and Amante, L., 1971, Immunoglobulins as cell receptors, *Ann. N.Y. Acad. Sci.* **190**:420–431.

Pierce, C. W., Asofsky, R., and Solliday, S. M., 1973, Immunoglobulin receptors on B lymphocytes: Shifts in immunoglobulin class during immune responses, *Fed. Proc. Fed. Am. Soc. Exp. Biol.* **32**:41–43.

Pierce, S. K., and Klinman, N. R., 1975, The allogeneic bisection of carrier-specific enhancement of monoclonal B-cell responses, *J. Exp. Med.* **142**:1165–1179.

Poljak, R. J., Amzel, L. M., Avery, H. P., Chen, B. L., Phizackerley, R. P., and Saul, F., 1973, Three-dimensional structure of the Fab′ fragment of a human immunoglobulin at 2.8-Å resolution, *Proc. Natl. Acad. Sci. U.S.A.* **70**:3305–3310.

Porter, R. R., 1967, The structure of antibodies, *Sci. Am.* **217**:81–90.

Press, J. L., Klinman, N. R., Henry, C., Wofsy, L., Delovitch, T. L., and McDevitt, H. O., 1975, Ia antigens on B cells: Relationship to B cell precursor function and to surface immunoglobulin, in: *Membrane Receptors of Lymphocytes* (M. Seligmann, J. L. Preud'homme, and F. M. Kourilsky, eds.), pp. 247–258, North-Holland, Amsterdam—Oxford, and American Elsevier, New York.

Raff, M. C., Owen, J. J. T., Cooper, M. D., Lawton, A. R., Megson, M., and Gathings, W. E., 1975, Differences in susceptibility of mature and immature mouse B lymphocytes to anti-immunoglobulin-induced immunoglobulin suppression *in vitro*: Possible implications for B cell tolerance to self, *J. Exp. Med.* **142**:1052–1064.

Raff, M. C., Megson, M., Owen, J. J. T., and Cooper, M. D., 1976, Early production of intracellular IgM by B-lymphocyte precursors in mouse, *Nature (London)* **259**:224–226.

Rowe, D. S., Hug, K., Forni, L., and Pernis, B., 1973, Immunoglobulin D as a lymphocyte receptor, *J. Exp. Med.* **138**:965–972.

Ryser, J.-E., and Vassalli, P., 1974, Mouse bone marrow lymphocytes and their differentiation, *J. Immunol.* **113**:719–728.

Salmon, S. E., and Smith, B. A., 1970, Immunoglobulin synthesis and total body tumor cell number in IgG multiple myeloma, *J. Clin. Invest.* **49**:1114–1121.

Scharff, M. D., and Laskov, R., 1970, Synthesis and assembly of immunoglobulin polypeptide chains, *Prog. Allergy* **14**:37–80.

Scheid, M. P., Goldstein, G., Hammerling, U., and Boyse, E. A., 1975, Induction of T and B lymphocyte differentiation *in vitro*, in: *Membrane Receptors of Lymphocytes* (M. Seligmann, J. L. Preud'homme, and F. M. Kourilsky, eds.), pp. 353–360, North-Holland, Amsterdam—Oxford, and American Elsevier, New York.

Shearer, G. M., 1974, Cell-mediated cytotoxicity to trinitrophenyl-modified syngeneic lymphocytes, *Eur. J. Immunol.* **4**:527–533.

Strober, S., and Dilley, J., 1973, Biological characteristics of T and B memory lymphocytes in the rat, *J. Exp. Med.* **137**:1275–1292.

Stutman, O., 1975, Humoral thymic factors influencing post-thymic cells, *Ann. N. Y. Acad. Sci.* **249**:89–105.

Talal, N., and Steinberg, A. D., 1974, The pathogenesis of autoimmunity in New Zealand black mice, *Curr. Top. Microbiol. Immunol.* **64**:79–103.

Taylor, R. B., 1965, Decay of immunological responsiveness after thymectomy in adult life, *Nature (London)* **208**:1334–1336.

Trenton, J., Wolf, N., Cheng, V., Fahlberg, W., Weiss, D., and Bonhag, R., 1967, Antibody production by mice repopulated with limited numbers of clones of lymphoid cell precursors, *J. Immunol.* **98**:1326–1337.

Vitetta, E. S., and Uhr, J. W., 1972, Cell surface immunoglobulin. V. Release from murine splenic lymphocytes, *J. Exp. Med.* **136**:676–696.

Vitetta, E. S., and Uhr, J., 1975, Immunoglobulin-receptors revisited, *Science* **189**:964–969.

Vogler, L. B., Crist, W. M., Bockman, D. E., Pearl, E. R., Lawton, A. R., and Cooper, M. D., 1978, Pre-B cell leukemia: A new phenotype of childhood lymphoblastic leukemia, *N. Engl. J. Med.* (in press).

Warner, N. L., 1974, Membrane immunoglobulins and antigen receptors on B and T lymphocytes, *Adv. Immunol.* **19**:67–216.

Weissman, I. L., 1967, Thymus cell migration, *J. Exp. Med.* **126**:291–304.

Winchester, R. J., Fu, S. M., Wernet, P., Kunkel, H. G., Dupont, B., and Jersild, C., 1975, Recognition by pregnancy serums of non-HL-A alloantigens selectively expressed on B lymphocytes, *J. Exp. Med.* **141**:924–929.

2

Regulation of the Immune Response

RICHARD K. GERSHON and CHARLES M. METZLER

1. Introduction

The virtually limitless number of foreign antigenic determinants that the immune system must be able to distinguish among and respond to allows for only a relatively small number of cells to be committed to recognizing any one determinant. Clonal expansion is therefore necessary to achieve amplification of the appropriate recognition unit. This process must be carefully regulated because of the severe consequences of excess proliferation of a single clone responding to one foreign determinant, and of the development of clones responding to self-determinants. As a result of this requirement for both amplification and precise regulation, there are a myriad of interactions, both positive and negative, that occur among the cells of the system. The nature and number of these interactions have been extremely hard to determine, principally because insufficient markers have been found to separate the interacting individual components of the system from one another for detailed analysis. Further, even when one of the system's components is isolated and studied, a Heisenberg-like principle of uncertainty exists: one can never be sure that the isolated component behaves in the same fashion in isolation as it does when being stimulated by signals from other parts of the interacting system.

The behavioral interdependence of individual components of the endocrine system prompted endocrinologists to think of an endocrine orchestra. A. J. S. Davies (1968) once suggested that immunologists might borrow this metaphor from the endocrinologists and think in terms of an immunological orchestra. At first, this orchestra was known to be composed of at least three major sections: T cells, B cells, and macrophages (Figure 1). Shortly thereafter, the orchestra grew in size when it became clear that the three major sections could be broken down into

RICHARD K. GERSHON and CHARLES M. METZLER • Laboratory of Cellular Immunology, Howard Hughes Medical Institute, and Department of Pathology, Yale University Medical School, New Haven, Connecticut 06510.

RICHARD K.
GERSHON AND
CHARLES M.
METZLER

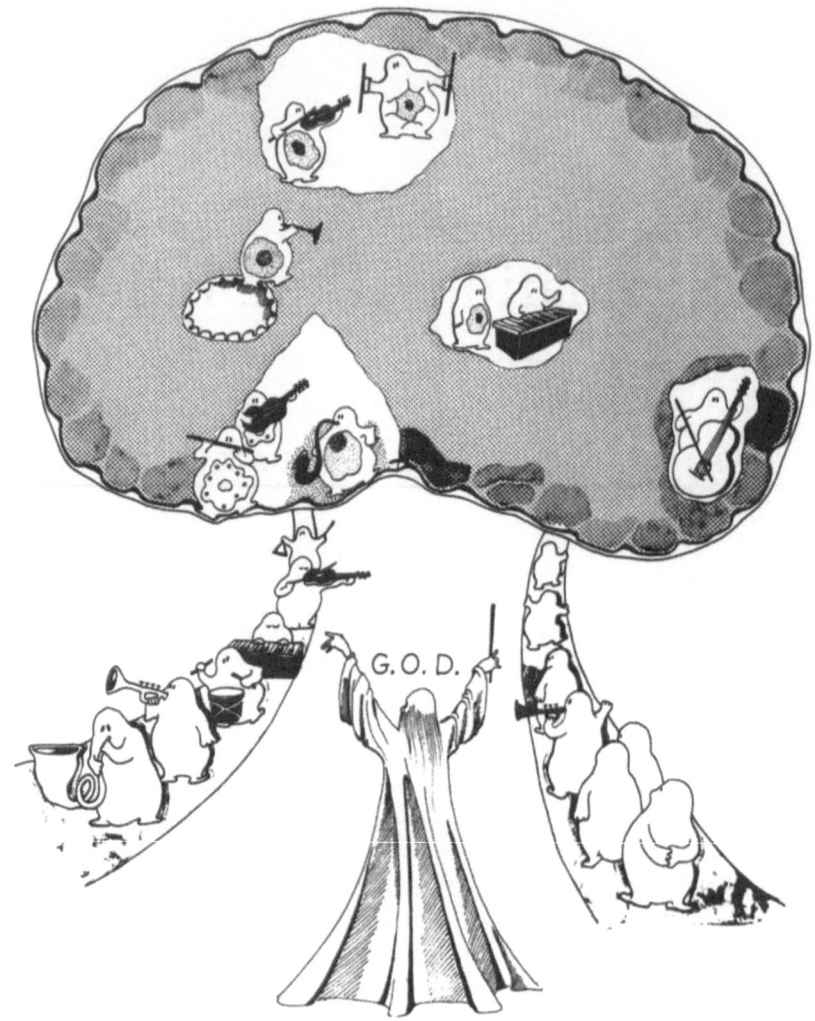

Figure 1. The Immunological Orchestra, *circa* 1968. At that time, the orchestra was known to be composed of at least three major sections: B cells (found in the follicles), T cells (found in the interfollicular cortex and migrating through postcapillary venules), and macrophages (dendritic cells in the follicles and sinusoidal lining cells). Plasma cells (found in the medullary cords) were known to be descended from B cells. At that time, the Generator of Diversity (G.O.D.) was the subject of intense curiosity, and thus was an ideal candidate for the conductor of the orchestra.

subsections—by both physical and anatomical methods of fractionation—and by function.

Most germane to the subject of control of the immune response was the observation that T cells could act as suppressor cells as well as helper cells (Gershon, 1973). This dual functional capability inherent in the T-cell pool made this cell population an excellent candidate for conductor of the immunological orchestra (Figure 2). Recently, Cantor and Boyse (1975a,b) employed antisera directed against the Ly differentiation antigens (described in Chapter 1) to show that helper *(Ly1)* and suppressor *(Ly23)* T cells belong to different stable cell populations. In addition, they defined a third subclass of T cells *(Ly123)* that cannot, as yet, be shown to be preprogrammed. Thus, the notion of a single conductor of the immunological orchestra is no longer tenable, and we have depicted the latest model of the orchestra in Figure 3. Most of the information that forms the basis for this model comes from studies of experimental rodents, but it is highly likely that the immune

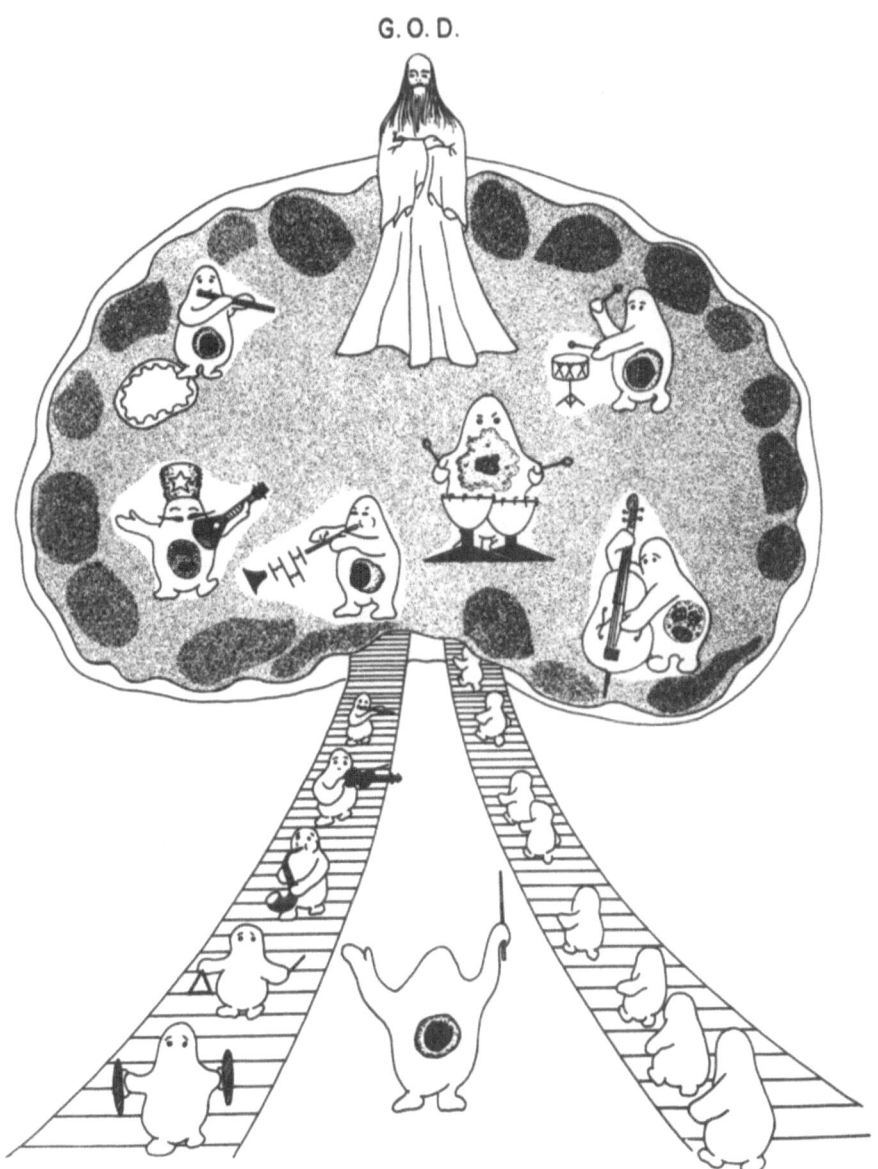

G. O. D.

Figure 2. The Immunological Orchestra, *circa* 1974. Around 1974, the orchestra had expanded to include basophils (lower right-hand corner) and eosinophils (lower left-hand corner), as well as monocytes, macrophages, B cells, and T cells. In addition, the recognition that T-cell regulation consists of both positive and negative signals resulted in the promotion of the regulatory T cell to conductor of the orchestra; the Generator of Diversity (G.O.D.) was relegated to emeritus status.

RICHARD K.
GERSHON AND
CHARLES M.
METZLER

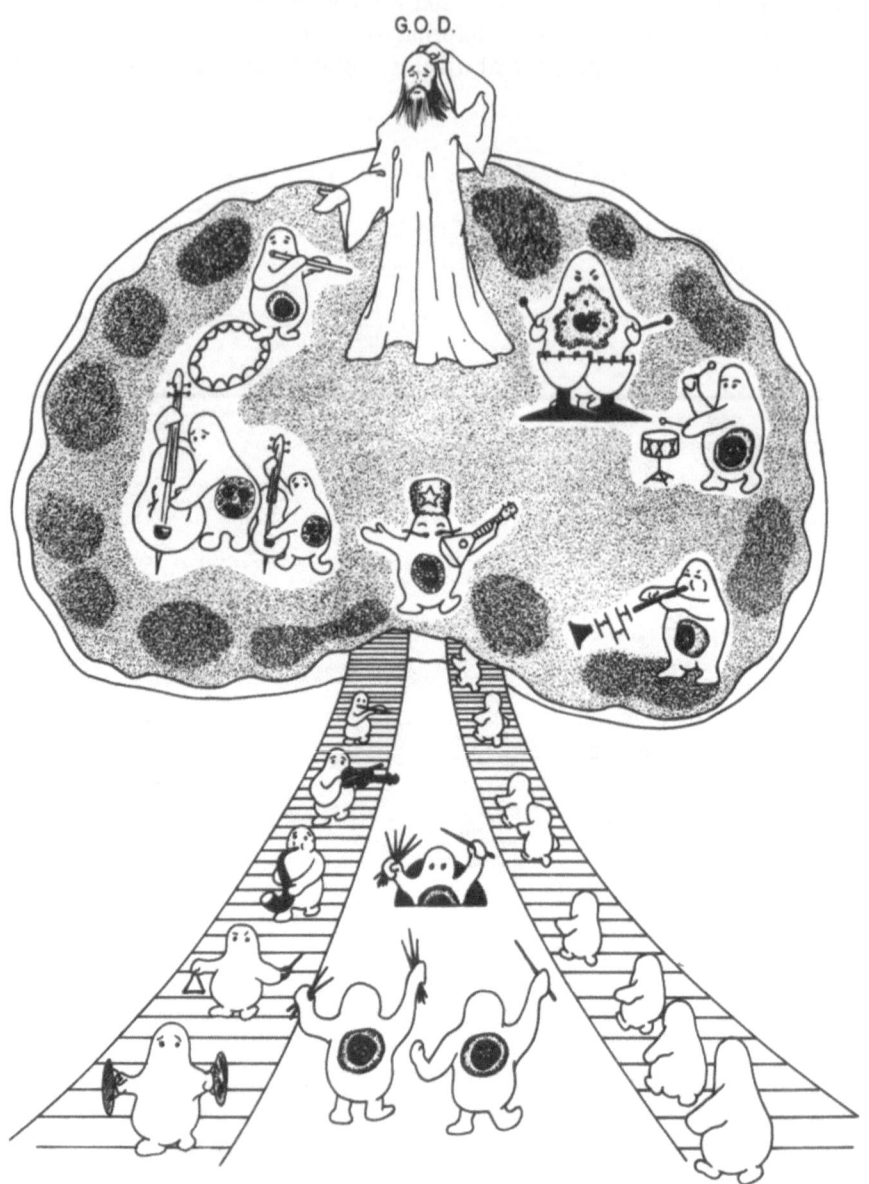

Figure 3. The Immunological Orchestra, *circa* 1978. The major change from the previous orchestra was brought about by the recognition that regulatory T cells are composed of three distinct subclasses: an *Ly1* helper cell (right-hand conductor), an *Ly23* suppressor cell (left-hand conductor), and an *Ly123* cell (in cue box), which regulates both the *Ly1* helper cell and the *Ly23* suppressor cell. The complexity of the interactions among the regulatory *Ly123* cell and the other two conductors is reflected by the change in the attitude of the Generator of Diversity (G.O.D.)

response of humans is similarly structured. In fact, a number of homologies have already been noted. In this chapter, we will try to describe some of the mechanisms by which the immune response is known to be controlled.

2. The T-Cell System

At present, the T-cell population can be subdivided into five functionally distinct classes: helper T cells, amplifier T cells, killer T cells, delayed-type-hypersensitivity-producing (DTH) T cells, and suppressor T cells. It is not yet known whether the T cells that mediate graft rejection, either graft-versus-host or host-versus-graft, are included in one of the five populations listed above or whether these cells belong to a separate subclass or subclasses. Each of these subclasses plays an important role in controlling the immune response.

2.1. Helper T Cells

The idea that thymus-derived lymphocytes (now called *T cells*) help non-thymus-derived lymphocytes (now called *B cells*) to make antibody was first suggested by the work of Claman and Chaperon (1969), and was firmly established by the studies of Davies (1969) and his colleagues and Miller and Mitchell (1969). Claman and Chaperon showed that thymus-derived lymphocytes could interact with lymphocytes from the bone marrow synergistically in the antibody response to sheep red blood cells (SRBC). Davies and his associates and Miller and Mitchell carried this work one step further. They mixed thymus-derived lymphocytes with antigenically different bone-marrow-derived lymphocytes so that one or the other of the two interacting cell populations could be removed after immunization. They found (as had Claman) synergistic interactions between the thymus-derived and bone-marrow-derived lymphocytes and also noted that the bone-marrow-derived lymphocyte was the producer of antibody.

The finding of cooperation between T and B cells in the production of an antibody response stimulated a reinvestigation of the earlier work of Ovary and Benacerraf (1963), who showed that hapten-specific anamnestic responses display marked carrier specificity. It was shown that this phenomenon was due to the interaction of two independent cell types, one of which reacted to the carrier and the other to the hapten (Rajewsky *et al.*, 1969; Katz *et al.*, 1970a,b; Mitchison, 1970, 1971). It could be inferred that the carrier-immune cell was a T cell and the antibody-producing, hapten-immune cell was a B cell. However, it was not until Raff (1971), following the lead of Reif and Allen (1964), showed that mouse T cells contained a distinctive surface differentiation antigen (originally called *Theta*, now called *Thy-1*) that distinguished them from other lymphocytes that this interpretation could be definitively established.

We emphasize this point because a recurring theme in immunology is that progress is made in dissecting the cellular basis of the immune response when new stable surface markers are discovered, which then allows further separation of lymphocyte subpopulations. Most of the discoveries of new lymphocyte subpopulations have been made in the mouse because of the finely understood genetics of this species and the availability of multiple inbred strains. Differentiation antigens often have allelic forms (i.e., they are similar to allotypes on immunoglobulins). Therefore, cross-immunization between closely related inbred strains can result in the production of antibodies that recognize one or the other alleles of the differentiation antigens. The lack of multiple inbred strains in other species has made the production of such antibodies in them more difficult. Nonetheless, human T cells can now be separated from other peripheral blood lymphocytes because of their peculiar affinity for SRBC, with which they form rosettes (Jondal *et al.*, 1973). This T-cell-rosette technique has allowed significant progress to be made in understanding the cellular basis for the human immune response. It is also important to point out that the finding that affinity to SRBC was a marker for human T cells probably could not have been understood or interpreted had not the dissection of T-cell responses been previously done in the mouse. It was the availability of murine models that made it feasible to define the human population of cells that form rosettes with SRBC.

The mechanism by which the T cell helped the B cell was obscure, but two general theories were put forward. One required intimate cell contact between the two interacting cell populations; the other suggested the production of humoral factors that operated at some distance. The humoral-factor theory was greatly enhanced by Feldmann's work, which showed that T and B cells could collaborate across a cell-impermeable membrane (Feldmann and Nossal, 1973). Since that time, a number of T-cell released factors with helper function have been described. Some of these factors are specific for the antigen that induces their production; i.e., they help only an immune response involving the antigen that induced their production, or they can be absorbed by the specific antigen, or both limitations obtain. Another group of helper factors has no demonstrable antigen specificity and is made in abundant amounts during mixed lymphocyte reactions *in vitro*. Marrack and Kappler (1976) showed that specific and nonspecific factors are made by different T cells during an *in vitro* immune response. It is not known how many different specific and nonspecific T-cell helper factors exist; however, there are probably more than one of each type.

2.1.1. Nonspecific Factors

Shimpl and Wecker (1975) described a non-antigen-specific factor called *thymus-replacing factor* (TRF) that is made by T cells, enhances the antibody response of thymus-depleted spleen cells, does not contain determinants that map to the major histocompatibility complex (MHC), and shows no genetic restriction (i.e., it can work on cells that are genetically disparate with the cells that make the factor, even though this incompatibility may lie within the MHC). TRF has significant affinity for Fc-like receptors on macrophage membranes (Gershon *et al.*, 1977). *Allogeneic effect factor* (AEF), which also augments immune responses nonspecifically, was first described by Katz (1972) and co-workers, and can produce effects similar to those produced by TRF. This factor, however, does contain MHC-coded antigens and does show genetic restriction, in that it will not augment the response of most cells bearing MHC antigens different from those found on cells that originally produced the factor. The affinity of AEF for macrophages is unknown.

2.1.2. Antigen-Specific Factors

Two classes of specific helper factors similar to the nonspecific helper factors mentioned above have been described: one that contains MHC-coded antigens and one that does not. Taussig *et al.* (1975) described an antigen-specific factor that contains antigens coded for by genes mapping in the MHC, but the activity of which is not totally restricted by the MHC of the target cells; i.e., it can help allogeneic or even xenogeneic cells. Feldmann described two antigen-specific helper factors. The initial factor he discovered was considered to be similar to monomeric IgM and had a reasonably high affinity for macrophages and did not contain MHC antigens (Feldmann and Nossal, 1973). More recently, Feldmann found another helper factor that is as specific as antibody, contains determinants coded for by the MHC, also has affinity for macrophages, and in fact requires the presence of macrophages in assay cultures for optimal activity (Feldmann *et al.*, 1975).

2.1.3. Other Factors

In addition to the factors listed above, numerous other T-cell-dependent factors that augment immune responses have been documented. These are generally referred to as *lymphokines* (see Section 2.4). In the recently published comprehensive review of the literature by Waksman and Namba (1976), some attempt has been made to organize and classify the factors made during the course of an immune response.

Thus, it is clear that helper T cells can make a battery of factors that can help B cells respond to antigen. Some of these factors have specificity for the stimulating antigen, some do not. The macrophage, by binding these factors, may act as an important intermediary in the transmission of signals from the helper cell to its target cell.

2.1.4. Fine-Tuning

The effect of helper T cells on B cells is more than a simple boost of activity. For example, helper T cells play an important role in determining the isotype of the antibody made (i.e., whether the antibody will be of the IgM, IgG, or IgE class) (Ishizaka, 1976; Press *et al.*, 1976). Generally, IgM antibodies tend to be less thymus-dependent than other classes (Davies, 1969). Helper T cells can also determine the allotype of the antibody made (Herzenberg *et al.*, 1975). In addition, the amount of T-cell help engendered by a given antigen is very important in determining the increase in affinity that occurs during the course of an immune response: the greater the helper activity, the more high-affinity antibody made (Gershon and Paul, 1971). Helper T cells may also play an important role in determining the heterogeneity of the immune response (Civin *et al.*, 1976), and sometimes even the net charge of the antibodies (Karniely *et al.*, 1973). Thus, the role of higher T cells is not only to increase the antibody response, but also to fine-tune its positive aspects.

2.1.5. Summary

In summary, the helper-T-cell pool is undoubtedly heterogeneous, although the exact amount of its heterogenity is not clear. Helper cells produce a battery of different factors, many of which are being elucidated at present. Some of the factors contain antigens coded for by the MHC and appear to be very important in regulating cell interactions. Macrophages are also extremely important in helping

RICHARD K.
GERSHON AND
CHARLES M.
METZLER

cell interactions take place. Gene products of the MHC expressed on macrophage membranes contribute to their ability to interact with helper T cells or helper-T-cell factors or both (Gershon et al., 1977; Rosenthal and Shevach, 1976). That some helper-T-cell factors work optimally when attached to macrophage membranes makes the old question whether helper T cells work by direct action on the B cell or via humoral factors somewhat obsolete, since humoral factors may be involved, but cell-to-cell contact may still be necessary.

2.2. Amplifier T Cells

Soon after the observation that synergistic interactions occurred between T and B cells, Cantor and Asofsky (1970), while studying graft-versus-host (GVH) responses, made the observation that there were similar synergistic interactions among cells within the T-cell pool. On the basis of this work, Raff and Cantor (1971) were able to divide T cells into two subpopulations. One subpopulation, found predominantly in the thymus and spleen, was called *T-1*. These cells were considered to be relatively immature and short-lived, generally noncirculating, radiosensitive, and insensitive to the effects of small doses of antilymphocyte serum (ALS) and thoracic duct drainage. T-1 activity declined considerably within a month after adult thymectomy. The second T-cell subpopulation, called *T-2*, is found predominantly in lymph nodes and the thoracic duct. This subpopulation contained more mature, long-lived cells that turned over their DNA very slowly, if at all (unless stimulated with antigen), and was relatively unaffected by adult thymectomy. Thus, workers were able to obtain enriched populations of T-1 cells by treating animals with limiting doses of ALS, and enriched populations of T-2 cells by performing an adult thymectomy and waiting a month or two.

With the use of these techniques to fractionate the T-cell pool, it was shown that interactions similar to those described in GVH responses occurred in the generation of cytotoxic effector T cells (see Section 2.3). In these interactions, it was shown that the helper effects came from the T-1 cell, while most of the cytotoxic effector cells came from the T-2 cell pool (Wagner, 1973; Cantor and Simpson, 1975). That the helper T cell for B-cell responses was found predominantly in the T-2 cell class (Cantor and Simpson, 1975) indicated that helper cells for cell-mediated immunity (CMI) might come from a different subclass than the T cells that helped B cells make antibody. However, with the development of the ability to further fractionate the T-2 subclass by means of the differential expression of Ly antigens on cells in this subclass, it was shown that the T-2 pool contains a helper cell for cytotoxic effector cells as well as for B cells (Cantor and Boyse, 1975a,b). In addition, it was shown that T-1 cells can augment the activity of the T-2 cell that acts as a helper for B cells, and that this augmentation can occur across a cell-impermeable membrane (Feldmann et al., 1975). Thus, T-1 cells can augment the generation of T helper cells of at least two different types: one that helps cytotoxic effector cells and another that helps B cells. Both types of helper T cells are found predominantly in the T-2 cell pool. Thus, it is probably most appropriate to refer to T-1 cells as amplifier cells that can increase helper-T-cell activity independently of the targets of the T-cell help.

2.3. Killer T Cells

Brunner and Cerottini (1971) were the first to establish that appropriately immunized T cells could lyse tumor cells or other cells that bore the antigens to which the T cells were immune. The lytic activity of these cells can be assayed *in vitro* using ^{51}Cr-labeled target cells (Cerottini and Brunner, 1971). This cell-mediated lympholysis (CML) test is used in clinical studies of T-cell function in humans as well as in experimental studies in rodents. The exact function of these *cytotoxic effector cells* (also referred to as *killer T cells*) in controlling the immune response is still not known, but because killer T cells have often been found to be present in animals at the height of graft rejection, it is generally assumed that they play an important role in the rejection process. Recent work also suggests that killer T cells are very important in antiviral immunity, since they kill virus-infected cells that express virally coded antigens on their surfaces (Doherty *et al.*, 1976). Killer T cells are subject to positive control by helper T cells in a fashion that seems quite similar to the way in which helper T cells enhance the antibody response of B cells (see Section 2.2). It is not known whether helper T cells for B cells form a distinct subclass from those that help killer T cells, but this would seem to our mind most probable, because either humoral immunity or cellular immunity may be individually expressed, depending on the type of immunization employed (Lagrange *et al.*, 1974). At present, however, no markers are available to fractionate helper-T-cell populations (they all have the same Ly phenotype); therefore, this point must remain conjectural.

2.4. Delayed-Type-Hypersensitivity-Producing T Cells

The classic prototype for a DTH response is the tuberculin reaction. It is called delayed because it usually takes 24–48 hr to develop after the eliciting antigen is inoculated into the skin. The reaction is sometimes preceded by the wheal and flare, which is called an immediate reaction, because it occurs in minutes and is mediated by reaginic antibody. It may also be preceded by another form of immediate hypersensitivity, the Arthus reaction, which takes about 3 hr to appear after the eliciting antigen is inoculated and is mediated by antibody and complement. DTH responses [which are clearly in a separate subclass from killer T cells (Huber *et al.*, 1976), although both are antibody- and complement-independent], are initiated by recirculating T cells (Johanovsky *et al.*, 1971). On contact with an antigen that they have previously seen, these recirculating T cells call forth other cells, such as the bone-marrow-derived monocytes, which normally do not recirculate (i.e., they do not get out of the blood and into the lymph with great ease) (Lubaroff and Waksman, 1968). At the site of the DTH reaction, these monocytes then differentiate into macrophages that ultimately cause the induration associated with this reaction (Lubaroff and Waksman, 1968).

There are other forms of DTH, however, in which the predominant cell called forth is not the monocyte. One such reaction, cutaneous basophil hypersensitivity (CBH), is usually produced by sensitizing either with low doses of antigen or with incomplete, instead of complete, Freund's adjuvant (Dvorak and Dvorak, 1974). CBH reactions are much less indurated than are classic DTH reactions. Immunization with many parasites also leads to the production of another form of DTH in which eosinophils are the predominant cells called forth (Warren *et al.*, 1967). Depending on the nature of the antigen and the mode of immunization, T cells therefore have the ability to call forth various types of effector cells from the blood to the site of the reaction. Thus, cells that do not ordinarily recirculate can enter the tissues and help to eliminate the foreign material. The mechanism by which T cells perform DTH functions is not fully understood. It has been shown, however, that T cells producing DTH, or associated with cells producing DTH, can make a battery of soluble products called lymphokines.

The initial lymphokine described by Bloom and Bennett (1966) as well as by David (1966) was called *migration-inhibition factor* (MIF) because this substance could inhibit the migration of macrophages out of capillary tubes *in vitro*. Since that time, a plethora of lymphokines have been described (see Waksman and Namba, 1976). Some act as chemotactic agents for the effector cells mentioned above. Others seem to be able to activate, arm, and generally enhance the functional capabilities of the effector cells brought to the site.

Besides calling forth effector cells from the blood and activating them at the site of the reaction with antigen, T cells mediating DTH either directly or indirectly cause contraction of the endothelial cells of small blood vessels, thus permitting entry of the effector cells into the site (Gershon *et al.*, 1975). At least one of the T-cell-released lymphokines has itself a direct effect on vascular permeability (David and David, 1972), but in addition, T cells can also cause tissue mast cells or basophils to release vasoactive substances. It was recently shown that without either the direct or the indirect action of T cells on vascular permeability, DTH responses will not occur because the effector macrophages cannot get out of the blood (Metzler and Gershon, 1978).

Activation of T cells that mediate DTH has many parallels with activation of helper T cells. For example, molecules that can serve as carriers in the helper-T-cell response can also produce DTH responses. In general, small molecules that function only as haptens cannot elicit DTH responses unless conjugated to a carrier.

Contact hypersensitivity is another example of a DTH response. It is probably produced in a fashion similar to other DTH responses, but there may be subtle differences. In contact hypersensitivity, it is assumed that when reactive haptens conjugate to self-proteins, they alter those proteins sufficiently for them to be recognized as foreign, allowing them to serve as carrier molecules. Reactive haptens are also known to alter proteins sufficiently so that these proteins can act as carriers in the antibody response. In fact, a good mechanism for breaking the tolerant state is to haptenize proteins to which experimental animals have been rendered tolerant (Weinbaum *et al.*, 1974).

2.5. Suppressor T Cells

The major T-cell functions heretofore discussed are all on the positive side. In addition to this positive control, T cells, or more precisely a subpopulation of T cells, exert negative control on the immune response. This subpopulation of T cells has been called *suppressor T cells* (Gershon *et al.*, 1972).

2.5.1. In Tolerance Induction and Maintenance

Suppressor-T-cell activity has been associated with many forms of immunological tolerance, including both high-zone (Gershon, 1973) and low-zone (Kolsch *et al.*, 1975) tolerance, and with tolerance induced by all types of antigens (Gershon, 1973). In these instances, tolerant animals have been shown to possess T cells that when mixed with normal cells, render the normal cells unresponsive to the specific antigen. Despite the plethora of recent demonstrations of suppressor-T-cell activity in tolerant animals, there are still a significant number of reports of experimentally produced tolerance in which exhaustive searches for suppressor T cells have proved fruitless (Weigle *et al.*, 1975). Of course, as the old saying goes, absence of proof is not proof of absence.

Since studies using Ly and MHC antisera to fractionate T cells indicate that suppressor T cells form a distinct subclass of cells that is always present (Herzenberg *et al.*, 1976; Murphy *et al.*, 1976), all immune responses must reflect a balance between helper and antagonizing suppressor-T-cell activity. Thus, although the mechanisms for making the suppressor effect dominant are not fully understood, some suppressor-T-cell activity is probably always present. Immunological experiments that fail to reveal their activity must therefore be interpreted with caution. We will quote one particular experiment to illustrate this point.

Chiller and Weigle (1973) studied mice made tolerant to human γ-globulin (HGG). They found that several months after tolerance induction, the mice remained completely unresponsive to HGG. However, B cells taken from these tolerant mice could respond as well as B cells taken from nontolerant mice when mixed with normal T cells. On the other hand, the T cells of the tolerant mice could not help normal B cells in the response to HGG. Thus, the authors concluded that at this stage, tolerance in the whole animal existed only at the T-cell level. They also looked for suppressor-T-cell activity by mixing cells from the tolerant animals with normal cells, then transferring this mixture to irradiated, neutral recipients. No suppressor-T-cell activity could be demonstrated in these experiments; therefore, one would predict that the tolerant state of these animals could be broken simply by restoration with normal T cells. Chiller and Weigle, however, were unable to restore the immune response by injecting up to 10^8 normal spleen cells into the tolerant animals. Why this inoculation failed to break the tolerant state is not clear. One possibility that must be considered is that suppressor-T-cell effects were dominant in the intact animal, but when the cells were removed and transferred to irradiated recipients, conditions were such that the suppressor-T-cell effect was circumvented. This interpretation is supported by the findings of Benjamin (1975), who used exactly the same tolerance induction model as Chiller and Weigle, but varied the assay technique for demonstrating suppressor-T-cell activity. He was able to show that specific suppressor T cells were indeed present at the time Chiller and Weigle were unable to find them.

For unknown reasons, it is easier to demonstrate suppressor-T-cell effects by injecting cells into a suppressive environment than by removing the suppressor cells from the suppressed mouse and assaying them *in vitro* or in adoptive transfer studies. In fact, one can sometimes find hidden memory cells in an unresponsive animal simply by taking the cells and testing them *in vitro* (Gershon, 1973). Recently, Eardley *et al.* (1976) defined some of the conditions necessary for demonstrating suppressor-T-cell activity. They found that the amount of helper activity in the assay population was a crucial determinant: the more active the helper T cells were, the greater was the suppressor activity in the test population. Thus, although it is highly likely that suppressor T cells are important in the induction or the maintenance of immunological tolerance, or in both, more information is needed to establish their exact role in the tolerance phenomenon.

Another question that has not yet been answered is whether tolerance to thymus-dependent antigens can be induced in mature B cells in the total absence of suppressor T cells. Now that antigenic markers that define suppressor T cells as a distinct subclass of cells have been discovered, these points can be tested. Preliminary evidence from Dr. Harvey Cantor's laboratory indicates that removal of the suppressor-T-cell subclass makes it extremely difficult and perhaps even impossible to produce tolerance (Cantor, H., personal communication). Although these results are based on very limited numbers of observations at this time, they seem to indicate that in some instances the association of suppressor-T-cell activity with immunological tolerance is more than fortuitous, and is probably causative. An interesting observation that might be interpreted to suggest that suppressor-T-cell activity is involved in the induction of self-tolerance is that T cells of newborn mice exert potent suppressor-T-cell activity in multiple assays (Mosier et al., 1975). Thus, it seems that functional suppressor activity precedes helper activity in ontogeny.

2.5.2. In Antigenic Competition

In the tolerance situations discussed above, suppressor-T-cell effects are highly specific; yet in other situations, suppressor T cells can also have nonspecific effects (compare these effects with the specific and nonspecific helper-T-cell effects discussed in Section 2.1). Thus, suppressor-T-cell activity can account for the phenomenon known as *antigenic competition* (Gershon and Kondo, 1971), which can be defined as a temporary state of anergy induced by immunization. It usually occurs after a strong immunization with a thymus-dependent antigen. Although it is known that in many cases this temporary period of anergy is due to suppressor-T-cell activity, the method through which it is effected is at present obscure. It seems likely, however, that in some human conditions, of which sarcoid is the classic prototype, there exists a state homologous with experimental antigenic competition (Kantor et al., 1976). Both are situations in which chronic persisting antigenic stimulation can keep nonspecific suppressor T cells continually active. If and when tolerance to the persisting antigen is induced, the suppressor-T-cell activity falls off and the anergic state disappears (Gershon, 1973; Kantor et al., 1976).

2.5.3. In Responses to Thymus-Independent Antigens

Some nonprotein antigens, which are poorly degradable and have multiple repeating determinants (such as the capsular polysaccharide of the pneumococcus bacillus or the artificial compound polyvinyl pyrrolidone), are called *thymus-independent antigens* because the immune response they elicit in T-cell-deprived animals is the same as the one they elicit in normal animals, indicating that they neither require nor benefit from significant amounts of T-cell help under normal circumstances. Furthermore, these antigens are unable to stimulate T-cell-dependent responses such as DTH. It has been shown that at least one of the reasons these antigens fail to elicit a thymus-dependent response is that they preferentially activate suppressor T cells that prevent the development of any helper cells. Thus, animals that are partially, but not totally, deprived of T cells make better responses than do normal animals, indicating that T cells with the potential to help the response can be found if suppression is alleviated (Baker, 1975). An interesting aspect of these antigens is that while they seem to activate specific suppressor T cells that prevent helper-T-cell effects from occurring, they are very poor at stimulating the nonspecific suppressor T cells that are responsible for antigenic competition (Moller, 1971). Thus, it may be that the reason these antigens seem to preferentially activate suppressor T cells is not that they are especially potent at activating suppressor T cells, but rather that they are poor at stimulating helper T cells. The administration of high doses of a thymus-dependent antigen, such as SRBC, can also produce a suppressor-cell predominance (Gershon *et al.*, 1974a). In this instance, however, a great deal of antigenic competition is produced, suggesting that suppression is effected by a different mechanism; i.e., these latter antigens activate lots of helper cells, but even more suppressor cells. Further evidence for this latter mechanism has been obtained by removing suppressor T cells either with cytotoxic drugs such as cyclophosphamide (Askenase *et al.*, 1975) or with Ly antisera (Weitzman *et al.*, 1976). Such treatments uncover a great deal of suppressed helper cells.

The preferential stimulation of suppressor T cells by polysaccharide antigens probably has significant survival value. Since the target of the suppressor T cell seems to be predominantly the helper T cell, which is important for the IgM-to-IgG switch (Davies, 1969) as well as for the production of high-affinity IgG antibody (Gershon and Paul, 1971), it is good that most polysaccharide antigens fail to produce such T-dependent antibodies. Were these antibodies produced, the maternal–fetal compatibility could be severely compromised, since the incidence of hemolytic disease of the newborn produced by maternal–paternal ABO incompatibility would be a severe problem. It is fortunate that most of the antibodies made against the ABO carbohydrate blood groups are IgM, which does not cross the placenta, or low-affinity IgG, which does not produce significant disease in the newborn, as do antibodies against the Rh blood group (see Pollack and Mollison, 1976).

2.5.4. In Autoimmunity

Dysfunction of suppressor-T-cell activity has been associated with several autoimmune disorders in experimental animals. The most striking one is the disease of New Zealand Black (NZB) mice, which mimics human lupus erythematosus in many ways. Long ago, it was noted that it was extremely difficult to make NZB mice tolerant to any experimental antigen (Staples and Talal, 1969). Later discoveries showed that when the mice were somewhere between the age of 6 weeks and 6 months, suppressor-T-cell activity became hard to detect in several assay systems (Dauphinee and Talal, 1973). Prior to 6 weeks of age, the suppressor activity seemed to be normal. Based on these observations, Steinberg *et al.* (1975) attempted to prevent the development of NZB disease, which usually occurs between the ages of 6 and 12 months, by injecting mice every 2 weeks with thymus cells from mice less than 1 month old. This regimen proved to be eminently successful and prevented the occurrence of autoantibodies and NZB disease in recipient mice. These results strongly suggest that suppressor-T-cell dysfunction may be an important cause of some autoimmune diseases. This contention is further supported by the role that suppressor T cells seem to play in some examples of *Ir*-gene-mediated control of the immune response.

We will discuss *Ir* genes at greater length in Section 5, but it is important to note at this juncture that many human diseases of suspected autoimmune etiology are significantly linked to certain *HLA* haplotypes. Most *Ir* genes in experimental animals are very closely linked to the MHC; therefore, it is not unreasonable to think that some human autoimmune diseases, particularly those that are linked to the human MHC, are due to some suppressor T cell dysfunction.

RICHARD K.
GERSHON AND
CHARLES M.
METZLER

2.5.5. In Fine-Tuning the Immune Response

Suppressor T cells have also been shown to play an important role in setting the level of an immune response, and in that sense it has been suggested that they could be thought of as "thymostats" (Gershon, 1974). It has been found that both immune B cells and immune T cells can trigger suppressor-T-cell activity in a non-immune-T-cell population (Gershon *et al.*, 1974c; Eardley and Gershon, 1975). When suppressor cells are triggered, they then act to prevent further recruitment of other cells into the response, but may not necessarily inhibit or shut off the memory cells that were previously generated and that were responsible for the suppressor-T-cell activation. In fact, some adjuvants have been shown to work by making memory helper T cells increasingly resistant to the effects of suppressor-T-cell activity (Gershon, 1973). Thus, there clearly seems to be some form of communication between helper and suppressor cells that is responsible, at least in part, for the level at which any given immune response is set.

2.5.6. In Chronic Allotype Suppression

Another interesting example of suppressor T cell activity is illustrated by the studies of the Herzenbergs and their co-workers on chronic allotype suppression (Herzenberg *et al.*, 1975, 1976). Many immunoglobulin (Ig) molecules exist in one of two allotypic forms. When an individual subject is heterozygous at the genetic locus that codes for the allotype, the phenomenon of allelic exclusion occurs; i.e., the subject will make both allotypic forms of the Ig, but an individual cell will make only one of the two possible forms. If the heterozygous subject is exposed to antibody against one of the two allotypes *in utero,* Ig bearing that allotypic marker becomes suppressed and usually remains suppressed for a short period after birth. In most cases, the allotype eventually reappears in normal amounts. In some special cases, however, the allotype starts to reappear and then disappears again, and remains absent for the life of the individual. This second disappearance is referred to as *chronic allotype suppression.* It has been shown that chronically allotype-suppressed mice have suppressor T cells that, when mixed with normal cells, can specifically suppress the response to antigen of Ig's bearing that allotypic marker. In this case, the suppressor T cells do not necessarily suppress the general antibody response to antigen, but suppress only the production of antibodies that bear the specific allotypic markers. The target of the chronic allotype suppressor T cell is the helper T cell, not the B cell. This is particularly interesting because there is no evidence that the helper T cell bears allotypic markers. The question therefore becomes: what marker on the helper T cell is the suppressor T cell seeing? The best hypothesis at present is that the *helper* T cell can recognize allotypic markers on the B cell, and that is how specific allotype cooperation is effected. The suppressor T cell sees the helper cell's recognition unit for the allotype, which could be considered to be an idiotypelike marker.

2.5.7. In Idiotype Suppression

The term *idiotype* refers to those specific amino acid sequences in the variable (V) region of Ig's that give them their unique ability to recognize antigen. For example, an antibody that reacts with a SRBC must have a different combining region than an antibody that recognizes bovine serum albumin (BSA). Because of this difference, their combining sites will be antigenically different, and antibodies can be raised against these unique sites. These antiidiotype antibodies have been made and can compete with antigen for the combining sites of the antibody. They have been shown to be able to suppress the production of idiotype (Cosenza and Kohler, 1972; Hart *et al.*, 1972; Eichmann, 1974), in a fashion similar to the way in which antiallotype antibodies can suppress the production of allotype. Another interesting parallel exists: under some circumstances, antiidiotypic antibody can lead to the generation of specific suppressor T cells that suppress only a given idiotype. For example, Eichmann (1975) showed that mice immunized with the carbohydrate moiety of *Streptococcus* A make a number of antibodies, one of which bears what is called the A5A idiotype. Under appropriate conditions, antibodies made against the A5A idiotype can suppress that idiotype and also cause the production of suppressor T cells, which also suppress the production of that specific idiotype. It should be emphasized that these suppressor T cells do not suppress the antibody response to *Streptococcus* A. All the other antibodies that can react with *Streptococcus* A but that *do not* bear the A5A idiotype are made in near-normal amounts. Only the given idiotype is suppressed. [It should also be pointed out that other regimens of giving antiidiotype antibody can cause the production of helper cells (Eichmann and Rajewsky, 1975).] This work has potentially far-reaching implications, and in a broad sense supports the network theory of Jerne (see Hoffmann, 1975). It may form a very important mechanism of immunoregulation. At the least, these idiotype-specific and allotype-specific suppressor T cells indicate that there are potentially many markers on lymphocytes that other lymphocytes can react with and can utilize for the fine regulation of the immune response.

2.5.8. In Human Immunological Disease

All the information discussed above comes from studies on experimental rodents. In 1975, Waldmann and his associates presented evidence that suppressor T cells may be involved in the pathogenesis of certain immunodeficiencies in humans (Waldmann *et al.*, 1975). They found that T lymphocytes isolated from some patients with common variable hypogammaglobulinemia could inhibit pokeweed mitogen-induced *in vitro* Ig production of normal cells. Recently, this work has been confirmed in other laboratories, and excess suppressor-T-cell activity has been implicated in other human diseases (Siegal *et al.*, 1976; Litwin and Zanjani, 1977). In addition, an animal model has been developed by Blaese *et al.* (1974) in which chickens rendered agammaglobulinemic by bursectomy and irradiation develop suppressor T cells that can produce agammaglobulinemia in normal birds.

2.5.9. Suppressor Factors

a. Specific Factors. Several groups of workers have isolated factors that can exert specific, potent suppressor activity. The best-characterized factor was initially isolated by Tada *et al.* (1975) from thymus cells and from splenic T cells of mice immunized with keyhole limpet hemocyanin (KLH). This factor is similar in many ways to the helper factor originally described by Taussig and Munro (see Section

2.1.2), in that it shows antigen specificity, is considerably smaller than Ig, and contains antigens coded for by the MHC. It differs in several respects in that it does not appear to be secreted into the medium by cultured cells; extraction procedures are required for its isolation. In addition, the activity shows strong genetic restriction; i.e., it will work optimally only on cells from mice with the same MHC haplotype as the cells that made it. Another important difference is that the MHC antigen it carries is coded for by a different subregion *(I-J)* than is the helper factor. Products of this particular MHC subregion are found only on T cells (Murphy *et al.,* 1976). Kapp and Benacerraf (1976) described an apparently identical factor in a different antigenic system, but their factor shows much less MHC restriction. Interestingly, these factors do not appear to work on helper cells or B cells. Rather, they seem to be part of a feedback loop in which suppressor cells recruit more suppressor cells from a cell pool that has not yet fully differentiated to a suppression path (Tada, T., and Benacerraf, B., personal communication). Thus, this factor is most likely a suppressor-inducer rather than a direct suppressor.

Asherson and Zembala (1976) described an antigen-specific factor that acts in suppressing contact hypersensitivity. This factor, like some of the helper factors mentioned above, has a relatively high affinity for macrophages. The molecular nature of this factor is not as well characterized as the factor described by Tada and Kapp and Benacerraf, although it does bear MHC antigens. One observation indicating that the factor may be different is that it is secreted into culture medium and does not need to be extracted.

b. Nonspecific Factors.   Another suppressor factor that bears MHC antigens was described by Rich and Rich (1976). The antigens on this factor, however, are coded for by a different subregion of the MHC *(I-C)* than are those on the factor described by Tada and Kapp and Benacerraf. This factor is secreted into culture medium during a mixed-lymphocyte reaction (MLR), as are the TRF and AEF helper factors described above. Like them, it lacks antigen specificity, and like AEF, its target cell must express antigens coded for by the same subregion of the MHC as the cells that made the factor for it to be optimally effective.

A number of other nonspecific suppressor factors of widely differing chemical compositions have been described (see Waksman and Namba, 1976). One of the most interesting of these is called soluble immune response suppressor factor (SIRS) and is released from suppressor T cells when they are stimulated with concanavalin A (Con A) (Pierce and Kapp, 1976). SIRS has many physical and chemical similarities to MIF and, like some of the other factors described above, has a significant affinity for macrophages. It does not contain MHC antigens. Interestingly, it has proved to be very difficult to obtain this factor after stimulating T cells from old NZB mice with Con A (Krakauer *et al.,* 1976). It would appear that measuring the ability of human cells to make this factor after stimulation with Con A could prove to be a very useful measure of suppressor-T-cell status in some diseases of immunological origin.

2.5.10.   Markers on Suppressor Cells

We mentioned in Section 2.5.9a that a factor extracted from suppressor T cells bears an antigen coded for by a special subregion of the MHC (the *I-J* subregion). This antigen can be found on the membrane of the suppressor cells.

One other interesting marker on suppressor T cells is a receptor that has a high affinity for histamine (Eichmann, 1975). Thus, it is quite possible (or perhaps even likely) that suppressor cells are capable of recognizing feedback signals from mast cells and basophils, and thus these cells are also important in the network that controls the immune response.

2.5.11. Amplification of Suppression

In Section 2.2, we described a classification of T cells into T-1 and T-2 categories. Both helper and suppressor T cells belong to the T-2 category. We also discussed amplifier cells that fall into the T-1 category. It turns out that T-1-like amplifier cells can increase not only helper activity, but also suppressor activity (Feldmann *et al.,* 1977). It is not known whether the same amplifier cell works on both helper cells and suppressor cells. Both types of amplifiers fall into the *Ly123*$^{+}$ class in mice.

It has often been noted that when T-1-cell activity is reduced, suppressor cell activity becomes much harder to demonstrate (Gershon, 1973). Although it is possible that this observation may be due to a loss of suppressor amplifier cells, the dramatic nature of the effects indicates that there may be cells in the T-1 population that can act directly as suppressors. Clearly, newborn mice have very few (if any) T-2-type cells (Raff and Cantor, 1971), yet their T cells can act as potent suppressor cells.

This brings us full circle to the Heisenberg-like principle mentioned at the beginning of this chapter. Since T-2 cells must be present in an assay culture for a response to occur, and since it has been shown that some cells make molecules that induce suppressor-cell activity, we cannot yet be absolutely certain that a T-1 cell can directly suppress helper T cells. More markers for T-cell subpopulations are required before this point can be made with certainty. Nonetheless, whether their mechanism of action is amplification, induction, or direct suppression, it is clear that T-1 cells can functionally produce strong immunosuppression.

2.5.12. Summary

In summary, although suppressor and helper T cells have distinct antigenic markers that define them as separate subpopulations, there is little else that distinguishes them. They both have amplifier cells that affect their function. They both make factors that have a number of similarities, including their specificity and absence of specificity, their affinity for macrophages, and the presence of MHC antigens in their factors. They intercommunicate in that the activity of one population affects the activity of the other. Thus, a "Newtonian transplant" performed by Gershon (1974) when he stated the "second law of thymodynamics" remains apropos: "For every helper T cell effect there seems to be an equal and opposite suppressor T cell effect." Whether tolerance or immunity results depends on numerous conditions that are slowly but surely being elucidated.

3. The B-Cell System

T cells or their products are not the only controlling factors in the immune response; B cells and macrophages also play an important role. The most important

RICHARD K.
GERSHON AND
CHARLES M.
METZLER

and best-studied mechanism of B-cell control of the immune response is via the production of antibody. Antibody may feed back and prevent the production of more antibody, and it may also interfere with CMI. This latter situation is the basis for the phenomenon known as *immunological enhancement,* by which passive transfer of serum from tumor-immune mice can lead to enhancement of the growth of transplanted tumors (Uhr and Moller, 1968). Antibody can enhance the growth of tumors or otherwise act as an immunosuppressive agent in at least three different ways: by an afferent, an efferent, or a central mechanism.

In the afferent mechanism, antibody reacts with antigen prior to the antigen's interacting with the cells of the immune system. This diverts the antigen to nonimmunological parts of the reticuloendothelial system (e.g., liver), and clears the antigen from the system before it has a chance to stimulate a response. In the efferent mechanism, antibodies that are incapable of either eliminating or inhibiting the stimulating antigen are made. These antibodies may be ineffective because the antigen-bearing cells or organisms are resistant to the lytic effects of antibody and complement, or because it may be non-complement-fixing antibody. In either case, the antibody can compete with more efficient antibodies or immune cells for antigenic sites, thus preventing the effective immune response from interacting with the target antigen. In the central mechanism of enhancement, the antibody alters the antigen's interaction with the immune system in such a way that suppressor elements dominate over helper effects.

The afferent, blocking effect of antibody is probably responsible for the inability to actively immunize newborn children, since the presence of passively acquired maternal antibodies blocks the antigen's path to the immune system. This mechanism is also operative in the suppression of the anti-Rh antibody response of Rh-negative mothers bearing Rh-positive offspring (see Pollack and Mollison, 1976). In this instance, Rh antigen is not released in significant amounts into the maternal circulation until the placenta separates. If anti-Rh antibodies are administered within 3 days following separation of the placenta, the maternal anti-Rh antibody response is completely suppressed. As a consequence of this ability to suppress the maternal Rh response with anti-Rh antibodies, the problem of erythroblastosis fetalis has been almost eliminated. In some instances, the afferent mechanism may act only at the B-cell level due to different antigen-dose requirements for triggering of T cells and B cells. Thus, it has been shown in some cases that when passive antibody completely blocks a primary antibody response, the generation of memory T cells can take place during the inhibited response (Gershon, 1973).

The most important area in which the efferent mechanism appears to be operative is tumor immunity (Uhr and Moller, 1968). Many tumors are resistant to antibody-mediated cytolysis, but are sensitive to cell-mediated killing. High titers of antibodies can successfully compete for antigenic sites on the tumors and, in so doing, prevent effector cells from killing the tumor. This mechanism is also probably operative in other instances in which organisms or cells are resistant to antibody-mediated killing, or in which a large amount of non-complement-fixing antibody is made.

Evidence for the central effect of antibody-mediated suppression is less strong. It has been shown, however, that passive antibody can cause some antigens to preferentially activate suppressor T cells, which those antigens would not have activated in the absence of passive antibody (Gershon *et al.,* 1974b). There are two possible mechanisms behind this preferential activation of suppressor cells. One is the ability of antibody to change the physical state of antigen. At some molar ratios of antigen to antibody, soluble complexes are formed. It is well known that soluble antigens are poor immunogens and can activate suppressor T cells. Another possible mechanism is via the antibody's interaction with Fc receptors on subsets of T cells; removal of the Fc fragment from antibody can markedly inhibit its suppressive effects (Sinclair, 1969).

In some instances, adoptive transfer of B cells that seem to be making very little antibody has been noted to produce immunosuppression (Gershon *et al.,* 1974c; Asherson and Zembala, 1976). Thus, it is possible that B cells may also regulate the immune response by means other than production of antibody. At the moment, however, because of the well-known highly suppressive effects of antibody, it must be assumed that it is via their production of antibody that these B cells produce immunosuppression. It is important to keep an open mind, however, because other mechanisms may also be operative. It has also been shown that the inhibitory capacity of antibody is quite dependent on its affinity; the higher its affinity, the more suppressive it is (Walker and Siskind, 1968). Thus, the passive administration of high-affinity antibody well after a primary immune response has started can suppress the maturation of the immune response that occurs over the course of many months.

Although the suppressive qualities of passively administered antibody (or even endogenously made antibody) have been emphasized, antibody can also act as an adjuvant. IgM and other low-affinity antibodies are particularly good at immunoaugmentation (Henry and Jerne, 1968). Although immunoenhancing effects of IgM antibody are best known, it has been shown that in thymus-independent responses, small amounts of IgM antibody can be highly suppressive and do not operate by the activation of suppressor T cells (Ordal *et al.,* 1976). Thus, the thymus-independent immune response seems to have an inherent regulatory capacity of its own, which differs from the regulation of thymus-dependent responses; i.e., the primary product of a thymus-independent response is IgM antibody, which can feed back and suppress a thymus-independent response much more effectively than it can suppress a thymus-dependent response.

It was recognized many years ago that at appropriate molar ratios, antigen–antibody complexes induced better delayed hypersensitivity than did antigen alone (Uhr *et al.,* 1957). In addition, hapten-mediated help for antibody responses to carriers has been described, and in some cases it has been shown that it is the antibody response against the hapten that is responsible for the hapten-mediated help (Janeway, 1973). Thus, immunological product (i.e. antibody) can exert both a positive and a negative feedback effect on the immune response both in the production of antibody and in CMI.

A number of investigators have noted an inverse correlation between DTH and antibody production. In some cases, it has been shown that the drug treatments that inhibit the production of antibody augment DTH (Lagrange *et al.,* 1974), causing many workers to think that the antibody feedback is an important mechanism for shutting off DTH responses. However, direct proof of this contention has not been obtained. In fact, several workers have reported opposite results: that passive antibody can augment delayed responses and suppress antibody (Liew and Parish,

1972; Zembala *et al.*, 1974). An alternative view has therefore been put forth: these drug treatments affect populations of T cells that determine whether antibody or DTH production will occur (Weitzman *et al.*, 1976).

4. The Reticuloendothelial System

Macrophages play a very important role in controlling the immune response in a number of different ways (see Unanue, 1972; Rosenthal and Shevach, 1976). One of their functions is to process antigen in a fashion that makes it more immunogenic. In addition, macrophages play a very important role in antigen presentation. Their role in antigen presentation is more than a passive one, since they have interaction structures on their membranes that facilitate the antigen-dependent triggering of T cells (Rosenthal and Shevach, 1976). These interaction structures contain MHC-coded antigens and have been shown to be shed in a form complexed with antigen. Thus, they are capable of activating T cells at some distance (Erb and Feldmann, 1975). In addition to their role in antigen processing and presentation, macrophages can act as important intermediaries in the transmission of T-cell-derived messages to other cells (Feldmann and Nossal, 1973; Ptak and Gershon, 1975). Macrophages are also capable of making immunostimulatory and immunosuppressive factors (Calderon and Unanue, 1975). The importance of suppressor macrophages in regulating the immune response is being increasingly recognized (Eggers and Wunderlich, 1975; Glaser *et al.*, 1975; Veit and Feldman, 1976). In addition to all these regulatory functions, macrophages are very important effector cells in the immune response to tumors and many parasitic organisms (see Nelson, 1976). In many instances, both the regulatory and the effector functions of macrophages are under T-cell control, and thus feedback loops between T cells and macrophages, similar to those between T cells and B cells described above, are an important part of the immunological network. Whether these many macrophage functions are mediated by different subsets of macrophages, as is the case with T cells, is not known. Preliminary evidence indicates, however, that suppressor and helper macrophages can be distinguished (Lee, K.-C., personal communication). It may be that the importance of macrophage-mediated control of the immune response has not been sufficiently appreciated or studied up to now. It would seem, however, that the importance of this cell in immunoregulation is beginning to achieve widespread recognition, and one would expect that in the next few years this situation will be rectified.

5. Immune Response Genes

The ability of persons to respond to specific antigen or specific determinants on complex antigens is under genetic control. There are at least two major classes of genes coding for proteins involved in the immune response that theoretically could determine whether an individual subject could or could not respond to a specific antigen. One class is composed of a group of structural genes that determine the amino acid sequences in the variable region of antibodies and T-cell receptors, thereby controlling idiotypic specificities. These genes are linked to allotypic markers (Pawlak and Nisonoff, 1973). There is little evidence that they or their products play a direct role in genetically determined unresponsiveness to specific antigens, since only one specific hereditary immunological deficiency has ever been mapped to allotype (Riblet *et al.*, 1975). Reports of regulatory autoantiidiotypic responses indicate, however, that antibody structural genes may have an important indirect role by serving as targets for regulatory molecules or cells (Anderson *et al.*, 1976).

Another class of immune response genes, called *H-linked Ir genes*, is closely linked to the MHC of experimental animals (McDevitt and Benacerraf, 1969; Benacerraf and McDevitt, 1972; Benacerraf and Katz, 1975). In some cases, individual animals lacking the relevant *H*-linked *Ir* gene may be totally unable to make an immune response to an antigen or an antigenic determinant. In other cases, they may only make a partial response, and in some cases, they may be unable to respond only when limiting amounts of antigen are used for immunization. Breeding studies indicate that the ability to respond to antigens under *H*-linked *Ir* gene control is inherited according to classic Mendelian genetics, with responsiveness being dominant. In some cases, however, matings of two nonresponder strains may yield responder offspring, which indicates that at least two different genes can control the response to some antigens, and that an individual animal must have responder alleles at both loci to generate an immune response (Dorf *et al.*, 1975; Melchers and Rajewsky, 1975; Munro and Taussig, 1975).

The products of the *H*-linked *Ir* genes are unknown, but seem to be inseparable from the cell-surface antigens that are responsible for MLR and GVH reactions (see Shreffler and David, 1975). In mice, it has been shown that these antigens are coded for in a distinct region of the MHC, named the *I* region because of its close relationship to *Ir* genes. This region is distinct from the regions coding for the classic histocompatibility antigens, which were originally defined by serological reactions. In mice, these latter regions are called *K* and *D*. Those *I*-region gene products that have been identified are expressed on a limited number of cell types, including some, but not all, lymphocytes, macrophages, and epithelial cells, while the classic histocompatibility antigens are expressed on almost all cells. In humans, the *HLA-D* region may be the homologue of the murine *I* region, and the *HLA-A*, *-B*, and *-C* regions may be the homologues of the murine *K* and *D* regions; at least there are a number of analogies between these respective pairs of loci.

Several studies indicate that *H*-linked *Ir* genes are unrelated to Ig *V*-region structural genes. For example, although individual subjects that lack a given *Ir* gene fail to give an antibody response on immunization with the relevant antigen, they can nevertheless be made to respond if the antigen is coupled to an appropriate carrier such as methylated-BSA (MBSA) (Green *et al.*, 1966; Gershon *et al.*, 1973). Thus, it is clear that nonresponders do have the appropriate structural genes for making antibody responses, and that their defect is expressed in the triggering or afferent arm of the immune response.

Another feature that distinguishes the *H*-linked *Ir* genes from Ig *V*-region genes is their specificity. Thus, the antibody response to some synthetic linear polypeptides made up of glutamic acid, lysine, and either tyrosine (GLT), phenylalanine (GLϕ), or proline (GLPro) is so cross-reactive that immunization with any of these polymers can be accurately measured by determining the antibody response to only one of them (Benacerraf and Katz, 1975). The *H*-linked *Ir* genes distinguish clearly among all three of these polymers, however, because the MHC haplotypes that determine responsiveness are quite distinct.

The cell type that is defective in individual subjects lacking *Ir* genes is not known, but there is some evidence implicating all three of the major cell types (i.e., macrophages, T cells, and B cells). Independently of the cell type directly affected, however, the functional expression of defectiveness is always exhibited at the T-cell level. That is to say, T-cell-dependent responses (such as carrier recognition, DTH, and antigen-mediated *in vitro* mitogenesis) are lacking. These defects may be a result of faulty interactions between T cells and B cells, or between T cells and macrophages, or both. Munro and Taussig (1975) presented evidence indicating that in cases in which there are two *H*-linked *Ir* genes controlling the immune response to a given antigen, one of the genes may be expressed in T cells and the other in B cells. Thus, matings between low-responder mice with T-cell defects and low-responder mice with B-cell defects yields responder mice, while matings between two different strains of low-responder mice with T-cell defects does not lead to responsiveness. In other situations, however, complementation between two *Ir* genes is required for a T-cell mitogenic response to occur (Benacerraf and Dorf, 1976). This indicates that interactions between two *Ir* genes may be required for optimal interactions between subclasses of T cells, or between T cells and macrophages, as well as for T-cell interactions with B cells. (It is also possible that *Ir* gene products might interact on the membrane of a single cell.)

It has been shown that the lack of appropriate *Ir* genes cannot be detected by antigen-binding studies. T and B cells of nonresponsive mice bind the relevant antigen in a manner indistinguishable from the way in which T and B cells from responder mice bind the antigen (Hammerling and McDevitt, 1974). This is compatible with the notion expressed above: that the lesion in nonresponders is in the triggering, not in the antigen-recognition phase.

The lack of triggering in some cases can be attributed to the activity of suppressor T cells. In these cases, it has been shown that immunization of nonresponder mice with the relevant antigen prevents their subsequent response to the antigen coupled to MBSA. Purified T cells from the immunized nonresponders can suppress the response of untreated animals to the antigen–MBSA complex (Kapp *et al.*, 1974).

The role of suppressor T cells in *H*-linked *Ir* gene control of the immune response has been shown in other situations. For example, no inbred mouse strain makes an antibody response after immunization with a simple polymer of glutamic acid and tyrosine (GT). All mice, however, make an anti-GT antibody response after immunization with GT coupled to MBSA. After immunization with free GT, some strains develop suppressor T cells that can inhibit the subsequent response to GT–MBSA, while other mice make a normal response to GT–MBSA after immunization with free GT (Debre *et al.*, 1975). The genes responsible for the development of suppressor T cells after immunization with GT have been called *Is genes*. Like *Ir* genes, these genes are linked to the *I* region of the murine MHC, are dominantly expressed, and show gene complementation between at least two loci. Although activation of suppressor T cells can explain some cases of *H*-linked *Ir* gene responsiveness, it probably cannot explain all. Defective interactions among different cell types are most likely also involved.

Studies in humans have shown that there is an association between HLA antigens and a variety of disease entities. In almost all studies, the main finding is the statistically significant increase in the incidence of a particular HLA antigenic type in the diseased patient population compared with an adequately matched control population. In many studies, the association is quite striking (Ritzmann, 1976). That many of the diseases that show a marked correlation with HLA antigenic type are diseases in which there is a suspected autoimmune etiology suggests that the association may be due to the presence or absence of human *Ir* or

Is genes. *H*-linked *Ir* genes are also playing a role in the generation of experimental autoimmune disorders in experimental animals (Tomazic *et al.*, 1974; Nossal, 1976; Rose *et al.*, 1976). Another relevant point is that most of the human disease associations with HLA antigens are with antigens coded for by the *HLA-B* locus. If the suspected homologies between the murine and human MHC discussed above are true, this association would be predicted, because the *HLA-B* locus is more like the murine *K* locus than the murine *D* locus, and murine-linked *Ir* genes are more closely associated with the *K* locus than with the *D* locus. Thus, there are enough analogies between the mapping of *Ir* and *Is* genes and human disease susceptibility genes to make one think that it is probable that human *H*-linked *Ir* or *Is* genes, or both, exist. Further, their presence or absence can predispose individuals to some types of disease. The ability to study human *H*-linked *Ir* or *Is* genes is extremely limited by ethical considerations. There is, however, some evidence suggesting that human *Ir* genes control the reagenic antibody response to ragweed pollen (Levine and Stember, 1972). The precise mechanism by which *H*-linked *Ir* genes work and their exact relationship to human disease susceptibility is a topic of great current immunological interest, and it is hoped that definitive answers to some of the questions raised in this section will be forthcoming in the near future.

6. Summary

This chapter has focused on the many interactions that take place among various subpopulations of leukocytes in the generation and regulation of both humoral and cell-mediated immune responses. The elucidation of many of these interactions over the past several years was made possible through the discovery and exploitation of cell-surface antigens on T lymphocytes of mice, which first enabled immunologists to distinguish between peripheral T cells and B cells using the Thy-1 (Θ) marker, and then enabled further breakdown of T cells into subpopulations based on the presence of the Ly-series antigens. Homeostasis within the immune system is achieved and maintained by these T-cell subpopulations, which, in concert, act as conductors of the "immunological orchestra." Suppressor T cells balance the effect of the well-known helper T cells in regulating antibody responses, and also play an important role in regulating the effect of effector cells in cell-mediated responses. Amplifier T cells, a subpopulation distinct from both helper T cells and suppressor T cells, are able to synergize with both these subpopulations to augment either the positive or the negative aspects of the response.

Many of the regulatory functions of T cells have been shown to be mediated through the production of a variety of helper or suppressor factors, some with specificity for antigen, some with no apparent specificity. The cell targets of these factors are almost as numerous as the factors themselves. T cells can be targets of factors produced by other T-cell subpopulations. Monocytes, and many classes of granulocytes, are called forth by T-cell factors to perform as effectors in different forms of delayed hypersensitivity. Finally, B cells can be activated or suppressed, specifically or nonspecifically, by factors produced by T cells. Macrophages are able to bind many of these factors and, in so doing, either "present" the factors to other lymphocytes or become "armed" in the process, thereafter serving as cytotoxic killers, particularly against many neoplasms.

Although antibody is the ultimate end product of a series of interactions among lymphocytes, it is also an important regulator of the immune response. One of the ways in which it performs this regulatory function is analogous to the way in which high enzyme levels feed back and suppress the production of more enzyme, i.e., by removing the inducer. Thus, high levels of antibody bind to antigen and prevent the subsequent interaction of antigen with lymphocytes. Alternatively, antigen–antibody complexes can activate suppressor T cells or block effector cells from interacting with antigen on the target cell.

Recently, immunologists have become aware that idiotype recognition is also an important mechanism through which immunoregulation is achieved. In the course of the immune response, antibodies can be made against idiotypes, those unique amino acid sequences of an antibody molecule that define its antigen-binding capacity. These antiidiotypic antibodies have been shown to induce both helper and suppressor T cells, depending on the mode of administration or class of antibody used, and may also alter the ability of antigens to trigger B or T lymphocytes by binding to the idiotype of the cell-surface antigen receptor.

The immune response is, of course, ultimately regulated by the gene pool. At this level, the ability to either respond or not respond to certain antigens has been shown to be controlled by immune response (Ir) genes located within the major histocompatibility complex (MHC). Whatever the primary defect might be, the functional defect is expressed at the T-cell level. In many cases, lack of a response to antigen is not due to lack of recognition on the part of genetically defective individuals. Rather, the recognition event triggers production of suppressor T cells, which in turn induce a state of specific unresponsiveness. Susceptibility to many human diseases is now found to be associated with particular haplotypes of the MHC, and it is not unreasonable to consider the possibility that these disease states may be caused or maintained by inappropriate immune responses under Ir gene control.

The myriad arcane interactions among the multiple classes and subclasses of leukocytes involved in the immune response make the deciphering of the hieroglyphics of their communication system extremely difficult. As Wald (1965) pointed out, however, systems that require a great deal of amplification (such as the blood-clotting system, the visual system, or the complement system) all have numerous interacting cascades of molecules. It would seem that the cells of the immune system are similar to the molecules Wald discussed. Since the other codes have been broken, students of cellular immunology can take heart; although the problem they are facing is difficult, it is not insurmountable.

ACKNOWLEDGMENTS

The authors' research reported in this chapter was supported by USPHS grants CA-08593 and CA-14216 from the NCI, AI-10497 from the NIAID, research contract CB-43994 from the NCI, and a fellowship to C.M.M. from the Cancer Research Institute.

We are particularly grateful to Ms. Astrid Swanson and to Ms. Tracy Hodson for help in the preparation of this manuscript.

References

Anderson, L. C., Binz, H., and Wigzell, H., 1976, Specific unresponsiveness to transplantation antigens induced by autoimmunization with syngeneic antigen-specific T lymphoblasts, *Nature (London)* **264**:778.

Asherson, G. L., and Zembala, M., 1976, Suppressor T cells in cell-mediated immunity, *Br. Med. Bull.* **32**:158–164.

Askenase, P. W., Hayden, B. J., and Gershon, R. K., 1975, Augmentation of delayed-type hypersensitivity by doses of cyclophosphamide which do not affect antibody responses, *J. Exp. Med.* **141**:697–702.

Baker, P. J., 1975, Homeostatic control of antibody responses: A model based on the recognition of cell-associated antibody by regulatory T cells, *Transplant. Rev.* **26**:3–20.

Benacerraf, B., and Dorf, M., 1976, The nature and function of specific *H*-linked immune response genes and immune suppression genes, in: *The Role of Products of the Histocompatibility Gene Complex in Immune Responses* (D. H. Katz and B. Benacerraf, eds.), pp. 225–256. Academic Press, New York.

Benacerraf, B., and Katz, D. H., 1975, The histocompatibility-linked immune response genes, *Adv. Cancer Res.* **21**:121–173.

Benacerraf, B., and McDevitt, H. O., 1972, Histocompatibility-linked immune response genes, *Science* **175**:273–279.

Benjamin, D., 1975, Evidence for specific suppression in the maintenance of immunologic tolerance, *J. Exp. Med.* **141**:635.

Blaese, R. M., Weiden, P. L., Koski, I., and Dooley, N., 1974, Infectious agammaglobulinemia transmission of immunodeficiency with grafts of agammaglobulinemic cells, *J. Exp. Med.* **140**:1097–1101.

Bloom, B. R., and Bennett, B., 1966, Mechanism of a reaction *in vitro* associated with delayed-type hypersensitivity, *Science* **153**:80–82.

Brunner, K. T., and Cerottini, J. C., 1971, Cytotoxic lymphocytes as effector cells of cell-mediated immunity, *Prog. Immunol.* **1**:385–398.

Calderon, J., and Unanue, E. R., 1975, Two biological activities regulating cell proliferation found in cultures of peritoneal exudate cells, *Nature (London)* **253**:359–361.

Cantor, H., and Asofsky, R., 1970, Synergy among lymphoid cells mediating the graft-versus-host response. II. Synergy in graft-versus-host reactions produced by Balb/c lymphoid cells of differing anatomic origin, *J. Exp. Med.* **131**:235–246.

Cantor, H., and Boyse, E. A., 1975a, Functional subclasses of T lymphocytes bearing different Ly antigens. I. The generation of functionally distinct T cell subclasses is a differentiative process independent of antigen, *J. Exp. Med.* **141**:1376–1389.

Cantor, H., and Boyse, E. A., 1975b, Functional subclasses of T lymphocytes bearing different Ly antigens. II. Co-operation between subclasses of Ly^+ cells in the generation of killer activity, *J. Exp. Med.* **141**:1390–1399.

Cantor, H., and Simpson, E., 1975, Regulation of the immune response by subclasses of T lymphocytes. I. Interactions between pre-killer T cells and regulatory T cells obtained from peripheral lymphoid tissues of mice, *Eur. J. Immunol.* **5**:330–336.

Cerottini, J. C., and Brunner, K. T., 1971, *In vitro* assay of target cell lysis by sensitized lymphocytes, in: *In Vitro Methods in Cell-Mediated Immunity* (B. R. Bloom and R. R. Glade, eds.), pp. 369–373, Academic Press, New York and London.

Chiller, J. M., and Weigle, W. O., 1973, Restoration of immunocompetency in tolerant lymphoid cell populations by cellular supplementation, *J. Immunol.* **110**:1051–1057.

Civin, C., Levine, H. B., Williamson, A. R., and Schlossman, S. F., 1976, The effects of antigen dose and adjuvant on the antibody response: Amplification of restricted B cell clones, *J. Immunol.* **116**:1400–1406.

Claman, H. N., and Chaperon, E. A., 1969, Immunologic complementation between thymus and marrow cells—A model for the two cell theory of immunocompetence, *Transplant. Rev.* **1**:92–113.

Cosenza, H., and Kohler, H., 1972, Specific suppression of the antibody response by antibodies to receptors, *Proc. Natl. Acad. Sci. U.S.A.* **69**:2701–2705.

Dauphinee, M. J., and Talal, N., 1973, Reversible restoration by thymosin of antigen-induced depression of spleen DNA synthesis in NZB mice, *J. Immunol.* **114**:1713–1716.

David, J., 1966, Delayed hypersensitivity *in vitro*: Its mediation by cell-free substances formed by lymphoid cell–antigen interaction, *Proc. Natl. Acad. Sci. U.S.A.* **56**:72–77.

David, J. R., and David, R. A., 1972, Cellular hypersensitivity and immunity, *Prog. Allergy* **16**:300–449.

Davies, A. J. S., 1968, The immunological orchestra, *Lancet* **1**:185.

Davies, A. J. S., 1969, The thymus and the cellular basis of immunity, *Transplant. Rev.* **1**:43–91.

Debre, P., Kapp, J. A., Dorf, M. E., and Benacerraf, B., 1975, Genetic control of specific immune suppression. II. *H-2* linked dominant genetic control of immune suppression by the random copolymer L-glutamic acid^{50}-L-tyrosine^{50} (GT), *J. Exp. Med.* **142**:1447–1454.

Doherty, P. C., Blanden, R. V., and Zinkernagel, R. M., 1976, Specificity of virus-immune effector cells for H-2K or H-2D compatible interactions: Implications for H-antigen diversity, *Transplant. Rev.* **29**:89–124.

Dorf, M. E., Stimpfling, J. H., and Benacerraf, B., 1975, Requirement for two *H-2* complex *Ir* genes for the immune response to the L-Glu, L-Lys, L-Phe terpolymer, *J. Exp. Med.* **141**:1459–1463.

Dvorak, H. F., and Dvorak, A. M., 1974, Cutaneous basophil hypersensitivity, *Prog. Immunol. II* **3**:171–181.

Eardley, D. D., and Gershon, R. K., 1975, Feedback induction of suppressor T cell activity, *J. Exp. Med.* **142**:524–529.

Eardley, D. D., Staskawicz, M. O., and Gershon, R. K., 1976, Suppressor cells: Dependence on assay conditions for functional activity, *J. Exp. Med.* **143**:1211–1219.

Eggers, A. E., and Wunderlich, J. R., 1975, Suppressor cells in tumor bearing mice capable of non-specific blocking of *in vitro* immunization against transplant antigens, *J. Immunol.* **114**:1554–1556.

Eichmann, K., 1974, Idiotype suppression. I. Influence of the dose and of the effector functions of anti-idiotypic antibody on the production of an idiotype, *Eur. J. Immunol.* **4**:296.

Eichmann, K., 1975, Idiotype suppression. II. Amplification of a suppressor T cell with anti-idiotypic activity, *Eur. J. Immunol.* **5**:511–517.

Eichmann, K., and Rajewsky, K., 1975, Induction of T and B cell immunity by anti-idiotypic antibody, *Eur. J. Immunol.* **5**:661–666.

Erb, P., and Feldmann, M., 1975, The role of macrophages in the generation of T helper cells. III. Influence of macrophage-derived factors in helper cell induction, *Eur. J. Immunol.* **5**:759–766.

Feldmann, M., and Nossal, G. J. V., 1973, Tolerance enhancement and the regulation of interactions between T cells, B cells and macrophages, *Transplant. Rev.* **13**:3–34.

Feldmann, M., Kilburn, D. G., and Levy, J., 1975, T interaction in the generation of helper cells *in vitro*, *Nature (London)* **256**:761.

Feldmann, M., Beverley, P., Erb, P., Howie, S., Kontiainen, S., Maoz, A., Mathies, M., McKenzie, I., and Woody, J., 1977, Current concepts of the antibody response: Heterogeneity of lymphoid cells, interactions and factors, *Cold Spring Harbor Symp. Quant. Biol.* **41**:113–118.

Gershon, R. K., 1973, T cell control of antibody production, in: *Contemporary Topics in Immunobiology*, Vol. 3 (M. D. Cooper and N. L. Warner, eds.), pp. 1–40, Plenum Press, New York.

Gershon, R. K., 1974, T cell regulation: The "Second Law of Thymodynamics," in: *The Immune System: Genes, Receptors, Signals* (E. E. Sercarz, A. R. Williamson, and C. F. Fox, eds.), pp. 471–484, Academic Press, New York.

Gershon, R. K., and Kondo, K., 1971, Antigenic competition between heterologous erythrocytes. I. Thymic dependency, *J. Immunol.* **106**:1524–1531.

Gershon, R. K., and Paul, W. E., 1971, Effect of thymus-derived lymphocytes on amount and affinity of anti-hapten antibody, *J. Immunol.* **106**:872–874.

Gershon, R. K., Cohen, P., Hencin, R., and Liebhaber, S. A., 1972, Suppressor T cells, *J. Immunol.* **108**:586–590.

Gershon, R. K., Maurer, P. H., and Merryman, C. F., 1973, A cellular basis for genetically controlled immunologic unresponsiveness in mice: Tolerance induction in T cells, *Proc. Natl. Acad. Sci. USA* **70**:250–254.

Gershon, R. K., Gery, T., and Waksman B. H., 1974a, Suppressive effects of *in vivo* immunization on PHA responses *in vitro*, *J. Immunol.* **112**:215–221.

Gershon, R. K., Mokyr, M. D., and Mitchell, M. S., 1974b, Activation of suppressor T cells by tumour cells and specific antibody, *Nature (London)* **250**:594–596.

Gershon, R. K., Orbach-Arbouys, S., and Calkins, C., 1974c, B cell signals which activate suppressor T cells, *Prog. Immunol. II* **2**:123.

Gershon, R. K., Askenase, P. W., and Gershon, M. D., 1975, Requirement for vasoactive amines for production of delayed-type hypersensitivity skin reactions, *J. Exp. Med.* **142**:732–747.

Gershon, R. K., Eardley, D. D., Naidorf, K. F. and Ptak, W. 1977, The hermaphrocyte: A suppressor-helper T cell, *Cold Spring Harbor Symp. Quant. Biol.* **41**:85–92.

Glaser, M., Kirchner, H., and Herberman, R. B., 1975, Inhibition of *in vitro* lymphoproliferative responses to tumor-associated antigens by suppressor cells from rats bearing progressively growing leukemia virus, *Int. J. Cancer* **16**:384–389.

Green, I., Paul, W. E., and Benacerraf, B., 1966, The behavior of hapten-poly-L-lysine conjugates as complete antigens in genetic responder and as haptens in non-responder guinea pigs, *J. Exp. Med.* **123**:859–879.

Hammerling, G. J., and McDevitt, H. O., 1974, Antigen binding T and B lymphocytes. II. Studies on the inhibition of antigen binding to T and B cells by anti-immunoglobulin and anti-*H-2* sera, *J. Immunol.* **112**:1734–1740.

Hart, D. A., Wang, A.-L., Pawlak, L. L., and Nisonoff, A., 1972, Suppression of idiotypic specificities in adult mice by administration of anti-idiotypic antibody, *J. Exp. Med.* **135**:1293–1300.

Henry, C., and Jerne, N. K., 1968, Competition of 19S and 7S antigen receptors in the regulation of the primary immune response, *J. Exp. Med.* **128**:133–152.

Herzenberg, L. A., Okumura, K., and Metzler, C. M., 1975, Regulation of immunoglobulin and antibody production by allotype suppressor T cells in mice, *Transplant. Rev.* **27**:57–83.

Herzenberg, L. A., Okumura, K., Cantor, H., Sato, V. L., Shen, F. W., Boyse, E. A., and Herzenberg, L. A., 1976, T-cell regulation of antibody responses: Demonstration of allotype specific helper T cells and their specific removal by suppressor T cells, *J. Exp. Med.* **144**:330–344.

Hoffmann, G. W., 1975, A theory of regulation and self–nonself discrimination in an immune network, *Eur. J. Immunol.* **5**:638–647.

Huber, B., Devinsky, O., Gershon, R. K., and Cantor, H., 1976, Cell-mediated immunity: Delayed-type hypersensitivity and cytotoxic responses are mediated by different T cell subclasses, *J. Exp. Med.* **143**:1534–1539.

Ishizaka, K., 1976, Cellular events in the IgE antibody response, *Adv. Immunol.* **23**:1–75.

Janeway, C. A., 1973, The mechanism of a hapten-specific helper effect in mice, *J. Immunol.* **111**:1250–1256.

Johanovsky, J., Pekarek, J., Svejear, J., Krejci, J., Barnet, K., Castrova, A., and Cech, K., 1971, Recent studies on manifestations of delayed cellular hypersensitivity *in vitro* and *in vivo*, *Prog. Immunol.* **1**:461–472.

Jondal, M., Wigzell, H., and Aiuti, F., 1973, Human lymphocyte subpopulations: Classification according to surface markers and/or functional characteristics, *Transplant. Rev.* **16**:163–195.

Kantor, F. S., Dwyer, J. M., and Mangi, R. J., 1976, Sarcoid, *J. Invest. Dermatol.* **67**:470–476.

Kapp, J. A., and Benacerraf, B., 1976, Immunosuppressive factor(s) extracted from lymphoid cells of non-responder mice primed with L-glutamic acid^{60}-L-alanine^{30}-L-tyrosine^{10} (GAT). I. Activity and antigenic specificity, *J. Immunol.* **116**:305–309.

Kapp, J. A., Pierce, C. W., Schlossman, S., and Benacerraf, B., 1974, Genetic control of immune responses *in vitro*. V. Stimulation of suppressor T cells in non-responder mice by the terpolymer L-glutamic acid^{60}-L-alanine^{30}-L-tyrosine^{10} (GAT), *J. Exp. Med.* **140**:648–659.

Karniely, Y., Mozes, E., Shearer, G. M., and Sela, M., 1973, The role of thymocytes and bone marrow cells in defining the response to the dinitrophenyl hapten attached to positively and negatively charged synthetic polypeptide carriers, *J. Exp. Med.* **137**:183–195.

Katz, D. H., 1972, The allogeneic effect on immune responses: Model for regulatory influences of T lymphocytes on the immune system, *Transplant. Rev.* **12**:141–179.

Katz, D. H., Paul, W. E., Goidl, E. A., and Benacerraf, B., 1970a, Carrier function in anti-hapten antibody responses. I. Enhancement of primary and secondary anti-hapten antibody responses by carrier preimmunization, *J. Exp. Med.* **133**:261–282.

Katz, D. H., Paul, W. E., Goidl, E. A., and Benacerraf, B., 1970b, Carrier function in anti-hapten antibody responses. II. Specific properties of carrier cells capable of enhancing anti-hapten antibody responses, *J. Exp. Med.* **133**:283–299.

Kolsch, E., Stumpf, R., and Weber, G., 1975, Low zone tolerance and suppressor T cells, *Transplant. Rev.* **26**:56–86.

Krakauer, R. S., Waldmann, T. A., and Strober, W., 1976, Loss of suppressor T cells in adult NZB/NZW mice, *J. Exp. Med.* **144**:662–673.

Lagrange, P. H., Mackaness, G. B., and Miller, J. E., 1974, Potentiation of T-cell-mediated immunity by selective suppression of antibody formation with cyclophosphamide, *J. Exp. Med.* **139**:1529–1539.

Levine, B. B., and Stember, R. H., 1972, Ragweed hay fever: Genetic control and linkage to *HLA* haplotypes, *Science* **178**:1201–1203.

Liew, F. Y., and Parish, C. R., 1972, Regulation of the immune response by antibody. I. Suppression of antibody formation and concomitant enhancement of cell-mediated immunity by passive antibody, *Cell. Immunol.* **4**:66–85.

Litwin, S. D., and Zanjani, E. D., 1977, Lymphocytes suppressing both immunoglobulin production and erythroid differentiation in hypogammaglobulinemia, *Nature (London)* **266**:57–58.

Lubaroff, D. M., and Waksman, B. H., 1968, Bone marrow as source of cells in reactions of cellular hypersensitivity. I. Passive transfer of tuberculin sensitivity in syngeneic systems, *J. Exp. Med.* **128**:1425–1432.

Marrack, P., and Kappler, J. W., 1976, Antigen-specific and non-specific mediators of T cell/B cell co-operation. II. Two higher T cells distinguished by their antigen sensitivities, *J. Immunol.* **116**:1373–1378.

McDevitt, H. O., and Benacerraf, B., 1969, Genetic control of specific immune responses, *Adv. Immunol.* **11**:31–74.

Melchers, I., and Rajewsky, K., 1975, Specific control of responsiveness by two complementing *Ir* loci in the *H-2* complex, *Eur. J. Immunol.* **5**:753–759.

Metzler, C. M., and Gershon, R. K., 1978, Dependence on vasoactive amines for the localization of leukocytes in DTH reaction sites and lymph nodes (submitted).

Miller, J. F. A. P., and Mitchell, G. F., 1969, Thymus and antigen-reactive cells, *Transplant, Rev.* **1**:3–42.

Mitchison, N. A., 1970, The carrier effect in the secondary response to hapten–protein conjugates. V. Use of anti-lymphocyte serum to deplete animals of helper cells, *Eur. J. Immunol.* **1**:68–75.

Mitchison, N. A., 1971, The carrier effect in the secondary response to hapten–protein conjugates. II. Cellular co-operation, *Eur. J. Immunol.* **1**:18–27.

Moller, G., 1971, Induction of antigenic competition with thymus dependent antigens: Effect on DNA synthesis in spleen cells, *J. Immunol.* **106**:1566–1571.

Mosier, D. E., Cohen, P. L., and Johnson, B. M., 1975, Suppressor cells in ontogeny of the immune response, in: *Suppressor Cells in Immunity* (S. K. Singhal and N. R. St. C. Sinclair, eds.), University of Western Ontario Press, pp. 28–32, London, Ontario, Canada.

Munro, A. J., and Taussig, M. J., 1975, Two genes in the major histocompatibility complex control immune response, *Nature (London)* **256**:103–106.

Murphy, D. B., Herzenberg, L. A., Okumura, K., Herzenberg, L. A., and McDevitt, H. O., 1976, A new *I* subregion *(I-J)* marked by a locus *(Ia-4)* controlling surface determinants on suppressor T lymphocytes, *J. Exp. Med.* **144**:699–712.

Nelson, D. S. (ed.), 1976, *Immunobiology of the Macrophage,* Academic Press, New York.

Nossal, G. J. V., 1976, General discussion—Session III: Immune response *(Ir)* gene systems, in: *The Role of Products of the Major Histocompatibility Gene Complex in Immune Responses* (D. H. Katz and G. Benacerraf, eds.), pp. 313–316, Academic Press, New York.

Ordal, J., Smith, S., Ness, D., Gershon, R. K., and Grumet, F. C., 1976, IgM-mediated, T cell-independent suppression of humoral immunity, *J. Immunol.* **116**:1182–1187.

Ovary, Z., and Benacerraf, B., 1963, Immunological specificity of the secondary response with dinitro-phenylated proteins, *Proc. Soc. Exp. Biol. Med.* **114**:72–76.

Pawlak, L. L., and Nisonoff, A., 1973, Distribution of a crossreactive idiotypic specificity in inbred strains of mice, *J. Exp. Med.* **137**:855–869.

Pierce, C. W., and Kapp, J. A., 1976, Regulation of immune response by suppressor T cells, *Contemp. Top. Immunobiol.* **5**:91–143.

Pollack, W., and Mollison, P. L. (eds.), 1976, *Rh Antibody Mediated Immunosuppression,* Ortho Research Institute of Medical Sciences, Raritan, New Jersey.

Press, J. L., Klinman, N. R., and McDevitt, H. O., 1976, Expression of Ia antigens on hapten-specific B cells. I. Delineation of B cell subpopulations, *J. Exp. Med.* **144**:414–427.

Ptak, W., and Gershon, R. K., 1975, Immunosuppression effected by macrophage surfaces, *J. Immunol.* **115**:1346–1350.

Raff, M. C., 1971, Surface antigenic markers for distinguishing T and B lymphocytes in mice, *Transplant. Rev.* **6**:52–80.

Raff, M. C., and Cantor, H., 1971, Subpopulations of thymus cells and thymus-derived lymphocytes, *Prog. Immunol.* **1**:83–93.

Rajewsky, K., Schirrmacher, V., Nase, S., and Jerne, N. K., 1969, The requirement of more than one antigenic determinant for immunogenicity, *J. Exp. Med.* **129**:1131–1143.

Reif, A. E., and Allen, J. M. V., 1964, The AKR thymic antigen and its distribution in leukemias and nervous tissues, *J. Exp. Med.* **120**:413–433.

Riblet, R., Blomberg, B., Weigert, M., Lieberman, R., Taylor, B. A., and Potter, M., 1975, Genetics of mouse antibodies. I. Linkage of the dextran response locus, V_h-*DEX,* to allotype, *Eur. J. Immunol.* **5**:775–777.

Rich, S. S., and Rich, R. R., 1976, Regulatory mechanisms in cell-mediated immune responses, *J. Immunol.* **143**:672–677.

Ritzmann, S. E., 1976, *HLA* patterns and disease associations, *J. Am. Med. Assoc.* **236**:2305–2309.

Rose, N. R., Bacon, L. D., and Sundick, R. S., 1976, Genetic determinants of thyroiditis in the 0S chicken, *Transplant. Rev.* **31**:264–285.

Rosenthal, A. S., and Shevach, E. M., 1976, The function of macrophages in T lymphocyte antigen recognition, in: *Contemporary Topics in Immunobiology,* Vol. 5 (W. O. Weigle, ed.), pp. 47–90, Plenum Press, New York.

Shimpl, A., and Wecker, E., 1975, A third signal in B cell activation given by TRF, *Transplant. Rev.* **23**:176–188.

Shreffler, D. C., and David, C. S., 1975, The *H-2* major histocompatibility complex and the immune response: Genetic variation, function and organization, *Adv. Immunol.* **20**:125–195.

Siegal, F. P., Siegal, M., and Good, R. A., 1976, Suppression of B-cell differentiation by leukocytes from hypogammaglobulinemic patients, *J. Clin. Invest.* **58**:109–122.

Sinclair, N. R. St. C., 1969, Regulation of the immune response. I. Reduction in ability of specific antibody to inhibit long-lasting IgG immunological priming after removal of the Fc fragment, *J. Exp. Med.* **129**:1183–1201.

Staples, P. J., and Talal, N., 1969, Relative inability to induce tolerance in adult NZB and NZB/NZWF₁ mice, *J. Exp. Med.* **129**:123–139.

Steinberg, A. D., Gerber, N. L., Gershwin, M. E., Morton, R., Goodman, D., Chused, T. M., Hardin, J. A., and Barthold, D. R., 1975, Loss of suppressor T cells in the pathogenesis of autoimmunity, in: *Suppressor Cells in Immunity* (S. K. Singhal and N. R. St. C. Sinclair, eds.), pp. 174–181, University of Western Ontario Press, London, Ontario Canada.

Tada, T., Taniguchi, M., and Takemor, T., 1975, Properties of primed suppressor T cells and their products, *Transplant. Rev.* **26**:106–129.

Taussig, M. J., Munroe, A. J., Campbell, R., David, C. S., and Staines, N. A., 1975, Antigen-specific T cell factor in co-operation: Mapping within the *I* region of the *H-2* complex and ability to co-operate across allogeneic barriers, *J. Exp. Med.* **142**:694–700.

Tomazic, V., Rose, N. R., and Shreffler, D. C., 1974, Autoimmune murine thyroiditis. IV. Localization of genetic control of the immune response, *J. Immunol.* **112**:965–969.

Uhr, J. W., and Moller, G., 1968, Regulatory effect of antibody on the immune response, *Adv. Immunol.* **8**:81–127.

Uhr, J. W., Salvin, S. B., and Pappenheimer, A. M., 1957, Delayed hypersensitivity. II. Induction of hypersensitivity in guinea pigs by means of antigen-antibody complexes, *J. Exp. Med.* **105**:11–24.

Unanue, E. R., 1972, The regulatory role of macrophages in antigenic stimulation, *Adv. Immunol.* **15**:95–166.

Veit, B. C., and Feldman, J. D., 1976, Altered lymphocyte functions in rats bearing syngeneic Moloney sarcoma tumors, *J. Immunol.* **117**:655–660.

Wagner, H., 1973, Synergy during *in vitro* cytotoxic allograft responses. I. Evidence for cell interactions between thymocytes and peripheral T cells, *J. Exp. Med.* **138**:1379.

Waksman, B. H., and Namba, Y., 1976, Commentary on soluble mediators of immunologic regulation, *Cell. Immunol.* **21**:161–176.

Wald, G., 1965, Visual excitation and blood clotting, *Science* **150**:1028–1030.

Waldmann, T. A., Broder, S., Krakauer, R., Durm, M., Goldman, C., and Meade, B., 1975, The role of suppressor T cells in immunodeficiency, in: *Suppressor Cells in Immunity* (S. K. Singhal and N. R. St. C. Sinclair, eds.), pp. 182–190, University of Western Ontario, London, Ontario, Canada.

Walker, J. G., and Siskind, G. W., 1968, Effect of antibody affinity upon its ability to suppress antibody formation, *Immunology* **14**:21–28.

Warren, K. S., Domingo, E. D., and Cowan, R. B. T., 1967, Granuloma formation around schistosome eggs as a manifestation of delayed hypersensitivity, *Am. J. Pathol.* **51**:735–756.

Weigle, W. O., Sieckmann, D. G., Doyle, M. V., and Chiller, J. M., 1975, Possible roles of suppressor cells in immunological tolerance, *Transplant. Rev.* **26**:186–205.

Weinbaum, F. I., Butchko, G. M., Lerman, S., Thorbecke, G. J., and Nisonoff, A., 1974, Comparison of cross-reactivities between albumins of various species at the level of antibody and helper T cells—studies in mice, *J. Immunol.* **113**:257.

Weitzman, S., Shen, F. W., and Cantor, H., 1976, Maintenance of hyporesponsiveness to antigen by a distinct subclass of T lymphocytes, *J. Immunol.* **117**:2209–2212.

Zembala, M., Ptak, W., and Hanczakowska, M., 1974, The induction of delayed hypersensitivity by macrophage-associated antigens, *Immunology* **26**:465–476.

3

Aging and Involution of the Immunological Apparatus

E. J. YUNIS, G. FERNANDES, and ROBERT A. GOOD

1. Introduction

Thymic involution and involution of the thymus-dependent system of cells responsible for cell-mediated immunity (CMI) occur in man as they do in all animals that possess a thymus. Specific thymic alterations related to aging were described and extensively discussed by Hammar (1926) and have been reviewed by many others (Good and Gabrielson, 1964). It has been known for many years that beginning at the time of sexual maturation, an apparent programmed involution begins in the central lymphoid organs. This is succeeded by a period of gradual involution of the peripheral lymphoid apparatus and declining vigor of immunological functions (Walford, 1969; Roberts-Thomson *et al.*, 1974; Yunis *et al.*, 1968, 1971a,b; Stutman *et al.*, 1968; Good and Yunis, 1974). In both man and mouse, the rate of immunological decline is highly variable. In aging research, fundamental questions to be answered focus on the determinants of variability in life span, i.e., longevity. The variability and thus the rate of immunological involution clearly implicate genetic determinants, as described later, but immunological involution, as with other aging processes, proceeds according to a schedule that fits a broad framework characteristic of the species.

In both animals and man, a progressive decrease in the mass of the lymphoid system generally begins after puberty and continues throughout adult life. Under normal circumstances, a good correlation exists between lymphoid mass and immunological functional capacity from birth until early adult life, during which time an equilibrium is established within the immune system. Decline in thymic size, however, followed by decline in cell-mediated immune function and progressive aging, occurs very rapidly in some persons and in some inbred mouse strains, whereas others may not show appreciable loss of immunological vigor until very

E. J. YUNIS • Sidney Farber Cancer Institute, Harvard Medical School, Boston, Massachusetts 02115. G. FERNANDES and ROBERT A. GOOD • Memorial Sloan-Kettering Cancer Center, New York, New York 10021.

much later in life. The nature of the immunodeficiency that occurs in some inbred strains of mice relatively early in life, as, for example, during the second half of the first year in NZB mice and (NZB × NZW) F_1 hybrid (B/W) mice, is strikingly similar to that produced or accelerated by neonatal thymectomy (Stutman *et al.*, 1968; Yunis *et al.*, 1968a,b, 1971a,b,; Teague *et al.*, 1970; Good and Yunis, 1974). CMI deteriorates spontaneously at an earlier age in autoimmune-prone strains than in autoimmune-resistant strains (Yunis *et al.*, 1968, 1969a,b, 1971a,b, 1975; Stutman *et al.*, 1968; Teague *et al.*, 1970; Good and Gabrielson, 1964; Good and Yunis, 1974).

Among inbred strains of mice, the rates of aging in general, and of immunological aging in particular, have clearly defined time constraints. CBA mice tend to be very long-lived and to maintain immunological function much longer than do certain other strains, such as NZB, B/W, A, and C57/BL/Ks. NZB and B/W mice are short-lived and develop immunodeficiencies and immunological abnormalities early in life. Indeed, these abnormalities usually occur during the second 6 months of life (Teague *et al.*, 1970; Rodey *et al.*, 1971). Note that we are discussing primarily age-related changes within the species without attempting to explain the possible evolutionary processes that determine the life-span differences among species. For instance, both survival and maintenance of immunological function are short in CBA mice in comparison with their duration in man, and survival and the temporal persistence of immunological functions of NZB mice may be long, compared with standards that could be applied to Snell–Bagg or Ames dwarf mice (Duquesnoy, 1975) and certain much shorter-lived animals, as, for example, shrews. In the same vein, the life span of the long-lived CBA mice may be very long when compared to that of the NZB and very short when compared to that of the turtle, elephant, or man.

2. Cellular Basis of Lymphoid Involution

2.1. Cellular Environment Changes

The decline of the immune system during aging is related to changes that include the cells themselves, characteristics of populations of such cells, and the environment in which these cells must function. Approximately 10% of the decline of the immune function has been attributed to factors of environment that are extrinsic to the cells (Makinodan and Adler, 1975). About 90% of the reduction of immunological vigor with aging as measured by antibody-forming capacity observed in old mice, however, appears to be a consequence of changes in the cells themselves (Perkins and Makinodan, 1971). The environmental changes in old mice that contribute to immunodeficiencies may be due to a number of factors of a systemic and noncellular nature, e.g., consequences of viral or bacterial infections, antigen–antibody complexes, products of other cells, hormones, and nutriments.

Another possible basis of defective immunological function with aging that still needs much study is the possibility that abnormalities of distribution of the lymphoid cells occur with aging. An abnormality of ecotaxis, the basis of which is considered in detail in Chapter 11, has been termed *ecotaxopathy*. Defects of distribution might come about as a consequence of either abnormalities intrinsic to the cells (and especially the surface membranes of the lymphoid cells) or factors extrinsic to the cells that represent changes in the environment provided by the several organs in which the cells reside. Changes in whole body or tissue or in environmental factors that alter the cell surfaces or change surface-dependent cell–cell interactions are also possible bases for defective immune function.

2.2. Cellular Changes

The ability to produce a humoral immune response is dependent on the interaction or collaboration of T lymphocytes (both helper T cells and suppressor T cells), macrophages, and B lymphocytes.

Three types of cellular changes could cause a decline in normal immune function: (1) An absolute decrease in cell number in which cell death exceeds cell generation. Such a decrease could be caused by any of a variety of factors, e.g., autoimmunity. (2) A relative decrease in cell number, such as might occur with a change in the proportion of one kind of lymphoid cell. An increase in the number of "suppressor cells" would be an example. (3) A decrease in functional efficiency of the individual cells such as might possibly be attributable to somatic mutation. Further, the decline in antibody-forming capacity that occurs with aging could be attributable to an alteration in the number or function of any of the three cell populations or to factors that interfered with their cooperative interactions. From experimental evidence, however, a predominant factor in immunological involution appears to be a decrease in T-helper-cell function, not a decrease in B-cell or macrophage function under ordinary circumstances (Heidrick and Makinodan, 1971). The decrease in immunologic vigor of the aged may be expressed quite differently in different persons, thus accounting for the variability of immunological performance of the old. In a system that is so dependent on interactions of several cellular components, perturbations of cell–cell communication could play crucial roles, and the opportunity for disturbance in efficient function might be attributable, not to one factor, but actually to several factors. For instance, merely an abnormal distribution of one subset of cells, e.g., helper or suppressor cells, without a real change in the effectiveness of any could very much disturb immunological adaptation.

2.2.1. Stem Cells

The total number of stem cells of the mouse bone marrow remains quite constant with age (Coggle and Proukakis, 1970; Chen, 1971); however, stem cells passaged *in vivo* can be exhausted (Siminovitch *et al.,* 1964; Lajtha and Schofield, 1971). Within the body, the stem cells do not appear to lose their lymphohemato-poietic ability with age (Harrison and Doubleday, 1975). The rate of B-cell formation appears to decline with age (Farrar *et al.,* 1974), and this change parallels certain kinetic parameters in spleen colony formation (Deitchman and Makinodan, 1975). It appears that the environment in which the stem cells find themselves induces changes in these cells that affect the responsiveness essential to their differentiation (Makinodan *et al.,* 1976).

2.2.2. Macrophages

Macrophages are not affected in their handling of antigens by aging. This is true not only during induction of immune responses, but also as measured by ingestion of antigenic aggregates or colloidal suspensions: (1) The *in vitro* phagocytic activity of old mice was equal to or better than that of young mice (Perkins and Makinodan, 1971). (2) the activity of at least three lysosomal enzymes in macrophages increased rather than decreased with age (Heidrick, 1972). This change was reflected in a diminution of the response of antigen-sensitive T cells or B cells to limiting doses of antigen (Lloyd and Triger, 1975). Also, a failure of antigens to localize in the follicles of lymphoid tissues of antigen-stimulated old mice (Metcalf *et al.*, 1966; Legge and Austin, 1968) has been described. These findings would indicate that the presentation of antigens may change with aging.

2.2.3. B Cells

The number of B cells in lymph nodes and spleen does not seem to change in any orderly fashion with age (Makinodan and Adler, 1975), but the number of plasma cells certainly increases with aging, especially in mice of certain autoimmune-prone strains (Good and Yunis, 1974). In humans, studies have been limited primarily to an analysis of relative and absolute numbers of circulating B cells, which appear to remain constant with age (Diaz-Jouanen *et al.*, 1975). B-cell responses to T-cell-independent antigens decrease with age (Price and Makinodan, 1972), however, as does the response to T-cell-dependent antigens (Makinodan and Peterson, 1962).

2.2.4. T Cells

The decline in immune functions that accompanies aging seems to be due mainly to changes in T cell populations. There is a decrease of germinal centers and an increase in numbers of plasma cells and macrophages, as well as an increase in the amount of connective tissue (Chino *et al.*, 1971; Peter, 1973; Good and Yunis, 1974). The number of circulating lymphocytes as well as the total and relative proportions that are T lymphocytes decrease progressively during or after middle age in man (Diaz-Jouanen *et al.*, 1975; Augener *et al.*, 1974; Alexopoulos and Babitis, 1976). Not all investigators, however, have encountered decline in absolute numbers of lymphocytes in the circulating blood of aged persons or even a decline in T lymphocytes (Hallgren and Yunis, 1977). Even though the decrease in number or proportion of T cells in both humans and mice could occur, the changes might not be sufficient to account for the changes in immunological functions that become very grossly defective with age. Functional studies include: (1) Age-related decrease in delayed hypersensitivity to skin test with antigens to which the subjects had not previously been sensitized, e.g., dinitrochlorobenzene (MacKay, 1972). (2) *In vivo* studies in mice that show that cells from old mice have decreased ability to mount a vigorous graft-versus-host (GVH) reaction (Stutman *et al.*, 1968; Teague *et al.*, 1970; Goodman and Makinodan, 1975). (3) Proliferative capacity of T cells of humans and rodents in response to lectins and allogeneic target cells (Pisciotta *et al.*, 1967; Heine, 1971; Hallgren *et al.*, 1973; Konen *et al.*, 1973; Mathies *et al.*, 1973; Roberts-Thomson *et al.*, 1974). (4) A decline in generation of cytotoxic cells against tumors, especially in short- and long-lived strains of mice. This decline is not so great in long-lived as it is in short-lived strains (Goodman and Makinodan, 1975; Fernandes *et al.*, 1976d). (5) Reports that declines in mixed lymphocyte reactions occur during aging. The data on this point are somewhat conflicting (Adler *et al.*,

1971; Hori *et al.*, 1973; Walters and Claman, 1975). In both mouse and man, however, substantial evidence of decrease in responses to allogeneic cells with no change in the stimulating capacity (Walford, 1969) has been generated. (6) The helper-cell function of T cells as is revealed by both studies in intact animals and *in vitro* assays (Price and Makinodan, 1972; Heidrick and Makinodan, 1971; Hardin *et al.*, 1973). (7) The suppressor-cell function of T cells on T-cell functions may also decline with age in man (Hallgren and Yunis, 1977), but in some systems, e.g., B/W mice, an increase in spontaneous nonspecific suppressor-cell activity that influences antibody production has been observed (Rodey *et al.*, 1971; Fernandes *et al.*, 1977).

2.3. Thymic Involution

Thymic involution precedes and is very likely largely responsible for the age-dependent decline in the ability of the immune system to generate functional T cells. It appears that the defect resides in a T-cell differentiation pathway (Yunis *et al.*, 1971a,b; Bach *et al.*, 1973; Hirokawa and Makinodan, 1975). The general pattern of age-related changes in thymus weight is similar in mice and man (Boyd, 1932; Shisa and Nishizuka, 1971). The thymus of long-lived strains increases in mass to a peak of approximately 70 mg at 6 weeks and then decreases rapidly up to 6 months of age, following which a gradual decrease in weight occurs, so that by 36 months, the thymus weighs less than 5 mg. The main features of the thymus changes with aging include decrease in the relative size of the thymic cortex, accompanied by increased numbers of macrophages in this organ. The medulla of the thymus of aged mice generally becomes infiltrated with plasma cells and mast cells (Figures 1A,B, 2A,B, and 3). Note that the thymus of the 25-month-old A mouse (Figures 2A,B) shows advanced involution as compared with the CBA strain of similar age (Figures 1A,B) (Yunis *et al.*, 1972, 1973).

The secretory activity of the mouse thymic epithelial cells was first suggested by Clark (1966), who found them to contain vesicles featured by dense granules. Hirokawa (1976) provided a splendid description of the electron-microscopic characteristics of the thymus at different ages. The young thymus is a spongy meshwork composed of epithelial cells, dense in the medulla as compared with the cortex, and the latter is packed with thymocytes. At the periphery and around the vascular areas, the parenchyma is separated by a thin basement membrane. In the atrophic thymus, 24 months or older, in long-lived mouse strains, a splitting of the meshwork of epithelial cells into small nests by infiltrating macrophages, plasma cells, lymphocytes, and fibroblasts is seen. These nests do not contain thymocytes and epithelial cells; instead, the epithelial cells are clustered, and are generally devoid of apparent contact with thymocytes.

The secretory epithelial cells of the thymus contain either vesicles with cilialike or microvillous structures packed with fine granular substance, or cells with vesicles having coarse granular structures or membranous substance of moderate electron density. The first kind of cell is found only in the medulla of the newborn thymus; the second kind is found mainly in the cortex of the thymus at all ages. The latter component is decreased so that at 24 months or later in long-lived strains of mice, these cells are very few and far between. In the same strains, irregular vesicles packed with coarse granular substances, electron-dense microbodies, or crystals can be found in the secretory cells after 16 months of age.

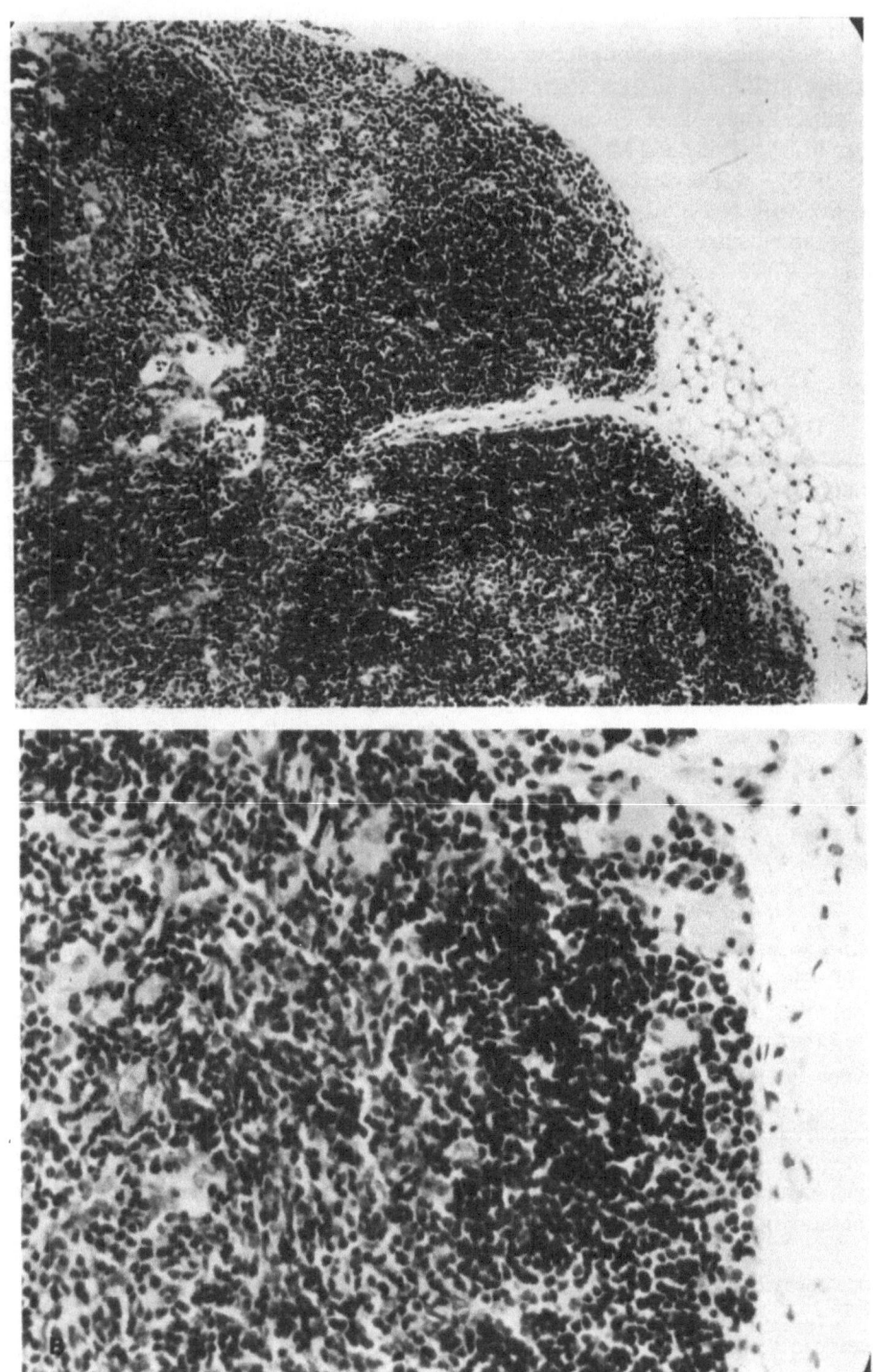

Figure 1 (A). Microscopic section of thymus from a 24-month-old CBA mouse showing remarkable preservation of normal histology, thinness of cortex, and increased number of blood vessels. Magnification × 100. Hematoxylin–eosin. (B). Section of thymus as in Figure 1A, but at higher magnification (× 375) to show large cells, such as histiocytes, and thin cortex.

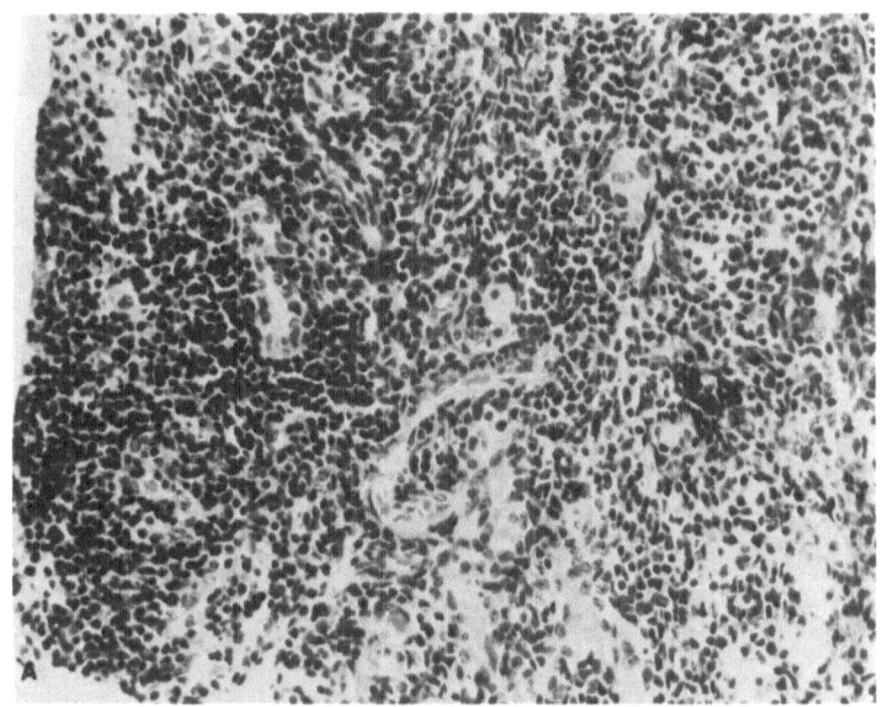

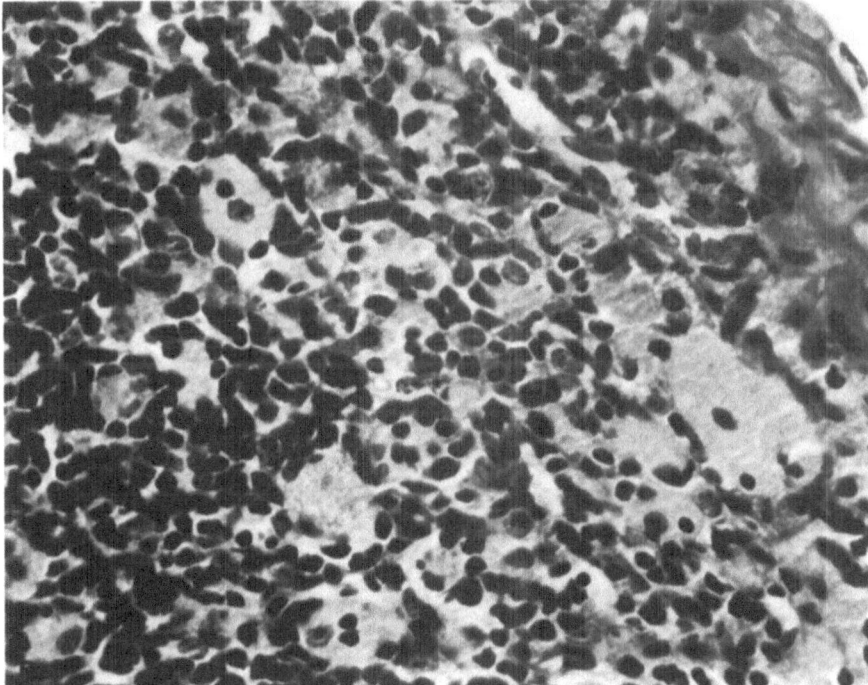

Figure 2 (A). Microscopic section of involuted thymus from a 25-month-old A strain mouse showing marked depletion of lymphocytes. Magnification × 250. Hematoxylin–eosin. (B). Cortex of thymus in Figure 2A, but at higher magnification (× 600) to show large number of large cells of granular cytoplasma and small nucleus and some lymphocytes and plasma cells. Hematoxylin–eosin.

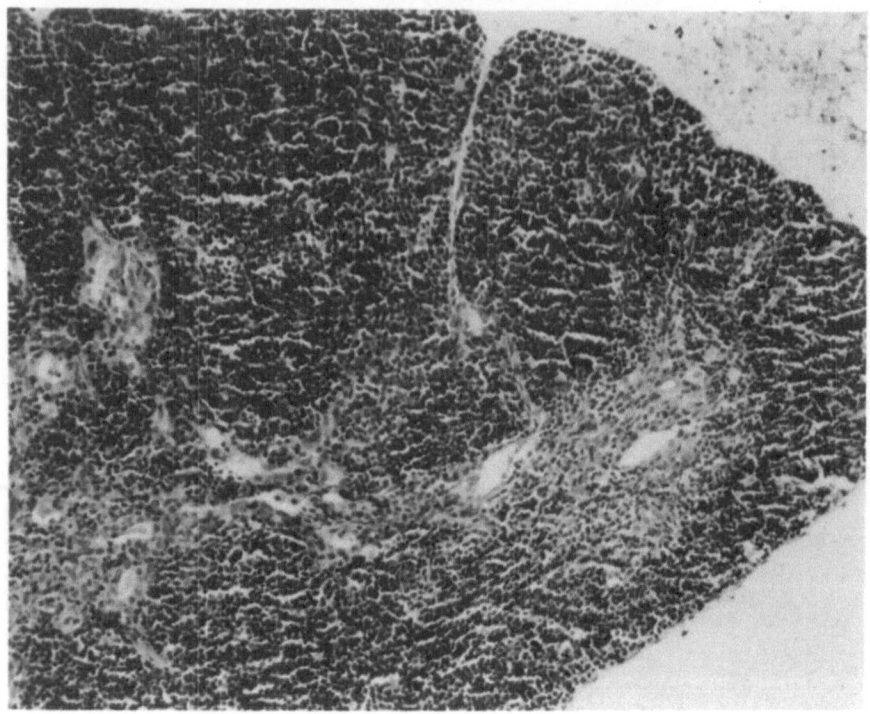

Figure 3. Microscopic section of thymus from a 12-month-old CBA mouse showing normal cortex and medulla. Magnification × 100. Hematoxylin–eosin.

Functionally, the progressive decline of thymic influence on T-cell differentiation results in progressive deficiencies with age of lymphocyte repopulation of T-cell-dependent areas of lymph nodes. Also, the mitogenic reactivity of spleen cells to T-cell-specific mitogens [phytohemagglutinin (PHA) and concanavalin A (Con A)], splenic T-cell helper function in a humoral response, and killer-cell activity of splenic T cells to allogeneic tumors (Fernandes *et al.,* 1976d) decline impressively with age, especially in certain mouse strains. It appears that three factors that determine the magnitude of immunological activity of the aged are the thymus, bone marrow, and humoral environment in which the lymphoid cells must function. Of these, the thymus seems to be by all odds the most limiting factor to immunological vigor in the aged man or mouse. It is of great interest that recent studies show that immunological capacity of aged animals can be strikingly reconstituted by transplantation of young thymus plus young bone marrow (Hirokawa and Makinodan, 1975).

3. Lymphoid Involution and the Diseases of Aging

Aging, diseases of aging, and thymic and immunological involution may occur early in certain inbred strains of mice and much later in others. In all strains studies, however, even the very long-lived strains, evidence of immunological involution may be found. In humans, involution of the thymus and the subsequent loss of immunological vigor also occur commonly, but in man, a large individual variation can be observed. It remains to be determined whether or not the decline of immunological vigor, which seems to be centrally and genetically determined, is directly or indirectly controlled by the major histocompatibility complex (MHC). The linkage group associated with the MHC is now considered as a "supergene," since it appears to control individuality in many ways. Cell-surface antigenicity, complement function, capacity to initiate and to produce antibody vigorously, recognition of foreign cells as in mixed leukocyte responses (Dupont *et al.*, 1975; Shreffler and David, 1975), immunological capacity to reject foreign cells, production of leukemia after injection with RNA tumor virus (Lilly and Pincus 1973), receptors for insulin (Rubinstein *et al.*, personal communication), and even sex-partner selection (Yamazaki *et al.*, 1976) seem to be controlled in a major way by the major histocompatibility region. It is also a major determinant of susceptibility or resistance to diseases that are commonly linked to aging, e.g., arthritis, diabetes mellitus, demyelinating disease of the CNS, malignancies, infections, vascular insufficiency, and renal and CNS malfunctions (Good and Yunis, 1974; Shreffler and David, 1975; Dupont *et al.*, 1975). Studies in both man and animals have provided much evidence for a relationship between diseases of adult life and a decline of immune function. In addition, congenital or adult-onset immunodeficiencies as well as immunodeficiency of the aged have been associated with malignancy and autoimmune pathology (Good and Yunis, 1974). Although the apparent linkage between the decline in immune function and age-associated disease is not mere coincidence, one still cannot assign the primary control of aging to the immune system. It is important to recognize at the outset that most of the major diseases of aging may be linked to perturbations of immunological functions. In this group, we would include inflammatory, cardiovascular renal disease, vasculitis and perhaps so-called degenerative vascular disease, autoimmunities, susceptibility to infection, cancer, and amyloidosis.

3.1. Immunological Theory of Aging

The association of immunological malfunction with aging has been analyzed in several ways. The immunological theory of aging, first clearly stated by Walford (1969), was extensively promulgated and developed by Burnet (1970b). This theory states that the immune system is essential to maintenance of health and that, to a major extent, the integrity of the immune system determines survival. Walford further suggested that aging results from somatic-cell variations of factors that determine self-recognition among cells. The progressive breakdown of this system results in the occurrence of autoimmunity and autoimmune disease. In our studies, the decline of vigorous immune function in man and mouse during aging has been associated with the same disases and immunological abnormalities found in man and animals that lack, on genetic grounds or from earlier thymic extirpation, normal T-cell immune systems (Good and Yunis, 1974). Observations provoked Burnet (1959) to maintain that clones of cells ordinarily forbidden expressiveness by an intact immune system appear by somatic mutation and persist when the immunity functions become defective. He concluded that this event explains the frequent autoimmunity observed in aging and immunodeficient man and animals (Burnet, 1970a).

On the other hand, Good and Yunis (1974) interpreted these associations to be more consistent with a forbidden-antigen theory of autoimmunity. We have argued that under several circumstances of immunodeficiency, antigens that otherwise would have been prohibited from entering the body, or else promptly eliminated from it, are permitted to enter or persist as infectious agents or antigens that can generate cross-reacting antibodies as a consequence of an inefficient or ineffective immune response (Yunis *et al.*, 1969a,b, 1972; Good and Yunis, 1974).

An interpretation of the immunological theory of aging based on thymic involution is that the primary events of aging are embodied in a chronological process that is genetically programmed to result in a decline in effective function and control of immunity through the T-dependent lymphoid system. The genetically programmed clock operates at a rate consistent with the median life span of the species, and for the longest-lived individuals or strains may adhere to limits imposed by the postulate of Hayflick (1965).

It is possible that the process of maturation of thymocytes ceases either through changes in CNS–endocrine control of the thymus or because of intrinsic temporal limitations of its function, which in turn bring about a progressive decline of thymic influence. An involution of the thymus would in turn impose an essential limit on the immunological vigor of the differentiation of B lymphocytes, which may also be necessary to explain fully the decline of humoral immunity during aging. The involution of either or both of these controlling lymphoid organs and loss of their generating and supportive functions with age impose restrictions on immunological vigor that are determined by the limited potentiality for differentiation or replication, or both, of the B and T lymphocytes, especially the latter.

The preceding discussion suggests that the primary age-related effect on the immune system is a decrease in T-cell functional capacity. The idea that this age-associated deficiency may be important in humans in the pathogenesis of diseases of the aged gained support by the finding that old people with defective CMI have decreased life expectancy (Roberts-Thomson *et al.*, 1974). The resulting imbalanced immune system in which the host is T-cell-deficient and B cells are more normal may be important in the pathogenesis of increased appearance of autoantibody and the autoimmune nature of a number of diseases associated with aging. This could be especially true if the balanced T-cell subpopulations become disordered or disorganized, as seems to be the case from our own studies (Hallgren and Yunis, 1977). The T-cell deficiency includes decrease of one kind of suppressor-cell function. This event might be one that allows autoimmune clones to arise or to be expressed. Conversely, loss of self-tolerance and the occurrence of autoimmunity could lead to the production of anti-T-cell autoantibodies and acceleration of the T-cell immunodeficiency with aging, and might thus permit expression of the destructive consequences of this T-cell immunodeficiency, as in neonatally thymectomized mice.

3.2. Immune Surveillance

Immunodeficiency or the decline of immune functions, autoimmunity, and appearance of malignancy go hand in hand. Cancer as a whole may be considered as a "disease of aging," but it is important at present not to draw conclusions from one or a few types of tumors. Ehrlich first postulated that immunological reactions may defend against cancer, and that cancers that occur frequently are usually eliminated from the body.

In 1959, Lewis Thomas (1961) suggested that protection against malignancy might be a major role played by cellular immune functions of the sort involved in allograft rejection and delayed hypersensitivity. The hypothesis of immune surveillance has since been restated and promulgated, especially by Burnet (1959, 1970a,b) and by Good and Finstad (1969), and many others. Failure of surveillance results in infections, autoimmune diseases, and cancer. This constellation of diseases closely resembles that produced by neonatal thymectomy and that which occurs with excessive frequency in immunosuppressed adults. It is a constellation that strikingly occurs with aging. Still, it is not clear whether a decline in normal immune capacity to threshold levels predisposes subjects to such diseases. As a basis for explanation of diseases of aging, this concept seems to us most favorable, since the onset of decline in thymus-derived T-cell-dependent immune functions is so strikingly and uniformly associated with age.

The concept of immunosurveillance is predicated on the possibility that tumor cells have antigens on their surfaces that can be recognized by the host as being foreign. Further, if immunosurveillance is to work in many or most instances, such antigens should be recognized as transplantation antigens, and the host should react to them with sufficient vigor to eliminate the cancer cells from the body. A corollary to this postulate is that failure of this mechanism for elimination of tumors is necessary to permit development of many or most cancers. This working hypothesis predicted a high frequency of malignancies in patients with primary immunodeficiencies, especially when the deficiencies involve the T-cell apparatus, a high frequency of malignancies in patients subjected to immunosuppression, a frequent immune response to malignant cells in all species studied, progressive evolution of spontaneous tumors composed of cells with low antigenicity, involution of the immunological system with aging, and difficulty with but ultimate ability to harness the immune response to resist cancer.

In almost all these predictions, the immunosurveillance concept has proved prophetic. Nonetheless, much evidence has been brought forward in opposition to this perspective. The antithesis of the immunosurveillance concept was stated repeatedly by Prehn (1970), Stutman (1974a), and Schwartz (1975). The essence of these arguments includes the following considerations:

1. Tumors of patients with primary and secondary immunodeficiencies represent not all cancers, but are selective for lymphoreticular malignances and certain GI tumors—few among many kinds of cancer (Kersey *et al.,* 1975).
2. *Nu/nu* mice, which lack a T-cell system, although they are extremely susceptible to virus-induced neoplasia, are not unusually susceptible to chemical-carcinogen-induced malignancy (Stutman, 1974).
3. Tumors of high antigenicity may grow to considerable size without generating effective immunity (Prehn, 1972).
4. Spontaneous cancers do not possess demonstrable tumor-specific antigens (Smith, 1972).
5. Under certain circumstances, immunostimulation may foster tumor spread (Prehn, 1972).
6. Chemical carcinogens, although both immunosuppressive and carcinogenic, exert their carcinogenic influences at doses far below those that are demonstrably immunosuppressive. There is clear dissociation of carcinogenic and immunosuppressive doses of agents that share capacity for those biological actions.
7. In some cancer, e.g., breast cancer in mice, immunity functions are essential to the development of the malignancy.

None of the arguments for or against the immunosurveillance concept is as yet definitive, and as is so often true with science, the controversy regarding this postulate has generated massive amounts of data and much greater understanding of both immunological function and pathogenesis of malignancy. The increasing incidence of cancers with aging could, for example, be the consequence of promoter or cofactors imposed by infection or autoimmunity or the long-term influence of chemical carcinogens, rather than the failure of immunosurveillance. Recently, Schwartz (1975) modified the immune surveillance theory to involve especially the malignancies of the lymphohematopoietic system. He reviewed his hypothesis based on experimental and clinical observations that the malignancies of the lymphohematopoietic system are the result of an immune imbalance involving the different subsets of lymphocytes, which, in the presence of continuous virus–host interaction, results in abnormal stimulus to proliferation favoring derivation of a clone of cells (likely a mutant) with consequent abnormal properties and survival advantage and thus capacity to develop malignancy. This concept is related in some way to the forbidden-antigen theory of autoimmunity and immunodeficiency previously stated by Good and Yunis (1974). According to the latter concept, it is the immunodeficiency that opens the door to excessive antigenic stimulation of remaining immunologically active lymphoid components. The stimulation derives from antigens that persist or infections that are not eliminated. The consequence is continued excessive proliferative activity in the lymphoid apparatus, increasing the chance for somatic-cell mutation and development of clones of cells with survival advantage in the individual.

Evidence exists for a relationship between autoimmunity and cancer. For instance, there is an increased frequency of tumors in association with known or suspected autoimmune disorders including thyroiditis, pernicious anemia, and ulcerative colitis (Blumenthal and Berns, 1964). Dermatomyositis is associated with several forms of malignancy (Page *et al.,* 1963). Autoimmune hemolytic anemia is frequently coexistent with lymphomas. Sjögren's syndrome predisposes greatly to lymphomatous malignancies (Talal and Bunim, 1966). In addition, autoimmune-susceptible strains and mice having chronic GVH reaction have a high propensity toward the development of lymphomas and other tumors. The immune surveillance theory, as currently conceived, does not explain the incidence of all forms of cancers in mice or man, but in autoimmune-susceptible strains and in aging might at least explain the association of early thymic involution, autoimmunity, and malignancy on the basis of lack of control of the B-cell system (loss in development of special classes of suppressor cells), as well as malignant proliferation of that system. For example, chronic lymphatic leukemia in man may be explained in this way (Yunis *et al.,* 1976a). Based on these observations, one might speculate that the thymic involution with disappearance of suppressor T cells and/or mutation in a single clone in the presence of continuous antigenic stimulation provided by the Gross leukemia virus and other viruses may be a major mechanism to explain proliferation of B cells and malignant B cells and malignant B cells. The ultimate role of development of malignant clones, e.g., among B lymphocytes, played by suppressor cells, killer cells, and even the newly defined natural killer cells (Kiessling *et al.,* 1975; Herberman *et al.,* 1975) in surveillance phenomena, if such exist, still needs to be analyzed.

On the other hand, in other forms of malignancy in mice, thymic involution may favor conditions of the host to bypass mechanisms of immunological resistance or to promote tumor development. A prime example of a condition in which normal thymic function favors tumor development is mammary adenocarcinoma in mice, in which removal of the thymus in the neonatal period is followed by very great prolongation of the latent period and decrease of the incidence of malignancy (Martinez, 1964; Yunis et al., 1969a).

3.3. Thymic Involution in Short-Lived Strains of Mice

Lymphoid neoplasms in general and lung tumors in mice occur at a younger age when shortening of life span is produced by irradiation (Alexander, 1957). From these studies, one might also postulate that thymus and thymic functions underlie processes that lead to both cancer development and short survival.

We have studied thymic involution in different inbred strains of mice. CBA mice tend to be very long-lived and to maintain immunological function longer than do mice of other strains when measured by several standards. By contrast, NZB and (B/W)F$_1$ mice are both short-lived and develop immunodeficiencies and immunological abnormalities early in life (Stutman et al., 1968; Teague et al., 1970; Rodey et al., 1971; Fernandes et al., 1977).

We (Good, 1954, 1973; Good et al., 1962; Good and Yunis, 1974) have been especially concerned with the consequences of deficiency and decline of the T-cell immunity system and its relationship to diseases of aging. The T-cell immunity system not only underlies delayed allergic responses and allograft rejection, but also is responsible for the vital defense of the body against facultative intracellular bacterial pathogens, fungi, and many viruses. It is essential for initiating humoral immunological responses to many antigens through the function of the subclass of helper T cells. It probably applies the damper to ongoing immunological processes with its class of specific suppressor T cells and inhibits accumulation of foreign organisms and perhaps malignant cells through the influence of killer T cells. Thus, the T-cell system is among the most vital and powerful components of the bodily defense. Through the lymphokines produced or generated by stimulated T cells, they can communicate with macrophages, eosinophils, and granulocytes. Thus, in many ways, the T cells act directly or indirectly in the bodily defense.

Shortly after a number of investigators (Archer and Pierce, 1961; Archer et al., 1962; Martinez et al., 1962; Good et al., 1962; Miller, 1961) independently discovered the essential role of the thymus in development and maintenance of the immunological functions, we encountered evidence that autoimmune phenomena, autoimmune disease, amyloidosis, wasting disease, hyalinization of vessels, vasculitis, and cardiovascular–renal diseases regularly accompany T-cell deficiency. Neonatally thymectomized rabbits with or without the addition of appendectomy or irradiation (Papermaster and Good, 1962; Sutherland et al., 1965; Kellum et al., 1965; Cooper et al., 1965; Yunis et al., 1965), like aging mice of certain strains (Teague et al., 1970) and immunodeficient man (Good, 1973a,b; Yunis and Greenberg, 1974), developed autoimmunities in high frequency. Furthermore, in both the immunological disturbances imposed by neonatal thymectomy and those occurring naturally with aging in several strains of mice, we found that when we corrected the immunodeficiency with thymus cells, thymus grafts, or fully differentiated syngeneic or even partially matched allogeneic T cells (Yunis et al., 1965, 1966, 1972), we could prevent many of these diseases. Indeed, we found it possible even to reverse (Yunis et al., 1971a,b, 1972) ongoing immunological and autoimmune disorders if the numbers of immunologically competent T cells given were sufficiently large or if several thymus transplants were given.

3.4. Autoimmune Strains of Mice

The New Zealand investigators Helyer and Howie (1963) found that the New Zealand Black (NZB) mice introduced into medical research by Bielschowsky in 1959 regularly showed spontaneous development of Coombs-positive hemolytic anemia. The autoimmune Coombs-positive hemolytic anemia that developed in these mice was originally attributed by Holmes and Burnet (1963, 1966) to an abnormality of thymic structure. Indeed, based on a study of very few animals, it was suggested that removal of the thymus might protect against the development of autoimmunity. Howie and Helyer (1968) could not confirm this preliminary finding, however, and the NZB mice as well as NZW and (NZB × NZW)F$_1$ hybrids were found to develop not only autoimmune hemolytic anemia, but also antinuclear antibodies. It then became clear that neonatal thymectomy in mice of autoimmune susceptible strains not only failed to protect against development of the autoimmune hemolytic anemia (Yunis et al., 1969a,b, 1972), but also shortened the incubation period of these autoimmune diseases and accelerated other apparent autoimmune phenomena such as anti-DNA and anti-nuclear antibody production and progressive renal disease that often occurred in such animals.

Teague and Friou (1969), and Teague et al. (1968), working with A/J mice, found that spontaneous development of antinuclear antibodies also characterized this strain. Teague then came to our laboratories, where in collaboration we studied the decline of immunological function with the influence of neonatal thymectomy in several strains of autoimmune-susceptible and autoimmune-resistant mice (Teague et al., 1969, 1970). In these studies, Teague et al. (1970) confirmed that two strains of A mice, A/J and Af/Umc, develop spontaneous autoimmune disease, and that the development of autoimmunity could be greatly facilitated by neonatal thymectomy. We noted that the pattern of autoimmune hemolytic anemia and antinuclear antibodies, renal pathology, and hyalin–amyloid disease (Figures 4A,B and 5A,B) that we observed after neonatal thymectomy early in life in certain strains of mice was similar to the changes that occurred with aging in these same inbred strains of animals. The autoimmune-susceptible strains of mice studied were NZB/Umc, NZW/Umc, A/J, Af/Umc, C57BL/KS/Umc, and the hybrids of these strains (Yunis et al., 1972). Neonatal thymectomy in these mice accelerated the development of the autoimmune phenomena and was accompanied by extraordinary plasma-cell proliferation in the lymphoid tissues. Plasma-cell proliferation in lymph nodes and spleen is also found frequently in these autoimmune-susceptible strains during aging (Yunis et al., 1969b, 1971a,b, 1972). In contrast, CBA/H/Umc and C3H/Umc mice, which do not develop autoimmunity spontaneously with aging, exhibit lymphoid tissue atrophy and show much less evidence of autoimmune phenomena following neonatal thymectomy (Yunis et al., 1972) (Figures 4A,B, 5A,B, 6, and 7). Even in CBA mice, however, autoimmunity accompanies the immunodeficiencies produced by neonatal thymectomy.

We then discovered that immunodeficiency develops with great frequency in the autoimmune-susceptible strains of mice during aging. Indeed, in NZB mice, a profound deficiency of CMIs could regularly be demonstrated early in the second half of the first year of life (Stutman et al., 1968; Yunis et al., 1967). These same phenomena were associated in the A/J and A/Umc strains of mice, but the defi-

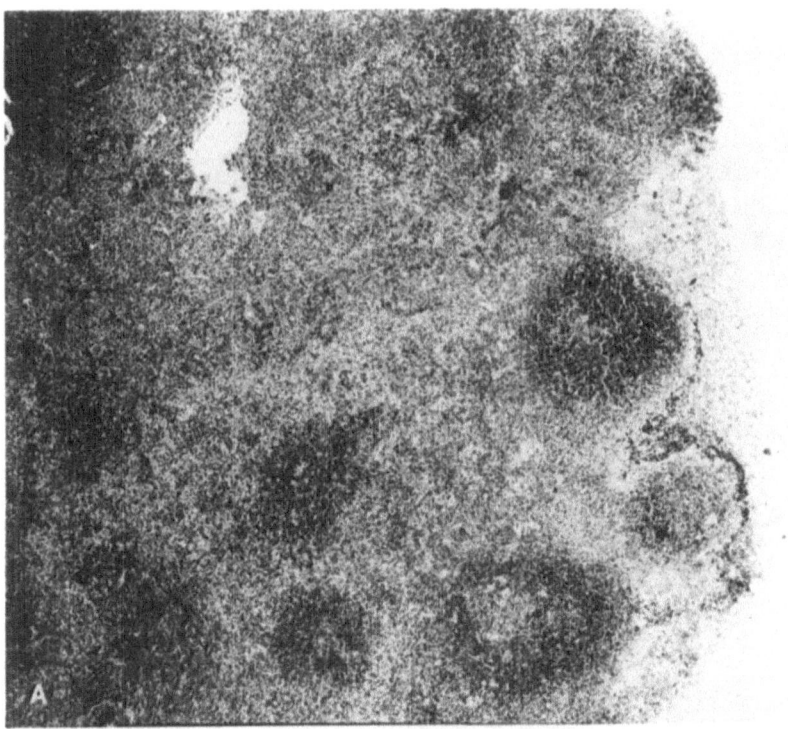

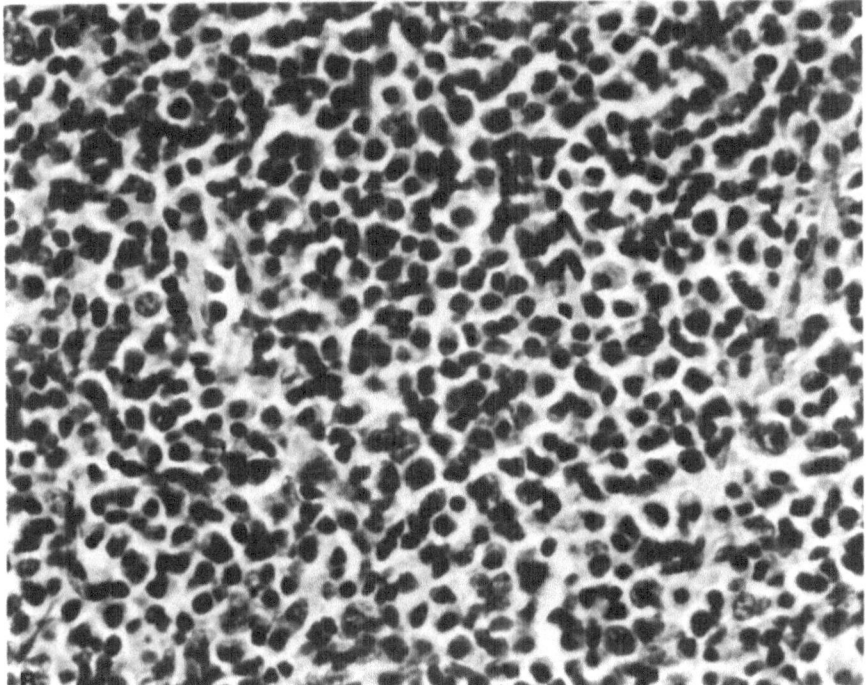

Figure 4 (A). Submaxillary lymph node of a 12-month-old A strain mouse showing enlargement with large number of lymphatic follicles and decrease of paracortical lymphocytes. Magnification ×40. Hematoxylin–eosin. (B). Same section as in Figure 4A, but at higher magnification (×600) to demonstrate the large number of plasma cells in the cortex of the lymph node (near marginal sinus). Hematoxylin–eosin.

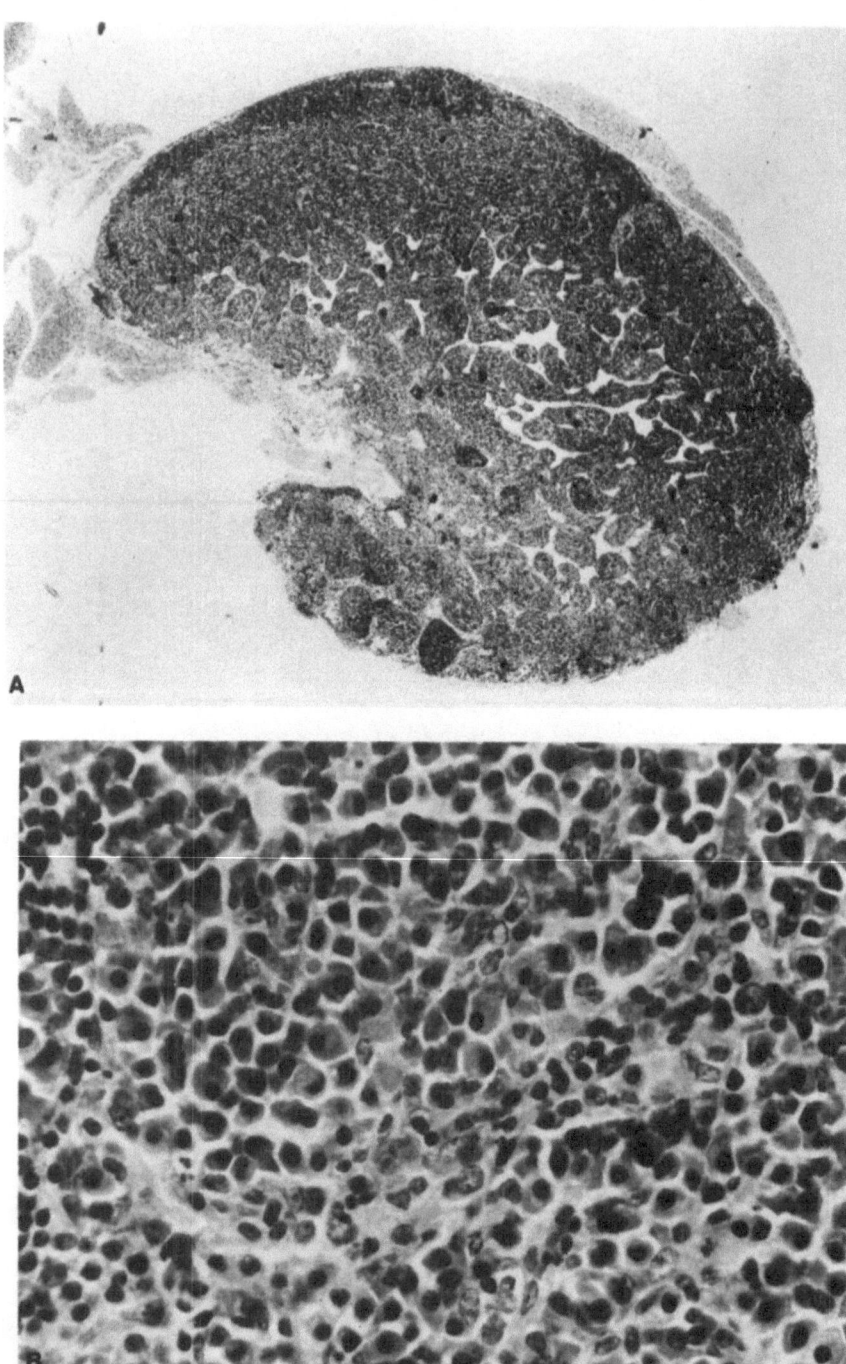

Figure 5 (A). Submaxillary lymph node from a 5-month-old neonatally thymectomized A strain mouse showing decrease of lymphocytes and size of lymphocyte follicles. Magnification × 40. Hematoxylin–eosin. (B). Same section as in Figure 5A, but at higher magnification (× 600) to demonstrate large number of plasma cells in the subcortical area. Hematoxylin–eosin.

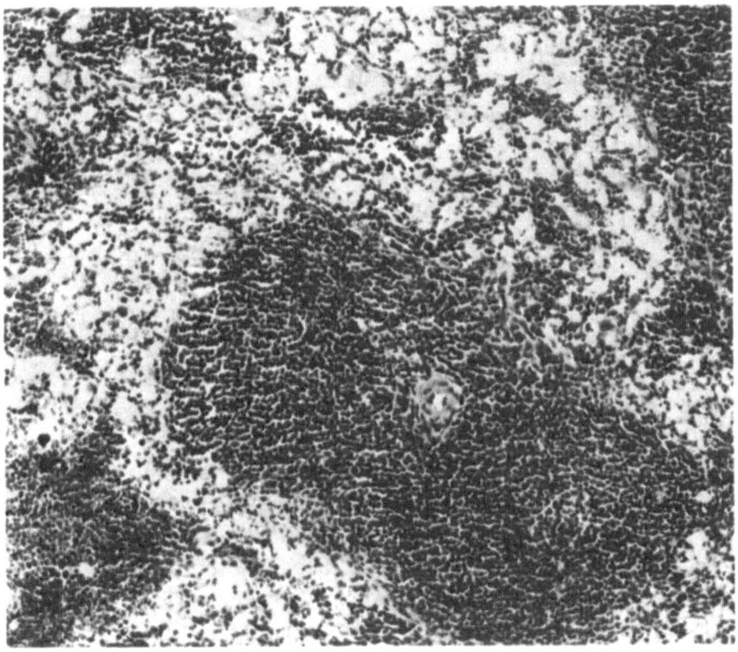

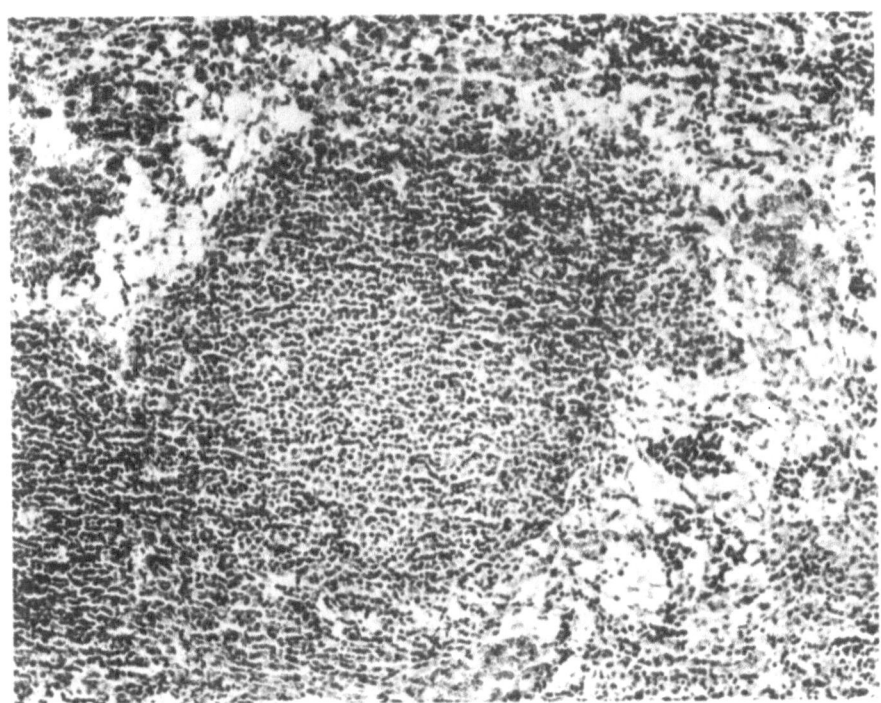

Figure 6. Spleen from a 5-month-old neonatally thymectomized A strain mouse to show perifollicular amyloid deposition. Magnification × 100. Hematoxylin–eosin.

Figure 7. Spleen from a 20-month-old A strain mouse showing perifollicular amyloid deposition. Magnification × 100. Hematoxylin–eosin.

ciency, like the autoimmunity, appeared earlier in the NZB/Umc mice than in mice of the A strains. The immunological deficiencies, autoimmune hemolytic anemia, antinuclear antibodies, and anti-DNA antibodies and the histological patterns of hematological, hepatic, splenic, and renal lesions that appeared early in life following neonatal thymectomy in autoimmune-susceptible mice reflected great acceleration of a process that has a propensity to develop in association with severe cellular immunodeficiency during aging in mice of these strains (Teague *et al.*, 1970).

Another line of evidence that seems to link the immunodeficiency with autoimmune phenomena is that represented by our efforts to correct the immunodeficiency in thymectomized animals. The development of immunodeficiency, autoimmunity, and the histological lesions including amyloidosis in Af/Umc mice is prevented by transplantation of syngeneic or allogeneic thymus from young mice. Another means of preventing the development of the entire spectrum of serological and histopathological lesions of autoimmune disease in these mice has been to inject either thymus lymphocytes or spleen lymphocytes from syngeneic, semiallogeneic, or allogeneic donors. To avoid a lethal GVH reaction, the thymus or peripheral lymphoid cells injected must be matched with those of the recipient at the major histocompatibility complex *(H-2)*. Even more impressive has been the influence on the autoimmune diseases in thymectomized mice of treatment with multiple thymus grafts or injection of large numbers of thymus cells or peripheral lymphoid cells, even after the wasting disease and autoimmune processes have appeared. It has been possible with each of these forms of cellular engineering to reverse the wasting processes and to improve autoimmune phenomena even after the latter have already appeared. Thus, cellular engineering by thymus transplantation or with appropriately matched thymus or peripheral lymphoid cells can be used to prevent and even to treat wasting disease and autoimmune phenomena in immunodeficient mice (Stutman *et al.*, 1967, 1968, 1969; Yunis *et al.*, 1965, 1967, 1971a,b, 1972).

3.5. Involution of the Lymphoid System and Amyloidosis

Several studies on the influence of central lymphoid tissue extirpation as a means of producing immunodeficiency in experimental animals (neonatal thymectomy, neonatal thymectomy plus irradiation, and others) led to a high frequency of both amyloidosis and autoimmune hemolytic anemia (Kellum *et al.*, 1965; Yunis *et al.*, 1967, 1969a,b, 1972). In these experimental animals, evidence of excessive stimulation of the remaining immunological system in the form of marked and disseminated plasmacytosis was "seen" as an indication of stimulation and differentiation of the B-lymphocyte population (Figures 4A,B and 5A,B). The immunodeficient animals also showed a high frequency of amyloidosis (Figures 6 and 7) and autoimmune hemolytic anemia (Yunis *et al.*, 1969a,b).

While we lack formal proof that the involution of the lymphoid system and consequent immunostimulation are directly responsible for the amyloidosis, it is appropriate to discuss several aspects that indicate that amyloidosis is a manifestation of immunological disturbance. The view that amyloidosis may reflect autoimmune disturbances was analyzed by Sutherland *et al.* (1965), Walford (1969), and Good and Yunis (1974). Besides having to do with immunological mechanisms, the condition is found in apparently all species of higher animals, generally in a large number of older members of each species. This disorder occurs in association with a number of disease conditions in man: chronic suppurative diseases, 10–25% of cases of rheumatoid arthritis, Hodgkin's disease, and multiple myeloma. When the amyloidosis appears to be secondary to another condition, it has been called *secondary amyloidosis*. When it occurs without apparent accompanying disease, it is called *idiopathic* or *primary amyloidosis*. Secondary amyloidosis is most frequently the consequence of multiple myeloma, a clonal malignant proliferation of plasma cells that is regularly accompanied by severe immunodeficiency. A distinguishing feature between the two forms of amyloidosis is the involvement of the CNS. This takes the form of so-called "senile plaques" that are a manifestation of generalized amyloidosis (Horst *et al.*, 1960).

Amyloidosis has been known for many years to be associated with frequent and persistent infections and rheumatoid diseases. Thus, it was of very real interest when Teilum (1968) showed that amyloidosis, like autoimmunity, occurs with inordinate frequency, and at an early age in patients with primary immunodeficiency diseases. The exact nature of this relationship remains to be elucidated. Nonetheless, the finding that amyloidosis of man is associated with both primary and secondary immunodeficiency, excessive infection, and probably excessive antigenic stimulation, as well as with aging, is most provocative. An attractive possibility is that amyloidosis is one consequence of excessive antigenic stimulation that is permitted by developing immunodeficiency with aging. The cells responsible for production of the amyloid are still a matter of dispute. In myeloma, as in aging, primary immunodeficiency diseases, and immunodeficiencies associated with other cancers and infection, one can visualize a circumstance in which antigenic stimulation could generate amyloid protein by stimulating cells of the immunity system to produce this interesting product. For this discussion, it is perhaps sufficient to consider that amyloidosis, like plasma-cell proliferation, is frequently a reflection of excessive stimulation consequent to immunodeficiency. Rapid progress in defining amyloidosis chemically by Glenner *et al.* (1973) and Franklin and Zucker-Franklin (1972) promises new approaches to understanding which cells produce amyloid in its several forms and why this substance or these substances are associated paradoxically with both immunological excesses and immunodeficiency.

Recently, the isolation of two major proteins which appear to be components of amyloid deposits, has brought a new dimension to the studies of age-related diseases. These proteins are chemically unrelated to the immunoglobulins, increase tenfold or more during the last decade of life, and are correlated with diseases of aging and the presence of several forms of cancer. It seems of great interest to investigate the role of these proteins in other disease processes associated with aging and perhaps aging itself (Franklin, 1975–1976). Of interest in the context of our considerations is that we have been able to prevent and possibly even to reverse amyloid deposition and autoimmune disease (Yunis *et al.*, 1965, 1972; Good and Yunis, 1974) by correcting immunodeficiency induced by neonatal thymectomy either by treatment with lymphoid cells or by thymus transplantation.

4. Thymus and Endocrine Organs

Recently, it has become evident that there is an intimate relationship between the thymus and the pituitary in very short-lived hypopituitary dwarf mice (Duquesnoy, 1975; Pierpaoli, 1975; Fabris *et al.*, 1972). These investigators showed that the immunological deficiencies of these prematurely aging mice can be corrected by injecting either growth hormone plus thyroxin or lymph node cells from normal hemiallogeneic donors. The hormonal manipulations were not effective, however, when the thymus had been removed prior to initiating the injections. These findings suggest that thymic function depends on normal production of growth hormone and thyrotropic hormone by the pituitary gland, and that thymic involution may be related to age changes of the pituitary and perhaps the hypothalamus. Hypothalmic control of endocrine function was studied by Dilman (1971), who proposed that the hypothalamus undergoes an age-associated elevation of the threshold of its response to feedback suppression. It is possible that these changes result in irreversible CNS–thymus abnormalities in the animal that contribute greatly to the breakdown of immunity, as well as other bodily functions, that is expressed as diseases of aging (Yunis *et al.*, 1977). It is possible that the thymus also interacts with the gonads (Nishizuka and Sakura, 1971), and that the complexities of immunodeficiency, immunological excesses, and autoimmunities may be understood only in terms of a complete analysis of the interactions of the endocrine organs and CNS with lymphoid differentiation and the maintenance of lymphoid cells and lymphoid functions. Indeed, even hormones like insulin may not only be essential to glucose metabolism in classic physiological terms, but may also play a crucial role in development and maintenance of immunological vigor, and consequently youthful integrity of the body and avoidance of diseases of aging.

5. Virus Infection and Lymphoid Involution

Several reports suggest a possible relationship between immunological deficits and viral infection (Yunis *et al.*, 1978). During the past several years, a great deal of attention has been placed on the possible role of viruses (endogenous and exogenous) in the pathogenesis of aging (Greenberg and Yunis, 1972) and of age-related diseases such as autoimmunity (Levy, 1974; Hotchin, 1971; Oldstone, 1971; Howie and Heyler, 1968) and malignancy (Gross, 1970). Based on studies in this perspective, Levy postulated a possible role for virus infection in the regulation of the thymic clock (Levy, 1974). Intimate relationships between persistent viral (slow virus) infection and autoimmune phenomena exist, and evidence for their existence has been summarized (Levy, 1974; Hotchin, 1971; Oldstone, 1971; Howie and Heyler, 1968). In considering these studies, one must emphasize the difficulties in separating the primary events from secondary events. The roles played by genetics in controlling thymic involution and the influence of environmental or intrinsic vertically transmitted factors such as viruses in these controls have not been worked out, but the findings demand extensive study.

One of the best animal models that reveal these intimate interrelationships among viral, genetic, and immunological determinants of disease is the NZB mouse (Talal, 1976). In this mouse, evidence exists for infection by one or up to three different RNA viruses—a Gross-type murine leukemia virus (Levy, 1974), a Moloney murine leukemia virus (Levy, 1974; Mellors, 1971), and a xenotropic C-type RNA virus (Levy, 1974). Since NZB mice have neonatal thymic abnormalities, it is attractive to think that the viral infections may play a major role in defining the immunological deficiencies and excesses of these mice and contribute not only to immune complex injury, amyloidosis, and autoimmunity, but also to the malignancies they develop.

6. Role of Nutrition in the Involution of the Lymphoid and Immune Systems

Walford *et al.* (1973–1974) showed that caloric restriction, which decreases both cellular and humoral immune functions early in life, may lead to preservation of immunological functions and immunological vigor late in life. In contrast, well-fed mice that show vigorous immunological function early in life are characterized by early decline of immunological function and earlier death.

We have studied the influence of moderate and severe chronic protein deprivation and of caloric restriction on the lymphoid system and the immune functions. Initially, we were concerned with the influence of diet on reproduction of NZB mice (Fernandes *et al.*, 1972). We found that dietary manipulations permitted, fostered, or inhibited reproduction and could shorten or lengthen life span. A high-fat diet favored expression of autoimmunity while it decreased expression of autoimmune phenomena in these animals. Recent studies with chronic moderate protein restriction in NZB mice achieved by reduction of dietary protein intake from the time of weaning to a level one third to one half that of the standard diet produced the following alterations of the lymphoid and immune systems: Mice fed the low-protein diet did not develop splenomegaly or experience thymic involution, which generally occurs by 7–10 months of age in NZB mice fed the usual amount of protein. Further, 7 to 10-month-old NZB mice fed low-protein (6%) diet maintained more vigorous antibody production to sheep red blood cells (SRBC), greater capacity of their lymphoid cells to produce GVH reactions, and more vigorous capacity to develop T-cell-mediated "killer"-cell immunity after immunization against DBA/2 mastocytoma cells than did NZB mice on a normal-protein (22%) diet. The decrease of proliferative response to PHA and Con A, which normally occurs with aging in NZB mice, was delayed by protein dietary restriction. Response to lipopolysaccharides, however, which also declines with age in NZB mice, did not appear to be influenced by diet. The low-protein diet also inhibited the rise of IgG_1 levels, prevented the increase in IgM levels, and inhibited the fall of IgA levels that usually occur with aging in NZB mice. The low-protein diet, although it delayed the onset of hemolytic anemia, did not prevent the development of this autoimmune disease, and did not significantly prolong life span (Fernandes *et al.*, 1976a).

The findings in NZB mice were somewhat different than those produced by protein deprivation in mice of other strains not so prone to develop autoimmunity. In the NZB mice, chronic moderate protein deprivation maintains ability to produce antibody to SRBC and inhibits involution of CMI functions (Fernandes *et al.*, 1976a). In C_3H mice, however, moderate protein or caloric restriction depresses ability to produce antibody to T-dependent antigens (Jose and Good, 1973; Fernandes *et al.*, 1976c). Several of our studies with moderate protein deprivation in mice, rats, and guinea pigs generally led to depression of ability to produce antibody while maintaining or even increasing expression of CMIs (Jose and Good, 1973a,b; Cooper *et al.*, 1974; Good *et al.*, 1976; Fernandes *et al.*, 1976a,b,c).

These data coupled with much earlier work (McCay *et al.*, 1939; Ross, 1969; Comfort, 1974), especially that of Walford *et al.* (1973–1974), showing that early caloric restriction can prolong life in long-lived mice led us to study the role of caloric restriction in immunity functions and longevity in (NZB × NZW)F_1 mice and mice of other strains. The results were nothing short of dramatic. The life span of these short-lived autoimmunity-prone mice was doubled when caloric food intake was cut to 50% of that ordinarily eaten by these mice when they are permitted *ad libitum* intake or given a higher caloric intake when fed a defined diet (Fernandes *et al.*, 1976b, 1977).

Our most recent work (Fernandes *et al.*, 1977) shows that this extraordinary prolongation of life of B/W mice, achieved by simple caloric restriction from weaning, results in maintenance of immunological vigor, inhibition of anti-DNA production, and inhibition of development of cardiovascular renal disease that is based on immunological assault, and inhibits perturbation in a spontaneous suppressor-T-cell population that occurs with aging in B/W mice.

7. Projections for Future Research and for Efforts to Prevent or Treat Diseases of Aging

Although research on prolongation of life is only beginning, it seems from experimental results already obtained that promising achievements are to be anticipated from investigations in this direction.

At the moment, it seems remote to anticipate prolongation of life far beyond limits imposed by ultimate genetic determinants. In short, it is unlikely that mice can be given the life span of man. In contrast, manipulations directed toward achieving expression of full genetic potential by forestalling appearance of the diseases of aging seem promising. Thus, even though the life span of a mouse cannot conceivably be converted to that of a horse, human, turtle, or elephant, the possibility of manipulating life span by permitting all or many members of a strain or individuals of an outbred species to reach the limitations of their genetic potentiality seems achievable.

In man, genetically superior persons may live as long as 95 to 110 years in vigorous good health. Arteriosclerosis, coronary vascular sclerosis, renal diseases, cancer, autoimmunities including arthritis, vasculitis, amyloidosis, and infections shorten life span below this potential. If these diseases of aging can be prevented or even reversed, the possibility of achieving much longer life with good health would be very real. Recent experimental observations suggest several directions in which such a goal can be realistically approached. By simple dietary protein or caloric restriction, it has been possible in NZB mice and more dramatically in B/W mice to very much delay the development of a whole set of diseases like those that shorten the lives of most persons. Even a delay of expression of cancer has already been possible (Fernandes *et al.*, 1976b). This achievement has been accomplished by procedures that in NZB or B/W mice restore or maintain immunological vigor that otherwise is lost with aging. Study of the mechanism by which diet accomplishes its influence may indeed yield approaches that permit greater flexibility and might enjoy greater acceptance than long-term caloric restriction. For example, Gabrielson *et al.* (1976) have already achieved dramatic influences on longevity of B/W mice using repetitive treatment with relatively low doses of actinomycin D, and Krakauer *et al.* (1976) have inhibited development of autoimmunity in B/W mice by injecting supernatant of lymphocytes that have been stimulated *in vitro* by Con A, a T-cell mitogen.

All this is merely a beginnning, especially since the involution of immunological function ties so closely to involution of the thymus. This avenue of investigation is especially encouraging, since some of the molecules responsible for thymus influence have already been defined in terms that permit one to anticipate synthesis of the hormone or hormones that in turn can be used as therapeutic agents. It will be of interest to determine soon whether or not such biologically active molecules can produce a prolongation of the life span of NZB or (NZB × NZW)F_1 mice as is produced by chronic caloric deprivation. Biological analyses may yield a number of additional approaches to accomplish this end. Further, developing methods to prevent or treat virus infections may interfere with accelerated thymic involution that is consequent to the influences of these agents.

Further efforts to use cellular, macromolecular-defined, small-molecular, or dietary manipulation to correct immunodeficiencies in neonatally thymectomized mice and short-lived autoimmune-prone mice, and even to delay the time of aging in the longer-lived strains, seems to be one of the approaches to diseases of aging most likely to be effective and thus most worthy of intensive investigation.

ACKNOWLEDGMENTS

The authors' research is supported by grants from the Public Health Service, National Institutes of Health, AI 11843, AI 08145, CA17404, CA05826, AI 06314, and CA21672, and the Department of Laboratory Medicine and Pathology, University of Minnesota.

References

Adler, W., Takiguchi, T., and Smith, R. T., 1971, Effect of age upon primary alloantigen recognition by mouse spleen cells, *J. Immunol.* **107**:1357–1362.

Alexander, P., 1967, The role of DNA lesions in processes leading to aging in mice, *Symp. Soc. Exp. Biol.* **21**:29–50.

Alexopoulos, C., and Babitis, P., 1976, Age dependence of T lymphocytes, *Lancet* **1**:426.

Archer, O. K., and Pierce, J. C., 1961, Role of thymus in development of the immune response, *Fed. Proc. Fed. Am. Soc. Exp. Biol.* **20**:26.

Archer, O. K., Pierce, J. C., Papermaster, B. W., and Good, R. A., 1962, Reduced antibody response in thymectomized rabbits, *Nature (London)* **195**:191–192.

Augener, W., Cohnen, G., Reuter, A., and Brittinger, G., 1974, Decrease of T lymphocytes during aging, *Lancet* **1**:1164.

Bach, F. J., Dardenne, M., and Salomon, J. C., 1973, Studies on thymus products. IV. Absence of serum "thymic activity" in adult NZB and (NZB × NZW) F_1 mice, *Clin. Exp. Immunol.* **14**:247–256.

Blumenthal, H.T., and Berns, A. W., 1964, Autoimmunity and aging, *Adv. Gerontol. Res.* **I**:289–307.

Boyd, E., 1932, The weight of the thymus gland in health and in disease, *Am. J. Dis. Child.* **43**:1162–1214.

Burnet, F. M., 1959, *The Clonal Selection Theory of Acquired Immunity*, Vanderbilt and Cambridge University Presses, Nashville, Tennessee.

Burnet, F. M., 1970a, *Immunological Surveillance*, Pergamon Press, New York.

Burnet, F. M., 1970b, An immunologic approach to ageing, *Lancet* **2**:358–360.

Chen, M. G., 1971, Age-related changes in hematopoietic stem cell populations of a long-lived hybrid mouse, *J. Cell. Physiol.* **78**:228–232.

Chino, F., Makinodan, T., Lever, W. H., and Peterson, W. J., 1971, The immune system of mice reared in clean and dirty conventional laboratory farms. I. Life expectancy and pathology of mice with long life spans, *J. Gerontol.* **26**:497–507.

Clark, S. L., Jr., 1966, Cytological evidences of secretion in the thymus, in: *Thymus—Experimental and Clinical Studies: Ciba Found. Symp.* (G. E. W. Wolstenholme and R. Porter, eds.), pp. 3–29, Churchill, London.

Coggle, J. E., and Proukakis, C., 1970, The effect of age on the bone marrow cellularity of the mouse, *Gerontologia* **16**:24–29.

Comfort, A., 1974, The position of aging studies, *Mech. Ageing Dev.* **3**:1–31.

Cooper, M. D., Peterson, R. D. A., and Good, R. A., 1965, Delineation of the thymic and bursal lymphoid systems in the chicken, *Nature (London)* **205**:143–146.

Cooper, W. C., Good, R. A., and Mariani, T., 1974, Effect of protein insufficiency on immune responsiveness, *Am. J. Clin. Nutr.* **27**:647–664.

Dietchman, J. W., and Makinodan, T., 1975, Effect of age on the rate of proliferation of lymphohemato-poietic stem cells, *Proc. 10th Int. Congr. Gerontol.* **2**:12.

Diaz-Jouanen, E., Williams, R. C., Jr., and Strickland, R. G., 1975, Age-related changes in T and B cells, *Lancet* **1**:688–689.

Dilman, V., 1971, Age associated elevation of hypothalamic threshhold to feedback control and its role in development, ageing and disease, *Lancet* **1**:1211–1219.

Dupont, B., Hansen, J., and Yunis, E. J., 1975, Human mixed-lymphocyte culture reaction: Genetics, specificity, and biological implications, *Adv. Immonol.* **23**:108–202.

Duquesnoy, R. J., 1975, The pituitary dwarf mouse: A model for study of endocrine immunodeficiency disease, in: *Immunodeficiency in Man and Animals* (D. Bergsma, R. A. Good, and J. Finstad, eds.), *Birth Defects: Orig. Art. Ser.,* Vol. XI, No. 1, pp. 536–543, Sinauer Associates, Sunderland, Massachusetts.

Fabris, N., Pierpaoli, W., and Sorkin, E., 1972, Lymphocytes, hormones, and ageing, *Nature (London)* **240**:557–559.

Fahey, J. L., Scoggins, R., Utz, J. P., and Szwed, C. F., 1963, Infection, antibody response and gammaglobulin components in multiple myeloma and macroglobulinemia, *Am. J. Med.* **35**:698.

Farrar, J. J., Loughman, B. E., and Nordin, A. A., 1974, Lymphopoietic potential of bone marrow cells from aged mice: Comparison of the cellular constituents of bone marrow from young and aged mice, *J. Immunol.* **112**:1244–1249.

Fernandes, G., Yunis, E. J., Smith, J., and Good, R. A., 1972, Dietary influence of breeding behavior, hemolytic anemia and longevity in NZB mice, *Proc. Soc. Exp. Biol. Med.* **139**:1189–1196.

Fernandes, G., Yunis, E. J., and Good, R. A., 1976a, Influence of protein restriction in immune functions in NZB mice, *J. Immunol.* **116**:782–790.

Fernandes, G., Yunis, E. J., and Good, R. A., 1976b, Influence of diet on survival of mice, *Proc. Natl. Acad. Sci. U.S.A.* **73**:1279–1283.

Fernandes, G., Yunis, E. J., and Good, R. A., 1976c, Suppression of adenocarcinoma by the immunolog-ical consequences of calorie restriction, *Nature (London)* **263**:504–507.

Fernandes, G., Yunis, E. J., and Good, R. A., 1976d, Age and genetic influence on immunity in NZB and autoimmunity resistant mice, *Clin. Immunol. Immunopathol.* **6**:318–333.

Fernandes, G., Friend, P., and Yunis, E. J., 1977, Influence of calorie restriction on autoimmune disease, *Fed. Proc.* **36**:1313a.

Franklin, E. C., 1975–1976, Amyloidosis, *Bull. Rheum. Dis.* **26**:832–836.

Franklin, E. C., and Zucker-Franklin, D., 1972, Current concepts of amyloidosis, *Adv. Immunol.* **15**:249–304.

Gabrielson, A. E., Luberst, A. S., and Olson, C. T., 1976, Suppression of murine lupus erythematosus by D actinomycin, *Nature* **264**:439.

Glenner, G. G., Terry, W. D., and Isersky, C., 1973, Amyloidosis: Its nature and pathogenesis, *Semin. Hematol.* **10**:65–86.

Good, R. A., 1954, Agammaglobulinemia—A provocative experiment of nature, *Bull. Univ. Minnesota Med. Found.* **26**:1–19.

Good, R. A., 1972a, Relations between immunity and malignancy, *Proc. Natl. Acad. Sci. U.S.A.* **69**:1026–1032.

Good, R. A., 1972b, Cellular engineering—An approach to treatment of genetically determined disease, in: *Advances in the Biosciences,* Vol. 8 (Gerhard Raspe and S. Bernhard, Eds.), pp. 411–431, Pergamon, New York.

Good, R. A., 1973a, Immunodeficiency in developmental perspective, *Harvey Lect.* **64**:1–107.

Good, R. A., 1973b, Overview of development, organization, function of lymphoid system and human disease, in: *Membranes and Viruses in Immunopathology* (S. B. Day and R. A. Good, eds.), pp. 425–436, Academic Press, New York.

Good, R. A., 1974, Cellular and macromolecular engineering—A vital new approach to disease, *Rush Presbyt. St. Luke's Med. Bull.* **13**:171–185.

Good, R. A., and Finstad, J., 1968, The development and involution of the lymphoid system and immunologic capacity, *Trans. Am. Clin. Climatol. Assoc.* **79**:69–107.

Good, R. A., and Gabrielson, A. E. (eds.), 1964, *The Thymus in Immunobiology,* Hoeber-Harper, New York.

Good, R. A., and Yunis, E. J., 1974, Association of autoimmunity, immunodeficiency, and aging in man, rabbits and mice, *Fed. Proc. Fed Am. Soc. Exp. Biol.* **33**:2040–2050.

Good, R. A., Dalmasso, A. P., Martinez, C., Archer, O. K., Pierce, J. C., and Papermaster, B. W., 1962, The role of the thymus in development of immunologic capacity in rabbits and mice, *J. Exp. Med.* **116**:773–796.

Good, R. A., Fernandes, G., Yunis, E. J., Cooper, W. C., Jose, D. C., Kramer, T. R., and Hansen, M. A., 1976, Nutritional deficiency, immunologic function and disease, *Am. J. Pathol.* **84**:599–614.

Goodman, S. A., and Makinodan, T., 1975, Effect of age on cell-mediated immunity in long-lived mice, *Clin. Exp. Immunol.* **19**:533–542.

Greenberg, L. J., and Yunis, E. J., 1972, Immunologic control of aging: A possible primary event, *Gerontologia* **18**:247–266.

Gross, L., 1970, *Oncogenic Viruses,* 2nd Ed., Pergamon Press, London.

Hallgren, H. M., and Yunis, E. J., 1977, Suppressor lymphocytes in young and aged humans, *J. Immunol.* **118**:204–208.

Hallgren, H. M., Buckley, C. E., III, Gilbertsen, V. A., and Yunis, E. J., 1973, Lymphocyte phytohemagglutinin responsiveness, immunoglobulins and autoantibodies in aging humans, *J. Immunol.* **111**:1101–1107.

Hammar, J. A., 1926, Die Menschen-Thymus in Gesundheit und Krankheit. I. Das normale Organ, *Z. Mikrosk.-Anat. Forsch.* **6**:1.

Hardin, J. A., Chused, T. M., and Steinberg, A. D., 1973, Suppressor cells in the graft versus host reaction, *J. Immunol.* **111**:650–651.

Harrison, D. E., and Doubleday, J. W., 1975, Normal function of immunologic stem cells from aged mice, *J. Immunol.* **114**:1314–1317.

Hayflick, L., 1965, The limited *in vitro* lifetime of human diploid cell strains, *Exp. Cell Res.* **37**:614–636.

Heidrick, M. L., 1972, Age-related changes in hydrolase activity of peritoneal macrophages, *Gerontologist* **12**:28.

Heidrick, M. L., and Makinodan, T., 1973, Nature of humoral immunologic deficiencies of the aged, in: *Proceedings of the Rocky Mountain Symposium on Aging,* Colorado State University, Fort Collins, Colorado, pp. 80–103.

Heine, K. R., 1971, Die Reaktionsfähigkeit der Lymphozyten im Alter, *Folia Haematol.* **96**:29–33.

Helyer, B. J., and Howie, J. B., 1963, Spontaneous autoimmune disease in NZB/Bl mice, *Br. J. Haematol.* **9**:119.

Herberman, R. B., Nunn, M. E., and Lavein, D. H., 1975, Natural cytotoxic reactivity of mouse lymphoid cells against syngeneic and allogeneic tumors. I. Distributing reactivity and specificity, *Int. J. Cancer* **16**:216–225.

Hirokawa, K., 1977, The thymus and aging, in: *Immunology and Aging* (T. Makinodan and E. J. Yunis, eds.), pp. 51–72, Plenum Press, New York.

Hirokawa, K., and Makinodan, T., 1975, Thymic involution: Effect on T cell differentiation, *J. Immunol.* **114**:1659–1664.

Holmes, M. C., and Burnet, F. M., 1963, The natural history of autoimmune disease in NZB mice, *Ann. Intern. Med.* **59**:265–276.

Holmes, M. C., and Burnet, F. M., 1966, Thymic changes in NZB mice and hybrids, in: *Thymus—Experimental and Clinical Studies: Ciba Found. Symp.* (G. E. W. Wolstenholme and R. Porter, eds.), pp. 381–390, Churchill, London.

Hori, Y., Perkins, E. H., and Halsall, M. K., 1973, Decline in phytohemagglutinin responsiveness of spleen cells from aging mice, *Proc. Soc. Exp. Biol. Med.* **114**:48–53.

Horst, L. v.d., Stam, F. C., and Wigboldus, J. M., 1960, Amyloidosis in senile and pre-senile involutional processes of the central nervous system, *J. Nerv. Ment. Dis.* **130**:578.

Hotchin, J., 1971, Virus, cell surface and self: Lymphocytic choriomeningitis of mice, *Am. J. Clin. Pathol.* **56**:333–349.

Howie, J. B., and Heyler, B. J., 1968, The immunology and pathology of NZB mice, *Adv. Immunol.* **9**:215–266.

Jose, D. G., and Good, R. A., 1973a, Quantitative effects of nutritional protein and calorie deficiency upon immune responses to tumors in mice, *Cancer Res.* **33**:807.

Jose, D. G., and Good, R. A., 1973b, Quantitative effects of nutritional essential amino acid deficiency upon immune responses to tumors in mice, *J. Exp. Med.* **137**:1.

Kellum, M. J., Sutherland, D. E. R., Eckert, E., Peterson, R. D. A., and Good, R. A., 1965, Wasting disease, Coombs positivity, and amyloidosis in rabbits subjected to central lymphoid tissue extirpation and irradiation, *Int. Arch. Allergy* **27**:6–26.

Kersey, J. H., and Good, R. A., 1972, Surveillance mechanisms and malignancy, in: *Membranes and Viruses in Immunopathology* (S. Day and R. A. Good, eds.), pp. 277–292, Academic Press, New York.

Kiessling, R., Klein, E., and Wigzell, H., 1975, Normal killer cells in the mouse. I. Cytotoxic cells with specificity for mouse Moloney leukemia cells: PTO specificity and distribution according to genotype, *Eur. J. Immunol.* **5**:112.

Konen, T. G., Smith, G. S., and Walford, R. L., 1973, Decline in mixed lymphocyte reactivity of spleen cells from aged mice of a long-lived strain, *J. Immunol.* **110**:1216–1221.

Krakauer, R. S., Strober, W., Rippeon, D. L., and Waldmann, T. A., 1976, Prevention of autoimmunity in experimental lupus erythematosus by soluble immune response suppressor, *Science* **194**:56–58.

Lajtha, L. J., and Schofield, R., 1971, Regulation of stem cell renewal and differentiation: Possible significance in aging, *Adv. Gerontol. Res.* **3**:131–146.

Legge, J. S., and Austin, C. M., 1968, Antigen localization and the immune response as a function of age, *Aust. J. Exp. Biol. Med. Sci.* **46**:361–365.

Levy, J. A., 1974, Autoimmunity and neoplasia: The possible role of C-type viruses, *Am. J. Clin. Pathol.* **62**:258–280.

Lilly, F., and Pincus, T., 1973, Genetic control of murine viral leukemogenesis, in: *Advances in Cancer Research,* Vol. 17 (G. Klein, S. Weinhouse, and A. Haddow, eds.), p. 231, Academic Press, New York.

Lloyd, R. S., and Triger, D. R., 1975, Studies on hepatic uptake of antigen. III. Studies of liver macrophage function in normal rats and following carbon tetrachloride administration, *Immunology* **29**:253–263.

MacKay, I. R., 1972, Ageing and immunological function in man, *Gerontologia* **18**:285–304.

Makinodan, T., and Adler, W. H., 1975, The effect of aging on the differentiation and proliferation potentials of cells of the immune system, *Fed. Proc. Fed. Am. Soc. Exp. Biol.* **34**:153–158.

Makinodan, T., and Peterson, W. J., 1962, Relative antibody-forming capacity of spleen cells as a function of age, *Proc. Natl. Acad. Sci. U.S.A.* **48**:234–238.

Makinodan, T., Albright, J. W., Good, P. I., Peter, C. P., and Heidrick, M. L., 1976, Reduced humoral immune activity in long-lived old mice: An approach to elucidating its mechanisms, *Immunology* **31**:903–911.

Martinez, C., 1964, Effect of early thymectomy on development of mammary tumor in mice, *Nature (London)* **203**:1188.

Martinez, C., Kersey, J., Papermaster, B. W., and Good, R. A., 1962, Skin homograft survival in thymectomized mice, *Proc. Soc. Exp. Biol. Med.* **109**:193–256.

Mathies, M., Lipps, L., Smith, G. S., and Walford, R. L., 1973, Age-related decline in response to phytohemagglutinin and pokeweed mitogen by spleen cells from hamsters and a long-lived mouse strain, *J. Gerontol.* **28**:425–430.

McCay, C. M., Maynard, L. A., Sperling, G., and Barnes, L. L., 1939, Retarded growth life span, ultimate body size and age changes in the albino rat after feeding diets restricted in calories, *J. Nutr.* **18**:1–13.

Mellors, R. C., 1971, Wild-type Gross leukemia virus and heritable autoimmune disease of New Zealand mice, *Am. J. Clin. Pathol.* **56**:270–278.

Metcalf, D., Moulds, R., and Pike, B., 1966, Influence of the spleen and thymus on immune responses in aging mice, *Clin. Exp. Immunol.* **2**:109–120.

Miller, J. F. A. P., 1961, Immunological function of the thymus, *Lancet* **2**:748–749.

Nishizuka, Y., and Sakura, T., 1971, Ovarian dysgenesis induced by neonatal thymectomy in the mouse, *Endocrinology* **89**:886–893.

Oldstone, M. B. A., 1971, Autoimmunity and viruses—Fact or fiction: Persistent LCM viral infection, anti-LCM viral immune response and tissue injury, *Am. J. Clin. Pathol.* **56**:299–302.

Page, A. R., Hansen, A. E., and Good, R. A., 1963, Occurrence of leukemia and lymphoma in patients with gammaglobulinemia, *Blood* **21**:197–206.

Papermaster, B. W., and Good, R. A., 1962, Relative contributions of the thymus and the bursa of Fabricius to the maturation of the lymphoreticular system and immunologic potential in the chicken, *Nature (London)* **196**:838–840.

Perkins, E. H., and Makinodan, T., 1971, Nature of humoral immunologic deficencies of the aged, in: *Proceedings of the 1st Rocky Mountain Symposium on Aging*, Colorado State University, Fort Collins, Colorado, pp. 80–103.

Peter, C. P., 1973, Possible immune origin of age-related pathological changes in long-lived mice, *Gerontologia* **28**:265–275.

Pierpaoli, W., 1975, Inability of thymus cells from newborn donors to restore transplantation immunity in athymic mice, *Immunology* **29**:465–468.

Pisciotta, A. V., Westring, D. W., Deprey, C., and Walsh, B., 1967, Mitogenic effect of phytohemagglutinin at different ages, *Nature (London)* **215**:193–194.

Prehn, R. T., 1970, in: *Immune Surveillance* (R. Smith and M. Landry, eds.), pp. 451–462, Academic Press, New York.

Prehn, R. T., 1972, The immune reaction as a stimulator of tumor growth, *Science* **176**:170.

Price, G. B., and Makinodan, T., 1972, Immunologic deficiencies in senescence. I. Characterization of intrinsic deficiencies, *J. Immunol.* **108**:403–412.

Roberts-Thomson, I., Whittingham, S., Youngchaiyud, U., and MacKay, I. R., 1974, Aging, immune response, and mortality, *Lancet* **2**:368–370.

Roder, J. C., Bell, D. A., and Singhal, S. K., 1975, Suppressor cells in New Zealand mice: possible role in the generation of autoimmunity, in: *Suppressor Cells in Immunity* (S. K. Singhal and N. R. St. C. Sinclair, eds.), pp. 164–173, University of Western Ontario, London, Ontario.

Rodey, G. E., Good, R. A., and Yunis, E. J., 1971, Progressive loss *in vitro* of cellular immunity with aging in strains of mice susceptible to autoimmune disease, *Clin. Exp. Immunol.* **9**:305–311.

Ross, M. H., 1969, Aging, nutrition and hepatic enzyme activity patterns in the rat, *J. Nutr.* **94**:565–601.

Schwartz, R. S., 1975, Viruses and systemic lupus erythematosus, *N. Engl. J. Med.* **293**:132–136.

Shisa, H., and Nishizuka, Y., 1971, Determining role of age and thymus in pathology of 7,12-dimethylbenzanthracene-induced leukemia in mice, *Gann* **62**:407–412.

Shreffler, D. C., and David, C. S., 1975, The *H-2* major histocompatibility complex and the immune response region: Genetic variation, function and organization, *Adv. Immunol.* **20**:125.

Siminovitch, L., Till, J. E., and McCulloch, E. A., 1964, Decline in colony-forming ability of marrow cells subjected to serial transplantation into irradiated mice, *J. Cell. Physiol.* **64**:23–31.

Smith, T. R., 1972, Possibilities and problems of immunologic intervention in cancer, *New Engl. J. Med.* **287**:439–450.

Stutman, O., 1972, Lymphocyte subpopulations in NZB mice: Deficit of thymus-dependent lymphocytes, *J. Immunol.* **109**:602–611.

Stutman, O., 1974a, Cell-mediated immunity and aging, *Fed. Proc. Fed. Am. Soc. Exp. Biol.* **33**:2028–2032.

Stutman, O., 1974b, Tumor development after 3-methylcholanthrene in immunologically deficient athymic-nude mice, *Science* **183**:534–536.

Stutman, O., 1974c, Immunodepression and malignancy, *Proc. XI Int. Cancer Congr.* **1**:275–279.

Stutman, O., Yunis, E. J., Smith, J. M., Martinez, C., and Good, R. A., 1967, Reversal of postthymectomy wasting disease in mice by multiple thymus grafts, *J. Immunol.* **98**:79–87.

Stutman, O., Yunis, E. J., and Good, R. A., 1968, Deficient immunologic functions of NZB/Bl mice, *Proc. Soc. Exp. Biol. Med.* **127**:1204–1207.

Stutman, O., Yunis, E. J., and Good, R. A., 1969, Thymus: An essential factor in lymphoid repopulation, *Transplant. Proc.* **1**:614–618.

Sutherland, D. E. R., Archer, O. K., Peterson, R. D. A., Eckert, E., and Good, R. A., 1965, Development of "autoimmune processes" in rabbits subjected to neonatal removal of central lymphoid tissue, *Lancet* **1**:130–133.

Talal, N., 1976, Disordered immunologic regulation and autoimmunity, *Transplant. Rev.* **31**:240–263.

Talal, N., and Bunim, J. J., 1966, The development of malignant lymphoma in the course of Sjögren's syndrome, *Am. J. Med.* **36**:529–540.

Teague, P. O., and Friou, G. J., 1969, Antinuclear antibodies in mice. II. Transformation with spleen cells, inhibition or prevention with thymus or spleen cells, *Immunology* **17**:665–675.

Teague, P. O., Friou, G. J., and Myers, L. L., 1968, Anti-nuclear antibodies in mice. I. Influence of age and possible genetic factors on spontaneous and induced responses, *J. Immunol.* **101**:791–798.

Teague, P. O., Yunis, E. J., Rodey, G., Fish, A. J., Stutman, O., and Good, R. A., 1970, Autoimmune phenomena and renal disease in mice: Role of thymectomy, aging and involution of immunologic capacity, *Lab. Invest.* **22**:121–130.

Teilum, G., 1968, Agammaglobulinemia and pathogenesis of amyloidosis, in: *Immunologic Deficiency Diseases in Man* (D. Bergsma and R. A. Good, eds.), *Birth Defects: Orig. Art. Ser.*, Vol. IV, No. 1, pp. 207–211, National Foundation Press, New York.

Thomas, L., 1961, Discussion, in: *Cellular and Humoral Aspects of the Hypersensitive States*, pp. 529–532, Hoeber-Harper, New York.

Walford, R. L., 1969, *The Immunologic Theory of Aging*, Munksgaard, Copenhagen.

Walford, R. L., Liu, R. K., Gerbase-deLima, M., Mathies, M., and Smith, G. S., 1973–1974, Long term dietary restriction and immune function in mice: Response to sheep red blood cells and to mitogenic agents, *Mech. Ageing Dev.* **2**:447–458.

Walters, C. S., and Claman, H. N., 1975, Age-related changes in cell-mediated immunity in Balb/C mouse, *J. Immunol.* **115**:1438–1443.

Yamazaki, K., Boyse, E. A., Mike, V., Thaler, H. T., Mathieson, B. J., Abbott, J., Boyse, J., Zayas, Z. A., and Thomas, L., 1976, Control of mating preferences in mice by genes in the major histocompatibility complex, *J. Exp. Med.* **144**:1324–1335.

Yunis, E. J., and Greenberg, L. J., 1974, Immunopathology of aging, *Fed. Proc. Fed. Am. Soc. Exp. Biol.* **33**:2017–2019.

Yunis, E. J., Hilgard, H., Martinez, C., and Good, R. A., 1965, Studies of immunologic reconstitution of thymectomized mice, *J. Exp. Med.* **121**:607–632.

Yunis, E. J., Martinez, C., Sjodin, K., and Good, R. A., 1966, Allograft tolerance in thymectomized mice injected with small doses of spleen cells, *Transplantation* **4**:582–586.

Yunis, E. J., Hong, R., Grewe, M. A., Martinez, C., Cornelius, E., and Good, R. A., 1967, Post-thymectomy wasting associated with autoimmune phenomena. I. Antiglobulin-positive anemia in A and C57BL/KsJ mice, *J. Exp. Med.* **125**:947–966.

Yunis, E. J., Martinez, C., Smith, J., Stutman, O., and Good, R. A., 1969a, Spontaneous mammary adenocarcinoma in mice: Influence of thymectomy and reconstitution with thymus grafts or spleen cells, *Cancer Res.* **29**:174–178.

Yunis, E. J., Teague, P. O., Stutman, O., and Good, R. A., 1969b, Post-thymectomy autoimmune phenomena in mice. II. Morphologic observations, *Lab. Invest.* **20**:46–61.

Yunis, E. J., Fernandes, G., and Stutman, O., 1971a, Susceptibility to involution of the thymus dependent lymphoid system and autoimmunity. *Am. J. Clin. Pathol.* **56**:280–292.

Yunis, E. J., Stutman, O., and Good, R. A., 1971b, Thymus, immunity and autoimmunity, *Ann. N.Y. Acad. Sci.* **183**:205–220.

Yunis, E. J., Fernandes, G., Teague, P. O., Stutman, O., and Good, R. A., 1972, The thymus, autoimmunity and the involution of the lymphoid system, in: *Tolerance, Autoimmunity and Aging* (M. Sigel and R. A. Good, eds.), pp. 62–120, Charles C. Thomas, Springfield, Illinois.

Yunis, E. J., Fernandes, G., Smith, J., Stutman, O., and Good, R. A., 1973, Involution of the thymus dependent lymphoid system, in: *Microenvironmental Aspects of Immunity* (B. D. Jaukovik and K. Isakovic, eds.), pp. 301–306, Plenum Press, New York.

Yunis, E. J., Fernandes, G., and Greenberg, L. J., 1975, Immune deficiency, autoimmunity and aging, in: *Immunodeficiency in Man and Animals* (D. Bergsma, R. A. Good, and J. Finstad, eds.), Sinauer Associates, Sunderland, Massachusetts.

Yunis, E. J., Fernandes, G., and Greenberg, L. J., 1976a, Tumor immunology, autoimmunity, and aging, *J. Am. Geriatr. Soc.* **24**:258–263.

Yunis, E. J., Fernandes, G., Smith, J., and Good, R. A., 1976b, Long survival and immunological reconstitution following transplantation with syngeneic or allogeneic fetal liver and neonatal spleen cells, *Transplant. Proc.* **8**:521–565.

Yunis, J. J., Greenberg, L. J., and Yunis, E. J., 1976c, Genetic, developmental, and evolutionary aspects of lifespan, in: *Immunology and Aging* (T. Makinodan and E. J. Yunis, eds.), pp. 91–98, Plenum Press, New York.

Yunis, E. J., Handwerger, B., Hallgren, H. M., Good, R. A., and Fernandes, G., 1978, Aging and immunity, in: *Mechanisms of Immunopathology* (Cohen, McCluskey, and Ward, eds.), John Wiley & Sons, New York (in press).

4

Experimental Models of Lymphoid Malignancies

RAYMOND D. A. PETERSON

1. Introduction

1.1. Historical Background

Thomas Hodgkin (1832) identified lymphoid neoplasia as a disease entity in man 146 years ago. His description served to focus attention on disorders arising within the lymphoid tissue as distinguished from those beginning elsewhere and only secondarily involving these areas. A very mixed assortment of diseases were first grouped together. Some were true lymphoid malignancies, others were not. In retrospect, at least three of Hodgkin's original patients had tuberculosis rather than tumors (Fox, 1926). Nonetheless, the process of identifying lymphoid malignancies was begun. The subsequent sorting, describing, and classifying continues today.

In the late 1800's, it was recognized that animals other than man also had lymphoid malignancies. Eberth (1878) first described leukemia in a mouse. Haaland (1905) expanded on the description, and since then both wild and laboratory animals with lymphomas have been the subject of widespread interest and study. Lymphoid malignancies have now been identified in virtually all vertebrate species that have been intensively scrutinized (Kaplan, H. S., 1974). Apparently comparable neoplasma are also being identified in invertebrates and poikilothermic vertebrates (Harshbarger and Dawe, 1973).

Experimental models of lymphoid malignancies were developed as soon as it became known that certain circumstances or events predispose an animal to develop a lymphoid neoplasm. This endeavor began with the observation that tumors, lymphoid and other types, occurred more frequently in successive generations of certain strains of mice (Slye, 1914). It advanced rapidly over the ensuing years with the realization that in addition to selective inbreeding of experimental animals, infectious agents, chemical substances, radiation, immunological reac-

---

RAYMOND D. A. PETERSON • Department of Pediatrics, University of South Alabama College of Medicine, Mobile, Alabama 36617.

tions, and combinations of these would predispose an animal to the development of a lymphoid malignancy. These predictable experimental models have provided the opportunity to study the pathogenesis of lymphoid malignancies and to incisively analyze specific events. The information derived from these experimental studies is now being brought to bear on the human lymphomas. The promise of a whole new approach to classifying, studying, and treating these malignancies is at hand.

1.2. Relationship of Normal to Malignant Lymphoid Tissue Development

The subject of normal lymphoid tissue development is appropriately reviewed in Chapter 1 (Cooper and Lawton, 1978). The available experimental studies clearly identify two distinct pathways of lymphocyte differentiation: one via the thymus ending in T lymphocytes, the other via the bursa of Fabricius or the bone marrow ending in B lymphocytes. The early conviction of a few investigators that parallels existed between the steps leading to normal and to malignant lymphocyte development has been borne out by experimental studies. These parallels and their implications will be presented early in this chapter.

1.3. Justification for Considering Lymphoid Malignancies as a Group of Related Diseases

The processes leading to malignancies of the cells comprising the lymphoid tissue are multifactorial, complex, and probably different for various types of tumors. It is unlikely that there is a common pathogenetic scheme of events applicable to all lymphoid malignancies. There may be no connection whatsoever between the sequence of events leading to a T-cell and to a B-cell malignancy. Even two malignancies of the same cell type, initiated by different inciting events, may lead to the malignant behavior of the cells by quite different mechanisms. Lymphoid malignancies may be an assortment of essentially unrelated diseases that only share the same location. It is furthermore possible that lymphoid malignancies are quite different from one species of animal to another, having in common only the homologous location.

Given all these unknowns, the only justification for continuing to consider these diseases as a group of related processes is that it is useful. To date, at least, more progress has been made by treating these malignancies as though they were somehow interrelated than by treating them as separate entities. The cells of the lymphoid tissue originate, differentiate, and function in intimate association. The notion of regulatory interactions among these cells is substantiated by numerous studies (Gershon and Metzler, 1978). It would be surprising if perturbations in these regulatory mechanisms did not underlie at least some of these malignancies. The interspecies differences regarding the development and functioning of the immune system and the pathogenesis of lymphoid malignancies appear to be minimal. Thus, it is reasonable and useful to consider lymphoid malignancies in various species as related phenomena.

1.4. Plan and Scope

The goal of this chapter is to provide an overview of the experimental models of lymphoid malignancies. This area of experimentation has expanded so rapidly in the past 10 years that more than such an overview would distort the balance of the book.

Section 2 will outline the clinical features of these neoplasms. Many models remain in essentially the descriptive phase of their development, similar to many of their human counterparts; therefore, the general clinical features remain important starting points for experimental studies.

Next, the classification of these malignancies based on the now well-established distinctions among the cell types constituting the lymphoid tissue will be introduced in Section 3. The inciting factors or etiological agents will then be discussed (Section 4), and finally, the scant data regarding the pathogenetic events that take place between the inciting events and the appearance of the malignancy will be addressed (Sections 5–7).

Table 1 presents the major experimental models of lymphoid malignancies together with some basic characteristics and references.

The scope of this presentation will thus be broad. The depth will be limited by the knowledge of the author and the anticipated level of interest of the reader. For those desiring further information regarding specific aspects of the problem, recent reviews will be cited whenever possible. Other references will be selective rather than comprehensive. They will attempt to identify original papers, pivotal experiments, and representative recent work.

2. Clinical Features

Lymphoid malignancies are by definition the malignant behavior of cells comprising the lymphoid tissue. The clinical features are determined by the consequences of this behavior. Solid tumors arising from within the major lymphoid tissues, i.e., thymus, spleen, and lymph nodes, dominate the picture. Later in the disease, malignant cells often move out from these sites and invade areas such as the CNS, liver, kidneys, and bone marrow.

Tumors may be dominated by lymphocytes, macrophages, reticulum–stromal cells, plasma cells, or combinations thereof. The nomenclature of these tumors has been a controversial, frustrating arena of activity for many years. Cell types may vary from one site to another, and appearances may change with the age of the tumor. The microscope permits only a limited number of variables with which to categorize a cell type or histological pattern. It is to the credit of those who have struggled with this most difficult subject that useful categories have been delineated: categories that correlate with prognosis, response to treatment regimens, and now with other methods of identifying cell types. These histopathological classifications continue to provide solid starting points for the design of experimental studies, as well as the basis for communication among investigators (Braylan et al., 1975; Dunn, 1954; Rappaport, 1966; Berard, 1972; Berard and Dorfman, 1974; Berard et al., 1969; Lukes and Butler, 1966; Lukes et al., 1966a,b; Lukes and Parker, 1978).

The terms leukemia and lymphoma are often used interchangeably, especially in the experimental lymphoid malignancy field. This is justifiable in many circumstances because peripheral blood involvement—leukemia—is a variable component of the lymphoid tissue malignancy (Dunn, 1954). Once the fundamental events underlying these malignancies are fully revealed, however, the meaning of this distinction should become clear and a knowledgeable decision can then be made regarding the nomenclature (Sheehan, 1971).

TABLE 1. Experimental Models of Lymphoid Malignancies

Species	Strain	Inciting factor	Cell type	Comments	References
Amphibia	*Xenopus*	Spontaneous	Lymphocytes, histiocytes	May be granulomas rather than "true" neoplasms.	Balls (1962), Balls and Ruben (1968), Ruben (1970), Ruben and Stevens (1970)
	Xenopus	Cell-free filtrate	Lymphocytes, histiocytes		Ruben et al. (1969), Nayar et al. (1970)
	Triturus pyrrhogaster	Spontaneous	Lymphosarcoma	May be granulomas rather than "true" neoplasms.	Inoue and Singer (1970a,b)
	Triturus pyrrhogaster	Mycobacteric?	Lymphosarcoma		Inoue and Singer (1970a)
	Ambystoma mexicanum	Skin graft rejection	Lymphosarcoma	Transplantable with cells. Tumor-specific antigens present. Extra chromosome.	DeLanney and Blackler (1969)
	Rana pipiens	Renal carcinoma implant	Plasma cell		Schochet and Lampert (1969)
Bovine		Spontaneous	Lymphoma–leukemia	Thymic tumor in 60% of sporadic cases. Multicentric type, common in enzootic form. Strong genetic influence. Serological studies.	Dungworth et al. (1964), W. F. H. Jarrett (1966), Cotchin (1960), Anderson and Jarrett (1968), Marshak et al. (1962), O. Jarrett (1970), Bendixen (1958), Clegg and Moss (1965), C. Olson (1974), Wittmann and Urbaneck (1969a,b) Croshaw et al. (1963), Marshak and Abt (1968), Weischer (1944) C. Olson et al. (1973), Datta et al. (1970), J. M. Miller and Olson (1972), Ferrer (1972), Paulsen et al. (1974)

Animal	Method	Cell type	Features	References
			Virus-associated.	Malmquist et al. (1969), Clarke and Attridge (1968), Ferrer et al. (1971, 1972), J. M. Miller et al. (1969), Callahan et al. (1976)
			Leukemia 10–75%.	Weber (1963), Marshak et al. (1962), Hyde et al. (1958)
			Epidemiology.	H. Olson (1961), Hugoson et al. (1968), Piper et al. (1975)
	Cell transplant		Incidence 70%, 2–14 years.	Rosenberger (1968), Marshak et al. (1967)
	Virus		C-type—calves; cattle to sheep.	L. D. Miller et al. (1972), C. Olson et al. (1972), Wittmann and Urbaneck (1969a)
Cat	Spontaneous	Pleiomorphic: T, B, and T & B.	9–15% of all cat malignancies virus-associated. Four anatomic forms: Multicentric Alimentary Thymic Leukemic	Cotchin (1952, 1957), W. Jarrett et al. (1964a,b, 1973a–c), Rickard et al. (1967), Laird et al. (1968a,b), Brodey et al. (1969), M. B. Gardner et al. (1971), W. Jarrett (1971), Holzworth (1960), Onions (1975)
	Virus		C-type. Incidence 50–100% in 2 mo to 4 yr. Same spectrum of neoplasms as in spontaneous disease. Membranous glomerulonephritis common. Occasional thymic atrophy. Can cross species barriers.	W. Jarrett et al. (1964a,b, 1973a,b), Rickard et al. (1968, 1969), Kawakami et al. (1967), Laird et al. (1968a,b), Theilen et al. (1970), Anderson and Jarrett (1971), Anderson et al. (1971), Essex (1975), O. Jarrett et al. (1971), Mackey et al. (1972), Hardy (1970), Hoover et al. (1972), Essex et al. (1971), Snyder and Theilen (1969), O. Jarrett (1970)

(Continued)

TABLE 1 (*continued*)

Species	Strain	Inciting factor	Cell type	Comments	References
Cat (*continued*)				Both vertical and horizontal transmission.	Hardy et al. (1975)
				Antibodies prevent horizontal transmission.	Essex et al. (1975a,b)
Chicken	Wild and inbred	Spontaneous	B	Serological diagnosis.	Sarma et al. (1971)
				Endemic, spreads horizontally, virus present.	H. Rubin et al. (1962), Gross (1970a), Burmester (1962), Conttral et al. (1954), Burmester et al. (1955), Burmester and Gentry (1954), Dmochowski et al. (1959), Dougherty and DiStefano (1967)
		Cell transfer		Dependent on age, route, genetic factors, immune status.	Burmester (1947), Pentimalli (1941), Furth (1932), C. Olson (1936), Burmester and Prickett (1945)
	Several, line 15 especially susceptible	Oncornavirus	B	Incidence 50–90% in 5–9 mo. Dose-dependent. Genetic factors important. Young chicks most susceptible. Prevented by bursectomy.	Furth (1933), Burmester et al. (1946, 1960a,b), Burmester and Gentry (1956) Peterson et al. (1963a, 1964, 1966), Cooper et al. (1968)
	Wild	Spontaneous	T	Marek's disease—neural lymphomatosis. Short incubation, endemic virus present.	Marek (1907), Pappenheimer et al. (1929), Biggs (1968), Powell et al. (1974)
		Herpes virus	T	Role of virus.	Biggs and Payne (1963, 1964), Churchill and Biggs (1967, 1968), Churchill (1968), Epstein et al. (1968), Nazerian et al. (1968), Nazerian and Witter (1970), Solomon et al. (1968), Witter et al. (1969a,b), Beasley et al. (1970), Calnek et al. (1970a,b), Purchase (1969)

Animal	No.	Origin	Type	Comments	References
			T	Thymic atrophy. Immune response impaired. Vaccine from turkey.	Purchase (1970), Purchase et al. (1968)
				T-cell character.	Purchase et al. (1971), Okazaki et al. (1970), Eidson et al. (1971), Purchase (1972); Hudson and Payne (1973), Powell et al. (1974), Nazerian and Sharma (1975), Rouse et al. (1973)
Dog		Spontaneous	Lymphoma	Peak incidence at 7 yr. <2% total incidence.	W. Jarrett et al. (1966), Dorn et al. (1968), Cohen (1968), Parodi et al. (1968)
				Virus seen in cultured cells.	Chapman et al. (1967)
				Transferred to mice. Simulates Hodgkin's.	Chin et al. (1968); Moulton and Bostick (1958), Squire (1969)
		Cell transfer	Lymphoma	20–100% incidence in 1–3 mo. Radiation of recipient generally required. Some regress.	Moldovanu et al. (1966, 1968), Kakuk et al. (1968), Rickard et al. (1968)
Fish	Salmon and others	Spontaneous	Lymphosarcomas	Thymus and kidney major sites.	Dawe (1969), C. E. Smith (1971)
	Pike	Spontaneous	Lymphoma	Epizootic pattern. Jaws often involved.	Mulcahy (1963, 1970), Mulcahy et al. (1970)
	Muskellunge	Cell-free filtrate	Lymphoma	Transplantable with cells. Jaws rarely involved.	Mulcahy and O'Leary (1970)
		Spontaneous	Lymphoma		Ritchie (1957), Sonstegard (1971)
Guinea pig	2	Spontaneous	B?	Associated oncornavirus. Thymus not affected. Associated herpes virus. Incidence 3.6%.	Shevach et al. (1972a), Nayak et al. (1975), Congdon and Lorenz (1954), Opler (1967a–c), Nadel et al. (1967), L. Gross and Feldman (1969), Hsiung and Kaplow (1969), Nayak and Murray (1973), Nayak (1974)
	13	Spontaneous		Incidence 6.7%.	Hsiung (1972)

(*Continued*)

TABLE 1 (continued)

Species	Strain	Inciting factor	Cell type	Comments	References
Guinea pig (continued)		Cell transfer		Local or systemic tumors in 12–15 days. Immunity develops.	Nadel (1957), Jungeblut and Kodza (1960, 1962), Jungeblut and Opler (1967), Miguez (1918), Snijders (1926), Congdon and Lorenz (1954), Ioachim and Berwick (1970), Feldman et al. (1974). L. Gross et al. (1970, 1973), Feldman and Gross (1970), L. Gross (1970a,b, 1971), L. Gross and Dreyfuss (1974), Nadel et al. (1970)
		Virus		Inconsistent results. Role of virus questionable.	Opler (1967b,c, 1968), Jungeblut and Kodza (1962), Ioachim and Berwick (1970), Gross et al. (1973), Tenser and Hsiung (1973)
		Radiation	Lymphocytes; stem-cells	Females > males. 7–12% incidence.	Van Pelt and Congdon (1972), Congdon and Lorenz (1954), Belousova and Strel'tsova (1967)
Hamster		Spontaneous	Reticulum sarcoma	0.2% incidence between 390 and 700 days.	van Hoosier et al. (1971)
		Cell transplant	Lymphoma	C-type virus observed. Immune response may eliminate.	Stenback et al. (1966), Carter and Gershon (1966), Gershon and Carter (1967), Gershon et al. (1967)
		Virus	Leukemia	Extracts from papillomas containing a papovavirus.	Graffi et al. (1968a,b)
		Rous virus Adenovirus	Sarcoma Lymphosarcomas Plasma cells		Ahlstrom and Forsby (1962), Trentin et al. (1968), Finkel et al. (1968), Fortner (1961), Garcia et al. (1961), Toth et al. (1961)
		Urethane	Pleiomorphic Some lymphoid		
Horse		Hydrocarbon Spontaneous	Lymphocytes	C-type virus isolated. Often alimentary tract involvement.	Freeman et al. (1971a,b), Wiseman et al. (1974), Roberts and Pinsent (1975)

	Strain	Induction	Cell type	Comments	References
Mouse	C58	Spontaneous	T	85% incidence in 5–18 mo. Thymic tumor uncommon. Virus recovered and transmitted.	MacDowell and Richter (1935), L. Gross (1956, 1970a), J. R. Tennant (1962)
	AKR	Spontaneous	T	90% incidence in 5–12 mo. Thymic tumor frequent, virus present.	Furth et al. (1933), L. Gross (1970a), Lowry et al. (1971), Kohn and Novak (1973)
	AKR	Spontaneous	T and B	One tumor line with double marker.	Greenberg and Zatz (1975)
	F	Spontaneous	Lymphoma	40% incidence in 6–18 mo.	Kirschbaum and Strong (1939), Kirschbaum (1944)
	DBA/2	Spontaneous	Lymphoma	40% incidence.	L. Gross (1970a)
	NZB	Spontaneous	T	Virus demonstrated by XC assay.	Levy and Pincus (1970), Proffitt et al. (1973)
	SJL/J	Spontaneous	Reticulum cells		Haran-Ghera et al. (1967, Murphy (1963), Dunn and Deringer (1968), Rubin (1968), Warren (1969), Yumoto and Dmochowski (1967), Shevach et al. (1972b,c)
	Balb/c and CDF	Spontaneous	M		
	SJL/J	Radiation	T	40% incidence, average 7 mo.	Haran-Ghera and Peled (1973), Rubin (1968), Haran-Ghera and Kotler (1968)
	C57BL/6	Radiation	T	100% incidence, thymic tumor, virus-associated.	H. S. Kaplan (1947, 1964), Haran-Ghera and Peled (1972), Nomura et al. (1972)
	Numerous	DMBA	T, B, and null cells	50–70% incidence.	Haran-Ghera (1973), Haran-Ghera et al. (1967, 1975), Haran-Ghera and Peled (1973), Tridente et al. (1964), Rask-Nielsen (1949), Huggins and Uematsu (1976), Law (1941)
		MC		RNA tumor virus expression induced.	Morton and Mider (1938, 1941), Tridente et al. (1964), McEndy et al. (1942), Whitmire et al. (1971), Price et al. (1971), Rhim et al. (1971)
	C57BL/6	BNU	T and B	75–96% in 3–6 mo.	Price et al. (1971), Rhim et al. (1971), Shisa et al. (1975)

(Continued)

TABLE 1 (*continued*)

Species	Strain	Inciting factor	Cell type	Comments	References
Mouse (*continued*)	Numerous	Urethan			Kawamoto et al. (1958), Doell and Carnes (1962), Fiore-Donati et al. (1961)
	Numerous	Nitrosourea			Joshi and Frei (1970)
		Nitroquinoline			Kinosita et al. (1964), Kinosita and Tanaka (1963)
		Triethylenemalamine			Conklin et al. (1963)
		Myleran			Upton et al. (1961), Nemeth (1963)
		Diphenylhydantoin			Krueger and Harris (1972), Krueger et al. (1972)
	Various	6-MP			Doell et al. (1967)
	Various	Azathioprine	Reticulum or lymphocytic		Krueger et al. (1971), Metcalf (1961)
		Allogeneic disease			Armstrong et al. (1970), Hirsch et al. (1970, 1972), Krueger and Heine (1972), L. J. Cole and Nowell (1970), Cornelius (1972a,b), Gleichmann et al. (1972), Schwartz et al. (1966), Schwartz and Beldotti (1965), Walford (1966), Krueger et al. (1971), Krueger (1974)
		Allogeneic disease		Virus-associated.	Armstrong et al. (1972, 1973), Cornelius (1972b, 1973)
	C3H and others	Gross virus	T	100% in 2–6 mo.	Boiron et al. (1967), L. Gross (1970a)
	Balb/c	B/TL virus		Epithelial and fibroblast cell lines produced.	J. R. Tennant (1962, 1969), J. R. Tennant et al. (1971), R. W. Tennant and Richter (1972)
	Various	Moloney virus	T	Origin from Sarcoma 37.	Moloney (1960, 1964)
	Balb/c	Moloney virus	M		Shevach et al. (1972b,c), L. Gross (1970a)
		Rauscher virus	T or B	Probably mixture of 2 viruses.	L. Gross (1970a), Rauscher (1962)
	C57BL/6	Radiation virus	T	80–100% incidence.	Haran-Ghera (1966), L. Gross (1958, 1959a)
Pig		Spontaneous	Lymphosarcoma	Very low incidence. Lymphocytosis, lymphosarcoma.	Anderson et al. (1969)
		Cell transplants			Case and Simon (1968)

Monkey		Strontium-90	Myeloid lymphoblasts	C-type particles associated.	Howard et al. (1968)
	Woolly	Spontaneous		Simian sarcoma virus associated (oncornavirus).	Theilen et al. (1971)
	Owl	Spontaneous		Herpes saimiri transmitted.	Hunt et al. (1975a)
	Marmoset	Simian sarcoma virus; Herpes ateles	Sarcoma; T		Wolfe et al. (1971a), Hunt et al. (1972b), Meléndez et al. (1972a)
		Herpes saimiri	T	100% incidence.	Wolfe et al. (1971b), Meléndez et al. (1972a), Deinhardt (1974)
		Epstein–Barr	B	50% incidence.	T. Shope et al. (1973), G. Miller et al. (1972), Falk et al. (1974), Werner et al. (1975)
				Receptor on B cell for EBV.	Jondal and Klein (1973)
	Owl	Herpes saimiri	T	Virus from squirrel monkey. 75% incidence.	Ablashi et al. (1971), Deinhardt et al. (1974), Wallen et al. (1973), Meléndez et al. (1973), Adamson et al. (1975)
	Spider	Epstein–Barr	Reticulum	30% incidence.	Epstein et al. (1973)
	Cebus albifrons	Herpes saimiri	T		Hunt et al. (1972a)
		Herpes saimiri	T		Meléndez et al. (1970)
Gibbon		Spontaneous and GaLV (oncornavirus)	Lymphosarcoma, myelogenous leukemia		Kawakami et al. (1972, 1975), Snyder et al. (1973), DePaoli and Garner (1968), Johnsen et al. (1971), DiGiacomo (1967)
Baboon		Probable virus	Reticulum		Lapin (1975b)
Rabbit	New Zealand	Herpes saimiri	Lymphosarcoma	Horizontal transmission. Both young and old are susceptible. 56% incidence. Brain involvement, occasional leukemia.	Daniel et al. (1974a,b), Hunt et al. (1975b)
	Cottontail (wild)	Spontaneous	Lymphoma	Low incidence.	Hinze (1971)
Rat	W/Fu	Spontaneous		C-type virus.	Kim et al. (1960), Sarma et al. (1973)
	W/Fu	Radiation	Leukemia	Low incidence, ≈2%.	Hunstein et al. (1963)

(Continued)

TABLE 1 (continued)

Species	Strain	Inciting factor	Cell type	Comments	References
Rat (continued)		Methylcholanthrene with or without radiation	Myeloblastic	24% myeloblastic leukemia with radiation + MC.	Svec and Hlavay (1961), Svejda et al. (1958). Shay et al. (1951)
	Long–Evans	DMBA	Stem cell	Prevented or reversed by hypophysectomy.	Huggins and Uematsu (1976), Huggins and Sugiyama (1966), Huggins et al. (1974), Uematsu and Huggins (1968, 1969), Prigozhina (1962)
		DMBA	Stem cell	Chromosomal abnormalities.	Kurita et al. (1968)
	W/Fu, Sprague–Dawley and others	TMBA	Leukemia osteopathy		Bird (1972)
		Gross virus	T	95% incidence in 2–4 mo. Adults not susceptible.	L. Gross (1961, 1963), Kirsten et al. (1962), Okano et al. (1963)
		Friend virus	Lymphoma		Mirand and Grace (1962), L. Gross (1964)
		Moloney virus	Lymphoma	70% incidence.	Moloney (1960)
		Graffi virus	Myeloid and lymphoid	10% incidence.	Graffi and Gimmy (1957), Graffi (1960)
		Rauscher virus			Rauscher (1962), L. Gross (1966), Cowan (1968), Frank and Schepky (1969)
Reptiles	Several snakes	Spontaneous	Lymphosarcoma		Zeigel and Clark (1969, 1970)
	Lizard	Spontaneous	Myxofibroma	C-type particles seen. DNA-polymerase.	Hatanaka et al. (1970)
	Boa	Rous virus	Lymphoma		Zwart and Harshbarger (1972)
	Lizard	Rous virus			Svet-Moldavsky et al. (1967), Veskova et al. (1970)
	Turtle	Rous virus			Svet-Moldavsky et al. (1967)

Even the early descriptive analyses of the animal lymphoid neoplasms heralded the later-to-be-discovered distinction between those malignancies that first appeared in the thymus and those that did not. Most spontaneous rodent lymphoid malignancies have a huge thymic tumor as the hallmark of the disease. The same is true for certain forms of lymphomas in other species and for many of the experimentally induced malignancies. The development of experimental models enabled sequential studies to be made of the processes leading to the ultimate generalized malignancies. These studies revealed that the "thymic-type" lymphoma first appears within the thymus, and only later are malignant cells found elsewhere (Kaplan, H. S., 1960; Siegler and Rich, 1963; Block, 1966; Block and Goodman, 1963). In contrast, the "nonthymic types" appear to begin in multifocal areas about the body, and only secondarily, if ever, do they involve the thymus.

Thymic-type lymphomas are composed of lymphocytes that appear immature by the criteria applied to normal cell maturation. Cells of the thymus cortex are the first to be involved, and preliminary evidence indicates they may be the ones possessing large numbers of H-2 alloantigens on their surfaces (Haran-Ghera et al., 1975). By more conventional criteria, these cells are called *lymphoblasts* and the tumors *lymphomas* or *lymphosarcomas*.

Abnormalities in chromosome number and morphology have been observed in several of these tumors (Ida et al., 1968; Tsuchida and Rich, 1964; Wakonig-Vaartaja, 1960; Pontén, 1963; Ottonen and Ball, 1973; Yosida and Law, 1968; Joneja and Stich, 1965; Kurita et al., 1968). Most of these studies were on cells from fully developed tumors. Generally, no chromosome abnormalities have been detected during the early pretumor period (Rich et al., 1964). Important clues to the molecular events responsible for the malignant behavior of these cells may be revealed by further analysis of these chromosomal abnormalities (German, 1974).

The cellular composition of the nonthymic lymphomas is often pleiomorphic. Some tumors are composed of a mixture of cell types; others, of immature-appearing lymphoblasts or plasma cells. Many have been described as reticulum-cell sarcomas, and others have been equated with Hodgkin's disease of man (Dunn, 1957; Dunn and Deringer, 1968; Haran-Ghera et al., 1967; Murphy, E. D., 1963; Rudali and Mogul, 1967). These latter tumors seem to preferentially involve the spleen, liver, and mesenteric lymph nodes. The plasma-cell tumors, both spontaneous and induced, are well characterized and are in every way comparable to myeloma of man (Potter, 1962; Potter and Kuff, 1961; Potter and Robertson, 1960).

Further clarification of the distinction between thymic-type and nonthymic-type lymphoid malignancies awaited experimental studies of two major animal models of lymphoma and the generation of knowledge regarding normal lymphoid tissue development.

3. Classification

3.1. T-Cell Lymphomas

The major discovery opening the way for a whole new concept of lymphoid malignancies—and, in retrospect, of the normal immune system—was the observation that thymectomy, performed during the preleukemic period in the AKR mouse, would prevent the development of the malignancy (McEndy et al., 1944). In succeeding years, other investigators reproduced this experiment, not only in the spontaneous lymphoma of the AKR, but also in numerous other experimental situations. Thymectomy prevents the development of lymphoma in another high-leukemic strain of mice, C58 (Law and Miller, 1950a), following radiation (Kaplan, H. S., 1950), hydrocarbon administration (Kaplan, H. S., 1950; Law and Miller, 1950b), and the injection of leukemogenic viruses (Miller, J. F. A. P., 1959; Gross, L., 1959b; Levinthal *et al.*, 1959).

The discovery that the thymus was the site of differentiation of a distinct population of lymphocytes (Cooper and Lawton, 1978; Archer and Pierce, 1961; Miller, J. F. A. P., 1961; Good *et al.*, 1962), now called *T cells,* reinforced the importance of Furth's original observation. Subsequent studies revealed that these normal T cells had surface markers that could serve to identify them after they left the thymus (Raff and Wortis, 1970; Raff, 1969; Takahashi *et al.*, 1971; Bach *et al.*, 1969; Brain *et al.*, 1970; Wybran *et al.*, 1972). These same markers are on the cells constituting those lymphomas that are prevented by thymectomy (Shevach *et al.*, 1972b,c; Haran-Ghera and Peled, 1973; Haran-Ghera *et al.*, 1975).

As a consequence of these two observations—(1) the effect of thymectomy on the pathogenesis of certain lymphomas and (2) the presence of T-cell markers on the cells of the same lymphomas—lymphomas can now be identified as belonging to the T-cell category or as being of another cell type.

One valid concern regarding this identification scheme is that the T-cell markers used for the identification of T cells are those present on normal lymphocytes. They may not necessarily be present on all malignant T cells, even though these cells originated in the thymus. The (C58NT) D Gross-virus-induced lymphoma is an example (Shellam, 1974). Conversely, it is known that malignant cells sometimes express genetic information not normally expressed in comparable normal cells (Coggin and Anderson, 1974; Dulbecco *et al.*, 1965; Hartwell *et al.*, 1965; Kit, 1968). Consequently, a T-cell marker might appear on a cell that was quite independent of the thymus during its differentiation. To date, however, the correlation generally remains valid.

3.2. B-Cell Lymphomas

The first lymphoid malignancy demonstrated to involve exclusively B cells, utilizing essentially the same criteria as just described for T cells, was chicken lymphoid leukosis (Peterson *et al.*, 1963a, 1964, 1966; Cooper *et al.*, 1968). This disease occurs spontaneously, and endemically, in flocks, and has been responsible for extensive financial losses to poultrymen. Consequently, it has been intensively studied, especially at the Regional Poultry Laboratory of the U.S. Department of Agriculture in East Lansing, Michigan (Purchase and Burmester, 1972).

The disease is recognized at the marketplace by a characteristic big liver, and hence was called *big liver disease* (Gross, L., 1970a). The liver and other organs are big and distorted because they are infiltrated with immature lymphocytes. The histopathology of the end-stage disease is a generalized lymphosarcoma, a designation that belies the true origin and significance of this lymphoid malignancy.

In 1954, Lucas *et al.*, (1954a,b) reported an important clue to the real biological significance of this tumor when they noted discrete lymphoid foci in the spleen, liver, and pancreas early in the disease, a pattern later lost when sheets of infiltrating lymphoblasts dominate the picture. Their observation was too early, however, to lead to the pivotal experiments conducted several years later.

The experimental model of chicken lymphoid leukosis was developed following two fundamental discoveries: the disease is caused by a virus (Furth, 1933; Burmester et al., 1946), and susceptibility is genetically determined (Burmester et al., 1960b). The definition of the malignancy as a B-cell disease occurred in tandem with the identification of the two major populations of lymphocytes in the chicken, T and B cells (Warner et al., 1962; Cooper et al., 1965a, 1966a), and later delineation of the same situation in mammals (Cooper and Lawton, 1978; Claman et al., 1966).

The B-cell character of chicken lymphoid leukosis was initially revealed by demonstrating that bursectomy, but not thymectomy, would prevent the disease (Peterson et al., 1963a, 1964, 1966). Later, the tumor cells were identified by their distinctive immunoglobulin surface markers (Cooper et al., 1974). These malignancies begin in B cells at an early stage of their differentiation within the bursa of Fabricius. Cells metastasize from there to the germinal centers within lymphoid tissue. The end-stage disease reveals a generalized lymphosarcoma with a loss of the follicular architectural pattern (Cooper et al., 1968). Unless the origin and pathogenesis were known, it would be impossible to distinguish this final disease picture from lymphomas with different origins. Nodular lymphoma in humans is clearly the counterpart of this experimental model (Jaffe et al., 1974).

It thus became established that the lymphoid malignancies could be composed exclusively of T cells or of B cells, and that a critical event in the pathogenesis of each occurs in the site of normal T- or B-cell differentiation. The early proposal that lymphoid neoplasms in essentially all animals could be so classified (Cooper et al., 1965b, 1966a,b, 1967) has been amply confirmed (Shevach et al., 1972b,c; Haran-Ghera and Peled, 1973; Haran-Ghera et al., 1975; Klein et al., 1968; Grey et al., 1971; Preud'Homme et al., 1971; Braylan et al., 1975; Green et al., 1975).

3.3. Other Cell Types

Several experimental lymphoid malignancies are composed of cells that do not possess characteristics of either T or B cells. Three such mouse tumors have been shown to be composed of cells with properties of the monocyte–macrophage line (Shevach et al., 1972b,c). Monocytes have receptors for C3 (Huber et al., 1968) and IgG (Huber and Fudenberg, 1968) that can be used to identify normal and malignant cells of this type (Shevach et al., 1973). The identification of yet other cell types within the lymphoid tissue capable of becoming malignant awaits further study— probably the development of techniques for identification of different cell lines and stages in the differentiation of the known ones.

4. Inciting Factors

4.1. Genetics

The genetic basis for the development of malignancies was recognized years ago, has been intensively studied, and is only now beginning to be clarified. As early as 1914, Slye called attention to the observation that tumors occurred more frequently in successive generations of certain families of mice (Slye, 1914, 1931). The recognition that inbred strains of animals would be valuable tools for the study of cancer, as well as other fundamental biological phenomena, led directly to the development of the inbred lines of animals available today.

Several strains were observed to have a high incidence of spontaneous lymphoma (MacDowell and Richter, 1935; Richter and MacDowell, 1929; Figge, 1954; Kirschbaum and Strong, 1939). One strain, AKR, was developed specifically for the study of lymphoma by selectively inbreeding animals from those families with the highest incidence of the disease (Furth *et al.*, 1933). The incidence of spontaneous lymphoid malignancies in these strains ranges from 50 to 90%, depending on a variety of variables, often unidentified.

Early studies provided clues regarding the character of the genetic mechanisms underlying these malignancies. Crosses of high- with low-lymphoma strains produced animals with an intermediate frequency of disease (MacDowell and Richter, 1935; MacDowell *et al.*, 1945; Cole, R. K., and Furth, 1941; Law, 1954). The incidence of lymphoma among F_2 and backcross progeny was roughly proportional to the fraction of their genetic material contributed by the high-lymphoma strain.

These early studies also indicated that simple genetic factors were not the only ones influencing the situation. A significant percentage of the inbred mice did not develop a lymphoid malignancy, although their progeny remained at the same high risk as progeny of animals developing leukemia (MacDowell and Richter, 1935). A maternal influence on the incidence was observed in certain models. Clearly, multigenic and nongenetic factors influence the process whereby a certain genetic configuration leads to a lymphoid malignancy.

A genetic predisposition to lymphoma development also exists in those situations in which the malignancy is incited by factors such as chemicals, viruses, radiation, and hormones (Kirschbaum and Mixer, 1947; Hirsch and Black, 1974). These factors produce disease only in genetically susceptible animals. A great deal of the new knowledge regarding the genetic factors has been learned from studies of these models.

Perhaps the most significant breakthrough in our understanding of genetic factors has been the consequence of new concepts and experimentation regarding viral-induced lymphoid malignancies. The difficult, but essential, struggle to arrive at a new concept of the cause of lymphoid malignancies that would integrate data from "genetic" and "viral" models of disease was the first step. Rowe (1973) summarized this effort in a highly recommended recent paper. In essence, he concludes that the differences between oncogenic viruses and genes is often only a semantic one, and that in this context it is appropriate to consider the terms as almost interchangeable.

These conclusions are based on considerable experimental data and some speculation, and are epitomized by the "oncogene theory" proposed by Huebner and Todaro (Huebner and Todaro, 1969; Todaro and Huebner, 1972). Briefly, the concept is that oncogenic viruses are an integral part of the genetic material of most animals. They are present as DNA copies of RNA viruses, or in the case of DNA viruses, as the viruses themselves. They are normally inherited together with all other genes, but only when "activated" by other factors do they express themselves in the form of infectious viruses, tumor-inducing agents, or identifiable antigenic products. The ultimate validity of this concept is probably not as important as are the experimental data derived in the process of assessing it.

An extensive series of studies support the contention that a DNA copy of at least one known RNA leukemogenic virus is incorporated in the genome of essentially all mouse cells. In the AKR mouse, there are three to four murine-leukemia-virus-specific nucleotide sequences on chromosome number 7 (Rowe, 1972, 1973; Rowe and Hartley, 1972, Rowe et al., 1972; Taylor et al., 1971; Lowry et al., 1974; Chattopadhyay et al., 1975). The expression of part of this oncogene results in the appearance on the cell surface of virus-specific antigenic markers such as the glycoprotein designated gp 70 (Lerner et al., 1976).

Regulation of this oncogene resides at two other identified chromosomal sites and perhaps more. One of these is on chromosome 4: a gene designated Fv-1 because it is one of two genes that regulate the development of Friend-virus-induced leukemia (Friend, 1957; Friend et al., 1958). Fv-1 regulates the lymphoid-leukosis-inducing component of Friend virus; Fv-2, the companion erythroid leukemia virus (Odaka, 1973). Fv-1 also determines susceptibility to several other lymphoid-malignancy-inducing viruses (Lilly, 1966a; Rowe et al., 1973; Rowe and Sato, 1973). It is probably the same locus designated Rgv-2 and postulated to regulate susceptibility to Gross virus. Two main alleles, $Fv-1^n$ and $Fv-1^b$, have been identified (Pincus et al., 1971a,b). They influence the rate of replication of the viruses, presumably by controlling processes occurring within, rather than on the surface of, host cells.

One other regulating locus has been identified on chromosome 17 of the mouse. This locus, Rgv-1, governs susceptibility to several leukemia-inducing viruses (Lilly, 1966a,b; Lilly et al., 1964; Lilly and Pincus, 1973). These include AKR, Gross, and radiation-induced leukemogenic virus. It is definitely within the H-2 locus, the major histocompatibility complex of the mouse. Mapping studies place it either in the K or the Ir segment of this complex. Genes in the Ir locus code for proteins known to be important for the functioning of the immune system, especially for the interaction of lymphoid tissue cells (Shreffler and David, 1975). Clarification of how Rgv-1 influences the pathogenesis of lymphoid tissue malignancies should be very revealing.

Although these representative experimental studies have all been in mice, similar situations have been described in many other species (Burmester et al., 1960b; Bendixen, 1963; Congdon and Lorenz, 1954; Jungeblut and Kodza, 1960). It seems reasonable to conclude that genetic factors govern the frequency and development of all lymphoid malignancies, including those occurring in man.

4.2. Viruses

The role of viruses as inciting factors in lymphoid malignancies is now a vast arena of intensive activity. Gross's comprehensive monograph on this subject is the best reference source to 1970 (Gross, L., 1970a). Other excellent reviews and symposia are available to update and amplify the subject (Kirsten and Panem, 1974; Kurstak and Maramorosch, 1974; Symposium on Fundamental Cancer Research, 1974; Cold Spring Harbor Symposia on Quantitative Biology, 1975; Deinhardt, 1975; Emmelot and Bentvelzen, 1972; Tooze, 1973).

It has been over 70 years since viruses were first observed to be associated with tumors (Sanarelli, 1898), but the full implications of the situation remain undisclosed. One aspect, the relationship of oncogenic viruses to the genetic material of the cell, was discussed in the preceding section. This section will focus on the virus *per se*.

The observation of Ellermann and Bang (1908) initiated the experimental studies linking viruses to malignancies. They demonstrated that a cell-free filtrate obtained from a chicken with erythromyeloblastic leukemia, when injected into another chicken, would activate a sequence of events leading to the same disease. The initial argument that diseases so transmitted were infections, rather than malignancies, has disappeared. There is no longer any question that virus-induced malignancies have all the characteristics of spontaneous tumors. Conversely, many "spontaneous" tumors can be demonstrated to have an associated virus, which, under appropriate circumstances, may transmit the malignancy to another animal.

The difficulties encountered in linking a virus to a malignancy have been numerous. The major hurdle has been the common experience of not being able to fulfill Koch's criteria. These criteria require that an infectious agent be present in the diseased animal and be capable of reproducing the same disease on transmission to another animal.

Several reasons for this difficulty have been identified. One, recognized early but blurred by the semantic arguments of the time, is that the age of the tumor may be important. Infectious virus is often obtained only from young tumors (Shope, R. E., 1933; Duran-Raynals and Freire, 1953; Noyes, 1959; Stone *et al.,* 1959; Carr, 1943). Even when infectious virus is obtained, other perplexing phenomena arise. A virus may elicit a tumor of quite different characteristics in another animal. For example, a commonly utilized lymphatic-leukemia-inducing virus was originally obtained from a sarcoma (Moloney, 1960). The age, species, strain, and sex of the host may also determine the outcome. For these and other reasons, investigators have generally dropped the requirement that viruses meet Koch's criteria before being considered oncogenic. Additional means of identifying viruses in tumors and attempting to establish their associations have been developed.

Electron microscopy offered a major tool (Dalton, 1962). The direct visualization of viruses in tumors has been almost too successful. Viruses have been seen in a wide variety of tumor cells, and in many nontumor cells as well. DNA viruses, such as adeno-, herpes-, papova-, and pox viruses have been identified by their structural characteristics in a variety of tumors (Fraenkel-Conrat, 1974; Dulbecco, 1975).

RNA viruses have been found even more often, and have required critical analysis to distinguish them from normal cellular structures. Bernhard (1960) developed a classification system for these tumor-associated RNA viruses that is used today with only a few modifications (Dalton *et al.,* 1966). The C-type particle, by this classification, is the one most often associated with lymphoid tissue malignancies.

Tumor viruses can also be identified by a variety of distinctive proteins that they encode (Black *et al.,* 1963; Habel and Eddy, 1963; Sjögren, 1974; Strand and August, 1974; Stromberg *et al.,* 1974; Lilly and Steeves, 1974). Some of these proteins are within the viral capsid; others are a part of the viral envelope. These latter are also on the surface membranes of those cells actively synthesizing viruses. Because of their antigenic properties, all these viral proteins can be identified by immunological techniques. The viral antigens on cell surfaces may act as transplantation antigens, for they determine the transplantability of tumor cells. Hence, they have been referred to as *tumor-specific transplantation antigens* (TSTA).

The nucleotide sequences of tumor viruses have also facilitated finding them in cells even when they are not actively synthesizing virus or their distinctive proteins. Despite the technical difficulty of identifying a very small nucleotide segment in a very large gene pool, competitive inhibition studies have disclosed these viruses in a variety of tumor cells (Spiegelman et al., 1973; Neiman, 1972; Varmus et al., 1974; Shoyab et al., 1974a,b; Gelb et al., 1971; Hehlmann et al., 1972).

Finally, the enzyme that permits the synthesis of a DNA copy of an RNA viral nucleotide sequence, reverse transcriptase, can be used as a marker of a presumptive oncornavirus (Temin and Mizutani, 1970; Baltimore, 1970). All oncornaviruses carry this enzyme. The most important consequence of reverse transcription is that it produces a double-stranded DNA copy of the viral RNA, which then becomes integrated into the cellular DNA. This *provirus,* as it has been called (Temin, 1976), has now been conclusively demonstrated not only to be a true copy of the RNA tumor virus, but also to be infectious and capable of transmitting the virus and its biological sequelae (Hill and Hillova, 1971, 1972; Svoboda et al., 1973; Montagnier and Vigier, 1972).

Tumor viruses may be acquired by an animal through the genetic material inherited from parents or by the more conventional mechanism whereby viruses enter and infect intact cells. The first has been called *vertical* transmission; the latter, *horizontal* transmission. Vertical transmission appears to be the major route. In some circumstances, both routes are possible. For example, feline leukemia is generally transmitted horizontally, although vertical transmission has also been demonstrated (Essex, 1975).

Vertical transmission may be the result of other than inheritance of genetic information. The fetus may be infected *in utero* by maternal virus or during the neonatal period via the milk. Characteristic C-type particles have been found in the placentas of several species (Gross, L., et al., 1975; Kalter et al., 1973a,b; Schidlovsky and Ahmed, 1973; Vernon et al., 1974; Dalton et al., 1974; Feldman, 1975). Leukemia has also been transmitted to suckling mice through the milk of virus-carrying mothers (Law and Moloney, 1961; Gross, L., 1962).

The molecular characterization of these viruses is today almost complete (*Cold Spring Harbor Symposia on Quantitative Biology,* 1975). The DNA tumor viruses, SV40, polyoma, adenovirus, and herpes (especially the Epstein–Barr virus) have been intensively studied. The details of how they replicate, integrate with the cellular genome, and express their genetic information are well described. In general, this extensive information may be summarized for our purposes here as follows: DNA tumor viruses are integrated into specific areas of the cellular genome. There, they express themselves by the production of a limited number of proteins plus, under certain conditions, by influencing the expression of host cell genes. How these proteins disturb the normal cellular regulatory mechanisms remains to be determined.

The RNA tumor viruses have also been extensively studied. They code for a DNA copy that is then integrated into the cellular genome and carried and replicated thereafter as an integral part of the genome. Four major parts of this viral genome have been identified. They can be schematically represented as in Figure 1.

The internal proteins confer antigenic markers on the virus that are useful in classifying them, but their functions are unknown. The envelope glycoprotein (designated gp70 because its molecular weight is about 70,000 daltons) is important for several reasons. It is on the surface of cells harboring and expressing the virus,

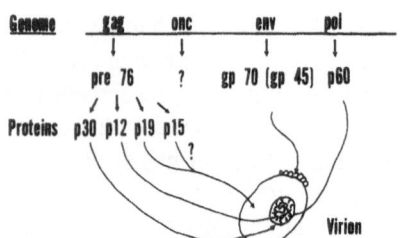

Figure 1. Genome and virion of a typical oncornavirus.

thus providing a useful marker. It is also the target for neutralizing antibodies. Its role in the malignant process, if any, is unknown. The onc portion of the viral genome can code for a protein or proteins with a molecular weight of approximately 40,000 daltons. The nature and role of this onc product are unknown. The RNA of the virion nucleus contains at least two and probably four identical subunits such as depicted in Figure 1. Two or more copies of this genome are present in infected cells.

A major breakthrough in unraveling the mechanisms whereby both RNA and DNA tumor viruses function was the discovery of "defective" viruses (Temin, 1962; Hanafusa *et al.*, 1963). It is clear, for example, that a "complete" Rous sarcoma virus has all the components necessary to transform a cell and lead to a tumor. The avian leukosis virus is a portion of the Rous sarcoma virus. It can incite leukemia, but can lead to a sarcoma only if the cell it invades already harbors an incomplete virus (Duesberg and Vogt, 1970). This general situation exists in mammals as well (Aaronson *et al.*, 1972; Steeves and Eckner, 1970; Brockman and Nathans, 1974; Chieco-Bianchi *et al.*, 1975), and may be an explanation for some of the complexities inherent in the experimental model systems. In addition, this situation has facilitated the development of a method to identify several murine leukemia viruses. The rat XC cell line, carrying defective Rous sarcoma virus, will transform if a rescuing murine leukemia virus is added to the culture (Klement *et al.*, 1969; Rowe *et al.*, 1970). At the moment, our knowledge of the molecular characteristics of tumor viruses far exceeds our knowledge of how they are related to tumors.

4.3. Radiation

The ability of ionizing radiations to incite cancer became apparent shortly after X-ray techniques were introduced into clinical medicine. In retrospect, irradiation had been an incitor of cancer long before this time. For several centuries, miners in certain areas of Czechoslovakia died of a strange lung disease now recognized as primary carcinoma. The radiation produced by uranium in those mines was the culprit (Peller, 1939; Rajewsky *et al.*, 1943).

The possible leukemogenic effect of radiation was also considered early and confirmed by a variety of tragic circumstances. Leukemia was observed among radiologists 8–10 times more frequently than among physicians not exposed to X rays (March, 1950; Ulrich, 1946; von Jagić *et al.*, 1911). The major catastrophic exposure of man to ionizing radiation was the consequence of the two atomic explosions in Japan. A high incidence of leukemia continues to occur in those persons near the center of these blasts (Folley *et al.*, 1952; Bizzozero *et al.*, 1966). These leukemias are predominantly myelocytic rather than lymphocytic.

Experimental animal models of radiation-induced lymphomas and leukemias have been extensively studied. A number of early studies clearly indicated that radiation would lead to leukemia in low-leukemia strains of mice (Krebs *et al.*, 1930; Henshaw, 1944; Hueper, 1934; Furth and Furth, 1936). The animal models were not really developed to a point of maximum usefulness, however, until the critical variables were identified and controlled. These included the genetic susceptibility of the host, age at irradiation, dose and frequency of the irradiation, and the sex of the animals. The details of these variables are clearly defined in a large series of important experiments (Kaplan, H. S., 1964, 1974; Kaplan, H. S., and Brown, 1952; Upton and Cosgrove, 1968) and will not be reviewed here.

A major discovery regarding radiation-induced lymphomas in the experimental animals was that the disease was transmissible to syngeneic animals via a cell-free filtrate of tumor tissue (Gross, L., and Feldman, 1968; Haran-Ghera, 1966; Haran-Ghera and Peled, 1967; Lieberman and Kaplan, 1959; Mathé and Bernard, 1958). The transmissible substance is an oncornavirus, similar, if not identical, to other murine leukemia viruses. X ray appears to "activate" this latent virus and result in the appearance of free infectious virus.

The mechanism whereby the radiation, or the associated oncornavirus, leads to the lymphoma is not known. The best-studied experimental models are all malignancies of the T-cell lymphocytes and are dependent for their inception on the presence of a thymus. What little is known regarding this situation is discussed in Section 5.

4.4. Chemical Carcinogens

Several chemically induced experimental models of leukemia and lymphoma are available for study. Hydrocarbons, alkylating agents, purine analogues, urethane, and nitroquinoline oxides have all been used successfully. They have been painted on the skin, administered orally, or injected into various sites about the rodent subjects. The genetic background, age, and sex of the animals play important determinant roles in the incidence and character of these malignancies, just as they do following other inciting events. References to representative examples are in Table 1.

A few chemically induced malignancies involve T cells, more involve B cells, and many affect cells identifiable only as stem cells or nonlymphoid cells.

There is some evidence to support the notion that a virus is implicated in the pathogenesis of chemically induced lymphomas (Igel *et al.*, 1969; Ball and McCarter, 1971; Colnaghi and Della Porta, 1973; Haran-Ghera, 1967; Irino *et al.*, 1963; Kinosita and Tanaka, 1963; Ribacchi and Giraldo, 1966; Toth, 1963; Zilber and Postnikova, 1966; Whitmire *et al.*, 1971; Yuspa *et al.*, 1973). Chemically induced lymphomas have been transmitted with cell-free filtrates, and viruses have been identified by other criteria.

The chemical activation of viruses *in vitro* is a subject of intensive study (Kaplan, J. C., *et al.*, 1971). Both DNA and RNA tumor viruses have been demonstrated to become induced to produce infectious viruses in such systems (Rothschild and Black, 1970; Lowry *et al.*, 1971). The halogenated pyrimidines have been most effective and studied in greatest detail (Teich *et al.*, 1973; Rowe and Hartley, 1972).

4.5. Immunological Inciting Events

Various manipulations of the immune system have led to an increased incidence of lymphoid malignancies. These have included excessive stimulation or suppression, or combinations of the two.

Chronic graft-versus-host, or allogeneic, disease is one of the best-studied situations (Hirsch *et al.*, 1970, 1972; Krueger and Heine, 1972; Gleichmann *et al.*, 1972; Schwartz *et al.*, 1966; Schwartz and Beldotti, 1965; Walford, 1966; Krueger *et al.*, 1971). The resultant tumors are generally reticulum-cell sarcomas. In some models, the malignant cells are derived from the host; in others, they are of donor origin. Allogeneic disease, both *in vivo* and *in vitro*, activates the expression of latent oncornaviruses (Hirsch *et al.*, 1970, 1972). These virus have all the characteristics of other murine leukemia viruses including the capacity to incite lymphoma when injected into appropriate recipient animals (Cornelius, 1972b; Armstrong *et al.*, 1973). Presumably, these viruses are involved in the process of lymphomogenesis in the allogeneic model.

Excessive antigenic stimulation by a variety of substances also promotes lymphomogenesis. *Salmonella* antigen, foreign protein, tubercle bacilli, zymosan, malaria parasites, and mineral oil injections have all been effectively utilized (Krueger *et al.*, 1971; Metcalf, 1961; McIntire and Princler, 1969; Jerusalem, 1968; Isliker *et al.*, 1973). The addition of immunosuppressive drugs to these models has occasionally further increased the frequency of lymphoid tumors (Casey, 1968; Burstein and Allison, 1970; Walker and Bole, 1973; Hirsch *et al.*, 1973).

Chronic viral infection may also promote to lymphoma. Lymphocytic choriomeningitis (LCM) virus activates murine leukemia antigen expression (Oldstone *et al.*, 1971; Riley and Fitzmaurice, 1973). This situation may be responsible for the increased incidence of lymphoma seen in LCM carriers (Sharon and Pollard, 1971). Chronic reovirus 3 infection has also been followed by the development of lymphoma, although the relationship remains to be clarified (Levy and Huebner, 1970).

There is some reason to suspect that certain DNA viruses may also somehow activate latent C-type oncornaviruses. The data are inconclusive, but the subject is worthy of direct study.

The high incidence of lymphoma in the NZB mouse strain may also be linked to these other "immunologically incited" lymphomas. The NZB mouse is known to carry type-C viruses (Lerner *et al.*, 1972), develop autoimmune disorders (Howie and Helyer, 1968; Shirai and Mellors, 1972; Mellors, 1965, 1966, 1969), and have a diminished cell-mediated immunity (Shirai and Mellors, 1972; Rodey *et al.*, 1971). Further suppression of their immune competence by cytotoxic agents increases even further the incidence of lymphoma (Walker and Bole, 1973).

Obviously, a much deeper understanding is required before these various immunological phenomena can be meaningfully related to the process of lymphomogenesis.

4.6. Hormones

A number of observations extending back many years indicate that hormones can incite, or at least significantly influence, lymphoid malignancies. Several experimental models are influenced by sex hormones (Silberberg and Silberberg, 1945; McEndy *et al.*, 1944; Law, 1947; Cole, R. K., and Furth, 1941; Kunii *et al.*, 1965; Murphy, J. B., 1944; Gardner, W. V., *et al.*, 1944). The general situation is that female gonadal hormones increase the incidence. Ovariectomy decreases the incidence, orichidectomy increases the incidence, and the administration of exogenous hormones produces results compatible with the extirpation experiments.

The mechanism whereby gonadal hormones influence the malignancies is not known. It may be direct, indirect, or both. For example, orchidectomy increases the incidence of lymphoma in the AKR mouse, but the same result can be obtained by housing males separately. It has been suggested that the constant fighting of AKR males housed together influences the process of leukemogenesis. A transmissible virus has also been obtained from an estrogen-induced lymphoma (Kunii *et al.*, 1965; Karande *et al.*, 1975).

Adrenal hormones were also noted early to influence the development of lymphomas as well as their behavior once present (Law, 1947; Murphy, J. B., and Sturm, 1944; Law and Speirs, 1947; Heilman and Kendall, 1944; Huggins and Uematsu, 1976; Huggins and Kuwahara, 1967). In general, adrenalectomy increases the incidence of lymphomas in appropriately selected strains of animals and increases the susceptibility to the growth of transplanted lymphomas from syngeneic animals. The administration of adrenal hormones, specifically corticosteroids, suppresses lymphoid malignancies (Upton and Furth, 1954; Woolley and Peters, 1953). The mechanisms responsible for these effects remain to be elucidated. This situation is particularly intriguing in light of recent observations indicating that glucocorticosteroids stimulate C-type virus production (Paran *et al.*, 1974).

The role of pituitary hormones has only recently been explored. Three separate studies conducted with four distinct experimental models all concluded that the pituitary is capable of significantly influencing the development of lymphoid tissue malignancies and perhaps even their behavior once they are established. Gross-virus-induced T-cell lymphoma in Sprague–Dawley rats is impaired by early hypophysectomy (Bentley *et al.*, 1974). Radiation and chemically induced leukemia in C57B1 and SJ/L mice is similarly stopped (Pierpaoli and Haran-Ghera, 1975). Chemically induced stem-cell leukemia in Long–Evans rats is impaired and even reversed by hypophysectomy of those animals (Huggins and Oka, 1972; Oka *et al.*, 1974).

Other humoral factors that appear to influence lymphoid malignancies have also been identified. These are substances such as chalones, thymic humoral factor, and other serum factors. Their roles remain to be fully defined (Metcalf, 1971).

Considerably more work is required before the hormone-dependent character of these malignancies can be clarified. In the meantime, it is reasonable to conclude that at least some lymphoid malignancies have hormonal dependence, an observation that links them to other well-defined hormonally dependent malignancies and may afford important approaches to both the study and the clinical management of these tumors.

5. Role of the Thymus

The central role of the thymus in the development of the immune system was appropriately emphasized earlier. So too was its role in the development of malignancies of the thymus-dependent lymphocytes.

Although more than 30 years have passed since the initial observation that thymectomy prevents the development of what we now know is a T-cell lymphoma, the nature of the role remains unknown. Numerous monographs and reviews summarize the vast experimental literature on this subject (Wolstenholme and Porter, 1966; Miller, J. F. A. P., 1959). The interested reader may turn to these for background and perhaps insight. This author suspects that the critical experiments remain to be devised and executed.

An experimental approach recently undertaken by Waksal (1976) may lead us closer to an understanding of the role of the thymus than we have been before. He demonstrated that thymic epithelial cells from animals with T-cell lymphoma will confer malignant behavioral characteristics on T lymphocytes from syngeneic animals. Thymic epithelial cells have been clearly shown to instruct lymphocytes how to behave as normal T cells. They may also be able to instruct them how to misbehave, perhaps as a consequence of the presence within the epithelial cell of a virus that is sending a faulty message to the developing T cell (Hays, 1968).

6. Role of the Bursa

Although the bursal role in the development of B-cell lymphoma of the chicken has been known for considerably less time than the thymus role in T-cell lymphomas, considerable data have been generated and insight gained. To a large degree, the reason is that the B cells have better-defined and identifiable characteristics than do T cells.

Studies of the B-cell population during the development of chicken lymphoid leukosis demonstrate a block in the normal sequence of events leading to full B-cell differentiation (Cooper *et al.*, 1974). The usual switch from IgM to IgG synthesis fails to occur in the malignant B cell, resulting in a population of B cells synthesizing a heterogeneous assortment of IgM molecules.

A recent study experimentally approaches the question of the role of bursal epithelial cells in the development of lymphoid leukosis (Purchase and Gilmour, 1975). Cyclophosphamide was used to deplete birds of their B-cell system while leaving intact the bursal epithelial cells. Such birds injected with a leukosis-inducing virus fail to develop lymphoma. Transplantation of normal B cells into such birds leads to the disease. This finding, coupled with the previous evidence showing the necessity of the bursa for leukemogenesis, suggests that the transforming target cell is exclusively in the bursa. Perhaps the bursal epithelium is misdirecting the differentiation of B cells. This situation may be analogous to the T cell–thymic epithelium relationship.

7. Immunological Considerations

There seems to be no question that immunological mechanisms can be effective deterrents to the development and survival of malignant cells (Smith, R. T., and Landy, 1970). Whether these mechanisms actually perform this act or perform it effectively is more open to question. In any event, the question of immunological surveillance and resistance to cancer is of special interest when the malignancy involves the cells of the immune system.

Early studies designed to analyze the immunological capacity of animals after the activation of the leukemogenic process but prior to the appearance of detectable malignant cells revealed an immunological deficiency involving both T- and B-cell function. The first of these studies revealed a diminished capacity to synthesize antibody to a bacteriophage and to reject skin grafts from allogenic animals differing at a non-*H-2* locus (Peterson *et al.*, 1963b; Dent *et al.*, 1965). Many other studies have amply confirmed this observation in many other experimental model systems (Doell *et al.*, 1967; Dent, 1972; Woodruff and Woodruff, 1975; Notkins *et al.*, 1970). The relationship of this early immunodeficiency to the subsequent development of lymphoma remains to be fully clarified.

Three major possibilities exist: (1) The immunodeficiency may be of no consequence, being merely an epiphenomenon and of no significance to the fundamental process. (2) The deficiency may be an essential first step wherein the animal's natural defense mechanism is incapacitated, thus rendering it unable to defend against malignant cells. (3) The immunodeficiency may be an indicator of a disturbance in the normal regulatory mechanisms that control cells of the lymphoid tissue, the latter being the critical step leading to lymphoma.

A fourth possibility also exists, although in a slightly different frame of reference. The tumors may produce substances that suppress the immune system. This latter subject has received considerable attention in the case of several nonlymphoid tumors (Kitagawa *et al.*, 1974, 1975; Takatsu *et al.*, 1972; Masaki *et al.*, 1972; Kennedy, 1975; Wong *et al.*, 1974).

Although immunodeficiencies can be identified in many experimental animals prior to the development of a lymphoma, there is no doubt that immunological reactions do occur in these animals and that they are directed at tumor-specific antigens. An extensive literature now attests to these immunological responses of lymphoma-bearing animals (Habel, 1969; Herberman, 1974; Cerottini and Brunner, 1974; Glaser *et al.*, 1976; Hellström and Hellström, 1974; Shellam, 1974). In some situations, these immunological reactions result in destruction of the malignant cells and recovery from the malignancy (Lamon *et al.*, 1972; Kobayashi, 1975). More often, the reactions proceed concurrently with the growth of the tumor, a situation that causes one to wonder whether the immune response is retarding or accelerating the process.

8. Conclusions

Experimental animal models of lymphoid malignancies are coming of age. The development phase has lasted over 50 years, but during that time, great strides have been taken in identifying the critical components of the models. Today, the study of these models should reveal many fundamental biological mechanisms involved in both the normal and the abnormal regulation of cells of the lymphoid tissue. Incisive analysis of these mechanisms will no doubt lead to the depth of understanding essential for the systematic treatment or prevention of the human counterparts.

ACKNOWLEDGMENTS

I wish to gratefully acknowledge the library services of Sarah Kelly and the secretarial talents of Judy Grafton and Mary Miller, plus the cooperation of my colleagues, whose work was delayed during the preparation of this manuscript.

RAYMOND D. A.
PETERSON

Aaronson, S. A., Bassin, R. H., and Weaver, C., 1972, Comparison of murine sarcoma viruses and S⁺ L⁻ transformed cells, *J. Virol.* **9**:701–704.

Ablashi, D. V., Loeb, W. F., Valerio, M. G., Adamson, R. H., Armstrong, G. R., Bennett, D. G., and Heine, U., 1971, Malignant lymphoma with lymphocytic leukemia in owl monkeys induced by Herpes virus saimiri, *J. Natl. Cancer Inst.* **47**:837–855.

Adamson, R. H., McIntire, K. R., Sieber, S. M., Correa, P., and Dalgard, D. W., 1975, Nonhuman primate models for lymphoma, leukemia, and other neoplasms, *Bibl. Haematol. (Pavia)* **40**:723–730.

Ahlstrom, C. G., and Forsby, N., 1962, Sarcomas in hamsters after injection with Rous chicken tumor material, *J. Exp. Med.* **115**:839–852.

Anderson, L. J., and Jarrett, W. F. H., 1968, Lymphosarcoma (leukemia) in cattle, sheep and pigs in Great Britain, *Cancer* **22**:398–405.

Anderson, L. J., and Jarrett, W. F. H., 1971, Membranous glomerulonephritis associated with leukemia in cats, *Res. Vet. Sci.* **12**:179–180.

Anderson, L. J., Jarrett, W. F. H., and Crighton, G. W., 1969, A classification of lymphoid neoplasms of domestic mammals, *Natl. Cancer Inst. Monogr.* **32**:343–353.

Anderson, L. J., Jarrett, W. F. H., Jarrett, O., and Laird, H. M., 1971, Feline leukaemia virus infection of kittens: Mortality associated with atrophy of the thymus and lymphoid depletion, *J. Natl. Cancer Inst.* **47**:807–817.

Archer, O. K., and Pierce, J. C., 1961, Role of the thymus in the development of immune response, *Fed. Proc. Fed. Am. Soc. Exp. Biol.* **20**:26.

Armstrong, M. Y. K., Gleichmann, E., Gleichmann, H., Beldotti, L., André-Schwartz, J., and Schwartz, R., 1970, Chronic allogeneic disease. II. Development of lymphomas, *J. Exp. Med.* **132**:417–439.

Armstrong, M. Y. K., Black, F. L., and Richards, F. F., 1972, Tumour induction by cell-free extracts derived from mice with graft versus host disease, *Nature (London) New Biol.* **235**:153–154.

Armstrong, M. Y. K., Ruddle, N. H., Lipman, M. B., and Richards, F. F., 1973, Tumor induction by immunologically activated murine leukemia virus, *J. Exp. Med.* **137**:1163–1179.

Bach, J. F., Dormont, J., Dardenne, M., and Balner, H., 1969, *In vitro* rosette inhibition by antihuman antilymphocyte serum: Correlation with skin graft prolongation in subhuman primates, *Transplantation* **8**:265–280.

Ball, J. K., and McCarter, J. A., 1971, Repeated demonstration of a mouse leukemia virus after treatment with chemical carcinogens, *J. Natl. Cancer Inst.* **46**:751–762.

Balls, M., 1962, Spontaneous neoplasms in amphibia: A review and description of six new cases, *Cancer Res.* **22**:1142–1154.

Balls, M., and Ruben, L. N., 1968, Lymphoid tumors in amphibia: A review, *Prog. Exp. Tumor Res.* **10**:238–260.

Baltimore, D., 1970, RNA-dependent DNA polymerase in virions of RNA tumor viruses, *Nature (London)* **226**:1209–1211.

Beasley, J. N., Patterson, L. T., and McWade, D. H., 1970, Transmission of Marek's disease by poultry dust and chicken dander, *Am. J. Vet. Res.* **31**:339–344.

Belousova, O. I., and Strel'tsova, V. N., 1967, Acute leukemia in guinea pigs in late periods after chornic irradiation, *Byull. Eksp. Biol. Med.* **64**:85–87.

Bendixen, H. J., 1958, Studies on bovine leukosis. II. Clinical diagnosis of bovine leukosis, *Nord. Veterinaermed.* **10**:273–301.

Bendixen, H. J., 1963, Preventive measures in cattle leukemia: Leukosis enzootica bovis, *Ann. N.Y. Acad. Sci.* **108**:1241–1267.

Bentley, H. P., Jr., Hughes, E. R., and Peterson, R. D. A., 1974, Effect of hypophysectomy on a virus-induced T-cell leukemia, *Nature (London)* **252**:747–748.

Berard, C. W., 1972, Histopathology of the lymphomas, in: *Hematology* (A. J. Ersler and R. W. Rundles, eds.), pp. 901–920, McGraw-Hill, New York.

Berard, C. W., and Dorfman, R. F., 1974, Histopathology of malignant lymphomas, *Clin. Haematol.* **3**:39.

Berard, C. W., O'Conor, G. T., Thomas, L. B., and Torloni, H. (eds.), 1969, Histopathological definition of Burkitt's tumor, *Bull. W.H.O.* **40**:601–607.

Bernhard, W., 1960, The detection and study of tumor viruses with the electron microscope, *Cancer Res.* **20**:717–727.

Biggs, P. M., 1968, Marek's disease—Current state of knowledge, *Curr. Top. Microbiol. Immunol.* **43**:92–125.

Biggs, P. M., and Payne, L. N., 1963, Transmission experiments with Marek's disease (fowl paralysis), *Vet. Res.* **75**:177–179.

Biggs, P. M., and Payne, L., 1964, Relationship of Marek's disease (neural lymphomatosis) to lymphoid leukosis, *Natl. Cancer Inst. Monogr.* **17**:83–98.

Bird, C., 1972, Leukemia induced by 7,8,12-trimethylbenz(a)anthracene in rats. II. Changes in bone marrow, *J. Natl. Cancer Inst.* **48**:429–439.

Bizzozero, O. J., Jr., Johnson, K. G., and Ciocco, A., 1966, Radiation-related leukemia in Hiroshima and Nagasaki, 1946–1964. I. Distribution, incidences and appearance time, *N. Engl. J. Med.* **274**:1095–1101.

Black, P. H., Rowe, W. P., Turner, H. C., and Huebner, R. J., 1963, A specific complement-fixing antigen present in SV 40 tumor and transformed cells, *Proc. Natl. Acad. Sci. U.S.A.* **50**:1148–1156.

Block, M., 1966, Prelymphomous or preleukemic state in mice: Relation to human preleukemia, *Natl. Cancer Inst. Monogr.* **22**:559–570.

Block, M., and Goodman, S. B., 1963, The histogenesis of Gross's viral induced mouse leukemia, *Cancer Res.* **23**:1634–1640.

Boiron, M., Lévy, J. P., and Périès, J., 1967, *In vitro* investigations on murine leukemia viruses, *Prog. Med. Virol.* **9**:341–391.

Brain, P., Gordon, J., and Willetts, W. A., 1970, Rosette formation by peripheral lymphocytes, *Clin. Exp. Immunol.* **6**:681–688.

Braylan, R. C., Jaffee, E. S., and Berard, C. W., 1975, Malignant lymphomas: Current classification and new observations, *Pathobiol. Annu.* **10**:213–270.

Brockman, W. W., and Nathans, D., 1974, The isolation of simian virus 40 variants with specifically altered genomes, *Proc. Natl. Acad. Sci. U.S.A.* **71**:942–946.

Brodey, R. S., McDonough, S. K., and Frye, F. L., 1969, Epidemiology of feline leukemia (lymphosarcoma), in: *Comparative Leukemia Research* (R. M. Dutcher, ed.), pp. 333–342, Karger, Basel.

Burmester, B. R., 1947, Studies on the transmission of avian visceral lymphomatosis. II. Propagation of lymphomatosis with cellular and cell-free preparations, *Cancer Res.* **7**:786–797.

Burmester, B. R., 1962, The vertical and horizontal transmission of avian visceral lymphomatosis, *Cold Spring Harbor Symp. Quant. Biol.* **27**:471–477.

Burmester, B. R., and Gentry, R. F., 1954, The transmission of avian visceral lymphomatosis by contact, *Cancer Res.* **14**:34–42.

Burmester, B. R., and Gentry, R. F., 1956, The response of susceptible chickens to graded doses of the virus of visceral lymphomatosis, *Poult. Sci.* **35**:17–26.

Burmester, B. R., and Prickett, C. O., 1945, The development of highly malignant tumor strains from naturally occurring avian lymphomatosis, *Cancer Res.* **5**:652–660.

Burmester, B. R., Prickett, C. O., and Belding, T. C., 1946, A filtrable agent producing lymphoid tumors and osteopetrosis in chickens, *Cancer Res.* **6**:189–196.

Burmester, B. R., Gentry, R. F., and Waters, N. F., 1955, The presence of the virus of visceral lymphomatosis in embryonated eggs of normal appearing hens, *Science* **34**:609–617.

Burmester, B. R., Gross, M. A., Walter, W. G. and Fontes, A. K., 1959, Pathogenecity of a viral strain (RAL12) causing avian visceral lymphomatosis and related neoplasms. II. Host–virus interrelations affecting response, *J. Natl. Cancer Inst.* **22**:103–127.

Burmester, B. R., Fontes, A. K., and Walter, W. G., 1960a, Pathogenicity of a viral strain (RPL12) causing avian visceral lymphomatosis and related neoplasms. III. Influence of host age and route of inoculation, *J. Natl. Cancer Inst.* **24**:1423–1442.

Burmester, B. R., Fontes, A. K., Waters, N. F., Bryan, W. R., and Groupé, V., 1960b, The response of several inbred lines of White Leghorns to inoculation with the viruses of strain RPL12 visceral lymphomatosis–erythroblastosis and of Rous sarcoma, *Poult. Sci.* **39**:199–215.

Burstein, N., and Allison, A. C., 1970, Effect of antilymphocytic serum on the appearance of reticular neoplasms in SJL-J mice, *Nature (London)* **225**:1139–1140.

Callahan, R., Lieber, M. M., Todaro, G. J., Graves, D. C., and Ferver, J. F., 1976, Bovine leukemia virus genes in the DNA of leukemic cattle, *Science* **192**:1005–1007.

Calnek, B. W., Adldinger, H. K., and Kahn, D. E., 1970a, Feather follicle epithelium: A source of enveloped and infectious cell-free herpesvirus from Marek's disease, *Avian Dis.* **14**:219–233.

Calnek, B. W., Ubertini, T., and Adldinger, H. K., 1970b, Viral antigen, virus particles, and infectivity of tissues from chickens with Marek's disease, *J. Natl. Cancer Inst.* **45**:341–351.

Carr, J. G., 1943, The relation between age, structure, and agent content of Rous No. 1 sarcomas, *Br. J. Exp. Pathol.* **24**:133–137.

Carter, R. L., and Gershon, R. K., 1966, Studies on homotransplantable lymphomas in hamsters. I. Histologic responses in lymphoid tissues and their relationship to metastasis, *Am. J. Pathol.* **49**:637–655.

Case, M. T. and Simon, J., 1968, Transmission studies of swine lymphosarcoma: Hematologic and pathologic changes in pigs inoculated with whole cell suspensions, *Am. J. Vet. Res.* **29**:263–269.

Casey, T. P., 1968, Azathioprine (Imuran) administration and the development of malignant lymphomas in NZB mice, *Clin. Exp. Immunol.* **3**:305–312.

Cerottini, J. C., and Brunner, K. T., 1974, Cell-mediated cytotoxicity, allograft rejection, and tumor immunity, *Adv. Immunol.* **18**:67–132.

Chapman, A. L., Bopp, W. J., Brightwell, A. S., Cohen, H., Nielsen, A. H., Gravelle, C. R., and Werder, A. A., 1967, Preliminary report on virus-like particles in canine leukemia and derived cell cultures, *Cancer Res.* **27**:18–25.

Chattopadhyay, S. K., Rowe, W. P., Teich, N. Y., and Lowy, D. R., 1975, Definitive evidence that the murine C-type virus inducing locus *AKV-1* is viral genetic material, *Proc. Natl. Acad. Sci. U.S.A.* **72**:906–910.

Chieco-Bianchi, L., Collavo, D., Colombatti, A., and Biasi, G., 1975, *In vivo* interactions between murine leukemia and sarcoma viruses, *Bibl. Haematol. (Pavia)* **40**:613–620.

Chin, T. D. Y., Chapman, A. L., Gravelle, C. R., Werder, A. A., and Nielsen, A. H., 1968, Studies of canine leukemia in tissue cultures and axenic mice, *Bibl. Haematol. (Pavia)* **30**:274–275.

Churchill, A. E., 1968, Herpes-type virus isolated in cell culture from tumors of chickens with Marek's disease. I. Studies in cell culture, *J. Natl. Cancer Inst.* **41**:939–950.

Churchill, A. E., and Biggs, P. M., 1967, Agent of Marek's disease in tissue culture, *Nature (London)* **215**:528–530.

Churchill, A. E., and Biggs, P. M., 1968, Herpes-type virus isolated in cell culture from tumors of chickens with Marek's disease. II. Studies *in vivo*, *J. Natl. Cancer Inst.* **41**:951–956.

Claman, H. N., Chaperon, E. A., and Triplett, R. F., 1966, Immunocompetence of transferred thymus–marrow cell combinations, *J. Immunol.* **97**:828–832.

Clarke, J. K., and Attridge, J. T., 1968, The morphology of simian foamy agents, *J. Gen. Virol.* **3**:185–190.

Clegg, F. G., and Moss, B., 1965, Skin leukosis in a heifer: An unusual clinical history, *Vet. Res.* **77**:271–272.

Coggin, J. H., and Anderson, N. G., 1974, Cancer, differentiation and embryonic antigens: Some central problems, *Adv. Cancer Res.* **19**:105–165.

Cohen, D., 1968, Exploitation of epidemiologic aspects of malignant lymphoma, *Bibl. Haematol. (Pavia)* **30**:268–270.

Cold Spring Harbor Symposia on Quantitative Biology, 1975, Vol. 39, Parts I and II, Cold Spring Harbor Laboratory, Cold Spring Harbor, New York.

Cole, L. J., and Nowell, P. C., 1970, Parental-F$_1$ hybrid bone marrow chimeras: High incidence of donor-type lymphomas, *Proc. Soc. Exp. Biol. Med.* **134**:653–657.

Cole, R. K., and Furth, J., 1941, Experimental studies on the genetics of spontaneous leukemia in mice, *Cancer Res.* **1**:957–965.

Colnaghi, M. I., and Della Porta, G., 1973, Evidence for virus related and unrelated antigens on murine lymphomas induced by chemical carcinogens, *J. Natl. Cancer Inst.* **50**:173–180.

Congdon, C. C., and Lorenz, E., 1954, Leukemia in guinea-pigs, *Am. J. Pathol.* **30**:337–359.

Conklin, J. W., Upton, A. C., Christenberry, K. W., and McDonald, T. P., 1963, Comparative late somatic effects of some radiomimetic agents and X-rays, *Radiat. Res.* **19**:156–168.

Conttral, G. E., Burmester, B. R., and Waters, N. F., 1954, Egg transmission of avian lymphomatosis, *Poult. Sci.* **33**:1174–1184.

Cooper, M. D., and Lawton, A. R., 1978, Development of lymphoid tissues, in: *The Immunopathology of Lymphoreticular Neoplasms* (J. J. Twomey and R. A. Good, eds.), Chapt. 1, Plenum Press, New York.

Cooper, M. D., Peterson, R. D. A., and Good, R. A., 1965a, Delineation of the thymic and bursal lymphoid systems in the chicken, *Nature (London)* **205**:143–146.

Cooper, M. D., Peterson, R. D. A., and Good, R. A., 1965b, A new perspective of the cellular basis of immunity and lymphocytic malignancies, *J. Clin. Invest.* **44**:1037–1038.

Cooper, M. D., Peterson, R. D. A., South, M. A., and Good, R. A., 1966a, The functions of the thymus system and the bursa system in the chicken, *J. Exp. Med.* **123**:75–102.

Cooper, M. D., Peterson, R. D. A., Gabrielsen, A. E., and Good, R. A., 1966b, Lymphoid malignancy and development, differentiation, and function of the lymphoreticular system, *Cancer Res.* **26**:1165–1169.

Cooper, M. D., Gabrielsen, A. E., and Good, R. A., 1967, Role of the thymus and other central lymphoid tissues in immunological disease, *Annu. Rev. Med.* **18**:113–138.

Cooper, M. D., Payne, L. N., Dent, P. B., Burmester, B. R., and Good, R. A., 1968, Pathogenesis of avian lymphoid leukosis. I. Histogenesis, *J. Natl. Cancer Inst.* **41**:373–378.

Cooper, M. D., Purchase, H. G., Bockman, D. E., and Gathings, W. E., 1974, Studies on the nature of the abnormality of B cell differentiation in avian lymphoid leukosis: Production of heterogeneous IgM by tumor cells, *J. Immunol.* **113**:1210–1222.

Cornelius, E. A., 1972a, Rapid viral induction of murine lymphomas in the graft-versus-host reaction, *J. Exp. Med.* **136**:1533–1544.

Cornelius, E. A., 1972b, Rapid immunological induction of murine lymphomas: Evidence for a viral etiology, *Science* **177**:524–525.

Cornelius, E. A., 1973, Development of tumors as a result of graft-versus-host reaction, *Exp. Hematol.* **1**:135–149.

Cotchin, E., 1952, Neoplasms in cats, *Proc. R. Soc. Med.* **45**:671–674.

Cotchin, E., 1957, Neoplasia in the cat, *Vet. Rec.* **69**:425–434.

Cotchin, E., 1960, Tumours of farm animals: A survey of tumours examined at the Royal Veterinary College, London, during 1950–1960, *Vet. Rec.* **72**:816–822.

Cowan, D. F., 1968, Diseases of captive reptiles, *J. Am. Vet. Med. Assoc.* **153**:848–859.

Croshaw, J. E., Jr., Abt, D. A., Marshak, R. R., Hare, W. C. D., Switzer, J., Ipsen, I., and Dutcher, R. M., 1963, Pedigree studies in bovine lymphosarcoma, *Ann. N.Y. Acad. Sci.* **108**:1193–1202.

Dalton, A. J., 1962, Micromorphology of murine tumor viruses and of affected cells, *Fed. Proc. Fed. Am. Soc. Exp. Biol.* **21**:936–941.

Dalton, A. J., Harven, E. D. E., Dmochowski, L., Feldman, D., Haguenau, F., Harris, W. W., Howatson, A. F., Moore, D., Pitelka, D., Smith, K., Uzman, B., and Ziegel, R., 1966, Suggestions for the classification of oncogenic RNA viruses, *J. Natl. Cancer Inst.* **37**:395–397.

Dalton, A. J., Hellmann, A., Kalter, S. S., and Helmke, R. J., 1974, Ultrastructural comparison of placental virus with several type-C-oncogenic viruses, *J. Natl. Cancer Inst.* **52**:1379–1381.

Daniel, M. D., Meléndez, L. V., and Hunt, R. D., 1974a, Herpes virus saimiri. VII. Induction of malignant lymphoma in New Zealand White rabbits, *J. Natl. Cancer Inst.* **53**:1803–1807.

Daniel, M. D., Meléndez, L. V., and Hunt, R. D., 1974b, Oncogenicity of Herpes virus saimiri in New Zealand White rabbits and recovery of the viral agent, *Bacteriol. Proc.* **141**:224.

Datta, S. K., Larson, V. L., Sorenson, D. K., Perman, V., Weber, A. L., Hammer, R. F., and Shope, R. F., 1970, Isolation of C-type particles from leukemia and lymphocytotic cattle, *Comp. Leuk. Res. Bibl. Haematol.* **36**:547.

Dawe, C. J., 1969, Neoplasms of blood cell origin in poikilothermic animals: A review, *Natl. Cancer Inst. Monogr.* **32**:7–28.

Deinhardt, F., 1974, Oncogenic Herpes viruses in species other than owl monkeys: A review, *J. Med. Primatol.* **3**:79–88.

Deinhard, F., 1975, Virus induced lymphoproliferative disease in non-human primates, *Br. J. Cancer* **31**:140–146.

Deinhardt, F., Falk, L. A., and Wolfe, L. G., 1974, Simian herpes viruses and neoplasia, *Adv. Cancer Res.* **19**:167–205.

DeLanney, L. E., and Blackler, K., 1969, Acceptance and regression of a strain specific lymphosarcoma in Mexican axolotls, in: *Biology of Amphibian Tumors* (H. Mizell, ed.), pp. 399–408, Springer-Verlag, New York.

Dent, P. B., 1972, Immunodepression by oncogenic viruses, *Prog. Med. Virol.* **14**:1–35.

Dent, P. B., Peterson, R. D. A., and Good, R. A., 1965, A defect in cellular immunity during the incubation period of Passage A leukemia in C3H mice, *Proc. Soc. Exp. Biol. Med.* **119**:869–871.

DePaoli, A., and Garner, F. M., 1968, Acute lymphocytic leukemia in a white-cheeked gibbon *(Hylobates concolor),* *Cancer Res.* **29**:2559–2561.

DiGiacomo, R. F., 1967, Burkitt's lymphoma in a white handed gibbon *(Hylobates lar),* *Cancer Res.* **27**:1178–1179.

Dmochowski, L., Grey, C. E., Burmester, B. R., and Gross, M. A., 1959, Submicroscopic morphology of avian neoplasms. III. Studies on visceral lymphomatosis, *Proc. Soc. Exp. Biol. Med.* **100**:514–516.

Doell, R. G., and Carnes, W. H., 1962, Urethan induction of thymic lymphoma in C57BL mice, *Nature (London)* **194**:588–589.

Doell, R. G., DeVaux St. Cyr, C., and Grabar, P., 1967, Immune reactivity prior to development of thymic lymphoma in C57BL mice, *Int. J. Cancer* **2**:103–108.

Dorn, C. R., Taylor, D. O. N., Schneider, R., Hibbard, H. H., and Klauber, M. R., 1968, Survey of animal neoplasms in Alameda and Contra Costa Counties, California. II. Cancer morbidity in dogs and cats from Alameda County, *J. Natl. Cancer Inst.* **40**:307–318.

Dougherty, R. M., and DiStefano, H. S., 1967, Sites of avian leukosis virus multiplication in congenitally infected chickens, *Cancer Res.* **27**:322–332.

Duesberg, P. H., and Vogt, P. K., 1970, Differences between the ribonucleic acids of transforming and nontransforming avian tumor viruses, *Proc. Natl. Acad. Sci. U.S.A.* **67**:1673–1680.

Dulbecco, R., 1975, Oncogenic viruses: The last 12 years, *Cold Spring Harbor Symp. Quant. Biol.* **39**:1–7.

Dulbecco, R., Hartwell, L. H., and Vogt, M., 1965, Induction of cellular DNA synthesis by polyoma virus, *Proc. Natl. Acad. Sci. U.S.A.* **53**:403–410.

Dungworth, D. L., Theilen, G. H., and Lengyel, J., 1964, Bovine lymphosarcoma in California. II. The thymic form, *Pathol. Vet.* **1**:323–350.

Dunn, T. B., 1954, Normal and pathologic anatomy of the reticular tissue in laboratory mice, with a classification and discussion of neoplasms, *J. Natl. Cancer Inst.* **14**:1281–1390.

Dunn, T. B., 1957, Plasma-cell neoplasms beginning in the ileocecal area in strain C3H mice, *J. Natl. Cancer Inst.* **19**:371–391.

Dunn, T. B., and Deringer, M. K., 1968, Reticulum cell neoplasm, type B, or the "Hodgkin's-like lesion" of the mouse, *J. Natl. Cancer Inst.* **40**:771–821.

Duran-Reynals, F., and Freire, P. M., 1953, The age of the tumor-bearing hosts as a factor conditioning the transmissibility of the Rous sarcoma by filtrates and cells, *Cancer Res.* **13**:376–382.

Eberth, C. J., 1878, Leukämie der Maus, *Arch. Pathol. Anat.* **72**:108–109.

Eidson, C. S., Fletcher, O. J., Kleven, S. H., and Anderson, D. P., 1971, Detection of Marek's disease antigen in feather follicle epithelium of chickens vaccinated against Marek's disease, *J. Natl. Cancer Inst.* **47**:113–120.

Ellermann, V., and Bang, O., 1908, Experimentelle Leukämie bei Hühnern, *Zentralbl. Bakteriol. Parasitenkd. Infektionskr. Hyg. Abt 1: Orig.* **46**:595–609.

Emmelot, P., and Bentvelzen, P. (eds.), 1972, *RNA Viruses and Host Genome in Oncogenesis*, American Elsevier, New York.

Epstein, M. A., Achong, B. C., Churchill, A. E., and Biggs, P. M., 1968, Structure and development of the herpes-type virus of Marek's disease, *J. Natl. Cancer Inst.* **41**:805–820.

Epstein, M. A., Hunt, R. D., and Rabin, H., 1973, Pilot experiments with EB virus in owl monkeys *(Aotus trivirgatus)*. 1. Reticuloproliferative disease in an inoculated animal, *Int. J. Cancer* **12**:309–318.

Essex, M., 1975, Horizontally and vertically transmitted oncornaviruses of cats, *Adv. Cancer Res.* **21**:175–248.

Essex, M., Klein, G., and Synder, 1971, Antibody to feline oncornavirus associated cell membrane antigen in neonatal cats, *Int. J. Cancer* **8**:384–390.

Essex, M., Hardy, W. D., Jr., Cotter, S. M., and Jakowski, R. M., 1975a, Immune response of healthy and leukemic cats to the feline oncornavirus-associated cell membrane antigen, *Bibl. Haematol. (Pavia)* **40**:483–488.

Essex, M., Sliski, A., Cotter, S. M., Jakowski, R. M., and Hardy, W. D., Jr., 1975b, Immunosurveillance of naturally occurring feline leukemia, *Science* **190**:790–792.

Falk, L., Wolfe, L., Deinhardt, F., Paciga, J., Dombos, L., Klein, G., Henle, W., and Henle, G., 1974, Epstein–Barr virus: Transformation of nonhuman primate lymphocytes *in vitro*, *Int. J. Cancer* **13**:363–376.

Feldman, D., 1975, An electron microscopic study of virus particles in Rhesus monkey placenta, *Proc. Natl. Acad. Sci. U.S.A.* **72**:118–121.

Feldman, D. G., and Gross, L., 1970, Electron microscopic study of the guinea pig leukemia virus, *Cancer Res.* **30**:2702–2711.

Feldman, D. G., Ehrenreich, T., and Gross, L., 1974, Electron microscopic study of the growth and regression of leukemic intradermal tumors in guinea pigs, *Cancer Res.* **34**:901–914.

Ferrer, J. F., 1972, Antigenic comparison of bovine type C virus with murine and feline leukemia viruses, *Cancer Res.* **32**:1871–1877.

Ferrer, J. F., Stock, N. D., and Lin, P., 1971, Detection of replicating C-type viruses in continuous cell cultures established from cows with leukemia: Effect of the culture medium, *J. Natl. Cancer Inst.* **47**:613–621.

Ferrer, J. F., Avila, L., and Stock, N. D., 1972, Serological detection of type C viruses found in bovine cultures, *Cancer Res.* **32**:1864–1870.

Figge, F. H. J., 1954, *Proc. Am. Assoc. Cancer Res.* **1**:13 (abstract).

Finkel, M. P., Biskis, B. O., and Farrell, C., 1968, Osteosarcomas appearing in Syrian hamsters after treatment with extracts of human osteosarcomas, *Proc. Natl. Acad. Sci. U.S.A.* **60**:1223–1230.

Fiore-Donati, L., Chieco-Bianchi, L., De Benedictis, G., and Maiorano, G., 1961, Leukemogenesis by urethan in newborn Swiss mice, *Nature (London)* **190**:278–279.

Folley, J. H., Borges, W., and Yamawaki, T., 1952, Incidence of leukemia in survivors of the atomic bomb in Hiroshima and Nagasaki, Japan, *Am. J. Med.* **13**:311–321.

Fortner, J. G., 1961, The influence of castration on spontaneous tumorigenesis in the Syrian (golden) hamster, *Cancer Res.* **21**:1491–1498.

Fox, H., 1926, Remarks on the presentation of microscopical preparations made from some of the original tissue described by Thomas Hodgkin, 1932, *Ann. Med. Hist.* **8**:370–374.

Fraenkel-Conrat, H., 1974, Descriptive catalogue of viruses, in: *Comprehensive Virology,* Vol. 1 (H. Fraenkel-Conrat and R. R. Wagner, eds.), Plenum Press, New York.

Frank, W., and Schepky, A., 1969, Metastasierendes Lymphosarkon bei einer Riesenschlange, *Eunectes murinus* (Linnaeus, 1758), *Pathol. Vet.* **6**:437–443.

Freeman, A. E., Price, P. J., and Bryan, R. J., 1971a, Transformation of rat and hamster embryo cells by extracts of city smog, *Proc. Natl. Acad. Sci. U.S.A.* **68**:445–449.

Freeman, A. E., Kelloff, G. J., Gilden, R. V., Lane, W. T., Swain, A. P., and Huebner, R. J., 1971b, Activation and isolation of hamster-specific C-type RNA viruses from tumors induced by cell cultures transformed by chemical carcinogens, *Proc. Natl. Acad. Sci. U.S.A.* **68**:2386–2390.

Friend, C., 1957, Cell free transmission in adult Swiss mice of a disease having the character of a leukemia, *J. Exp. Med.* **105**:307–318.

Friend, C., and Rossi, G. B., 1968, Transplantation immunity and the suppression of spleen colony formation by immunization with murine leukemia virus preparations (Friend), *Int. J. Cancer* **3**:523–529.

Furth, J., 1932, Studies on the nature of the agent transmitting leukosis of fowls. I. Its concentration in blood cells and plasma and relation to the incubation period, *J. Exp. Med.* **55**:465–478.

Furth, J., 1933, Lymphomatosis, myelomatosis, and endothelioma of chickens caused by filterable agent. I. Transmission experiments, *J. Exp. Med.* **58**:253–275.

Furth, J., and Furth, O. B., 1936, Neoplastic disease produced in mice by general irradiation with X-rays. I. Incidence and type of neoplasms, *Am. J. Cancer* **28**:54–65.

Furth, J., Seibold, H. R., and Rathbone, R. R., 1933, Experimental studies on lymphomatosis of mice, *Am. J. Cancer* **19**:521–604.

Garcia, H., Baroni, C., and Rappaport, H., 1961, Transplantable tumors of the Syrian golden hamster (*Mesocricetus auratus*), *J. Natl. Cancer Inst.* **27**:1323–1333.

Gardner, M. B., Rongey, R. W., and Johnson, E. Y., 1971, C-type tumor virus particles in salivary tissue of domestic cats, *J. Natl. Cancer Inst.* **47**:561–568.

Gardner, W. U., Dougherty, F. T., and Williams, W. L., 1944, Lymphoid tumors in mice receiving steroid hormones, *Cancer Res.* **4**:73–87.

Gelb, L. D., Kohne, D. E., and Martin, M., 1971, Quantitation of simian virus 40 sequences in African green monkey, mouse and virus-transformed cell genomes, *J. Mol. Biol.* **57**:129–145.

German, J. (ed.), 1974, *Chromosomes and Cancer,* John Wiley & Sons, New York.

Gershon, R. K., and Carter, R. L., 1967, Studies on homotransplantable lymphomas in hamsters. II. The specificity of the histologic responses in lymphoid tissues and their relationship to metastasis, *Am. J. Pathol.* **50**:137–157.

Gershon, R. K., and Metzler, C. M., 1978, Regulation of the immune response, in: *The Immunopathology of Lymphoreticular Neoplasms* (R. A. Good and J. J. Twomey, eds.), Chapt. 2, Plenum Press, New York.

Gershon, R. K., Carter, R. L., and Lane, N. J., 1967, Studies on homotransplantable lymphomas in hamsters. IV. Observation on macrophages in the expression of tumor immunity, *Am. J. Pathol.* **51**:1111–1125.

Glaser, M., Lavrin, D. H., and Herberman, R. B., 1976, *In vivo* protection against syngeneic Gross virus-induced lymphoma in rats: Comparison with *in vitro* studies of cell-mediated immunity, *J. Immunol.* **16**:1507–1511.

Gleichmann, E., Gleichmann, H., and Schwartz, R. S., 1972, Immunologic induction of malignant lymphoma: Genetic factors in the graft-versus-host model, *J. Natl. Cancer Inst.* **49**:793–804.

Good, R. A., Dalmasso, A. P., Martinez, C., Archer, O. K., Pierce, J. C., and Papermaster, B. W., 1962, The role of the thymus in development of immunologic capacity in rabbits and mice, *J. Exp. Med.* **116**:733–796.

Graffi, A., 1960, Neuere Untersuchungen über das Virus der myeloischen Leukämie der Maus, in: *Progress in Experimental Tumor Research* (F. Hamburger, ed.), pp. 112–161, S. Karger, Basel, and J.B. Lippincott, Philadelphia.

Graffi, A., and Gimmy, J., 1957, Erzeugung von Leukosen bei der Ratte durch ein leukämogenes Agens der Maus, *Naturwissenschaften* **44**:518.

Graffi, A., Schramm, T., Bender, E., Graffi, I., Horn, K. H., and Bierwolf, D., 1968a, Cell-free transmissible leukoses in Syrian hamsters, probably of viral etiology, *Br. J. Cancer* **22**:577–581.

Graffi, A., Schramm, T., Graffi, I., Bierwolf, D., and Bender, E., 1968b, Virus-associated skin tumors of the Syrian hamster: Preliminary note, *J. Natl. Cancer Inst.* **40**:867–868.

Green, I., Jaffe, E. S., Shevach, E. M., Edelson, R. L., Frank, M. M., and Berard, C. W., 1975, Determination of the origin of malignant reticular cells by the use of surface membrane markers, in: *The Reticuloendothelial System: International Academy of Pathology Monograph 16*, pp. 282–300, Williams and Wilkins, Baltimore.

Greenberg, R. S., and Zatz, M. M., 1975, Spontaneous AKR lymphoma with T and B cell characteristics, *Nature (London)* **257**:314–316.

Grey, H. M., Rabellino, E., and Pirofsky, B., 1971, Immunoglobulins on the surface of lymphocytes. IV. Distribution in hypogammaglobulinemia, cellular immune deficiency and chornic lymphatic leukemia, *J. Clin. Invest.* **50**:2368–2375.

Gross, L., 1956, Viral (egg-borne) etiology of mouse leukemia: Filtered extracts from leukemic C59 mice, causing leukemia (or parotid tumors) following inoculation into newborn C57 Brown, or C3H mice, *Cancer* **9**:778–791.

Gross, L., 1958, Attempt to recover filterable agent from X-ray induced leukemia, *Acta. Haematol.* **19**:353–361.

Gross, L., 1959a, Serial cell-free passage of a radiation-activated mouse leukemia agent, *Proc. Soc. Exp. Biol. Med.* **100**:102–105.

Gross, L., 1959b, Effect of thymectomy on development of leukemia in C3H mice inoculated with "passage" virus, *Proc. Soc. Exp. Biol. Med.* **100**:325–328.

Gross, L., 1961, Induction of leukemia in rats with mouse leukemia (passage A) virus, *Proc. Soc. Exp. Biol. Med.* **106**:890–893.

Gross, L., 1962, Transmission of mouse leukemia virus through milk of virus-injected C3H female mice, *Proc. Soc. Exp. Biol. Med.* **109**:830–836.

Gross, L., 1963, Serial cell-free passage in rats of the mouse leukemia virus: Effect of thymectomy, *Proc. Soc. Exp. Biol. Med.* **112**:939–945.

Gross, L., 1964, Attempt at classification of mouse leukemia viruses, *Acta Haematol.* **32**:81–88.

Gross, L., 1966, The Rauscher virus: A mixture of the Friend virus and of the mouse leukemia virus (Gross)?, *Acta Haematol.* **35**:200–213.

Gross, L., 1970a, *Oncogenic Viruses*, 2nd Ed., Pergamon Press, New York.

Gross, L., 1970b, Specific, active, intradermal immunization against leukemia in guinea pigs, *Acta Haematol.* **44**:1–10.

Gross, L., 1971, Studies on the nature of acquired immunity against leukemia in guinea pigs, *Acta Haematol.* **45**:218–231.

Gross, L., and Dreyfuss, Y., 1974, The role of the skin in active specific immunization against leukemia in guinea pigs, *Proc. Natl. Acad. Sci. U.S.A.* **71**:3550–3554.

Gross, L., and Feldman, D. G., 1968, Electron microscopic studies of radiation-induced leukemia in mice: Virus release following total-body X-ray irradiation, *Cancer Res.* **28**:1677–1685.

Gross, L., and Feldman, D. G., 1969, Virus particles in guinea pig leukemia and in cat mammary carcinoma, *Proc. Am. Assoc. Cancer Res.* **10**:128.

Gross, L., Dreyfuss, Y., Ehrenreich, T., and Moore, L. A., 1970, Experimental studies on leukemia in guinea pigs, *Acta Haematol.* **43**:193–209.

Gross, L., Feldman, D. G., Ehrenreich, T., Dreyfuss, Y., and Moore, L. A., 1973, Comparative studies of subcutaneous and intradermal leukemic tumors in guinea pigs, *Cancer Res.* **33**:293–301.

Gross, L., Schidlovsky, G., Feldman, D., Dreyfuss, Y., and Moore, L. A., 1975, C-type virus particles in placenta of normal healthy Sprague–Dawley rats, *Proc. Natl. Acad. Sci. U.S.A.* **72**:3240–3244.

Gross, P. A., Fong, C. K. Y., and Hsiung, G. D., 1973, Characterization of guinea pig C-type virus, *Proc. Soc. Exp. Biol. Med.* **143**:367–370.

Haaland, M., 1905, Les tumeurs de la souris, *Ann. Inst. Pasteur* **19**:165–208.

Habel, K., 1969, Antigens of virus-induced tumors, *Adv. Immunol.* **10**:229–250.

Habel, K., and Eddy, B. E., 1963, Specificity of resistance to tumor challenge of polyoma and SV40 virus-immune hamsters, *Proc. Soc. Exp. Biol. Med.* **113**:1–4.

Hanafusa, H., Hanafusa, T., and Rubin, H., 1963, The defectiveness of Rous sarcoma virus, *Proc. Natl. Acad. Sci. U.S.A.* **49**:572–580.

Haran-Ghera, N., 1966, Leukemogenic activity of centrifugates from irradiated mouse thymus and bone marrow, *Int. J. Cancer* **1**:81–87.

Haran-Ghera, N., 1967, A leukemogenic filtrable agent from chemically induced lymphoid leukemia in C57BL mice, *Proc. Soc. Exp. Biol. Med.* **124**:697–699.

Haran-Ghera, N., 1973, Relationship between tumour cell and host in chemical leukaemogenesis, *Nature (London) New Biol.* **246**:84–86.

Haran-Ghera, N., and Kotler, M., 1968, A leukemogenic filterable agent from reticular cell neoplasms in the SJL-J strain of mice, *Bibl. Haematol. (Pavia)* **30**:70–72.

Haran-Ghera, N., and Peled, A., 1967, The mechanism of radiation action in leukemogenesis: Isolation of a leukaemogenic filtrable agent from tissues of irradiated and normal C57BL mice, *Br. J. Cancer* **21**:730–737.

Haran-Ghera, N., and Peled, A., 1972, Leukemogenic virus release in mice by irradiation, *Proc. Am. Assoc. Cancer Res.* **13**:10.

Haran-Ghera, N., and Peled, A., 1973, Thymus and bone marrow derived lymphatic leukemia in mice, *Nature (London)* **241**:396–398.

Haran-Ghera, N., Kotler, M., and Meshorer, A., 1967, Studies in leukemia development in the SJL/J strain of mice, *J. Natl. Cancer Inst.* **39**:653–661.

Haran-Ghera, N., Ben-Yaakov, M., Chazan, R., and Peled, A., 1975, Pathways in thymus- and bone marrow-derived lymphatic leukemia in mice, *Bibl. Haematol. (Pavia)* **30**:133–141.

Hardy, W. D., 1970, Immunodiffusion studies of feline leukemia and sarcoma, *J. Am. Vet. Med. Assoc.* **158**:1060–1069.

Hardy, W. D., Jr., Hess, P. W., Essex, M., Cotter, S., McClelland, A. J., and MacEwen, G., 1975, Horizontal transmission of feline leukemia virus in cats, *Bibl. Haematol. (Pavia)* **40**:67–74.

Harshbarger, J. C., and Dawe, C. J., 1973, Hematopoietic neoplasms in invertebrate and poikilothermic vertebrate animals, *Bibl. Haematol. (Pavia)* **39**:1–25.

Hartwell, L. H., Vogt, M., and Dulbecco, R., 1965, Induction of cellular DNA synthesis by polyoma virus, *Virology* **27**:262–272.

Hatanaka, M., Huebner, R. J., and Gilden, R. V., 1970, DNA polymerase activity associated with RNA tumor viruses, *Proc. Natl. Acad. Sci. U.S.A.* **67**:143–147.

Hays, E. R., 1968, The role of thymus epithelial reticular cells in viral leukemogenesis, *Cancer Res.* **28**:21–26.

Hehlmann, E., Kufe, D., and Spiegelman, S., 1972, RNA in human leukemic cells related to the RNA of a mouse leukemia virus, *Proc. Natl. Acad. Sci. U.S.A.* **69**:435–439.

Heilman, F. R., and Kendall, E. C., 1944, The influence of 11-dehydro-17-hydroxycorticosterone (compound E) on the growth of a malignant tumor in the mouse, *Endocrinology* **34**:416–420.

Hellström, K. E., and Hellström, I., 1974, Lymphocyte-mediated cytotoxicity and blocking serum activity to tumor antigens, *Adv. Immunol.* **18**:209–277.

Henshaw, P. S., 1944, Leukemia in mice following exposure to X-rays, *Radiology* **43**:279–285.

Herberman, R. B., 1974, Cell-mediated immunity to tumor cells, *Adv. Cancer Res.* **19**:207–263.

Hill, M., and Hillova, J., 1971, Production virale dans les fibroblastes de poule traités par l'acide désoxyribonucléique de cellules XC de rat transformées par le virus de Rous, *C. R. Acad. Sci.* **272**:3094.

Hill, M., and Hillova, J., 1972, Virus recovery in chicken cells treated with Rous sarcoma cell DNA, *Nature (London) New Biol.* **237**:35–39.

Hinze, H. C., 1971, New members of the herpesvirus group isolated from wild cottontail rabbit, *Infect. Immun.* **3**:350–354.

Hirsch, M. S., and Black, P. H., 1974, Activation of mammalian leukemia viruses, *Adv. Virus Res.* **19**:265–313.

Hirsch, M. S., Black, P. H., Tracy, G. S., Liebowitz, S., and Schwartz, R. S., 1970, Leukemia virus activation in chronic allogeneic disease, *Proc. Natl. Acad. Sci. U.S.A.* **67**:1914–1917.

Hirsch, M. S., Phillips, S. M., Solnik, C., Black, P. H., Schwartz, R. S., and Carpenter, C. B., 1972, Activation of leukemia viruses by graft-versus-host and mixed lymphocyte reactions *in vitro*, *Proc. Natl. Acad. Sci. U.S.A.* **69**:1069–1072.

Hirsch, M. S., Black, P. H., Wood, M. L., and Monaco, A. P., 1973, Effects of pyran copolymer on leukemogenesis in immunosuppressed AKR mice, *J. Immunol.* **111**:91–95.

Hodgkin, T., 1832, On some morbid appearances of the absorbent glands and spleen, *Med.-Chir. Trans.* **17**:68–114.

Holzworth, J., 1960, Leukemia and related neoplasms in the cat. I. Lymphoid malignancies, *J. Am. Vet. Med. Assoc.* **136**:47–69.

Hoover, E. A., McCullough, C. G., and Griesemer, R. A., 1972, Intranasal transmission of feline leukemia, *J. Natl. Cancer Inst.* **48**:973–983.

Howard, E. B., Clarke, W. J., and Hackett, P. L., 1968, Experimental myeloproliferative and lympho-proliferative diseases of swine, *Bibl. Haematol. (Pavia)* **30**:255–262.

Howie, J. B., and Helyer, B. J., 1968, The immunology and pathology of NZB mice, *Adv. Immunol.* **9**:215–266.

Hsiung, G. D., 1972, Activation of guinea pig C-type virus in cultured spleen cells by *S*-bromodeoxyuri-dine, *J. Natl. Cancer Inst.* **49**:567–570.

Hsiung, G. D., and Kaplow, L. S., 1969, Herpeslike virus isolated from spontaneously degenerated tissue culture derived from leukemia-susceptible guinea pigs, *J. Virol.* **3**:355–357.

Huber, H., and Fudenberg, H. H., 1968, Receptor sites of human monocytes for IgG, *Int. Arch. Allergy Appl. Immunol.* **34**:18–31.

Huber, H., Polley, M. J., Linscott, W. D., Fudenberg, H. H., and Muller-Eberhard, H. J., 1968, Human monocytes: Distinct receptor sites for the third component of complement and for immunoglobulin G, *Science* **162**:1281–1283.

Hudson, L., and Payne, L. N., 1973, An analysis of the T and B cells of Marek's disease lymphomas of the chicken, *Nature (London) New Biol.* **241**:52–53.

Huebner, R. J., and Todaro, G. J., 1969, Oncogenes of RNA tumor viruses as determinants of cancer, *Proc. Natl. Acad. Sci. U.S.A.* **64**:1087–1094.

Hueper, W. C., 1934, Leukemoid and leukemic conditions in white mice with spontaneous mammary carcinoma, *Folia Haematol.* **52**:167–178.

Huggins, C., and Kuwahara, I., 1967, Effect of dexamethasone on stem-cell leukemias of rat, in: *Endogenous Factors Influencing Host–Tumor Balance* (R. W. Wissler, T. L. Dao, and S. Wood, Jr., eds.), p. 9, University of Chicago Press.

Huggins, C., and Oka, H., 1972, Regression of stem-cell erythroblastic leukemia after hypophysectomy, *Cancer Res.* **32**:239–242.

Huggins, C. B., and Sugiyama, T., 1966, Induction of leukemia in rat by pulse-doses of 7,12-dimethyl-benz(a)anthracene, *Proc. Natl. Acad. Sci. U.S.A.* **55**:74–81.

Huggins, C. G., and Uematsu, K., 1976, Induction of lymphatic leukemia in non-inbred mice and its control with glucocorticoids, *Cancer* **37**:177–180.

Huggins, C. G., Yoshida, H., and Bird, C. C., 1974, Hormone-dependent stem-cell rat leukemia evoked by a series of feedings of 7,12-dimethylbenz(a)anthracene, *J. Natl. Cancer Inst.* **52**:1301–1304.

Hugoson, G., Vennstrom, R., and Henriksson, K., 1968, The occurrence of bovine leukosis following the introduction of babesiosis vaccination, *Bibl. Haematol. (Pavia)* **31**:157–161.

Hunstein, V. W., Stutz, E., and Reincke, U., 1963, Strahleninduzierte Leukämien bei Wistar-Ratten nach fraktionierter Ganzkörperbestrahlung, *Blut* **9**:389–404.

Hunt, R. D., Meléndez, L. V., King, N. W., and Garcia, F. G., 1972a, *Herpesvirus saimiri* malignant lymphoma in spider monkeys, *J. Med. Primatol.* **1**:114.

Hunt, R. D., Meléndez, L. V., Garcia, F. G., and Trum, B. F., 1972b, Pathologic features of *Herpesvirus ateles* lymphoma in cotton-topped marmosets *(Saguinus oedipus)*, *J. Natl. Cancer Inst.* **49**:1631–1639.

Hunt, R. D., Barahona, H. H., King, N. W., Fraser, C. E. O., Garcia, F. G., and Meléndez, L. V.,

1975a, Spontaneous Herpesvirus saimiri lymphoma in owl monkeys, *Bibl. Haematol. (Pavia)* **40**:351–355.

Hunt, R. D., Daniel, M. D., Baggs, R. B., Blake, B. J., Silva, D., DuBose, D., and Meléndez, L. V., 1975b, Clinicopathologic characterization of Herpesvirus saimiri malignant lymphoma in New Zealand white rabbits, *J. Natl. Cancer Inst.* **54**:1401–1412.

Hyde, J. L., King, J. M., and Bentinck-Smith, J., 1958, A case of bovine myelogenous leukemia, *Cornell Vet.* **48**:269–276.

Ida, N., Ohba, Y., Fukuhara, A., and Kohno, M., 1968, Chromosome conditions of hypodiploid Moloney virus-induced leukemia, its transplantability and inductivity, *J. Natl. Cancer Inst.* **40**:97–110.

Igel, H. J., Huebner, R. J., and Tuner, H. C., 1969, Mouse leukemia virus activation by chemical carcinogens, *Science* **166**:1624–1626.

Inoue, S., and Singer, M., 1970a, Experiments on a spontaneously originated visceral tumor in the newt, *Triturus pyrrhogaster, Ann. N.Y. Acad. Sci.* **174**:729–764.

Inoue, S., and Singer, M., 1970b, Lymphosarcomatous disease of the newt, *Triturus pyrrhogaster, Bibl. Haematol. (Pavia)* **36**:640–641.

Ioachim, H. L., and Berwick, L., 1970, Leukemia of guinea pigs, *Bibl. Haematol. (Pavia)* **36**:566–573.

Irino, S., Ota, Z., Sezaki, T., Suzaki, M., and Hiraki, K., 1963, Cell-free transmission of 20-methylcholanthrene-induced Rf mouse leukemia and electron microscopic demonstration of virus particles in its leukemia tissue, *Gann* **54**:225–237.

Isliker, H., Leuchtenberger, C., and Kliem, U., 1973, Effects of prolonged RES stimulation on the frequency of malignant tumors and lymphomatous disorders in mice, *J. Reticuloendothel. Soc.* **13**:459–466.

Jaffe, E. S., Shevach, E. M., Frank, M. M., Berard, C. W., and Green, I., 1974, Nodular lymphoma: Evidence for origin from follicular B lymphocytes, *N. Engl. J. Med.* **290**:813–819.

Jarrett, O., 1970, Evidence for the viral etiology of leukemia in the domestic mammals, *Adv. Cancer Res.* **13**:39–62.

Jarrett, O., Pitts, J. D., and Whalley, J. M., 1971, Isolation of the nucleic acid of feline leukaemia virus, *Virology* **43**:317–320.

Jarrett, W. F. H., 1966, Experimental studies of feline and bovine leukemia, *Proc. R. Soc. Med.* **59**:661–662.

Jarrett, W. F. H., 1971, Feline leukemia, *Int. Rev. Exp. Pathol.* **10**:243–263.

Jarrett, W. F. H., Martin, W. B., Crighton, G. W., Dalton, R. G., and Stewart, M. F., 1964a, Leukemia in the cat: Transmission experiments with leukaemia (lymphosarcoma), *Nature (London)* **202**:566–567.

Jarrett, W. F. H., Crawford, E. M., Martin, W. B., and Davie, F., 1964b, Leukemia in the cat: A virus-like particle associated with leukemia (lymphosarcoma), *Nature (London)* **202**:567–568.

Jarrett, W. F. H., Crighton, G. W., and Dalton, R. G., 1966, Leukemia and lymphosarcoma in animals and men. I. Lymphosarcoma or leukemia in the domestic animals, *Vet. Res.* **79**:693–699.

Jarrett, W. F. H., Essex, M., and Mackey, L., 1973a, Antibodies in normal and leukemic cats to feline oncornavirus-associated cell membrane antigens, *J. Natl. Cancer Inst.* **51**:261–263.

Jarrett, W. F. H., Jarrett, O., Mackey, L., Laird, H., Hardy, W., and Essex, M., 1973b, Horizontal transmission of leukemia virus and leukemia in the cat, *J. Natl. Cancer Inst.* **51**:833–841.

Jarrett, W. F. H., Mackey, L. J., Jarrett, O., and Laird, H. M., 1973c, Feline leukaemie virus infection— The spectrum of associated disease and its relevance to the pathogenesis and immunology of leukaemie, *Bibl. Haematol. (Pavia)* **39**:93–101.

Jerusalem, C., 1968, Relationship between malaria infection *(Plasmodium berghei)* and malignant lymphoma in mice, *Z. Tropenmed. Parasitol.* **19**:94–108.

Johnsen, D. O., Wooding, W. L., Tanticharoenyos, P., and Bourgeois, C. H., 1971, Malignant lymphoma in the gibbon, *J. Am. Vet. Med. Assoc.* **159**:563–566.

Jondal, M., and Klein, G., 1973, Surface markers on human B and T lymphocytes. II. Presence of Epstein–Barr virus receptors on B lymphocytes, *J. Exp. Med.* **138**:1365–1378.

Joneja, M. G., and Stich, H. F., 1965, Chromosome aberrations in virus-induced murine leukemia, *Exp. Cell Res.* **40**:148–151.

Joshi, V. V., and Frei, J. V., 1970, Gross and microscopic changes in the lymphoreticular system during genesis of malignant lymphoma induced by a single injection of methylnitrosourea in adult mice, *J. Natl. Cancer Inst.* **44**:379–387.

Jungeblut, C. W., and Kodza, H., 1960, Attempts to adapt leukemia L₂C from inbred to noninbred guinea pigs, *Am. J. Pathol.* **37**:191–201.

Jungeblut, C. W., and Kodza, H., 1962, Studies of leukemia L₂C in guinea pigs, *Arch. Gesamte Virusforsch.* **12**:537–551.

Jungeblut, C. W., and Opler, S. R., 1967, On the pathogenesis of cavian leukemia, *Am. J. Pathol.* **51**:1153–1160.

Kakuk, T. J., Hinz, R. W., Langham, R. F., and Conner, G. H., 1968, Experimental transmission of canine malignant lymphoma to the beagle neonate, *Cancer Res.* **28**:716–723.

Kalter, S. S., Helmke, R. J., Heberling, R. L., Panigel, M., Fowler, A. K., Strickland, J. E., and Hellman, A., 1973a, Brief communication: C-type particles in normal human placentas, *J. Natl. Cancer Inst.* **50**:1081–1084.

Kalter, S. S., Helmke, R. J., Panigel, M., Heberling, R. L., Felsburg, P. J., and Axelrod, L. R., 1973b, Observation of apparent C-type particles in baboon *(Papio cynocephalus)* placentas, *Science* **179**:1332–1333.

Kaplan, H. S., 1947, Observations on radiation-induced lymphoid tumors of mice, *Cancer Res.* **7**:141–147.

Kaplan, H. S., 1950, Influence of thymectomy, splenectomy, and gonadectomy on incidence of radiation-induced lymphoid tumors in strain C57 Black mice, *J. Natl. Cancer Inst.* **11**:83–90.

Kaplan, H. S., 1960, Early microscopic diagnosis of lymphosarcoma *in situ* in thymus of irradiated mice, *Fed. Proc. Fed. Am. Soc. Exp. Biol.* **19**:399.

Kaplan, H. S., 1964, The role of radiation in experimental leukemogenesis, *Natl. Cancer Inst. Monogr.* **14**:207–220.

Kaplan, H. S., 1974, Leukemia and lymphoma in experimental and domestic animals, *Ser. Haematol.* **7**:94–163.

Kaplan, H. S., and Brown, M. B., 1952, A quantitative dose–response study of lymphoid-tumor development in irradiated C57 Black mice, *J. Natl. Cancer Inst.* **13**:185–208.

Kaplan, J. C., Black, P. H., and Rothschild, H., 1971, Induction of virogenic mammalian cells with chemical and physical agents, *Proc. Can. Cancer Res. Conf.* **9**:143–158.

Karande, K. A., Raskar, S. P., and Ranadive, K. J., 1975, Activation of murine leukaemie virus under different physiological conditions, *Br. J. Cancer* **31**:434–442.

Kawakami, T. G., Theilen, G. H., Dungworth, D. L., Beall, S. G., and Munn, R. J., 1967, "C"-type viral particles in plasma of feline leukemia, *Science* **158**:1049–1050.

Kawakami, T. G., Huff, S. D., Buckley, P. M., Dungworth, D. L., Snyder, S. P., and Gilden, R. V., 1972, C-type virus associated with gibbon lymphosarcoma, *Nature (London) New Biol.* **235**:170–171.

Kawakami, T. G., Buckley, P. M., DePaoli, A., Noll, W., and Bustad, L. K., 1975, Studies on the prevalence of Type C virus associated with gibbon hematopoietic neoplasms, *Bibl. Haematol. (Pavia)* **40**:385–389.

Kawamoto, S., Ida, N., Kirschbaum, A., and Taylor, G., 1958, Urethan and leukemogenesis in mice, *Cancer Res.* **18**:725–729.

Kennedy, J. C., 1975, *In vitro* and *in vivo* effects of immunosuppressive and toxic material produced and released by cancer cells, in: *Host Defense Against Cancer and Its Potentiation* (D. Mizuno, G. Chihara, F. Fukuoka, T. Yamamoto, and Y. Yamamura, eds.), pp. 67–82, University of Tokyo Press, Tokyo, and University Park Press, Baltimore.

Kim, U., Clifton, K. H., and Furth, J., 1960, A highly inbred line of Wistar rats yielding spontaneous mammo-somatotropic pituitary and other tumors, *J. Natl. Cancer Inst.* **24**:1031–1055.

Kinosita, R., and Tanaka, T., 1963, Lymphoma in ICR mice treated with 4-nitroquinoline oxide (4 NQO), in: *Viruses, Nucleic Acids, and Cancer; A Collection of Papers,* pp. 571–574, Williams and Wilkins, Baltimore.

Kinosita, R., Tanaka, T., and Kakefuda, T., 1964, Experimental carcinogenesis by 4-nitroquinoline *N*-oxide (4 NQO), *Proc. Am. Assoc. Cancer Res.* **5**:34.

Kirschbaum, A., 1944, Genetic and certain non-genetic factors with reference to leukemia in the F strain of mice, *Proc. Soc. Exp. Biol. Med.* **55**:147–149.

Kirschbaum, A., and Mixer, H. W., 1947, Induction of leukemia in eight inbred stocks of mice varying in susceptibility to the spontaneous disease, *J. Lab. Clin. Med.* **32**:720–731.

Kirschbaum, A., and Strong, L. C., 1939, Leukemia in the F strain of mice: Observation on cytology, general morphology, and transmission, *Am. J. Cancer* **37**:400–413.

Kirsten, W. H., and Panem, S. B., 1974, Some aspects of viral oncogenesis, in: *The Physiopathology of Cancer*, Vol. 1, *Biology and Biochemistry* (P. Shubik, ed.), pp. 226–333, Karger, Basel.

Kirsten, W. H., Platz, C. E., and Flocks, J. S., 1962, Lymphoid neoplasms in rats after inoculation with cell-free extracts of leukemic AKR mice, *J. Natl. Cancer Inst.* **29**:293–319.

Kit, S., 1968, Viral-induced enzymes and the problem of viral oncogenesis, *Adv. Cancer Res.* **11**:73–221.

Kitagawa, M., Hamaoka, T., Takatsu, K., Haba, S., Yamashita, U., and Masaki, H., 1974, Disturbance of immune surveillance in tumor-bearing host, *Gann Monogr.: Cancer Res.* **16**:45–52.

Kitagawa, M., Hamaoka, T., Haba, S., Takatsu, K., and Masaki, H., 1975, Selective suppression of T-cell activity in tumor-bearing host and attempt for its improvement, in: *Host Defense Against Cancer and Its Potentiation* (D. Mizuno, G. Chihara, F. Fukuoka, T. Yamamoto, and Y. Yamamura, eds.), pp. 31–39, University Park Press, Baltimore.

Klein, E., Klein, G., Nadkarni, J. S., Nadkarni, J. J., Wigzell, H., and Clifford, P., 1968, Surface IgM-kappa specificity on a Burkitt lymphoma cell *in vivo* and in derived culture lines, *Cancer Res.* **28**:1300–1310.

Klement, V., Rowe, W. P., Hartley, J. W., and Pugh, W. E., 1969, Mixed culture cytopathogenicity: A new test for growth of murine leukemia viruses in tissue culture, *Proc. Natl. Acad. Sci. U.S.A.* **63**:753–758.

Kobayashi, H., 1975, Lymphomas and immunological tolerance in the rat induced by murine leukemia viruses, *Bibl. Haematol. (Pavia)* **40**:291–300.

Kohn, R. R., and Novak, D., 1973, Variability in AKR mouse leukemia mortality, *J. Natl. Cancer Inst.* **51**:683–685.

Krebs, K., Task-Nielsen, H. C., and Wagner, A., 1930, Origin of lymphosarcomatosis and its relation to other forms of leucosis in white mice, *Acta Radiol. Suppl.* **10**:1–53.

Krueger, G. R. F., 1974, Lymphoreticular neoplasia in immonosuppression: Facts and fancies, *Beitr. Pathol.* **151**:221–233.

Krueger, G. R. F., and Harris, D., 1972, Is phenytoin carcinogenic?, *Lancet* **1**:323.

Krueger, G. R. F., and Heine, U. I., 1972, Morphogenesis of two immunologically induced mouse lymphomas, *Cancer Res.* **32**:573–582.

Krueger, G. R. F., Malmgren, R. A., and Berard, C. W., 1971, Malignant lymphomas and plasmacytosis in mice under prolonged immunosuppression and persistent antigenic stimulation, *Transplantation* **11**:138–144.

Krueger, G. R. F., Harris, D., and Sussman, E., 1972, Effect of Dilantin in mice, *Z. Krebsforsch.* **78**:290–302.

Kunii, A., Takemoto, H., and Furth, J., 1965, Leukemogenic filterable agent from estrogen-induced thymic lymphoma in RF mice, *Proc. Soc. Exp. Biol. Med.* **119**:1211–1215.

Kurita, Y., Sugiyami, T., and Nishizuka, Y., 1968, Cytogenetic studies on rat leukemia induced by pulse doses of 7,12-dimethylbenz(a)anthracene, *Cancer Res.* **28**:1738–1752.

Kurstak, E., and Maramorosch, K. (eds.), 1974, *Viruses, Evolution and Cancer: Basic Considerations*, Academic Press, New York.

Laird, H. M., Jarrett, O., Crighton, G. W., and Jarrett, W. F. H., 1968a, An electron microscopic study of virus particles in spontaneous leukemia in the cat, *J. Natl. Cancer Inst.* **41**:867–878.

Laird, H. M., Jarrett, O., Crighton, G. W., Jarrett, W. F. H., and Hay, D., 1968b, Replication of leukemogenic-type virus in cats inoculated with feline lymphosarcoma extracts, *J. Natl. Cancer Inst.* **41**:879–893.

Lamon, E. W., Skurzak, H. M., and Klein, E., 1972, The lymphocyte response to a primary viral neoplasm (MSV) through its entire course in Balb/c mice, *Int. J. Cancer* **10**:581–588.

Lapin, B. A., 1975, Possible ways viral leukemia spreads among the Hamadryas baboons of the Sukhumi monkey colony, *Bibl. Haematol. (Pavia)* **40**:75–84.

Law, L. W., 1941, The induction of leukemia in mice following percutaneous applications of 9,10-dimethyl-1,2-benzanthracene, *Cancer Res.* **1**:564–571.

Law, L. W., 1947, Effect of gonadectomy and adrenalectomy on the appearance and incidence of spontaneous lymphoid leukemia in C58 mice, *J. Natl. Cancer Inst.* **8**:157–159.

Law, L. W., 1954, Genetic studies in experimental cancer, *Adv. Cancer Res.* **2**:281–352.

Law, L. W., and Miller, J. H., 1950a, Observations on the effect of thymectomy on spontaneous leukemias in mice of the high-leukemia strains, RIL and C58, *J. Natl. Cancer Inst.* **11**:253–262.

Law, L. W., and Miller, J. H., 1950b, The influence of thymectomy on the incidence of carcinogen-induced leukemia in strain DBA mice. *J. Natl. Cancer Inst.* **11**:425–438.

Law, L. W., and Moloney, J. B., 1961, Studies of congenital transmission of leukemia virus in mice, *Proc. Soc. Exp. Biol. Med.* **108**:715–723.

Law, L. W., and Speirs, R., 1947, The response of spontaneous leukemias to adrenal cortical extracts, *Proc. Soc. Exp. Biol. Med.* **66**:226–230.

Lerner, R. A., Jensen, F., Kennel, S. J., Dixon, F. J., DesRoches, G., and Francke, U., 1972, Karyotypic, virologic, and immunologic analyses of two continuous lymphocyte lines established from New Zealand Black mice: Possible relationship of chromosomal mosaicism to autoimmunity, *Proc. Natl. Acad. Sci. U.S.A.* **69**:2965–2969.

Lerner, R. A., Wilson, C. B., DelVillano, B. C., McConahey, P. J., and Dixon, F. J., 1976, Endogenous oncornaviral gene expression in adult and fetal mice: Quantitative, histologic, and physiologic studies of the major viral glycoprotein, gp 70, *J. Exp. Med.* **143**:151–166.

Levinthal, J. D., Buffett, R. F., and Furth, J., 1959, Prevention of viral lymphoid leukemia of mice by thymectomy, *Proc. Soc. Exp. Biol. Med.* **100**:610–614.

Levy, J. A., and Huebner, R. J., 1970, Association of murine leukaemia virus from a mouse lymphoma (2731-L) with reovirus type 3 infection, *Nature (London)* **225**:949–950.

Levy, J. A., and Pincus, T., 1970, Demonstration of biological activity of a murine leukemia virus of New Zealand Black mice, *Science* **170**:326–327.

Lieberman, M., and Kaplan, H. S., 1959, Leukemogenic activity of filtrates from radiation-induced lymphoid tumors of mice, *Science* **130**:387–388.

Lilly, F., 1966a, The inheritance of susceptibility to the Gross leukemia virus in mice, *Genetics* **53**:529–539.

Lilly, F., 1966b, The histocompatibility-2 locus and susceptibility to tumor indication, *Natl. Cancer Inst. Monogr.* **22**:631–642.

Lilly, F., and Pincus, T., 1973, Genetic control of murine viral leukemogenesis, *Adv. Cancer Res.* **17**:231–277.

Lilly, F., and Steeves, R., 1974, Antigens of murine leukemia virus, *Biochim. Biophys. Acta* **355**:105–118.

Lilly, F., Boyse, E. A., and Old, L. J., 1964, Genetic basis of susceptibility to viral leukemogenesis, *Lancet* **2**:1207–1209.

Lowry, D. R., Rowe, W. P., Teich, N., and Hartley, J. W., 1971, Murine leukemia virus: High frequency activation *in vitro* by 5-iododeoxyuridine and 5-bromodeoxyuridine, *Science* **174**:155–156.

Lowry, D. R., Chattopadhyay, S. K., Teich, N. M., Rowe, W. P., and Levine, A. S., 1974, AKR murine leukemia virus genome: Frequency of sequences in DNA of high-, low-, and non-virus-yielding mouse strains, *Proc. Natl. Acad. Sci. U.S.A.* **71**:3555–3559.

Lucas, A. M., Denington, E. M., Cottral, G. E., and Burmester, B. R., 1954a, Production of so-called normal lymphoid foci following inoculation with lymphoid tumor filtrate. I. Pancreas, *Poult. Sci.* **33**:562–570.

Lucas, A. M., Denington, E. M., Cottral, G. E., and Burmester, B. R., 1954b, Production of so-called normal lymphoid foci following inoculation with lymphoid tumor filtrate. II. Liver and spleen, *Poult. Sci.* **33**:571–584.

Lukes, R. J., and Parker, J. W., 1978, The pathology of lymphoreticular neoplasms, in: *The Immunopathology of Lymphoreticular Neoplasms* (R. A. Good, and J. J. Twomey, eds.), Chapt. 9, Plenum Press, New York.

Lukes, R. J., and Butler, J. J., 1966, The pathology and nomenclature of Hodgkin's disease, *Cancer Res.* **26**:1063–1083.

Lukes, R. J., Butler, J. J., and Hicks, E. B., 1966a, Natural history of Hodgkin's disease as related to its pathologic picture, *Cancer* **19**:317–344.

Lukes, R. J., Craver, L. F., Hall, T. C., Rappaport, H., and Ruben, P., 1966b, Report of the nomenclature committee, *Cancer Res.* **26**:1311.

MacDowell, E. C., and Richter, M. N., 1935, Mouse leukemia, IX. The role of heredity in spontaneous cases, *Arch. Pathol.* **20**:709–724.

MacDowell, E. C., Potter, J. S., and Taylor, M. J., 1945, Mouse leukemia: Role of genes in spontaneous cases, *Cancer Res.* **5**:65–83.

Mackey, L. J., Jarrett, W. F., and Jarrett, O., 1972, An experimental study of virus leukemia in cats, *J. Natl. Cancer Inst.* **48**:1663–1670.

Malmquist, W. A., Van Der Maaten, M. J., and Boothe, A. D., 1969, Isolation, immunodiffusion, immunofluorescence, and electron microscopy of a syncytial virus of lymphosarcomatous and apparently normal cattle, *Cancer Res.* **29**:188–200.

March, H. C., 1950, Leukemia in radiologists in a 20 year period, *Am. J. Med. Sci.* **220**:282–286.

Marek, J., 1907, Multiple Nervenentzündung (Polyneuritis) bei Hühnern, *Dtsch. Tieraerztl. Wochenschr.* **15**:417–421.

Marshak, R. R., and Abt, D. A., 1968, Epidemiology of bovine leukosis, *Bibl. Haematol. (Pavia)* **30**:166–182.

Marshak, R. R., Coriell, L. L., Lawrence, W. C., Croshaw, J. E., Jr., Schryver, H. F., Altera, K. P., and Nichols, W. W., 1962, Studies on bovine lymphosarcoma. I. Clinical aspects, pathological alterations, and herd studies, *Cancer Res.* **22**:202–217.

Marshak, R. R., Hare, W. C. D., Dodd, D. C., McFeely, R. A., Martin, J. E., and Dutcher, R. M., 1967, Transplantation of lymphosarcoma in calves, *Cancer Res.* **27**:498–504.

Masaki, H., Takatsu, K., Hamaoka, T., and Kitagawa, M., 1972, Immunosuppressive activity of chromatin fraction derived from nuclei of Ehrlich ascites tumor cells, *Gann* **63**:633–635.

Mathé, G., and Bernard, J., 1958, Fréquence de leucémies et de tumeurs chez des souris C57BL/6 ayant recu à la naissance du plasma d'animaux irradiés, *Rev. Fr. Etud. Clin. Biol.* **3**:257–258.

McEndy, D. P., Boon, M. C., and Furth, J., 1942, Induction of leukemia in mice by methylcholanthrene and X-rays, *J. Natl. Cancer Inst.* **3**:227–247.

McEndy, D. P., Boon, M. C., and Furth, J., 1944, On the role of the thymus, spleen, and gonads in the development of leukemia in a high-leukemia stock of mice, *Cancer Res.* **4**:377–383.

McIntire, K. R., and Princler, G. L., 1969, Prolonged adjuvant stimulation in germ-free BALB/c mice: Development of plasma cell neoplasia, *Immunology* **17**:481–487.

Meléndez, L. V., Hunt, R. D., Daniel, M. D., Fraser, C. E. O., Garcia, F. H., and Williamson, F. D., 1970, Lethal reticuloproliferative disease induced in *Cebus albifrons* monkeys by *Herpesvirus saimiri*, *Int. J. Cancer* **6**:431–435.

Meléndez, L. V., Hunt, R. D., Daniel, M. D., Blake, B. J., and Garcia, F. G., 1971, Acute lymphocytic leukemia in owl monkeys *(Aotus trivirgatus)* inoculated with *Herpesvirus saimiri*, *Science* **171**:1161–1163.

Meléndez, L. V., Hunt, R. D., Daniel, M. D., Fraser, C. E. O., Barahona, H. H., Garcia, F. G., and King, N. W., 1972a, Lymphoma viruses of monkeys: *Herpesvirus saimiri* and *Herpesvirus ateles,* the first oncogenic herpesviruses of primates—A review, in: *Oncogenesis and Herpesviruses: Proceedings of a Symposium,* Christ's College, Cambridge, England, 20–25 June 1971 (P. M. Biggs, G. de-The, and L. N. Payne, eds.), pp. 451–461, Lyon.

Meléndez, L. V., Hunt, R. D., King, N. W., Barahona, H. H., Daniel, M. D., Fraser, C. E. O., and Garcia, F. G., 1972b, A new lymphoma virus of monkeys: *Herpesvirus ateles, Nature (London) New Biol.* **235**:182–184.

Mellors, R. C., 1965, Autoimmune disease in NZB/BL mice. I. Pathology and pathogenesis of a model system for spontaneous glomerulonephritis, *J. Exp. Med.* **122**:22–37.

Mellors, R. C., 1966, Autoimmune disease in NZB/B1 mice. II. Autoimmunity and malignant lymphoma, *Blood* **27**:435–448.

Mellors, R. C., 1969, Murine leukemia-like virus and the immunopathological disorders of New Zealand Black mice, *J. Infect. Dis.* **120**:480–487.

Metcalf, D., 1961, Reticular tumours in mice subjected to prolonged antigenic stimulation, *Br. J. Cancer* **15**:769–779.

Metcalf, D., 1971, Humoral regulators in the development and progression of leukemia, *Adv. Cancer Res.* **14**:181–230.

Miguez, C., 1918, Sarcoma espontáneo transplantable en el cobayo, *Rev. Inst. Bacteriol. Buenos Aires* **1**:147–154.

Miller, G., Shope, T., Lisco, H., Stitt, D., and Lipman, M., 1972, Epstein–Barr virus: Transformation, cytopathic changes and viral antigens in squirrel monkey and marmoset leukocytes, *Proc. Natl. Acad. Sci. U.S.A.* **69**:383–387.

Miller, J. F. A. P., 1959, Role of the thymus in murine leukemia, *Nature (London)* **183**:1069.

Miller, J. F. A. P., 1961, Immunological function of the thymus, *Lancet* **2**:748–749.

Miller, J. M., and Olson, C., 1972, Precipitating antibody to an internal antigen of the C-type virus associated with bovine lymphosarcoma, *J. Natl. Cancer Inst.* **49**:1459–1461.

Miller, J. M., Miller, L. D., Olson, C., and Gillette, K. G., 1969, Virus-like particles in phytohemagglutinin stimulated lymphocyte cultures with reference to bovine lymphosarcoma, *J. Natl. Cancer Inst.* **43**:1297–1302.

Miller, L. D., Miller, J. M., and Olson, C., 1972, Inoculation of calves with the C-type virus associated with bovine lymphosarcoma, *J. Natl. Cancer Inst.* **48**:423–428.

Mirand, E. A., and Grace, J. T., Jr., 1962, Induction of leukemia in rats with Friend virus, *Virology* **17**:364–366.

Moldovanu, G., Moore, A. E., Friedman, M., and Miller, D. G., 1966, Cellular transmission of lymphosarcoma in dogs, *Nature (London)* **210**:1342–1343.

Moldovanu, G., Moore, A. E., Friedman, M., and Miller, D. G., 1968, Canine lymphosarcoma maintained in serial passage, *Bibl. Haematol. (Pavia)* **30**:276–278.

Moloney, J. B., 1960, Biological studies on a lymphoid leukemia virus extracted from sarcoma 37. I. Origin and introductory investigations, *J. Natl. Cancer Inst.* **24**:933–951.

Moloney, J. B., 1964, The rodent leukemias: Virus induced murine leukemias, *Annu. Rev. Med.* **15**:383–392.

Montagnier, L., and Vigier, P., 1972, Un intermédiaire ADN infectieux et transformant du virus du sarcome de Rous dans les cellules de poule transformées par le virus, *C. R. Acad. Sci.* **274**:1977–1980.

Morton, J. J., and Mider, G. B., 1938, The production of lymphomatosis in mice of known genetic constitution, *Science* **87**:327–328.

Morton, J. J., and Mider, C. B., 1941, Some effects of carcinogenic agents on mice subject to spontaneous leukoses, *Cancer Res.* **1**:95–98.

Moulton, J. E., and Bostick, W. L., 1958, Canine malignant lymphoma simulating Hodgkin's disease in man, *J. Am. Vet. Med. Assoc.* **132**:204–209.

Mulcahy, M. F., 1963, Lymphosarcoma in the pike, *Esox lucius* L. (Pisces; Esocidae), in Ireland, *Proc. R. Ir. Acad. Ser. B.* **63**:103–129.

Mulcahy, M. F., 1970, The thymus glands and lymphosarcoma in the pike, *Esox lucius* L. (Pisces; Esocidae). in Ireland, *Bibl. Haematol. (Pavia)* **36**:600–609.

Mulcahy, M. F., and O'Leary, A., 1970, Cell-free transmission of lymphosarcoma in the northern pike *Esox lucius* L. (Pisces; Esocidae), *Experimentia* **26**:891.

Mulcahy, M. F., Winqvist, G., and Dawe, C. J., 1970, The neoplastic cell type in lymphoreticular neoplasms of the northern pike, *Esox lucius* L., *Cancer Res.* **30**:2712–2717.

Murphy, E. D., 1963, SJL/J, a new inbred strain of mouse with a high, early incidence of reticulum-cell neoplasms, *Proc. Am. Assoc. Cancer Res.* **4**:46.

Murphy, J. B., 1944, The effect of castration, theelin and testosterone on the incidence of leukemia in a Rockefeller Institute strain of mice, *Cancer Res.* **4**:622–624.

Murphy, J. B., and Sturm, E., 1944, The effect of adrenal cortical and pituitary adrenotropic hormones on transplanted leukemia of rats, *Science* **99**:303.

Nadel, E. M., 1957, Transplantation of leukemia from inbred to non inbred guinea pigs, *J. Natl. Cancer Inst.* **19**:351–359.

Nadel, E., Banfield, W., Burstein, S., and Tousimis, A. J., 1967, Virus particles associated with strain 2 guinea pig leukemia (L_2C/N-B), *J. Natl. Cancer Inst.* **83**:979–982.

Nadel, E., Lui, P., Grill, F., and Burstein, S., 1970, Transplantability of cell-free L_2C/13BN leukemia in strain 13 guinea pigs, *Fed. Proc. Fed. Am. Soc. Exp. Biol.* **29**:449.

Nayak, D. P., 1974, Endogenous guinea pig virus: Equability of virus-specific DNA in normal, leukemia and virus-producing cells, *Proc. Natl. Acad. Sci. U.S.A.* **71**:1164–1168.

Nayak, D. P., and Murray, P. R., 1973. Induction of type C viruses in cultured guinea pig cells, *J. Virol.* **12**:177–187.

Napak, D. P., Murray, P., Goldblatt, D., and Karpov, K., 1975, An endogenous oncornavirus of guinea pigs: Its expression in leukemic cells, *Bibl. Haematol. (Pavia)* **40**:545–559.

Nayar, K. K., Arthur, E., and Balls, M., 1970, Transmission of an amphibian lymphosarcoma to and through insects, *Oncology* **24**:370–377.

Nazerian, K., and Sharma, J. M., 1975, Detection of T-cell surface antigens in a Marek's disease lymphoblastoid cell line, *J. Natl. Cancer Inst.* **54**:277–279.

Nazerian, K., and Witter, R. L., 1970, Cell-free transmission and *in vivo* replication of Marek's disease virus, *J. Virol.* **5**:388–397.

Nazerian, K., Solomon, J. J., Witter, R. L., and Burmester, B. R., 1968, Studies on the etiology of Marek's disease. II. Finding of a herpesvirus in cell culture, *Proc. Soc. Exp. Biol. Med.* **127**:177–182.

Neiman, P. E., 1972, Rous sarcoma virus nucleotide sequences in cellular DNA: Measurement by RNA–DNA hybridization, *Science* **178**:750–753.

Nemeth, L., 1963, A comparative study of the late effects of certain radiomimetic drugs and X-rays, in: *Cellular Basis and Aetiology of Late Somatic Effects of Ionizing Radiation* (R. J. C. Harris, ed.), pp. 57–58, Academic Press, New York.

Nomura, S., Bassin, R. H., and Fischinger, P. J., 1972, Replication of radiation-induced murine leukemia virus in normal and transformed mouse cells, *J. Virol.* **9**:494–502.

Notkins, A. L., Mergenhagen, S. E., and Howard, R. J., 1970, Effect of virus infections on the function of the immune system, *Annu. Rev. Microbiol.* **24**:525–538.

Noyes, W. F., 1959, Studies on the Shope rabbit papilloma virus. II. The location of infective virus in papillomas of the cottontail rabbit, *J. Exp. Med.* **109**:423–428.

Odaka, T., 1973, Inheritance of susceptibility to Friend mouse leukemia virus. X. Separate genetic control of two viruses in Friend virus preparation, *Int. J. Cancer* **11**:567–574.

Oka, H., Aida, M., Yamada, S., Hayama, K., and Oda, T., 1974, Effect of hypophysectomy on rat leukemia cells, *Cancer Res.* **34**:1926–1929.

Okano, H., Kunii, A., and Furth, J., 1963, An electron microscopic study of leukemia induced in rats with Gross virus, *Cancer Res.* **23**:1169–1175.

Okazaki, W., Purchase, H. G., and Burmester, B. R., 1970, Protection against Marek's disease by vaccination with a herpesvirus of turkeys, *Avian Dis.* **14**:413–429.

Oldstone, M. B. A., Aoki, T., and Dixon, F. J., 1971, Activation of spontaneous murine leukemia virus-related antigen by lymphocytic choriomeningitis virus, *Science* **174**:843–845.

Olson, C., Jr., 1936, A study of transmissible fowl leukosis, *J. Am. Vet. Med. Assoc.* **89**:681–705.

Olson, C., 1974, Bovine lymphosarcoma (leukemia)—A synopsis, *J. Am. Vet. Med. Assoc.* **165**:630–632.

Olson, C., Miller, L. D., Miller, J. M., and Hoss, H. E., 1972, Transmission of lymphosarcoma from cattle to sheep, *J. Natl. Cancer Inst.* **49**:1463–1467.

Olson, C., Hoss, H. E., Miller, J. M., and Baumgartener, L. E., 1973, Evidence of bovine C-type (leukemia) virus in dairy cattle, *J. Am. Vet. Med. Assoc.* **163**:355–357.

Olson, H., 1961, Studien über das Autfreten und die Verbreitung der Rinderleukose in Schweden, *Acta. Vet. Scand.* **2** (Suppl. 2):13–46.

Onions, D. E., 1975, B- and T-cells in canine lymphosarcoma, *Vet. Rec.* **97**:108.

Opler, S. R.,1967a, Pathology of cavian viral leukemia, *Am. J. Pathol.* **51**:1135–1141.

Opler, S. R., 1967b, Observation of a new virus associated with guinea pig leukemia: Preliminary note, *J. Natl. Cancer Inst.* **38**:797–800.

Opler, S. R., 1967c, Animal model of viral oncogenesis, *Nature (London)* **215**:184.

Opler, S. R., 1968, Transmission of viral induced cavian leukemia by the oral route, *Oncology* **22**:273–280.

Ottonen, P. O., and Ball, J. K., 1973, Lack of correlation between gross chromosome abnormalities and carcinogenesis with 7,12-dimethylbenz(a)anthracene, *J. Natl. Cancer Inst.* **50**:497–501.

Pappenheimer, A. M., Dunn, L. C., and Cone, V., 1929, Studies on fowl paralysis (neurolymphomatosis gallinarum): Clinical features and pathology, *J. Exp. Med.* **49**:63–86.

Paran, M., Wu, A. M., Richardson, L. A., and Gallo, R. C., 1974, Glucocorticosteroids and RNA tumor viruses, *Haematol. Bluttransfus.* **14**:197–205.

Parodi, A., Wyers, M., and Paris, J., 1968, Incidence of canine lymphoid leukosis: Age, sex, and breed distribution; results of a necropsic survey, *Bibl. Haematol. (Pavia)* **30**:263–267.

Paulsen, J., Rudolph, R., and Miller, J. M., 1974, Antibodies common to ovine and bovine C-type virus specific antigen in serum from sheep with spontaneous leukosis and from inoculated animals, *Med. Microbiol. Immunol.* **159**:105.

Peller, S., 1939, Lung cancer among mine workers in Joachimsthal, *Hum. Biol.* **11**:130–143.

Pentimalli, F., 1941, Transplantable lymphosarcoma of chicken, *Cancer Res.* **1**:69–70.

Peterson, R. D. A., Burmester, B. R., Fredrickson, T. N., and Good, R. A., 1963a, Prevention of lymphatic leukemia in the chicken by the surgical removal of the bursa of Fabricius, *J. Lab. Clin. Med.* **62**:1000.

Peterson, R. D. A., Hendrickson, R., and Good, R. A., 1963b, Reduced antibody forming capacity during the incubation period of Passage A leukemia in C3H mice, *Prod. Soc. Exp. Biol. Med.* **114**:517–520.

Peterson, R. D. A., Burmester, B. R., Fredrickson, T. N., Purchase, H. G., and Good, R. A., 1964, Effect of bursectomy and thymectomy on the development of visceral lymphomatosis in the chicken, *J. Natl. Cancer Inst.* **32**:1343–1354.

Peterson, R. D. A., Purchase, H. G., Burmester, B. R., Cooper, M. D., and Good, R. A., 1966, Relationships among visceral lymphomatosis, bursa of Fabricius, and bursa-dependent lymphoid tissue of the chicken, *J. Natl. Cancer Inst.* **36**:585–598.

Pierpaoli, W., and Haran-Ghera, N., 1975, Prevention of induced leukemia in mice by immunological inhibition of adenohypophysis, *Nature (London)* **254**:334–335.

Pincus, T., Hartley, J. W., and Rowe, W. P., 1971a, A major genetic locus affecting resistance to infection with murine leukemia viruses. I. Tissue culture studies of naturally occurring viruses, *J. Exp. Med.* **133**:1219–1233.

Pincus, T., Rowe, W. P., and Lilly, F., 1971b, A major genetic locus affecting resistance to infection with murine leukemia viruses. II. Apparent identity of a major locus described for resistance to Friend murine leukemia virus, *J. Exp. Med.* **133**:1234–1241.

Piper, C. E., Abt, D. A., Ferrer, J. F., and Marshak, R. R., 1975, Seroepidemiological evidence for horizontal transmission of bovine C-type virus, *Cancer Res.* **35**:2714–2716.

Pontén, J., 1963, Chromosome analysis of three virus-associated chicken tumors: Rous sarcoma, erythroleukemia, and RPL12 lymphoid tumor, *J. Natl. Cancer Inst.* **30**:897–921.

Potter, M., 1962, Plasma cell neoplasia in a single host: A mosaic of different protein-producing cell types, *J. Exp. Med.* **115**:339–356.

Potter, M., and Kuff, E. L., 1961, Myeloma globulins of plasma-cell neoplasms in inbred mice. I. Immunoelectrophoresis of serum, with rabbit antibodies prepared against microsome fractions of the neoplasms, *J. Natl. Cancer Inst.* **26**:1109–1137.

Potter, M., and Robertson, C. L., 1960, Development of plasma-cell neoplasms in Balb/c mice after intraperitoneal injection of paraffin-oil adjuvant, heat-killed staphylococcus mixtures, *J. Natl. Cancer Inst.* **25**:847–861.

Powell, P. C., Payne, L. N., Frazier, J. A., and Rennie, M., 1974, T lymphoblastoid cell lines from Marek's disease lymphomas, *Nature (London)* **251**:79–80.

Preud'Homme, J. L., Klein, M., Verroust, P., and Seligmann, M., 1971, Immunoglobulines monoclonales de membrane dans les leucémies lymphoides chroniques, *Rev. Eur. Etud. Clin. Biol.* **16**:1025–1031.

Price, P. J., Freeman, A. E., and Lane, W. T., 1971, Morphological transformation of rat embryo cells by the combined action of 3-methylcholanthrene and Rauscher leukemia virus, *Nature (London) New Biol.* **230**:144–146.

Prigozhina, E., 1962, Induction of leukoses in rats with dimethylbenzanthracene and its transplantation, *Vopr. Onkol.* **8**:64–70.

Proffitt, M. R., Hirsch, M. S., and Black, P. H., 1973, Murine leukemia: A virus-induced autoimmune disease?, *Science* **182**:821–823.

Purchase, H. G., 1969, Immunofluorescence in the study of Marek's disease. I. Detection of antigen in cell cultures and an antigenic comparison of eight isolates, *J. Virol.* **3**:557–565.

Purchase, H. G., 1970, Virus-specific immunofluorescent and precipitin antigens and cell-free virus in the tissue of birds infected with Marek's disease, *Cancer Res.* **30**:1898–1908.

Purchase, H. G., 1972, Role of herpesviruses in Marek's disease, a malignant lymphoma of chickens, *Fed. Proc. Fed. Am. Soc. Exp. Biol.* **31**:1634–1638.

Purchase, H. G., and Burmester, B. R., 1972, The leukosis/sarcoma group, in: *Diseases of Poultry* (M. S. Hofstad, ed.), pp. 502–568, Iowa State University Press, Ames.

Purchase, H. G., and Gilmour, D. G., 1975, Lymphoid leukosis in chickens chemically bursectomized and subsequently inoculated with bursa cells, *J. Natl. Cancer Inst.* **55**:851–855.

Purchase, H. G., Chubb, R. C., and Biggs, P. M., 1968, Effect of lymphoid leukosis and Marek's disease on the immunological responsiveness of the chicken, *J. Natl. Cancer Inst.* **40**:583–592.

Purchase, H. G., Okazaki, W., and Burmester, B. R., 1971, Field trials with the herpes virus of turkeys (HVT) strain FC126 as a vaccine against Marek's disease, *Poult. Sci.* **50**:775–783.

Raff, M. C., 1969, Theta isoantigen as a marker of thymus-derived lymphocytes in mice, *Nature (London)* **224**:378–379.

Raff, M. C., and Wortis, H. H., 1970, Thymus dependence of Θ (theta)-bearing cells in the peripheral lymphoid tissue of mice, *Immunology* **18**:931–942.

Rajewsky, B., Schraub, A., and Kahlau, G., 1943, Experimentelle Geschwulsterzeugung durch Einatmung von Radiumemanation, *Naturwissenschaften* **31**:170–171.

Rappaport, H., 1966, Tumors of the hematopoietic system, in: *Atlas of Tumor Pathology,* Sect. III, Armed Forces Institute of Pathology, Washington, D.C.

Rask-Nielsen, R., 1949, Investigations into the varying manifestations of leukaemic lesions following injections of 9 : 10-dimethyl-1 : 2-benzanthracene into different subcutaneous sites in Street mice, *Br. J. Cancer* **3**:549–556.

Rauscher, F. J., 1962, A virus-induced disease of mice characterized by erythropoiesis and lymphoid leukemia, *J. Natl. Cancer Inst.* **29**:515–543.

Rhim, J. S., Vass, W., and Cho, H. Y., 1971, Malignant transformation induced by 7,12-dimethylbenz(a)anthracene in rat embryo cells infected with Rauscher leukemia virus, *Int. J. Cancer* **7**:65–74.

Ribacchi, R., and Giraldo, G., 1966, Leukemia virus release in chemically or physically induced lymphomas in Balb/c mice, *Natl. Cancer Inst. Monogr.* **22**:701–711.

Rich, M. A., Tsuchida, R., and Siegler, R., 1964, Chromosome aberrations: Their role in the etiology of murine leukemia, *Science* **146**:252–253.

Richter, M. N., and MacDowell, E. C., 1929, The experimental transmission of leukemia in mice, *Proc. Soc. Exp. Biol. Med.* **26**:362–364.

Rickard, C. G., Barr, L. M., Noronha, F., Dougherty, E., and Post, J. E., 1967, C-type virus particles in spontaneous lymphocytic leukemia in a cat, *Cornell Vet.* **57**:302–307.

Rickard, C. G., Gillespie, J. H., Lee, K. M., Noronha, F., Post, J. E., and Savage, E. L., 1968, Transmission and electron microscopy of lymphocytic leukemia in the cat, *Bibl. Haematol. (Pavia)* **31**:282–284.

Rickard, C. G., Post, J. E., Noronha, F., and Barr, L. M., 1969, A transmissible virus-induced lymphocytic leukemia of the cat, *J. Natl. Cancer Inst.* **42**:987–1014.

Riley, V., and Fitzmaurice, M. A., 1973, "Helper" influence of the LDH-virus in the production of leukemia by attenuated Rauscher virus, *Fed. Proc. Fed. Am. Soc. Exp. Biol.* **64**:112.

Ritchie, R. C., 1957, cited in Schlumberger, H. G., Tumors characteristic for certain animal species: A review, *Cancer Res.* **17**:823–832.

Roberts, M. C. and Pinsent, P. V. N., 1975, Malabsorption in the horse associated with alimentary lymphosarcoma, *Equine Vet. J.* **7**:166–172.

Rodey, G. E., Good, R. A., and Tunis, E. J., 1971, Progressive loss *in vitro* of cellular immunity with ageing in strains of mice susceptible to autoimmune disease, *Clin. Exp. Immunol.* **9**:305–311.

Rosenberger, G., 1968, Successful experimental transmission of bovine leukosis, *Bibl. Haematol. (Pavia)* **30**:136–139.

Rothschild, H., and Black, P. H., 1970, Analysis of SV40-induced transformation of hamster kidney tissue *in vitro*. VII. Induction of SV40 virus from transformed hamster cell clones by various agents, *Virology* **42**:251–256.

Rouse, B. T., Wells, R. H., and Warner, N. L., 1973, Proportion of T and B lymphocytes in lesions of Marek's disease: Theoretical implications for pathogenesis, *J. Immunol.* **110**:534–539.

Rowe, W. P., 1972, Studies of genetic transmission of murine leukemia virus by AKR mice. I. Grosses with F_v-1^n strains of mice, *J. Exp. Med.* **136**:1272–1285.

Rowe, W. P., 1973, Genetic factors in the natural history of murine leukemia virus infection, G. H. H. Clowes Memorial Lecture, *Cancer Res.* **33**:3061–3068.

Rowe, W. P., and Hartley, J. W., 1972, Studies of genetic transmission of murine leukemia virus by AKR mice. II. Grosses with F_v-1^b strains of mice, *J. Exp. Med.* **136**:1286–1301.

Rowe, W. P., and Sato, H., 1973, Genetic mapping of the *Fv-1* locus of the mouse, *Science* **189**:640–641.

Rowe, W. P., Pugh, W. E., and Hartley, V. W., 1970, Plaque assay techniques for murine leukemia viruses, *Virology* **42**:1136–1139.

Rowe, W. P., Hartley, J. W., and Bremner, T., 1972, Genetic mapping of a murine leukemia virus-inducing locus of AKR mice, *Science* **178**:860–862.

Rowe, W. P., Humphrey, J. B., and Lilly, F., 1973, A major genetic locus affecting resistance to infection with murine leukemia viruses. III. Assignment of the *Fv-1* locus to linkage group VIII of the mouse, *J. Exp. Med.* **137**:850–853.

Ruben, L. N., 1970, Lymphoreticular disorders and responses in *Xenopus laevis*, the South African clawed toad, *Bibl. Haematol. (Pavia)* **36**:638–639.

Ruben, L. N., and Stevens, J. M., 1970, A comparison between granulomatosis and lymphoreticular neoplasia in *Diemictylus viridescens* and *Xenopus laevis*, *Cancer Res.* **30**:2613–2619.

Ruben, L. N., Balls, M., Stevens, J., and Rafferty, N. S., 1969, A new transmissible disease in the South African clawed toad, *Xenopus laevis*, *Oncology* **23**:228–237.

Rubin, H., Franshier, L., Cornelius, A., and Hughes, W. F., 1962, Tolerance and immunity in chickens after congenital and contact infection with an avian leukosis virus, *Virology* **17**:143–156.

Rubin, P., 1968, Hodgkin's-like reticulum cell sarcoma in SVL/J mouse: An animal model of lymphoma to solve clinical problems, *Radiol. Clin. North Am.* **6**:25–44.

Rudali, G., and Mogul, M. R., 1967, Sur quelques caractères de la maladie spontanée des souris SUL/J, *Eur. J. Cancer* **3**:217.

Sanarelli, G., 1898, Das myxomatogene Virus. Beitrag zum Studium der Krankheitserreger ausserhalb des Sichtbaren, *Zentralbl. Bakteriol. Parasitenkd. Infektionskr. Hyg. Abt 1* **23**:865.

Sarma, P. S., Gilden, R. V., and Huebner, R. J., 1971, Complement-fixation test for Felini leukemia and sarcoma viruses (the COCAL test), *Virology* **44**:137–145.

Sarma, P. S., Dejkunchorn, P., Vernon, M. L., Gilden, R. V., and Bergs, V., 1973, Wistar–Furth rat C type virus—Biologic and antigenic characterization, *Proc. Soc. Exp. Biol. Med.* **142**:461–465.

Schidlovsky, G., and Ahmed, M., 1973, C-type virus particles in placentas and fetal tissues of rhesus monkeys, *J. Natl. Cancer Inst.* **51**:225–233.

Schochet, S. S., Jr., and Lampert, P. W., 1969, Plasmocytoma in a *Rana pipiens*, in: *Biology of Amphibian Tumors* (M. Mizell, ed.), pp. 204–214, Springer-Verlag, New York.

Schwartz, R. S., and Beldotti, L., 1965, Malignant lymphomas following allogeneic disease: Transition from an immunological to a neoplastic disorder, *Science* **149**:1511–1514.

Schwartz, R., André-Schwartz, V., Armstrong, M. Y. K., and Beldotti, L., 1966, Neoplastic sequelae of allogeneic disease. I. Thoretical considerations and experimental design, *Ann. N.Y. Acad. Sci.* **129**:804–821.

Sharon, N., and Pollard, M., 1971, LCM virus is oncogenic, *Bacteriol. Proc.* **61**:178.

Shay, H., Gruenstien, M., Marx, H. E., and Glazer, L., 1951, The development of lymphatic and myelogenus leukemia in Wistar rats following gastric instillation of mythylcholanthrene, *Cancer Res.* **11**:29–34.

Sheehan, W. W., 1971, The relationship between lymphocytic leukemias and lymphomas, in: *Current Concepts in the Management of Leukemia and Lymphoma*, Vol. 36, *Recent Results in Cancer Research* (J. E. Ultmann, M. L. Griem, W. H. Kirsten, and R. W. Wissler, eds), p. 24, Springer-Verlag, Berlin.

Shellam, G. R., 1974, Studies on a Gross-virus-induced lymphoma in the rat. I. The cell-mediated immune response, *Int. J. Cancer* **14**:65–82.

Shevach, E. M., Ellman, L., Davie, J. M., and Green, I., 1972a, L$_2$C guinea pig lymphatic leukemia: A ''B'' cell leukemia, *Blood* **39**:1–12.

Shevach, E., Herberman, R., Lieberman, R., Frank, M. M., and Green, I., 1972b, Receptors for immunoglobulin and complement on mouse leukemias and lymphomas, *J. Immunol.* **108**:325–328.

Shevach, E. M., Stobe, J. D., and Green, I., 1972c, Immunoglobulin and theta bearing murine leukemia and lymphomas, *J. Immunol.* **108**:1146–1151.

Shevach, E. M., Jaffe, E. S., and Green, I., 1973, Receptors for complement and immunoglobulins on human and animal lymphoid cells, *Transplant. Rev.* **16**:3–28.

Shirai, T., and Mellors, R. C., 1972, Natural cytotoxic autoantibody against thymocytes in NZB mice, *Clin. Exp. Immunol.* **12**:133–152.

Shisa, H., Matsudaira, Y., Hiai, H., and Nishizuka, Y., 1975, Origin of leukemic cells in mouse leukemia induced by *N*-butylnitrosourea, *Gann* **66**:37–42.

Shope, R. E., 1933, Infectious papillomatosis of rabbits, *J. Exp. Med.* **58**:607–624.

Shope, T., Dechario, D., and Miller, G., 1973, Malignant lymphoma in cottontop marmosets after inoculation with Epstein–Barr virus, *Proc. Natl. Acad. Sci. U.S.A.* **70**:2487–2491.

Shoyab, M., Baluda, M. A., and Evans, R., 1974a, Acquisition of new DNA sequences after infection of chicken cells with avian myeloblastosis virus, *J. Virol.* **13**:331–339.

Shoyab, M., Markham, P. D., and Baluda, M. A., 1974b, Reliability of RNA–DNA filter hybridization for the detection of oncornavirus specific DNA sequences, *J. Virol.* **14**:225–230.

Shreffler, D. C., and David, C. S., 1975, The *H-2* major histocompatibility complex and the *I* immune response region: Genetic variation, function, and organization, *Adv. Immunol.* **20**:125–195.

Siegler, R., and Rich, M. A., 1963, Unilateral histogenesis of AKR thymic lymphoma, *Cancer Res.* **23**:1669–1678.

Silberberg, M., and Silberberg, R., 1945, Significance of the age factor and sex glands in experimental leukemia of mice, *Proc. Soc. Exp. Biol. Med.* **58**:347–348.

Sjögren, H. O., 1974, Studies on specific transplantation resistance to polysma virus-induced tumors. I–IV, *J. Natl. Cancer Inst.* **32**: 361–74.

Slye, M., 1914, The incidence and inheritability of spontaneous tumors in mice, *J. Med. Res.* **30**:281–298.

Slye, M., 1931, The relation of heredity to the occurrence of spontaneous leukemia, pseudo-leukemia, lymphosarcoma and allied diseases in mice: Preliminary report, *Am. J. Cancer* **15**:1361–1368.

Smith, C. E., 1971, An undifferentiated hematopoietic neoplasm with histologic manifestations of leukemia in a cut throat trout *(Salmo clarki)*, *J. Fish. Res. Board Can.* **28**:112–113.

Smith, R. T., and Landy, M. (eds), 1970, *Immune Surveillance*, Academic Press, New York.

Snijders, E. P., 1926, Over een overentbare leukaemie bij cavia's, *Ned. Tijdschr. Geneeskd.* **70**:1256–1262.

Snyder, S. P., and Theilen, G. H., 1969, Transmissible feline fibrosarcoma, *Nature (London)* **221**:1074–1075.

Snyder, S. P., Dungworth, D. L., Kawakami, T. G., Callaway, E., and Lau, D. T.-L., 1973, Two cases of lymphosarcoma in gibbons *(Hylobates lar)* with associated C-type virus, *J. Natl. Cancer Inst.* **51**:89–94.

Solomon, J. J., Witter, R. L., Nazerian, K., and Burmester, B. R., 1968, Studies on the etiology of Marek's disease. I. Propagation of the agent in cell culture, *Proc. Soc. Exp. Biol. Med.* **127**:173–177.

Sonstegard, R., 1971, Description and epizootiological studies of infectious pancreatic necrosis virus of salmonids and lymphosarcoma of *Esox masquinongy,* Ph.D. dissertation, Gvelph, Ontario.

Spiegelman, S., Kufe, D., Hehlmann, R., and Peters, W. P., 1973, Evidence for RNA tumor viruses in human lymphomas inducing Burkitt's disease, *Cancer Res.* **33**:1515–1526.

Squire, R. A., 1969, Spontaneous hematopoietic tumors of dogs, *Natl. Cancer Inst. Monogr.* **32**:97–116.

Steeves, R. A., and Eckner, R. J., 1970, Host induced changes in infectivity of Friend spleen focus-forming virus, *J. Natl. Cancer Inst.* **44**:587–594.

Stenback, W. A., VanHoosier, G. L., Jr., and Tretin, J. J., 1966, Virus particles in hamster tumors as revealed by electron microscopy, *Proc. Soc. Exp. Biol. Med.* **122**:1219–1223.

Stone, R. S., Shope, R. E., and Moore, D. H., 1959, Electron microscope study of the development of the papilloma virus in the skin of the rabbit, *J. Exp. Med.* **110**:543–546.

Strand, M., and August, J. T., 1974, Structural proteins of mammalian oncogenic RNA viruses: Multiple antigenic determinants of the major internal protein and envelope glycoprotein, *J. Virol.* **13**:171–80.

Stromberg, K., Hurley, N. E., Davis, N. L., Rueckert, R. R., and Fleissner, E., 1974, Structural studies of avian myeloblastosis virus: Comparison of polypeptides in viron and core component by dodecyl sulfate–polyacrylamide gel electrophoresis, *J. Virol.* **13**:513–528.

Svec, F., and Hlavay, E., 1961, Transmission of a filterable agent from rat leukemia induced by X-irradiation and treatment with methylcholanthrene, *Acta Haematol.* **26**:252–260.

Svejda, J., Kossey, P., Hlavayová, E., and Svec, F., 1958, Histological picture of the transplantable rat leukaemia induced by X-irradiation and methylcholanthrene, *Neoplasma* **5**:123–131.

Svet-Moldavsky, G. J., Trubeheninova, L., and Ravkina, L., 1967, Pathogenicity of the chicken sarcoma virus (Schmidt–Ruppin) for amphibians and reptiles, *Nature (London)* **214**:300–302.

Svoboda, J., Hložanek, I., Mach, O., Michlová, A., Říman, J., and Urbánková, M., 1973, Transfection of chicken fibroblasts with single exposure to DNA from virogenic mammalian cells, *J. Gen. Virol.* **21**:47–55.

Symposium on Fundamental Cancer Research, 1974, Molecular studies in viral neoplasia: A collection of papers presented at the 25th annual symposium on fundamental cancer research, 1972, published for the University of Texas M. D. Anderson Hospital and Tumor Institute at Houston, Williams & Wilkins, Baltimore.

Takahashi, T., Old, L. J., McIntire, K. R., and Boyse, E. A., 1971, Immunoglobulin and other surface antigens of cells of the immune system, *J. Exp. Med.* **134**:815–832.

Takatsu, K., Hamaoka, T., Yamaskita, U., and Kitaqawa, M., 1972, Suppressed activity of thymus-derived cell in tumor-bearing host, *Gann* **63**:273–275.

Taylor, B. A., Meier, H., and Myers, D. D., 1971, Host-gene control of C-type RNA tumor virus: Inheritance of the group-specific antigen of murine leukemic virus, *Proc. Natl. Acad. Sci. U.S.A.* **68**:3190–3194.

Teich, N., Lowy, D. R., Hartley, J. W., and Rowe, W. P., 1973, Studies of the mechanism of induction of infectious murine leukemia virus from AKR mouse embryo cell lines by 5-iododeoxyuridine and 5-bromodeoxyuridine, *Virology* **51**:163–173.

Temin, H. M., 1962, Separation of morphological conversion and virus production in Rous sarcoma virus infection, *Cold Spring Harbor Symp. Quant. Biol.* **27**:407–414.

Temin, H. M., 1976, The DNA provirus hypothesis, *Science* **192**:1075–1080.

Temin, H. M., and Mizutani, S., 1970, RNA-dependent DNA polymerase in virions of Rous sarcoma virus, *Nature (London)* **226**:1211–1213.

Tennant, J. R., 1962, Derivation of a murine lymphoid leukemia virus, *J. Natl. Cancer Inst.* **28**:1291–1303.

Tennant, J. R., 1969, Characterization of two Balb/c infant thymus cell lines infected with lympholeukemogenic virus, *J. Natl. Cancer Inst.* **42**:739–748.

Tennant, J. R., Lambertenghi, G., Kingsley, S., and deHarven, E., 1971, Correlation between presence of leukemia virus in cultured cells and their immunogenicity in a leukemia isotransplant system, *J. Natl. Cancer Inst.* **47**:781–788.

Tennant, R. W., and Richter, C. B., 1972, Murine leukemia virus: Restriction in fused permissive and nonpermissive cells, *Science* **178**:516–518.

Tenser, R. B., and Hsiung, G. D., 1973, Infection of thymus cells *in vivo* and *in vitro* with a guinea pig herpes-like virus and the effect of antibody on virus replication in organ culture, *J. Immunol.* 110:552–560.

Theilen, G., Dungworth, D. L., Kawakami, T. G., Munn, R. J., Wand, J. M., and Harroed, J. B., 1970, Experimental induction of lymphosarcoma in the cat with "C"-type virus, *Cancer Res.* 30:401–408.

Theilen, G. H., Gould, D., Fowler, M., and Dungsworth, D. L., 1971, C-type virus in tumor tissue of a Wodly monkey (*Lagothrix* sp.) with fibrosarcoma, *J. Natl. Cancer Inst.* 47:881–889.

Todaro, G., and Huebner, R. J., 1972, The viral oncogene hypothesis: New evidence, *Proc. Natl. Acad. Sci. U.S.A.* 69:1009–1015.

Tooze, J. (ed.), 1973, *The Molecular Biology of Tumour Viruses,* Cold Spring Harbor Laboratory, Cold Spring Harbor, New York.

Toth, B., 1963, Development of malignant lymphomas by cell-free filtrates prepared from a chemically induced mouse lymphoma, *Proc. Soc. Exp. Biol. Med.* 112:873–875.

Toth, B., Tomatis, L., and Shubik, P., 1961, Multipotential carcinogenesis with urethan in the Syrian golden hamster, *Cancer Res.* 21:1537–1541.

Trentin, J. J., VanHoosier, G. L., and Samper, L., 1968, The oncogenicity of human adenoviruses in hamsters, *Proc. Soc. Exp. Biol. Med.* 127:683–689.

Tridente, G., Pennelli, N., Mazzarella, L., and Fiore-Donati, L., 1964, Studies on the oncogenic response of newborn mice to various carcinogenic chemical agents. I. Leukemogenesis by 9,10-dimethyl-1,2-benzanthracene and 20-methycholanthrene in Swiss, C57BL, and C3Hf/Gs mice, *Boll. Soc. Ital. Biol. Sper.* 40:604–608.

Tsuchida, R., and Rich, M. A., 1964, Chromosomal aberrations in viral leukemiogenesis. 1. Friend and Raucher leukemia, *J. Natl. Cancer Inst.* 33:33–47.

Uematsu, K., and Huggins, C., 1968, Induction of leukemia and ovarian tumors in mice by pulse-doses of polycyclic aromatic hydrocarbons, *Mol. Pharmacol.* 4:427–434.

Uematsu, K., and Huggins, C., 1969, Hydrocarbon-induced leukemie in adolescent and adult mice, *Gann* 60:545–555.

Ulrich, H., 1946, The incidence of leukemia in radiologists, *N. Engl. J. Med.* 234:45–46.

Upton, A. C., and Cosgrove, G. E., Jr., 1968, Radiation induced leukemia, in: *Experimental Leukemie* (M. A. Rich, ed.), pp. 131–158, North-Holland, Amsterdam.

Upton, A. C., and Furth, J., 1954, The effects of cortisone on the development of spontaneous leukemia in mice and on its induction by irradiation, *Blood* 9:686–695.

Upton, A. C., Wolff, F. F., and Sniffen, E. P., 1961, Leukemogeneic effect of myleran on the mouse thymus, *Proc. Soc. Exp. Biol. Med.* 108:464–467.

Van Hoosier, G. L., Jr., Spjut, H. J., and Trentin, J. J., 1971, Spontaneous tumors of the syrian hamster: Observations in a closed breeding colony and a review of the literature, in: *Defining the Laboratory Animal,* National Academy of Sciences, Washington, D.C.

Van Pelt, A., and Congdon, C. C., 1972, Radiation leukemia in guinea pigs, *Radiat. Res.* 52:68–81.

Varmus, H. E., Heasley, S., and Bishop, J. M., 1974, Use of DNA–DNA annealing to detect new virus-specific DNA sequences in chicken embryo fibroblasts after infection by avian sarcoma virus, *J. Virol.* 14:895–903.

Vernon, M. L., McMahon, J. M., and Hackett, J. J., 1974, Additional evidence of type-C particles in human placentas, *J. Natl. Cancer Inst.* 52:987–989.

Veskova, T. K., Trubcheninova, L. P., and Dook, J. L., 1970, Tumors in reptiles inoculated with chicken Rous sarcoma material, *Folia Biol. (Prague)* 16:353–366.

von Jagić, N., Schwartz, G., and V. Siebenrock, L., 1911, Blutbefunde bei Röntgenologen, *Berl. Klin. Wochenschr.* 48:1220–1222.

Wakonig-Vaartaja, R., 1960, Chromosomes in leukemia induced by 537 and Friend viruses, *Br. J. Cancer* 15:120–122.

Waksal, S. D., 1976, Leukemic transformation of thymus-derived lymphocytes *in vitro, Fed. Proc. Fed. Am. Soc. Exp. Biol.* 35:737 (abstract).

Walford, R. L., 1966, Increased incidence of lymphoma after injection of mice with cells differing at weak histocompatibility loci, *Science* 152:78–80.

Walker, S. E., and Bole, G. G., 1973, Augmented incidence of neoplasia in NZB-NZW mice treated with long-term cyclophosphamide, *J. Clin. Med.* 82:619–633.

Wallen, W. C., Neubauer, R. H., Rabin, H., and Cicmanec, J. L., 1973, Non-immune rosette formation by lymphoma and leukemic cells from herpes virus saimiri-infected owl monkeys, *J. Natl. Cancer Inst.* 51:967–975.

Warner, N. L., Szenberg, A., and Burnet, F. M., 1962, The immunological role of different lymphoid organs on the chicken. I. Dissociation of immunological responsiveness, *Aust. J. Exp. Biol. Med. Sci.* **40**:373–387.

Warren, K. S., 1969, Inhibition of granuloma formation around *Schistosoma mansoni* eggs. V. "Hodg-kin's-like lesion" in SJL/J mice, *Am. J. Pathol.* **56**:293–303.

Weber, W. T., 1963, Hematologic aspects of bovine lymphosarcoma, *Ann. N.Y. Acad. Sci.* **108**:1270–1283.

Weischer, F., 1944, Erbbedingtheit und Bekämpfung der Rinderleukose. *Dtsch. Tiéraerztl. Wochenschr.* **52**:83–84.

Werner, J., Wolf, H., Apodaca, J., and Zur Hausen, H., 1975, Lymphoproliferative disease in a cotton-top marmoset after inoculation with infectious mononucleosis-derived Epstein–Barr virus, *Int. J. Cancer* **15**:1000–1008.

Whitmire, C. E., Salerno, R. A., Rabstein, L. S., Huebner, R. J., and Turner, H. C., 1971, RNA tumor-virus antigen expression in chemically induced tumors: Virus-genome-specified common antigens detected by complement fixation in mouse tumors induced by 3-methylcholanthrene, *J. Natl. Cancer Inst.* **47**:1255–1265.

Wiseman, A., Petrie, L., and Murray, M., 1974, Diarrhoea in the horse as a result of alimentary lymphosarcoma, *Vet. Rec.* **95**:454–457.

Witter, R. L., Solomon, J. J., and Burgoyne, G. H., 1969a, Cell culture techniques for primary isolation of Marek's disease-associated herpes virus, *Avian Dis.* **13**:101–118.

Witter, R. L., Burgoyne, G. H., and Solomon, J. J., 1969b, Evidence for a herpesvirus as an etiologic agent of Marek's disease, *Avian Dis.* **13**:171–184.

Wittmann, W., and Urbaneck, D., 1969a, *Leukose des Rindes: Handbuch der Virus-Infektionen bei Tieren*, Vol. V/1, pp. 41–74, Gustav Fisher, Vienna.

Wittmann, W., and Urbeneck, D., 1969b, Untersuchungen zur Ätiologie der Rinderleukose. 8. Übertra-gungsversuche mit Blut leukoseerkranter Rinder auf Schäflammer (Kurzmitteilung), *Arch. Exp. Vet. Med.* **23**:709–713.

Wolfe, L. G., Deinhardt, F., Theilen, G. H., Rabin, H., Kawakami, T., and Bustad, L. K., 1971a, Induction of tumors in marmoset monkeys by simian sarcoma virus, type I (Lagothix): A prelimi-nary report, *J. Nat. Cancer Inst.* **47**:115–120.

Wolfe, L. G., Falk, L. A., and Deinhardt, F., 1971b, Oncogenicity of *Herpesvirus saimiri* in marmoset monkeys, *J. Natl. Cancer Inst.* **47**:1145–1162.

Wolstenholme, G. E. W., and Porter, R. (eds), 1966, *The Thymus: Experimental and Clinical Studies: Ciba Foundation Symposium*, Little, Brown, Boston.

Wong, A., Mankovitz, R., and Kennedy, J. C., 1974, Immunosuppressive and immunostimulatory factors produced by malignant cells *in vitro*, *Int. J. Cancer* **13**:530–542.

Woodruff, J. F., and Woodruff, J. J., 1975, The effect of viral infections on the function of the immune system, in: *Viral Immunology and Immunopathology* (A. L. Notkins, ed.), pp. 393–418, Academic Press, New York.

Woolley, G. W., and Peters, B. A., 1953, Prolongation of life in high-leukemic AKR mice by cortisone, *Proc. Soc. Exp. Biol. Med.* **82**:286–287.

Wybran, J., Carr, M. C., and Fudenberg, H. H., 1972, The human rosette-forming cell as a marker of a population of thymus-derived cells, *J. Clin. Invest.* **51**:2537–2543.

Yosida, T. H., and Law, L. W., 1968, Chromosomal alteration and the development of tumors. XVII. Chromosomes of the mouse leukemia induced by Moloney leukemogenic virus (MLV) infection, *Cytologia* **33**:256–268.

Yumoto, T., and Dmochowski, L., 1967, Light and electron microscopic studies of organs and tissues of SJL/J strain of mice with reticulum cell neoplasma resembling Hodgkin's disease, *Cancer Res.* **27**:2098–2112.

Yuspa, S. H., Morgan, D. L., and Levy, J. A., 1973, *In vitro* cultivation of a chemically induced epidermal carcinoma: Establishment of three cell lines and isolation of murine leukemic virus, *J. Natl. Cancer Inst.* **50**:1561–1570.

Zeigel, R. F., and Clark, H. F., 1969, Electron microscopic observations on a "C"-type virus in cell cultures derived from a tumor-bearing viper, *J. Natl. Cancer Inst.* **43**:1097–1102.

Zeigel, R. F., and Clark, H. F., 1970, Current studies on a new "C"-type virus of presumed reptilian origin, *Bibl. Haematol. (Pavia)* **36**:643.

Zilber, L. A., and Postnikova, Z. A., 1966, Induction of a leukemogenic agent by a chemical carcinogen in inbred mice, *Natl. Cancer Inst. Monogr.* **22**:397–403.

Zwart, P., and Harshbarger, J. C., 1972, Hematopoietic neoplasms in lizards: Report of a typical case in *Hydrosaurus ambionensis* and of a probable case in *Varanus salvator*, *Int. J. Cancer* **9**:248–253.

5

Epidemiology of Primary Neoplasms of Lymphoid Tissues in Animals

WILLIAM D. HARDY, JR.

1. Introduction

This chapter will discuss the occurrence of lymphoid tumors of animals other than man to acquaint the interested reader with the epidemiology and etiology of these tumors. The term *lymphosarcoma* (LSA) will be used to describe tumors arising from lymphoid tissues that result in either discrete solid tumor masses or the diffuse infiltration of tissues and organs by neoplastic lymphocytes. The presence of neoplastic lymphocytes in the peripheral blood will be considered a manifestation of LSA, and will be termed a *leukemic blood profile*. This usage is somewhat different from the common usage in human medicine.

In man, hematopoietic neoplasms may be present at birth, are the most prevalent neoplasms in prepubertal children, and account for one half of all childhood malignant neoplasms (*Vital Statistics,* 1966; Burkitt and O'Conor, 1961). Human leukemias and lymphomas may occur at any age, but the incidence of most types increases with age. Hematopoietic neoplasms of domesticated mammals, most of which are nonleukemic lymphosarcomas, occur most frequently in mature animals, although they have also been observed in bovine fetuses and calves, kittens, and young swine (Squire, 1963). Some authors have reported differences in the anatomical sites of involvement and in the cytomorphological types of lymphomas as a function of age in cattle (Dungworth *et al.,* 1964; Theilen and Dungworth, 1965) and kittens. Age-dependent differences have also been observed in hematopoietic neoplasms of mice (Dunn, 1954) and of chickens (Burmester, 1968).

LSA is the most common tumor of "lower" animals, and has been reported in fish, reptiles, birds, and mammals. In addition to being found in domestic animals,

WILLIAM D. HARDY, JR. • Laboratory of Veterinary Oncology, Memorial Sloan-Kettering Cancer Center, New York, New York 10021.

lymphoid tumors have been found in feral cold-blooded animals such as the northern pike, muskellunge, goldfish, trout, salmon, cobra, anaconda, timber rattlesnake, lizard, and toad, and in feral warm-blooded animals such as the mouse, rat, hamster, sea lion, buffalo, skunk, squirrel, civet, opossum, kangaroo rat, monkey, deer, and elephant. Fish are the "lowest" animals in the animal kingdom to have lymphocytes, and thus only animals from fish and above can have true lymphoid tumors (Table 1). Lymphoidlike tumors, however, have been reported in mollusks, including three species of oysters and one species of mussel.

The site of normal lymphopoiesis varies somewhat in different animal phyla (Table 2). While lymphopoiesis occurs in the spleen, thymus, bone marrow, and intestine of all animals from amphibians and above, only mammals have lymph nodes (Harshbarger and Dawe, 1973). Fish produce lymphocytes in all the sites listed except for the bone marrow, but they compensate for this by producing lymphocytes in the mesonephros. The localization of LSA varies in different animals according to the sites of normal lymphocyte production.

1.1. Epidemiology

Epidemiology is the study of the occurrence and distribution of diseases with the object of discovering their cause so that preventative measures can be developed. Obviously, all such studies in animals are hampered by the fact that the animal populations at risk are unknown, and that the cause of death is not determined for most animals. Thus, it is impossible to obtain accurate incidence figures for naturally occurring animal LSA. Most of the information concerning LSA in animals is obtained from studies of experimental animals, rather than from studies of naturally occurring disease. Only the naturally occurring LSAs of cats, cow, and chickens have been adequately studied epidemiologically. The etiology of many animal LSAs is unknown, and the only etiological agents that have been discovered to date are viruses.

In general, epidemiological methods often cannot detect the contagious or infectious nature of chronic diseases or diseases with long latent periods. For example, no epidemiological evidence was obtained to suggest that hepatitis and infectious mononucleosis in man or LSA in cats were contagious diseases (Schneider, 1972). It was only after the development of serological and virological methods to detect the etiological agents that their modes of transmission were discovered. The physician should keep this in mind when considering epidemiological evidence for or against the contagious nature of human lymphoid tumors.

TABLE 1. Presence (+) or Absence (−) of Hemic and Reticular Cells in Animals[a]

Phylum	Hemo-blasts	Erythro-cytes	Lympho-cytes	Neutro-phils	Eosino-phils	Baso-phils	Mono-cytes	Plasma cells
Mollusks	+[b]	−	−	−	?	−	+	−
Fish	+[b]	+	+[b]	+	+	+	+	+
Amphibians	+[b]	+	+	+	+	+	+	+
Reptiles	+[b]	+	+	+	+	+	+	+
Birds	−	+[b]	+[b] ·	+[b]	+[b]	+	+	+
Mammals	−	+[b]	+[b]	+[b]	+[b]	+[b]	+[b]	+[b]

[a]Adapted from Harshbarger and Dawe (1973).   [b]Neoplasms are known for the indicated cell type.

131

EPIDEMIOLOGY OF
PRIMARY
NEOPLASMS OF
LYMPHOID TISSUES
IN ANIMALS

TABLE 2. Presence (+) or Absence (−) of Lymphopoiesis in
Various Sites in Animals[a]

Phylum	Mesonephros	Lymph nodes	Spleen	Thymus	Intestine	Bone marrow
Fish	+	[b]	+	+	+	−
Amphibians	−	[b]	+	+	+	+
Birds	−	[b]	+	+	+	+
Mammals	−	+	+	+	+	+

[a]Adapted from Harshbarger and Dawe (1973).
[b]Fish, amphibians, and birds do not have lymph nodes.

1.2. Influence of Man on Naturally Occurring Lymphosarcoma in Animals

Man has markedly altered the ways in which animals are able to distribute themselves in the environment (ecodistribution). He has hunted many wild species to extinction, or near to extinction, and has limited their natural habitats by farming and by urban expansion. Because of diminished habitats for wildlife, the population density of some wild animals has become higher than before. When man has domesticated animals for his use, he has often severely crowded them into small geographical units for easier management. The pollution resulting from man's industrial activities has also altered the ecodistribution of wild animals, and has had a general effect on the incidence of cancer in all animals (Hardy, 1976a).

This chapter will review the epidemiology and etiology of LSA in animals. It must be remembered that the different animal species are exposed to different selection pressures by man, and for this and other reasons have different frequencies of naturally occurring LSA. There are four classes of animals to consider: (1) wild animals; (2) domesticated food-producing animals; (3) domesticated pet animals; and (4) laboratory animals (Table 3).

Very little is known about the epidemiology of naturally occurring LSA in wild animals. For example, although man has produced inbred laboratory strains of mice, some of which have artificially high and others artificially low occurrences of LSA, very little is known about the occurrence of LSA in wild mice. There is very little or no epidemiological information about LSA in other wild animal species, since man does not observe these animals unless they are captured and crowded together in zoological parks.

Animals that man has domesticated for food-production purposes, such as

TABLE 3. Ecodistribution of Animals That Develop Naturally
Occurring Lymphosarcomas

Wild	Domesticated	Laboratory
Mollusks	Food-producing	Mouse
Fish	Chicken	Rat
Amphibians	Cow	Hamster
Reptiles	Sheep	Guinea pig
Rodents	Pig	Primates
Mouse	Pets	
	Cat	
	Dog	

chickens, pigs, sheep, and beef cattle, are crowded together and kept until they are suitable for slaughter. Thus, studies of "natural" epidemiology of LSA in these animals are biased because of crowding and because of the slaughter of relatively young animals, which eliminates the possibility of the development of LSA in old age. The dairy cow is an exception, since these animals are often kept until a fairly old age for the production of milk. There have been excellent epidemiological studies of LSA in dairy cattle that show that an infectious agent causes bovine lymphosarcoma.

The ecodistribution of domesticated pet animals is very similar if not identical to the demography of the human population, and these animals are therefore excellent models for the study of human diseases. Extensive and well-executed epidemiological studies of feline and canine LSA have been done. Feline lymphosarcoma is caused by the feline leukemia virus (FeLV), and this virus is spread contagiously among pet cats. In contrast, there is no evidence that canine lymphosarcoma is contagious, and it is not known what causes LSA in dogs.

1.3. Etiology

The only known causes of naturally occurring LSA in animals are oncogenic viruses, which are divided into two groups: (1) those containing RNA and (2) those containing DNA. All oncogenic viruses either contain DNA or, in the case of RNA viruses, produce DNA by an enzyme called *RNA-dependent DNA polymerase (reverse transcriptase)*. This enzyme uses the viral RNA to make DNA copies, which are then inserted into, and interact with, the infected cell's DNA (genes) (Baltimore, 1970). The viral, or virally specified, DNA may contain the information necessary for both viral production (virogene) and cellular transformation (oncogene).

1.3.1. Oncogenic RNA Viruses (Oncornaviruses)

Various names such as leukovirus, Thylaxoviridae, C-type viruses, and oncogenic RNA viruses have been used to denote this class of virus, but the name *oncornavirus* [*onco*(genic)*rna*(RNA)*virus*] is now widely accepted (Nowinski *et al.,* 1970; Dalton *et al.,* 1974). Oncornaviruses have been isolated from leukemias and sarcomas of snakes, chickens, mice, rats, guinea pigs, hamsters, cats, cattle, pigs, woolly monkeys, and gibbon apes (Table 4).

TABLE 4. Leukemogenic Oncornaviruses of Animals

Animal	Oncornavirus[a]
Pike	Pike leukemia virus
Chicken	Avian leukosis virus (ALV)
Mouse	Murine leukemia virus (MuLV)
Rat	Rat leukemia virus
Guinea pig	Guinea pig leukemia virus
Hamster	Hamster leukemia virus (HaLV)
Cat	Feline leukemia virus (FeLV)
Cattle	Bovine leukemia virus (BLV)
Gibbon ape	Gibbon ape leukemia virus (GaLV)

[a]The abbreviations in parentheses here and in Tables 7 and 8 are those that are used in the text.

133

EPIDEMIOLOGY OF
PRIMARY
NEOPLASMS OF
LYMPHOID TISSUES
IN ANIMALS

TABLE 5. Transmission of Oncornaviruses

Mode	Route
Infectious (horizontal)	
Contact	Saliva
	Urine
	Blood
Epigenetic	*In utero* via blood
	Milk
Genetic (vertical)	Gene (virogene)

Oncornaviruses are spherical, about 90–100 nm in diameter, with a centrally located symmetrical electron-dense nucleoid about 70 nm in diameter (Gallo and Todaro, 1976). The viral surface usually possesses short spikes and knobs. Viral assembly is by budding from the infected cell membrane. Oncornavirus genomes are composed of a poly A containing single-stranded RNA that is complexed with a DNA polymerase (reverse transcriptase) in the electron-dense viral core. The presence of an antigenically specific reverse transcriptase enzyme is unique to a number of RNA-containing viruses, and the proposed name for these viruses is *Retraviridae* (Dalton *et al.*, 1974). Oncornaviruses constitute three genera of the family Retraviridae.

a. Transmission of Oncornaviruses. Oncornaviruses can be transmitted vertically via the genes or horizontally by contagion (Table 5) (Gross, L., 1970a). In the past, the term *vertical* transmission included congenital transmission of complete oncornaviruses *in utero* to the fetus as well as genetic transmission of viral-specified DNA in the genes. The term *vertical* transmission is more correctly used to denote only *genetic* transmission, while congenital transmission of complete virus should be considered a form of *horizontal* or *contagious* transmission. Genetic, or vertical, transmission of oncornaviruses from parent to offspring via the germ line is the way in which viral genes have been maintained in animal populations (Huebner and Todaro, 1969). The evidence for vertical transmission is that "virus-free" cell cultures from the chicken, mouse, rat, hamster, pig, and baboon can produce endogenous oncornaviruses (which are present in every cell of the body as virally coded DNA) after treatment with chemical inducing agents (Table 6) (Gallo and Todaro, 1976). Cocultivation of cell cultures with permissive heterospecies cell cultures results in the production of endogenous oncornaviruses. Avian and mammalian cells are resistant to superinfection with, and replication of, their own endogenous oncornaviruses. In some instances, endogenous oncornaviruses have escaped from their hosts' control mechanisms and have become infectious for the species from which they arose, and in some cases have even infected other

**TABLE 6. Species That Carry a
Complete Endogenous Oncornavirus in
Normal Cells**[a]

Chicken	Rat
Chinese hamster	Cat
Syrian hamster	Pig
Mouse *(Mus musculus)*	Baboon
Mouse *(Mus caroli)*	

[a]Adapted from Gallo and Todaro (1976).

TABLE 7. Species That Have Infectious
Oncornaviruses (Horizontal Transmission)[a,b]

Species	Oncornavirus
Pike	Pike leukemia virus
Mouse	Laboratory strains
	Murine leukemia virus (MuLV)
	Murine sarcoma virus (MuSV)
Cat	Feline leukemia virus (FeLV)
	Feline sarcoma virus (FeSV)
Cattle	Bovine leukemia virus (BLV)
Woolly monkey	Simian sarcoma virus (SSV)
Gibbon ape	Gibbon ape leukemia virus (GaLV)

[a] Adapted from Gallo and Todaro (1976).
[b] Viral genomes are not found in normal cells.

species (Gallo and Todaro, 1976). An example of this is the FeLV, a contagious oncornavirus of cats, which originated from the rat and is now an exogenous cat oncornavirus (Benveniste and Todaro, 1974).

Feline, gibbon ape, and bovine leukemia viruses are transmitted horizontally by contagion (Table 7). After entry into the animal, the oncornavirus penetrates the susceptible cell, uncoats, and synthesizes a DNA copy of the viral RNA genome with the catalytic assistance of the reverse transcriptase enzyme. After the viral DNA copy (provirus) is synthesized, it integrates into the DNA of the cell's chromosomes. The second phase of the oncornavirus replication cycle begins when the integrated genome synthesizes viral RNA. Once new viral RNA has been made, viral proteins can be synthesized and complete virions can then be assembled. One of the viral proteins produced may transform the lymphocyte into a neoplastic cell and thus produce LSA. In some instances, transformation occurs even though there is incomplete or no virus expression (i.e., no viral production); in other instances, it occurs with complete virus production.

Infectious or horizontal transmission can be divided into two modes: (1) contact and (2) epigenetic. Contact transmission requires that the oncornaviruses be excreted or secreted from the infected animal. This is the major mode by which FeLV is spread among cats living in their natural (household) environment, and is also thought to be significant for the avian, bovine, and gibbon leukemia viruses. The routes of transmission include saliva, urine, feces, and blood. Epigenetic transmission is a form of horizontal transmission, not vertical (genetic) transmission, since the viral genome is not transmitted as part of the host's genome. Epigenetic transmission occurs when oncornaviruses are transmitted to the embryo *in utero* via the maternal blood, via the egg in chickens, or to the newborn animal shortly after birth via the milk. This mode of transmission appears to be important for avian leukemia viruses, since these viruses are transmitted via the egg as complete viruses. It is also a significant mode for the spread of the FeLV.

b. Oncornavirus Antigens. There are one glycoprotein and five protein structural molecules of oncornaviruses. Different antigenic determinants, which can be divided into three classes, are present on these molecules: (1) Type-specific determinants are those present only in a single virus serotype (e.g., FeLV serotype A, not FeLV serotypes B or C). (2) Group-specific (species-specific) determinants are those shared by various serotypes of oncornaviruses from a single species (i.e., all FeLV serotypes have the same group-specific determinants). (3) Interspecies

135

EPIDEMIOLOGY OF
PRIMARY
NEOPLASMS OF
LYMPHOID TISSUES
IN ANIMALS

determinants are those that are shared among viruses originating from different mammalian species (e.g., murine, feline, and simian oncornaviruses).

The structural molecules are named for their protein (p) or glycoprotein (gp) composition and their molecular weight (August *et al.*, 1974). Thus, the major internal viral protein, which has a molecular weight of 30,000 daltons, is called the p30 molecule, and the major envelope glycoprotein, which has a molecular weight of 71,000 daltons, is called the gp71 molecule.

The major glycoprotein is a structural component of the viral envelope, and antibodies produced against its antigenic determinants will neutralize the virus. The p30 molecule of mammalian oncornaviruses possesses all three classes of antigenic determinants: type, group, and—except for the bovine leukemia virus—the shared identical interspecies antigenic determinants (Gilden *et al.*, 1971). Thus, high-titered antibody to the interspecies antigen of the p30 molecule can be used to detect all mammalian oncornaviruses except the bovine leukemia virus. The major group-specific antigenic determinant of p30 is unique to all oncornaviruses of a single species, and is considered a species-specific antigen. Thus, all murine oncornavirus p30 molecules contain the same group-specific antigen, which is different from the major p30 group-specific antigens of other species' oncornaviruses (Geering *et al.*, 1968, 1970). Detection of the species-specific antigen can be used to determine the species of origin of an oncornavirus, and antibodies to this antigen have been used in seroepidemiological studies of the occurrence of various animal oncornaviruses under natural conditions. The cat and nonhuman primates have two oncornaviruses, one of which is a nononcogenic endogenous oncornavirus that has a species-specific group antigen that differs from that found in the oncogenic (exogenous) oncornaviruses of each species. The endogenous and exogenous oncornaviruses of cats and nonhuman primates can be distinguished serologically, and it is only the exogenous oncornaviruses that induce LSA in these species.

c. Detection of Oncornaviruses. There are numerous techniques available for detecting oncornaviruses. The first technique to be used was electron microscopy, but this technique has limitations and is not now used as a routine method of searching for these viruses.

Immunological and biochemical techniques have replaced electron microscopy. The following immunological methods are employed at present: immunodiffusion, immunofluorescence, complement-fixation, cytotoxicity, and the very sensitive radioimmunoprecipitation technique. Another sensitive assay is the biochemical technique for detecting the oncornavirus reverse transcriptase enzyme. Detection of the viral reverse transcriptase from culture fluids or in tumor homogenates is equivalent to detection of the oncornavirus.

The isolation of oncornaviruses in tissue-culture-grown cells is also possible. Leukemogenic oncornaviruses grow well in fibroblasts and do not cause a cytopathological effect in these cells, nor do they transform cells *in vitro*. In contrast, sarcomagenic oncornaviruses do transform normal fibroblasts in culture.

1.3.2. Oncogenic DNA Viruses—Herpesviruses

Examples of naturally occurring oncogenic DNA viruses are the poxviruses of monkeys and rabbits, the papillomaviruses of dogs, horses, cattle, and rabbits, and the herpesviruses of chickens, primates, and frogs. Herpesviruses are the only DNA viruses associated with lymphoid tumors (Table 8), and I will restrict my discussion to these viruses.

WILLIAM D. HARDY, JR.

TABLE 8.   Leukemogenic Herpesviruses of Animals

Representative virus	Natural host	Oncogenic in: Natural host	Oncogenic in: Experimental host	Experimental hosts
Marek's disease virus (MDV)	Chicken	Yes	Yes	Chicken
Herpesvirus saimiri (HVS)	Squirrel monkey	No	Yes	Marmoset and other monkeys
Herpesvirus ateles (HVA)	Spider monkey	No	Yes	Marmoset and other monkeys

Herpesviruses exist in almost every species including man. They have the ability to persist in the host in a latent form after a primary infection, and often persist and cause disease in the presence of neutralizing antibody titers (Rapp, 1976). Productive herpesvirus infections cause cell death. In contrast, malignant transformation occurs only in nonproductively infected cells that are able to divide and grow.

Herpesviruses are relatively large, complex viruses consisting of structural elements arranged in concentric layers. The innermost layer is known as the *core* and contains the DNA genome. The core is surrounded by a *capsid,* which is composed of multiple protein layers arranged in the form of an icosahedron containing 162 hollow cylindrical capsomers. The capsid is surrounded, in turn, by the *tegument* and *envelope.* The capsid is a rigid structure 100 nm in diameter, whereas the envelope is less rigid and gives the complete virus a diameter of 150–200 nm (Nahmias and Roizman, 1973). The enveloped viral particles are infectious, while the nonenveloped particles are usually not infectious.

a. Transmission of Herpesviruses.   Herpesviruses are present in many organs of the body and can be shed into the environment via the saliva, urine, and feces (Rosato *et al.,* 1970). Contagious transmission can occur as a result of close contact between animals or by the dissemination of contaminated dust particles in the air (Porter and Daughman, 1965; Servoian *et al.,* 1963). Transplacental transmission of herpesviruses also occurs in several animal species; however, there is no evidence of genetic transmission of herpesviruses (Nahmias *et al.,* 1970).

b. Fate of Infected Cells.   Infection of a cell with a herpesvirus can result in either productive or nonproductive infection (Roizman, 1971). Productive infection results in the synthesis of infectious virions with concomitant cell death, while nonproductive infection results in the perpetuation of the viral genome in the living cell. Little is known about the mechanism(s) of nonproductive infection, but nonproductively infected cells may undergo malignant transformation, divide, and produce tumors (Klein, 1972).

c. Antigens.   Until recently, immunological studies of herpesviruses were restricted by difficulties in obtaining pure virus. A common antigen of herpesviruses was found by immunodiffusion and is thought to be a component of the viral capsid (Kirkwood *et al.,* 1969). Type-specific antigens were also found by neutralization and membrane immunofluorescent tests (Nahmias *et al.,* 1971).

d. Detection of Herpesviruses.   Seroepidemiological studies of the occurrence of herpesviruses in the natural environment have been done by assaying serum for neutralizing antibody.

137

EPIDEMIOLOGY OF
PRIMARY
NEOPLASMS OF
LYMPHOID TISSUES
IN ANIMALS

I will now discuss the epidemiology of naturally occurring LSA in "lower" animal species (see Table 3), emphasizing, where possible, the incidence, clinical findings, tissues involved, etiology, epidemiology, seroepidemiology, prevention, and public health aspects of LSA in each animal.

2. Lymphosarcoma in Cold-Blooded Animals

2.1. Mollusks

Mollusks do not have lymphocytes; thus, they do not develop LSA. Hematopoietic tumors can originate from hyaline hemocytes, however, and have been found in three species of oysters and one species of mussel (Harshbarger and Dawe, 1973). These tumors are very rare, but have been found in mollusks living in four widely separated bodies of water. No epidemiological studies of these hematopoietic tumors have been reported.

2.2. Fish—Northern Pike

LSA has been reported in 21 species of fish (Dawe, 1969). Nearly half the cases have occurred in fish of the order Salmoniformes. The kidney and thymus are usually the primary organs involved, although the liver and spleen are also involved in many cases. Fish do not possess lymph nodes, but a leukemic blood profile is occasionally present.

2.2.1. Incidence

Lymphoreticular tumors have been most thoroughly studied in northern pike in Ireland, where these tumors occur in epizootics. The occurrence of pike LSA varies from year to year, from season to season, and from lake to lake, suggesting the presence of an infectious etiological agent. Epidemics in some lakes were so extensive that 1 of 8 pikes caught had LSA, compared with an overall tumor frequency of 1 tumor per 800 fish (Dawe, 1969). Similar epidemics have been reported in Canada and in the northern United States (Dawe, 1969). In one study, 20% of the pike from certain lakes had LSA (Papas *et al.*, 1976).

2.2.2. Tissues Involved

Tumors were found in the jaws of 60% of the fish studied, with the trunk, thymus, tongue, gill bars, nostrils, pharynx, head, stomach, tail, kidney, and other sites being involved less frequently. The frequency of involvement of the jaws is similar to that found for Burkitt's lymphoma of African children. Morphologically, the tumor cells are classified as atypical hemocytoblasts or immunoblasts (Mulcahy *et al.*, 1970).

2.2.3. Etiology

Electron-microscopic examination of tumors from Irish pike did not reveal any virus particles (Mulcahy and O'Leary, 1970), but cell-free filtrates prepared from a LSA of the jaw of a female pike induced widely disseminated LSA in a young pike.

This tumor was successfully transmitted, by cell-free filtrates, to 4 other pike (Mulcahy and O'Leary, 1970). In another study, 89 of 100 pike that were inoculated with cell-free tumor homogenates developed LSA within 7 weeks (Brown et al., 1975). Recently, evidence of oncornavirus particles in pike LSA was obtained by analyzing tumor tissues for reverse transcriptase activity associated with a particulate fraction comparable to an oncornavirus density of 1.16 g/cm³. Electron-microscopic studies of the particulate fractions revealed numerous oncornaviruslike particles (Papas et al., 1976).

2.2.4. Epidemiology

The occurrence of pike LSA in nature exhibits marked seasonal periodicity, with most tumors developing during the cold-water months of fall and winter, when the mean water temperatures are 12 and 4°C, respectively. Epidemiological studies revealed that the tumors frequently regress spontaneously during the summer months, when the water temperatures vary between 21 and 30°C (Papas et al., 1976). Another study reported that 11% of pike caught in the polluted waters of the Fox River in Illinois had LSA (Brown et al., 1975).

2.3. Amphibians

There are no reports of naturally occurring LSA in free-living amphibians. There are, however, several reports describing LSA occurring in the laboratory-housed South African clawed toad, *Xenopus laevis,* and of the transmissibility of these tumors by cell-free filtrates (Dawe, 1969; Balls, 1965a,b; Balls and Ruben, 1967; Ruben and Balls, 1967). The lesions in these toads involved mainly the liver, spleen, kidneys, and muscles of the head. There is some controversy as to the actual histological interpretation of these lesions. One reviewer suggested that the lesions may in fact have been acid-fast bacilli granulomas (Dawe, 1969). Similar lesions, caused by these bacilli, are known to occur in various amphibians.

LSA was induced in toads with tumor homogenates that had been filtered through 100-nm pore filters. In one experiment, 9 of 10 uninoculated control toads kept in the same tank with filtrate-inoculated toads developed the disease (Balls and Ruben, 1967; Ruben and Balls, 1967). An oncornavirus has not been found in toads with LSA.

2.4. Reptiles

Primitive reptiles are thought to have given rise to birds and primitive mammals (Dawe, 1969). It is interesting that no lymphoid tumors have been reported in reptiles, while lymphoid tumors are among the most frequently occurring tumors in birds and mammals. The lack of reported reptilian lymphoid tumors is probably a result of inadequate investigation of this disease in these animals. This seems a likely explanation, since there are reports that the Rous sarcoma virus can produce tumors in reptiles, and since oncornaviruses have been isolated from two naturally occurring sarcomas, those of a viper and a corn snake (Svet-Moldavsky et al., 1967; Zeigel and Clark, 1969; Lunger et al., 1974).

3.1. Chicken

3.1.1. Introduction

The most common neoplastic diseases of domestic fowl are leukosis and Marek's disease. Both diseases are lymphoproliferative, but avian leukosis is caused by an oncornavirus, while Marek's disease is caused by a cell-associated herpesvirus. The two diseases also have different pathological manifestations; e.g., avian leukosis is primarily a B-cell neoplasm of lymphoid tissues, whereas Marek's disease is a T-cell LSA with an unusual predilection for nervous tissue. Since there are many differences between these two diseases, they will be considered separately.

3.1.2. Avian Leukosis Complex

a. Incidence. Avian leukosis is a complex group of diseases, caused by the avian leukosis virus (ALV), that cause major economic losses to the poultry industry. They are the most common forms of neoplastic disease in the domestic chicken. The diseases of the avian leukosis complex can reach epizootic proportions, and in some areas, some of the diseases are considered to be enzootic. Most of the diseases of this complex are disseminated proliferative processes. They include lymphoid leukosis, myelocytomatosis, osteopetrosis, solid tumors, erythroblastosis, and myeloblastosis.

b. Lymphoid Leukosis. This is a neoplastic disease of the lymphoreticular tissues. In most cases, lymphocytes are involved.

Occurrence. Lymphoid leukosis is a chronic disease of adult chickens that can result in heavy losses. It is now the single most common type of avian neoplasm, but it rarely occurs in chickens less than 6 months old and usually does not become evident until after sexual maturity (Crittenden, 1976). Males appear to be affected less frequently than females (Olson and Bullis, 1942).

Clinical Findings. There are no specific clinical pathological signs associated with avian lymphoid leukosis, and birds can die of the disease with no outward indication of ill health. The most common nonspecific signs seen in birds with the disease are listlessness, inappetence, emaciation, ruffling of the feathers, paling and shrivelling of the comb, and sometimes postural changes (Purchase, 1976; Feldman and Olson, 1965). In addition, there may also be signs associated with the anatomical location of lesions. For example, GI involvement may cause diarrhea or constipation, and nerve involvement may result in paralysis.

Tissues Involved. Lymphoid leukosis can occur in nearly every tissue and organ of the body, and in most birds, more than one site is involved. The primary lesion occurs in the bursa of Fabricius, the liver and spleen are almost invariably affected, and tumors occur frequently in the heart, lungs, kidneys, and ovaries (Purchase, 1976; Feldman and Olson, 1965). The brain is only rarely involved, however, and since birds do not have lymph nodes, there can be no lymph node involvement. There are three forms of the disease: diffuse, nodular, and combined (Feldman and Olson, 1965). In the diffuse form, neoplastic lymphocytes diffusely infiltrate the affected organs; in the nodular form, the tumor cells are arranged in a follicular pattern and are surrounded and isolated by connective tissue. In the combined form, both the diffuse and nodular forms of the disease can exist in a single organ or in different organs in a single bird. Organs affected by the diffuse form of lymphoid leukosis are uniformly enlarged and may develop the overall gray-white color of the tumor. In contrast, organs affected by nodular leukosis contain discrete gray-white tumor masses. Lymphoid leukosis is a B-cell disease.

c. Myelocytomatosis. This is a neoplastic disease involving the myelocytes.

Occurrence. The disease occurs sporadically in young adult birds (Purchase, 1976).

Clinical Findings. There are few clinical signs associated with this disease. In most cases, only a slight indisposition is noticed about a week before death. Sudden death without noticeable signs sometimes occurs, suggesting that the course of the disease is rapid. In rare cases, the tumor can be detected externally on the head or in the region of the sternum (Feldman and Olson, 1965).

Tissues Involved. Nearly every tissue or organ of the body may be affected, although there is a tendency for tumors to develop on the surface of bones associated with the periosteum (Feldman and Olson, 1965). The tumors have a characteristic cream-colored appearance and a consistency resembling that of congealed cream.

d. Osteopetrosis. This is a progressive diaphyseal dysplasia of the bones.

Occurrence. The disease occurs sporadically in nature and affects males more often than females (Purchase, 1976).

Clinical Findings. Diseased leg bones can be identified by abnormal thickenings and irregularities in the diaphyseal or metaphyseal regions due to disordered new bone formation. The affected areas are hard and insensitive.

Tissues Involved. Osteopetrosis occurs chiefly in the long bones, but can also occur in the pelvis, shoulder girdle, and, rarely, in the spine. The phalanges and skull bones are not affected (Purchase, 1976).

e. Solid Tumors. Many avian solid tumors such as fibrosarcoma, endothelioma, hemangioma, and nephroma are caused by ALV. The only solid tumors known not to be caused by ALV are ovarian carcinoma, astrocytoma, and melanoma (Helmboldt and Frederickson, 1969).

f. Erythroblastosis and Myeloblastosis. These are diseases in which precursors of erythrocytes or granulocytes are found in the bloodstream. Both diseases are primarily laboratory phenomena, and occur only rarely in chickens in their natural environment (Helmboldt and Frederickson, 1969). They will therefore not be discussed in this chapter.

g. Etiology. The first animal oncornavirus was discovered by Rous (1911). The Rous sarcoma virus is closely related to ALV, and it is now known that the diseases of the avian leukosis complex are caused by this group of oncornaviruses. The ALVs have a similar morphology to, and share many of the characteristics of, other oncornaviruses. ALVs are classified into seven major subgroups (A–G) based on their host range, interference pattern, and antigenic character (Crittenden, 1976). Subgroups A–D are exogenous chicken oncornaviruses, subgroup E is an endogenous chicken virus, and subgroups F and G are found only in pheasants (Fujita *et al.*, 1974). Viral isolates that are the primary cause of a single disease, such as the avian myeloblastosis virus (AMV), may belong to any of the subgroups or may consist of mixtures of viruses belonging to different subgroups. The presence of viruses of different subgroups in flocks of chickens has been studied by examining birds for the presence of antibody to ALV and by isolating virus from tissues and tumors.

141

EPIDEMIOLOGY OF
PRIMARY
NEOPLASMS OF
LYMPHOID TISSUES
IN ANIMALS

h. Epidemiology of Avian Leukosis Virus. The infection of chickens with subgroup A ALV is widespread in the natural environment (Shimizu, 1972). Subgroup B virus is also found among commercial chicken flocks, but much less commonly than subgroup A virus. It is unlikely that the other subgroups of ALV are important as etiological agents of naturally occurring disease (Shimizu, 1972). Epidemiological studies showed that ALV is transmitted contagiously (horizontally) among chickens living in the natural environment (Burmester and Gentry, 1954a). Virus is excreted in the saliva and feces, and infection can also occur as a result of aerosolization (Burmester, 1956; Burmester and Gentry, 1954b). Congenital infection of chicken embryos, via the egg, is of primary importance for the dissemination of ALV, since congenitally infected birds are immunologically tolerant to ALV infection. Infected birds, tolerant to ALV, are ideal carriers and shedders of the virus, and are probably the major source of contact infection for other birds (Rubin *et al.,* 1961, 1962; Burmester and Purchase, 1969).

Susceptibility to ALV infection is controlled by a single pair of dominant autosomal genes (Crittenden *et al.,* 1967). In farm flocks, four types of mature birds can be identified (Burmester and Purchase, 1970): (1) Genetically susceptible viremic birds with no ALV antibody. These birds were infected *in ovo,* and females of this type shed the virus continuously in their eggs. (2) Genetically susceptible nonviremic birds with ALV antibody. Some birds in this category intermittently shed virus. (3) Genetically susceptible nonviremic birds with no antibody. (4) Genetically resistant nonviremic birds with no antibody. Birds in this category have never been infected with ALV, and are rarely found in most flocks of chickens. Day-old chicks belonging to all four classes are found, but their neutralizing antibody is maternal in origin. After about 2½ months, maternal neutralizing antibody is lost, and between 3 and 5 months of age, they become susceptible and can be infected with ALV from birds shedding the virus (Shimizu, 1972).

Congenitally infected birds and birds infected very early in life have the greatest chance of developing disease. Genetic resistance or maternal antibodies can prevent or delay infection and thus reduce the incidence of disease. Dams that are genetically resistant to infection, however, can have susceptible progeny sired by a bird with a dominant gene for susceptibility. These chicks will not be protected by maternal antibodies, and will thus be susceptible to early infection, will shed the virus during their entire lifetime, and are likely to develop disease.

i. Control. There is at present no effective treatment for the diseases caused by ALV. It is now possible, however, to establish "breeder" flocks that are free of the virus (Hughes *et al.,* 1963). Three basic steps are involved: (1) Eggs laid by hens with ALV-neutralizing antibody are tested for the virus. (2) Chicks hatched from virus-free eggs are reared in isolation and are tested for virus antibody at 16 weeks of age. (3) Chickens without antibody are then used as breeders for a virus-free stock. By the use of this technique, an ALV-free flock can be obtained in a single generation. Some hens with antibody intermittently shed ALV into their eggs, however, making it difficult and expensive to develop ALV-free flocks on a commercial scale. Thus, to date, ALV has been eradicated only from small flocks used for research purposes.

j. Public Health. Lymphoid leukosis is known to occur in turkeys and Japanese quail (McKee *et al.,* 1963; Wight, 1963). Experimental attempts to transmit the avian leukosis diseases to doves and guinea fowl have been unsuccessful (Helmboldt and Frederickson, 1969). There is no evidence that ALV can induce any diseases in humans (Priester and Mason, 1974).

3.1.3. Marek's Disease

a. Incidence. Marek's disease is a multifocal lymphoproliferative disease that almost always affects the nervous system. Before vaccination became available, Marek's disease was one of the most common naturally occurring neoplasms of the domestic chicken. It occurs primarily in young birds between the ages of 2 and 5 months, although it has been observed in birds as young as 3 weeks old and in birds 2 years old (Jungherr and Hughes, 1965). Both sexes and all breeds are susceptible to the disease, although different lines of chickens differ greatly in their susceptibility (Jungherr and Hughes, 1965; Purchase, 1976). The mortality in affected flocks may exceed 50% (Bruner and Gillespie, 1973).

b. Clinical Findings. The most common clinical sign is an asymmetrical spastic or flaccid paralysis of the wing, leg, or neck (Jungherr and Hughes, 1965; Campbell, 1969). In the initial stages of the disease, there is paralysis of the limb muscles and bunching of the digits. Incoordination of the flexor and extensor muscles may result in a jerky gait. In advanced stages of the disease, the leg or wing trails and the perching reflex is impaired. Paralysis of the neck may result in torticollis, and if the deep muscles and nerves are affected, there may be respiratory distress, distension of the crop, and intestinal stasis (Jungherr and Hughes, 1965; Campbell, 1969).

c. Tissues Involved. Unlike lymphoid leukosis, Marek's disease localizes primarily in the nervous system, although visceral organs and other tissues may also be involved. The brachial, celiac, and lumbar plexuses are frequently swollen, the sciatic nerve is often thickened and edematous, the dorsal ganglia may be enlarged, and the vagus nerve is often involved. Tumor masses may also occur in the feather follicles, gonads, and, to a lesser extent, in the alimentary tract, lungs, heart, and kidneys (Jungherr and Hughes, 1965; Campbell, 1969). The gross lesions frequently appear as discrete grayish-white swellings, but diffuse infiltrative growths are also seen. The nerve trunks may be infiltrated by small round cells indistinguishable from lymphocytes, and myelin degeneration of the nerve sheath may occur (Jungherr and Hughes, 1965; Bruner and Gillespie, 1973). Marek's disease is a T-cell LSA.

d. Etiology. Marek's disease is caused by a cytomegalovirus that is one of the B group of cell-associated herpesviruses (Bruner and Gillespie, 1973). The viral particle is 85–100 nm in diameter, and has a DNA genome and a capsid with 162 hollow cylindrical capsomeres. All field isolates of the virus appear to be antigenically identical.

e. Epidemiology. Under natural conditions, the Marek's disease virus (MDV) is spread contagiously among chickens. The virus enters through the respiratory tract and infects lymphocytes. About 2 weeks after infection, enveloped infectious virions are released from the feather-follicle epithelium (Purchase, 1976). The virus is then shed in the dust and dander and contaminates the environment (Beasley *et al.*, 1970). MDV is stable in the environment and can be transmitted over great distances by airborne dust (Servoian *et al.*, 1963). Most chicks have protective maternal antibodies until they are 3 weeks of age that not only delay infection but also decrease the severity of the subsequent disease (Purchase, 1976). Once a bird is infected with MDV, however, it remains viremic, and sheds infectious virus, for the rest of its life (Purchase, 1976; Sharma, 1976). Congential transmission (via the egg) is not known to occur and is not involved in the natural spread of the disease.

143

EPIDEMIOLOGY OF
PRIMARY
NEOPLASMS OF
LYMPHOID TISSUES
IN ANIMALS

f. Prevention. There is no cure for Marek's disease, and controlling the disease by the development of genetically resistant strains of chickens and by isolation and eradication procedures was, at best, only partially successful. In 1969, the first Marek's disease vaccine was produced using live attenuated MDV. Effective vaccines composed of attenuated MDV are difficult to produce, however, since the yield of virus is quite low. Thus Marek's disease is now prevented by vaccination with a herpesvirus derived from turkeys (HVT) (Purchase, 1975). HVT is antigenically related to MDV, but has little or no pathogenicity in any animal yet tested. The HVT vaccine is highly effective and has resulted in a reduction of 82% in the condemnation rates for Marek's disease in the USA over the 4-year period 1970–1974 (Purchase, 1976). Since birds vaccinated with HVT vaccine can be infected with and can shed MDV into the environment, immunity appears to be directed against nonvirion viral-induced antigens that occur on the tumor-cell surface (Purchase, 1976). The vaccine does not prevent the spread of virulent MDV in the environment, and it must be administered to every chicken; these disadvantages are offset, however, by its effectiveness.

Marek's disease and its prevention by HVT vaccine is an excellent model for the study and control of tumorigenesis induced by other herpesviruses. In particular, the prevention of Marek's disease by cell-membrane fragments free of the virus would be an excellent model for possible immunoprophylaxis for cancer in humans.

g. Public Health. Marek's disease occurs in other members of the order Galliformes. It has been observed in Japanese quail, pigeons, ducks, geese, swans, canaries, and budgerigars (Wight, 1963). Mammals and mammalian cells are refractory to MDV infection, and no MDV-related disease has been reported in humans (Sharma, 1976).

3.2. Mouse

3.2.1. Introduction

Mus musculus, the common house mouse, is one of man's most commensal animal associates. *Mus musculus* originated in Asia and the Middle East, then spread to all parts of the world and moved into grain-storage containers, which were often attached to man's domicile. Grain-storage containers have large rodent populations that excrete large amounts of urine and feces into both human and animal feeds. Huebner (1963) reviewed studies investigating the spread of murine viruses to grain-eaters.

WILLIAM D. HARDY, JR.

3.2.2. Incidence

a. Wild Mice. There have only been two studies of wild mouse LSAs. The first study, from the National Cancer Institute, involved trapping 15 female and 15 male mice and observing the tumors that developed in their noninbred laboratory-raised descendants over a 10-year period (Andervont and Dunn, 1962; Dunn and Andervont, 1963). A total of 225 mice were observed, and 98 (43.5%) developed tumors. Pulmonary tumors were the most frequent tumors, followed by reticulum-cell tumors (type B or Hodgkin's-like lymphoid tumors). Only 2 lymphocytic tumors were reported, which is in marked contrast to the occurrence of LSA in some inbred strains of laboratory mice such as the AKR and C58 strains (Dunn and Andervont, 1963). The reticular tumors developed in wild mice at about 2 years of age, while similar tumors, which occur in "high-incidence" laboratory mice, develop in mice less than 1 year of age (Andervont and Dunn, 1962).

A more recent study of the tumor occurrence in wild mice entailed trapping mice from several areas of southern California and housing them individually in Mason jars for the rest of their lives (Gardner *et al.,* 1971a, 1973a). Naturally occurring tumors developed in 28 of 293 (9.5%) of these mice (Gardner *et al.,* 1973a). LSA was the most common tumor, accounting for 15 of the 28 tumors. The mice that developed LSA were estimated, on the basis of body weight at the time of capture, to be over 2 years of age.

b. Laboratory Mice. The laboratory mouse has been the most extensively studied animal in regard to LSA. Shortly after World War I, a small group of geneticists recognized the need to develop uniformly susceptible strains of mice for certain biological studies, principally for experimental cancer research. The development of inbred strains of mice was begun by C. C. Little and a few other geneticists (Gross, L., 1970a). Successive generations of mating brother to sister resulted in inbred strains after 15–20 successive generations. Animals in inbred strains are, for all practical purposes, as alike as identical twins. Maud Slye (1914) reported that tumors occurred much more frequently in successive generations of mice of certain families. The development of high-, moderate-, and low-leukemia-incidence strains of mice made possible the discovery of the murine leukemia virus (MuLV). Of the high-incidence leukemia strains, the AKR is probably the most representative. AKR LSA occurs more frequently in females (70–90%) than in males (52–77%), and develops by 6–8 months of age (Slye, 1914). It was noticed that almost all AKR mice with LSA had involvement of the thymus, and it was thought that the thymus was the target gland for this disease. This was proven when removal of the thymus early in life increased the latent period for the development of LSA and also increased the incidence of myeloid leukemia (Gross, L., 1970a). Some strains of mice such as the BALB/c and C57BL have naturally low incidences (10%) of LSA.

3.2.3. Clinical Findings

a. Wild Mice. No clinical findings were reported in the studies of descendants of wild mice reared in the laboratories at the National Cancer Institute or in the mice trapped in southern California. It can be surmised from the distribution of

145

EPIDEMIOLOGY OF
PRIMARY
NEOPLASMS OF
LYMPHOID TISSUES
IN ANIMALS

gross lesions, however, that the mice experienced general malaise, weight loss, anemia, and occasional respiratory difficulty due to tumor localization in the anterior mediastinum. There was no mention of a leukemic blood profile in wild mice with LSA. Many mice from one colony in southern California developed a fatal hindlimb paralysis due to neuronal degeneration caused by the MuLV (Gardner *et al.*, 1973b, 1976a,b).

b. Laboratory Mice. The AKR mouse develops LSA within the first year of life. The signs are loss of weight, roughened hair coat, inappetence, enlargement of lymph nodes, anemia, and respiratory difficulty due to thymic involvement. A leukemic blood profile ranging from 23,000 to 125,000/mm^3 develops in 38% of AKR mice.

3.2.4. Tissues Involved

a. Wild Mice. The majority of the tumors that developed in wild mice in the National Cancer Institute study and in mice from most of the trapping areas of southern California were histologically classified as reticulum-cell tumors (type B, or the Hodgkin's-like lesions) (Andervont and Dunn, 1962; Dunn and Andervont, 1963; Gardner *et al.*, 1973a,b). Most of these tumors involved the thymus gland, with the spleen, Peyer's patches, and liver occasionally being involved. It is not known whether the peripheral blood was invaded by neoplastic cells.

Mice obtained from one trapping area in southern California had a much higher incidence of LSA than did mice from other areas. Histologically, these tumors were diffuse, poorly differentiated, and lymphocytic, and were usually accompanied by a leukemic blood profile (Gardner *et al.*, 1973b). The tumors were widely distributed, with marked enlargement of peripheral, mesenteric, and mediastinal lymph nodes and involvement of spleen, liver, kidneys, intestines, and bone marrow. In contrast to the reticular type B tumors of wild mice from other trapping areas and the LSA of the AKR mouse, the thymus gland was not involved. Numerous MuLV particles were seen in all tumor tissues.

b. Laboratory Mice. In laboratory mice, the "naturally occurring" LSA is caused by the Gross or AKR serotype of MuLV. This virus induces lymphoid tumors with widespread involvement of lymphoid organs. Other laboratory-derived MuLVs, including Friend and Rauscher leukemia viruses, induce neoplasia of a different cell type, the erythroid cell.

The "naturally occurring" LSA of AKR mice involves the thymus in almost all cases, along with spleen, lymph nodes, and occasionally the intestinal tract (Gross, L., 1970a). In 35% of AKR mice with LSA, there is a leukemic blood profile. Nonlymphoid organs such as the lungs, kidneys, liver, and salivary glands are often infiltrated with tumor cells. Numerous MuLV particles can be seen in lymphoid, erythroid, and even some epithelial cells of AKR mice with LSA.

Friend and Rauscher MuLVs induce neoplastic proliferations of the red-blood-cell series, resulting in erythroleukemia. Mice experimentally infected with these viruses develop splenomegaly and involvement of the bone marrow and the peripheral blood. The Moloney strain of MuLV induces lymphoid neoplasia. There are numerous other laboratory isolates of MuLV, but they will not be discussed.

WILLIAM D. HARDY,
JR.

3.2.5. Etiology

LSA of wild and laboratory mice is caused by an oncornavirus, the MuLV. Factors that modify the expression of the MuLV in mice are immunological responsiveness, genetic susceptibility or resistance, age, chemicals, and radiation (Gross, L., 1970a).

Murine C-type oncornaviruses are classified into three categories according to the tumors or lesions induced in mice: the MuLVs, the spleen focus-forming viruses (SFFVs), and the murine sarcoma viruses (MuSVs) (Steeves, 1974). Only the MuLVs will be discussed, since only they induce LSA in mice, while SFFVs (Friend and Rauscher viruses) induce erythroleukemia and MuSVs induce sarcomas. The first MuLV was isolated in 1951 by Gross from AKR LSAs and embryos (Gross, L., 1951). In neonatally infected mice, most MuLVs induce LSA in 2–6 months, but the degree to which mice are susceptible is controlled by several genes (Steeves, 1974). In AKR mice, MuLV may behave as an inheritable component (genetic vertical transmission) with its expression genetically controlled. MuLV produces severe immunosuppression, which may enable the few MuLV-transformed lymphoid cells to grow and spread into massive tumors. It is also known that MuLV can be transmitted horizontally via contact and epigenetically by passage *in utero* or via milk (Rongey *et al.,* 1973). Genetic transmission is, however, the most common mode of transmission of MuLV in laboratory mice (Gross, L., 1970a; Aoki *et al.,* 1968).

Typical Gross or AKR MuLV has been isolated from wild mice, and it is known that this virus is oncogenic in feral mice (Aoki *et al.,* 1968). Since the incidence of LSA differs markedly among wild mice colonies, however, the mode of transmission is not clear. Both genetic (vertical) and contagious or epigenetic (horizontal) transmission may be equally important in wild mice.

3.2.6. Epidemiology

a. Wild Mice. In general, wild mice from most trapping areas in southern California are cancer-resistant (Gardner *et al.,* 1973a). Mice from two colonies located 40 miles apart showed a tenfold increased incidence of LSA with aging, however, when compared with similar mice from other colonies (Gardner *et al.,* 1973b, 1976a). After the wild mice reached 1 year of age, 2% of the mice from these colonies also showed a high incidence of a fatal hindlimb paralytic disease of neurogenic origin caused by MuLV (Gardner *et al.,* 1976a).

It must be remembered that wild mice in these studies were trapped in the wild but kept in the laboratory for observation of LSA development. There have not been any studies of the occurrence of LSA in wild mice living in their natural habitat. Of recently trapped mice from an area with the high incidence of LSA, however, 80% had MuLV in their tissues at the time of their capture. These findings are very similar to those that are described in Section 3.11.5 for the FeLV. Certain cat households, like certain high-incidence wild-mouse-trapping areas, have very high frequencies of FeLV infection and LSA development.

b. Laboratory Mice. No epidemiological studies have been performed on laboratory mice, since they are by definition experimental animals. Several research groups have shown that MuLV can be transmitted contagiously by contact and epigenetically (Gross, L., 1970a; Aoki *et al.*, 1968). It is generally agreed, however, that genetic vertical transmission is the most important mode of MuLV transmission in some strains of laboratory mice (Gross, 1970a).

147

EPIDEMIOLOGY OF
PRIMARY
NEOPLASMS OF
LYMPHOID TISSUES
IN ANIMALS

3.2.7. Prevention

In laboratory mice, LSA can be prevented by producing genetically resistant inbred strains or by MuLV vaccination (Steeves, 1974; Huebner *et al.*, 1976). However, since LSA occurs only infrequently in wild mice and since there is little interest in preventing its spread, no similar studies of wild mice have been attempted.

3.2.8. Public Health

MuLV does not efficiently infect and replicate in human cultured cells, and there are no data to suggest that MuLV infects and causes diseases in man. It must be remembered, however, that wild mice live, urinate, and defecate extensively in grain-storage areas (Huebner, 1963), and this source of contamination should be considered, since a number of investigators have found antigens or reverse transcriptase activity in human tumors that are partially related to MuLV. The significance of these observations is at present unresolved, although most researchers do not consider MuLV a threat to human health.

3.3. Rat

3.3.1. Incidence

There is a low incidence of naturally occurring tumors, including LSA, in wild rats (McCoy, 1909). There is considerable variation in the type and frequency of tumors among different strains of laboratory rats. In one study of 31,868 laboratory rats, only 521 primary tumors occurred in 489 rats (Bullock and Curtis, 1930). Mammary tumors are the most frequently occurring rat tumors, followed by LSA (McCoy, 1909; Bullock and Curtis, 1930; Crain, 1958; Kim *et al.*, 1960). Three studies showed that 210 (21%) of a total of 955 rats developed LSA, and that most of the rats that developed LSA were aged, i.e., 1½–2 years old (Bullock and Curtis, 1930; Crain, 1958; Saxton *et al.*, 1948).

3.3.2. Clinical Findings

Clinical signs were not described in any of the reports of rat LSA. However, since the cecal lymph nodes and GI tract were often infiltrated with tumor cells, signs referable to the GI system probably occurred.

3.3.3. Tissues Involved

The tissues involved with naturally occurring LSA of rats vary with the strains of rats studied. There are no reports concerning the sites of involvement for wild rats. In one study, the cecal lymph nodes were involved in 23 of 41 Wistar rats with

LSA (Crain, 1958). Some of these rats also had involvement of pulmonary lymphoid tissue, and 18 had LSA originating in the peribronchial lymph nodes. In some rats, the tumor was widely disseminated to the peritoneal surfaces, stomach, pancreas, kidneys, liver, and spleen.

In another study of naturally occurring LSA of highly inbred Wistar rats, 9% of the animals had severe leukemic blood profiles (Kim *et al.*, 1960). The white blood cell counts in these rats ranged from 100,000 to 500,000/mm^3, and 50–90% of the cells were lymphoblasts. The LSA was associated with progressive anemia, and large numbers of nucleated red blood cells appeared in the blood in the terminal stages of the disease. There was marked splenomegaly, and moderate hepatomegaly with or without generalized lymphadenopathy. The liver, spleen, and bone marrow were extensively infiltrated with leukemic cells. In the same study, 2 rats developed LSA without a leukemic blood profile.

3.3.4. Etiology

LSA can be experimentally induced in rats with the MuLVs, particularly with the wild-type AKR or Gross leukemia virus. Since this discovery, rat oncornaviruses have been isolated from normal rat cells as well as from cultured rat tumor cells induced by MuSVs (Ting, 1968; Teitz *et al.*, 1971; Lieber *et al.*, 1973). The rat oncornavirus possesses the major interspecies (gs-3) antigen of mammalian oncornaviruses as well as its own unique rat species-specific (gs-1) antigen (Geering *et al.*, 1968, 1970; Oroszlan *et al.*, 1972). There is no evidence that the rat oncornavirus induces naturally occurring LSA or any other tumors in the rat or in any other species.

3.3.5. Epidemiology

There have been no studies of the epidemiology of naturally occurring rat LSA.

3.3.6. Prevention

There have been no studies of methods for prevention of naturally occurring rat LSA. Immunization of rats against MuLV can, however, prevent the induction of experimentally induced LSA (Ioachim *et al.*, 1973).

3.3.7. Public Health

There have been no public health studies of rat LSA or of the rat oncornavirus. This virus, however, is generally considered not to be dangerous to man.

3.4. Hamster

There are only a few reports of naturally occurring LSA in hamsters kept in colonies. Three different hamster LSAs will be reviewed separately: (1) the contagious TM hamster LSA; (2) the hamster leukemia virus (HaLV)-induced LSA; and (3) the epizootics of hamster LSA that occurred at the University of Tennessee.

3.4.1. Contagious TM Hamster Lymphosarcoma

149

EPIDEMIOLOGY OF
PRIMARY
NEOPLASMS OF
LYMPHOID TISSUES
IN ANIMALS

a. Incidence. The initial occurrence of the contagious LSA of the hamster was reported in 1961 (Brindley and Banfield, 1961). This tumor occurred in the upper lip of a 2-year old male Syrian hamster.

b. Clinical Findings. Although no clinical signs were reported, the tumor developed first in the larynx, and it is therefore probable that the affected hamsters showed respiratory signs.

c. Tissues Involved. After transmission via cannibalism, the larynx was the first site of tumor growth, but the GI tract was never involved. Neoplastic lymphocytes appeared in the blood 5 days after the tumor was first seen in the larynx, and the white blood cell count increased to above 100,000/mm^3.

d. Etiology. The etiological agent of the TM hamster LSA is unknown. No virus has been found to be associated with this tumor. Spread of the tumor among hamsters occurs by the transplantation and growth of the tumor cells, although this does not preclude the possibility of a subcellular etiological agent (Banfield, 1969). The tumor has a characteristic male karyotype (the original tumor occurred in a male hamster) regardless of the sex of the recipient with LSA, which confirms that the transplanted cells, not the recipient's cells, are the tumor cells.

e. Epidemiology. The epidemiology of the TM hamster lymphoma was studied in hamsters caged together. Tumor cells were transmitted directly by cannibalism and by the mosquito, *Aides aegypti* (Brindley and Banfield, 1961; Banfield, 1969; Banfield *et al.*, 1965, 1966). This was the first time that mammalian tumor cells were shown to be transferred to a susceptible animal by an insect vector.

3.4.2. Hamster-Leukemia-Virus-Induced Lymphosarcoma

a. Incidence. The HaLV has been isolated from hamster tumors induced by the MuSV and from normal cultured hamster cells, and has been observed by electron microscopy in naturally occurring hamster LSAs (Lieber *et al.*, 1973; Stenback *et al.*, 1966, 1968; Klement *et al.*, 1969; Graffi *et al.*, 1968).

Stenback *et al.* (1966) were the first to report finding C-type oncornavirus (HaLV) particles in 9 transplantable tumors, 5 of which were LSA. C-type oncornaviruses were observed in all 5 of the LSAs. One of these LSAs arose spontaneously in an untreated hamster, and this tumor was designated the D-9 hamster LSA. The D-9 LSA is readily transplantable in hamsters.

Graffi *et al.* (1968) observed C-type oncornaviruses in LSA of Syrian hamsters that were being used in transmission studies of papovavirus-containing epithelial skin tumors. No previous hamsters had developed LSA in this colony. A total of 99 of 239 (41.5%) newborn hamsters inoculated with skin tumor extracts developed LSA. Cell-free filtrates of skin tumors also induced LSA in recipient hamsters.

b. Etiology. Numerous HaLV particles were observed in the D-9 hamster LSA (Stenback *et al.*, 1966). The tumor grew rapidly after transplantation by trocar and caused death within 12–14 days. The plasma of hamsters with LSA contained a large number of HaLVs. HaLV derived from hamster LSAs is immunologically distinct from the oncornaviruses of other species, and has been found experimentally to be a leukemogenic oncornavirus of the hamster.

In the report of Graffi *et al.* (1968), the original hamster epithelial skin tumors were found by electron microscopy to contain papovavirus particles, but no C-type oncornaviruses were found. In contrast, LSA cells had no detectable papovavirus, but did contain C-type oncornaviruses. It is probable that there were a few C-type oncornaviruses in the skin tumors that induced LSA when they were transferred to newborn susceptible hamsters.

Recent studies indicate that HaLV has a hamster-species-specific antigen that identifies its origin from hamster (Nowinski *et al.*, 1971). It is not known, however, whether HaLV causes naturally occurring hamster LSA.

3.4.3. Epizootic Hamster Lymphosarcoma at the University of Tennessee

a. Incidence. In 1975, three epizootics of naturally occurring LSA developed in hamsters kept in the University of Tennessee colony, which contained both inbred and random-bred Syrian hamsters (Ambrose and Coggin, 1975). The tumors developed in 20% of the colony-born hamsters, and were naturally horizontally transmitted to 17% of the nonrelated hamsters introduced into the colony.

b. Clinical Findings. No clinical signs were described for the hamsters with LSA in this epizootic. Since 45% of the LSAs occurred in the small intestine, however, GI signs probably occurred.

c. Tissues Involved. Most (45%) of the LSAs arose along the small intestine as single or multiple lesions (Ambrose and Coggin, 1975). Other major sites of involvement in hamsters with LSA were the mesenteric lymph nodes (19%), liver (11%), kidneys (10%), and spleen (6%).

d. Etiology. The etiological agent of this highly contagious LSA has not been elucidated. The transfer of an exogenous oncogenic virus by direct or indirect contact seems to be the most plausible explanation.

e. Epidemiology. No previous cases of LSA had occurred in the colony or in the colony of the commercial supplier during the preceding 5 years. In the first year of the epizootic, half the hamsters developed LSA. Over the entire duration of the three epizootics, tumors developed in 61 (20%) of 309 hamsters born in the colony, and in 122 (17.6%) of 637 hamsters born outside the colony but later introduced into the colony. The average length of stay in the colony for those hamsters that were introduced into the colony and that developed LSA was 8 weeks. Thus, LSA developed in random-bred hamsters very shortly after exposure to the etiological agent. Two attempts to stop the epizootic of LSA by eliminating all hamsters followed by a thorough disinfection and repopulation failed. A separate epizootic occurred in hamsters at the Yale School of Medicine after the introduction of hamsters with LSA from the University of Tennessee (Ambrose and Coggin, 1975). The transmission of the etiological agent was apparently airborne, since the LSA developed among caged hamsters that had had no direct contact with any hamster with LSA.

f. Prevention. Attempts to prevent the epizootic of hamster LSA, using ordinary sanitation procedures, failed, possibly because of the survival of the etiological agent in the air.

3.4.4. Public Health

There have been no studies of the public health aspects of hamster LSAs or of the HaLV. The HaLV is not considered to be a hazardous agent to humans.

3.5. Guinea Pig

3.5.1. Incidence

Naturally occurring LSA was observed in middle-aged guinea pigs as early as 1918 (Miguez, 1918). LSA with a leukemic blood profile could be induced in inbred guinea pigs by cell-graft transplantation (Miguez, 1918; Gross, L., 1970a). In fact, transmission of guinea pig LSA was reported prior to successful transplantation of mouse leukemia. There were, however, no reports of the occurrence of guinea pig LSA from the 1920's until 1954, when naturally occurring LSA was observed in 10 (3.3%) of 303 guinea pigs at the National Cancer Institute (Congdon and Lorenz, 1954). In this study, 4 of 112 "strain 2" guinea pigs, 2 of 30 "strain 13" guinea pigs, and 4 of 161 hybrid guinea pigs developed LSA.

3.5.2. Clinical Findings

The clinical findings were not described in any of the studies of naturally occurring or transplantable guinea pig LSA.

3.5.3. Tissues Involved

Naturally occurring and transmissible LSA of guinea pigs is a disseminated disease in which tumor cells infiltrate various internal organs (Gross, L., et al., 1970). A leukemic blood profile develops, characterized by a large number of white blood cells, mainly lymphocytes and immature blast cells.

After inoculation of leukemic cells, LSA first develops at the subcutaneous inoculation site, then metastasizes to the axillary and cervical lymph nodes, followed by the development of a leukemic blood profile (Gross, L., et al., 1970). The peripheral white blood cell count usually increases to 200,000/mm³ and consists principally of large primitive blast cells. In the advanced stages of the disease, the bone marrow is heavily infiltrated with leukemic cells. There is considerable enlargement of the spleen and liver, but involvement of the thymus has not been reported.

3.5.4. Etiology

Guinea pig LSA is a transplantable tumor in strain 2 and hybrid guinea pigs. LSA developed in the inoculated young guinea pigs after a latent period of only 15–30 days. Transmission was accomplished by inoculation of either blood, plasma, serum, or leukemic cells (Nadel, 1957; Jungeblut and Kodza, 1962). Cell-free preparations and filtrates were also reported to induce LSA in guinea pigs (Jungeblut and Kodza, 1962). Other investigators, however, have been unable to repeat transmission of the tumor by cell-free filtrates (Gross, L., et al., 1970).

Although there is some dispute as to the leukemogenic activity of cell-free filtrate preparations, the etiological agent is thought to be a virus, since three different virus particles have been observed in LSA cells and in normal spleen cells from strain 2 and Hartley guinea pigs. Opler (1967) was the first to observe "C-type-like" virus associated with the guinea pig LSA, and this observation was quickly confirmed by other investigators (Nadel et al., 1967). The site of production of this virus, and its morphology, differed from those of known C-type oncornaviruses. The virus particle is smaller than C-type oncornaviruses, measuring between 70 and 90 nm in diameter. A central nucleoid is surrounded by a fuzzy outer coat, which differs from the smooth viral envelope of C-type oncornaviruses. Virus particles are seen in the perinuclear cisterna (nuclear envelope) as well as in the cisternae of the endoplasmic reticulum (Opler, 1967; Nadel et al., 1967). These sites of virus localization also differ from those of C-type oncornaviruses, which are found in the extracellular spaces, intracellular vacuoles, and budding from the plasma membrane of infected cells. None of the guinea pig viral particles was seen budding from the cell plasma membrane. These particles were initially called C-type virus, but this designation appears to be incorrect, since the morphological and physical properties are different from those of C-type oncornaviruses. The relationship of "C-type-like" viral particles to the etiology of guinea pig leukemia is unknown.

Il Ma et al. (1969) reported, for the first time, a typical C-type oncornavirus in the germinal centers of lymph nodes, Peyer's patches, and spleens from 6 of 6 normal adult Hartley guinea pigs. C-type oncornaviruses were also observed in normal spleen cells after treatment with 5-bromo-2'-deoxyuridine (Hsiung, 1972; Nayak and Murray, 1973; Gross, P. A., et al., 1973; Rhim et al., 1975). These particles were typical of known oncornaviruses, since they had a density of 1.16–1.17 g/ml, a 65–70 S RNA, and a viral reverse transcriptase. Rhim et al. (1975) reported that there was no antigenic cross-reaction of guinea pig C-type oncornaviruses with other mammalian oncornaviruses. Thus, it appears that the guinea pig oncornavirus is an endogenous virus of normal and leukemic guinea pigs, but its relationship to the etiology of guinea pig LSA is unclear.

The third type of virus to be isolated from guinea pig LSA and normal cells was a herpesvirus, the guinea pig herpeslike virus (GPHLV) (Hsiung and Kaplow, 1969; Nayak, 1971). GPHLV was not found in leukocytes taken directly from infected animals, but was induced from these cells after they had been in culture for 3 days (Hsiung and Kaplow, 1969). This virus has been shown to transform guinea pig leukocytes in vitro; however, when these transformed leukocytes were injected back into guinea pigs, they did not induce leukemia (Hsiung et al., 1973).

Whether the "C-type-like" virus, the C-type oncornavirus, or the GPHLV alone causes guinea pig LSA is unknown. It is possible that any two or all three of these viruses may interact to cause LSA in guinea pigs.

3.5.5. Epidemiology

There have been no studies of the epidemiology of LSA among guinea pigs. Opler (1967) reported that guinea pig LSA could be transmitted by oral feeding of spleen cells from leukemic guinea pigs. This raises the possibility of cannibalistic transmission of the disease among guinea pigs, although guinea pigs are not as cannibalistic as hamsters or mice.

153

EPIDEMIOLOGY OF
PRIMARY
NEOPLASMS OF
LYMPHOID TISSUES
IN ANIMALS

3.5.6. Prevention

L. Gross (1970b, 1971) was able to immunize guinea pigs against their transplantable leukemia by the intradermal inoculation of small doses of leukemic cell suspensions. The resulting intracutaneous tumors regress in 50% of the inoculated animals, and the majority of these guinea pigs are immune to challenge with large numbers of leukemic cells (Gross, L., 1970b). The active immunity appears to be cell-mediated, since protection cannot be transferred by serum (Gross, L., 1971).

3.5.7. Public Health

There is no known public health danger from guinea pig LSA or from the three viruses isolated from guinea pigs with LSA.

3.6. Cattle

3.6.1. Incidence

Bovine LSA occurs in cattle of all ages and breeds, but it occurs predominantly in 5- to 8-year-old animals and most frequently in dairy breeds. The higher occurrence in dairy breeds can be partly accounted for by slaughter practices. Beef cattle are slaughtered at early ages and do not live to 5–8 years, the age at which LSA develops in the dairy breeds. LSA is the most common tumor of dairy cattle, accounting for 50% of all tumors in cattle. The occurrence of LSA in slaughtered cattle is 19 per 100,000 adult cattle (bulls and cows), 48 per 100,000 cows, and 2 per 100,000 calves (Hare *et al.*, 1964; Migaki, 1969).

3.6.2. Clinical Findings

The clinical signs of LSA depend on the location of the major lesions. The usual clinical syndrome is emaciation; normocytic, normochromic anemia; weight loss; a decrease in milk production; and enlargement of one or more of the peripheral lymph nodes. Posterior paresis or paralysis occurs in about 50% of cases. A leukemic blood profile is not common, occurring in only 5–10% of cattle with LSA (Toit, 1916; Weber, 1963).

3.6.3. Tissues Involved

There are four forms of bovine LSA based on sites of gross tumor localization and the age of occurrence.

a. Adult Multicentric Form. This is the most common form of LSA in cattle, and is characterized by internal lymphadenopathy and involvement of various other organ systems. Right heart failure and infiltration of the spinal cord and eye may also occur. The majority of cattle with adult multicentric LSA are 6–9 years old. The course of the disease is variable, but the mean duration from the time of diagnosis is 61 days.

b. Calf Multicentric Form. This form is characterized by a rapid enlargement of lymph nodes with bone marrow involvement, and occurs in calves between 3 and 6 months of age. Anemia due to bone marrow infiltration is common. Neoplastic lymphocytes infiltrate various internal organs in the advanced stages of the disease.

c. Thymic Form. This form is relatively rare, occurs in young cattle 1–2 years old, and is characterized by massive enlargement of the thymus accompanied by swelling of the neck, bloat, and cardiovascular distress. If the animal survives long enough, there may be generalized enlargement of lymph nodes.

d. Skin Form. This form is very rare, and is characterized by lymphosarcomatous lesions of the skin, especially on the neck, back, rump, and thighs. There may be enlargement of lymph nodes. The skin lesions and lymph node enlargements may regress completely, although there is usually recurrence of the disease with subsequent tumor involvement in many organ systems.

In general, bovine LSA is a disease of all lymphoid organs. Lymph nodes were involved in 95%, heart in 50%, spleen in 19%, kidneys in 18%, liver in 10%, intestinal tract in 8%, lung in 9%, thymus in 2%, and blood in 10% of slaughtered cattle with LSA (Migaki, 1969).

3.6.4. Etiology

The bovine leukemia virus (BLV), which causes bovine LSA, is an oncornavirus member of the family Retroviridae. BLV is enveloped, matures by budding from the cell membrane, and has an RNA genome and a viral reverse transcriptase. However, BLV has several unique features. All mammalian oncornaviruses share a common interspecies antigen on the viral p30 protein molecule, but extensive studies of BLV by various groups have failed to detect this common antigen in BLV (Ferrer, 1972; Ferrer *et al.*, 1975; Gilden *et al.*, 1975). Another unique feature of BLV is the cell-associated nature of the virus. BLV tends to stick to cells that produce it, and a large yield of virus in culture fluids is hard to obtain (Ferrer *et al.*, 1971). Finally, cattle infected with BLV under natural conditions produce large amounts of antibody to an internal virion antigen (Miller, J. M., and Olson, 1972; Ferrer *et al.*, 1972). In general, other animals infected with their oncornaviruses do not produce antibodies to the internal virion antigens, or do so only in low amounts.

It was reported recently that the DNA copy of the BLV genome is found only in tissues of cattle with the adult form of LSA, not in cattle with the thymic form or in healthy cattle (Callahan *et al.*, 1976). This finding, along with the seroepidemiological and epidemiological studies, shows conclusively that BLV is an infectious agent for cattle, and that it is not inherited as a gene in normal noninfected cattle.

3.6.5. Epidemiology

Bovine LSA can occur sporadically or enzootically. The sporadic type includes the thymic and calf multicentric forms and some of the adult multicentric cases. The enzootic type includes a majority of the adult multicentric cases. The sporadic type occurs more or less at random in most cattle-raising countries, while the enzootic form occurs as multiple cases in certain areas. For example, only the sporadic form occurs in the United Kingdom and on the Danish island of Jutland, while the enzootic form occurs in other parts of Denmark, in Germany, and in the United States (Anderson and Jarrett, 1968).

155

EPIDEMIOLOGY OF
PRIMARY
NEOPLASMS OF
LYMPHOID TISSUES
IN ANIMALS

It was noted that LSA appeared in LSA-free herds several years after the introduction of unrelated breeding animals from high-incidence herds (Marshak and Abt, 1968; Olson, 1974). Certain areas in Denmark had a tenfold higher incidence of LSA in cattle than did other areas. These high-incidence areas had a LSA rate of 28.7 cases per 100,000 cattle, while the low-incidence areas had a rate of 1.5 cases per 100,000 cattle (Bendixen, 1960). Similar observations were made in other European countries and in the United States, and these findings suggested that an infectious or contagious agent was the cause of bovine LSA. It was not until 1969, when Miller and her colleagues reported finding oncornaviruslike particles in phytohemagglutinin (PHA)-stimulated lymphocyte cultures from cattle with LSA, that elucidation of the contagious nature of this disease began (Miller, J. M., *et al.*, 1969). Miller's group and others began to grow and isolate BLV, and also to perform transmission studies (Ferrer *et al.*, 1971; Olson *et al.*, 1972; Miller, L. D., *et al.*, 1972). Sheep and cattle with induced LSA produced strong precipitating antibody to BLV, which was then used as an immunological reagent for detecting BLV (Miller, J. M., and Olson, 1972).

3.6.6. Seroepidemiology

Immunodiffusion, complement-fixation, and immunofluorescent serological methods were employed in field studies to determine the prevalence of BLV in cattle under natural conditions (Miller, J. M., and Olson, 1972; Ferrer and Bhatt, 1973; Miller, J. M., and Van Der Maaten, 1972). With the immunodiffusion test, over 7000 cattle from the north central United States were tested for antibody to the internal antigens of BLV (Baumgartener *et al.*, 1975). Sera from 4394 dairy cattle in 100 herds and from 2792 beef cattle in 50 herds were tested. Antibody to BLV was found in 66% of the 100 dairy herds and in 10.2% of the 4394 dairy cattle in these herds. In contrast, a much lower number of reactions was found in beef herds. Only 14% of the 50 beef herds and 2.3% of the 2792 cattle in these herds had antibody. Few of the cattle with antibody were less than 2 years old, which suggests that transmission of BLV is slow. The prevalence of BLV infection appears to be the same for both bulls and cows.

There was a striking difference in the occurrence of BLV antibody in healthy cattle from herds with a history of LSA compared with cattle from herds with no history of LSA (Olson *et al.*, 1973). In 5 herds in which no animals had developed LSA during the past 13–33 years, the percentage of healthy cattle with antibody (2–16%) was lower than that in 6 herds in which 24 cattle had developed LSA during the previous 7 years. Of the cattle in these 6 herds, 24–40% had BLV antibody. No BLV antibody was found in 100 dairy cattle from 10 herds on the isolated Island of Jersey or in 126 dairy cattle from an isolated herd in the United States, both of which were free of LSA (Olson and Baumgartener, 1975).

At birth, most calves in herds in which LSA has occurred previously are not infected with BLV and do not have BLV antibodies. Foster nursing experiments showed that BLV is only rarely transmitted through the milk, and that calves acquire BLV contagiously from infected cattle with which they are housed (Piper *et al.*, 1975). BLV does not seem to have a reservoir in animals other than cattle. Sera from over 2000 pigs, goats, sheep, ponies, and 17 species of wild animals were tested for BLV antibody, but none was found (Olson and Baumgartener, 1975).

3.6.7. Prevention

The epidemiological data indicate that methods of preventing bovine LSA by detecting those cattle that are most likely to develop LSA or by detecting BLV-infected cattle are feasible. Prevention may be accomplished by (1) hematological detection and slaughter of cattle with persistent lymphocytosis or (2) serological detection and slaughter of cattle with BLV antibody.

Persistent lymphocytosis is defined as an increase in the absolute lymphocyte count of 3 or more standard deviations above the normal mean as determined for the respective breed and age group of animals in LSA-free herds (Miller, J. M., and Olson, 1972). There has been much controversy concerning the use of hematological detection and slaughter of cattle with persistent lymphocytosis. Some investigators feel that detection of persistent lymphocytosis is a preleukemic finding, and that many of these animals will develop LSA (Knuth and Volkman, 1916; Bendixen, 1963, 1967). Others feel that persistent lymphocytosis is not an accurate indication of impending LSA development (Marshak, 1968; Abt *et al.*, 1970). The control method consists of hematological detection of cattle with persistent lymphocytosis, followed by isolation of the herd and slaughter of those cattle with lymphocytosis. If there are many cattle with lymphocytosis in a herd, the entire herd is slaughtered. Bendixen reported that the control measures have reduced the incidence of bovine LSA in Denmark from 28.7 to 3.0 cases per 100,000 cattle in 11 years (Bendixen, 1963, 1967, 1969, 1973). These results are impressive, since this preventive procedure has reduced the bovine LSA incidence by about tenfold in Denmark.

Another possible method of control is the serological detection of BLV-infected cattle. Although these techniques are well established, no country has adopted them in a formal control program. It might be possible to use the immuno-diffusion or immunofluorescent antibody tests to detect BLV-infected cattle for the purpose of removing them from contact with uninfected susceptible herd members.

3.6.8. Public Health

Since BLV is shed in cow's milk, and since it can experimentally infect both goats and sheep, with about 20% of the infected sheep developing LSA in 2–4 years, the question whether BLV is a hazard to man has been raised (Olson *et al.*, 1972; Olson and Baumgartener, 1975). In one study, two chimpanzees developed erythroleukemia after being fed cow's milk suspected of containing BLV (McClure *et al.*, 1974). There was also a recent report of a cluster of seven people who were associated with a powdered-milk plant who developed LSA (Bartsch *et al.*, 1975).

At present, there is no serological evidence of transmission of BLV to man. Tests of well over 500 laboratory personnel working with BLV, dairymen, veterinarians, and patients with leukemia detected no antibody to BLV (Olson and Baumgartener, 1975; Gilden *et al.*, 1975; Caldwell *et al.*, 1976). Also, when BLV is added to cow's milk, the infectivity is destroyed by commercial pasteurization at

74°C for 16 sec (Olson and Baumgartener, 1975). Thus, to date, there is no evidence that directly links BLV to human infection or disease. It seems advisable, however, to stress that all milk for human consumption should be pasteurized.

157

EPIDEMIOLOGY OF
PRIMARY
NEOPLASMS OF
LYMPHOID TISSUES
IN ANIMALS

3.7. Sheep

3.7.1. Incidence

Sheep LSA is the most common form of neoplasm in sheep, occurring at a frequency of 0.5–1 sheep per 100,000 slaughtered sheep per year (Migaki, 1969; Marshak, 1968; Brandly and Migaki, 1963).

3.7.2. Tissues Involved

Several organs are usually involved in sheep with LSA. Lymph nodes are always affected, and the liver, spleen, and kidneys are involved in 40% of the animals (Migaki, 1969). The thymus is rarely involved.

3.7.3. Etiology

Oncornavirus particles were found by electron microscopy in PHA-stimulated lymphocyte cultures from sheep with LSA. Virus was observed in cultured cells from 7 sheep with either LSA or lymphocytosis, but not in cultures from 38 healthy sheep from the same flock (Paulsen *et al.*, 1972). Many sheep from this flock had previously developed LSA. Virus was seen in sheep cells grown in culture in which the medium was supplemented with fetal calf serum as well as in medium supplemented with sheep serum or plasma, but as in BLV-infected cultures, budding virus was rarely observed.

The virus isolated from sheep with LSA has the typical characteristics of other oncornaviruses. It labels with [^{3}H]uridine, has a density of 1.16–1.18 g/cm^3, and has a reverse transcriptase (Paulsen *et al.*, 1976). Virus isolated from sheep lymphocyte cultures produced LSA when injected into sheep (Paulsen *et al.*, 1976). Thus, experimental evidence now indicates that the ovine leukemia virus (OLV) can induce LSA in sheep. Recent antigenic analysis of the OLV and BLV indicates that a similar if not identical antigen is shared by both viruses, as shown by the cross-reactivity with both bovine and ovine sera (Paulsen *et al.*, 1976). There is no antigenic cross-reactivity of OLV with any other mammalian oncornaviruses.

3.7.4. Epidemiology

There have been several epidemiological studies of sheep LSA in Germany (Enke *et al.*, 1964; Ulbrich *et al.*, 1970; Paulsen *et al.*, 1971). Enzootic occurrence of sheep LSA, similar to enzootic bovine LSA, has been reported in certain flocks. These findings along with the finding that OLV can experimentally induce LSA in sheep, show that naturally occurring sheep LSA is caused by a contagious oncornavirus.

Since both sheep and cattle often inhabit the same farm, it is possible that the same virus is responsible for LSA in both species. It is known that BLV can induce LSA in sheep, and studies to determine whether OLV can induce LSA in cattle are in progress (Paulsen *et al.*, 1976). Additional studies of the enzymes and antigens of both viruses may determine the relationship between OLV and BLV.

3.8. Horses

3.8.1. Incidence

The incidence of LSA in slaughtered horses is 6.2 cases per 100,000. This incidence is high for a farm animal, and is second only to the contagiously spread BLV LSA of cattle (Migaki, 1969). Most horses that develop LSA are between 6 and 9 years old, although the disease has occurred in foals.

3.8.2. Clinical Findings

LSA in the horse is often localized, producing a variety of clinical signs (Squire, 1963). Generalized lymph node involvement was reported in only 5 of 17 cases (Cotchin, 1960; Runnells and Benbrook, 1944; Theilen and Fowler, 1962; Schalm, 1975). Anemia is usually absent, although a leukemic blood profile is common even though the disease is often localized (Squire, 1963).

3.8.3. Tissues Involved

There is generalized lymph node involvement in about one third of the horses with LSA, and also invasion of the major parenchymal organs (Runnells and Benbrock, 1944; Theilen and Fowler, 1962). The thymus, skin, heart, and eye may also be involved. Some tumors arise locally in the stomach and intestines and disseminate to other organs.

3.8.4. Etiology

There is no known cause of equine LSA.

3.8.5. Epidemiology

There have been no epidemiological studies of equine LSA.

3.9. Swine

3.9.1. Incidence

LSA is the most common tumor of swine, although it is rare in swine in the United States (Koller *et al.*, 1970). Based on three studies, the incidence rate is approximately 0.88 case per 100,000 pigs slaughtered (Monlux *et al.*, 1956; Renier *et al.*, 1966; Anderson and Jarrett, 1968). A 10-year study showed, however, that 1.58 pigs with LSA were found in every 100,000 pigs slaughtered (Migaki, 1969). The age at which swine are slaughtered must be considered when analyzing this low incidence figure, since 92% of all swine are slaughtered at 6 months of age and since a higher incidence was noted for 1-year-old swine in another study (Migaki, 1969; Renier *et al.*, 1966).

3.9.2. Clinical Findings

LSA is seldom diagnosed clinically in swine, and is usually apparent only at necropsy. The disease usually occurs without a leukemic blood profile.

159

EPIDEMIOLOGY OF
PRIMARY
NEOPLASMS OF
LYMPHOID TISSUES
IN ANIMALS

3.9.3. Tissues Involved

The lymph nodes, spleen, and liver are often involved, while the kidneys, thymus, and bone marrow are less frequently affected (Migaki, 1969; Anderson and Jarrett, 1968). Histologically, the affected tissues are invaded by neoplastic lymphoblasts and lymphocytes, which disrupt the normal tissue architecture.

3.9.4. Etiology

There is no known etiological agent for swine LSA. No virus has been associated with swine LSA, but an oncornavirus was found in four pig cell culture lines (Armstrong *et al.*, 1971). The relationship of this virus to swine LSA is unknown.

3.9.5. Epidemiology

There have been no epidemiological studies of swine LSA, and there are no reports of multiple occurrences in herds to suggest the presence of a contagious agent.

3.10. Dog

3.10.1. Incidence

LSA accounts for 5–7% of all canine tumors and is the third most common tumor after mammary and skin tumors (Dorn *et al.*, 1967). The annual incidence is 24 cases for every 100,000 dogs in the population at risk (Dorn *et al.*, 1967, 1968a,b). There is no sex predilection, and 85% of cases occur in mature dogs between 5 and 10 years old (Hardy, 1974a; Squire, 1963, 1969). LSA does occur in dogs less than 1 year of age, however, and is often accompanied by a severe leukemic blood profile. One veterinary school clinic reported that LSA occurred in 2% of all dogs admitted and that 22% of all tumors diagnosed were LSA (Jarrett, W. F. H., *et al.*, 1966). Certain breeds of dogs such as boxers, cocker spaniels, and fox terriers develop LSA more frequently than do other breeds, while the beagle has a lower incidence than most breeds (Cohen *et al.*, 1959, 1974; Howard and Nielsen, 1965; Morris, 1968). Canine LSA is similar to human LSA in its response to drugs and in the lack of a known viral etiology.

3.10.2. Clinical Findings

The most characteristic and frequent clinical finding is a generalized enlargement of the peripheral lymph nodes. Peripheral lymphadenopathy occurs more constantly in the dog than in any other species (Squire, 1963; Van Pelt and Conner, 1968). Many dogs with LSA appear relatively healthy, although fever, anorexia, depression, and emaciation may be present. The major signs depend on the organ system(s) in which there is gross tumor localization. Splenomegaly, tonsillar enlargement (in approximately 50% of cases), bone marrow, and other organ involvement usually occur in advanced stages of the disease. Respiratory distress, uremia, anemia, icterus, and even paraplegia may occur. A hematological feature in about 50% of cases is a granulocytic leukemoid reaction of 20,000–30,000/mm³; the cause of this marrow response is unknown (Squire, 1963). Of dogs with LSA, 60% have a moderate normocytic, normochromic anemia.

A leukemic blood profile occurs in only 20% of dogs in the early stages of LSA. Leukemic cells appear in the blood in more than 50% of dogs with advanced disease, however, and this finding is usually associated with extensive tumor dissemination. The total leukocyte count may be greatly elevated, but more often, there is a relative lymphocytosis with a normal or only slightly elevated leukocyte count (Squire, 1963). The staging of canine LSA is based on gross tumor localization, hematological findings, and constitutional signs (Table 9) (Hardy, 1974a).

Of all the animals that develop LSA only the dog has been routinely treated for this disease. There are numerous therapy protocols, and the drugs of choice are corticosteroids, cyclophosphamide, vincristine, vinblastine, and L-asparaginase (Hardy, 1974a; Squire, 1963). The mean survival time of untreated dogs with LSA is only 27 days, and therapy can extend survival to an average of 173 days (Hardy and Old, 1970; MacEwen and Hess, 1975; Brick et al., 1968). The author treated two lymphosarcomatous dogs with L-asparaginase; the dogs survived for 5 and 6 years, and died of causes unrelated to their tumors (Hardy and Old, 1970). Canine LSA is an excellent animal model in which to study new forms of therapy such as combination chemotherapy.

TABLE 9. **Stages of Canine Lymphosarcoma**[a]

Parameter	I	II	III	IV
Peripheral lymph-adenopathy	Present	Present	Present	Present
Hepatosplenomeg-aly	Absent	Present	Present	Present
Hemogram[b]	Normal	Normal	1. Slight anemia (PCV 20–37%) 2. 10% abnormal lymphocytes	1. Moderate to severe anemia 2. 10% abnormal lymphocytes
Bone marrow	Normal	Normal	Slight marrow involvement	Moderate to extensive marrow involvement
Constitutional signs	None	Lethargy	1. Lethargy 2. Depression 3. Anorexia 4. Signs referable to sites of tumor involvement	1. Lethargy 2. Depression 3. Anorexia 4. Signs referable to sites of tumor involvement

[a]From Hardy (1974a).

[b]Of dogs with lymphosarcoma, 50% have a moderate leukocytosis of 20,000–30,000/mm³ with a neutrophilia and left shift.

3.10.3. Tissues Involved

161

EPIDEMIOLOGY OF
PRIMARY
NEOPLASMS OF
LYMPHOID TISSUES
IN ANIMALS

Canine LSA is considered to be of unifocal origin, and multiple lesions are considered to be metastatic (Squire, 1963). In the terminal stages, virtually all groups of lymph nodes are involved, and the spleen, liver, kidney, and intestines are often infiltrated with neoplastic lymphocytes. In contrast to other animals, thymic involvement occurs only rarely in dogs. Four forms of the disease are recognized, based on gross tumor localization: (1) the multicentric form, which occurs about as frequently as the alimentary form and is characterized by generalized lymph node enlargement along with involvement of other major viscera; (2) the alimentary form, which involves the intestinal tract and mesenteric lymph nodes; (3) the thymic form, which occurs only rarely in dogs; and (4) the unclassified form, which is rare and is characterized by tumor localization in the CNS, skin, and eyes.

3.10.4. Etiology

There is no known cause of naturally occurring LSA in dogs. No oncornaviruses have been isolated from dogs, and there is only one report of an oncornavirus occurring in a dog with LSA (Jarrett, W. F. H., *et al.,* 1966). This finding has not been confirmed, and it must therefore be concluded that there is no known canine leukemia virus.

Since the boxer and cocker spaniel have high occurrences of LSA, some authors have suggested that these breeds may transmit oncogenic viruses via their genes, although there is no experimental support for this hypothesis (Cohen *et al.,* 1974). There is recent evidence that dogs with LSA produce antibodies to antigens found in their tumors. This reactivity is similar to that found in cattle that react to the BLV, and suggests that a virus may be causing canine LSA (Winters and Snow, 1974a,b). Further work is needed to support or refute this concept.

3.10.5. Epidemiology

Experimental induction of LSA in dogs by strontium-90, plutonium, and FeLV has been reported (Casarett, 1965; Lebel *et al.,* 1970; Rickard *et al.,* 1969). There is no evidence, however, that these radioactive materials or FeLV cause naturally occurring LSA in pet dogs. There have not been many detailed epidemiological studies of canine LSA, and clusters of LSA have not been reported among unrelated dogs. Thus, there appears to be no evidence, to date, for a contagious etiological agent for canine LSA.

3.11. Cat

3.11.1. Incidence

The annual incidence of LSA in cats is 200 cases per 100,000 cats in the population at risk, which is the highest incidence of naturally occurring LSA in any animal (Essex and Francis, 1976). LSA accounts for one third of all feline tumors and for 90% of all feline hematopoietic neoplasms. Nearly half (42%) of cats with LSA are less than 3 years old, and the disease occurs equally in both sexes and in all breeds (Meincke *et al.,* 1972).

WILLIAM D. HARDY, JR.

3.11.2. Clinical Findings

The clinical signs of LSA in cats are nonspecific and include (in decreasing frequency of occurrence) anemia, abdominal mass, hydrothorax, peripheral lymphadenopathy, pyrexia, enlarged kidneys, and cachexia. The signs shown by individual cats vary and depend on the localization of the tumor. Of cats with LSA, however, 50% usually have severe normocytic, normochromic (nonregenerative) anemias, and 30 to 40% have a leukemic blood profile (Meincke *et al.*, 1972).

3.11.3. Tissues Involved

Feline LSA is classified into four main forms according to the anatomical distribution of the major lesions (Crighton, 1969). In order of decreasing occurrence, they are:

a. Alimentary Lymphosarcoma. The main tumor sites are the abdominal lymph nodes, the GI tract, and the kidneys. In some cats, all these sites are simultaneously involved; in other cats, tumors occur at only one or two sites. Other organs are rarely involved. Cats with this form of the disease tend to be older than cats with other forms of LSA. We have found that LSAs of the intestinal tract are of B-cell origin with immunoglobulins on the tumor-cell surfaces.

b. Thymic (Anterior Mediastinal) Lymphosarcoma. In this form of LSA, tumors are found in the thymus and lymph nodes of the anterior mediastinum. Young cats, often less than 1 year old, tend to develop this form of the disease more often than other forms of LSA. We have found that thymic LSA cells are T cells, since they form rosettes with guinea pig erythrocytes and do not have surface immunoglobulins.

c. Multicentric Lymphosarcoma. The characteristic feature of this form of LSA is superficial, abdominal, and thoracic lymphadenopathy either alone or in combination. Often, there is also liver and spleen enlargement.

d. Unclassified Lymphosarcoma. This is a rare form of LSA characterized by localization in the skin, eyes, nasopharynx, and CNS. In some cats, there are neoplastic cells in the circulating blood, but no organ involvement which is similar to acute lymphoblastic leukemia in humans.

3.11.4. Etiology

Feline LSA and several nonneoplastic feline diseases are caused by the FeLV (Jarrett, W. F. H., *et al.*, 1964; Hardy *et al.*, 1969, 1976a). FeLV is also indirectly responsible for numerous other diseases. Since FeLV exerts an immunosuppressive effect, it makes the FeLV-infected cat more susceptible to secondary infections (Cotter *et al.*, 1975; Hardy *et al.*, 1976a). The immunosuppressive effects of FeLV were shown in infected laboratory cats, which were able to maintain skin grafts longer than did noninfected cats (Perryman *et al.*, 1972). These experiments showed that FeLV depresses the cell-mediated immune response of cats. It is not known whether FeLV also depresses the humoral immune response.

FeLV is an exogenous oncornavirus; i.e., its genome is not found integrated in the chromosomes of normal uninfected cat cells. Viral antigens are associated with the viral envelope and viral core. The envelope antigens are type-specific and distinguish three different strains of FeLV (FeLV-A, -B, and -C)(Sarma and Log,

1973). The core (internal) antigens are identical for all strains of FeLV, and are therefore termed *group-specific* (gs) antigens (Hardy *et al.*, 1969; Hardy, 1974b). The major gs-1 antigen is unique to FeLV, and detection of this antigen is the basis of the fluorescent antibody test for FeLV in peripheral leukocytes of cats (Geering *et al.*, 1968; Hardy *et al.*, 1973b). In addition to the viral antigens, FeLV induces a feline oncornavirus-associated cell-membrane antigen (FOCMA) in the plasma membrane of cells transformed by FeLV regardless of whether they replicate FeLV or not (Essex *et al.*, 1971; Hardy, 1976a). This is a true transformation or tumor-specific antigen, and its discovery is a major finding in cancer biology.

Cats can produce antibodies to all three classes of FeLV antigens. Antibody against the viral envelope antigens neutralizes FeLV infection, antibody against gs antigens has no known biological function, and antibody against FOCMA can prevent the development of LSA (Hardy, 1976a; Essex *et al.*, 1975a).

3.11.5. Epidemiology

The contagious nature of FeLV was suspected from the early observations by veterinarians that feline LSA tended to occur in clusters (Schneider *et al.*, 1967; Brodey *et al.*, 1970; Hardy *et al.*, 1973a). The first epidemiological study of feline LSA examined the question of whether or not the occurrence of LSA was significantly higher in multiple-cat households than in single-cat households (Schneider, 1970). No association between LSA and multiple-cat households was found. From this study, it was concluded that feline LSA was not a contagious disease. However, the development of a simple, but sensitive, test for FeLV gs antigens in peripheral blood leukocytes enabled thousands of cats living in their natural environment to be tested for the virus (Hardy *et al.*, 1973a, Hardy, 1976a). Approximately 33% of the healthy cats living in the same household as cats with FeLV-related diseases (such as LSA) were infected with FeLV, whereas all healthy cats living in households with no history of FeLV-related diseases were uninfected, and only 0.31% of stray cats, with an unknown FeLV exposure, were FeLV-infected (Hardy *et al.*, 1973a). FeLV was detected in the urine, saliva, and peripheral blood of infected cats, and is probably spread among cats via the litterbox, by mutual grooming, and possibly by bloodsucking parasites such as the cat flea (Hardy *et al.*, 1973a; Gardner *et al.*, 1971b). In one study, 336 veterinary hospital blood-donor cats were tested for FeLV, and 43 (12.8%) were found to be infected (Hardy, 1976b). The virus is therefore probably spread iatrogenically in addition to the natural methods of transmission. FeLV is also found in the milk and fetuses of infected queens, which is evidence that FeLV is spread congenitally (epigenetically) as well as by contact (Hardy, 1976a).

Once infected, healthy cats were found to have a much greater chance of developing the FeLV-caused diseases than cats in the general cat population, in which the occurrence of FeLV is low (0.1%) (Hardy *et al.*, 1973a). These results, which were confirmed by studies of laboratory cats, prove conclusively that FeLV is a contagious virus and show that surveys of disease development alone are inadequate for determining whether or not the etiological agent is contagious (Schneider, 1970; Jarrett, W. H. F., *et al.*, 1973). There is no evidence for the vertical (genetic) transmission of FeLV from one generation of cats to the next.

163

EPIDEMIOLOGY OF
PRIMARY
NEOPLASMS OF
LYMPHOID TISSUES
IN ANIMALS

WILLIAM D. HARDY,
JR.

3.11.6. Seroepidemiology

The distribution of FeLV-neutralizing antibody and of antibody to FOCMA among cats living in their natural household environments has been found to depend on the environmental exposure of cats to FeLV. These seroepidemiological studies have confirmed the epidemiological suggestions that FeLV is a contagious virus.

a. Distribution of FeLV-Neutralizing Antibody. Of 34 non-FeLV-infected cats with no exposure to FeLV, none was found to have neutralizing antibody. Of 212 FeLV-exposed but uninfected cats, however, 94 (44%) were found to have protective ($\geqslant 1:10$) neutralizing antibody titers. Of 40 uninfected stray cats, with an unknown history of FeLV exposure, only 2 (5%) had neutralizing antibody, while none of the 141 diseased or healthy FeLV-infected cats had developed neutralizing antibody. The development of neutralizing antibody is thus clearly associated with environmental exposure to FeLV (Hardy *et al.*, 1976a).

b. Distribution of FOCMA Antibody. FOCMA antibody is an excellent example of immune surveillance against a naturally occurring tumor. Both FeLV-infected and uninfected cats with protective titers ($\geqslant 1:8$) of FOCMA antibody are resistant to the development of LSA. FeLV-infected cats with protective FOCMA antibody titers will not develop LSA but will be FeLV carriers and shedders for the rest of their lives (Essex *et al.*, 1975a,b). A low incidence of nonprotective titers of FOCMA antibody is found in healthy cats from single-cat households, in which the cat is not usually exposed to other cats, and in healthy cats from multiple-cat households in which there has been no FeLV diseases. The occurrence of protective titers of FOCMA antibody is high, however, in healthy cats from households in which FeLV-related diseases have occurred. These results are further evidence of the contagious nature of FeLV.

3.11.7. Prevention

There is no effective treatment for the diseases caused by FeLV, but the spread of the virus, and its related diseases, in the natural environment can be prevented by the use of a simple FeLV test-and-removal program (Hardy *et al.*, 1974a, 1976b). In this program, all cats living in a household are tested for FeLV, and any infected cats are removed (by euthanasia or isolation) from contact with uninfected healthy cats. The uninfected cats are then quarantined and retested 3 months later. If the uninfected cats are still uninfected in the second test, the cats in the household are considered FeLV-free. If any of the initially uninfected cats are found to be infected in the second FeLV test, they are removed, and a third test is done on the remaining cats 3 months after the second test. When all the cats in a household are negative in two consecutive FeLV tests, done 3 months apart, the cats in the household are considered to be virus-free. This program has been successful in preventing the spread of FeLV and the diseases it causes among pet cats (Hardy *et al.*, 1976b).

The prospects for the development of an FeLV vaccine are excellent. Some cats have already been experimentally vaccinated with a low-dose live virus, with inactivated virus, and with inactivated tumor cells (Hardy *et al.*, 1976a; Jarrett, W., *et al.*, 1974; Olsen *et al.*, 1976). It is likely that FeLV diseases will be prevented in the near future by a combination of the FeLV test-and-removal program and vaccination.

3.11.8. Public Health

165

EPIDEMIOLOGY OF
PRIMARY
NEOPLASMS OF
LYMPHOID TISSUES
IN ANIMALS

FeLV can replicate in human and canine tissue culture cells, and when it is injected into newborn puppies, it causes LSA (Jarrett, O., *et al.*, 1969; Rickard *et al.*, 1969). There is no evidence, however, that FeLV infects people living with FeLV-infected cats (Hardy *et al.*, 1976a). Over 500 people, including some with cancer, have been tested for FeLV and none has been found to be infected. In addition, 100 people have been tested for FeLV-neutralizing antibody, and no antibody has been found in any individual. It is still too early, however, to conclude that there is no danger from FeLV, and immunosuppressed persons and pregnant women should not be exposed to cats infected with this virus (Hardy *et al.*, 1974b). Persons who are frequently exposed to FeLV, such as veterinarians and laboratory personnel, should take all precautions necessary for handling a moderate-risk biohazardous agent.

3.12. Primates

3.12.1. Introduction

There is no information regarding the occurrence of lymphoid tumors in feral nonhuman primates. In a review of spontaneous hematopoietic neoplasms of adult captive nonhuman primates, Lingeman (1969) reported 21 lymphoid tumors and 1 myeloid leukemia. Since Lingeman's report, 98 additional lymphoid tumors have been reported in 87 monkeys and 11 gibbon apes (Lapin, 1973, 1975, 1976; Kawakami *et al.*, 1972; Jones *et al.*, 1972; Snyder *et al.*, 1973; Johnsen *et al.*, 1971; Schneider, 1976). These reports (excluding the 1 case of myeloid leukemia reported by Lingeman) are summarized in Table 10. Three striking epidemics of primate LSA have occurred: (1) In an epidemic at the California Primate Research Center in Davis, California, 43 of 1400 rhesus monkeys developed LSA (Schneider, 1976). (2) In another epidemic at a primate colony in Sukhumi, Russia, 43 of 1480 *Hamadryas* baboons developed lymphatic leukemia (Lapin, 1973, 1975, 1976). (3) In the third epidemic, at the SEATO primate colony, 4 of 120 gibbon apes developed LSA, while 5 other gibbons developed granulocytic leukemia (Kawakami *et al.*, 1972; Johnsen *et al.*, 1971). LSA has occurred in members of 5 of the 11 nonhuman primate families, including Old World rhesus and cynomolgus monkeys and New World woolly, tamarin, and marmoset monkeys (Table 10). Reports of lymphoid tumors in apes are very rare, and these tumors have been observed only in gibbons (Lingeman, 1969; Kawakami *et al.*, 1972, 1973, 1975, 1976; Jones *et al.*, 1972; Snyder *et al.*, 1973; Johnsen *et al.*, 1971; DePaoli and Garner, 1968; DiGiacomo, 1967). Not many gibbons are in captivity compared with the numbers of captive monkeys and other apes, but the occurrence of lymphoid tumors among captive gibbons is extraordinarily high (Walker, 1968). Gibbons are smaller and more agile than other apes, mature sexually in 6–10 years, and have survived as long as 30 years in captivity (Walker, 1968). Gibbons are considered to be man's fourth closest animal relative, and the finding that gibbon LSA is spread contagiously is highly significant. Compared with the number of other types of neoplasms, only a small number of lymphoid neoplasms have been observed in monkeys and apes (Lingeman, 1969).

TABLE 10. Lymphoid Tumors Reported in Subhuman Primates

Primate common name	Number of animals	Average age[a]	Sex[a]	Diagnosis
Monkeys				
Cynomologus	2	NR	1 F, 1 NR	Lymphatic leukemia; lymphosarcoma
Green monkey	4	NR	1 F, 3 NR	Reticulosis, 3; lymphatic leukemia, 1
Stair's monkey	1	NR	NR	Lymphatic leukemia
Rhesus monkey	45	1, 5 yr; 44 NR	1 F, 44 NR	Lymphosarcoma
Woolly monkey	1	NR	NR	Lymphatic leukemia
Galago monkey	1	NR	NR	Lymphatic leukemia
Marmoset monkey	1	NR	NR	Lymphatic leukemia
Tamarin	1	NR	NR	Lymphatic leukemia
Sooty mangabey	1	NR	NR	Lymphosarcoma
Baboon	46	45, >5 yr; 1 NR	2 F	Hodgkin's sarcoma, 1; round-cell sarcoma, 1
			1 M	Reticulosarcoma, 1
			43 NR	Lymphosarcoma, 43
Unspecified	1	NR	NR	Lymphosarcoma
Subtotal:	104			
Apes				
Gibbon ape	15	2 NR: 13 avg 4.1 yr	7 F, 8 M	Lymphosarcoma
Subtotal:	15			
Total:	119			

[a](NR) Not reported.

Tumors have not often been observed in young primates. For example, 800,000 young monkeys, most of them rhesus monkeys, were imported into the United States between 1957 and 1960 for the production and testing of polio vaccine. Many of these animals were retained for only a few weeks, were used as donors for kidneys for cell cultures, and were subjected to extensive clinical examinations and necropsies. Only 1 solid tumor and 1 possible LSA were noted in this large group of young monkeys (Newberne and Robinson, 1960; Jungherr, 1963).

Both oncornaviruses and herpesviruses cause LSA in primates, although in many of the cases, no etiological agent is known. For the sake of convenience, I will divide my discussion of LSA into the naturally occurring LSAs of monkeys and gibbon apes and the experimentally induced herpesvirus LSAs.

3.12.2 Naturally Occurring Lymphosarcoma

a. Rhesus Monkey. *Incidence.* Stowell *et al.* (1971) reported that in a 25-month period, 24 rhesus monkeys living at the National Center for Primate Biology in Davis, California, had developed LSA. This is an incidence rate of 1200 cases per 100,000 adult rhesus monkeys. Of the 24 monkeys, 21 were adults, 17 were females, and all but 5 were imported from India. There was no known exposure to chemical carcinogenic agents, but 10 of the 24 monkeys had been used in experiments involving the inoculation of malaria parasites *(Plasmodium cynomolgi)*, followed by successful antimalarial therapy.

167

EPIDEMIOLOGY OF
PRIMARY
NEOPLASMS OF
LYMPHOID TISSUES
IN ANIMALS

Additional data on the outbreak of LSA in rhesus monkeys at the California Primate Research Center were recently reported (Schneider, 1976). During the 5-year period from February 1969 to May 1974, the average rhesus monkey population at the center was 1000. A total of 43 cases of LSA were observed during this period; 7 of the animals who developed LSA were born in the colony, 36 were not. Reanalysis of the outbreak indicated that the incidence rate was 1000 cases per 100,000 rhesus monkeys per year. This is an unusually high occurrence of LSA, and to this author it suggests that a contagious etiological agent may be involved.

Tissues Involved. Tumors were found in several different organs, including the heart, lymph nodes, kidneys, intestines, spleen, liver, lungs, CNS, muscle, retroorbital tissue, and skeletal muscle. The tumors were classified as LSA composed of differentiated lymphoid cells.

Etiology. Herpeslike virus was isolated from the tumor cells or peripheral leukocytes from 3 animals. The disease was transmitted to an immunosuppressed rhesus monkey by inoculation of tumor cells. Disseminated LSA developed 3 months later, but there has been no cell-free transmission of the disease to date.

Comparison with Burkitt's Lymphoma. The LSA of the rhesus monkey resembles Burkitt's lymphoma of man in that both diseases occur in many of the same organs, there is an identical histopathological appearance, a reticuloendothelial reaction is associated with malaria infection, and there appears to be an association with herpes-type viruses. There are also some differences between the diseases; for instance, rhesus LSA does not primarily affect juveniles, does not involve the mandible, and involves the peripheral lymph nodes more often than does Burkitt's tumor.

b. *Hamadryas* **Baboons**. *Incidence.* Lapin (1973, 1975, 1976) has repeatedly reported on a continuing outbreak of LSA in *Hamadryas* baboons kept at the Institute of Experimental Pathology and Therapy of the USSR Academy of Medical Sciences in Sukhumi. The outbreak began at the end of 1967 and has continued to the present time. Of 1480 baboons, 43 (2.9%) developed the disease.

Clinical Findings. LSA in the baboons at the Sukhumi colony developed without clinical signs and became evident only in its terminal stage. The reports gave only a cursory description of the clinical or pathological features of the disease. However, lymphoblasts appeared in the peripheral blood and there was involvement of the spleen, lymph nodes, bone marrow, and intestinal tract.

Etiology. The etiological agent was reported to be an oncornavirus. Lapin (1973, 1975, 1976) observed numerous oncornavirus particles in plasma, urinary sediments, kidneys, lungs, salivary glands, bone marrow, and tumor tissue. He inoculated 8 monkeys with urine sediment from a baboon with LSA, and 4 have subsequently developed LSA (Lapin, 1976).

Recently, a herpesvirus, immunologically similar to Epstein–Barr virus, was also isolated from cells of a continuous lymphoblastoid cell line established from a baboon with LSA (Lapin, 1976). Healthy baboons in contact with baboons with LSA have antibodies to this herpesvirus, but the etiological significance of the herpesvirus is unknown.

Epidemiology. The baboons of the colony have been inbred, and 80% of them are descendants of 3 breeders. The disease appears to spread via contact, since all animals that developed LSA did so after being in contact with a baboon who had developed the disease. Genetic transmission seems unlikely because some nonrelated baboons introduced into the colony after the beginning of the outbreak also developed disease (Lapin, 1973, 1975, 1976). A few newborn baboons had LSA at birth. It appears that horizontal contagious transmission of an infectious agent by contact and by the epigenetic route occurred in this colony.

c. **Gibbon Apes.** *Incidence.* All reported lymphoid tumors of apes have occurred in one species, *Hyobates,* the gibbon. Only 3 cases were reported in gibbons up until 1969, and Lingeman concluded from these 3 cases that the frequency of LSA in gibbon apes was exceptionally high for the number of gibbons in captivity (Lingeman, 1969). Newberne and Robinson (1960) first described LSA in a male gibbon of unknown age. DiGiacomo (1967) described a LSA that was indistinguishable from Burkitt's lymphoma in a female gibbon, and DePaoli and Garner (1968) reported acute lymphocytic leukemia in a 1½-year-old male gibbon. Additional lymphoid and myeloid tumors have occurred in captive gibbons, and recent articles report that gibbon hematopoietic neoplasms have occurred in clusters in some colonies. Johnsen *et al.* (1971) reported that 4 gibbons in a total population of 120 developed LSA at the SEATO colony in Bangkok, Thailand, in a period of 16 months. More recently, DePaoli *et al.* (1973) reported that 5 other gibbons from the same colony developed granulocytic leukemia. In a different colony at the San Francisco Medical Center, 2 cases of LSA were found in 6 gibbons that had all been imported at the same time (Snyder *et al.,* 1973). The tumor cells were found in the lymph nodes, liver, and bone marrow, and were predominantly prolymphocytes.

Etiology. Electron microscopy revealed typical C-type oncornaviruses in lymph nodes, spleen, liver, and bone marrow. Primary cell cultures initiated from these gibbon tumor cells produced numerous oncornavirus particles that had a density of 1.16 g/ml, a 70 S RNA, and a reverse transcriptase, and which incorporated [^{3}H]uridine (Kawakami *et al.,* 1972, 1975, 1976). Immunological analysis of the virus revealed a unique p30 species-specific antigen (gs-1), which is not found in the known mammalian C-type oncornaviruses of the cat, mouse, rat, or hamster (Kawakami *et al.,* 1975; Parks *et al.,* 1973). The gibbon virus does possess, however, the interspecies p30 antigen (gs-3), which is common to most mammalian C-type oncornaviruses (Parks *et al.,* 1973). Antigenic analysis of the p30 (gs-1) antigens of the gibbon leukemia virus and the simian sarcoma virus (SSV), previously isolated from a naturally occurring fibrosarcoma of a pet woolly monkey, showed that these antigens were identical (Kawakami *et al.,* 1975; Parks *et al.,* 1973; Theilen *et al.,* 1971; Kawakami and Buckley, 1974). Thus, for the first time, two oncogenic oncornaviruses from the same species (although two different primates) were found to have identical p30 gs-1 species-specific antigenic determinants. The gibbon leukemia virus was subsequently isolated from or detected in tumor tissues of 6 leukemic gibbons, but not from tissues of 16 normal gibbons or from 3 LSAs and 3 sarcomas of rhesus monkeys (Kawakami *et al.,* 1975; Parks *et al.,* 1973).

Seroepidemiology. Kawakami *et al.* (1975) found naturally occurring neutralizing antibody to the gibbon leukemia virus in 13 of 89 gibbons from colonies in which animals had previously developed LSA, but in only 2 of 44 gibbons from colonies in which the disease had not previously occurred. This is strong evidence, along with the clustering of cases of gibbon leukemia, for the contagious nature of the gibbon ape leukemia virus.

169

EPIDEMIOLOGY OF
PRIMARY
NEOPLASMS OF
LYMPHOID TISSUES
IN ANIMALS

Kawakami *et al.* (1976) also studied the response of 3 young gibbons to inoculation of the gibbon leukemia virus. All 3 gibbons developed plasma viremia, 1 week after the first inoculation, that persisted for 4 weeks. Neutralizing antibody was detectable after the second week, and reached a maximum between the fourth and sixth weeks before diminishing. Of the 3 gibbons, 2 subsequently developed plasma viremia, which has persisted for over a year in the absence of neutralizing antibody. Although the gibbons initially developed neutralizing antibody, they were unable to clear the virus and became persistently viremic. Kawakami *et al.* (1976) concluded that LSA occurred, not because of an inherent absence of an immune response to the virus, but because of an inability to maintain a virus-free state following the initial immune response.

3.12.3. Experimentally Induced Herpesvirus Lymphosarcomas

During the last few years, two oncogenic simian herpesviruses, Herpesvirus saimiri and Herpesvirus ateles, have been found experimentally to induce LSA in a variety of nonhuman primates. It must be emphasized that the oncogenicity of these viruses has been demonstrated only by experimental inoculation into other nonhuman primate species, and that there is no evidence that these viruses induce LSA in any nonhuman primate under natural conditions.

a. Incidence in Natural Hosts. *Herpesvirus saimiri (HVS).* HVS was first isolated in 1968 from a normal squirrel monkey kidney-cell culture (Meléndez *et al.*, 1968). Since then, many different isolates of HVS have been made from other squirrel monkey kidney cultures. It has also been found that 50–70% of recently captured feral squirrel monkeys have neutralizing antibody to HVS (Fraser and Meléndez, 1974). HVS induces a latent infection in the squirrel monkey, but no naturally occurring LSA has been found in this species, even though a high percentage of these monkeys are chronically infected (Falk *et al.*, 1972a,b). HVS infection is transmitted horizontally, probably via oropharyngeal secretions (Fraser and Meléndez, 1974).

It is unlikely that interspecies (primate) spread of HVS occurs in nature because squirrel monkeys, the natural host species, and owl monkeys and marmosets, the LSA-susceptible species, occupy different ecological niches. Natural HVS infection and LSA development occurred, however, in a group of imported owl monkeys (Hunt *et al.*, 1973). The explanation for this rare occurrence is that trappers frequently mix small lots of primates of different species, and the owl monkeys that developed LSA were probably kept together with squirrel monkeys shortly after their capture.

Herpesvirus ateles (HVA). HVA was isolated from kidney-cell cultures from a healthy spider monkey (Meléndez *et al.*, 1972). Numerous HVA isolates were subsequently made from kidney-cell cultures and from peripheral lymphocytes of spider monkeys (Fraser and Meléndez, 1974). The distribution of HVA in its natural host, the spider monkey, has not been studied.

b. Experimental Oncogenicity. HVS and HVA cause LSA after experimental infection of several primate species that are closely related to the natural hosts. Some HVS-infected marmosets as well as some HVS-infected owl monkeys developed LSA with a leukemic blood profile (Meléndez *et al.*, 1973; Wolfe *et al.*, 1971). The disease is disseminated, with LSA involving the liver, kidneys, spleen, lymph nodes, thymus, bone marrow, and other organs. Not all marmosets or owl monkeys develop LSA after inoculation with HVS or HVA; some develop only a latent infection.

The disease can be transmitted by inoculating pure HVS or HVA or blood from a monkey with LSA into a susceptible monkey. Koch's postulates have been fulfilled, since virus can be reisolated from the monkeys that develop LSA (Laufs and Fleckenstein, 1973; Laufs, 1976). Whereas HVS regularly caused a latent infection in common marmosets, HVA induced LSA in the same species. After dual infection with HVS and HVA, common marmosets developed LSA (Laufs, 1976). A host-specific factor appeared to modify the effects of HVS in these animals.

Both HVS and HVA are lymphotropic viruses, and infected monkeys carry the HVS and HVA genomes in their circulating lymphocytes in a repressed form. Oncogenic HVS or HVA can be isolated from their natural hosts, from latently infected monkeys, and from tumor-bearing animals by cocultivation of overtly or latently infected cells with permissive cells from marmosets or owl monkeys (Laufs, 1976). The T lymphocyte is probably the target cell for infection and transformation by these viruses (Laufs, 1976). HVS is also oncogenic in a nonprimate species, the New Zealand white rabbit, in which it produces LSA.

c. **Prevention.** Two types of experimental HVS and HVA vaccines have been developed and are effective in preventing LSA induction by these viruses. Killed vaccines were prepared by heat or formaldehyde inactivation of HVS and HVA (Laufs, 1976; Laufs and Steinke, 1975a). These vaccines proved to be safe in 121 vaccinated monkeys of four different species (Laufs and Steinke, 1975a). The protection against HVS can be passively transferred by serum from a vaccinated monkey (Laufs and Steinke, 1975b).

Attenuated live HVS was isolated after several passages of wild-type HVS in cell culture at 39°C. This attentuated virus was inoculated into cotton-top marmosets and squirrel monkeys, and none of the vaccinated monkeys developed LSA after challenge, even though they became persistently infected with the vaccine HVS (Laufs, 1976).

d. **Relevance to Man.** There is strong evidence that herpesviruses cause Burkitt's lymphoma and nasopharyngeal carcinoma in man (Klein, 1973). The experimental manipulation of nonhuman primate LSA induced by herpesvirus will certainly add to our understanding of human oncogenic herpesviruses. For example, the use of killed HVS and HVA vaccines as well as DNA-free viral membrane vaccines will yield data on the safety and efficiency of these vaccines that may be useful in the possible development of similar human herpesvirus vaccines. Also, a complete understanding of the immune response and host factors in HVS- and HVA-infected monkeys may aid similar studies in man. The study of these oncogenic herpesviruses in nonhuman primates raises expectations for the eventual understanding and control of viral-induced lymphoid cancers in man.

3.13. Human

Although I have reviewed LSA in animals other than man, a few general comments comparing the disease in different species are in order. The discovery that oncogenic viruses are contagious in cats, cattle, and primates is of basic importance to our concepts concerning the possibility that some tumors in humans

171

EPIDEMIOLOGY OF
PRIMARY
NEOPLASMS OF
LYMPHOID TISSUES
IN ANIMALS

may also be contagious. There are epidemiological studies (see other chapters in this volume) that suggest that Burkitt's lymphoma, Hodgkin's disease, and some leukemias may be caused by a contagious agent or agents. It is encouraging that test-and-removal control methods in cats and cattle are able to reduce the spread of oncornaviruses and prevent the development of LSA in these species. Also, studies of animals show that the DNA-herpesvirus-induced LSA in chickens and the FeLV-induced LSA of cats can be prevented by vaccination. It is thus possible that vaccination against a putative oncogenic virus of humans may be feasible.

ACKNOWLEDGMENTS

This work was supported by National Cancer Institute Grants CA-16599, CA-18488, and CA-08748, and the Cancer Research Institute. Dr. Hardy is a Scholar of the Leukemia Society of America, Inc.

The author thanks Dr. A. J. McClelland for assistance in the preparation of this manuscript.

References

Abt, D. A., Marshak, R. R., Kulp, H. W., and Pollock, R. J., Jr., 1970, Studies on the relationship between lymphocytosis and bovine leukosis, in: *Comparative Leukemia Research* (R. M. Dutcher, ed.), pp. 527–536, Karger, Basel.

Aoki, T., Boyse, E. A., and Old, L. J., 1968, Wild-type Gross leukemia virus. III. Serological tests as indicators of leukemia risk, *J. Natl. Cancer Inst.* 41:103–110.

Ambrose, K. R., and Coggin, J. H., Jr., 1975, An epizootic in hamsters of lymphomas of undetermined origin and mode of transmission, *J. Natl. Cancer Inst.* 54:877–880.

Anderson, L. J., and Jarrett, W. F. H., 1968, Lymphosarcoma (leukemia) in cattle, sheep and pigs in Great Britain, *Cancer* 22:398–405.

Andervont, H. B., and Dunn, T. B.: 1962, Occurrence of tumors in wild house mice, *J. Natl. Cancer Inst.* 28:1153–1163.

Armstrong, J. A., Porterfield, J. S., and DeMadrid, A. T., 1971, C-type virus particles in pig kidney cell lines, *J. Gen. Virol.* 10:195–198.

August, J. T., Bolognesi, D. P., Fleissner, E., Gilden, R. V., and Nowinski, R. C., 1974, A proposed nomenclature for the virion proteins of oncogenic RNA viruses, *Virology* 60:595–600.

Balls, M., 1965a, Lymphosarcoma in the South African clawed toad, *Xenopus laevis:* A virus tumor, *Ann. N. Y. Acad. Sci.* 126:256–273.

Balls, M., 1965b, The incidence of pathologic abnormalities including spontaneous lymphosarcomas in a laboratory stock of *Xenopus* (the South African clawed toad), *Cancer Res.* 25:3–6.

Balls, M., and Ruben, L. N., 1967, The transmission of lymphosarcoma in *Xenopus laevis,* the South African clawed toad, *Cancer Res.* 27:654–659.

Baltimore, D., 1970, Viral RNA-dependent DNA polymerase, *Nature (London)* 226:1209–1211.

Banfield, W. G., 1969, Hamster lymphoma, TM, *Natl. Cancer Inst. Monogr.* 32:335–336.

Banfield, W. G., Woke, P. A., MacKay, C. M., and Cooper, H. L., 1965, Mosquito transmission of a reticulum cell sarcoma of hamsters, *Science* 148:1239–1240.

Banfield, W. G., Woke, P. A., and MacKay, C. M., 1966, Mosquito transmission of lymphomas, *Cancer* 19:1333–1336.

Bärtsch, D. C., Springher, F., and Falk, H., 1975, Acute nonlymphocytic leukemia, *J. Am. Med. Assoc.* 232:1333–1336.

Baumgartener, L. E., Olson, C., Miller, J. M., and Van Der Maaten, M. J., 1975, Survey for antibodies to leukemia (C-type) virus in cattle, *J. Am. Vet. Med. Assoc.* 166:249–251.

Beasley, J. N., Patterson, L. T., and McWade, D. H., 1970, Transmission of Marek's disease by poultry house dust and chicken dander, *Am. J. Vet. Res.* 31:339–344.

Bendixen, H. J., 1960, Untersuchungen über die Rinderleukose in Dänemark, *Dtsch. Tieraerztl. Wochenschr.* 67:4–7.

Bendixen, H. J., 1963, Preventive measures in cattle leukemia: Leukosis enzootic bovis, *Ann. N. Y. Acad. Sci.* **108**:1241–1267.

Bendixen, H. J., 1967, Epizootiology, diagnosis, and control of bovine leukosis, *Bull. Off. Int. Epizoot.* **68**:73–99.

Bendixen, H. J., 1969, Preventive measures in cattle leukemia: Leukosis enzootic bovis, *Natl. Cancer Inst. Monogr.* **39**:1241–1267.

Bendixen, H. J., 1973, Epidemiological studies of enzootic bovine leukosis associated with the public control program in Denmark, 1959–1971, in: *Unifying Concepts of Leukemia* (R. M. Dutcher and L. Chieco-Bianchi, eds.), pp. 215–219, Karger, Basel.

Benveniste, R. E., and Todaro, G. J., 1974, Evolution of type-C viral genes: Inheritance of exogenously acquired viral genes, *Nature (London)* **252**:456–459.

Brandly, P. J., and Migaki, G., 1963, Types of tumors found by Federal meat inspectors in an eight-year survey, *Ann. N. Y. Acad. Sci.* **108**:872–879.

Brick, J. O., Roenigk, W. J., and Wilson, G. P., 1968, Chemotherapy of malignant lymphoma in dogs and cats, *J. Am. Vet. Med. Assoc.* **153**:47–52.

Brindley, D. C., and Banfield, W. G., 1961, A contagious tumor of the hamster, *J. Natl. Cancer Inst.* **26**:949–957.

Brodey, R. S., McDonough, S., Frye, F. L., and Hardy, W. D., Jr., 1970, Epidemiology of feline leukemia, in: *Comparative Leukemia Research* (R. M. Dutcher, ed.), pp. 333–342, Karger, Basel.

Brown, E. R., Keith, L., Hazdra, J. J., and Arndt, T., 1975, Tumors in fish caught in polluted waters: Possible explanations, in: *Comparative Leukemia Research 1973* (Y. Ito and R. M. Dutcher, eds.), pp. 47–57, Karger, Basel.

Bruner, D. W., and Gillespie, J. H., 1973, *Hagan's Infectious Diseases of Domestic Animals,* 6th Ed., Cornell University Press, Ithaca and London.

Bullock, F. D., and Curtis, M. R., 1930, Spontaneous tumors of the rat, *J. Cancer Res.* **14**:1–115.

Burkitt, D., and O'Conor, G. T., 1961, Malignant lymphoma in African children. I. A clinical syndrome, *Cancer* **14**:258–269.

Burmester, B. R., 1956, The shedding of the virus of visceral lymphomatosis in the saliva and the feces of normal and lymphomatous chickens, *Poult. Sci.* **35**:1089–1099.

Burmester, B. R., 1968, Current status of avian leukosis complex, *Southwest Vet.* **21**:131–138.

Burmester, B. R., and Gentry, R. F., 1954a, The transmission of avian visceral lymphomatosis by contact, *Cancer Res.* **14**:34–42.

Burmester, B. R., and Gentry, R. F., 1954b, A study of possible avenues of infection with virus of avian visceral lymphomatosis, *Proc. Am. Vet. Med. Assoc.* 311–316.

Burmester, B. R., and Purchase, H. G., 1970, Occurrence, transmission and oncogenic spectrum of the avian leukosis viruses, in: *Comparative Leukemia Research 1969* (R. M. Dutcher, ed.), pp. 83–95, Karger, Basel.

Caldwell, G. G. Baumgartener, L., Carter, C., Cotter, S., Currier, R., Essex, M., Hardy, W., Olson, C., and Olsen, R., 1976, Seroepidemiologic testing in man for evidence of antibodies to feline leukemia virus and bovine leukemia virus, in: *Comparative Leukemia Research 1975* (J. Clemmesen and D. S. Yohn, eds.), pp. 238–241, Karger, Basel.

Callahan, R., Lieber, M. M., Todaro, G. J., Graves, D. C., and Ferrer, J. F., 1976, Bovine leukemia virus genes in the DNA of leukemic cattle, *Science* **192**:1005–1007.

Campbell, J. G., 1969, *Tumours of the Fowl,* J. B. Lippincott, Philadelphia.

Casarett, G. W., 1965, Experimental radiation carcinogenesis, *Prog. Exp. Tumor Res.* **7**:49–76.

Cohen, D., Booth, S., and Sussman, O., 1959, An epidemiological study of canine lymphoma and its public health significance, *Am. J. Vet. Res.* **20**:1026–1031.

Cohen, D., Reif, J. S., Brodey, R. S., and Keiser, H., 1974, Epidemiological analysis of the most prevalent sites and types of canine neoplasia observed in a veterinary hospital, *Cancer Res.* **34**:2859–2868.

Congdon, C. C., and Lorenz, E., 1954, Leukemia in guinea pigs, *Am. J. Pathol.* **30**:337–359.

Cotchin, E., 1960, Tumours of farm animals, *Vet. Rec.* **72**:816–823.

Cotter, S. M., Hardy, W. D., Jr., and Essex, M., 1975, Association of feline leukemia virus with lymphosarcoma and other disorders in the cat, *J. Am. Vet. Med. Assoc.* **166**:449–454.

Crain, R. C., 1958, Spontaneous tumors in the Rochester strain of the Wistar rat, *Am. J. Pathol.* **34**:311–335.

Crighton, G. W., 1969, Lymphosarcoma in the cat, *Vet. Rec.* **84**:329–331.

Crittenden, L. B., 1976, The epidemiology of avian lymphoid leukosis, *Cancer Res.* **36**:570–573.

173

EPIDEMIOLOGY OF
PRIMARY
NEOPLASMS OF
LYMPHOID TISSUES
IN ANIMALS

Crittenden, L. B., Stone, H. A., Reamer, R. H., and Okazaki, W., 1967, Two loci controlling genetic cellular resistance to avian leukosis-sarcoma viruses, *J. Virol.* **5**:898–904.

Dalton, A. J., Melnick, J. L., Bauer, H., Beaudreau, G., Bentzvelzen, P., Bolognesi, D., Gallo, R., Graffi, A., Haguenau, F., Heston, W., Huebner, R., Todaro, G., and Heine, U. I., 1974, The case for a family of reverse transcriptase viruses: Retraviridae, *Intervirology* **4**:201–206.

Dawe, C. J., 1969, Neoplasms of blood cell origin in poikilothermic animals—A review, *Natl. Cancer Inst. Monogr.* **32**:7–28.

DePaoli, A., and Garner, F. M., 1968, Acute lymphocytic leukemia in a white-cheeked gibbon *(Hylobates concolor)*, *Cancer Res.* **28**:2559–2561.

DePaoli, A., Johnsen, D. O., and Noll, W. W., 1973, Granulocytic leukemia in whitehanded gibbons, *J. Am. Vet. Med. Assoc.* **163**:624–628.

DiGiacomo, R. F., 1967, Burkitt's lymphoma in a whitehanded gibbon *(Hylobates lar)*, *Cancer Res.* **27**:1178–1179.

Dorn, C. R., Taylor, D. O. N., and Hibbard, H. H., 1967, Epizootic characteristics of canine and feline leukemia and lymphoma, *Am. J. Vet. Res.* **28**:993–1001.

Dorn, C. R., Taylor, D. O. N., Frye, F. L., and Hibbard, H. H., 1968a, Survey of animal neoplasma in Alameda and Contra Costa counties, California. I. Methodology and description of cases, *J. Natl. Cancer Inst.* **40**:295–305.

Dorn, C. R., Taylor, D. O. N., Schneider, R., Hibbard, H. H., and Klauber, M. R., 1968b, Survey of animal neoplasms in Alameda and Contra Costa counties, California. II. Cancer morbidity in dogs and cats from Alameda county, *J. Natl. Cancer Inst.* **40**:307–318.

Dungworth, D. L., Theilen, G. H., and Lengyel, J., 1964, Bovine lymphosarcoma in California. II. The thymic form, *Pathol. Vet.* **1**:323–350.

Dunn, T. B., 1954, Normal and pathologic anatomy of the reticular tissue in laboratory mice, with a classification and discussion of neoplasms, *J. Natl. Cancer Inst.* **14**:1281–1433.

Dunn, T. B., and Andervont, H. B., 1963, Histology of some neoplasms and non-neoplastic lesions found in wild mice maintained under laboratory conditons, *J. Natl. Cancer Inst.* **31**:873–885.

Enke, K. H., Jungwitz, M., and Rossger, M., 1964, Ein kasuistischer Beitrag zur lymphatischen Leukose des Schafes, *Dtsch. Tieraerztl. Wochenschr.* **68**:359–364.

Essex, M., and Francis, D. P., 1976, The risk to humans from malignant diseases of their pets: An unsettled issue, *J. Am. Anim. Hosp. Assoc.* **12**:386–390.

Essex, M., Klein, G., Snyder, S. P., and Harrold, J. B., 1971, Feline sarcoma virus (FSV) induced tumors: Correlation between humoral antibody and tumor regression, *Nature (London)* **233**:195–196.

Essex, M., Sliski, A., Cotter, S. M., Jakowski, R. M., and Hardy, W. D., Jr., 1975a, Immunosurveillance of naturally occurring feline leukemia, *Science* **190**:790–792.

Essex, M., Jakowski, R. M., Hardy, W. D., Jr., Cotter, S. M., Hess, P., and Sliski, A., 1975b, Feline oncornavirus-associated cell membrane antigen. III. Antibody titers in cats from leukemia cluster households, *J. Natl. Cancer Inst.* **54**:637–641.

Falk, L. A., Wolfe, L. G., and Deinhardt, F., 1972a, Herpesvirus saimiri (HVS): Incidence of latent infection in squirrel monkeys, *Fed. Proc. Fed. Am. Soc. Exp. Biol.* **31**:806.

Falk, L. A., Wolfe, L. G., and Deinhardt, F., 1972b, Isolation of *Herpesvirus saimiri* from blood of squirrel monkeys *(Saimiri sciureus)*, *J. Natl. Cancer Inst.* **48**:1499–1505.

Feldman, W. H., and Olson, C., 1965, Neoplastic diseases of the chicken, in: *Diseases of Poultry* (H. E. Biester and L. H. Schwarte, eds.), pp. 863–924, The Iowa State University Press, Ames.

Ferrer, J. F., 1972, Antigenic comparison of bovine type-C virus with murine and feline leukemia viruses, *Cancer Res.* **32**:1871–1877.

Ferrer, J. F., and Bhatt, D. M., 1973, Occurrence of fluorescent and precipitin antibodies to a bovine C-type virus (BLV) among the cattle population, *Proc. Am. Assoc. Cancer Res.* **14**:118.

Ferrer, J. F. Stock, N. D., and Lin, P. S., 1971, Detection of replicating C-type viruses in continuous cell cultures established from cows with leukemia: Effect of the culture medium, *J. Natl. Cancer Inst.* **27**:613–621.

Ferrer, J. F., Avila, L., and Stock, N. D., 1972, Serological detection of type-C viruses found in bovine cultures, *Cancer Res.* **32**:1864–1870.

Ferrer, J. F., Bhatt, D. M., Marshak, R. R., and Abt, D. A., 1975, Further studies on the antigenic properties and distribution of the putative bovine leukemia virus, in: *Comparative Leukemia Research 1973* (Y. Ito and R. M. Dutcher, eds.), pp. 59–66, University of Tokyo Press, Tokyo/Karger, Basel.

Fraser, C. E. O., and Meléndez, L. V., 1974, The oncogenic herpesviruses, in: *Handbook of Laboratory Animal Science* (E. C. Melby, Jr., and N. H. Altman, eds.), pp. 48–60, CRC Press, Cleveland.

Fujita, D. J., Chen, Y. C., Friis, R. R., and Vogt, P. K., 1974, RNA tumor viruses of pheasants: Characterization of avian leukosis subgroups F and G, *Virology* **60**:558–571.

Gallo, R. C., and Todaro, G. J., 1976, Oncogenic RNA viruses, *Semin. Oncol.* **3**:81–95.

Gardner, M. B., Officer, J. E., Rongey, R. W., Estes, J. D., Turner, H. C., and Huebner, R. J., 1971a, C-type RNA tumour virus genome expression in wild house mice, *Nature (London)* **232**:617–620.

Gardner, M. B., Rongey, R. W., Johnson, E. Y., De Journett, R., and Huebner, R. J., 1971b, C-type virus particles in salivary tissue of domestic cats, *J. Natl. Cancer Inst.* **47**:561–565.

Gardner, M. B., Henderson, B. E., Rongey, R. W., Estes, J. D., and Huebner, R. J., 1973a, Spontaneous tumors of aging wild house mice: Incidence, pathology, and C-type virus expression, *J. Natl. Cancer Inst.* **50**:719–726.

Gardner, M. B., Henderson, B. E., Estes, J. D., Menck, H., Parker, J. C., and Huebner, R. J., 1973b, Unusually high incidence of spontaneous lymphomas in wild house mice, *J. Natl. Cancer Inst.* **50**:1571–1575.

Gardner, M. B., Klement, V., Rasheed, S., Rongey, R. W., Brown, J. C., Pike, M., Henderson, B. E., and Huebner, R. J., 1976a, The pathogenesis of lymphoma and paralysis in wild mice, in: *Comparative Leukemia Research 1975* (J. Clemmesen and D. S. Yohn, eds.), pp. 204–208, Karger, Basel.

Gardner, M. B., Henderson, B. E., Estes, J. D., Rongey, R. W., Casagrandre, J., Pike, M., and Huebner, R. J., 1976b, The epidemiology and virology of C-type virus-associated hematological cancers and related diseases in wild mice, *Cancer Res.* **36**:574–581.

Geering, G., Hardy, W. D., Jr., Old, L. J., DeHarven, E., and Brodey, R. S., 1968, Shared group-specific antigen of murine and feline leukemia viruses, *Virology* **36**:678–680.

Geering, G., Aoki, T., and Old, L. J., 1970, Shared viral antigen of mammalian leukemia viruses, *Nature (London)* **226**:265–266.

Gilden, R. V., Oroszlan, S., and Huebner, R. J., 1971, Coexistance of intraspecies and interspecies specific antigenic determinants on the major structural polypeptide of mammalian C-type viruses, *Nature (London)* **231**:107–108.

Gilden, R. V., Long, C. W., Hanson, M., Toni, R., Charman, H. P., Oroszlan, S., Miller, J. M., and Van Der Maatan, M. J., 1975, Characteristics of the major internal protein and RNA dependent DNA polymerase of bovine leukemia virus, *J. Gen. Virol.* **29**:305–314.

Graffi, A., Schramm, T., Bender, E., Graffi, I., Horn, K.-H., and Bierwolf: D., 1968, Cell-free transmissible leukoses in Syrian hamsters, probably of viral aetiology, *Br. J. Cancer* **22**:577–581.

Gross, L., 1951, Pathogenic properties, and "vertical" transmission of the mouse leukemia agent, *Proc. Soc. Exp. Biol. Med.* **78**:342–348.

Gross, L., 1970a, *Oncogenic Viruses*, 2nd Ed., Pergamon Press, New York.

Gross, L., 1970b, Specific, active, intradermal immunization against leukemia in guinea pigs, *Acta Haematol.* **44**:1–10.

Gross, L., 1971, Studies on the nature of acquired immunity against leukemia in guinea pigs, *Acta Haematol.* **45**:218–231.

Gross, L., Dreyfuss, Y., Ehrenreich, T., and Moore, L. A., 1970, Experimental studies on leukemia in guinea pigs, *Acta. Haematol.* **43**:193–209.

Gross, P. A., Fong, C. K. Y., and Hsiung, G. D., 1973, Characterization of guinea pig C-type virus, *Proc. Soc. Exp. Biol. Med.* **143**:367–370.

Hardy, W. D., Jr., 1974a, Management of lymphosarcoma, in: *Current Veterinary Therapy*, Vol. V (R. W. Kirk, ed.), pp. 381–387, W. B. Saunders, Philadelphia.

Hardy, W. D., Jr., 1974b, Immunology of oncornaviruses, *Vet. Clin. North Am.* **4**:133–146.

Hardy, W. D., Jr., 1976a, The etiology of canine and feline tumors, *J. Am. Anim. Hosp. Assoc.* **12**:313–334.

Hardy, W. D., Jr., 1976b, (unpublished).

Hardy W. D., Jr., and Old L. J., 1970, L-Asparaginase in the treatment of neoplastic diseases of the dog, cat and cow, *Recent Results Cancer Res.* **33**:131–139.

Hardy, W. D., Jr., Geering, G., Old, L. J., DeHarven, E., Brodey, R. S., and McDonough, S., 1969, Feline leukemia virus: Occurrence of viral antigen in the tissues of cats with lymphosarcoma and other diseases, *Science* **166**:1019–1021.

Hardy, W. D., Jr., Old, L. J., Hess, P. W., Essex, M., and Cotter, S. M., 1973a, Horizontal transmission of feline leukemia virus, *Nature (London)* **244**:266–269.

175

EPIDEMIOLOGY OF
PRIMARY
NEOPLASMS OF
LYMPHOID TISSUES
IN ANIMALS

Hardy, W. D., Jr., Hirshaut, Y., and Hess, P., 1973b, Detection of the feline leukemia virus and other mammalian oncornaviruses by immunofluorescence, in: *Unifying Concepts of Leukemia* (R. M. Dutcher and L. Chieco-Bianchi, eds.), pp. 778–799, Karger, Basel.

Hardy, W. D., Jr., McClelland, A. J., Hess, P. W., and MacEwen, E. G., 1974a, Veterinarians and the control of feline leukemia virus, *J. Am. Anim. Hosp. Assoc.* **10**:367–372.

Hardy, W. D., Jr., McClelland, A. J., Hess, P. W., and MacEwen, E. G., 1974b, Feline leukemia virus and public health awareness, *J. Am. Vet. Med. Assoc.* **165**:1020–1021.

Hardy, W. D., Jr., Hess, P. W., MacEwen, E. G., McClelland, A. J., Zuckerman, E. E., Essex, M., Cotter, S. M., and Jarrett, O., 1976a, Biology of feline leukemia virus in the natural environment, *Cancer Res.* **36**:582–588.

Hardy, W. D., Jr., McClelland, A. J., Zuckerman, E. E., Hess, P. W., Essex, M., Cotter, S. M., MacEwen, E. G., and Hayes, A. A., 1976b, Prevention of the contagious spread of feline leukemia virus and the development of leukemia in pet cats, *Nature (London)* **263**:326–328.

Hare, W. C. D., Marshak, R. R., Abt, D. A., Dutcher, R. M., and Crowshaw, J. E., Jr., 1964, Bovine lymphosarcoma: A review of studies on cattle in the eastern United States, *Can. Vet. J.* **5**:180–198.

Harshbarger, J. C., and Dawe, C. J., 1973, Hematopoietic neoplasms in invertebrate and poikilothermic vertebrate animals, in: *Unifying Concepts of Leukemia* (R. M. Dutcher and L. Chieco-Bianchi, eds.), pp. 1–25, Karger, Basel.

Helmboldt, C. F., and Frederickson, T. N., 1969, The avian leukosis complex, *Natl. Cancer Inst. Monogr.* **32**:29–39.

Howard, E. B., and Nielsen, S. W., 1965, Neoplasia of the boxer dog, *Am. J. Vet. Res.* **26**:1121–1131.

Hsiung, G. D., 1972, Activation of guinea pig C-type virus in cultured spleen cells by 5-bromo-2'-deoxyuridine, *J. Natl. Cancer Inst.* **49**:567–570.

Hsiung, G. D., and Kaplow, L. S., 1969, Herpes-like virus isolated from spontaneously degenerated tissue culture derived from leukemia susceptible guinea pigs, *J. Virol.* **3**:355–357.

Hsiung, G. D., Fong, C. K. Y., and Lam, K. M., 1973, *In vitro* transformation of leukocytes with a guinea pig herpes-like virus, in: *Unifying Concepts of Leukemia* (R. M. Dutcher and L. Chieco-Bianchi, eds.), pp. 401–409, Karger, Basel.

Huebner, R. J., 1963, Tumor virus study systems, *Ann. N. Y. Acad. Sci.* **108**:1129–1148.

Huebner, R. J., and Todaro, G. J., 1969, Oncogenesis of RNA tumor viruses as determinants of cancer, *Proc. Natl. Acad. Sci. U.S.A.* **64**:1087–1094.

Huebner, R. J., Gilden, R. V., Lane, W. T., Toni, R., Trimmer, R. W., and Hill, P. R., 1976, Suppression of murine type-C RNA virogenes by type-specific oncornavirus vaccines: Prospects for prevention of cancer, *Proc. Natl. Acad. Sci. U.S.A.* **73**:620–624.

Hughes, W. F., Watanabe, D. H., and Rubin, H., 1963, The development of a chicken flock apparently free of leukosis virus, *Avian Dis.* **7**:154–165.

Hunt, R. D., Garcia, F. G., Barahona, H. H., King, N. W., Fraser, C. E. O., and Meléndez, L. V., 1973, Spontaneous *Herpesvirus saimiri* lymphoma in an owl monkey, *J. Infect. Dis.* **127**:723–725.

Il Ma, B., Swartzendruber, D. C., and Murphy, W. H., 1969, Detection of virus-like particles in germinal centers of normal guinea pigs, *Proc. Soc. Exp. Biol. Med.* **130**:586–590.

Ioachim, H. L., Gimovsky, M. L., and Keller, S. E., 1973, Maternal vaccination with formalin-inactivated Gross lymphoma virus in rats and transfer of immunity to offspring, *Proc. Soc. Exp. Biol. Med.* **144**:376–379.

Jarrett, O., Laird, H. M., and Hay, D., 1969, Growth of feline leukemia virus in human cells, *Nature (London)* **224**:1208–1209.

Jarrett, W. F. H., Crawford, E. M., Martin, W. B., and Davie, F., 1964, A virus-like particle associated with leukemia (lymphosarcoma), *Nature (London)* **202**:567–569.

Jarrett, W. F. H., Crighton, G. W., and Dalton, R. G., 1966, Leukemia and lymphosarcoma in animals and man, *Vet. Rec.* **79**:693–699.

Jarrett, W. F. H., Jarrett, O., Mackey, L., Laird, H., Hardy, W. D., Jr., and Essex, M., 1973, Horizontal transmission of leukemia virus and leukemia in the cat, *J. Natl. Cancer Inst.* **51**:833–841.

Jarrett, W., Mackey, L., Jarrett, O., Laird, H., and Hood, C., 1974, Antibody response and virus survival in cats vaccinated against feline leukemia, *Nature (London)* **248**:230–232.

Johnsen, D. O., Wooding, W. L., Tanticharoenyos, P., and Bourgeous, C. H., Jr., 1971, Malignant lymphoma in the gibbon, *J. Am. Vet. Med. Assoc.* **159**:563–566.

Jones, M. D., Lan, D. T., and Warthen, J., 1972, Lymphoblastic lymphosarcoma in two white-handed gibbons, *Hylobates lar, J. Natl. Cancer Inst.* **49**:599–601.

Jungeblut, C. W., and Kodza, H., 1962, Studies of leukemia L₂C in guinea pigs, *Arch. Gesamte Virusforsch.* **12**:537–551.

Jungherr, E., 1963, Tumors and tumor-like conditions in monkeys, *Ann. N. Y. Acad. Sci.* **108**:777–792.

Jungherr, E., and Hughes, W. F., 1965, The avian leukosis complex, in: *Diseases of Poultry* (H. E. Biester and L. H. Schwarte, eds.), pp. 512–567, Iowa State University Press, Ames.

Kawakami, T. G., and Buckley, P. M., 1974, Antigenic studies on gibbon type-C viruses, *Transplant. Proc.* **6**:193–196.

Kawakami, T. G., Huff, S. D., Buckley, P. M., Dungworth, D. L., Snyder, S. P., and Gilden, R. V., 1972, C-type virus associated with gibbon lymphosarcoma, *Nature (London) New Biol.* **235**:170–171.

Kawakami, T. G., Buckley, P. M., McDowell, T. S., and DePaoli, A., 1973, Antibodies to simian C-type virus antigen in sera of gibbons *(Hylobates* sp.), *Nature (London) New Biol.* **246**:105–107.

Kawakami, T. G., Buckley, P. M., DePaoli, A., Noll, W., and Bustad, L. K., 1975, Studies on the prevalence of type-C virus associated with gibbon hematopoietic neoplasms, in: *Comparative Leukemia Research 1973* (Y. Ito and R. M. Dutcher, eds.), pp. 385–389, University of Tokyo Press, Tokyo/Karger, Basel.

Kawakami, T. G., McDowell, T. S., Johnson, D. L., Breznock, A. L., and Harrold, J. B., 1976, Oncornavirus–host interactions in gibbons, in: *Comparative Leukemia Research 1975* (J. Clemmesen and D. S. Yohn, eds.), pp. 184–186, Karger, Basel.

Kim, U., Clifton, K. H., and Furth, J., 1960, A highly inbred line of Wistar rats yielding spontaneous mammo-somatotropic pituitary and other tumors, *J. Natl. Cancer Inst.* **24**:1031–1047.

Kirkwood, J. M., Geering, G., Old, L. J., Mizell, M., and Wallace, J., 1969, A preliminary report on the serology of Lucké and Burkitt Herpes-type viruses: A shared antigen, in: *Biology of Amphibian Tumors* (M. Mizell, ed.), pp. 365–367, Springer-Verlag, New York.

Klein, G., 1972, Herpesviruses and oncogenesis, *Proc. Natl. Acad. Sci. U.S.A.* **69**:1056–1064.

Klein, G., 1973, The Epstein–Barr virus, in: *The Herpesviruses* (A. S. Kaplan, ed.), pp. 521–550, Academic Press, New York.

Klement, V., Hartley, J. W., Rowe, W., and Huebner, R. J., 1969, Recovery of a hamster-specific, focus-forming, and sarcomagenic virus from a "noninfectious" hamster tumor induced by the Kirsten mouse sarcoma virus, *J. Natl. Cancer Inst.* **43**:925–934.

Knuth, P., and Volkman, O., 1916, Untersuchungen über die Lymphozytomatose des Rindes, *Z. Inftionskr. Haustiere* **17**:393–467.

Koller, L. D., Olson, C., and Gillette, K. G., 1970, Attempted transmission of bovine lymphosarcoma to swine, *Am. J. Vet. Res.* **31**:285–289.

Lapin, B. A., 1973, The epidemiologic and genetic aspects of an outbreak of leukemia among *Hamadryas* baboons of the Sukhumi monkey colony, in: *Unifying Concepts of Leukemia* (R. M. Dutcher and L. Chieco-Bianchi, eds.), pp. 263–268, Karger, Basel.

Lapin, B. A., 1975, Possible ways viral leukemia spreads among the *Hamadryas* baboons of the Sukhumi monkey colony, in: *Comparative Leukemia Research 1973* (Y. Ito and R. M. Dutcher, eds.), pp. 75–84, University of Tokyo Press, Tokyo/Karger, Basel.

Lapin, B. A., 1976, Epidemiology of leukemia among baboons of Sukhumi monkey colony, in: *Comparative Leukemia Research 1975* (J. Clemmesen and D. S. Yohn, eds.), pp. 212–215, Karger, Basel.

Laufs, R., 1976, Nonhuman primate oncogenic herpesviruses: Virus–host relationships, in: *Comparative Leukemia Research 1975* (J. Clemmesen and D. S. Yohn, eds.), pp- 331–335, Karger, Basel.

Laufs, R., and Fleckenstein, B., 1973, Malignant lymphoma induced by partially purified *Herpesvirus saimiri* and recovery of infectious virus from tumorous lymph nodes, *Med. Microbiol. Immunol.* **158**:135–146.

Laufs, R., and Steinke, H., 1975a, Vaccination of non-human primates against malignant lymphoma, *Nature (London)* **253**:71–72.

Laufs, R., and Steinke, H., 1975b, Passive immunization of marmoset monkeys against neoplasia induced by a herpesvirus, *Nature (London)* **255**:226–228.

Lebel, J. L., Bull, E. H., Johnson, L. J., and Watters, R. L., 1970, Lymphosarcoma associated with nodal concentration of plutonium in dogs: A preliminary report, *Am. J. Vet. Res.* **31**:1513–1516.

Lieber, M. M., Benveniste, R. E., Livingston, D. M., and Todaro, G. J., 1973, Mammalian cells in culture frequently release type-C viruses, *Science* **182**:56–59.

Lingeman, C. H., 1969, Spontaneous hematopoietic neoplasms of nonhuman primates: Review, case report, and comparative studies, *Natl. Cancer Inst. Monogr.* **32**:157–170.

177

EPIDEMIOLOGY OF
PRIMARY
NEOPLASMS OF
LYMPHOID TISSUES
IN ANIMALS

Lunger, P. D., Hardy, W. D., Jr., and Clark, H. F., 1974, C-type virus particles in a reptilian tumor, *J. Natl. Cancer Inst.* **52**:1231–1235.

MacEwen, E. G., and Hess, P. W., 1975, Management of hematopoietic neoplasms in the canine, *J. Am. Anim. Hosp. Assoc. Proceed.* **2**:109–125.

Marshak, R. R., 1968, Criteria for the determination of the normal and leukotic state in cattle, *J. Natl. Cancer Inst.* **41**:243–263.

Marshak, R. R., and Abt, D. A., 1968, Bovine leukemia, in: *Experimental Leukemia* (M. Rich, ed.), pp. 191–204, Appleton-Century-Crofts, New York.

McClure, H. M., Keeling, M. E., Custer, R. P., Marshak, R. R., Abt, D. A., and Ferrer, J. F., 1974, Erythroleukemia in two infant chimpanzees fed milk from cows naturally infected with bovine C-type virus, *Cancer Res.* **34**:2745–2757.

McCoy, G. W., 1909, A preliminary report of tumors found in wild rats, *J. Med. Res.* **21**:285–296.

McKee, G. S., Lucas, A. M., Denington, E. M., and Lover, F. C., 1963, Separation of leukotic and non-leukotic lesions in turkeys on the inspection line, *Avian Dis.* **7**:19–30.

Meincke, J. E., Hobbie, W. V., and Hardy, W. D., Jr., 1972, Lymphoreticular malignancies in the cat: Clinical findings, *J. Am. Vet. Med. Assoc.* **160**:1093–1099.

Meléndez, L. V., Daniel, M. D., Hunt, R. D., and Garcia, F. G., 1968, An apparently new herpesvirus from primary kidney cultures of the squirrel monkey, *Lab. Anim. Care* **18**:374–381.

Meléndez, L. V., Hunt, R. D., King, N. W., Barahona, H. H., Daniel, M. D., Fraser, C. E. O., and Garcia, F. G., 1972, A new lymphoma virus of monkeys: Herpesvirus ateles, *Nature (London) New Biol.* **235**:182–184.

Meléndez, L. V., Hunt, R. D., Daniel, M. D., Blake, B. J., and Garcia, F. G., 1973, Acute lymphocytic leukemia in owl monkeys inoculated with *Herpesvirus saimiri, Science* **171**:1161–1163.

Migaki, G., 1969, Hematopoietic neoplasms of slaughter animals, *Natl. Cancer Inst. Monogr.* **32**:121–139.

Miguez, C., 1918, Sarcoma espontáneo transplantable en al cobayo, *Rev. Inst. Bacteriol. Buenos Aires* **1**:147–154.

Miller, J. M., and Olson, C., 1972, Precipitating antibody to an internal antigen of the C-type virus associated with bovine lymphosarcoma, *J. Natl. Cancer Inst.* **49**:1459–1462.

Miller, J. M., and Van Der Maaten, M. J., 1972, A complement fixation test for the bovine leukemia (C-type) virus, *J. Natl. Cancer Inst.* **53**:1699–1702.

Miller, J. M., Miller, L. D., Olson, C., and Gillette, K. G., 1969, Virus-like particles in phytohemagglu-tinin stimulated lymphocyte cultures with reference to bovine lymphosarcoma, *J. Natl. Cancer Inst.* **43**:1297–1305.

Miller, L. D., Miller, J. M., and Olson, C., 1972, Inoculation of calves with particles resembling C-type virus from cultures of bovine lymphosarcoma, *J. Natl. Cancer Inst.* **48**:423–428.

Monlux, A. W., Anderson, W. A., and Davis, C. L., 1956, A survey of tumors occurring in cattle, sheep and swine, *Am. J. Vet. Res.* **17**:646–677.

Morris, W. P., 1968, Neoplasms and spontaneous diseases in a beagle colony, *J. Am. Vet. Med. Assoc.* **152**:1085.

Mulcahy, M. F., and O'Leary, A., 1970, Cell-free transmission of lymphosarcoma in the northern pike *Esox lucius* L. (Pisces; Esocidae), *Experientia* **8**:891.

Mulcahy, M. F., Winguist, G., and Dawe, C. L., 1970, The neoplastic cell type in lymphoreticular neoplasms of northern pike, *Esox lucius* L., *Cancer Res.* **30**:2712–2717.

Nadel, E. M., 1957, Transplanation of leukemia from inbred to non-inbred guinea pigs, *J. Natl. Cancer Inst.* **19**:351–359.

Nadel, E., Banfield, W., Burstein, S., and Tousimis, A. J., 1967, Virus particles associated with strain 2 guinea pig leukemia (L₂C/N-B), *J. Natl. Cancer Inst.* **38**:979–981.

Nahmias, A. J., and Roizman, B., 1973, Infection with herpes-simplex viruses 1 and 2, *N. Engl. J. Med.* **289**:667–674.

Nahmias, A. J., Alford, C. A., and Korones, A. B. , 1970, Infection of the newborn with *Herpesvirus hominis, Adv. Pediatr.* **17**:185–226.

Nahmias, A. J., delBuono, I., Schneweis, K. E., Gordon, D. S., and Thies, D., 1971, Type-specific surface antigens of cells infected with herpes simplex virus (1 and 2), *Proc. Soc. Exp. Biol. Med.* **138**:21–27.

Nayak, D. P., 1971, Isolation and characterization of a herpesvirus from leukemic guinea pigs, *J. Virol.* **8**:579–588.

Nayak, D. P., and Murray, P. R., 1973, Induction of type C viruses in cultured guinea pig cells, *J. Virol.* **12**:177–187.

Newberne, J. W., and Robinson, V. B., 1960, Spontaneous tumors in primates—A report of two cases with notes on the apparent low incidence of neoplasms in subhuman primates, *Am. J. Vet. Res.* **21**:150–155.

Nowinski, R. C., Old, L. J., Sarkar, N. H., and Moore, D. H., 1970, Common properties of the oncogenic RNA viruses (oncornaviruses), *Virology* **42**:1152–1157.

Nowinski, R. C., Old, L. J., O'Donnell, P. V. O., and Sanders, F. K., 1971, Serological identification of hamster oncornaviruses, *Nature (London)* **230**:282–284.

Olsen, R. G., Schaller, J. P., Hoover, E. A., and Yohn, D. S., 1976, Experimental oncornavirus vaccines in the cat, in: *Comparative Leukemia Research 1975* (J. Clemmesen and D. S. Yohn, eds.), pp. 515–517, Karger, Basel.

Olson, C., 1974, Bovine lymphosarcoma (leukemia)—A synopsis, *J. Am. Vet. Med. Assoc.* **165**:630–632.

Olson, C., and Baumgartener, L. E., 1975, Lymphosarcoma (leukemia) of cattle, *Bovine Pract.* **10**:15–22.

Olson, C., and Bullis, K. L., 1942, A survey and study of spontaneous neoplastic diseases in chickens, *Mass. Agr. Exp. Stn. Bull.* 391.

Olson, C., Miller, L. D., Miller, J. M., and Hoss, H. E., 1972, Transmission of lymphosarcoma from cattle to sheep, *J. Natl. Cancer Inst.* **49**:1463–1467.

Olson, C., Hoss, H. E., Miller, J. M., and Baumgartener, L. E., 1973, Evidence of bovine C-type (leukemia) virus in dairy cattle, *J. Am. Vet. Med. Assoc.* **163**:355–357.

Opler, S. R., 1967, Observations on a new virus associated with guinea pig leukemia: Preliminary note, *J. Natl. Cancer Inst.* **38**:746–798.

Oroszlan, S., Bova, D., Huebner, R. J., and Gilden, R. V., 1972, Major group-specific protein of rat type-C viruses, *J. Virol.* **10**:746–750.

Papas, T. S., Dahlberg, J. E., and Sonstegard, R. A., 1976, Type-C virus in lymphosarcoma in northern pike *(Esox lucius), Nature (London)* **261**:506–508.

Parks, W. P., Scolnick, E. M., Noon, M. C., Watson, C. J., and Kawakami, T. G., 1973, Radioimmunoassay of mammalian type-C polypeptides. IV. Characterization of woolly monkey and gibbon viral antigens, *Int. J. Cancer* **12**:129–137.

Paulsen, J., Best, E., Frese, K., and Rudolph, R., 1971, Enzootische lymphatische Leukose bei Schafen-Lymphocytose, pathologische Anatomie und Histologie, *Zentralbl. Vetinaer-Med. Reihe B* **18**:33–43.

Paulsen, J., Rudolph, R., Hoffmann, R., Weiss, E., and Schliesser, T., 1972, C-type virus particles in phytohemagglutinin-stimulated lymphocyte cultures with reference to enzootic lymphatic leukosis in sheep, *Med. Microbiol. Immunol.* **158**:105–112.

Paulsen, J., Rohde, W., Pauli, G., Harms, E., and Bauer, H., 1976, Comparative studies on ovine and bovine C-type particles in: *Comparative Leukemia Research 1975* (J. Clemmesen and D. S. Yohn, eds.), pp. 190–192, Karger, Basel.

Perryman, L. E., Hoover, E. A., and Yohn, D. S., 1972, Immunologic reactivity of the cat: Immunosuppression in experimental feline leukemia, *J. Natl. Cancer Inst.* **49**:1357–1365.

Piper, C. E., Abt, D. A., Ferrer, J. F., and Marshak, R. R., 1975, Seroepidemiological evidence for horizontal transmission of bovine C-type virus, *Cancer Res.* **35**:2714–2716.

Porter, P. S., and Baughman, R. D., 1965, Epidemiology of herpes simplex among wrestlers, *J. Am. Med. Assoc.* **194**:998–1000.

Priester, W. A., and Mason, T. J., 1974, Human cancer mortality in relation to poultry population by county, in 10 southeastern states, *J. Natl. Cancer Inst.* **53**:45–49.

Purchase, H. G., 1975, Progress in the control of Marek's disease, *Am. J. Vet. Res.* **36**:587–590.

Purchase, H. G., 1976, Marek's disease: Epizootology, control, and relationship to oncornaviruses, in: *Comparative Leukemia Research 1975* (J. Clemmesen and D. S. Yohn, eds.), pp. 199–203, Karger, Basel.

Rapp, F., 1976, Viruses as an etiologic factor in cancer, *Semin. Oncol.* **3**:49–63.

Renier, F., Chevrel, L., Friedman, J. C., Gaquiere, G., and Guelfi, J., 1966, Quelque considérations sur les leucoses porcines, *Nouv. Rev. Fr. Hématol.* **6**:239–252.

Rhim, J. S., Cho, H. Y., Duh, F. G., and Vernon, M. L., 1975, Characterization of murine sarcoma virus, transformation of guinea pig cells and activation of an RNA tumor-like virus from nonproducer

179

EPIDEMIOLOGY OF
PRIMARY
NEOPLASMS OF
LYMPHOID TISSUES
IN ANIMALS

guinea pig cells, in: *Comparative Leukemia Research 1973* (Y. Ito and R. M. Dutcher, eds.), pp. 153–164, University of Tokyo Press, Tokyo/Karger, Basel.

Rickard, C. G., Post, J. E. , Noronha, F., and Barr, L. M. A., 1969, Transmissible virus-induced lymphocytic leukemia of the cat, *J. Natl. Cancer Inst.* **42**:987–1014.

Roizman, B., 1971, Herpesviruses, man and cancer—or the persistence of the viruses of love, in: *Of Microbes and Life* (J. Monod and E. Borek, eds.), pp. 189–214, Columbia University Press, New York.

Rongey, R. W., Hlavackova, A., Lara, S., Estes, J., and Gardner, M. B., 1973, Type B and C RNA virus in breast tissue and milk of wild mice, *J. Natl. Cancer Inst.* **50**:1581–1589.

Rosato, F. E., Rosato, E. F., and Plotkin, S. A., 1970, Herpetic paronychia—An occupational hazard of medical personnel, *N. Engl. J. Med.* **283**:804–805.

Rous, P., 1911, A sarcoma of the fowl transmissible by an agent separable from the tumor cells, *J. Exp. Med.* **13**:397–411.

Ruben, L. N., and Balls, M., 1967, Further studies of a transmissible amphibian lymphosarcoma, *Cancer Res.* **27**:293–296.

Rubin, H., Cornelius, A., and Fanshier, L., 1961, The pattern of congenital transmission of an avian leukosis virus, *Proc. Natl. Acad. Sci. U.S.A.* **47**:1058–1069.

Rubin, H., Fanshier, L., Cornelius, A., and Hughes, W. F., 1962, Tolerance and immunity in chickens after congenital infection with an avian leukosis virus, *Virology* **17**:143–156.

Runnells, R. A., and Benbrook, E. A., 1944, Malignant lymphoid tumors in horses, *J. Am. Vet. Med. Assoc.* **104**:148–150.

Sarma, P. S., and Log, T., 1973, Subgroup classification of feline leukemia and sarcoma viruses by viral interference and neutralization tests, *Virology* **54**:160–169.

Saxton, J. A., Jr., Sperling, G. A., Barnes, L., and McCay, C. M., 1948, The influence of nutrition upon the incidence of spontaneous tumors of the albino rat, *Acta Unio Int. Contra. Cancrum* **6**:423–431.

Schalm, O. W., 1975, *Veterinary Hematology,* Lea & Febiger, Philadelphia.

Schneider, R., 1970, The natural history of malignant lymphoma and sarcoma in cats and their assocaition with cancer in man and dog, *J. Am. Vet. Med. Assoc.* **157**:1753–1758.

Schneider, R., 1972, Human cancer in households containing cats with malignant lymphoma, *Int. J. Cancer* **10**:338–344.

Schneider, R., 1976, Comparative epidemiological aspects of naturally occurring malignant lymphoma in domestic cats and rhesus monkeys, in: *Comparative Leukemia Research 1975* (J. Clemmesen and D. S. Yohn, eds.), pp. 227–231, Karger, Basel.

Schneider, R., Frye, F. L., Taylor, D. O. N., and Dorn, C. R., 1967, A household cluster of feline malignant lymphoma, *Cancer Res.* **27**:1316–1322.

Servoian, M., Chamberlain, D. M., and Larose, R. N., 1963, Avian lymphomatosis. V. Air-borne transmission, *Avian Dis.* **7**:102–105.

Sharma, J. M., 1976, Marek's disease, Lucké frog carcinoma and other animal oncogenic herpesviruses, in: *Comparative Luekemia Research 1975* (J. Clemmesen and D. S. Yohn, eds.), pp. 343–347, Karger, Basel.

Schimizu, T., 1972, Natural transmission of avian leukosis viruses among chickens, *Gann Monogr. Cancer Res.* **12**:3–9.

Slye, M., 1914, The incidence and inheritability of spontaneous tumors in mice, *J. Med. Res.* **30**:281–298.

Snyder, S. P., Dungworth, D. L., Kawakami, T. G., Callaway, E., and Lau, D. T.-L., 1973, Lymphosarcomas in two gibbons *(Hylobates lar)* with associated C-type virus, *J. Natl. Cancer Inst.* **51**:89–94.

Squire, R. A., 1963, Hematopoietic tumors of domestic animals, *Cornell Vet.* **54**:97–150.

Squire, R. A., 1969, Spontaneous hematopoietic tumors of dogs, *Natl. Cancer Inst. Monogr.* **32**:97–109.

Steeves, R., 1974, Murine oncornaviruses, in: *Handbook of Laboratory Animal Science,* Vol. 2 (E. C. Melby, Jr., and N. H. Altman, eds.), pp. 4–11, CRC Press, Cleveland.

Stenback, W. A., Van Hoosier, G. L., Jr., and Trentin, J. J., 1966, Virus particles in hamster tumors as revealed by electron microscopy, *Proc. Soc. Exp. Biol. Med.* **122**:1219–1223.

Stenback, W. A., Van Hoosier, G. L., Jr., and Trentin, J. J., 1968, Biophysical, biological, and cytochemical features of a virus associated with transplantable hamster tumors, *J. Virol.* **2**:1115–1121.

Stowell, R. E., Smith, E. K., Espana, C., and Nelson, V. G., 1971, Outbreak of malignant lymphoma in rhesus monkeys, *Lab. Invest.* **25**:476–479.

Svet-Moldavsky, G. J., Trubcheninova, L., and Ravkina, L. I., 1967, Pathogenicity of the chicken sarcoma virus (Schmidt–Ruppin) for amphibians and reptiles, *Nature (London)* **214**:300–302.

Teitz, Y., Lennette, E. H., Oshiro, L. S., and Cremer, N. E., 1971, Release of C-type particles from normal rat thymus cultures and those infected with Moloney leukemia virus, *J. Natl. Cancer Inst.* **46**:11–21.

Theilen, G. H., and Dungworth, D. L., 1965, Bovine lymphosarcoma in California. III. The calf form, *Am. J. Vet. Res.* **26**:696–709.

Theilen, G. H., and Fowler, M. E., 1962, Lymphosarcoma (lymphocytic leukemia) in the horse, *J. Am. Vet. Med. Assoc.* **140**:923–930.

Theilen, G. H., Gould, D., Fowler, M., and Dungworth, D. L., 1971, C-type virus in tumor tissue of woolly monkey *(Lagothrix spp.)* with fibrosarcoma, *J. Natl. Cancer Inst.* **47**:881–889.

Ting, R. C., 1968, Biological and serological properties of viral particles from a nonproducer rat neoplasm induced by murine sarcoma virus (Moloney), *J. Virol.* **2**:865–868.

Toit, P. J. du, 1916, Beitrag zur Morphologie des normalen und leukämischen Rinderblutes, *Arch. Tierheilk.* **43**:144–203.

Ulbrich, F., Best, E., Paulsen, J., Nitzschke, E., and Fritzsche, K., 1970, Beobachtungen an einer von der Leukose befallenen Schafherde, *Tieraerztl. Umsch.* **25**:277–283.

Van Pelt, R. W., and Conner, G. H., 1968, Clinicopathologic survey of malignant lymphoma in the dog, *J. Am. Vet. Med. Assoc.* **152**:976–989.

Vital Statistics of the United States—1964, 1966, U.S. Department of Health, Education and Welfare, Washington, D.C.

Walker, E. P., 1968, *Mammals of the World,* 2nd Ed., Johns Hopkins University Press, Baltimore.

Weber, W. T., 1963, Hematologic aspects of bovine lymphosarcoma, *Ann. N. Y. Acad. Sci.* **108**:1270–1283.

Wight, P. A. L., 1963, Lymphoid leukosis and fowl paralysis in the quail, *Vet. Rec.* **75**:685–687.

Winters, W. D., and Snow, H. D., 1974a, Immunodiffusion studies of canine lymphosarcoma antigens, *J. Natl. Cancer Inst.* **53**:1027–1031.

Winters, W. D., and Snow, H. D., 1974b, Precipitating antibodies to canine lymphosarcoma-associated antigens, *Am. J. Vet. Res.* **35**:1333–1335.

Wolfe, L. G., Falk, L. A., and Deinhardt, F., 1971, Oncogenicity of Herpesvirus saimiri in marmoset monkeys, *J. Natl. Cancer Inst.* **47**:1145–1162.

Zeigel, R. F., and Clark, H. F., 1969, Electron microscopic observations on a "C"-type virus in cell culture derived from a tumor-bearing viper, *J. Natl. Cancer Inst.* **46**:309–321.

6

Epidemiology of Lymphoreticular Malignancies in Man

NICHOLAS J. VIANNA

it's important to trace
both person and place
time is not everything
just an important something

1. Introduction

In recent years, rapid advances have been made in lymphoma research. These advances are due in large part to a more complete understanding of basic immunological concepts and to our growing realization that some alteration in host immunity might be a prerequisite for the development of many lymphoreticular malignancies. Epidemiological investigations, which of necessity must consider the elements of person, place, and time, have also been directed at certain fundamental issues: What is the importance of environmental and genetic factors in these diseases? Do both play a role? How do the various lymphomas differ, and what are these differences telling us? In some instances, notably Hodgkin's disease and Burkitt's lymphoma, specific etiological hypotheses have been advanced. Our knowledge of the other lymphomas is more limited.

In this chapter, selected topics of epidemiological interest are presented. These topics include the relevance of age, sex, marital status, geography, and socioeconomic class. The relationship between lymphomas and other diseases, particularly aberrations of immunological function, are alluded to herein and are reviewed in Chapters 7 and 8. Attention is also drawn to the association among lymphomas, immunodeficiency states, and certain histocompatibility antigens. The significance of these observations is discussed.

NICHOLAS J. VIANNA • Cancer Control Bureau, New York State Department of Health, Albany, New York 12237.

NICHOLAS J. VIANNA

2. Importance of Environmental Factors

It is exceedingly difficult to separate man's environment from genetic factors. The evaluation of potentially important environmental factors in the etiology or pathophysiology of a disease requires the application of all available epidemiological methods. Since any single approach has limitations, the strength of the conclusion(s) lies in the consistency of the results.

3. International and Regional Differences

Despite limitations, geographic distributions of pathology have played an important role in suggesting that environmental influences might be important in the etiology of certain lymphoreticular disorders. Perhaps the most striking example of this is Burkitt's lymphoma. Although this lymphoma occurs sporadically in the United States, Canada, Great Britain, and Brazil, it is endemic in tropical countries, such as Uganda in Africa (Burkitt and Davies, 1961) and New Guinea (Booth et al., 1967). Even within the African continent, there appear to be belts of high and low prevalence. These observations focus attention on differences among these regions that might be relevant to this lymphoma. This was one of the first approaches to investigating this disorder.

In contrast to Burkitt's lymphoma, Hodgkin's disease and the other lymphomas occur with greater regularity throughout the world. Obvious international and regional variations in incidence patterns have been observed, however, and these variations suggest that environmental factors might also be important in these disorders.

In developed Western countries, Hodgkin's disease is characterized by a bimodal age–incidence curve (MacMahon, 1966) (Figure 1) that distinguishes it from other lymphoreticular malignancies. This contrasts with Japan, where the young adult mode is absent and the incidence of Hodgkin's disease increases with age in a fashion similar to that observed for lymphosarcoma and reticulum-cell sarcoma in Western countries (MacMahon, 1966). In less developed countries such as Peru and Lebanon, a bimodality is observed, but the first peak occurs in childhood (Correa and O'Conor, 1971). There is also a remarkably high frequency of lymphomas during the first two age decades (El-Gazayerli et al., 1962). Chronic stimulation of reticuloendothelial elements in lymphoid tissues related to endemic bilharziasis may be a factor in this distribution pattern.

Regional differences have also been observed within countries. In the United States, mortality rates among young adults from Hodgkin's disease in 11 contiguous Southern states were significantly lower than in Northern states between 1949–1954 and 1959–1961 (Cole et al., 1968). Even among counties in the United States, mortality rates appear to vary markedly (Mason, T. J., et al., 1975), and within certain counties, rates may differ appreciably if observations are made over long periods (Vianna et al., 1972).

In the United States and most European countries, non-Hodgkin's lymphomas increase in frequency with age (MacMahon, 1966). In Egypt, however, these lymphomas tend to occur at earlier ages (El-Gazayerli et al., 1962). In Japan and Uganda, there is a high rate of reticulum-cell sarcoma and low rates of lymphosarcoma and Hodgkin's disease relative to the United States (Anderson *et al.*, 1970). In contrast, Latin American countries seem to have a higher frequency of Hodgkin's disease (Besuschio, 1974).

4. Socioeconomic and Urban–Rural Factors

Available evidence suggests that lymphomas are most prevalent among the more prosperous segments of society (MacMahon, 1966). This pattern of prevalence might be particularly true of Hodgkin's disease. In the United States, this apparent association between Hodgkin's disease and socioeconomic status is most apparent after the age of 15 years. Perhaps the most compelling evidence suggesting an association between socioeconomic factors and Hodgkin's disease comes from the work of Correa and O'Conor (1971). These investigators identified three distinct age–incidence patterns for this disorder, each apparently associated with a different level of economic development. One pattern is found in developing countries, and is characterized by high childhood (primarily males), low young adult, and high adult rates. In well-developed countries, rates are low in childhood, but high in both young adult and older age groups (Figure 1). An intermediate pattern is found in rural areas of developing countries. During the war years 1949–1953, Hodgkin's disease occurred most often among the upper class in England and Wales (Mac-

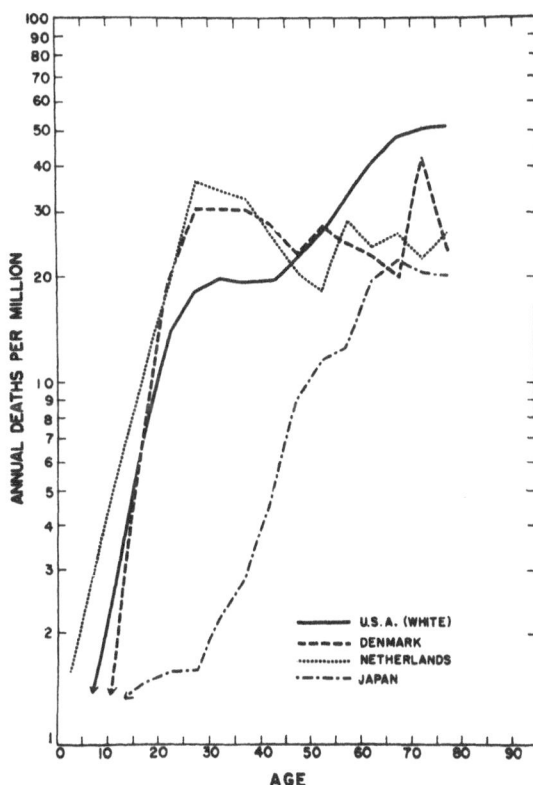

Figure 1. Age-specific death rates from Hodgkin's disease in four countries, 1950–1953. Reprinted with permission from MacMahon (1966).

Mahon, 1966). This pattern was not observed in the period 1959–1963 after relative economic recovery from World War II (Registrar-General's Decennial Supplement, 1961; Alderson and Nayak, 1972).

The malignant lymphomas as a group also appear to be characterized by higher rates in urban than in rural areas (MacMahon, 1966). While overall rates for Hodgkin's disease would indicate that it is primarily an urban disorder, male children may be the exception. In Denmark, the incidence of this disease in males under 15 years of age is higher in rural than in urban areas (Clemmesen, 1964). A similar observation was made in rural regions of Germany for males under 30 years of age (Dörken and Singer-Bakker, 1972). In farm residents of California, both incidence and mortality rates for Hodgkin's disease appear to be significantly higher for males than for females (Fasal *et al.*, 1968). Unfortunately, there is little information on urban–rural factors for the different non-Hodgkin's lymphomas.

5. Migration Studies

Environmental factors also appear to be important in the epidemiology of lymphomas among migrant groups. Mortality rates from Hodgkin's disease are higher among Japanese-Americans than among native Japanese, especially in the 15–34 and over-50 age groups (Mason, T. J., and Fraumeni, 1974). The importance of environmental vs. racial factors is illustrated by the comparable mortality rate from Hodgkin's disease among Japanese and Caucasians living in Hawaii (Blaisdell and Boxer, 1971). Neither was any significant difference in the incidence of Hodgkin's disease observed among various Israeli migrant populations, although the classic bimodality appeared to be more pronounced for patients born in the United States, Europe, and Asia than for those born in Africa (Meytes and Modan, 1969). Finally, standard lymphoma mortality ratios for Isei males and females are similar to those for the white population in the United States (Meytes and Modan, 1969).

6. Gender and Marital Status

Lymphomas are more prevalent among males than among females in the United States (MacMahon, 1966 (Figure 2), and sex-related differences in survival are most apparent among young adults. Bjelke (1969) reported that marital status influences the incidence of lymphomas among young Norwegian women, being higher among those who had married than among those who had not. This pattern is supported by our observations in New York State (excluding New York City) from 1951 through 1960 and 1961 through 1970 (Vianna *et al.*, 1976). Marital status appeared to influence the frequency of Hodgkin's disease specifically, however, and not that of other primary tumors of lymphoid tissues. We recorded much lower rates of Hodgkin's disease among young married females than among either young unmarried females (Figure 3) or young males regardless of marital status (Figure 4). Marital history had no apparent relevance to the frequency of Hodgkin's disease among older population groups irrespective of their sex.

These preliminary findings require further evaluation using incidence data. It will be necessary to distinguish the direct role of marriage from the occurrence and frequency of pregnancy and, perhaps, the chronic use of oral contraceptives.

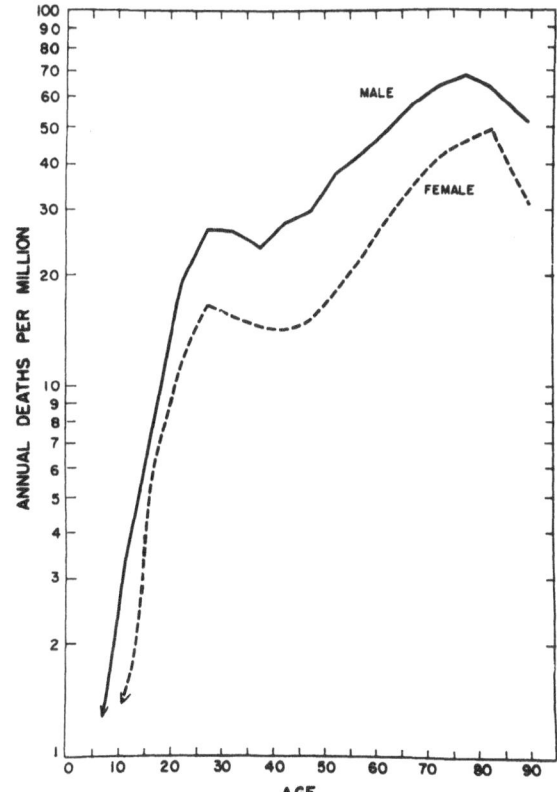

Figure 2. Age-specific mortality rates from Hodgkin's disease by sex in the United States, 1958–1962 (data from National Center for Health Statistics). Reprinted with permission from Mac-Mahon (1966).

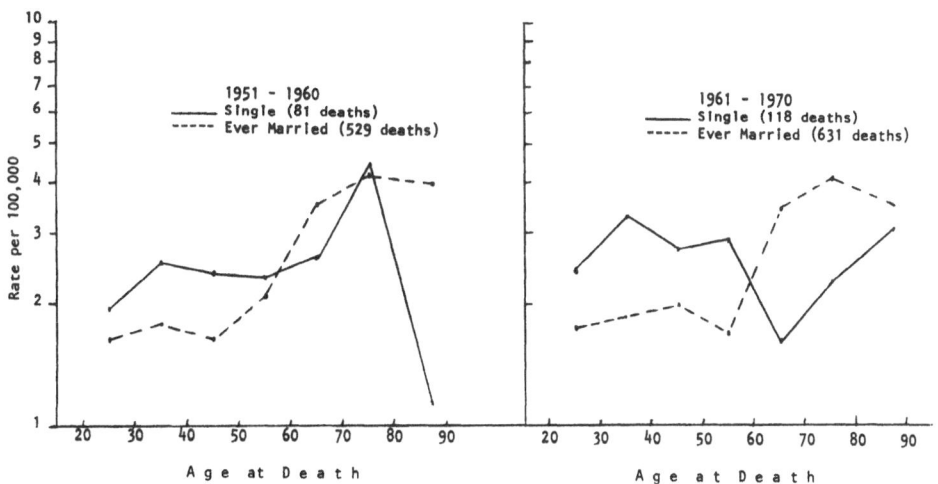

Figure 3. Age-specific mortality rates for females with Hodgkin's disease in New York State (excluding New York City) for the periods 1951–1960 and 1961–1970.

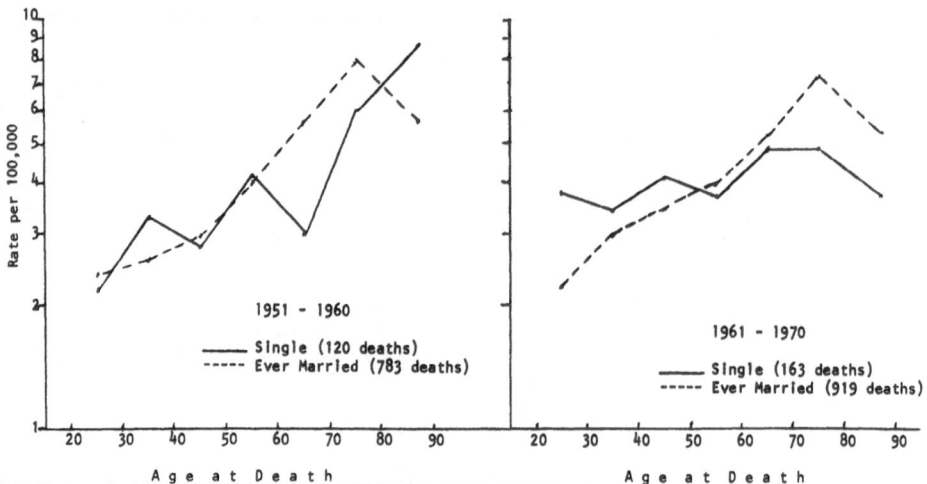

Figure 4. Age-specific mortality rates for males with Hodgkin's disease in New York State (excluding New York City) for the periods 1951–1960 and 1961–1970.

Differences in life style associated with marriage (Fry *et al.*, 1976) may be a contributing factor to the findings presented in the preceding paragraph. For example, marriage at a young age might be indicative of popularity at an early age. Young single females, however, are likely to have a wider circle of acquaintances than their married counterparts in the future. Thus, if gregariousness is a factor in Hodgkin's disease, there might be two distinct age–incidence peaks for young adult females, the earlier one occurring among those married. Alternatively, the relatively low mortality rates of Hodgkin's disease among young married females may wholly reflect incidence and be indicative of increased resistance to this disease. Reproduction could have a role in such resistance. Reduced activity of thymus-derived lymphocytes during the late stages of pregnancy (Finn *et al.*, 1972) may generate some resistance to Hodgkin's disease. It also seems important to evaluate the risk of developing Hodgkin's disease among young females with spouses who have this disease.

Other potentially important considerations arise from this apparent difference associated with marital status. If a marital factor is important for Hodgkin's disease alone, is this importance indicative of susceptibility to different etiologies or reflective of environmental factors that modify expression of the disease? Does marital status have bearing on the high rate of nodular sclerotic Hodgkin's tumors among young females (Thomas and Berard, 1973)? The frequency of nodular sclerotic tumors, which carry a relatively favorable prognosis, would have bearing on survival among different patient groups. It seems clear that future investigations should take a three-dimensional view of Hodgkin's disease by considering the simultaneous influence of age, sex, and marital status on the incidence and expression of this disorder.

7. Geographic Variations in Tumor Presentation

Reports from different areas of the world suggest that the frequency and anatomical site of various lymphomas differ geographically. Intestinal lymphoma is remarkably frequent in certain Arab countries (Ramot and Many, 1972); chronic parasitic infestations may contribute to this finding. Reference has already been made to the geographic localization of Burkitt's lymphoma. Chronic stimulation of the reticuloendothelial system may create a favorable environment for the development of this tumor (Daldorf *et al.*, 1964). If so, the remarkable sparing of the spleen with this lymphoma (see Chapter 13) remains to be explained. Other related observations include: (1) the high frequency of abdominal Burkitt's lymphoma in regions in which this tumor occurs sporadically (Cohen *et al.*, 1969); (2) the apparent high frequency of splenic and nasal lymphomas in certain South American countries (Weiss and Morón, 1962; Andrade and Waldeck, 1971); and (3) the predominance of histological types of Hodgkin's tumors that are usually associated with a relatively unfavorable prognosis among children from certain African (Burn *et al.*, 1971) and South American countries (Correa and O'Conor, 1971).

The fundamental question underlying all these observations is whether certain environmental factors such as chronic infection, might influence both the type and the primary anatomical site of certain lymphoreticular malignancies.

8. Epidemiology of Burkitt's Lymphoma

There are several features that distinguish this lymphoma from other primary tumors of lymphoid tissues. These features facilitate epidemiological investigation. Burkitt's lymphoma can be distinguished from other lymphomas on histological, cytological, and histochemical grounds (Wright, 1963; Berard, 1969). The obvious jaw tumors in African patients with this disease enabled Burkitt (1958) to map its geographic distribution in Uganda. This mapping led, in turn, to the unique observation that there are belts of high and low prevalence of Burkitt's lymphoma in Africa, and that this lymphoma occurred with a particularly high frequency around lakes, but was relatively infrequent in mountain regions with altitudes above 5000 feet (Burkitt and Davies, 1961). The prevalence of the tumor was greatest in regions that had a mean temperature of 60°F or greater during the coolest season of the year and an average annual rainfall in excess of 20 inches (Haddow, 1963). E. H. Williams *et al.* (1974) reported that peak diagnosis of this neoplasm in the West Nile district of Uganda occurs during the second half of the year. Similar climatic conditions have been associated with a high rate of Burkitt's lymphoma in New Guinea (Booth *et al.*, 1967). The apparent coincidence of these geographic and climatic conditions with this disease is an association that is unique among the lymphomas. These observations led to the suggestion that some vector-borne biological agent might be important in the etiology of this tumor. There ensued an intensive search for viruses from this tumor, a search from which the Epstein–Barr virus (EBV) has emerged as the most likely candidate (Epstein *et al.*, 1965).

Immediate difficulties were encountered, since the EBV is a ubiquitous member of the herpes virus family (Diehl *et al.*, 1968), which makes it difficult to hold the EBV totally accountable for Burkitt's lymphoma. One explanation might be that this virus is not a causal agent, but merely a passenger. An alternative possibility is that other factors alter host immunological responses to the EBV, an alteration that, in some way, then predisposes to Burkitt's lymphoma in areas in which this disease is endemic. While the list of possible cofactors is large and possibly includes social and genetic influences, interest has centered around the suggestion that malaria might predispose to this lymphoma (Daldorf *et al.*, 1964). This hypothesis is attractive on several counts: (1) A close geographic association has been demonstrated between the incidence of Burkitt's lymphoma and malariometric indices (Burkitt, 1969). Furthermore, the incidence of this tumor may have declined in areas in which adequate malaria control has been instituted (Baikie *et al.*, 1972). (2) That malaria gametocytes cannot develop successfully within mosquitos when the average temperature is below 60°F (Herms and James, 1961) fits well with the climatic conditions associated with this tumor. (3) There is experimental evidence that the incidence of lymphomas is increased in Swiss mice that are chronically infected with Plasmodium berghei malaria (Jerusalem *et al.*, 1971).

Available evidence strongly suggests that the EBV and malarial parasites play an etiological role in Burkitt's lymphoma. Nevertheless, that this tumor occasionally occurs in countries in which malaria is exceedingly rare indicates that malaria is not essential to the occurrence of this neoplasm. Furthermore, no significant difference in EBV titers has been observed between Burkitt's lymphoma cases in the United States and seemingly healthy persons. In fact, EBV antibody titer could not be detected in certain American cases (Hirshaut *et al.*, 1973). Several hypotheses can be raised to explain these apparent discrepancies: (1) African and American Burkitt's lymphoma could be histologically similar lymphomas with distinct etiologies; this possibility could explain certain clinical differences observed in these countries (Cohen *et al.*, 1969). (2) Environmental factors other than malaria might predispose to a Burkitt-like tumor in countries such as the United States, Great Britain, and Canada, with or without contribution by the EBV. (3) Time–space cluster analyses have produced variable data. Significant findings were reported from the West Nile district and Bwamba (Pike *et al.*, 1967), but not from the North Mara district of Tanzania (Brubaker *et al.*, 1973); it remains to be determined how this difference might be related to the phenomenon of epidemic drift, in which disease clusters may move from county to county. (4) The timing of exposure, particularly to the EBV, might be an important factor. Burkitt's lymphoma is primarily a disease of African children, with a mean age-peak of about 8 years, which suggests a relatively brief induction period for this disease. It would be helpful to determine whether any seasonality (month of birth or onset or both) is present.

9. Hodgkin's Disease Aggregates

Unlike Burkitt's lymphoma, Hodgkin's disease has been recognized as a distinct entity for well over a century. It is also a disorder that has been embedded in controversy, a fact that is undoubtedly related to its many heterogeneous features. Epidemiological evidence has been presented that is consistent with the possibility that Hodgkin's disease might be two or more entities (MacMahon, 1966), and reference has already been made to the influence of factors such as race, socioeconomic status, and possibly marital status on overall incidence and age-specific incidence rates. Clinically, this disease can progress rapidly or it can assume a more indolent character. Histological variants of prognostic import have also been recognized (see Chapter 9).

Hodgkin's disease has long been suspected of having an infectious etiology; in 1938, the fifth revision of the International Classification of Diseases listed it with mumps and other disease under "other infectious and parasitic communicable diseases." While epidemiology alone can never fully resolve this issue, it can determine whether this disease has features that are consistent with an infectious etiology. To do this effectively, however, one must study Hodgkin's disease within the community. One approach to this subject is to see whether patient aggregates of Hodgkin's disease have features consistent with a communicable hypothesis. It is important to undertake such studies using as reference the behavior of classic diseases known to have an infectious etiology. This importance holds particularly true with regard to the concept of "transmission."

It is well established that each case of tuberculosis generally gives rise to less than one other new case, and that its incubation period is highly variable. Failure to demonstrate apparent transmission does not rule out an infectious etiology. The state of infectivity may be past with the onset of symptoms, particularly in the case of certain viral disorders. For example, polioviremia appears to be limited to the period of minor illness, and measles and rubella viruses disappear rapidly from tissues after the onset of antibody responses. The same may be true for infectious mononucleosis, in which transmission of the EBV and clinical disease is difficult to establish. Subclinical infection is a condition that abounds in the world of infectious diseases and can confound even well-structured epidemiological investigations, such as time–space cluster analysis.

These considerations underline the necessity to initially conduct an open-ended investigation that allows for a broader transmission pattern than directly from case to case and a variable but long latent period. One must realize, however, both the merits and the limitations of this approach, which is an important step toward developing etiological hypotheses, but does not constitute formal objective proof.

An effort was made to determine whether students diagnosed with Hodgkin's disease in Albany County, New York, between 1950 and 1970 were associated by prior social contact, be it direct (case–case) or indirect (through some healthy intermediary), with other patients with Hodgkin's disease. "Social links" were considered established only if the persons involved had the opportunity for repetitive contact (e.g., classmates, teammates). A total of 34 patients (31 with Hodgkin's disease) were linked with other patients in this fashion (Vianna *et al.,* 1972). Subsequent investigations in other parts of New York (Vianna *et al.,* 1972) and other states (Klinger and Minton, 1973; Dworsky and Henderson, 1974; Schimpff *et al.,* 1975) uncovered similar patient groupings of Hodgkin's disease.

Demonstration of these disease aggregates is consistent with the possibility that environmental factors, and possibly infectious factors, contribute to the etiology of Hodgkin's disease. Of greater importance are the epidemiological features that these studies uncovered: (1) Aggregates were primarily school-based. (2) Case-to-case contact was clearly demonstrable, but a healthy intermediary was more frequently needed to link Hodgkin's disease patients. (3) The time interval between diagnoses was long and variable, with a mean of about 3 years. (4) Although most of the linked patients were young adults, all age groups were represented, and there did not appear to be any predominant sex pattern. (5) There were several instances in which students who attended the same class with a diagnosed case remained healthy but Hodgkin's disease developed in a relative living in the same household. In Albany, 9 of the 15 linked cases who were not student cases lived in the same household with a school-age contact who had a well-defined association with at least one school-based case (Vianna *et al.*, 1972. (6) Where it was possible to follow the time–space activities of cases and contacts from a defined patient aggregate, these persons became associated with other people who subsequently developed Hodgkin's disease. (7) Both favorable and unfavorable Rye subtypes were observed in most groupings.

Taken collectively, the observations described above suggest that in those instances in which a patient with Hodgkin's disease attends a school, a greater than expected number of additional cases might subsequently occur if the hypothetically exposed group could be followed for a sufficiently long period of time. Stated in this fashion, the hypothesis of transmission in Hodgkin's disease takes a more specific form that allows expression of many infectious disease characteristics (e.g., variable transmission, a carrier state, and a long but variable latent period). Transmission can be tested objectively.

An epidemiological search for Hodgkin's aggregates was undertaken in the 777 public schools located in Nassau and Suffolk Counties, New York (Vianna and Polan, 1973). The study centered around students and teachers with Hodgkin's disease. The data suggested that a greater than expected number of secondary cases were found in schools with index cases. This observation is consistent with some continuous common source exposure or horizontal transmission. The latter possibility is favored by the fact that in those instances in which an institution had more than one contiguous school, the index–secondary case phenomenon was usually limited to one building (Vianna and Polan, 1973). This preliminary evidence, the rarity of Hodgkin's disease, the apparent existence of an asymptomatic carrier state, and the childhood peak observed only in poorly developed countries suggest that Hodgkin's disease might be a rare manifestation of a relatively common infectious agent. Additional studies of this type will be required to evaluate further the possibility that Hodgkin's disease has an infectious component.

10. Prior Tonsillectomy and Hodgkin's Disease

R. W. Miller (1966) suggested that the rapid rise in mortality from Hodgkin's disease among children might coincide with physiological involution of the tonsils. This observation, the rarity with which Hodgkin's disease involves the pharyngeal tonsils (Al-Saleem *et al.*, 1970; Bonadonna and Fossari-Bellani, 1968), and the fact that the tonsils are immunocompetent tissues (Ogra, 1971) suggested that prior tonsillectomy might be a predisposing factor to Hodgkin's disease.

The first investigation of this hypothesis was a case–control study conducted in Nassau and Suffolk Counties, New York (Vianna *et al.*, 1971). This study, which was limited to all cases of Hodgkin's disease diagnosed among residents of these counties who were 40 years of age or less, suggested that prior tonsillectomy increased the risk of developing Hodgkin's disease by a factor of 2.9. A subsequent study failed to confirm these results, which could reflect the small number of patients evaluated and the fact that all age groups were included (Ruuskanen *et al.*, 1971). Additional studies have been undertaken using siblings of patients as the control group. This methodology minimizes the possibility that differences in socioeconomic status will influence the data. It must be appreciated, however, that sibling controls introduce a number of biases, including the likelihood that siblings, especially those close in age to the patients, will have similar tonsillectomy histories. Despite this possibility, the four studies that have employed sibling controls (Newell *et al.,* 1973; Pike and Smith, 1973; Gutensohn *et al.,* 1975; Vianna *et al.,* 1974b) suggest that a positive association exists. The wide range of risk ratios (1.2–3.6) observed indicates, however, the need for more precise evaluation of this hypothesis.

Future studies should give particular attention to the following considerations: (1) the source of study patients, since it is well established that the selection of cases from a single medical facility can introduce a bias arising from selective factors that lead patients to that institution (a geographically based study is therefore preferable); (2) the age and sex composition of study patients, since it is possible that prior tonsillectomy is an important factor only for certain age groups; (3) the histological subtypes and status of patients, since this factor might influence survival; and (4) the age and reasons for tonsillectomy.

11. Importance of the Altered Immune State

Evidence derived from a variety of studies suggests that alteration of man's immune system might be important in the pathogenesis of certain neoplastic disorders. An increased incidence of lymphomas has been found in congenital immunological deficiency disorders (including hypogammaglobulinemia, ataxia-telangiectasia and Wiskott–Aldrich syndrome) (Doll and Kinlen, 1970; Page *et al.,* 1963) (see Chapter 7). Furthermore, a 200-fold increased frequency of malignancy, particularly of histiocytic lymphomas, has been documented in homograft recipients (Hoover and Fraumeni, 1973) (see Chapter 8).

The collagen vascular diseases can generally be defined as disorders in which autoantibodies or sensitized lymphocytes react with host tissue. It has been suggested that a selective or generalized immunological deficiency might contribute to the pathogenesis of these disorders (Fudenberg, 1968). There are several lines of experimental evidence that disturbances of the thymus and other lymphoid tissues might underlie all three phenomena, namely, immunodeficiency, autoimmunity, and lymphoreticular proliferative disorders:

1. Neonatally thymectomized animals are immunologically deficient (Miller, J. F. A. P., 1962), develop reticuloendothelial hyperplasia, have a high incidence of autoimmune phenomena (DeVries *et al.,* 1964), manifest terminal lymphoid hypoplasia (Miller, J. F. A. P., and Howard, 1964), and become wasted.
2. The thymus involutes prematurely in NZB mice. These mice develop Coomb's-positive hemolytic anemia (Burnet and Holmes, 1964; Holmes and Burnet, 1963), and about 20% of the longer survivors develop lymphoma (Mellors, 1966).
3. About 30% of F_1 hybrid mice that survive graft-versus-host reactions by transplanted parental lymphoid cells develop lymphoma (Schwartz and Beldotti, 1965).
4. C3H mouse recipients of isogeneic spleen transplants have a high incidence of lymphoma after an interval of 1 year (Walford and Hildemann, 1965).

These experimental models raise the exciting possibility that a counterpart exists in man. Autoimmune disease and immunological perturbations occur in almost 50% of patients with certain primary immunodeficiency syndromes (Goldberg *et al.*, 1974). Furthermore, there appears to be a high incidence of lymphoreticular disorders with many of these syndromes:

1. Bruton-type hypogammaglobulinemia has been associated with leukemia (Gatti and Good, 1971; Reisman *et al.*, 1964), lymphoma (Page *et al.*, 1963), chronic arthritis suggestive of rheumatoid arthritis, and dermatomyositis (Rosen and Janeway, 1966). Several patients with selective IgA deficiency have developed leukemia (Recant and Hartroft, 1962) or lymphoma (Binder and Reynolds, 1967). This dysgammaglobulinemia has also been coicidentally associated with rheumatoid arthritis, systemic lupus erythematosus, and thyroiditis (Ammann and Hong, 1971).
2. Autoimmune hemolytic anemia (South and Starling, 1969), lymphosarcoma (Lamvik and Moe, 1969), Hodgkin's disease (Bermuth *et al.*, 1970), and leukemia (Kadowaki *et al.*, 1965) have been documented in patients with combined immunodeficiency.
3. In ataxia–telangiectasia, the whole spectrum of lymphoreticular disorders has been observed (Gatti and Good, 1971; Smeby, 1966; Boder and Sedgwick, 1963; Hecht *et al.*, 1966; Dunn *et al.*, 1964). Anti-smooth-muscle antibodies, antimitochondrial antibodies, and autoimmune endocrinopathies are also present in some patients with this syndrome (Goldberg *et al.*, 1974).
4. Lymphocytic and histiocytic lymphomas have occurred with Wiskott–Aldrich syndrome (TenBensel *et al.*, 1966; Kildeberg, 1963; Pearson *et al.*, 1966), and autoimmune hemolytic disease may occur in 5% of cases (Ballow *et al.*, 1973).

There is considerable evidence to support the concept that immunoregulatory deficits contribute to the pathogenesis of autoimmunity, which in turn is coincidentally related to lymphoreticular malignancy. Patients with hypogammaglobulinemia have a high incidence of rheumatoid arthritis (Hijmans *et al.*, 1961). Bowdler and Glick (1966) reported a patient with autoimmune hemolytic anemia who developed Hodgkin's disease 3 years later, and Pirofsky (1968) studied 234 patients with this type of anemia and found that 114 patients developed reticuloendothelial neoplasia. It is generally accepted that patients with Sjögren's syndrome have an increased frequency of certain lymphomas (Doll and Kinlen, 1970; Talal and Bunin, 1964; Talal *et al.*, 1967, 1970; Azzopardi and Evans, 1971). A similar association might be true of other collagen vascular disorders, including lupus erythematosus, rheumatoid arthritis, scleroderma, dermatomyositis, chronic thyroiditis, and periarteritis nodosum (Cammarata *et al.*, 1963; Williams, R. C., 1959; Cox, 1964; Howqua and MacKay, 1963).

D. G. Miller (1967) examined the association of various collagen vascular disorders with lymphomas in 264 patients and found that 17 patients had both processes and 5 patients had autoimmune disease followed by the development of lymphoma. Unfortunately, the results of larger surveys of this possible association have been conflicting; one study (Oleinick, 1967) showed no significant increase in the incidence of lymphoreticular malignancies in patients with lupus erythematosus or rheumatoid arthritis, whereas another survey (Lea, 1964) of 1356 male patients with lymphoma found a statistically significant excess of antecedent rheumatic disease when compared with a randomly selected control group. All these reports suggest that some association among immune deficiency, autoimmunity, and lymphoma might exist, but the variability with regard to which process precedes the other makes interpretation difficult. The immune deficiency or autoimmune conditions or both could be the result of an unrecognized lymphoma, or, alternatively, autoimmune disorders could predispose to neoplasia. Neither hypothesis explains satisfactorily the temporal variations in onset of the different components or the fact that disease activities of these conditions are frequently dissociated in the same patient (Pirofsky, 1969).

A more likely possibility is that these disorders are the result of the same underlying defect (Pirofsky, 1968). In man, heredity appears to play a role in the occurrence of systemic lupus erythematosus, rheumatoid arthritis, and Sjögren's syndrome (Leonhardt, 1967; Bloch et al., 1965). There are numerous reports of the occurrence of systemic lupus erythematosus in two or more family members, including identical twins, and extending to more than one generation (Blumenfeld et al., 1963; Harvey et al., 1954, Fudenberg et al., 1962). There also appears to be some relationship, but not a fully delineated one, between certain collagen vascular disorders, such as lupus erythematosus and Sjögren's syndrome (Heaton, 1959), in individual patients. Genetic factors may also be important in the apparent association between autoimmune disease and lymphomas. Preliminary evidence suggests that patients with Hodgkin's disease (Jeannet and Magnin, 1971) and systemic lupus erythematosus (Waters et al., 1971) might have an excess of the W15 histocompatibility antigen. Rotstein and Good (1962) reported a high incidence of immunological abnormalities in the family of a patient with hypogammaglobulinemia. A. M. S. Mason and Golding (1971) found that 7 of 19 relatives of a patient with multiple immunological abnormalities had both an abnormality of serum immunoglobulins and various autoantibody responses. There are several close relatives (usually sibs) of patients with various lymphoreticular malignancies, including chronic lymphatic leukemia, lymphosarcoma (Fraumeni et al., 1969), reticulum-cell sarcoma (Potolsky et al., 1971), and Hodgkin's disease (Creagan and Fraumeni, 1972), who also have the malignancies. Furthermore, the occurrence of all three entities (immune deficiency, autoimmunity, and lymphoma) has been reported in certain families. The most provocative report (Wolf, 1962) describes a family in which systemic lupus erythematosus, idiopathic thrombocytopenic purpura, leukemic reticuloendotheliosis, Hodgkin's disease, and common variable hypogammaglobulinemia were manifested. There is experimental evidence to support the clinical suggestion that genetic factors may be important to the pathogenesis of these diseases (Fudenberg, 1968).

Although genetic factors appear to be important, the possibility that environmental influences might precipitate one or more of these disorders must also be considered. In experimental animals, there is evidence suggesting that a virus might be responsible for autoimmune disease, immunosuppression, and lymphomas (Mellors et al., 1968; Farrow et al., 1970). In man, elevated EBV antibody titers have been reported in lupus erythematosus (Evans et al., 1971) and certain lymphomas, most notably Burkitt's lymphoma (Epstein et al., 1965). Tubuloreticular structures, morphologically resembling viral nucleocapsids, have been observed in lupus erythematosus, other collagen vascular disorders, and certain lymphomas (Prunieras et al., 1972). Furthermore, in a study of EBV antigen in relatives of cancer patients (including lymphomas), Levine et al. (1974) found significantly higher levels of capsid and early antigen among members of multiple-case families than in controls.

While the observations described above strongly suggest that some relationship between certain connective tissue disorders and various lymphoreticular malignancies might exist, it is important to realize that most of the available evidence comes from case reports. Accordingly, the underlying hypothesis requires detailed objective evaluation before being accepted. In designing a test system, however, attention must be given to the various jokers in the pack. Rheumatoid diseases frequently mimic malignancy, and the lymphomas may be clinically indistinguishable from certain connective tissue diseases (Miller, D. G., 1967). These phenomena underlie the need for histological confirmation. In addition, immunosuppressive agents, which might predispose to certain neoplastic disorders (Doll and Kinlen, 1970; Hoover and Fraumeni, 1973), are often employed in the treatment of many collagen vascular diseases. One method of overcoming this problem would be to study the incidence of lymphoreticular malignancies in blood- and non-blood-related relatives of patients with well-documented connective tissue disorders. This approach seems to be quite reasonable, since autoimmune, immunological, and lymphoreticular disorders have been observed among members of the same family.

12. The Histocompatibility Antigen System and the Malignant Lymphomas

Lilly (1968) showed that susceptibility to murine leukemia induced with Gross virus is influenced by at least two major genes, one of which is closely associated with the H-2 locus. Other experimental studies have demonstrated that there are genes that control the immune response to certain antigens that are closely linked to the major histocompatibility locus (McDevitt and Bodmer, 1974). These observations led to the suggestion that histocompatibility-linked genes might effect susceptibility to certain tumors and viruses through their influence on the immune system (McDevitt and Bodmer, 1972, 1974).

There is growing evidence that the major histocompatibility genetic locus (HLA system) in man may be important in determining disease susceptibility. The first significant association between the HLA system and a lymphoma was reported by Amiel (1967). This study showed an increased incidence of 4C antigen among patients with Hodgkin's disease relative to other, healthy subjects. Numerous reports of a correlation between this lymphoma and various cross-reacting HLA antigens (5, W5, W15, and W18) (Forbes and Morris, 1970; Morris and Forbes, 1971, VanRood and VanLeeuwen, 1971), which are closely related to 4C, have been published. Other studies (Coukell et al., 1971; Dick, 1972), however, have failed to show a significant association between the 4C antigen complex and Hodgkin's disease. Among the various factors that might account for this discrepancy are the small number of patients in most series, variability in their racial composition and in the selection of control populations, the possible influence of therapy on HLA antigens, and the possibility that an association exists, not with the HLA system, but rather with some closely related locus.

The histological type of Hodgkin's tumors in individual patients may have bearing on the frequency of specific HLA antigens: Falk and Osoba (1971) observed an excess frequency of HLA-A1 in 8 patients with mixed-cellularity and lymphocyte-depleted tumors. Graff et al. (1974) found an increased frequency of HLA-A5 with mixed-cellularity or lymphocyte-predominant tumors, whereas HLA-A1 and 8 and W18 antigens were significantly more prevalent with mixed-cellularity Hodgkin's disease. Forbes and Morris (1970) reported that W5 occurred primarily in female patients with mixed-cellularity disease, and were uncommon with nodular-sclerotic tumors. Coukell *et al.*, (1971) and Dick (1972) reported an increased incidence of HLA-A7 in patients with nodular-sclerotic lymphomas. One study on leukocyte antigens with other lymphomas (Rege *et al.*, 1971) suggested that the association between HLA-A5 antigen and Hodgkin's disease might extend to other types of lymphomas as well.

The Rye histological subtypes may reflect interactions between host immune responses and Hodgkin's disease. Perhaps the histopathological pattern of this disease is determined in part by the influence of histocompatibility type on immune responsiveness. Two lines of evidence lend some indirect support to this hypothesis: (1) In a recent study of familial Hodgkin's disease (Vianna *et al.*, 1974a), many blood-related pairs had concordant Rye subtypes. This observation suggested that genetic factors, possibly related to the HLA system, might influence host reactivity. (2) Sybesma (1972) found a significantly higher frequency of HLA-A12 antigen among untreated patients with Hodgkin's disease who could not mount an antibody response to influenza A Hong Kong vaccine.

Racial factors are another important consideration in malignant lymphomas. While differences in disease experience might be due to variability in customs or environmental exposures or both, it is also clear that members of a specific ethnic group share many genetically determined traits. Thus, both the environmental and the genetic ends of the spectrum must be viewed in examining ethnicity.

With the possible exception of multiple myeloma, the incidence of lymphoreticular malignancies in the black population is considerably lower than that in whites (MacMahon, 1966). The reasons for these differences are unknown, but certain avenues of approach would seem to be available. For example, we know that poorly developed countries have a bimodal incidence curve for Hodgkin's disease that is characterized by a peak in childhood and another in the elderly. An important question is whether the pattern for the black population in the United States more closely resembles this distribution or the classic bimodal curve, with modes in the young adult and elderly age groups. Observation of patterns similar to those found in poorly developed countries would be consistent with some environmental influence, and would also raise the possibility that age at exposure is an important factor. In view of the reported association between certain HLA antigens and Hodgkin's disease, however, some consideration must also be given to the fact that the frequency of some antigens differs markedly among Caucasians and Negroes (Terasaki, 1971) (e.g., Te 57 is considerably more common in the Negro population). If certain HLA phenotypes were associated with an increased frequency of this lymphoma, it would be reasonable to expect that the others would be associated with a decrease and might, in fact, be protective. Consider the following: Hodgkin's disease is rare in Japan, particularly in young adults. The highest frequency of HLA-A9 has been observed in Orientals, while other antigens such as HLA-A1 and 8, which have been associated with an increased frequency of Hodgkin's disease, are virtually absent (Terasaki, 1971). Certain viral infections may be most prevalent in subjects with specific histocompatibility antigens (Morris and Forbes, 1971) (e.g., infectious mononucleosis and W5 antigen). Only a small number of persons infected with a virus such as rubella might have a high potential for spreading the disease

(Hattis *et al.*, 1973). It has been further suggested that persons who harbor certain viruses (e.g., rubella) have a relatively high genotypic frequency of HLA-A1 and 8 haplotypes. These observations raise the possibility that the histocompatibility system influences susceptibility, retention, and transmission of certain viruses in man (Honeyman and Menser, 1974).

In keeping with this concept, Honeyman and Menser (1974) suggested that the incidence of Hodgkin's disease in several ethnic groups correlates significantly with the gene frequency of HLA-A1 and 8 antigens. We therefore come full circle. Evidence derived from a variety of epidemiological studies suggests that environmental factors are important in the etiology of Hodgkin's disease, and it seems clear that factors such as socioeconomic development and possibly marital status might markedly influence the age-specific incidence curve for this disorder. It is equally possible that the HLA system or some closely related genetic system modulates the effect of these factors. A similar interaction might hold true for other malignant lymphomas.

There is additional evidence suggesting that genetic factors might be important in the etiology of malignant lymphomas. Certain chromosomal aberrations, such as the Chediak–Higashi syndrome, and congenital immunological disorders are associated with an increased incidence of lymphomas (Doll and Kinlen, 1970). An extra band of fluorescence has been frequently observed on chromosome 14qT in Burkitt's lymphoma (Rowley, 1974), but the specific nature of this defect remains unknown. Milham and Hesser (1967) suggested that Italian surnames appear more commonly among Hodgkin's disease patients, and MacMahon (1966) found a high rate for this disorder among Jews in Brooklyn, New York. All these observations require further evaluation.

13. Concluding Remarks

The field of lymphoma research is in a state of rapid flux—a state that is likely to continue into the future. At present, however, some important signposts are visible. We can no longer speak of "all" lymphomas (or leukemias); too many essential differences exist among and within certain subgroups of these disorders. While this is most dramatically exemplified with Hodgkin's disease, it might also hold true for Burkitt's lymphoma (African vs. American types) and lymphosarcoma. Available evidence also suggests that both environmental and genetic factors are of etiological importance for most of the lymphomas. This seems to be a central theme that underlies all the major lymphomas. Here, too, we are faced with a variety of dichotomies. It seems clear that our major efforts in the future should be directed at a better understanding of these differences.

References

Alderson, M. R., and Nayak, R., 1972, Epidemiology of Hodgkin's disease, *J. Chronic Dis.* **25**:253–259.

Al-Saleem, T., Hartwich, R., Robins, R., and Blady, J. V., 1970, Malignant lymphomas of the pharynx, *Cancer* **26**:1383–1387.

Amiel, J. L., 1967, Study of leukocyte phenotypes in Hodgkin's disease, in: *Histocompatibility Testing 1967* (P. L. Mattiuz and R. M. Tose, eds.), pp. 78–81, Munksgaard, Copenhagen.

Ammann, A. J. and Hong, R., 1971, Selective IgA deficiency: Presentation of 30 cases and review of the literature, *Medicine (Baltimore)* **50**:223–236.

Anderson, R. E., Ishida, K., and Li, Y., 1970, Geographic aspects of malignant lymphoma and multiple myeloma, *Am. J. Pathol.* **61**:85–96.

Andrade, Z., and Waldeck, N. A., 1971, Follicular lymphoma of the spleen in patients with hepatosplenic schistosomiasis mansoni, *Am. J. Trop. Med. Hyg.* **20**:237–245.

Azzopardi, J. G., and Evans, D. J., 1971, Malignant lymphomas of parotid associated with Mikuliez disease, *J. Clin. Pathol.* **24**:744–752.

Baikie, A. G., Kinlen, L. J., and Pike, M. C., 1972, Detection and assessment of case clustering in Burkitt's lymphoma and Hodgkin's disease, in: *Current Problems in the Epidemiology of Cancer and Lymphomas* (E. Grundmann and H. Tullinius, eds.), pp. 201–207, Springer-Verlag, Berlin, Heidelberg, New York.

Ballow, M., Dupont, B., and Good, R. A., 1973, Autoimmune hemolytic anemia in Wiskott–Aldrich syndrome during treatment with transfer factor, *J. Pediatr.* **83**:772–780.

Berard, C. W., 1969, Histopathologic definition of Burkitt's tumor, *Bull. W.H.O.* **40**:601.

Bermuth, G. V., Minielly, J. A., and Logan, G. B., 1970, Hodgkin's disease and thymic alymphoplasia in a 5 month old infant, *Pediatrics* **45**:792–798.

Besuschio, S. C., 1974, Geographic pathology of lymphomas in Latin America, *Medicina (Mexico City)* **34**:31–38.

Binder, H. J., and Reynolds, R. D., 1967, Control of diarrhea in secondary hypogammaglobulinemia by fresh plasma infusions, *N. Engl. J. Med.* **277**:802–803.

Bjelke, E., 1969, Hodgkin's disease in Norway, *Acta Med. Scand.* **185**:73–79.

Blaisdell, R. K., and Boxer, G. J., 1971, Scientific Contributions, Second Meeting of the Asian–Pacific Division of the International Society of Haematology, Melbourne.

Bloch, K. J., Buchanan, W. W., and Wohl, M. J., 1965, Sjögren's syndrome: A clinical, pathologic and serological study of sixty-two cases, *Medicine (Baltimore)* **44**:187–231.

Blumenfeld, H. B., Kaplan, S. B., and Mills, D. M., 1963, Disseminated lupus erythematosus in identical twins, *J. Am. Med. Assoc.* **185**:667–669.

Boder, E., and Sedgwick, R. P., 1963, Ataxia–telangiectasia—Review of 101 cases, in: *Little Club Clinics in Developmental Medicine*, No. 8, *Cerebellum, Posture and Cerebral Palsy* (G. E. Walsh, ed.), pp. 110–118, The National Spastics Society and Heinemann Books, London.

Bondonna, G., and Fossari-Bellani, F., 1968, The spread of malignant lymphomas in children, *Tumori* **54**:311–320.

Booth, K., Burkitt, D. P., Bassett, D. J., Cook, R. A., and Biddulph, T., 1967, Burkitt lymphoma in Papua, New Guinea, *Br. J. Cancer* **21**:657–664.

Bowdler, A. J., and Glick, J. W., 1966, Autoimmune hemolytic anemia as the herald state of Hodgkin's disease, *Ann. Intern. Med.* **65**:761–767.

Brubaker, G., Geser, A., and Pike, M., 1973, Burkitt's lymphoma in the North Mara district of Tanzania, 1964–1970: Failure to find evidence of time–space clustering in a high risk isolated rural area, *Br. J. Cancer* **28**:469–472.

Burkitt, D. P., 1958, A sarcoma involving the jaws in African children, *Br. J. Surg.* **46**:218–223.

Burkitt, D. P., 1969, Etiology of Burkitt's lymphoma—An alternative hypothesis to a vectoral virus, *J. Natl. Cancer Inst.* **42**:19–27.

Burkitt, D. P., and Davies, J. N. P., 1961, Lymphoma syndrome in Uganda and tropical Africa, *Afr. Med. Press* **245**:367–371.

Burn, C., Davies, J. N. P., Dodge, O. G., and Nias, B. C., 1971, Hodgkin's disease in English and African children, *J. Natl. Cancer Inst.* **46**:37–46.

Burnet, F. M., and Holmes, M. C., 1964, Thymic changes in the mouse strain NZB in relation to the autoimmune state, *J. Pathol. Bacteriol.* **88**:229–241.

Cammarata, R. J., Rodman, G. P., and Jensen, W. N., 1963, Systematic rheumatic disease and malignant lymphoma, *Arch. Intern. Med.* **111**:330–337.

Clemmesen, J., 1964, *Statistical Studies in the Aetiology of Malignant Neoplasms*, Vol. II, *Basic Tables, Denmark 1943–57*, Munksgaard, Copenhagen.

Cohen, M. H., Bennett, J. M., Berard, C. W., and Ziegler, J. L., 1969, Burkitt's tumor in the United States, *Cancer* **23**:1259–1272.

Cole, P., MacMahon, B., and Aisenberg, A., 1968, Mortality from Hodgkin's disease in the United States, *Lancet* **2**:1371–1374.

Correa, P., and O'Conor, G. T., 1971, Epidemiologic patterns of Hodgkin's disease, *Int. J. Cancer.* **8**:192–201.

Coukell, A., Bodmer, J. G., and Bodmer, W. F., 1971, *HL-A* types of 44 Hodgkin's patients, *Transplant. Pro.* **3**:1291–1293.

Cox, M. T., 1964, Malignant lymphoma of thyroid, *J. Clin. Pathol.* **17**:591–601.

Creagan, E. T., and Fraumeni, J. F., 1972, Familial Hodgkin's disease, *Lancet* **2**:547.

Daldorf, G., Linsell, C. A., and Barnhart, F. E., 1964, An epidemiologic approach to lymphomas of African children and Burkitt's sarcoma of the jaws, *Perspect. Biol. Med.* **7**:435–439.

DeVries, M. J., VanPutten, L. M., and Balner, H., 1964, Lésions sugerant une reactivité auto-immune chez des souris atteintes de la "runt disease" après thymectomie néonatale, *Rev. Fr. Etud. Clin. Biol.* **9**:381.

Dick, F. R., 1972, *HL-A* and lymphoid tumors, *Cancer Res.* **32**:2608–2611.

Diehl, V., Henle, G., Henle, L., and Kohn, G., 1968, Demonstration of a herpes group virus in cultures of peripheral leukocytes from patients with infectious mononucleosis, *J. Virol.* **2**:663–671.

Doll, R., and Kinlen, L., 1970, Immunosurveillance and cancer: Epidemiologic evidence, *Br. Med. J.* **4**:420–423.

Dörken, H., and Singer-Bakker, H., 1972, Hodgkin's disease in childhood—An epidemiologic study in Northern Germany, in: *Current Problems in the Epidemiology of Cancer and Lymphomas* (E. Grundmann and H. Tullinius, eds.), pp. 235–239, Springer-Verlag, Berlin, Heidelberg, New York.

Dunn, H. G., Meuwissen, H., and Livingston, C. S., 1964, Ataxia–telangiectasia. *Can. Med. Assoc. J.* **91**:1106–1118.

Dworsky, R. L., and Henderson, B. E., 1974, Hodgkin's disease clustering in families and communities, *Cancer Res.* **34**:1161.

El-Gazayerli, M., Khalil, H., and Abdel, A., 1962, Observations on some bilharzial reactions, *Alexandria Med. J.* **8**:434–438.

Epstein, M. A., Barr, Y. M., and Achong, B. G., 1965, Studies with Burkitt's lymphoma, *Wistar Inst. Symp. Monogr.* **4**:69–75.

Evans, A. S., Rothfield, N. F., and Niederman, J. C., 1971, Raised antibody titers to EV virus in systemic lupus erythematosus, *Lancet* **1**:167–168.

Falk, T., and Osoba, D., 1971, *HL-A* antigens and survival in Hodgkin's disease, *Lancet* **2**:1118.

Farrow, L. J., Holborow, E. J., and Johnson, G. D., 1970, Auto-antibodies and the hepatitis associated antigen in acute infective hepatitis, *Br. Med. J.* **2**:693–695.

Fasal, E., Jackson, E. W., and Klauber, M. R., 1968, Leukemia and lymphoma mortality and farm residence, *Am. J. Epidemiol.* **87**:267–274.

Finn, R., St. Hill, C. A., and Govan, A. J., 1972, Immunologic responses in pregnancy and survival of fetal homograft, *Br. Med. J.* **3**:150–152.

Forbes, J. F., and Morris, P. J., 1970, Leucocyte antigens in Hodgkin's disease, *Lancet* **2**:849–851.

Fraumeni, J. F., Vogel, C. L., and DeVita, V. T., 1969, Familial chronic lymphocytic leukemia, *Ann. Intern. Med.* **71**:279–284.

Fry, R. A., Meersschaert, A., Linder, L., and Dunham, D., 1976, *Men, Women and Change: A Sociology of Marriage and Family*, p. 156, McGraw-Hill, New York.

Fudenberg, H. H., 1968, Are autoimmune diseases immunologic deficiency states?, *Hosp. Pract.* **3**:43–53.

Fudenberg, H. H., German, J. L., and Kunkel, H. G., 1962, The occurrence of rheumatoid factor and other abnormalities in families of patients with aggamoglobulinemia, *Arthritis Rheum.* **5**:565–588.

Gatti, R. A., and Good, R. A., 1971, Occurrence of malignancy in immunodeficiency disease, *Cancer* **28**:89–98.

Goldberg, L. S., Bluestone, R., and Stiehm, E. R., 1974, Human autoimmunity, with pernicious anemia as a model, *Ann. Intern. Med.* **81**:372–380.

Graff, K. S., Simon, R. M., Yankee, R. A., DiVita, V. T., and Rogetine, G. N., 1974, *HL-A* antigens in Hodgkin's disease: Histopathologic and clinical correlations, *J. Natl. Cancer Inst.* **52**:1087–1090.

Gutensohn, N., Li, F. P., Johnson, R. E., and Cole, P., 1975, Hodgkin's disease, tonsillectomy and family size, *N. Engl. J. Med.* **292**:22–25.

Haddow, A. J., 1963, An improved map for the study of Burkitt's lymphoma syndrome in Africa, *East Afr. Med. J.* **40**:429–436.

Harvey, A. M., Shulman, L. E., and Tumulty, P. A., 1954, Systemic lupus erythematosus: Review of the literature and clinical analysis of 138 cases, *Medicine (Baltimore)* **33**:291–437.

Hattis, R. P., Halstead, S. B., Herrmann, K. L., and Witte, J. J., 1973, Rubella in an immunized island population. *J. Am. Med. Assoc.* **223**:1019–1021.

Heaton, J. M., 1959, Sjögren's syndrome and systemic lupus erythematosus, *Br. Med. J.* 1:466–469.

Hecht, F., Koler, R. D., and Rigas, D. A., 1966, Leukemia and lymphocytes in ataxia telangiectasia, *Lancet* 2:1193.

Herms, W. B., and James, M. T., 1961, Mosquitoes as vectors of disease, in: *Medical Entomology*, p. 195, Macmillan Co., New York.

Hijmans, W., Doniach, D., and Roitt, J. M., 1961, Serologic overlap between lupus erythematosus, rheumatoid arthritis and thyroid auto-immune disease, *Br. Med. J.* 2:909–914.

Hirshaut, Y., Cohen, M. H., and Stevens, D. A., 1973, Epstein–Barr virus antibodies in American and African Burkitt's lymphoma, *Lancet* 2:114-118.

Holmes, M. C., and Burnet, F. M., 1963, The natural history of autoimmune disease in NZB mice, *Ann. Intern. Med.* 59:265–276.

Honeyman, M. C., and Menser, M. A., 1974, Ethnicity is a significant factor in the epidemiology of rubella and Hodgkin's disease, *Nature (London)* 251:441–442.

Hoover, R., and Fraumeni, J. F., 1973, Risk of cancer in renal transplant recipients, *Lancet* 2:55–57.

Howqua, J., and MacKay, I. R., 1963, LE cells in lymphoma, *Blood* 22:191–198.

Jeannet, M., and Magnin, C., 1971, *HL-A* antigens in hematological malignant disease, *Tranplant Proc.* 3:1301–1303.

Jerusalem, C., Jap, P., and Eling, W., 1971, Virus induced malignant lymphoma in mice dependent on a RES "conditioned" by chronic parasitic infection (P. berghei), in: *The Reticuloendothelial System and Immune Phenomena* (N. R. DiLuzio and K. Flemming, eds.), pp. 319–399, Plenum Press, New York.

Kadowaki, J. I., Thompson, R., and Zuelzer, W. W., 1965, XX/XY lymphoid chimaerism in congenital immunological deficiency syndrome with thymic alymphoplasia, *Lancet* 2:1152–1156.

Kildeberg, P., 1963, A case of Aldrich's syndrome, *Acta Pediatr. Scand. (Suppl.)* 140:120–121.

Klinger, R. J., and Minton, J. P., 1973, Case clustering of Hodgkin's disease in a small rural community with associations among cases, *Lancet* 1:168–170.

Lamvik, J., and Moe, P. J., 1969, Thymic dysplasia with immunologic deficiency, *Acta Pathol. Microbiol. Scand.* 76:349–360.

Lea, A. J., 1964, An association between rheumatic diseases and the reticuloses, *Ann. Rheum. Dis.* 23:480–484.

Leonhardt, E. T. G., 1967, Familial studies in systemic lupus erythematosus, *Clin. Exp. Immunol.* 2:743.

Levine, P. H., Fraumeni, F. F., and Reisher, J. I., 1974, Antibodies to Epstein–Barr virus associated antigen in relatives of cancer patients, *J. Natl. Cancer Inst.* 52:1037–1040.

Lilly, F., 1968, The effect of histocompatibility 2 type in response to the Friend leukemia virus in mice, *J. Exp. Med.* 127:465–473.

MacMahon, B., 1966, Epidemiology of Hodgkin's disease, *Cancer Res.* 26:1189–1200.

Mason, A. M. S., and Golding, P. L., 1971, Multiple immunologic abnormalities in a family, *J. Clin. Pathol.* 24:732–735.

Mason, T. J., and Fraumeni, J. F., Jr., 1974, Hodgkin's disease among Japanese Americans, *Lancet* 1:215.

Mason, T. J., McKay, F. W., Hoover, R., Blot, W., and Fraumeni, J. F., 1975, *Atlas of Cancer Mortality for U.S. Counties: 1950–1969,* U.S. Department of Health, Education and Welfare (DHEW Publ. No. NIH 75-780), pp. 58–59.

McDevitt, H. O., and Bodmer, W. F., 1972, Histocompatibility antigens, immune responsiveness and susceptibility to disease, *Am. J. Med.* 52:1–8.

McDevitt, H. O., and Bodmer, W. F., 1974, *HL-A* immune-response genes and disease, *Lancet* 1:1269–1274.

Mellors, R., 1966, Autoimmune disease in NZB/BL mice. II. Autoimmunity and malignant lymphoma, *Blood* 27:435–448.

Mellors, R. C., Aoki, T., and Huebner, R., 1968, Further implications of murine leukemia-like virus in the disorders of NZB mice, *J. Exp. Med.* 129:1045–1062.

Meytes, D., and Modan, B., 1969, Selected aspects of Hodgkin's disease in a whole community, *Blood* 34:91–98.

Milham, S., and Hesser, J., 1967, Hodgkin's disease in woodworkers, *Lancet* 2:136–139.

Miller, D. G., 1967, The association of immune disease and malignant lymphoma, *Ann. Intern. Med.* 66:507–521.

Miller, J. F. A. P., 1962, Effect of neonatal thymectomy on immunologic responsiveness of the mouse, *Proc. R. Soc. London* 156:415–428.

Miller, J. F. A. P., and Howard, J. G., 1964, Some similarities between the neonatal thymectomy syndrome and graft-versus-host disease, *J. Reticuloendothel. Soc.* **1**:369–392.

Miller, R. W., 1966, Mortality in childhood Hodgkin's disease. An etiologic clue, *J.A.M.A.* **198**:216–218.

Morris, P. J., and Forbes, J. F., 1971, *HL-A* and Hodgkin's disease, *Transplant, Proc.* **3**:1275–1276.

Newell, G. R., Rawlings, W., and Kinnear, B. K., 1973, Case control study of Hodgkin's disease. I. Results of the interview questionnaire, *J. Natl. Cancer Inst.* **51**:1437–1441.

Ogra, P., 1971, Effect of tonsillectomy and adenoidectomy on nasopharyngeal antibody response to poliovirus, *N. Engl. J. Med.* **284**:59–64.

Oleinick, A., 1967, Leukemia or lymphoma occurring subsequent to an autoimmune disease, *Blood* **29**:144–153.

Page, A. R., Hanson, A. E., and Good, R., 1963, Occurrence of leukemia and lymphoma in patients with agammaglobulinemia, *Blood* **21**:197–206.

Pearson, H. A., Shulman, N. R., and Oski, F. A., 1966, Platelet survival in Wiskott–Aldrich syndrome, *J. Pediatr.* **68**:754–760.

Pike, M. C., and Smith, P. G., 1973, Tonsillectomy and Hodgkin's disease, *Lancet* **1**:434.

Pike, M. C., Williams, E. H., and Wright, D., 1967, Burkitt's tumor in the West Nile district of Uganda 1961–1965, *Br. Med. J.* **2**:395.

Pirofsky, B., 1968, Autoimmune hemolytic anemia and neoplasia of the reticuloendothelium, *Ann. Intern. Med.* **68**:109–121.

Pirofsky, B., 1969, *Autoimmunization and the Autoimmune Hemolytic Anemias,* pp. 96–146, William and Wilkins Co., Baltimore.

Potolsky, A. I., Heath, C. W., and Buckley, C. E., 1971, Lymphoreticular malignancies and immunologic abnormalities in a sibship, *Am. J. Med.* **50**:42–48.

Prunieras, M., Grupper, C., and Durepaire, R., 1972, Les inclusions type lupus la peau—valeur diagnostique. *Nouv. Presse Med.* **1**:1133.

Ramot, B., and Many, A., 1972, Primary intestinal lymphoma, in: *Current Problems in the Epidemiology of Cancer and Lymphomas* (E. Grundmann and H. Tullinius, eds.), pp. 194–198, Springer-Verlag, Berlin, Heidelberg, New York.

Recant, L., and Hartroft, W. S., 1962, Clinicopathologic conference: Rademacher's disease, *Am. J. Med.* **32**:80–95.

Rege, V., Patel, R., and Briggs, W. A., 1971, Leukocyte antigens and disease. II. Association of HL-A5 and lymphomas, *Am. J. Clin. Pathol.* **58**:14–16.

The Registrar-General's Decennial Supplement, England and Wales, 1961, Occupational Mortality Tables, p. 148, Her Majesty's Stationery Office, London (1971).

Reisman, L. E., Mitani, M., and Zuelzer, W. W., 1964, Chromosome studies in leukemia. I. Evidence for the origin of leukemic stem lines from aneuploid mutants, *N. Engl. J. Med.* **270**:591–597.

Rosen, F. S., and Janeway, C. A., 1966, The gammaglobulins. III. The antibody deficiency syndromes, *N. Engl. J. Med.* **275**:709–715.

Rotstein, J., and Good, R., 1962, Significance of simultaneous occurrence of connective tissue disease and agammaglobulinemia, *Ann. Rheum. Dis.* **21**:202–206.

Rowley, J. D., 1974, Do human tumors show a chromosome pattern specific for each etiologic agent?, *J. Natl. Cancer Inst.* **52**:315–319.

Ruuskanen, O., Vanha-Pertulla, T., and Kouvalainen, K., 1971, Tonsillectomy, appendectomy and Hodgkin's disease, *Lancet* **1**:1127–1128.

Schimpff, S. C., Schimpff, C., and Barger, D., 1975, Leukemia and lymphoma patients interlinked by prior social contact, *Lancet* **1**:124–129.

Schwartz, R. S., and Beldotti, L., 1965, Malignant lymphomas following allogenic disease: Transition from an immunologic to a neoplastic disorder, *Science* **149**:1511–1514.

Smeby, B., 1966, Ataxia–telangiectasia, *Acta Paediatr. Scand.* **55**:239.

South, M. A., and Starling, K. A., 1969, Anti-LW antibody production in a child with combined immune deficiency disease, *N. Engl. J. Med.* **280**:94–95.

Sybesma, J. P., 1972, Antibody response related to *HL-A* antigens in Hodgkin's disease and other lymphomas, *Lancet* **2**:884–886.

Talal, N., and Bunin, J. J., 1964, The development of malignant lymphoma in the course of Sjögren's syndrome, *Am. J. Med.* **36**:529–540.

Talal, N., Sokoloff, L., and Bath, W. F., 1967, Extrasalivary lymph node abnormalities in Sjögren's syndrome, *Am. J. Med.* **43**:50–65.

Talal, N., Asofsky, R., and Lightbody, P., 1970, Immunoglobulin synthesis by salivary gland lymphoid cells in Sjögren's syndrome, *J. Clin. Invest.* **49**:49–54.

Talal, N., and Bunin, J. J., 1964, The development of malignant lymphoma in the course of Sjögren's syndrome, *Am. J. Med.* **36**:529–540.

Talal, N., Sokoloff, L., and Bath, W. F., 1967, Extrasalivary lymph node abnormalities in Sjögren's syndrome, *Am. J. Med.* **43**:50–65.

TenBensel, R. W., Stadlan, E. M., and Krivit, W., 1966, The development of malignancy in the course of the Aldrich syndrome, *J. Pediatr.* **68**:761–767.

Terasaki, P. I., 1971, *HL-A* histocompatibility discriminants, *Dis.-Mon.,* December.

Thomas, L. B., and Berard, C. W., 1973, Relationship of histopathologic type at diagnosis to clinical parameters and to histologic distribution at autopsy, *Gann* **15**:253–273.

VanRood, J. J., and VanLeeuwen, A., 1971, *HL-A* and the group five system in Hodgkin's disease, *Transplant. Proc.* **3**:1283–1286.

Vianna, N. J., and Polan, A. K., 1973, Epidemiologic evidence for transmission of Hodgkin's disease, *N. Engl. J. Med.* **289**:499–504.

Vianna, N. J., Greenwald, P., and Davies, J. N. P., 1971, Tonsillectomy and Hodgkin's disease: The lymphoid tissue barrier, *Lancet* **1**:431–432.

Vianna, N. J., Greenwald, P., Brady, J., Polan, A., Dwork, A., Mauro, J., and Davies, J. N. P., 1972, Hodgkin's disease: Cases with features of a community outbreak, *Ann. Intern. Med.* **77**:169–180.

Vianna, N. J., Davies, J. N. P., Polan, A. K., and Wolfgang, P., 1974a, Familial Hodgkin's disease: An environmental and genetic disorder, *Lancet* **2**:854–858.

Vianna, N. J., Greenwald, P., and Polan, A., 1974b, Tonsillectomy and Hodgkin's disease, *Lancet* **2**:168–169.

Vianna, N. J., Polan, A., and Kirmss, V., 1976, Lymphoma mortality and marital status, Vital Records Data, New York State Health Department, Albany, New York.

Walford, R. L., and Hildemann, W. H., 1965, Life span and lymphoma incidence of mice injected at birth with spleen cells across a weak histocompatibility locus, *Am. J. Pathol.* **47**:713–721.

Waters, H., Konrad, P., and Walford, R. L., 1971, The distribution of *HL-A* histocompatibility factors and genes in patients with systemic lupus erythematosus, *Tissue Antigens* **1**:68–73.

Weiss, P., and Morón, J., 1962, Linfomas (reticulosarcomas) nasales, *Dermatol. Rev. Mex.* **6**:34–38.

Williams, E. H., Day, N. E., and Geser, A. G., 1974, Seasonal variation in onset in Burkitt's lymphoma in the West Nile district of Uganda, *Lancet* **2**:19–21.

Williams, R. C., 1959, Dermatomyositis and malignancy: A review of the literature, *Ann. Intern. Med.* **50**:1174–1181.

Wolf, J. K., 1962, Primary acquired agammoglobulinemia with a family history of collagen disease and hematologic disorders, *N. Engl. J. Med.* **266**:473–480.

Wright, D. H., 1963, Cytology and histochemistry of the Burkitt lymphoma, *Br. J. Cancer* **17**:50–58.

7

Immunodeficiency Diseases and Malignancy

BEATRICE D. SPECTOR, GUY S. PERRY III,
ROBERT A. GOOD, and JOHN H. KERSEY

1. Introduction

Genetically induced immunodeficiencies, drug-induced immunodeficiencies, and several lymphoreticular malignancies constitute a group of disorders in which immunodeficiency and malignancy are frequently related. Chronic lymphatic leukemia and multiple myeloma are malignant proliferations of the lymphoreticular system associated with specific abnormalities of T or B cells that were recognized as immunologically related disorders in the 1950's and early 1960's (Cone and Uhr, 1964). The discovery of an association between these malignancies and immunodeficiency was some of the earliest evidence implicating immunological factors in some forms of human oncogenesis (Good, 1972). Recent evidence that renal transplant recipients on immunosuppressive regimens are at increased risk for developing malignancies has provided additional insight into this complex problem of the nature of the association between cellular abnormalities and malignancy (Hoover and Fraumeni, 1973; Penn, 1975).

Genetically induced immunodeficiencies are rare disorders. Data on the cancer experience of patients with these disorders provide the basis for this review of immunodeficiency and malignancy. Over 200 cases of cancer occurring in patients with diagnosed immunodeficiency diseases have been collected by the Immunodeficiency-Cancer Registry (ICR), a tumor registry established in 1971 under the aegis of the World Health Organization Committee on Primary Immunodeficiencies (Fudenberg et al., 1971). Compilation of data on numbers of diagnosed immunodeficiency patients with and without malignancy provides evidence that immunodeficiency diseases predispose to malignancy, since mortality rates for cancer in

BEATRICE D. SPECTOR, GUY S. PERRY III, and JOHN H. KERSEY • Department of Laboratory Medicine and Pathology, University of Minnesota, Minneapolis, Minnesota 55455. ROBERT A. GOOD • Memorial Sloan-Kettering Cancer Center, New York, New York 10021.

immunodeficiency groups are 100-fold greater than rates expected for the general population (Kersey *et al.*, 1974). This chapter presents discussions of the types of immunodeficiencies that predispose to malignancy, the patterns of malignancies by reported morphology and site, and suggested models or hypotheses of the role of immune deficiency in oncogenesis.

2. Identification of Genetically Induced Immunodeficiencies That Predispose to Malignancy

Immunologists have identified a wide range of immunodeficiency disorders that have been classified according to several criteria: inheritance, association with certain well-defined clinical and histological abnormalities, and estimation of circulating antibodies, immunoglobulins, B cells, and T cells. A list of those immunodeficiency disorders associated with relatively well-characterized features and classified according to the suggested nature of the cellular defect as ascertained by enumeration and function of T and B cells was published by Cooper *et al.* (1973). Criteria for this list provided the ICR with means to classify each case report into an appropriate immunodeficiency disease category. The 227 cases registered at present in the ICR constitute seven immunodeficiency states: X-linked (Bruton's) hypogammaglobulinemia (12 cases), IgA deficiency (13 cases), IgM deficiency (7 cases), variable immunodeficiency (70 cases), severe combined immunodeficiency (SCID) (11 cases), ataxia–telangiectasia (79 cases), and Wiskott–Aldrich syndrome (35 cases).

For a number of years, it appeared that each of these disorders was associated with an increased cancer risk, ranging from 2 to 10%, depending on the type of immunodeficiency disease in question (Table 1) (Gatti and Good, 1971; Good, 1972; Kersey *et al.*, 1973a). Newly obtained data from a nationwide survey that collected over 800 cases of various immunodeficiency diseases provide additional insight into this association (Spector *et al.*, 1977). These data suggest that patients with X-linked (Bruton's) hypogammaglobulinemia may not have an increased predisposition to develop cancer, and that these with other immunodeficiency diseases, such as ataxia–telangiectasia and Wiskott–Aldrich syndrome, may have higher cancer risks than previously estimated. These preliminary observations are currently undergoing further analysis.

TABLE 1.   Estimated Incidence of Malignancy in Primary Immunodeficiency Syndromes[a]

Disease	Approximate incidence of malignancy	Estimated risk (%)
X-linked (Bruton's) hypogammaglobulinemia	6/100	6
Severe combined immunodeficiency	9/400	2
IgM deficiency	6/70	8
Wiskott–Aldrich syndrome	24/300	8
Ataxia–telangiectasia	52/500	10
Variable immunodeficiency	41/500	8
TOTALS:	138/1870	7

[a]From Kersey *et al.* (1973a).

A brief, general description of these seven primary immunodeficiency diseases follows (see also Bergsma, 1975). X-linked (Bruton's) hypogammaglobulinemia, isolated IgA deficiency, and isolated IgM deficiency have a primary defect of the humoral B-cell system. Defects of both B- and T-cell immune components occur with variable immunodeficiency, SCID, ataxia–telangiectasia, and Wiskott–Aldrich syndrome. Increased susceptibility to infection is the cardinal symptom of severe primary immunodeficiency disorders; GI disturbance and autoimmunity have also been reported in patients with particular immunodeficiency diseases.

Boys with X-linked hypogammaglobulinemia are severely compromised immunologically, since they generally have very few B lymphocytes and no Ig-secreting plasma cells (Kersey and Gajl-Peczalska, 1975). They have an inordinately high susceptibility to infections with encapsulated organisms, e.g., *Hemophilus influenzae, Pseudomonas aeruginosa,* and *Diplococcus pneumoniae.* These clinical problems have been treated with some success with γ-globulin or plasma therapy. To date, 12 cancer cases have been identified in this disorder.

Isolated IgA deficiency is responsible for recurrent infections and coincides with autoimmune disease and GI disorders in some patients, while others with comparably severe IgA deficiency are asymptomatic (Amman and Hong, 1971). The incidence of isolated IgA deficiency ranges between 1 in 500 and 1 in 700 persons, which is considerably higher than the frequency of such recessively inherited diseases as X-linked hypogammaglobulinemia, Wiskott–Aldrich syndrome, and ataxia–telangiectasia (Huntley and Stephenson, 1968; Amman and Hong, 1971). Of patients with IgA deficiency, 13 are known to have developed malignancies; 2 patients developed multiple primary neoplasms.

Isolated IgM deficiency occurs in approximately 1 in 1000 persons. Some persons remain asymptomatic, while others are highly susceptible to upper respiratory infections, particularly by gram-negative bacteria and bacteremia (Hobbs, 1975). To date, malignancies have been found in 7 persons with IgM deficiency.

Variable immunodeficiency probably encompasses several syndromes that remain to be clearly distinguished. Included are cases previously classified as "congenital" and non-X-linked (or sporadic) hypogammaglobulinemia, primary dysgammaglobulinemia, and "acquired" primary hypogammaglobulinemia (Good, 1972). Enumeration of Ig-bearing lymphocytes in such patients has led to the delineation of at least two different patterns that likely reflect different underlying mechanisms (Cooper *et al.,* 1973). Cell-mediated (T-cell) immune competence is usually adequate (Kersey and Gajl-Peczalska, 1975), although deficits of this component of the immune response have been identified (Gellman and Vietti, 1970; Kopp *et al.,* 1968; Twomey *et al.,* 1970). Cancer diagnoses have been reported in 70 patients with this disease classification; 16 are known to have developed their malignancy before the age of 20, and 50 others after age 20. Three patients had multiple primary neoplasms.

SCID consists of a heterogeneous group of disorders that begin in the neonatal period or shortly thereafter. Deficits of stem-cell differentiation to functional T and B cells appear to be responsible for the immunological abnormalities in these patients. Adenosine deaminase deficiency is a concomitant enzyme deficiency identified with one form of SCID (Pollara *et al.,* 1975). Without immunological reconstitution through organ transplantation (e.g., bone marrow, fetal liver), affected children usually die within the first 2 years of life. Eleven children with this disorder are known to have developed malignancy. One of these 11 had received transfer factor prior to the onset of malignancy (Gelfand *et al.,* 1974). To our knowledge, no child who has been reconstituted has developed a malignancy.

Ataxia–telangiectasia is a multisystem disease that presents as cerebellar ataxia, ocular telangiectasia, and recurrent sinopulmonary infections (Sedgwick and Boder, 1972). In addition, hormonal abnormalities have been observed in many girls who reach puberty (Boder, 1975). IgA and IgE are frequently at low levels or absent (Good, 1972). Cell-mediated responses are abnormal during life, and at autopsy, children affected with this disease are found to have hypoplastic thymus glands. Ataxia–telangiectasia is transmitted in an autosomally recessive pattern, and the gene frequency for this disorder has been estimated to be as high as 1 in 100 (Swift *et al.,* 1976). Swift and colleagues observed that probable carriers of the ataxia-telangiectasia gene have higher than expected frequencies of several types of neoplasms—including lymphomas and gall bladder, biliary, and pancreatic carcino-mas—than do other family members less likely to be carriers of the defective gene. The largest number of cancers reported in any single immunodeficiency group is the 79 cases identified with ataxia–telangiectasia.

Wiskott–Aldrich syndrome is a multisystem disorder, inherited as an X-linked trait. It is characterized by eczema, thrombocytopenia, and increased susceptibility to infections. Many patients with this disease have progressive deficits of cell-mediated immunity, low serum IgM levels, and elevated serum concentrations of IgA and IgE. They fail to develop antibodies to polysaccharide antigens (e.g., pneumococcus polysaccharide, Vi antigen, blood group antigens), but are capable of producing IgM and IgG antibodies to protein antigens (Good, 1972). Immuno-globulin catabolism is accelerated with this disorder, and isohemagglutinin titers are almost always low or absent (Krivit and Good, 1959; Blaese *et al.,* 1975). Boys with Wiskott–Aldrich syndrome usually die of severe infections or cerebral hemorrhage by the second age decade. There have been 35 reports of cancer in Wiskott–Aldrich patients.

3. Malignancy Patterns in the Genetically Induced Immunodeficiencies

3.1. General Histopathological Categories

Table 2 groups the 227 reported cases of primary immunodeficiency and cancer by disease diagnosis and tumor pathology. Each of the 6 cases with multiple primary tumors is grouped by the histology of the cancer that was diagnosed first. The immunodeficiencies are listed in order of increasing frequency of lymphoreticu-lar tumors. Lymphoreticular tumors dominate the overall proportions of histologi-cally identified neoplasms (57% of total cases), and are the most prevalent neo-plasms in five of the seven primary immunodeficiencies: variable immunodeficiency (49%), SCID (55%), ataxia–telangiectasia (61%), IgM deficiency (71%), and Wis-kott–Aldrich syndrome (83%) (Table 2). In the two remaining disorders, IgA deficiency and X-linked hypogammaglobulinemia, lymphoreticular tumors account for 31 and 33%, respectively, of total.

Differences in malignancy patterns are found in the distribution of epithelial cancers (carcinomas) and leukemias (all types): with isolated IgA deficiency, 54% of

TABLE 2. Immunodeficiency-Cancer Registry: Summary of Cases

Disease	Histological type										Total cases
	Lymphoreticular[a]		Leukemia		Epithelial		Mesenchymal		Nervous system		
	%	N	%	N	%	N	%	N	%	N	
IgA deficiency	31	4	—	—	54	7	7.5	1	7.5	1	13
X-linked (Bruton's) hypogammaglobulinemia	33	4	58	7	—	—	—	—	8	1	12
Variable immunodeficiency	49	34	6	4	43	30	1	1	1	1	70
Severe combined immunodeficiency	55	6	45	5	—	—	—	—	—	—	11
Ataxia–telangiectasia	61	48	23	18	11	9	1	1	4	3	79
IgM deficiency	71.4	5	—	—	14.3	1	—	—	14.3	1	7
Wiskott–Aldrich syndrome	80	28	5	2	3	1	3	1	9	3	35
TOTALS:	57	129	16	36	21	48	2	4	4	10	227

[a]Malignant lymphomas and malignant reticuloendothelioses.

all cancers are epithelial, while leukemias comprise 58% of all reported cancers with X-linked hypogammaglobulinemia (Table 2). Epithelial cancers occur almost as frequently as lymphoreticular tumors in patients with variable immunodeficiency (43 and 49%, respectively), and are relatively less prevalent than lymphoreticular neoplasms with IgM deficiency (14.3 vs. 71.4%) or ataxia–telangiectasia (11 vs. 61%). Leukemias account for a large percentage of neoplasms with SCID (45%), less with ataxia–telangiectasia (23%), and even less with variable immunodeficiency (6%) and Wiskott–Aldrich syndrome (5%). Mesenchymal tumors (e.g., sarcomas) and nervous system tumors (neuroblastoma, primary tumors of the brain) are reported in very small numbers (i.e., 1 or 2 cases) of patients with immunodeficiency diseases; these malignancies represent 2 and 4%, respectively, of all reported tumors in the registry file.

3.2. Age and Sex

Cancers occurring in an immunodeficiency population, as with those occurring in the presumed immunologically normal general population, have unique sex- and age-related characteristics that may provide additional etiological clues to oncogenesis. Table 3 lists 191 cases by sex, age at cancer diagnosis, and primary site of the tumor, and 36 cases by age unknown (21 cases) or sex and age unknown (15 cases) and primary site of the tumor, except for the lymphoreticular tumors, which include several cases originating in nonlymphoid organs, e.g., skin, bladder, bone, small intestine, and brain. The most common tumors occur in childhood in both sexes and are mainly of lymphoreticular origin; these malignancies include lymphomas, reticuloendothelioses, and leukemias that develop in patients with immunodeficiencies that become evident at a very early age, e.g., X-linked (Bruton's) hypogammaglobulinemia, SCID, Wiskott–Aldrich syndrome, and ataxia–telangiectasia (Kersey *et al.*, 1973a) (see Table 2). Conversely, the bulk of epithelial malignancies, i.e., those in the stomach, other digestive organs, and other sites, occur later in life, as reflected in the relatively high frequency of these particular neoplasms with IgA deficiency and variable immunodeficiency, diseases known to have a more varied age of onset (Table 2).

The 2:1 male/female ratio can be attributed to the inclusion of patients with X-linked disorders. Sex becomes a less significant variable after childhood.

3.3. Specific Histopathological Categories

3.3.1. Malignant Lymphomas and Reticuloendothelioses

Malignant lymphomas and reticuloendothelioses comprise 129 (57%) of the 227 cases registered with the ICR (Table 2), making them the most frequently reported tumors in cases of genetically induced immunodeficiency disease and cancer. The earliest case reports of this association appeared in 1961 with the Wiskott–Aldrich syndrome (Coleman *et al.*, 1961) and in 1963 with ataxia–telangiectasia (Boder and Sedgwick, 1963) and X-linked hypogammaglobulinemia (Page *et al.*, 1963). A review of the world's literature in 1971 revealed that 44 of 80 neoplasms reported in immunodeficient patients were malignant lymphomas or reticuloendothelioses. Waldmann *et al.* (1972) reported that these tumors accounted for 6 of 10 malignan-

TABLE 3. Immunodeficiency-Cancer Registry: Distribution of Cancers by Primary Tumor Site and Sex and Age (191 Cases), Age Unknown (21 Cases), and Sex and Age Unknown (15 Cases)

Age (yr):	Males										Females										Sex and age unk.
	0-9	10-14	15-19	20-29	30-39	40-49	50-59	60-74	Unk.	Total	0-9	10-14	15-19	20-29	30-39	40-49	50-59	60-74	Unk.	Total	
Lymphoreticular	38	15	7	5	3	1	3	1	10	83	17	7	2	—	1	6	2	3	1	39	7
Leukemias	12	5	1	1	2	—	2	—	5	25	5	1	—	—	—	—	—	1	—	7	4
Stomach	—	—	—	1	2	2	5	1	—	12	—	1	1	1	—	—	3	1	—	7	1
Other digestive organs	—	—	—	—	—	—	—	—	—	—	—	—	—	—	—	—	—	—	—	—	—
Lung	—	—	—	—	—	1	1	1	1	4	—	—	1	—	—	1	1	1	—	5	1
Breast	—	—	—	—	—	—	—	—	—	—	—	—	—	—	1	1	1	—	—	3	1
Genitourinary	—	—	—	—	—	—	—	—	—	—	—	—	2	—	—	1	—	1	—	4	—
Nervous system	3	1	—	1	2	1	—	1	3	7	1	2	1	—	1	—	—	—	—	3	—
Skin	—	—	—	—	—	—	—	1	1	5	—	—	1	—	—	—	1	—	—	1	—
Other sites	1	—	—	—	—	—	—	—	1	2	—	—	—	1	—	1	1	—	—	4	1[a]
TOTALS:	54	21	8	8	7	5	11	4	20	138	24	12	7	1	3	11	8	7	1	74	15

[a] Liposarcoma.

cies diagnosed in immunodeficiency patients studied at the NIH. The histopathological classification of these and other cases collected by the ICR appears in Table 4.

All 129 tumors are listed by the histopathological diagnosis used by the reporting physician, and are classified into the following five groups:

Hodgkin's disease	21 cases
Lymphosarcoma or lymphocytic lymphoma	25 cases
Reticulum-cell sarcoma or histiocytic lymphoma	29 cases
Malignant reticuloendotheliosis	14 cases
Other	40 cases

The "Other" category includes 37 cases in which no specific cell type was reported

TABLE 4. Immunodeficiency-Cancer Registry: Histopathological Classification of 129 Malignant Lymphomas

Malignancy	Cases	Immunodeficiency[a]						
		AT	WAS	V	SCID	IgA	IgM	X
Histiocytic lymphomas	29	10	8	5	1	2	3	—
Reticulum-cell sarcoma	21							
Reticulosarcoma	1							
Reticulum-cell lymphoma	1							
Reticular lymphosarcoma	1							
Histocytosarcoma	1							
Histocytic lymphoma	2							
Undifferentiated lymphoma	2							
Lymphocytic lymphomas	25	14	—	9	1	1	—	—
Lymphosarcoma	20							
Malignant lymphosarcoma	1							
Small-cell lymphosarcoma	1							
Lymphoblastic lymphosarcoma	1							
Lymphocytic lymphosarcoma	1							
Disseminated lymphosarcoma	1							
Hodgkin's disease	21	8	3	6	1	1	1	1
Malignant reticuloendothelioses	14	1	10	3	—	—	—	—
Malignant reticuloendotheliosis	9							
Generalized reticuloendotheliosis	1							
Generalized malignant reticuloendotheliosis	1							
Malignant reticulosis	1							
Malignant histocytosis	1							
Histiocytic reticulosis	1							
Others[b]	40	15	7	11	3	—	1	3
Lymphoma (NOS)	23							
Malignant lymphoma(NOS)	7							
Lymphoreticular (NOS)	5							
Non-Hodgkin's lymphoma (NOS)	2							
Burkitt's lymphoma	1							
Undifferentiated round-cell sarcoma	1							
Plasmacytoma (lung)	1							

[a](AT) Ataxia–telangiectasia; (WAS) Wiskott–Aldrich syndrome; (V) variable immunodeficiency; (SCID) severe combined immunodeficiency; (IgA) IgA deficiency (selective); (IgM) IgM deficiency (selective); (X) X-linked (Bruton's) hypogammaglobulinemia.
[b](NOS) Not otherwise specified.

and 3 cases in which the histopathological diagnosis did not fit into any of the other four groups: 1 Burkitt's lymphoma, 1 undifferentiated round-cell sarcoma, and 1 plasmacytoma of the lung. A summary of the numbers of each cell type for specific immunodeficiency diseases appears in the right-hand section of Table 4. The relative frequencies of three cell types—histiocytic and lymphocytic lymphomas and Hodgkin's disease—are approximately the same for ataxia–telangiectasia, variable immunodeficiency, and IgA deficiency. At least half the tumors that occur with SCID and X-linked hypogammaglobulinemia are nonspecified tumors, which makes accurate description of cell types for these immunodeficiency disorders difficult at this time. The most frequently reported cell type for IgM deficiency is histiocytic lymphoma. Wiskott–Aldrich syndrome, with which IgM responses are usually impaired, is clustered in the histiocytic lymphomas and is the immunodeficiency diagnosis in 10 of 14 cases with malignant reticuloendotheliosis. In addition, there are 3 cases of Hodgkin's disease but no lymphocytic lymphomas reported in boys with Wiskott–Aldrich syndrome.

Available data on the age, sex, and primary site, or histology, of malignancies occurring in the immunologically competent general population indicate that, in comparison, our ICR population of immunodeficiency patients with cancer, diagnosed prior to age 15, is represented by more children, especially males (Cutler and Young, 1975). This observation suggests that the distribution of tumor cell types, specifically those of the lymphoreticular system, might also differ in these two cancer populations. Estimates of the proportional distribution of three lymphoma cell types—Hodgkin's disease and lymphocytic and histiocytic lymphomas—in cancer patients from the immunologically competent general population were compared with the observed numbers of the same cell types in immunodeficient patients (Table 5). The data show that histiocytic lymphomas account for a larger percentage of malignant lymphomas in immunodeficiency patients than they do for either the

TABLE 5. Percentage Distribution and Ratios of Three Lymphoma Cell Types in Patients with Immunodeficiency Diseases[a] and in the General Population[b]

Cell type[c]	Percentage distribution			Ratios			
	Immuno-deficiency population		General population estimates (%)		Immunodeficiency population	General population	Relative difference
	%	N					
All ages							
HD	28	21	35	HD/LL	0.85	0.78	1.09
LL	33	25	45	HL/LL	1.18	0.44	2.68
HL	39	29	20	HL/HD	1.39	0.57	2.44
Children less than 15 years old							
HD	26	12	52	HD/LL	0.68	1.27	0.54
LL	38	18	41	HL/LL	0.95	0.17	5.59
HL	36	17	7	HL/HD	1.38	0.13	10.62

[a]Immunodeficiency-Cancer Registry Data, University of Minnesota, 1976.
[b]All ages: Rundles (1972); children less than 15 years old: Young and Miller (1975).
[c](HD) Hodgkin's disease; (LL) Lymphocytic lymphoma; (HL) histiocytic lymphoma.

"All ages" or the "Children less than 15 years old" group in the general population (39 vs. 20% and 36 vs. 7%, respectively). Correspondingly, Hodgkin's disease and lymphocytic lymphomas are underrepresented to varying degrees in both immunodeficiency series in comparison with general population figures. The difference is especially noticeable in children, in whom Hodgkin's disease accounts for 52% of all of these neoplasms in the general childhood cancer population, but only 26% among children with genetically induced immunodeficiency diseases who developed similar malignancies.

Table 5 also shows the ratios between any two cell types based on their observed percentages. These ratios were computed for each cancer population as a numerical statement of the frequency of the reporting of specific cell types with respect to each other in each population. Comparisons of these ratios show generally that the greatest differences occur when the ratios of histiocytic lymphomas to Hodgkin's disease in the two populations are compared, and that this difference is greatest in the childhood populations (10.62). In every ratio comparison that includes histiocytic lymphomas, the differences observed are quite large, ranging from 2.44 to 10.62, depending on the cell type with which histiocytic lymphoma is compared and the ages of the population (Table 5). The Hodgkin's disease/lymphocytic lymphoma ratios are almost parity in the comparison of subjects at all ages. The higher frequency of Hodgkin's disease with general childhood cancer relative to children with primary immunodeficiency accounts for the difference between these two populations in the Hodgkin's disease/lymphocytic lymphoma ratios (0.54).

The observed differences in the percentage distribution and ratios of malignant lymphoma cell types appearing in Table 5 may have several explanations. It is possible that the frequency of primary immunodeficiency disease for any particular type of neoplasm may be too small for meaningful comparisons with general population figures, and that the observed differences may be due mainly to errors introduced by the size of the series; unfortunately, the cell types of 37 malignant lymphomas in immunodeficient patients remain unknown at present. However, this lack of information concerning the cell identity of tumors is not likely to alter interpretation of data significantly because of the way patients with these unidentified neoplasms are distributed among the various immunodeficiency diseases (see Table 4).

On the other hand, the increased reporting of histiocytic lymphomas (Table 5) may indicate an increased predisposition to lymphoreticular malignancies of this type in patients with several primary immunodeficiency diseases who develop neoplasms. Histiocytic lymphomas accounted for the largest number of specified malignant lymphomas among the primary immunodeficiency disease–cancer population and, in addition, included most of the IgM-deficiency cases and a large number of cases of Wiskott–Aldrich syndrome, an immunological disorder that is characterized, in part, by low serum IgM. There were 14 cases of malignant reticuloendotheliosis in the primary immunodeficiency disease series that were not included in the comparison studies. Like histiocytic lymphoma, malignant reticuloendotheliosis is characterized by malignant histiocytic proliferation. The combined total of these two neoplastic disorders (43 cases) obtained from patients with primary immunodeficiency is large enough to suggest that together they hold a unique place in the association between immunodeficiency and oncogenesis. When we are able to assert the relative risk of various cell types of malignancy in immunodeficiency-disease populations, we will be able to confirm or revise the preliminary observations suggested by the data in Table 5.

3.3.2. Epithelial Malignancies of the Gastrointestinal Tract

The distribution of cancers in our primary immunodeficiency patient series (see Table 3) reveals that a surprisingly large number of primary immunodeficiency patients have developed GI malignancies, particularly stomach cancers. The series of GI tumors, compiled from literature reports and unpublished cases submitted to the ICR, is presented in Table 6. There are 20 cases of stomach cancer (Nos. 1–20) and 5 cases of primary malignancies of other digestive organs (Nos. 21–25), the latter including 3 sigmoid colon tumors (Nos. 22, 24, 25) and 1 each of the parotid gland (No. 21) and the buccal cavity (No. 23). Stomach cancers occurred in 3 females with ataxia–telangiectasia (Nos. 1–3), ages 16, 21, and 19; 4 females (Nos. 10, 13, 15, 16), 9 males (Nos. 4–9, 11, 12, 14), and 1 of unknown sex (No. 20) with variable immunodeficiency, ages 15–72; and 3 males with IgA deficiency (Nos. 17–19), ages 40, 53, and 72.

As indicated in Table 6, several clinical problems, besides immunodeficiency, preceded the development of stomach carcinomas, including 3 cases of nodular lymphoid hyperplasia (Nos. 6, 10, 13), 4 cases of pernicious anemia (Nos. 8, 13, 17, 19), 4 cases of malabsorption or atrophic gastritis or both (Nos. 5, 13, 14, 18), and 5 cases of *Giardia lamblia* or *Trichomonas hominis* cysts (Nos. 4, 6, 11, 13, 14). Symptoms of clinical problems were found in several cases (Nos. 6, 13, 14). Studies on autoimmune disorders in immunodeficiency diseases indicate that pernicious anemia occurs earlier in life in patients with variable immunodeficiency than in the general population (Twomey *et al.*, 1970, 1976). Serum IgA was at low levels or absent in several cases; these data may have etiological significance regarding oncogenesis (Walker and Hong, 1973). Cancer was reported in families of 3 cases, including stomach cancer in the mother of Case Nos. 2 and 3 and unspecified tumors in the mother and 2 siblings in Case No. 16. An interesting association between immunodeficiency and gastrointestinal cancer was observed in Case No. 24, in which the patient's brother died of a histiocytic lymphoma. The brother was found to have no quantitative IgA in his serum (Hamoudi *et al.*, 1974). In summary, in an age-matched population, we would expect bowel cancers to occur more frequently than stomach cancers (Cutler and Young, 1975). The opposite situation is found in our series.

It is possible that subclinical or compartmentalized immunological abnormalities play a role in the development of gastric carcinomas in both the immunodeficient and the general population. A recent study of surviving members of a large kindred in which 12 members in 4 generations died of gastric cancer showed that immunological abnormalities were present in at least 5 members (Creagan and Fraumeni, 1973). The observation of a series of GI tumors occurring in patients with primary immunodeficiency disease suggests that an intimate association exists between immunodeficiency and carcinomas involving tissues of entodermal origin. On the other hand, breast and cervical cancers, lung tumors, and skin carcinomas, which to date have been reported only in small numbers in primary immunodeficiency disease patients, may be due to other, nonimmunological factors.

TABLE 6. Gastrointestinal Tumors in Immunodeficiency Diseases

Case No.	Sex	Immunodeficiency		Malignancy		Associated conditions/ comments	Ref. Nos.[c]
		Age of onset	Diagnosis[a]	Age at diagnosis	Cell type[b]/primary site		
1	F	Newborn	AT	16	Colloid ca./pylorus	Absent serum IgA.	1
2	F	2	AT	21	Mucin Adenocarcinoma/ stomach	Maternal history of adenocarcinoma of stomach, sister of Case No. 3.	2
3	F	Early childh.	AT	19	Adenocarcinoma/ stomach	Sister of Case No. 2.	2
4	M	8	V	15	Adenocarcinoma/ stomach	*Giardia lamblia* cysts; absent serum IgA.	3
5	M	12	V	27	Carcinoma (NOS)/ stomach	Nontropical sprue, age 12; poliomyelitis, age 22; furunculosis, atrophic gastritis, malabsorption.	4
6	M	22	V	31	Scirrhous adenocarcinoma/ stomach	Nodular lymphoid hyperplasia, small bowel; splenomegaly; *G. lamblia* in stools.	5
7	M	Infancy	V	33	Carcinoma (NOS)/ stomach	Steatorrhea; brother has similar immunodeficiency.	6
8	M	41	V	47	Carcinoma (NOS)/ stomach	Pernicious anemia, age 28.	7, 8
9	M	Unk.	V	50	Carcinoma (NOS)/ stomach		9
10	F	39	V	54	Carcinoma (NOS)/ stomach	Diarrhea, steatorrhea, nodular lymphoid hyperplasia, small bowel.	5
11	M	29	V	55	Adenocarcinoma/ stomach	*G. lamblia*.	10
12	M	Unk.	V	57	Carcinoma (NOS)/ stomach		8
13	F	31	V	56	Adenocarcinoma/ stomach	Pernicious anemia; malabsorption, atrophic gastritis; nodular lymphoid hyperplasia; *G. lamblia*; splenomegaly.	5
14	M	26	V	59	Scirrhous adenocarcinoma/ stomach	Mild malabsorption; myxedema; *Trichomonas hominis* in stool; emphysema.	5
15	F	24	V	53	Carcinoma (NOS/ stomach	Persistent diarrhea from age 41; serum IgA nil.	6, 8
16	F	16	V	67	Carcinoma (NOS)/ stomach	Steatorrhea; serum IgA nil; mother, 2 siblings died of cancer, >60 years.	6, 8
17	M	Unk.	IgA	40	Carcinoma (NOS)/ stomach	Pernicious anemia, age 25; repeated infections 4 years before cancer; absent serum IgA.	11

(Continued)

TABLE 6. (*continued*)　　　　　　　　　　　　　**215**

IMMUNODEFICIENCY
DISEASES AND
MALIGNANCY

Case No.	Sex	Immunodeficiency		Malignancy		Associated conditions/ comments	Ref. Nos.
		Age of onset	Diagnosis[a]	Age at diagnosis	Cell type[b]/primary site		
18	M	Unk.	IgA	53	Anaplastic cancer/ stomach	Malabsorption, age 55; vitiligo, 57; absent IgA at autopsy.	12
19	M	Unk.	IgA	72	Adenocarcinoma/ stomach	Pernicious anemia, age 64.	13
20	Unk	Unk.	V	Unk.	Carcinoma (NOS)/ stomach		14
21	F	Unk.	AT	17	Mucoepidermoid/ parotid gland		15
22	F	27	V	47	Carcinoma(NOS)/ sigmoid colon	Diarrhea, nodular lymphoid hyperplasia, small bowel; toxic thyroid nodule.	5
23	F	Unk.	V	59	Carcinoma (NOS)/ buccal cavity		16
24	F	3	IgA	12	Adenocarcinoma/ sigmoid colon	Hereditary spherocytic anemia; recurrent polyps at 10; benign cavernous hemangioma, 14; malignant thymoma, 15.5; epidermoid carcinoma, scalp, 17; primary malignant astrocytoma, 20; brother with IgA deficiency and histiocytic lymphoma.	17
25	F	Unk.	IgA	46	Carcinoma/sigmoid colon	Absent serum IgA 14 years post.	18

[a] Abbreviations as in Table 4.
[b] (NOS) Not otherwise specified.
[c] (1) Schuler *et al.* (1971); (2) Haerer *et al.* (1969); Jackson (1972); (3) Shackelford and McAlister (1975); (4) Forssman and Herner (1964); (5) Hermans *et al.* (1976); (6) Medical Research Council (1970); (7) Rolles (1973); (8) Rees-Jones (1976); (9) Morell (1973); (10) Chaplin (1975); (11) Leikola (1973); (12) Fraser and Rankin (1970); (13) Hanson (1975); (14) Siegal (1976); (15) Ochs (1973): (16) Kirkpatrick (1976); (17) Hamoudi *et al.* (1974); (18) M. V. Miller *et al.* (1970).

3.4.　Estimates of Cancer Risk

The distribution of cancers by age and primary site indirectly supports the conclusion that immunodeficient patients are at greatly increased risk for developing cancer, despite a shortened life span (2–20 years). Four years ago, a survey of physicians was done to estimate the prevalence of childhood immunodeficiency diseases. The results showed that approximately 700 children, up to 15 years of age, had been diagnosed with various primary immunodeficiency diseases during a 12-year period (1960–1972) when 69 immunodeficient children had died of cancer. It was estimated that the median life span was 10 years. These figures indicate that the cancer mortality rate for children with primary immunodeficiency is about 0.8% per year (Kersey *et al.*, 1974). R. W. Miller (1969) noted that the national childhood cancer mortality rate is 0.007% per year. The relative cancer mortality risk for immunodeficient children, then, is approximately 100 times that of the general

TABLE 7. Mortality from Cancer of Various Types in Children Less Than 15 Years of Age[a]

Tumor type	Unselected children[b]	Primary immunodeficiency children[c]	
		All countries	U.S. only
Leukemias	48%	25% (16)	25% (10)
Central nervous system	16%	4% (2)	3% (1)
Lymphoreticular (e.g., reticulum-cell sarcoma, lymphosarcoma, Hodgkin's disease)	8%	67% (40)	69% (27)
Bone	4%	2% (1)	0%
Other	24%	2% (1)	3% (1)
TOTALS:		60	39

[a]From Kersey *et al.* (1974).
[b]Death certificates of 29,457 children in the United States, 1960–1966 (Miller, R. W., 1969).
[c]Immunodeficiency-Cancer Registry; number of cases in parentheses.

childhood population. A comparison of malignancy patterns for immunodeficient children and "unselected" children in the general population who died of cancer appears in Table 7. The data show significantly different patterns of tumor prevalence between the two groups. Most significantly, while only 8% of tumors were lymphoreticular in origin in unselected children, 67% were lymphoreticular in immunodeficient children. While leukemias accounted for 48% of malignancies in unselected children, they accounted for only 25% of neoplasms in immunodeficient patients. Although Wilms's tumor and neuroblastoma occur quite frequently in the general childhood population, only single cases of these cancers (associated with IgA deficiency and IgM deficiency, respectively) have been reported to the ICR (Young and Miller, 1975).

4. Possible Mechanisms Linking Human Immunodeficiency and Malignancy: Hypotheses

These data on patients with genetically induced immunodeficiency diseases who have developed malignancies suggest the possibility of genetic influences on malignancy, since the lymphoid apparatus in persons with these disorders is both the site of genetic aberration and the principal site of cancer development. Epidemiological data, such as the association among primary disease, age, and tumor histology, collected on this series strongly implicate abnormalities of the immune system as a major factor in oncogenesis. Hypotheses of the mechanisms of oncogenesis involving the lymphoid system fall into at least two general categories: (1) the immune system in persons with genetically induced immunodeficiencies has increased likelihood of establishing lines of malignant cells, and (2) the immune system in these diseases has decreased ability to eliminate malignant cells as they do develop (Kersey and Spector, 1975).

Several pathogenic mechanisms may be responsible for the increased malignant transformation of lymphoid cells, including (1) intrinsic defects in lymphoid cells and (2) chronic antigenic stimulation (including graft-versus-host diseases), resulting in enhanced lymphoid proliferation with increased opportunity for development of malignant cells; (3) the activation of endogenous viruses or, perhaps, infection with exogenous viruses that have oncogenic potential; and (4) the lack of regulatory feedback mechanisms, resulting in enhanced lymphoid proliferation.

Evidence supporting an etiological role of intrinsic defects in lymphoid cells in oncogenesis is available on at least one primary immunodeficiency disease, ataxia–telangiectasia, in which chromosomal instability of lymphoid populations has been frequently observed (Bochkov et al., 1974; Hecht et al., 1973; McCaw et al., 1975). The most frequently observed abnormality in both fibroblasts and lymphocytes was translocation of the long-arm portion of the chromosome to the 14 homologue or to chromosome 6, 7, or X. Other chromosomal abnormalities have been observed in ataxia–telangiectasia, including increased breakage, as well as gain or loss of chromatid material. Case reports of ataxia–telangiectasia patients include several notable examples. A 19-year-old male, whose two siblings had fatal ataxia–telangiectasia and acute lymphocytic leukemia, initially had translocation at chromosome 14 in 1% of his lymphoid cells, which increased to 80% translocation by the time of his death 4 years later. No malignancy was ever observed (Hecht et al., 1973). Another case, a woman in her third age decade, whose lymphocytes exhibited a balanced translocation of chromosome 14 before and after her development of chronic lymphatic leukemia, also showed a dramatic increase in the percentage of translocated lymphocytes (eventually 100%) (McCaw et al., 1975).

In other studies, an extra band on chromosome 14 has been seen in several individuals with lymphoproliferative malignancies, such as Burkitt's lymphoma, multiple myeloma, plasma cell leukemia, Hodgkin's disease, and lymphocytic lymphoma (Manolova and Manolova, 1972; Petit et al., 1972; Wurster-Hill et al., 1973; Reeves, 1973). It is of interest that many of these same lymphoproliferative malignancies have frequently been observed in patients with ataxia–telangiectasia and other primary immunodeficiencies (see Table 2).

The role of intrinsic defects of lymphoid cells in the pathogenesis of malignancy is supported by results of a study in which fibroblasts from 3 ataxia–telangiectasia donors and 2 normal controls were exposed to gamma radiation and then measured for DNA repair. The level of DNA repair in the ataxia–telangiectasia fibroblasts was about half that found with normal fibroblasts (Paterson et al., 1976). These data may explain the enhanced radiosensitivity (e.g., radiation dermatitis) seen in those patients with tumors who are treated with radiotherapy (Gotoff et al., 1967; Morgan et al., 1968; Cunliffe et al., 1975). Another ataxia–telangiectasia patient developed basal-cell carcinoma of the scalp following radiation treatment to the area for a *Tinea* infection (Levin and Perlov, 1971).

Impaired DNA repair mechanisms have also been found in xeroderma pigmentosum (XP), a genetic disorder that predisposes to skin tumors. Like ataxia–telangiectasia, this disorder is inherited in an autosomal recessive manner. Persons with XP have increased skin sensitivity to UV light, and DNA repair by these fibroblasts is defective after exposure to UV light (Cleaver, 1968). It is possible that defective DNA repair due to either UV or gamma radiation may have an as yet unexplained etiological role in some forms of neoplastic transformation since skin cancers have not been reported in large numbers in either ataxia–telangiectasia or XP. The data do suggest, however, that immune deficiency may be another manifestation of the lymphoid defect, but would not be causally related to tumor development.

Some evidence exists for the role of exogenous or endogenous viruses as a pathogenic mechanism of malignancy in primary immunodeficiencies. In a recent study, virological and cell analyses were performed on tissue from a histiocytic lymphoma of the brain in a boy with Wiskott–Aldrich syndrome; a virus was isolated that resembled the BKV papovavirus previously found by others (Takemoto *et al.*, 1974). BKV has also been isolated from the urine of several renal transplant recipients on immunosuppressive therapy (Gardner *et al.*, 1971) and from the brains of 2 patients with progressive multifocal leukoencephalopathy (Padgett *et al.*, 1971; Weiner *et al.*, 1972), a demyelinating disorder with concomitant immunological abnormalities. The relationship between the new virus (called MMV by the authors) and BKV was established both morphologically and immunologically. For example, MMV produced hemagglutin when tumor cells were cultivated with human fetal brain tissue and a continuous line from African green monkey kidney (VERO), and the hemagglutin could be inhibited by the addition of anti-BKV rabbit serum to the brain isolate culture. MMV was also isolated from urine pellets, and papovirus particles were observed by electron microscopy in brain tissue and urine of this boy. Serum from the patient had high antivirus antibody at least 1 year before the tumor was detected. In this patient with Wiskott–Aldrich syndrome, the MMV may have been a passenger virus having no causative role in tumor production. Viruses that were serologically identical to BKV were isolated from 2 additional patients with Wiskott–Aldrich syndrome, however, although neither of these 2 boys had a malignancy at the time the virus studies were performed (Takemoto *et al.*, 1974). The various papovavirus studies suggest that papovaviruses may be common in renal transplant recipients, in whom the risk of developing lymphoma is also high (see Chapter 8), as well as in patients with immunodeficiency diseases. Further investigation is needed into the role of viruses in the increased incidence of malignancies in the immunologically compromised host.

Data supporting the role of impaired regulatory feedback mechanisms in oncogenesis are available from studies on experimental animals. Suppressor T lymphocytes act as regulators of proliferative responses to several antigens in the mouse. The New Zealand mouse, an inbred strain that spontaneously develops autoimmune disease (i.e., Coombs-positive hemolytic anemia and immune complex glomerulonephritis), also develops lymphoreticular malignancies (Gershwin and Steinberg, 1973). These New Zealand mice appear to be defective in generation of suppressor cells. By analogy, in humans with abnormal immune systems, a lack of suppressor function could allow an increased lymphoproliferative response due to any one of a variety of mechanisms. This in turn could result in increased risk of mutation and abnormal lymphoid clones that would lead to a malignant cell population. To date, no data on humans are available to support this hypothesis. In fact, recent data suggest that certain forms of immunodeficiency are associated with increased (rather than decreased) suppressor activity. The role of increased suppressor activity in oncogenesis remains unclear.

The second category of hypotheses, i.e., those that suggest decreased ability of the lymphoid system to recognize and destroy malignant lymphoid cells, includes several aspects. These include the possibilities of defective recognition or defective response following recognition. Defective recognition of malignant cells may be due to defective receptors for tumor cells; defective response could be a result of inability to generate effector mechanisms that normally destroy malignant lymphoid cells.

Finally, the possible role of immunological surveillance mechanisms in the defense against malignant cells has become a matter of increasing skepticism. The immunological surveillance theory predicts that a major role of the immune system (especially the cell-mediated system) is host defense against malignant cells. Premises of this theory are that malignant cells develop frequently, and that under normal conditions they are destroyed by immunological mechanisms. Therefore, immunodeficiency, which is due to abnormal immune function, would be expected to be associated with earlier and more frequent cancers of all types (Kersey *et al.,* 1973b). Our data suggest a different emphasis, however. Most tumors common to the general childhood population, i.e., nervous system tumors, rhabdomyosarcoma, Wilms's tumor, Ewing's sarcoma, and retinoblastoma have rarely been reported in immunodeficient children (Young and Miller, 1975). The proportion of tumors that arise in the lymphoid system (lymphoreticular tumors and leukemias, 74% of total tumors) is simply too large and too selective to be explained by the immunological surveillance theory. If the immune surveillance theory could explain the increased malignancy rate in primary immunodeficiencies (Melief and Schwartz, 1975), then it would also predict a greater than expected rate of multiple primaries. In the registry series of 227 cancer cases, however, only 6 patients have developed multiple primaries; the expected rate is 2% (Cutler and Young, 1975), which indicates that the risk for developing multiple primary neoplasms is not increased among persons with primary immunodeficiencies.

5. Conclusions

It appears that there is much work ahead to define the nature of the association between genetic and drug-induced cellular defects, immunodeficiency, and cancer. The data on patients with primary immunodeficiency who develop cancer are useful in the development of models interrelating the immune system and cancer, but the association between immune function and oncogenesis is so complex as to defy precise analysis. Future studies will undoubtedly be directed by more subtle genetic and drug- and chemically induced defects in the general population that result in lymphoid malignancy and immune deficiency. Analyses of these defects should allow a more enlightened understanding of the function of the lymphoid system in normal and pathological states.

References

Amman, A. J., and Hong, R., 1971, Selective IgA deficiency: Presentation of 30 cases and a review of the literature, *Medicine* **50**:223–236.

Bergsma, D. (ed.), 1975, *Immunodeficiency in Man and Animals, Birth Defects: Orig. Artic. Ser.,* Vol. XI, No. 1, Sinauer Associates, Sunderland, Massachusetts.

Blaese, R. M., Strober, W., and Waldmann, T. A., 1975, Immunodeficiency in the Wiskott–Aldrich syndrome, in: *Immunodeficiency in Man and Animals* (D. Bergsma, ed.), *Birth Defects: Orig. Artic. Ser.,* Vol. XI, No. 1, pp. 250–254, Sinauer Associates, Sunderland, Massachusetts.

Bochkov, N. P., Lopukhin, Y. M., Kuleshov, N. P., and Kovalchuk, L. V., 1974, Cytogenetic study of patients with ataxia–telangiectasia, *Humangenetik* **24**:115–128.

Boder, E., 1974, Ataxia–telangiectasia: Some historic, clinical, and pathologic observations, in: *Immunodeficiency in Man and Animals* (D. Bergsma, ed.), *Birth Defects: Orig. Artic. Ser.,* Vol. XI, No. 1, pp. 255–270, Sinauer Associates, Sunderland, Massachusetts.

Boder, E., and Sedgwick, R., 1963, Ataxia–telangiectasia: A review of 101 cases, in: *Cerebellum Posture and Cerebral Palsy* (G. Walsh, ed.), Vol. 8, pp. 110–118, Little Club for Clinical and Developmental Medicine, National Spastics Society, Medical, Education and Information Unit, London.

Chaplin, H., 1975, Department of Medicine, Washington University, St. Louis (personal communication to ICR).

Cleaver, J. E., 1968, Defective repair replication of DNA in xeroderma pigmentosum, *Nature (London)* **218**:652–656.

Coleman, A., Leikin, S., and Guin, G. H., 1961, Aldrich's syndrome, *Clin. Proc. Child. Hosp. Natl. Med. Cent.* **17**:22–27.

Cone, L., and Uhr, J. W., 1964, Immunological deficiency diseases associated with chronic lymphatic leukemia and multiple myeloma, *J. Clin. Invest.* **43**:2241–2248.

Cooper, M. D., Faulk, W. P., Fudenberg, H. H., Good, R. A. Hitzig, W., Kunkel, H., Rosen, F., Seligmann, M., Soothill, J., and Wedgwood, R. J., 1973, Classification of primary immunodeficiencies, *N. Engl. J. Med.* **288**:966–967.

Creagan, E. T., and Fraumeni, J. F., Jr., 1973, Familial gastric cancer and immunologic abnormalities, *Cancer* **32**:1325–1331.

Cunliffe, P. N., Mann, J. R., Cameron, A. H., and Roberts, K. D., 1975, Radiosensitivity in ataxia-telangiectasia, *Br. J. Radiol.* **48**:374–376.

Cutler, S. J., and Young, J. L., Jr., 1975, Incidence data, in: *Third National Cancer Survey,* National Cancer Institute Monograph 41, U.S. Department of Health, Education and Welfare, Washington, D.C.

Forssman, O., and Herner, B., 1964, Acquired agammaglobulinemia and malabsorption, *Acta Med. Scand.* **176**:779–786.

Fraser, K. J., and Rankin, J. G., 1970, Selective deficiency of IgA immunoglobulins associated with carcinoma of the stomach, *Australas. Ann. Med.* **19**:165–167.

Fudenberg, H. H., Good, R. A., Goodman, H. C., Hitzig, W., Kunkel, H., Roitt, I., Rosen, F., Rowe, D., Seligmann, M., and Soothill, J., 1971, Primary immunodeficiencies: Report of a World Health Organization Committee (special article), *Pediatrics* **47**:927–946.

Gardner, S. D., Field, S. M., Coleman, D., and Hulme, B., 1971, New human papovavirus (B. K.) isolated from urine after renal transplantation, *Lancet* **1**:1253–1257.

Gatti, R. A., and Good, R. A., 1971, Occurrence of malignancy in immunodeficiency disease, *Cancer* **28**:89–98.

Gelfand, E. W., Baumal, R., Huber, J., Crookston, M. C., and Shumak, K. H., 1974, Polyclonal gammopathy and lymphoproliferation following transfer factor in severe combined immunodeficiency disease, *N. Engl. J. Med.* **289**:1385–1389.

Gellman, E. F., and Vietti, T. J., 1970, Congenital hypogammaglobulinemia preceding Hodgkin's disease: A case report and review of the literature, *J. Pediatr.* **76**:131–133.

Gershwin, M. E., and Steinberg, A. D., 1973, Loss of suppressor function as a cause of lymphoid malignancy, *Lancet* **2**:1174–1176.

Good, R. A., 1972, Relations between immunity and malignancy, *Proc. Natl. Acad. Sci. U.S.A.* **69**:1026–1032.

Gotoff, S. O., Amirmokri, E., and Liebner, E. J., 1967, Ataxia–telangiectasia: Neoplasia, untoward response to X-irradiation, and tuberous sclerosis, *Am. J. Dis. Child.* **114**:617–625.

Haerer, A. F., Jackson, J. F., and Evers, C. G., 1969, Ataxia–telangiectasia with gastric carcinoma, *J. Am. Med. Assoc.* **210**:1884–1887.

Hamoudi, A. B., Ertel, I., Newton, W. A., Jr., Reiner, C. G., and Clatworthy, H. W., 1974, Multiple neoplasms in an adolescent child associated with IgA deficiency, *Cancer* **33**:1134–1144.

Hanson, L. A., 1975, Department of Immunology, Institute of Medical Microbiology, University of Göteborg, Göteborg, Sweden (personal communication to ICR).

Hecht, F. McCaw, B., and Koler, R. D., 1973, Ataxia–telangiectasia: Clonal growth of translocation lymphocytes, *N. Engl. J. Med.* **289**:286–291.

Hermans, P. E., Diaz-Buxo, J. A., and Stobo, J. D., 1976, Idiopathic late-onset immunoglobulin deficiency: Clinical observations in 50 patients, *Am. J. Med.* **61**:221–237.

Hobbs, J., 1975, IgM deficiency, in: *Immunodeficiency in Man and Animals* (D. Bergsma, ed.), *Birth Defects: Orig. Artic. Ser.,* Vol. XI, pp. 112–116, Sinauer Associates, Sunderland, Massachusetts.

Hoover, R. N., and Fraumeni, J. F., Jr., 1973, Risk of cancer in renal-transplant recipients, *Lancet* **2**:55–57.

Huntley, C. C., and Stephenson, R. L., 1968, IgA deficiency: Family studies, *N. C. Med. J.* **29**:325–331.

Jackson, J. F., 1972, Ataxia–telangiectasia, in: *Skin, Heredity, and Malignant Neoplasms* (H. T. Lynch, ed.), pp. 94–103, Medical Examination Publishing Co., Flushing, New York.

Kersey, J. H., and Gajl-Peczalska, K. J., 1975, T and B lymphocytes in humans: A review, *Am. J. Pathol.* **81**:446–458.

Kersey, J. H., and Spector, B. D., 1975, Immune deficiency diseases, in *Persons at High Risk of Cancer: An Approach to Cancer Etiology and Control* (J. F. Fraumeni, Jr., ed.), pp. 55–67, Academic Press, New York.

Kersey, J. H., Spector, B. D., and Good, R. A., 1973a, Primary immunodeficiency diseases and cancer: The Immunodeficiency-Cancer Registry, *Int. J. Cancer* **12**:333–347.

Kersey, J., Spector, B. D., and Good, R. A., 1973b, Immunodeficiency and cancer, in: *Advances in Cancer Research* (S. Weinhouse and G. Klein, eds.), Vol. 18, pp. 211–230, Academic Press, New York.

Kersey, J. H., Spector, B. D., and Good, R. A., 1974, Cancer in children with primary immunodeficiency diseases, *J. Pediatrics* **84**:263–264.

Kirkpatrick, C., 1976, NIAID–NIH, Bethesda, Maryland (personal communication to ICR).

Kopp, W. L., Trier, J. S., Stiehm, E. R., and Foroozan, P., 1968, Acquired agammaglobulinemia with defective delayed hypersensitivity, *Ann. Intern. Med.* **69**:309–317.

Krivit, W., and Good, R. A., 1959, Aldrich's syndrome (Thrombocytopenia, eczema, and infection in infants), *Am. J. Dis. Child.* **97**:137–153.

Leikola, J., Koistinen, J., Lehtinen, J., and Virolainen, M., 1973, IgA-induced anaphylactic transfusion reactions: A report of 4 cases, *Blood* **42**:111–119.

Levin, S., and Perlov, S., 1971, Ataxia–telangiectasia in Israel with observations on its relationship to malignant disease, *Isr. J. Med. Sci.* **7**:1535–1541.

Manolova, G., and Manolova, Y., 1972, Marker band in one chromosome 14 from Burkitt's lymphomas, *Nature (London)* **237**:33–34.

McCaw, B. K., Hecht, F., Harnden, D. G., and Teplitz, R., 1975, Somatic rearrangement of chromosome 14 in human lymphocytes, *Proc. Natl. Acad. Sci. U.S.A.* **72**:2071–2075.

Medical Research Council, 1970, *Hypogammaglobulinaemia in the United Kingdom,* Her Majesty's Stationery Office, London.

Melief, C. J. M., and Schwartz, R. S., 1975, Immunocompetence and malignancy, in: *Cancer: A Comprehensive Treatise* (F. F. Becker, ed.), Vol. 1, pp. 121–160, Plenum Press, New York.

Miller, R. W., 1969, Fifty-two forms of childhood cancer: United States mortality experience, 1960–1966, *J. Pediatr.* **75**:685–689.

Miller, M. V., Holland, P. V., Sugarbaker, E., Strober, W., and Waldmann, T. A., 1970, Anaphylactic reactions to IgA: A difficult transfusion problem, *Am. J. Clin. Pathol.* **54**:618–621.

Morell, A., 1973, Institute for Clinical and Experimental Cancer Research, Tiefenau Hospital, University of Berne, Berne, Switzerland (personal communication to ICR).

Morgan, J. L., Holcomb, T. M., and Morrissey, R. W., 1968, Radiation reaction in ataxia–telangiectasia, *Am. J. Dis. Child.* **116**:537–538.

Ochs, H., 1975, University Hospital, University of Washington, Seattle, Washington (personal communication to ICR).

Padgett, B. L., Walker, D. L., Zurhein, G. M., and Eckroade, R. J., 1971, Cultivation of papova-like virus from human brain with progressive multifocal leucoencephalopathy, *Lancet* **1**:1257–1260.

Page, A. R., Hansen, A. E., and Good, R. A., 1963, Occurrence of leukemia and lymphoma in patients with agammaglobulinemia, *Blood* **21**:197–206.

Paterson, M. C., Smith, B. P., Lohman, P. H. M., Anderson, A. K., and Fishman, L., 1976, Defective excision repair of gamma ray-damaged DNA in human (ataxia–telangiectasia) fibroblasts, *Nature (London)* **260**:444–446.

Penn, I., 1975, The incidence of malignancies in transplant recipients, *Transplant. Proc.* **7**:323.

Petit, P., Verhest, A., Lecluse van der Bilt, F., and Jongsma, A., 1972, The chromosomes of the EB virus-positive Burkitt cell line PsJ.HRlK studied by the fluorescent staining technique, *Pathol. Eur.* **7**:17–21.

Pollara, B., Moore, J. J., Jr., Pickering, R. J., Gabrielsen, A. E., and Meuwissen, H. J., 1975, Combined immunodeficiency disease, in: *Immunodeficiency in Man and Animals* (D. Bergsma, ed.), *Birth Defects: Orig. Artic. Ser.,* Vol. XI, No. 1, pp. 120–123, Sinauer Associates, Sunderland, Massachusetts.

Rees-Jones, A., 1976, Regional Immunology Laboratory, E. Birmingham Hospital, Birmingham, England (personal communication to ICR).

Reeves, B. R., 1973, Cytogenetics of malignant lymphomas: Studies using a Giemsa-banding technique, *Humangenetik* **20**:231–250.

Rolles, T. E., 1973, Regional Immunology Laboratory, E. Birmingham Hospital, Birmingham, England (personal communication to ICR).

Rundles, R. W., 1972, Lymphosarcoma, in: *Hematology* (W. J. Williams, E. Beutler, A. Erslev, and R. W. Rundles, eds.), Chapter 110, pp. 927–937, McGraw-Hill, New York.

Schuler, D., Schöngut, L., Cserháti, E., Siegler, J., and Gács, G., 1971, Lymphoblastic transformation, chromosome pattern and delayed-type skin reaction in ataxia–telangiectasia, *Acta Paediatr. Scand.* **70**:66–72.

Sedgwick, R. P., and Boder, E., 1972, Ataxia–telangiectasia, in: *Handbook of Clinical Neurology* (P. J. Vinken and G. W. Bruyen, eds.), pp. 267–339, North-Holland, Amsterdam.

Shackelford, G. D., and McAlister, W. H., 1975, Primary immunodeficiency disease and malignancy, *Am. J. Roentgenol. Radium Ther. Nucl. Med.* **123**:144–153.

Siegal, F., 1976, Sloan-Kettering Memorial Institute, New York, New York (personal communication to ICR).

Spector, B. D., Kersey, J. H., and Perry, G. S., III, 1977 (unpublished).

Swift, M., Sholman, L., Perry, M., and Chase, C., 1976, Malignant neoplasms in the families of patients with ataxia–telangiectasia, *Cancer Res.* **36**:209–215.

Takemoto, K. K., Rabson, A. S., Mullarkey, M. F., Blaese, R. M., Garon, C. F., and Nelson, D., 1974, Isolation of papovavirus from brain tumor and urine of a patient with Wiskott–Aldrich syndrome, *J. Natl. Cancer Inst.* **53**:1205–1207.

Twomey, J. J., Jordan, P. H., Laughter, A. H., Meuwissen, H. J., and Good, R. A., 1970, The gastric disorder in immunoglobulin patients, *Ann. Intern. Med.* **72**:499–504.

Twomey, J. J., Jordan, P. H., Jarrold, T., Trubowitz, S., Ritz, N. D., and Conn. H. O., 1976, The syndrome of immunoglobulin deficiency and pernicious anemia, *Am. J. Med.* **47**:340–350.

Waldmann, T. A., Strober, W., and Blaese, R. M., 1972, Immunodeficiency disease and malignancy: Various immunologic deficiencies of man and the role of immune processes in the control of malignant disease, *Ann. Intern. Med.* **77**:605–628.

Walker, W. A., and Hong, R., 1973, Immunology of the gastrointestinal tract, Part I, *J. Pediatr.* **83**:517–530.

Weiner, L. P., Herndon, R. M., Narayan, O., Johnson, R. T., Shar, K., Rubinstein, L. J., Preziosk, T. J., and Conley, F. K., 1972, Isolation of virus related to SV40 from patients with progressive multifocal leukoencephalopathy, *N. Engl. J. Med.* **286**:385–390.

Wurster-Hill, D. H., McIntyre, O. R., Cornell, G. G., and Maurer, L. H., 1973, Marker-chromosome 14 in multiple myeloma and plasma-cell leukaemia, *Lancet* **2**:1031.

Young, J. L., and Miller, R. W., 1975, Incidence of malignant tumors in U.S. children, *J. Pediatr.* **86**:254–258.

8

Immunosuppression and Malignant Disease

ISRAEL PENN

1. Introduction

In recent years, great progress has been made in the field of immunology. As part of this process, there has been a recrudescence of interest in the relationship between immunity and cancer. In experimental animals and in man, tumor-specific antigens have been demonstrated in at least some neoplasms, as well as cellular and humoral immune responses to these antigens. An important advance in our knowledge was the finding that states of immune deficiency are associated with an increased incidence of malignancies, particularly of lymphomas. This increase has been observed both in naturally occurring diseases (Gatti and Good, 1971; Kersey *et al.*, 1973) and in conditions produced by iatrogenic manipulations of immunity (Penn, 1970, 1973, 1974a,b, 1976, 1978; Penn and Starzl, 1972, 1973; Penn et al., 1969). Important among the latter conditions is the immunosuppression produced in organ-transplant recipients. In 1968, we first drew attention to an increased incidence of neoplasms in this group of patients (Penn *et al.,* 1969). Since then, we have maintained an informal registry to which physicians from many countries have generously contributed data. The cases reported up to January 1, 1976, provide the clinical material on which this chapter is based.

2. Incidence of Malignancies in Organ-Transplant Recipients

A carefully followed series of a large number of renal-transplant recipients, such as that of the University of Colorado Medical Center and Denver Veterans Administration Hospital, provides accurate information on the frequency of cancer in these patients. In the first 556 recipients, there were 31 who developed malignancies after transplantation, an incidence of 5.6%. Thus, cancer occurs at a frequency

---

ISRAEL PENN • Department of Surgery, University of Colorado School of Medicine, and Veterans Administration Hospital, Denver, Colorado 80220.

approximately 100 times greater than it does in the general population in the same age range (Penn, 1970).

3. Varieties of Neoplasms in Organ-Transplant Recipients

The Denver Transplant Tumor Registry has data on 357 patients who developed 375 tumors after organ transplantation. Of these patients, 352 were recipients of kidney homografts, 4 had cardiac transplants, and 1 had a liver homograft. Nonlymphomatous tumors occurred in 265 patients, solid lymphomas in 87, and both a nonlymphomatous neoplasm and a solid lymphoma in each of 5 patients (Table 1).

4. Lymphomas in Organ-Transplant Recipients

4.1. Incidence

In the spontaneously occurring immune deficiency states, the majority of neoplasms reported are lymphoreticular (Gatti and Good, 1971; Kersey *et al.*, 1973). In the organ-transplant recipients, there has been a similar disproportionately high incidence of solid lymphomas: In the series being discussed, 92 of the 357 patients (25.8%) developed these neoplasms, whereas lymphomas ordinarily consti-

TABLE 1. Varieties of Neoplasms in Organ-Homograft Recipients

Type of tumor	Number of patients
Cancers of skin and lips	147
Solid lymphomas	93
Carcinomas of uterus	28
Cervix (26)	
Body (2)	
Carcinomas of lung	15
Metastatic carcinomas	
(primary site unknown)	13
Carcinomas of colon and rectum	9
Carcinomas of kidney	8
Host kidney (5)	
Homograft kidney (3)	
Carcinomas of breast	6
Leukemias	6
Carcinomas of liver and bile ducts	6
Carcinomas of urinary bladder	6
Carcinomas of thyroid	4
Carcinomas of testis	4
Cancers of stomach (1 carcinoid tumor)	4
Soft-tissue sarcomas	4
Miscellaneous cancers	22
TOTAL:	375[a]

[a]Several of the 357 patients had more than one type of cancer. See Section 3 of the text.

tute only about 3% of all malignant tumors in man (Silverberg and Holleb, 1974). In a study at the National Cancer Institute, the risk among renal-transplant recipients of developing lymphoma was about 35 times higher than normal (Hoover and Fraumeni, 1973).

4.2. Types

Table 2 summarizes the primary neoplasms of lymphoid tissues that have been reported. The classification of lymphomas is fraught with pitfalls (Lukes and Collins, 1974). In this chapter, an attempt has been made to keep the terminology as simple as possible, although it is recognized that some of the nomenclature used is obsolescent. The diagnosis of reticulum-cell sarcoma includes cases labeled as "histiocytic lymphoma," "cerebral microglioma," "reticulosarcoma," and "immunoblastic sarcoma." The "Lymphoma" category in Table 2 includes cases in which the pathologist was not prepared to make a more specific diagnosis. There has been much controversy about the identity of the primary cell of Kaposi's sarcoma. It is included among the lymphomas because some physicians regard it as belonging to this class of neoplasms (Moertel and Hagedorn, 1957; Ormsby and Montgomery, 1954; Warner and O'Loughlin, 1975).

In the general population, Hodgkin's disease makes up 34% of solid lymphomas (Silverberg and Holleb, 1974), and it is the most common lymphoma in any age group (Levin et al., 1974). The series being discussed is most unusual in that only 1 of 93 tumors ($\approx$1%) was diagnosed as Hodgkin's disease; the bulk of the lymphomas were reticulum-cell sarcomas. Hoover and Fraumeni (1973) pointed out that these neoplasms are 350 times more common in renal-transplant recipients than in the general population. The preponderance of reticulum-cell sarcomas, most of which are probably the "immunoblastic sarcomas" of Lukes and Collins (1974), may well reflect an abnormal immune response to the foreign histocompatibility antigens of the homograft, which will be discussed in Section 6.1.3d.

Are the lymphoma cells of donor or recipient origin? A substantial number of donor lymphocytes are inevitably transplanted with the homograft. In animal experiments, some of the lymphomas were of donor-cell origin, though the majority were composed of host lymphocytes (Armstrong, M. Y. K., et al., 1973; Gleich-

TABLE 2. Solid Lymphomas in 92 Organ-Homograft
Recipients

Type of lymphoma	Number of patients
Reticulum-cell sarcoma	65[a]
Kaposi's sarcoma	11[a]
Lymphoma (includes 1 plasma cell lymphoma)	8
Lymphosarcoma	5
Lymphoreticular malignancy	2
Hodgkin's disease	1
?Histiocytic reticulosis	1

[a]The total number of tumors is 93 because one patient had both a reticulum-cell sarcoma and a Kaposi's sarcoma.

mann, E., *et al.*, 1975). The origin of the cells in the human lymphomas was studied in 3 cases; all were of host origin (Brown *et al.*, 1974; Penn, 1974a; Portmann *et al.*, 1976).

4.3. Clinical Features

4.3.1. Age of Patients

At the time of transplantation, the average age of the patients who later developed nonlymphomatous neoplasms was 40 years (range 8–64 years). Recipients who developed lymphomas were slightly younger at transplant, averaging 36 years (range 8–70 years). Of patients who developed nonlymphomatous tumors, 50% were over the age of 40, compared with 33% of those who developed lymphomas.

4.3.2. Sex of Patients

In the series of 357 patients, males outnumbered females by approximately 1.75 to 1 (226 males to 131 females). Among the patients with nonlymphomatous lesions, there were 167 males and 98 females; with lymphomas, 56 males and 31 females; and with both types of tumors, 3 males and 2 females.

4.3.3. Time of Appearance after Transplantation

In the overall series, tumors were diagnosed an average of approximately 32 months after transplantation. The nonlymphomatous lesions appeared 35 months postoperatively on the average (range 1–154 months), whereas the lymphomas appeared at a considerably earlier stage, averaging 23 months (range 2–146 months).

4.3.4. Organs Affected by Lymphomas

Of 11 patients with Kaposi's sarcoma, 6 had lesions involving the skin of one or more extremities, with involvement of the left tonsil in one and the mucosa of the mouth and nose in another. The other 5 had visceral involvement, particularly of the alimentary tract and lungs.

The 82 patients with other lymphomas (see Table 2) can be divided into two groups—those with widespread lesions and those with the disease localized to a single viscus. There were 39 recipients in the disseminated-disease group, in which the distribution of tumor was similar to that in the general population; tumor was most often present in the liver, spleen, lymph nodes, bone marrow, and lungs.

Of 43 patients with localized lymphomas, the organs affected were the brain (29), spinal cord (1), bone marrow (1), liver (3), small bowel (2), esophagus (1), vagina (1), stomach (1), lung (2), kidney homograft (1), and submandibular area (1). The frequency of involvement of the CNS was most unusual: in the 82 patients with non-Kaposi's lymphomas, the brain or spinal cord was affected in 38 instances (46%) (Table 3), whereas in the general population, these structures are involved in

TABLE 3. Lymphomas Involving the Brain or Spinal Cord

Patients with lymphoma (excluding Kaposi's sarcoma)	82
Brain or spinal cord involvement	38
Brain only	29
Spinal cord only	1
Brain and skin	1
Brain and lungs	2
Brain and lymph nodes	1
Brain and multiple organs	4[a]

[a]Excludes two patients with widespread tumor in whom the only CNS involvement
was the pituitary gland in one and the pia mater in the other.

less than 2% (Richmond *et al.*, 1962; Rosenberg *et al.*, 1961). Possible reasons the CNS was so frequently involved are discussed by Schneck and Penn (1971).

The homograft was involved by lymphoma in 17 instances (kidney 16, liver 1). This figure (21%) is not surprising in view of the 34% incidence of renal involvement by lymphoma found in the general population (Richmond *et al.*, 1962). Neoplastic involvement of the homograft ranged from incidentally discovered microscopic lesions to clinically obvious tumors. In planning treatment of patients with lymphomas, the possibility of homograft involvement should be borne in mind.

4.3.5. Possibility of Transmission from Organ Donors

The 357 patients received their organs from 404 donors, of whom 133 (33%) were related living donors and 271 (67%) were unrelated donors (usually cadavers). Almost the same percentages were noted in the recipients who developed lymphomas. We must consider the possibility that malignant cells could have been inadvertently transplanted with the homograft in instances in which donors with cancer were used. Of the recipients, 6 received organs from cancerous donors but in no instance did they develop tumors of the same type as those in the donors. Of these 6, 2 developed reticulum cell sarcomas, whereas their respective donors had a carcinoma of the colon and a medulloblastoma.

4.3.6. Preexisting Neoplasms in the Recipients

Among the 357 patients, there were 8 who had known neoplasms prior to transplantation, including 2 recipients who subsequently developed lymphomas. In only one instance, however, was there any morphological relationship between the earlier and later tumors. This was in a patient who was treated for multiple myeloma and subsequently developed a pulmonary immunoblastoma. The possibility could not be excluded in this instance that the lesion developing after transplantation was a poorly differentiated plasmacytoma.

It is possible that some of the 375 tumors were present at the time of transplantation but were not diagnosed. A total of 21 patients (8%) with nonlymphomatous lesions and 7 (8%) with lymphomas manifested their neoplasms within the first 4 months after transplantation. We have previously discussed the possibility that the immunosuppressive affect of chronic uremia *per se* contributed to the development of at least some of these tumors (Penn and Starzl, 1972).

4.3.7. Immunosuppressive Measures Used

The immunosuppressive measures used are summarized in Table 4. There was very little difference in the treatments given to patients with lymphomas as compared with those given to recipients with other neoplasms, except that in the former group a greater percentage (36 vs. 24%) received treatment with antilymphocyte globulin (ALG). The development of malignancies could not be related to the use of any particular immunosuppressive measure, but the malignancies appeared to be associated with immunosuppression in general.

4.3.8. Treatment of Lymphomas

We have previously reported (Penn, 1970; Wilson, R. E., and Penn, 1975) a series of organ-homograft recipients who developed neoplasms following inadvertent transmission of malignant cells from donors with cancer. In several patients, treatment of the main tumor mass and discontinuation of immunosuppressive therapy was followed by disappearance of metastases. Presumably, the patients' depressed immune systems recovered and destroyed the transplanted foreign malignant cells. Is this form of therapy applicable to the patients with lymphomas in whom the tumor cells were presumably of host origin? Thus far, experience has been limited, since many lymphomas were diagnosed only at autopsy, or treatment was initiated when the patient was already *in extremis*. Several recipients, however, have responded well to conventional therapy of the lymphomas following reduction or cessation of immunosuppressive therapy. One of our patients is still alive with good renal function 8 years after radiotherapy to a cerebral lymphoma and reduction of immunosuppressive therapy, and shows no evidence of residual disease. Should the physician choose to continue with the patient's usual dose of immunosuppressive agents, however, there is a risk of excessive depression of the bone marrow if chemotherapeutic agents, such as cyclophosphamide or vincristine, are used concomitantly to treat the lymphoma. Since many of the chemotherapeutic agents used in the treatment of lymphomas have immunosuppressive side effects,

TABLE 4. Immunosuppressive Measures Used[a]

Agent	Number of patients
Prednisone	355
Azathioprine	355
ALG	94[b]
Local irradiation of the homograft	111
Splenectomy	81
Actinomycin	72
Cyclophosphamide	17
Thoracic duct fistula	11
Thymectomy	8

[a]Other treatments included thymic irradiation (2), endolymphatic irradiation (3), total-body irradiation (2), extracorporeal irradiation of the peripheral blood (1), 6-mercaptopurine (1), methotrexate (1), and azaserine (1).
[b]Two patients received ALG after the appearance of the tumors.

reduction or cessation of immunosuppressive therapy does not inevitably result in rejection of the organ homograft. If the kidney homograft nevertheless undergoes rejection, it should be removed and the patient maintained on dialysis.

4.3.9. Prognosis

The prognosis for patients with lymphomas is dismal. Only 14% are currently alive, compared with 58% of recipients with other types of neoplasms. Of the lymphoma survivors, 30% are patients with nonvisceral Kaposi's sarcoma.

5. Neoplasms in Nontransplant Patients Treated with Immunosuppressive and Cancer Chemotherapeutic Agents

We have provided unequivocal evidence of an increased incidence of neoplasms, particularly of lymphomas, in organ-homograft recipients treated with immunosuppressive agents. Does the same problem exist in nontransplant patients treated with immunosuppressive agents for diseases such as glomerulonephritis, psoriasis, rheumatoid arthritis, systemic lupus erythematosus, and other disorders of uncertain etiology? We have data on 70 such patients with 72 cancers that appeared after the commencement of this treatment (Penn, 1974b, 1978). Of these tumors, 20 (28%) were lymphomas, a figure similar to that observed in organ-homograft recipients. Is there an increased incidence of these tumors related to the immunosuppressive therapy? Alternatively, are these neoplasms merely a reflection of the increased incidence of malignancies, particularly of lymphomas, that occurs with autoimmune diseases (Hoerni and Laporte, 1970; Oleinick, 1976; Talal and Bunim, 1964)? Since there are currently no accurate statistics available on the numbers of patients at risk, it will be necessary to conduct carefully controlled prospective trials of immunosuppressive therapy to answer these questions.

As mentioned in Section 4.3.8, many of the cancer chemotherapeutic compounds have immunosuppressive side effects. In previous reports (Penn, 1974b, 1978; Penn and Starzl, 1973), we alluded to the paradox that agents used to treat cancer may themselves be oncogenic. At present, we have data on 185 patients who were treated with chemotherapy for neoplasms, mostly of the lymphohemopoietic system, and who subsequently developed 194 new malignancies. Of these new tumors, 36 (19%) were lymphomas. None of the patients in whom these tumors occurred had preexisting tumors of this type. A total of 27 of the lymphomas occurred in patients who had received chemotherapy for chronic *granulocytic* leukemia.

Even if we take into account that patients with one cancer are more prone to additional neoplasms (Moertel *et al.*, 1961), that some malignancies may represent transitions of one form of cancer into another related type, and that patients may have been treated with other potentially oncogenic agents such as radiotherapy (*New England Journal of Medicine,* 1972; Castro *et al.*, 1973), the evidence suggests that chemotherapy is responsible for the development of at least some of the new malignancies. A statistically significant increased incidence of additional cancers was reported in patients with chronic lymphocytic leukemia (Manusow and Weinerman, 1975), Hodgkin's disease (Arseneau *et al.*, 1972; Sieber, 1975), and multiple myeloma (Sieber, 1975), all of which are subject to vigorous therapy. In addition, Greenspan and Tung (1974) reported a 15% incidence of second cancers in patients with Stage III ovarian carcinomas who had complete regression of their neoplasms for more than 5 years after intensive maintenance chemotherapy.

6. Possible Causes of Neoplasms

The increased incidence of malignancies under the conditions described above raises fundamental questions regarding the cause or causes of these neoplasms. We can only speculate on these causes, since there are still large gaps in our knowledge in this area. In all probability, the cancers develop as a result of a complex interplay of multiple factors, to which we will now turn our attention.

6.1. Alterations in Immunity

6.1.1. Preexisting Disease

Some of the diseases that result in chronic failure of the kidney, liver, or heart and necessitate transplantation are autoimmune disorders. As noted in Section 5, an increased incidence of malignancies has been described with some autoimmune diseases (Hoerni and Laporte, 1970; Oleinick, 1967; Talal and Bunim, 1964). The question therefore arises whether the increased incidence of malignancies in organ-homograft recipients is related to the original disease. Relevant to this question, a study of 290 renal-transplant recipients who developed malignancies indicated little relationship between the cause of renal failure and the development of neoplasia (Bergan, 1976).

6.1.2. Depressed Immunity in Uremia

Chronic renal failure is associated with depression of immune responses (Kasakura and Lowenstein, 1967; Morrison et al., 1963; Wilson, W. E. C., and Kirkpatrick, 1964). In a previous report (Penn and Starzl, 1972), we discussed the possibility that chronic uremia might be responsible for the development of some tumors manifesting themselves before or in the first few months after transplantation. Matas et al. (1975) recently reported a statistically significant increase in cancer in patients with end-stage renal failure.

6.1.3. Therapeutic Manipulation

Therapeutic manipulation of immune reactivity may facilitate the growth of cancer through several possible mechanisms, which are discussed below.

a. Immune Surveillance. In the course of daily "wear and tear," millions of cells are lost and require replacement. Mutations, some of which are potentially malignant, arise either spontaneously or under the influence of environmental oncogens. The immune surveillance hypothesis (Burnet, 1971; Ehrlich, 1957; Thomas, 1959) states that a major function of the lymphoreticular system is to recognize such cells and to destroy them or inhibit their growth. If this function is impaired by immunosuppressive therapy, an increased incidence of tumors should occur. This attractive theory was widely accepted at first, but in recent years has come under increasing criticism, in part because of conflicting results from animal experiments (Andrews, 1974; Baldwin, 1976; Gleichmann, H., and Gleichmann, 1973; Haughton and Whitmore, 1976; Kripke and Borsos, 1974; Melief and Schwartz, 1975; Möller and Möller, 1976; Prehn, 1976; Prehn and Lappe, 1971; Rygaard and Povlsen, 1976; Schwartz, 1972, 1975; Simpson and Nehlsen, 1971). Current views can be summarized as follows: Immunosuppression facilitates the ease with which malignant cells can be transplanted and accelerates metastatic growth. Viral oncogenesis is markedly potentiated by immunosuppression in many systems, but whether this potentiation represents decreased surveillance or lowered resistance to the virus *per se* is not always clear. The influence of immunosuppression on chemical oncogenesis is equivocal. Apparently, immunosuppressive therapy does not increase the susceptibility to "spontaneous" tumors. In man, several observations contradict the immune surveillance hypothesis. In some diseases, such as leprosy and sarcoidosis, there is pronounced immunosuppression, but no increased cancer incidence. If the surveillance theory is correct, we would expect an increased frequency of all types of malignancies, yet we have found a disproportionately high incidence of lymphomas. Obviously, some other mechanism must be responsible for their development.

b. Immune Stimulation. In contrast to the immune surveillance hypothesis, Prehn (Prehn, 1976; Prehn and Lappe, 1971) believes that a very weak immune reaction, rather than inhibiting tumor growth, may actually stimulate it. He regards the effects of immunological reactions on their target tissues as biphasic, stimulating cell division and growth at one level and inhibiting growth and destroying cells at another. This theory fails to explain the high incidence of lymphomas that we have observed.

c. Immunoregulation. Feedback processes, either cellular or humoral, are recognized as important in controlling the extent of immune reactions. On the basis of these mechanisms, two theories have been formulated that may explain the unusually high incidence of lymphomas with autoimmune diseases, in naturally occurring immune deficiency states, or in organ-homograft recipients. In the first theory, there is believed to be a reduction of thymic suppressor function (Gershwin and Steinberg, 1973), which normally retards continued lymphoid proliferation. If unregulated proliferation is thus allowed to continue, it could ultimately progress to lymphoreticular malignancy. Furthermore, once the loss of regulation occurs, the defensive state of the immune system is upset and other nonlymphoid tumors have an opportunity to develop.

The second hypothesis is based on the discovery that latent oncogenic viruses can be activated immunologically (Hirsch *et al.*, 1970, 1973; Schwartz, 1972, 1975). The theory is based on findings in experimental models indicating that continuous antigenic stimulation of partially immunodeficient mice can trigger the development of lymphoreticular neoplasms (Armstrong, M. Y. K., *et al.*, 1973; Krueger, 1972). In patients with congenital or acquired immunodeficiency, the immune response is only partially suppressed. It is postulated that there is defective antibody production, which fails to suppress lymphocyte transformation and proliferation, and leads to derepression of the virogene and assemblage of oncogenic viruses in an environment favoring their replication. Viruses shed from lymphoblasts infect cells in the microenvironment of the immunological reaction. These cells undergo malignant transformation and eventually give rise to a neoplasm.

d. Chronic Antigenic Stimulation. In a wide variety of animal experiments, chronic exposure to foreign antigens has resulted in a high incidence of malignant lymphomas (Armstrong, M. Y. K., *et al.*, 1970; Balls and Ruben, 1968; Gleichmann, E., *et al.*, 1975; Jerusalem, 1968; Metcalf, 1963; Suciu-Foca *et al.*, 1970; Walford and Hildemann, 1965). Whether these tumors are caused by the liberation of oncogenic viruses, as described above, or by chronic stimulation of lymphoid tissue, leading to hyperplasia and ultimately neoplasia, is unknown. The high incidence of lymphomas in transplant patients could be related to the chronic presence of the homograft with its foreign histocompatibility antigens. As mentioned in Section 4.2, reticulum-cell sarcoma is the most common form of lymphoma observed in immunosuppressed patients. Lukes and Collins (1974) state that the cells making up this tumor have all the morphological features of an antigen-stimulated lymphocyte and prefer to call the neoplasm an "immunoblastic sarcoma." Their interpretation is consistent with the notion that antigenic stimulation can be a factor in the development of lymphomas.

Warner and O'Loughlin (1975) suggested that Kaposi's sarcoma is the result of a chronic immunological reaction between antigenically altered or transformed lymphoid cells and normal lymphocytes. In the course of this local graft-versus-host (GVH)-type activity, an angiogenesis factor is liberated, and intense proliferation of mesenchymal and endothelial cells ensues. During the GVH-like activity, an oncogenic virus is either transferred to or induced in the cells responsive to the angiogenesis factor. Thus, the stage is set for neoplastic transformation of these cells in an environment that is conducive to the progressive growth of the virally transformed vasoformative mesenchyme.

e. Oncogenic Viruses. There are two mechanisms by which oncogenic viruses can be activated in organ-transplant recipients. (1) Episodes of threatened homograft rejection are common in these patients. As mentioned in the preceding section, antigenic stimuli can activate latent endogenous oncornaviruses (Hirsch *et al.*, 1970). This activation can occur after a process as seemingly innocuous as rejection of a skin homograft (Hirsch *et al.*, 1973). Such immunologically activated viruses can be oncogenic (Armstrong, M. Y. K., *et al.*, 1973). (2) Impaired immune defense mechanisms are responsible for a high incidence of virus infections in immunosuppressed patients (Allen and Cole, 1972; Armstrong, D., 1973; Coleman *et al.*, 1973; Spencer and Andersen, 1970; Stevens, 1973). Some infections are with viruses that are potentially oncogenic in man, including the Epstein–Barr, herpes hominis I and II, and polyoma viruses. The common kinds of malignancy observed in these patients—lymphomas and cancers of the skin, lip, and uterine cervix—are precisely those for which oncogenic viruses are suspected to be etiological.

f. Oncogenicity of the Immunosuppressive Agents. Immunosuppressive and cancer chemotherapeutic agents have caused chromosome breaks, nuclear abnormalities, cytological dysplasia, and teratogenic effects in man and animals. Nevertheless, a direct oncogenic effect of these compounds in man has been demonstrated with only one substance: the alkylating agent chlornaphazine (Penn, 1974b, 1976; Penn and Starzl, 1973).

g. Co-oncogenic Effects of the Immunosuppressive Agents. Another possible mechanism through which immunosuppressive agents may contribute to the development of malignancy is by potentiating the effects of environmental carcinogens such as tobacco and radiation. In experiments with hairless mice, chronic azathioprine administration enhanced the oncogenic effects of ultraviolet light in causing skin cancers (Koranda *et al.*, 1975). If these results can be extrapolated to man, they might explain the high incidence of skin cancers observed in organ-homograft recipients.

6.2. Role of Other Factors

Why do cancers develop in some organ-transplant recipients but not in others treated in precisely the same way? Perhaps genetic factors account, at least in part, for this difference in behavior. For example, the combined action of several genes determines the ultimate balance between resistance and susceptibility to the induction of leukemia in mice by either endogenous or exogenous viruses (Lilly, 1972). Much more needs to be learned about genetic factors, which may operate through immunological or nonimmunological mechanisms, or both, and which determine resistance or susceptibility to cancer.

Besides the immunosuppressive agents, organ-transplant recipients are occasionally treated with other potentially oncogenic drugs. These drugs include isoniazid (Miller, 1974), which is used in the prevention and treatment of tuberculosis, and diphenylhydantoin (Dilantin) (*Lancet*, 1971; Li *et al.*, 1975), which is used to prevent convulsions in patients who have had hypertensive encephalopathy and other cerebral disorders.

7. Implications for the Future Use of the Immunosuppressive and Cancer Chemotherapeutic Agents

Because of the risks of infection and malignancy and other side effects (Penn, 1973), the immunosuppressive agents should be used only when strongly indicated. In nontransplant patients, their administration should be limited to situations in which other forms of therapy have failed to control the patient's disorders. Immunosuppressive therapy is essential in the management of organ-homograft recipients. The 5.6% risk of malignancy should not serve as a deterrent to transplantation, since many of the cancers are of low grade and can be easily treated by conventional methods. Nevertheless, we should not be complacent about current therapy, but should strive to replace our nonspecific blunderbuss attack on the immune system with methods for the induction of specific immune unresponsiveness limited to the antigens of the homograft. Advantage should also be taken of this clinical model to learn more about factors that lead to oncogenesis in man.

Cancer chemotherapy is worthwhile in patients with advanced or widespread malignancies, since the potential control of the neoplasms for months or years far outweighs the risk of development of additional tumors. This hazard appears to be less with intermittent therapy than with continuous prolonged administration, since the lymphoreticular system tends to recover between the courses of treatment (George *et al.*, 1972; Hersh *et al.*, 1973). Chemotherapy as an adjuvant to surgery or radiotherapy in the management of localized cancers has produced encouraging results with some malignancies. There is a possibility, however, that it may impair the host's immune defenses and actually promote the growth of tumor cells. Careful monitoring of humoral and cellular immunity before and after institution of chemotherapy may ultimately provide the answer to this question.

8. Summary

There is a markedly increased incidence of cancer in organ-homograft recipients. Many of the tumors are low-grade lesions of the skin, lip, and uterine cervix. Almost 26% of the neoplasms, however, are highly lethal lymphomas, as compared with a 3% incidence in the general population. The lymphomas occur at a young age (average 36 years) and after a relatively short induction time following transplantation (average 23 months). Unlike the distribution seen in the general population, Hodgkin's disease is rare, and the preponderant type of lymphoma is reticulum-cell sarcoma. Many of these tumors have the morphological features of antigen-activated lymphocytes and can be classified as "immunoblastic sarcomas." Whereas lymphomas in the general population seldom involve the CNS, the CNS is involved in nearly half the organ-homograft patients with lymphomas other than Kaposi's sarcoma, and in many instances the lesions are confined only to the brain and spinal cord. The homograft is involved by lymphoma in 21% of cases.

The cause of the increased incidence of malignancies in organ-homograft recipients is unclear, but a complex interplay of multiple factors is probably responsible. One hypothesis is that the immunosurveillance function of the lymphoreticular system is depressed so that mutant cells can develop into neoplasms. If this is true, we would expect an increased incidence of cancer of the breast, lung, pancreas, and colon. Such an increase has not been observed, nor does the theory explain the high incidence of lymphomas. It is also unlikely that the immunosuppressive agents alone are responsible for the increased incidence of cancer. We must also consider the role of viruses in the immunosuppressed patients, since viruses can cause both cancer and infection under different circumstances. In addition, chronic antigenic stimulation of the lymphoid system by foreign histocompatibility antigens of the homograft may play a role in the unusually high incidence of lymphomas.

ACKNOWLEDGMENTS

The author wishes to thank his numerous colleagues, working in transplant and cancer chemotherapy centers throughout the world, for their generous contribution of data concerning their patients.

The author's research is supported in part by research grant 6985 from the Veterans Administration, by grants AI-AM-08898 and AM-07772 from the National Institutes of Health, and by grants RR-00051 and RR-00069 from the General Clinical Research Centers Program of the Division of Research Resources, National Institutes of Health.

References

Allen, D. W., and Cole, P., 1972, Viruses and human cancer, *N. Engl. J. Med.* **286**:70–82.

Andrews, E. J., 1974, Failure of immunosurveillance against chemically induced *in situ* tumors in mice, *J. Natl. Cancer Inst.* **52**:729–732.

Armstrong, D., 1973, Infectious complications in cancer patients treated with chemical immunosuppressive agents, *Transplant. Proc.* **5**:1245–1248.

Armstrong, M. Y. K., Gleichmann, E., Gleichmann, H., Beldotti, L., and Andre-Schwartz, R. S., 1970, Chronic allogeneic disease. II. Development of lymphomas, *J. Exp. Med.* **132**:417–439.

Armstrong, M. Y. K., Ruddle, N. H., Lipman, M. B., and Richards, F. F., 1973, Tumor induction by immunologically activated murine leukemia virus, *J. Exp. Med.* **137**:1163–1179.

Arseneau, J. C., Sponzo, R. W., Levine, D. L., Schnipper, L. E., Bonner, H., Young, R. C., Cannellos, G. P., Johnson, R. E., and DeVita, V. T., 1972, Nonlymphomatous malignant tumors complicating Hodgkin's disease: Possible association with intensive therapy, *N. Engl. J. Med.* **287**:1119–1122.

Baldwin, R. W., 1976, Role of immunosurveillance against chemically induced rat tumors, *Transplant, Rev.* **28**:62–74.

Balls, M., and Ruben, L. N., 1968, Lymphoid tumors in amphibia: A review, *Prog. Exp. Tumor Res.* **10**:238–260.

Bergan, J. J., 1976, A.C.S.–N.I.H. Organ Transplant Registry, February *Newsletter.*

Brown, R. S., Schiff, M., and Mitchell, M. S., 1974, Reticulum cell sarcoma of host origin arising in a transplanted kidney, *Ann. Intern. Med.* **80**:459–463.

Burnet, F. M., 1971, Immunological surveillance in neoplasia, *Transplant. Rev.* **7**:3–25.

Castro, E. B., Rosen, P. P., and Quan, S. H. Q., 1973, Carcinoma of large intestine in patients irradiated for carcinoma of cervix and uterus, *Cancer* **31**:45–52.

Coleman, D. V., Gardner, S. D., and Field, A. M., 1973, Human polyomavirus infection in renal allograft recipients, *Br. Med. J.* **3**:371–375.

Ehrlich, P., 1957, Über den jetzigen Stand der Karzinomforschung, in: *The Collected Papers of Paul Ehrlich,* Vol. 2, p. 550, Pergamon Press, London.

Gatti, R. A., and Good, R. A., 1971, Occurrence of malignancy in immunodeficiency diseases: A literature review, *Cancer* **28**:89–98.

George, R. P., Poth, J. L., Gordon, D., and Schrier, S. L., 1972, Multiple myeloma—Intermittent combination chemotherapy compared to continuous therapy, *Cancer* **29**:1665–1670.

Gershwin, M. E., and Steinberg, A. D., 1973, Loss of suppressor function as a cause of lymphoid malignancy, *Lancet* **2**:1174–1176.

Gleichmann, E., Gleichmann, H., Schwartz, R. S. Weinblatt, A., and Armstrong, M. Y. K., 1975, Immunologic induction of malignant lymphoma: Identification of donor and host tumors in the graft-versus-host model, *J. Natl. Cancer Inst.* **54**:107–116.

Gleichmann, H., and Gleichmann, E., 1973, Immunosuppression and neoplasia. I. Critical review of experimental carcinogenesis and the immunosurveillance theory, *Klin. Wochenschr.* **51**:255–259.

Greenspan, E. M., and Tung, B. G., 1974, Acute myeloblastic leukemia after cure of ovarian cancer, *J. Am. Med. Assoc.* **230**:418–420.

Haughton, G., and Whitmore, A. C., 1976, Genetics, the immune response and oncogenesis, *Transplant, Rev.* **28**:75–97.

Hersh, E. M., Gutterman, J. U., Mavligit, G., McCredie, K. B., Bodey, G. P., Freireich, E. J., Rossen, R. D., and Butler, W. T., 1973, Host defense, chemical immunosuppression and the transplant recipient—Relative effects of intermittent versus continuous immunosuppressive therapy with reference to the objectives of treatment, *Transplant. Proc.* **5**:1191–1195.

Hirsch, M. S., Black, P. H., Tracy, G. S., Leibowitz, S., and Schwartz, R. S., 1970, Leukemia virus activation in chronic allogeneic disease, *Proc. Natl. Acad. Sci. U.S.A.* **67**:1914–1917.

Hirsch, M. S., Ellis, D. A., Black, P. H., Monaco, A. P., and Wood, M. L., 1973, Leukemia virus activation during homograft rejection, *Science* **180**:500–502.

Hoerni, B., and Laporte, G., 1970, Immunological disorders in the aetiology of lymphoreticular neoplasms, *Rev. Eur. Etud. Clin. Biol.* **15**:841–850.

Hoover, R., and Fraumeni, J. F., Jr., 1973, Risk of cancer in renal-transplant recipients, *Lancet* **2**:55–57.

Jerusalem, C., 1968, Relationship between malaria infection *(Plasmodium berghei)* and malignant lymphoma in mice, *Z. Tropenmed. Parasitol.* **19**:94–108.

Kasakura, S., and Lowenstein, L., 1967, The effect of uremic blood on mixed lymphocyte reactions and on cultures of leukocytes with phytohemagglutinin, *Transplantation* **5**:283–289.

Kersey, J. H., Spector, B. D., and Good, R. A., 1973, Primary immunodeficiency diseases and cancer: The immunodeficiency–Cancer Registry, *Int. J. Cancer* **12**:333–347.

Koranda, F. C., Loeffler, R. T., Koranda, D. M., and Penn, I., 1975, Accelerated induction of skin cancers by ultraviolet radiation in hairless mice treated with immunosuppressive agents, *Surg. Forum* **26**:145–146.

Kripke, M. L., and Borsos, T., 1974, Immune surveillance revisited, *J. Natl. Cancer Inst.* **52**:1393–1395.

Krueger, G. R. F., 1972, Chronic immunosuppression and lymphomagenesis in man and mice, in: *Conference on Immunology of Carcinogensis,* National Cancer Institute Monograph No. 35, p. 138, National Cancer Institute, Bethesda, Maryland.

Lancet, 1971, Is phenytoin carcinogenic? (editorial), **2**:1071–1072.

Levin, D. L., Devesa, S. S., Godwin, J. D., II, and Silverman, D. T., 1974, *Cancer Rates and Statistics,* 2nd Ed., U.S. Department of Health, Education and Welfare, Washington, D.C.

Li, F. P., Willard, D. R., Goodman, R., and Vawter, G., 1975, Malignant lymphoma after diphenylhydantoin (Dilantin) therapy, *Cancer* **36**:1359–1362.

Lilly, F., 1972, Mouse leukemia: A model of multiple gene disease, *J. Natl. Cancer Inst.* **49**:927–934.

Lukes, R. J., and Collins, R. D., 1974, Immunologic characterization of human malignant lymphomas, *Cancer* **34**:1488–1503.

Manusow, D., and Weinerman, B. H., 1975, Subsequent neoplasia in chronic lymphocytic leukemia, *J. Am. Med. Assoc.* **232**:267–269.

Matas, A. J., Simmons, R. L., Kjellstrand, C. M., Buselmeier, T. J., and Najarian, J. S., 1975, Increased incidence of malignancy during chronic renal failure, *Lancet* **1**:883–886.

Melief, C. J. M., and Schwartz, R. S., 1975, Immunocompetence and malignancy, in: *Cancer: A Comprehensive Treatise* (F. F. Becker, ed.) Vol. 1, pp. 121–159, Plenum Press, New York.

Metcalf, D., 1963, Induction of reticular tumours in mice by repeated antigenic stimulation, *Acta Unio Int. Contra Cancrun* **19**:657–659.

Miller, C. T., 1974, Isoniazid and cancer risks (letter to the editor), *J. Am. Med. Assoc.* **230**:1254.

Moertel, C. G., and Hagedorn, A. B., 1957, Leukemia or lymphoma and coexistent primary malignant lesions: A review of the literature and a study of 120 cases, *Blood* **12**:788–803.

Moertel, C. G., Dockerty, M. B., and Baggenstoss, A. H., 1961, Multiple primary malignant neoplasms. I. Introduction and presentation of data, *Cancer* **14**:221–230.

Möller, G., and Möller, E., 1976, The concept of immunological surveillance against neoplasia, *Transplant. Rev.* **28**:3–16.

Morrison, A. B., Maness, K., and Tawes, R., 1963, Skin homograft survival in chronic renal insufficiency, *Arch. Pathol.* **75**:139–143.

New England Journal of Medicine, 1972, Case records of the Massachusetts General Hospital: Case 47-1972, **287**:1085–1091.

Oleinick, A., 1967, Leukemia or lymphoma occurring subsequent to an auto-immune disease, *Blood* **29**:144–153.

Ormsby, O. S., and Montgomery, H., 1954, *Diseases of the Skin*, 8th Ed., p. 913, Lea and Febiger, Philadelphia.

Penn, I., 1970, *Malignant Tumors in Organ Transplant Recipients*, Springer-Verlag, New York.

Penn, I., 1973, Transplantation, in: *Outpatient Surgery* (G. J. Hill, II., ed.), pp. 872–906, W. B. Saunders, Philadelphia.

Penn, I., 1974a, Malignancies in recipients of organ transplants, in: *The Role of Immunological Factors in Viral and Oncogenic Processes*, Seventh Miles International Symposium (R. F. Beers, Jr., R. C. Tilghman, and E. G. Bassett, eds.), pp. 211–221, *Johns Hopkins Med. J. (Suppl. 3)*, Baltimore.

Penn, I., 1974b, Chemical immunosuppression and human cancer, *Cancer* **34**:1474–1480.

Penn, I., 1976, Second malignant neoplasms associated with immunosuppressive medications, *Cancer* **37**:1024–1032.

Penn, I., 1978, Cancer associated with immunosuppression, in: *Handbook of Clinical Immunology, CRC Handbook Series in Clinical Laboratory Science* (A. Baumgarten and F. F. Richards, eds.), CRC Press, Cleveland (in press).

Penn, I., and Starzl, T. E., 1972, Malignant tumors arising *de novo* in immunosuppressed organ transplant recipients, *Transplantation* **14**:407–417.

Penn, I., and Starzl, T. E., 1973, The effect of immunosuppression on cancer, in: *Seventh National Cancer Conference Proceedings*, pp. 425–436, J. B. Lippincott, Philadelphia.

Penn, I., Hammond, W. Brettschneider, L., and Starzl, T. E., 1969, Malignant lymphomas in transplantation patients, *Transplant. Proc.* **1**:106–112.

Portmann, B., Schindler, A.-M., Murray-Lyon, I. M., and Williams, R., 1976, Histological sexing of a reticulum cell sarcoma arising after liver transplantation, *Gastroenterology* **70**:82–84.

Prehn, R. T., 1976, Do tumors grow because of the immune response of the host?, *Transplant. Rev.* **28**:34–42.

Prehn, R. T., and Lappe, M. A., 1971, An immunostimulation theory of tumor development, *Transplant Rev.* **7**:26–54.

Richmond, J., Sherman, R. S., Diamond, H. D., and Craver, L. F., 1962, Renal lesions associated with malignant lymphomas, *Am. J. Med.* **32**:184–207.

Rosenberg, S. A., Diamond, H. D., Jaslowitz, B., and Craver, L. F., 1961, Lymphosarcoma: A review of 1269 cases, *Medicine (Baltimore)* **40**:31–84.

Rygaard, J., and Povlsen, C. O., 1976, The nude mouse vs. the hypothesis of immunological surveillance, *Transplant. Rev.* **28**:43–61.

Schneck, S. A., and Penn, I., 1971, *De novo* cerebral neoplasms in renal transplant recipients, *Lancet* 1:983–986.

Schwartz, R. S., 1972, Immunoregulation, oncogenic viruses and malignant lymphomas, *Lancet* 1:1266–1269.

Schwartz, R. S., 1975, Another look at immunologic surveillance, *N. Engl. J. Med.* **293**:181–184.

Sieber, S. M., 1975, Cancer chemotherapeutic agents and carcinogenesis, *Cancer Chemother. Rep.* **59**:915–918.

Silverberg, E., and Holleb, A. I., 1974, Cancer Statistics 1974—Worldwide Epidemiology, *Cancer* **24**:2–21.

Simpson, E., and Nehlsen, S. L., 1971, Prolonged administration of antithymocyte serum in mice. I. Histopathological investigations, *Clin. Exp. Immunol.* **9**:79–98.

Spencer, E. S., and Andersen, H. K., 1970, Clinically evident, non-terminal infections with herpes viruses and the wart virus in immunosuppressed renal allograft recipients, *Br. Med. J.* **3**:251–254.

Stevens, D. A., 1973, Immunosuppression and virus infections, *Transplant. Proc.* **5**:1259–1262.

Suciu-Foca, N., Dumitrescu, V., Lazar, C., and Nachtigal, M., 1970, Host and tumor modifications associated with serial heterotransplantation of tumors through immunologically tolerant animals, *Cancer Res.* **30**:1681–1691.

Talal, N., and Bunim, J. J., 1964, The development of malignant lymphoma in the course of Sjögren's syndrome, *Am. J. Med.* **36**:529–540.

Thomas, L., 1959, Discussion of Medawar, P. B.: Reactions to homologous tissue antigens in relation to hypersensitivity, in: *Cellular and Humoral Aspects of the Hypersensitive States* (H. S. Lawrence, ed.), pp. 529–532, Paul Hoeber, New York.

Walford, R. L., and Hildemann, W. H., 1965, Life span and lymphoma-incidence of mice injected at birth with spleen cells across a weak histocompatibility locus, *Am. J. Pathol.* **47**:713–721.

Warner, T. F. C. S., and O'Loughlin, S., 1975, Kaposi's sarcoma: A byproduct of tumour rejection, *Lancet* **2**:687–689.

Wilson, R. E., and Penn, I., 1975, Fate of tumors transplanted with a renal allograft, *Transplant. Proc.* **7**:327–331.

Wilson, W. E. C., and Kirkpatrick, C. H., 1964, Immunologic aspects of renal homotransplantation, in: *Experience in Renal Transplantation* (T. E. Starzl, ed.), pp. 239–261, W. B. Saunders, Philadelphia.

9

The Pathology of Lymphoreticular Neoplasms

ROBERT J. LUKES and JOHN W. PARKER

1. Introduction*

The malignant lymphomas are now acknowledged to be neoplasms of the immune system. The traditional terminology and classifications of the past, including the clinically useful classification of Rappaport (Rappaport *et al.*, 1956), were proposed before the recent dramatic developments in immunology and therefore have no relationship to our modern understanding of immunology. Beginning in 1971, we proposed a conceptually new approach to the understanding of malignant lymphomas (Collins and Lukes, 1971; Lukes and Collins, 1973, 1974a,b). This approach was based on (1) the newly appreciated existence of the T- and B-lymphocytic systems; (2) our hypothesis that lymphomas may arise from aberrations in lymphocyte transformation; and (3) the availability of techniques to identify cells as belonging to the T- or the B-lymphocytic system. In this approach, lymphoma cells are regarded as immune cells that, although defective, function, migrate, "home" to, and reside in tissue sites in ways similar to their normal counterparts. Funda-

---

*Abbreviations used in this chapter: (ALL) Acute lymphocytic leukemia; (CLL) chronic lymphocytic leukemia; (EA) erythrocyte–antibody complex; (EAC) erythrocyte–antibody–complement complex; (FCC) follicular center cell(s); (HBLA) human B-lymphocyte antigen; (H chain) heavy chain; (HTLA) human T-lymphocyte antigen; (IBL) immunoblastic lymphadenopathy; (IBS) immunoblastic sarcoma; (Ig) immunoglobulin; (L chain) light chain; (MGP) methyl green–pyronin stain; (MLR) mixed-lymphocyte reaction; (NSE) nonspecific esterase; (PAS) periodic acid–Schiff stain; (PHA) phytohemagglutinin; (PWM) pokeweed mitogen; (SIg) surface Ig; (SLE) systemic lupus erythematosus; (SRBC) sheep erythrocyte(s); (U cell) undefined cell.

ROBERT J. LUKES and JOHN W. PARKER • Department of Pathology, University of Southern California School of Medicine, Los Angeles, California, and Los Angeles County–University of Southern California Medical Center.

ROBERT J. LUKES AND
JOHN W. PARKER

mental to our new functional approach is the follicular center cell (FCC) concept, which has the following bases: (1) FCC are plasma-cell precursors; (2) the follicular center is a site of B-cell transformation; (3) lymphomas of FCC type are observed with both follicular and diffuse histological patterns; and (4) these lymphomas are a group of different cytological types, rather than one lymphoma of follicular structures, previously termed "follicular lymphoma."

From our initial morphological studies of several large case populations, we were able to relate the malignant lymphomas to subpopulations of the T- and B-cell systems, and proposed that the majority of large-cell lymphomas, diagnosed as reticulum-cell sarcoma or histiocytic lymphoma in the past, were, instead, large transformed lymphocytes of either the T- or the B-cell system. A multiparameter approach employing a variety of techniques including special morphology, cytochemistry, electron microscopy, cell culture, immunoperoxidase identification of intracellular immunoglobulin (Ig) and muramidase, and immunological surface-marker methods was proposed as a means of redefining malignant lymphomas in modern immunological terms (Lukes and Collins, 1974a,b, 1975). The results of our combined study of 384 cases of non-Hodgkin's lymphomas and related leukemias from Vanderbilt University, in collaboration with Dr. Robert Collins and his co-workers, and ours from the LAC–USC Medical Center* reveal that lymphomas, with few exceptions, mark as T or B cells, and rarely as histiocytes (Lukes and Collins, 1977). These studies are supported by the reports of other workers on small groups of cases of various cytological types, many using terminology we have proposed.

In this presentation, we will briefly review the immunological background and the conceptual and morphological basis of our approach to a better understanding of lymphomas. In addition, we will discuss the results of our multiparameter studies, using illustrative cases to demonstrate their application; emerging clinical–morphological–immunological entities; and the immediate and future implications of this functional approach.

2. Immunological Background

Our redefinition of malignant lymphomas as neoplasms of the immune system has been based on (1) the development of malignant lymphomas in abnormal immune disorders; (2) the existence of T- and B-cell systems in man; (3) our proposal that most lymphomas develop with a block or a "switch on" (derepression) of lymphocyte transformation; and (4) the availability of techniques for the characterization of T- and B-cell systems in man. In this approach, we have attempted to relate lymphoma cells to their normal counterparts, according to their morphological features, anatomical distribution and spread, and immunological surface markers. It appears that lymphoma cells frequently develop, in abnormal immune states, in T- or B-cell areas and migrate and function in varying degree in ways similar to their normal counterparts. In reviewing the immunological basis of our approach to the malignant lymphomas, we will concentrate primarily on the role of alterations in lymphocyte transformation, and only briefly on the other areas, since they are discussed in detail in other chapters.

---

*The studies at LAC–USC Medical Center were performed by the authors and their colleagues—Clive Taylor, Barbara Tindle, Paul Pattengale, Thomas Lincoln, Adelbert Cramer, and Arthur Williams.

2.1. Development of Malignant Lymphomas in Abnormal Immune States

Malignant lymphomas have been observed in a variety of congenital immunological disorders by a number of authors. These observations provided the basis for the proposal by Good and Finstad (1968) of the existence of a fundamental immunological abnormality as a mechanism for developing malignant lymphomas. Similarly, lymphomas have been observed to arise in a variety of acquired immunological abnormalities at various ages, e.g., Sjögren's syndrome, α-chain disease, and therapeutic immunosuppression. We noticed that these lymphomas were proliferations of transformed lymphocytes (immunoblasts), developing in a wide variety of disorders, and proposed that the basic mechanism involved the "switch on" of lymphocyte transformation in a defective immune state. In addition to the immunological abnormalities enumerated above, we have observed immunoblastic sarcomas developing in the thyroid in Hashimoto's disease, in systemic lupus erythematosus (SLE), glutin-sensitive malabsorption disease, Waldenström's macroglobulinemia, chronic lymphocytic leukemia (CLL), and senescence. From these observations, it appears that a patient with an abnormal immune state, whether congenital or acquired, is vulnerable to the development of lymphoma, either because of the appearance of an abnormal clone of cells or because of defective control of lymphocyte transformation.

2.2. Lymphocyte Systems

The recent progress in immunology has been the subject of numerous reviews, and its relationship to malignant lymphomas was recently emphasized by Hansen and Good (1974). The T- and B-lymphocyte systems originally discovered through ablation experiments in animals were confirmed in man through studies of various immune deficiency states. A progenitor cell for the T and B lymphocytes also exists, possibly a marrow stem cell. We have previously proposed the term *U cell* (undefined or unmarked) to indicate that the cell lacks both T- and B-cell markers. The term U cell, as we use it, includes uncommitted progenitor cells that lack T or B differentiating markers as well as those lymphocytes that may fall into either class, but are as yet unrecognized by the marker techniques currently in use. In all three systems (T, B, and U), lymphocyte transformation apparently occurs. In the case of the B- and T-cell systems, this transformation from small lymphocytes to proliferating blast cells occurs as an amplification mechanism in response to antigens. In the case of the progenitor cells, a similar transformation and proliferation may occur, in response to depletion of the T- and B-cell systems, to maintain the stem-cell compartment, rather than to direct antigenic stimulation. Since lymphocyte transformation is an active phenomenon involving morphological, biochemical, and functional changes, there is a range of cells at different stages in each system. This range of cells resulting from lymphocyte transformation in the B, T, and U systems accounts for the remarkable diversity of the morphological and functional expressions of both normal lymphocytes and their lymphomatous counterparts.

The development of the T- and B-cell systems is well documented in experimental animals. The T cell acquires its particular membrane and functional characteristics, when the progenitor cell migrates to the thymus, during a series of maturational events accompanied by changes in surface markers, response to mitogens, and functional capacity, under the influence of thymic epithelial cells. In a similar manner, in the avian species, the progenitor cell, after migrating to the bursa of Fabricius, acquires its B-cell characteristics. The precise location of the bursal equivalent in man has not been identified, although the liver, spleen, bone marrow, and GI lymphoid tissues have been proposed as candidates.

The T-cell or thymus-dependent system is involved in cellular immunity and is measured clinically by delayed hypersensitivity responsiveness and several *in vitro* tests. These tests include the lymphocyte transformation response to mitogens and certain antigens including tissue antigens, release of a variety of soluble mediators (lymphokines) on exposure to antigen, and a range of cellular activities that identify subpopulations of T lymphocytes, i.e., suppressor, helper, and killer T cells. The diversity and complexity of functioning T-cell subpopulations are appreciated but their morphological expressions are unknown. It appears that malignant lymphomas of T cells may at times possess some of these differentiated functions. Broder *et al.* (1976) reported that Sézary cells are helper T cells and Yoshida *et al.* (1975), that these cells produce migration-inhibition factor.

The B-cell system (bursal equivalent, bone marrow) functions in Ig and antibody production, and is evaluated clinically by measurement of serum Ig levels and antibody response to antigens. The functioning of neoplastic cells of this system is well known, e.g., Ig production in Waldenström's macroglobulinemia and multiple myeloma.

The topographical distribution of the T- and B-lymphocyte systems is now well established and is important in the understanding of normal immune reactions and the morphological interpretation of malignant lymphomas. From ablation experiments in animals and parallel findings in congenital immune defects in man, it has become apparent that the B-cell system resides primarily in the follicular centers of lymphoid tissues, where B cells are produced through active proliferation. However, descendants from these cells, immunoblasts and plasma cells, are found in interfollicular areas and medullary cords. The T-cell system is distributed in the paracortical areas of lymph nodes, in perivascular regions of the spleen, and in small foci in the GI tract. B cells are found in primary and secondary follicles wherever they exist in the lymphoid tissue throughout the body, in the Malpighian bodies of the spleen, and in the lamina propria of the GI tract, and are interspersed in the bone marrow. These lymphocyte systems are not static. The T lymphocytes circulate 4–6 times a day and account for approximately 60–70% of normal peripheral blood lymphocytes. It has been estimated that 20–25% of the peripheral blood lymphocytes are B cells, though recent studies suggest that this percentage may be considerably lower. There is an extremely complex circulating traffic of lymphocytes through blood and tissues, with highly selective "homing" of the T and B cells to preferential anatomical sites throughout the body. Our morphological studies have shown that lymphomas are distributed in a highly predictable fashion that parallels the migration and distribution characteristics of their normal lymphocyte counterparts. This localization has assisted in the identification of specific cytological features for the different lymphomas.

2.3. Lymphocyte Transformation

Lymphocyte transformation as an *in vitro* phenomenon, first described by Nowell and co-workers (Hungerford *et al.*, 1959; Nowell, 1960), has resulted in intensive research aimed at defining the mechanisms involved and in determining the role of this striking phenomenon in immunology. Over the past two decades, it has been used as a model for the study of the control mechanisms involved in cellular proliferation and the expression of differentiated immunological features, for biochemical studies of normal lymphoid cells, for *in vitro* studies of immune responses, and as a genetic tool. The morphological changes that occur when a small lymphocyte is stimulated to change into a dividing blast cell following exposure to a nonspecific (polyclonal) mitogenic agent or a specific antigen have been documented by light and electron microscopy by many investigators. That this *in vitro* phenomenon relates to normal *in vivo* immunological reactions and possibly to the evolution of malignant lymphomas has been largely unexplored, however, until recently (Lukes and Collins, 1973, 1974a,b, 1975).

A broad variety of "nonspecific" reagents will stimulate lymphocyte transformation *in vitro*. Commonly used representatives of this group include phytohemagglutinin (PHA), pokeweed mitogen (PWM), and concanavalin A (Con A), but there are a large number of other plant lectins that will also stimulate transformation (Parker *et al.*, 1969; Toyoshima *et al.*, 1970). Most specifically tested mitogen lectins stimulate human T lymphocytes (O'Brien *et al.*, 1978), although PWM stimulates both B and T lymphocytes (Waxdal and Basham, 1974). Mitogens specific for human B lymphocytes have not been available until recently, although high-molecular-weight polymers such as dextran and bacterial lipopolysaccharides specifically stimulate murine B lymphocytes. An aqueous extract of *Nocardia opaca* was recently reported to be a specific human B-lymphocyte mitogen (Brochier *et al.*, 1976) and offers promise for clarifying the morphological alterations that occur in B-lymphocyte transformation. In addition to the mitogenic plant lectins, there are also a variety of chemical agents that stimulate transformation, including mercury and zinc ions (Schöpf *et al.*, 1967; Berger and Skinner, 1974; Caron *et al.*, 1970), cyclic GMP (Weinstein *et al.*, 1974, 1975), a calcium ionophore A23187 (Maino *et al.*, 1974; Hovi *et al.*, 1976), proteolytic enzymes (Vischer, 1974; Kaplan and Bona, 1974), and the oxidizing agents sodium periodate and galactose oxidase (O'Brien and Parker, 1976). The immunological importance of these "nonspecific" lymphocyte stimulants lies in the observation that specific antigens will stimulate lymphocytes from sensitized donors (Pearmain *et al.*, 1963), and that lymphocyte transformation occurs when lymphocytes from two nonidentical donors are mixed in culture, i.e., the mixed-lymphocyte reaction (MLR) (Bain *et al.*, 1964).

The mechanisms of initiating transformation are complex and poorly understood, involving cellular interactions among T and B lymphocytes, macrophages, and subpopulations of each. These interactions have been reviewed recently elsewhere (Oppenheim and Rosenstreich, 1976; O'Brien *et al.*, 1978), and we will confine ourselves to a discussion of the morphological changes that occur and relate them to our discussion of lymphomas.

In brief, on mitogenic treatment of lymphocytes, a characteristic and well-studied sequence of events occurs. There are striking early increases in the flux of cations, anions, amino acids, nucleosides, carbohydrates, and other substrates for cell metabolism across the plasma membrane. Some of these increased fluxes begin almost immediately after the stimuli are applied. This increased flux is accompanied and followed by increased incorporation of exogeneously provided substrates into cellular metabolic pathways and into synthetic products. The metabolic activation is accompanied by a sequence of morphological changes, including nuclear enlargement and increasing cytoplasm. Cytoplasmic organelles increase in variety and number, and after 2 or 3 days, many cells are "blasts." After variable periods of time, the activated cells elaborate products and acquire properties related to differentiated immune functions. Many of the blast cells in the population undergo replication of chromosomes and cell division. This transformation is followed by reversion of the transformed cells to small lymphocytes resembling those originally stimulated, or, if mitogen remains in the medium, repeat stimulation of some of these cells may occur. In addition to reversion to small lymphocytes, some plasma-cytoid cells appear, and it has been demonstrated that there is Ig production by lymphocytes stimulated with PWM. Cytotoxic activity by cells resulting from T-lymphocyte stimulation in the MLR also occurs. Thus, the transformation phenom-enon appears to be a modulation or recycling from small lymphocytes to blast cells that divide to give rise to daughter cells. These daughter cells may then function as memory cells or effector cells in both the T- and B-cell systems.

The transformed lymphocyte is 4–6 times the size of a small lymphocyte [Figure 1(2),(4)]; it has finely distributed chromatin, one or more prominent nucleoli, and abundant deeply basophilic cytoplasm in Romanowsky-stained prepa-rations. The cytoplasm is also intensely pyroninophilic. The *in vitro* transformed lymphocytes grow in cohesive clusters, as seen in sections of cell buttons from cultures (Figure 2A,B). The cells show wide variations in size, depending on the mitogen used, and resemble a primitive-appearing neoplastic process with numer-

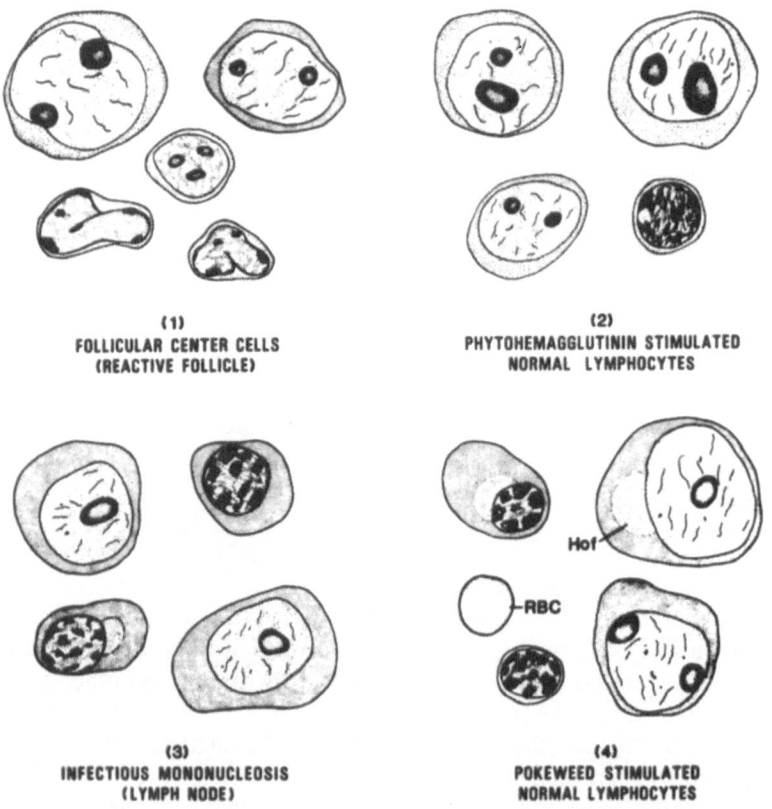

(1)
FOLLICULAR CENTER CELLS
(REACTIVE FOLLICLE)

(2)
PHYTOHEMAGGLUTININ STIMULATED
NORMAL LYMPHOCYTES

(3)
INFECTIOUS MONONUCLEOSIS
(LYMPH NODE)

(4)
POKEWEED STIMULATED
NORMAL LYMPHOCYTES

Figure 1. Comparison of *in vivo* and *in vitro* transformed lymphocytes. The camera lucida drawings in this figure and in Figures 3 and 4 were all made at uniform magnification, so that cell sizes are all relative. Diagnoses were verified by multiparameter studies.

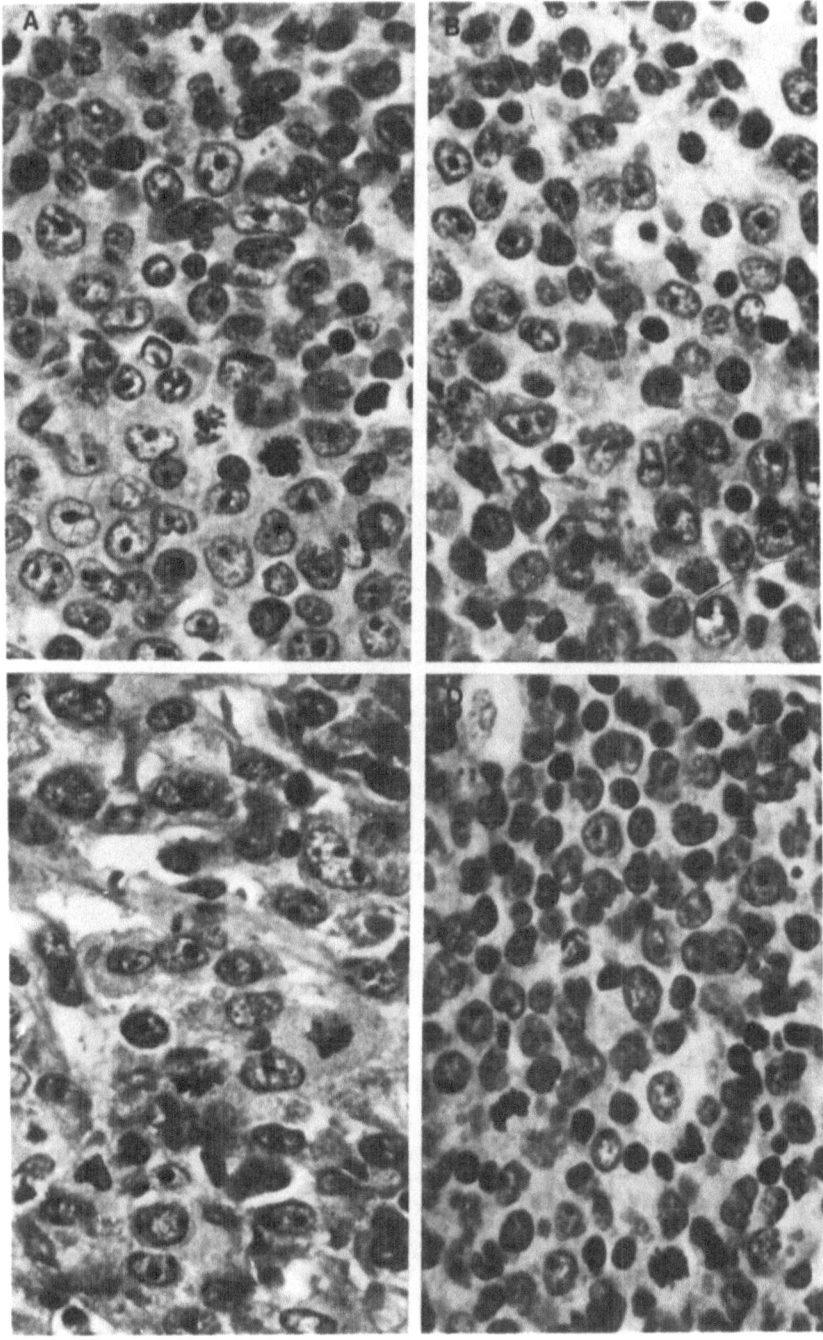

Figure 2. Photomicrographs of paraffin sections stained with hematoxylin–eosin. All magnifications ×800. (A) Cell pellet from a 3-day PHA-stimulated human lymphocyte culture; (B) PWM-stimulated culture; (C) tissue section of immunoblastic sarcoma, T-cell type; (D) tissue section of immunoblastic sarcoma, B-cell type.

ROBERT J. LUKES AND
JOHN W. PARKER

ous mitotic figures. On comparing these sections of transformed lymphocytes with sections of lymphoid tissues, we were impressed by the remarkable resemblance of the lymphocytes transformed *in vitro* to the large cells both in normal reactive lymphoid tissues [Figure 1(1),(3)] and in malignant lymphomas of B- [Figure 4(4)–(6)] and T-cell [Figure 3(3)] types, as shown in camera lucida drawings. Large transformed lymphocytes (immunoblasts) are identified in small numbers in the interfollicular tissues in benign reactions and in larger numbers in severe reactions, as seen in infectious mononucleosis [Figure 1(3)] and in regional lymph nodes draining smallpox vaccinations. Variable numbers of transformed lymphocytes with the same morphological features are seen in paraffin sections of reactive follicular centers [Figure 1(1)], and apparently reflect the state of reactivity. Since the follicular center appears to be the site of B-cell proliferation and production, we regard the large transformed lymphocytes in follicular centers as transformed B cells. Transformed lymphocytes (immunoblasts) of both T- and B-cell types appear to occur in the interfollicular tissue and, with experience, can be differentiated in histological sections. The B immunoblast is larger, possesses more intensely staining pyroninophylic cytoplasm, and at times may have plasmacytoid features. This ability to distinguish between actively proliferating T and B lymphocytes was confirmed in a morphological study of T- and B-lymphoblastoid cell lines (Parker *et al.*, 1977).

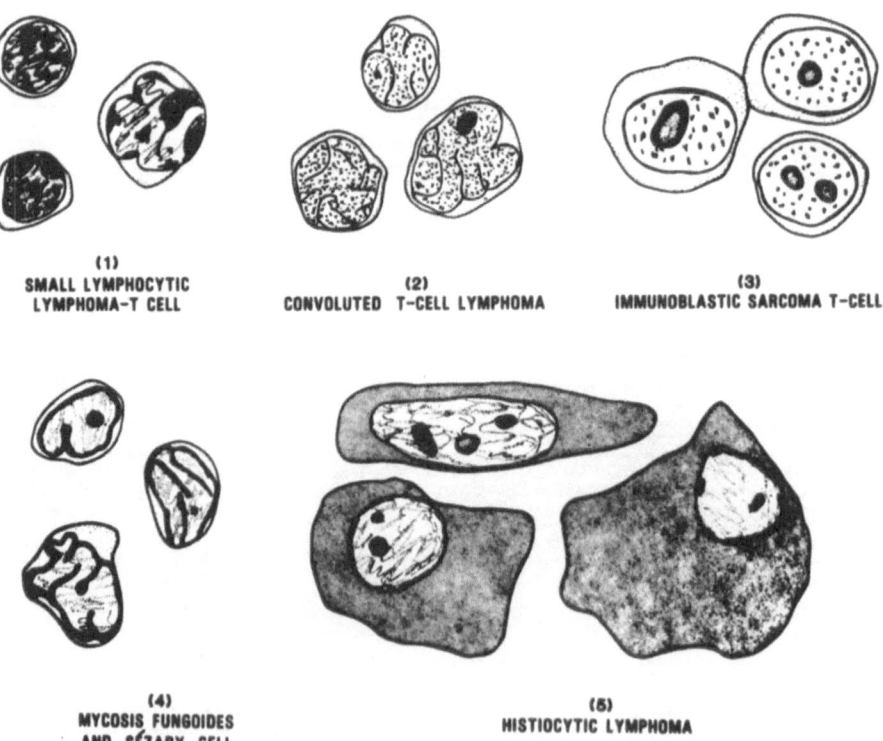

(1)
SMALL LYMPHOCYTIC
LYMPHOMA-T CELL

(2)
CONVOLUTED T-CELL LYMPHOMA

(3)
IMMUNOBLASTIC SARCOMA T-CELL

(4)
MYCOSIS FUNGOIDES
AND SÉZARY CELL

(5)
HISTIOCYTIC LYMPHOMA

Figure 3. Camera lucida drawings of T-cell and histiocytic lymphomas.

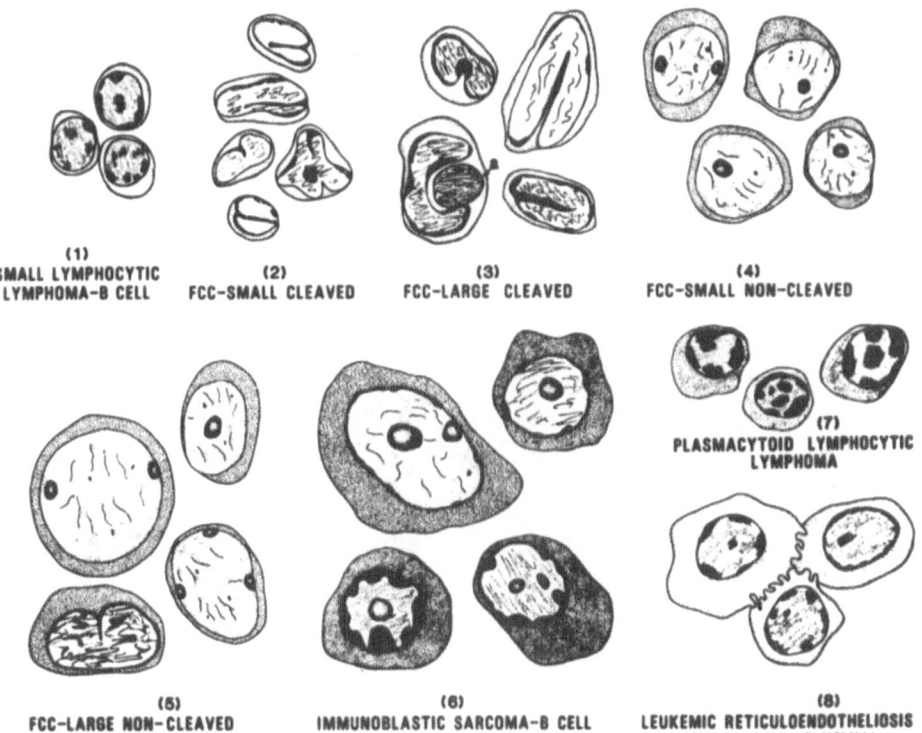

(1)
SMALL LYMPHOCYTIC
LYMPHOMA-B CELL

(2)
FCC-SMALL CLEAVED

(3)
FCC-LARGE CLEAVED

(4)
FCC-SMALL NON-CLEAVED

(5)
FCC-LARGE NON-CLEAVED

(6)
IMMUNOBLASTIC SARCOMA-B CELL

(7)
PLASMACYTOID LYMPHOCYTIC
LYMPHOMA

(8)
LEUKEMIC RETICULOENDOTHELIOSIS
(HAIRY CELL LEUKEMIA)

Figure 4. Camera lucida drawings of B-cell lymphomas.

2.4. *In Vivo* B-Cell Transformation

Following the recognition of transformed B cells in follicular centers, we proposed the FCC concept (Lukes and Collins, 1973, 1974a,b, 1975). Camera lucida studies of normal follicular centers revealed four cell types: (1) cleaved FCC; (2) noncleaved FCC; (3) tingible body macrophages; and (4) dendritic reticulum cells. The wide range in size of both cleaved and noncleaved cells revealed by the camera lucida drawings [see Figures 1(1) and 6] of normal FCC was attributed to stages in B-cell transformation.

Identification of nuclear cleavage planes depends on the technical quality of the fixing, processing, and histological sectioning. In the average formalin-fixed, thick lymph node section, the cytological features, particularly nuclear cleavage planes, are not readily discernible. These cleavage planes can be readily seen, however, in 4-μm sections of tissues fixed in B5 (Lillie and Fullmer, 1976) or Zenker's fixative (Figure 5A), and are even more convincingly demonstrated in electron micrographs (Figure 5C). Methyl green–pyronin (MGP)-stained, well-fixed tissues demonstrate the character of the noncleaved (transformed) FCC most ideally.

As illustrated by the camera lucida drawings (Figure 6), the FCC transformation concept involves a sequence in B-cell transformation from the small B lymphocyte of the lymphocytic mantle to the large noncleaved FCC. In this concept, antigen trapped in the follicular center on the surface of dendritic reticulum cells,

ROBERT J. LUKES AND
JOHN W. PARKER

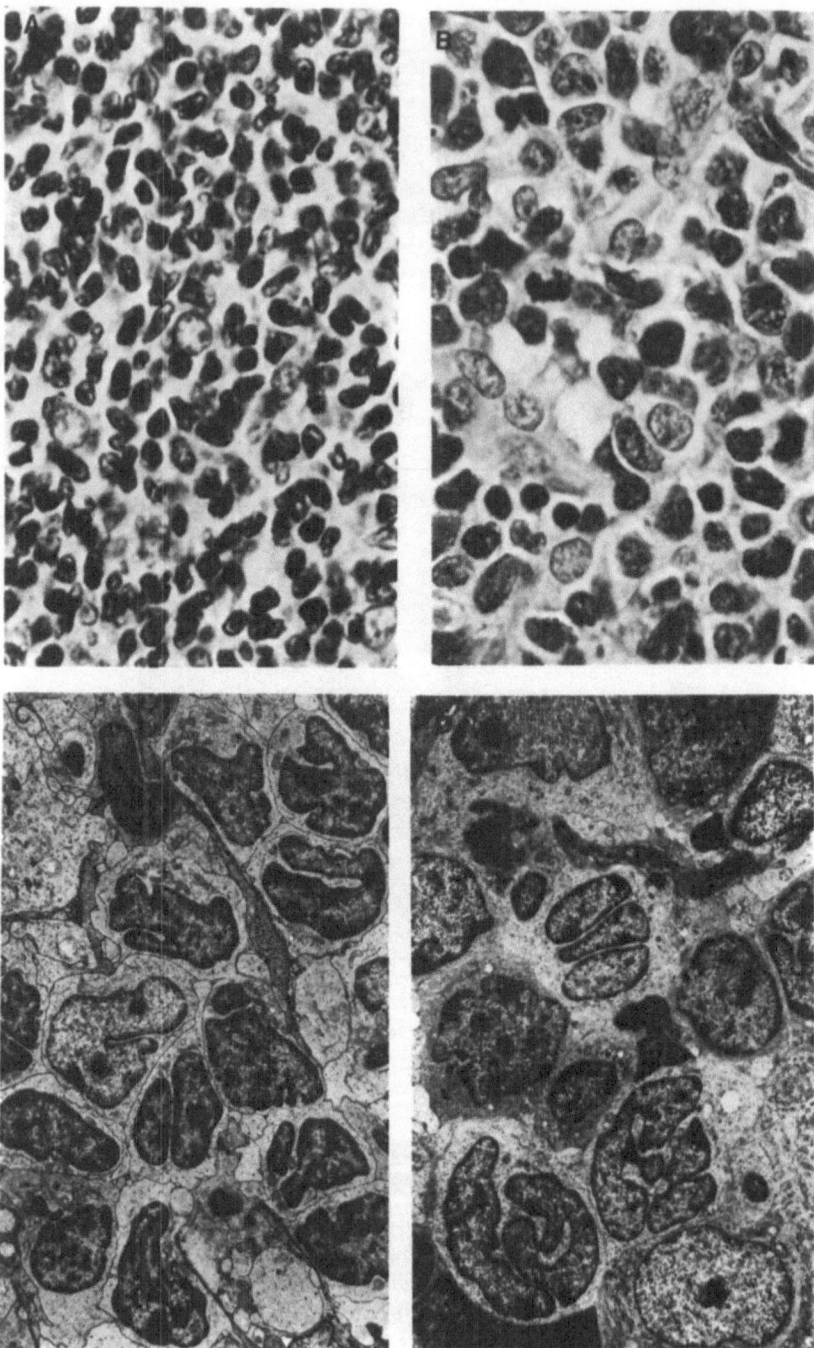

Figure 5. (A) Paraffin section of small cleaved FCC lymphoma. Hematoxylin–eosin. ×800. (B) Paraffin section of convoluted T-cell lymphoma. Hematoxylin–eosin. ×800. (C) Electron micrograph of small cleaved FCC lymphoma. ×1900. (D) Electron micrograph of convoluted T-cell lymphoma. ×1000.

CLEAVED   NON-CLEAVED

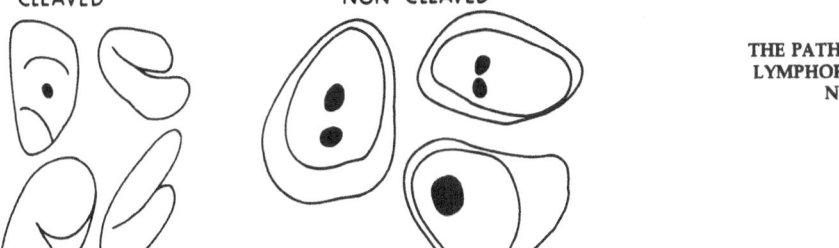

Figure 6. Camera lucida drawings of normal FCC illustrating the range of variation in size and configuration of cleaved cells and in the size and amount of cytoplasm of the noncleaved cells.

illustrated schematically as a perifollicular cell, induces a lymphocyte to undergo transformation, as reported by Nossal *et al.* (1968).

In the first stage, the small lymphocyte changes to the small cleaved FCC. By gradual enlargement and acquisition of a small amount of pyroninophilic cytoplasm, it reaches a second stage, the large cleaved FCC. In the third stage, the small noncleaved FCC, the nucleus becomes round and the nuclear chromatin finely dispersed, and a small nucleolus appears. The cytoplasm is prominently pyroninophilic. In the fourth stage, the large noncleaved FCC is similar, but larger, has more abundant pale acidophilic cytoplasm and one to three more prominent nucleoli, often situated on the nuclear membrane. The cleaved cells of the follicular center are essentially nondividing cells, whereas all the noncleaved cells are part of a proliferating population.

From the immunoperoxidase studies of Dr. Clive Taylor, of our group, cytoplasmic Ig is seen first in the large cleaved FCC in small amounts and increases in the small and large noncleaved FCC stages (Taylor, 1976a). Surface Ig (SIg), however, is seen on small lymphocytes and small cleaved cells. From studies of large numbers of histological sections, it appears that large noncleaved FCC migrate from the follicular center into the interfollicular tissue, where we have designated it an immunoblast of B-cell type. This apparent migration is supported by the recent ultrastructural studies of the follicular centers of tonsils by Kojima and Tsunoda (1976), also using the immunoperoxidase technique. The demonstration of cytoplasmic Ig in FCC and some immunoblasts of the interfollicular tissue further suggests that these cells are related and indicates that they are B cells. The proposed direction of *in vivo* transformation of B cells in the follicular center contradicts previous views that held that large "stem" cells gave rise to "differentiated" small lymphocytes. Our concept is based on our studies of *in vitro* lymphocyte transformation, and emphasizes the dormant nature of the small lymphocyte as a progenitor cell, which gives rise to the large transformed "blast" cells or immunoblasts. These cells may revert to small dormant lymphocytes (modulation) or become plasma cells. Although we have not as yet observed the nuclear "cleaving"

ROBERT J. LUKES AND
JOHN W. PARKER

in *in vitro* transformation studies of peripheral blood lymphocytes, "cleaving" may be a feature only of FCC in a particular microenvironment. Also, a pure B-cell mitogen for human lymphocytes has not been available until recently. The *Nocardia opaca* extract may help to resolve this apparent inconsistency.

The proposed sequence in the FCC concept parallels the evolution observed in FCC lymphomas. A lymphoma that is initially a small cleaved FCC type with limited aggressiveness may later change to the highly aggressive noncleaved FCC type. Thus, the FCC concept provides the basis for relating the cytological types of FCC neoplasms to their normal counterparts, and permits an understanding of the evolution of the neoplastic process in the B-cell system.

2.5. *In Vivo* T-Cell Transformation

The transformed lymphocytes (immunoblasts) of the T- and B-cell systems are generally similar, but the B immunoblast appears to be larger and have more abundant, dense, and pyroninophilic cytoplasm, and may show plasmacytoid features. The demonstration of cytoplasmic Ig by the immunoperoxidase technique (Taylor and Mason, 1974) is a helpful method for distinguishing transformed T- and B-cell types in the interfollicular tissue, because of the cytoplasmic content of Ig in B cells. Transformation of T cells *in vivo* appears to occur in a fashion somewhat parallel to that of B cells, but outside the follicular center in the paracortical region, without the formation of cells with cleaved nuclei or plasma cells. The intermediate cells in T-cell transformation have round nuclei, finely dispersed chromatin, small nucleoli, and a moderate amount of pyroninophilic cytoplasm. The T-cell lymphomas with distinctive morphological features observed thus far may represent expansions of defective counterparts of normal cells that ordinarily occur only in small numbers and thus have not yet been described. The convoluted T-cell lymphoma that we described in children (Barcos and Lukes, 1975) and young adults (Rosen *et al.*, 1975) [see Figures 4(2) and 5B,D] may arise from a pre-T cell (Stein *et al.*, 1976). The cerebriform cell of Sézary syndrome was proposed as a lymphoma of helper cells by Broder *et al.* (1976). There is also some suggestion that it has a morphological counterpart in normal PHA-transformed lymphocytes *in vitro* (Yeckley *et al.*, 1975). Both cells will be described in some detail in the following description of cytological types of lymphomas.

3. A Functional Cytological Classification of Malignant Lymphomas

Our functional classification of malignant lymphomas is based on the following considerations and observations: (1) malignant lymphomas are neoplasms of the immune system; (2) they primarily involve T- and B-cell and U-cell (undefined) systems, and rarely histiocytes and monocytes; (3) malignant lymphomas may develop as a block or a "switch on" (derepression) of lymphocyte transformation in the various lymphocytic systems; and (4) the cytological types of lymphoma are morphologically and functionally similar to normal cell counterparts. The cytological types of lymphoma relate to B- and T-cell transformation stages, as shown in Figure 7, with the exception of the true histiocytic lymphoma, the convoluted lymphocyte that has been proposed to be a pre-T cell (Stein *et al.*, 1976), and the cerebriform cell of Sézary's syndrome and mycosis fungoides. The nature of the neoplastic cell in Hodgkin's disease is still unclear.

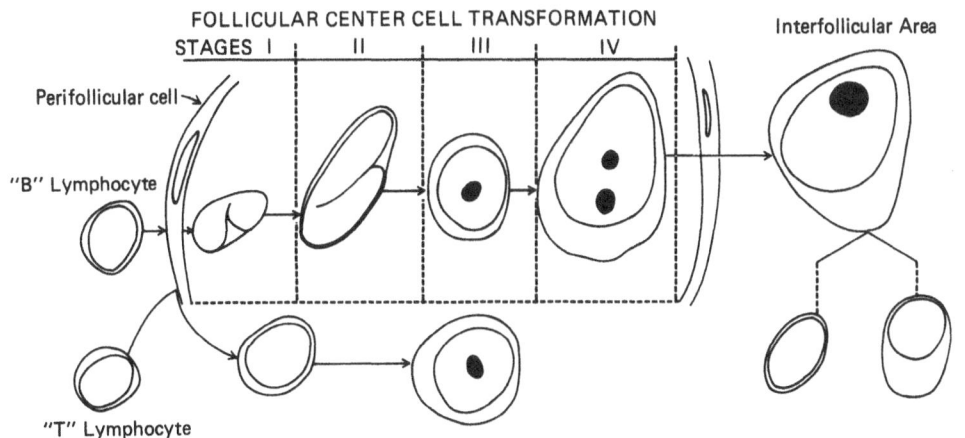

Figure 7. Schematic representation of normal transformation of FCC in comparison with the transformation of T cells. (I) Small cleaved cell; (II) large cleaved cell; (III) small noncleaved transformed cell; (IV) large noncleaved transformed cell. The latter gives rise to a B immunoblast, which may revert to a small lymphocyte or become a plasma cell. A T immunoblast results from T-lymphocyte transformation. Lymphomas appear to develop from either a "block" in or a "switch on" of this *in vivo* lymphocyte transformation.

Although the functional classification was proposed before the use of immunological surface-marker studies in human malignant lymphomas, our recent report of multiparameter studies on 384 cases of lymphomas and related leukemias (Lukes and Collins, 1977) confirmed the value of the immunological approach and the reality of the cytological types. Since our initial proposal of this classification, only the lymphoma of small T lymphocytes has been added. Final acceptance of any classification is dependent on the soundness of the conceptual basis, the clinical relevance in terms of prognostic and therapeutic significance, and the effectiveness of its application. Acceptance by pathologists is dependent on ease of application and reproducibility in its use. Unfortunately, the complexity of the immune system and the diversity of its expressions eliminates the possibility of a simple classification.

The functional classification of malignant lymphomas is presented in Table 1. The major groups are: (1) U-cell (undefined); (2) T-cell; (3) B-cell; (4) histiocytic; (5) Hodgkin's disease; (6) unclassifiable. The U-cell (undefined) type is hypothetical and was proposed for cellular proliferations with primitive morphological features that are not distinctive and in which identifying immunological or cytochemical markers are absent, using presently available techniques. It includes the so-called "null" cell, true stem cells of the bone marrow, and the cells of acute lymphocytic leukemia (ALL) of childhood, which lack specific markers. Increasing numbers of the latter, however, appear to be marking as B and T cells using specific antisera (Schlossman *et al.,* 1976; Kaplan *et al.,* 1977). The unclassifiable category is used for lymphomatous-appearing proliferations in which the findings are indistinct or obscured for technical reasons, so that the process cannot be classified precisely.

Examination of the general features of this functional classification reveals that there is a small lymphocyte type and a large transformed lymphocyte type or immunoblastic sarcoma in both the T- and the B-cell group. The T-cell group also includes cytological types with extraordinary nuclear configurations—the primitive-

ROBERT J. LUKES AND
JOHN W. PARKER

TABLE 1. Functional Classification of Malignant Lymphomas

U-cell (undefined)
T-cell
    Small lymphocyte
    Convoluted lymphocyte
    Sézary–mycosis fungoides
    Immunoblastic sarcoma of T cells
B-cell
    Small lymphocyte
    Plasmacytoid lymphocyte
    Follicular center cell (FCC)
      Follicular, diffuse, follicular and diffuse, and with or without sclerosis
        Small cleaved
        Large cleaved
        Small noncleaved (transformed)
        Large noncleaved (transformed)
    Immunoblastic sarcoma of B cells
    Hairy-cell leukemia
Histiocytic
Cell of uncertain origin
    Hodgkin's disease—origin of neoplastic cell uncertain
      Lymphocyte predominance
      Mixed cellularity
      Lymphocyte depletion
      Nodular sclerosis
Unclassifiable

appearing convoluted T cell and the cerebriform cell of Sézary's syndrome and mycosis fungoides. The B-cell group includes the FCC and the plasmacytoid lymphocytic types, the latter frequently associated with dysglobulinemia, as in Waldenström's syndrome. The histiocytic class refers to lymphomas of macrophages, those disorders that exhibit the cytochemical features of histiocytes, as demonstrated by the presence of cytoplasmic nonspecific esterase (NSE) activity using an α-naphthyl butyrate substrate (Yam et al., 1971a) and muramidase activity as detected by the immunoperoxidase technique (Mason and Taylor, 1975). These lymphoma cells also fail to mark as B or T cells.

Hodgkin's disease is classified according to the well-established Rye classification (Lukes et al., 1966a), which is a condensed version of the original Lukes–Butler classification (Lukes et al., 1966b).

We will first briefly describe each cytological type of lymphoma using this functional classification, and then discuss the histopathological evolution of the follicular center lymphomas, compare the functional classification with other lymphoma classifications, present in general the results of our immunological and cytochemical studies, and finally describe several cases that illustrate the correlation of morphological diagnosis within this classification with T- and B-cell markers.

Our goals in the studies we are currently pursuing are to identify specific cytoclinical entities for therapeutic and prognostic purposes and to isolate homogeneous cell populations for cell kinetic investigations, design of therapy, determination of retained differentiated functions, and illumination of the biology of lymphoma development.

3.1.1. Small Lymphocyte (T Cell)

A lymphoma–leukemia of small T cells [see Figure 3(1)] has been demonstrated by multiparameter studies in a small group of cases, but the distinctiveness of the morphological features has not been established. The cytological features we have observed in the limited sample available to us resemble the normal small lymphocyte. The nucleus has compact nuclear chromatin and a small amount of pale-staining cytoplasm. The nucleus at times has a somewhat irregular nuclear configuration. The distinctiveness of this configurational change is uncertain at the present time.

3.1.2. Convoluted Lymphocyte

This process is a diffuse proliferation of primitive-appearing noncohesive cells [see Figures 3(2) and 5B,D] occurring in widely infiltrated masses or in partially or totally involved lymph nodes. The lymphoma cells vary in size, ranging from that of a small lymphocyte to 4–5 lymphocyte nuclear diameters. The nucleus has distinctive, evenly distributed, finely stippled chromatin and a small or inconspicuous nucleolus. The nuclei of the smaller cells are round, while the larger cells show dense irregular lines penetrating from the surface of the nucleus and subdividing it. The nuclear subdivisions usually suggest the convolutions of the brain (verified by electron microscopy), but some nuclei are irregular and almost lobated from the deep indentations (Figure 5B). The proportion of small and large cells varies from case to case. The frequency of mitoses typically ranges from 5 to 7 per high power field and relates directly to the number of large cells. The cytoplasm is indistinct or scanty, and appears to relate to the noncohesive character of the cells. Occasionally, reactive ''starry-sky'' phagocytes are interspersed among the lymphoma cells and present a histological appearance that may be mistaken for a Burkitt's lymphoma in overly thick sections.

3.1.3. Immunoblastic Sarcoma of T Cells

We are just learning to recognize this cytological type [see Figure 3(3)]. It exhibits a spectrum, from lymphocytes with small, irregular, twisted-appearing nuclei to fully transformed lymphocytes. The medium-size and large cells resemble *in vitro* transformed lymphocytes, and in histological sections have pale-staining to almost water-clear cytoplasm with well-defined, cohesive, interlocking cytoplasmic membranes (see Figure 2C). The nucleus is round to oval, with finely distributed chromatin and usually one central prominent nucleolus. The process generally extends throughout the lymph node, and is not associated with follicle or nodule formation. The small, distinctive lymphocyte with the irregular nucleus appears to be a significant component of an abnormal evolving T-cell proliferation.

3.1.4. Cerebriform Cell of Sézary's Syndrome and Mycosis Fungoides

The lymphoma cells in these closely related conditions [see Figure 3(4)] are of medium size and approximately 2–3 normal lymphocytes in diameter. They have

ROBERT J. LUKES AND
JOHN W. PARKER

barely discernible linear subdivisions in cells found in the peripheral blood and tissues, but in the late aggressive stages, the cells may be large, the chromatin finely dispersed, and the nuclear configuration remarkably abnormal. The cytoplasm typically contains numerous small periodic acid–Schiff (PAS)-positive globules, at times in a "necklace" distribution around the nucleus. Ultrastructural studies demonstrate dramatically the deep nuclear indentations responsible for the cerebri-form appearance (Lutzner *et al.*, 1975). In paraffin sections, however, in compari-son with the primitive convoluted lymphocyte, the cerebriform cell in these entities has compact chromatin, less obvious nuclear irregularity, and few mitoses.

3.1.5. T Cell Associated with Histiocytes

Another type of T-cell lymphoma is emerging from the heterogeneous group of disorders described by Lennert and Mestdagh (1968). It is a medium-size lympho-cyte with a distinctive distorted, twisted-appearing nucleus with dispersed chroma-tin, a small nucleolus, and scanty cytoplasm. Typically, there is an associated component of reactive histiocytes occurring in small clusters regularly interspersed through the lymph node. Immunoblasts are usually infrequent, although in two cases, a subsequent biopsy showed a predominance of immunoblasts of T cells—an immunoblastic sarcoma (IBS). Plasma cells are infrequent or absent. In a small group of our cases, these cells have, for the most part, marked as T cells. Lennert (Lennert *et al.*, 1975) called this lymphoma the *lymphoepithelioid* cell type.

3.2. B-Cell Types

3.2.1. Small Lymphocytes of B Cells

This lymphoma is a diffuse proliferation of noncohesive small lymphocytes closely resembling normal lymphocytes [see Figure 4(1)]. They have uniform round nuclei with compact basophilic chromatin, inapparent nucleoli, and a narrow rim of pale-staining cytoplasm. Large transformed lymphocytes and mitoses are usually infrequent, and plasma cells are rare. Lymphomatous follicles or nodules are not a feature of this proliferation.

3.2.2. Plasmacytoid Lymphocyte

This lymphomatous proliferation [see Figure 4(7)] is generally similar to the small lymphocyte of B cells, with the exception of an abnormal plasma-cell compo-nent of variable prominence. The latter cells possess cytoplasm that resembles that of the plasma cell, but a nucleus more like a lymphocyte. There is also a component of cells intermediate between the small lymphocyte and the abnormal plasma cell. A large, pale, acidophilic-staining globule that is PAS-positive is occasionally found overlying the nucleus (Dutcher body) in Waldenström's macroglobulinemia (Dutcher and Fahey, 1959), a representative of this group. A similar cellular proliferation without Dutcher bodies is found with other types of dysglobulinemias. At times, the proliferation may be present without any detectable serum gammopathy.

The FCC types of lymphomas may be observed with follicular, follicular and diffuse, or diffuse histological patterns, with or without sclerosis. In the small cleaved FCC type, there is usually some degree of lymphomatous follicle (nodular) formation, while follicle formation is found in approximately half of large cleaved FCC lymphomas and only occasionally (10%) in the noncleaved FCC types.

a. Small Cleaved FCC. The small cleaved FCC [see Figures 4(2) and 5A,C] exhibits a wide range of sizes, varying from the diameter of a small lymphocyte to that of a reactive histiocyte nucleus. The nuclei have an irregular configuration, and typically, a portion of the cells have identifiable nuclear cleavage planes similar to those seen in normal FCC. The frequency of nuclear cleavage in general is related to the size of the nucleus. The nuclear chromatin is compact and basophilic, nucleoli are inconspicuous, and mitotic figures are rare. The cytoplasm is scanty or indistinct. Noncleaved (transformed) FCC are intermixed with the cleaved cells in small numbers, and are demonstrated most easily with the MGP stain. Occasionally, they are numerous, comprising 10–20% of the population. Typically, the small cleaved FCC are not limited to lymphomatous follicles, but extend throughout the interfollicular tissue and commonly infiltrate the capsule (see Section 3.2.3e).

b. Large Cleaved FCC. The nucleus of the large cleaved FCC [see Figure 4(3)] is larger than the nucleus of a reactive histiocyte and exhibits prominent irregularity of nuclei. With exaggeration of nuclear cleavage, the nuclei may present unusually large, polyploid forms that at times resemble Reed–Sternberg cells. The frequency of mitoses is variable, but appears to relate to the number of large noncleaved cells accompanying the large cleaved FCC. The cytoplasm is moderate in amount and pyroninophilic, and this proliferation is frequently associated with a deposit of pale-staining intercellular material and early sclerosis. A small cleaved FCC component commonly accompanies the large cleaved FCC proliferation, particularly when there is a sclerosing component. In a small proportion of our cases, the large cleaved FCC contain cytoplasmic globular inclusions that have been identified as Ig with immunoperoxidase staining [Figure 4(3)a]. When small and large cleaved FCC are found in the same specimen, this process is designated as the large cleaved FCC type whenever the large cleaved FCC component predominates.

c. Small Noncleaved (Transformed) FCC. This lymphoma [see Figure 4(4)] is composed of medium-size cells resembling small transformed lymphocytes [see Figure 1(1),(2)]. The nuclei are usually round, and although variable in size, generally do not exceed the size of a histiocyte nucleus. The nuclear chromatin is finely dispersed, and there are one to three small nucleoli. There is a moderate amount of pyroninophilic cytoplasm with cohesive cellular borders in well-fixed tissue. Commonly, reactive phagocytes of "starry-sky" type are interspersed throughout the tumor. This lymphoma fulfills the criteria of Burkitt's lymphoma of Africa when the nuclei are uniform in size and configuration and the nucleoli are small (Berard et al., 1969). In tissue imprints, the small noncleaved FCC lymphoma has nuclei with finely dispersed acidophilic chromatin and one to three small nucleoli. There is a moderate amount of deeply basophilic cytoplasm, which usually contains a number of small clear vacuoles. The small noncleaved FCC lymphoma seen in the United States usually exhibits considerably more variation in nuclear size and nucleolar prominence than Burkitt's lymphoma of Africa. This type has commonly been referred to as the *undifferentiated* Burkitt's type. We have observed a follicular (nodular) pattern in approximately 10% of the cases of the small noncleaved FCC, usually in minimal degree. The recent report of follicle (nodule) formation in several cases of Burkitt's lymphoma by Mann *et al.* (1976) provides support for our proposal that Burkitt's lymphoma is of FCC type (Lukes and Collins, 1973, 1974a,b, 1975). The process, however, is generally a diffuse lymphomatous proliferation extending throughout a lymph node or lymphoid mass, leaving little evidence of normal architectural features.

d. Large Noncleaved (Transformed) FCC. This lymphoma [see Figure 4(5)] in general possesses cytological features similar to those of the small non-cleaved FCC type, with the exception that the cells and their nuclei are larger and have more abundant, but lightly staining, cytoplasm. The nuclei are round or oval but often irregular in configuration, and the nucleoli are prominent. Frequently, two nucleoli are found situated at the nuclear membrane, on the short axis of an oval nucleus, in a characteristic pattern. Mitoses are numerous. Both individual cell necrosis and areas of necrosis are common. Evidence of FCC nature is provided by the presence of small or large cleaved FCC and lymphomatous follicle formation in approximately 10% of the cases.

e. Evolution of FCC Lymphomas. In our experience, lymphomas of FCC are the most common types of lymphomas and exhibit the greatest variation in expression. There is a definite relationship, however, between the cytological type and the frequency of lymphomatous follicles. The variation in follicular patterns is illustrated in Figure 8, and the relationship of FCC types to follicular pattern in

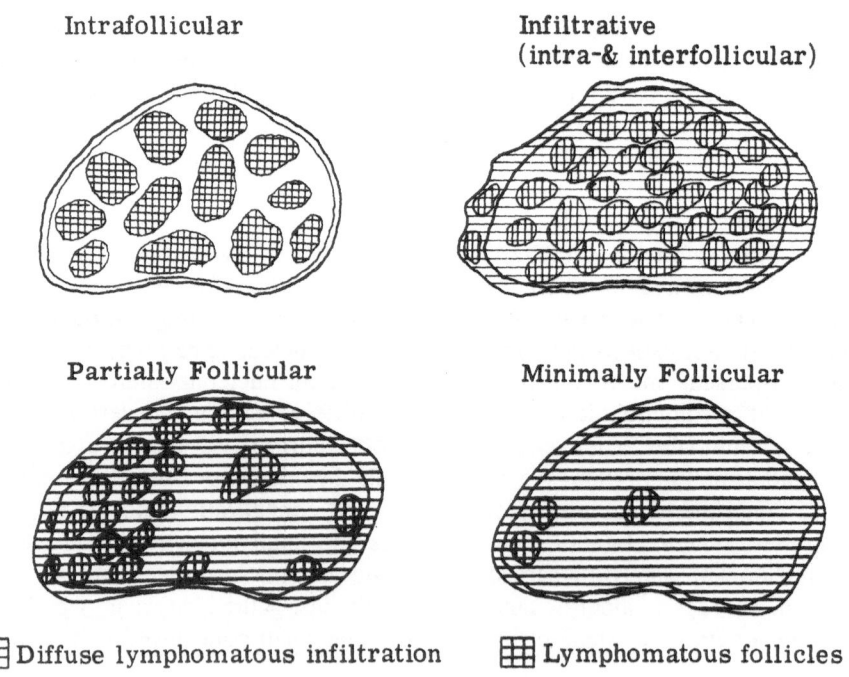

Figure 8. Variations in follicular pattern in FCC lymphomas.

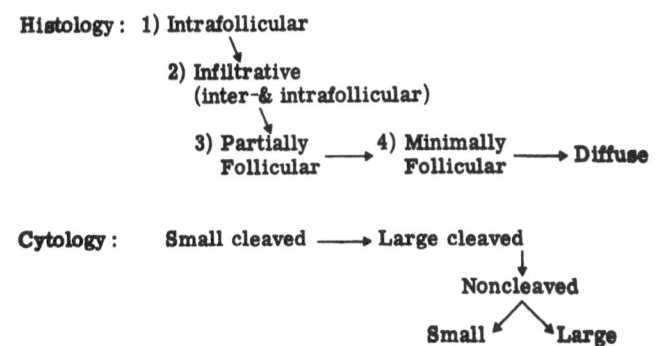

Figure 9. Evolution of FCC lymphomas—relationship of histological pattern and cytological types.

Figure 9. FCC may be limited to the follicular centers or extend throughout the lymph node in both intrafollicular and interfollicular tissues, with variations only in the frequency of follicle formation. The distribution patterns of FCC lymphomas (Figure 8) are categorized as (a) *intrafollicular* when the FCC are limited to follicular centers; (b) *infiltrative follicular* when follicles extend throughout the node and into the capsule; (c) *partially follicular* when the FCC involve the entire node, but follicles are limited to less than 50% of the node; and (d) *minimally follicular* when only one or a few follicles are identified, although FCC involve the entire node. All FCC types also occur as diffuse processes without any discernible follicular structures. This wide range in follicle formation and FCC distribution may be encountered in any FCC type, but it is most common with the small cleaved FCC type. The small cleaved FCC found in the interfollicular tissue is smaller and less cohesive than the small cleaved FCC of the follicular center. It infiltrates through the interfollicular tissue and throughout broad areas of the capsule in a distinctive manner. This infiltrative feature is associated with "seeding" to the marrow and a high incidence of bone marrow involvement, possibly in excess of 70%, occasional leukemic manifestation, and associated involvement of the spleen and retroperitoneal lymph nodes. The small cleaved FCC is commonly found in association with the large cleaved FCC and in residual foci in the large noncleaved FCC type. The frequency of follicle formation relates to the cytological type (see Figure 9). The small cleaved FCC usually (approximately 75%) exhibits some degree of follicle formation, primarily in the infiltrative follicular pattern; the large cleaved FCC commonly (approximately 50%) shows some follicle formation, usually in partial or minimal degree; and the noncleaved FCC types only occasionally (approximately 10%) show follicles, most often in partial or minimal degree. Thus, the FCC types with apparent low proliferative rates (small and large cleaved FCC with few or rare mitoses) exhibit follicle formation, while those with numerous mitoses and apparently high proliferative rates (noncleaved FCC) show the least follicle formation. These observations on the relationship of FCC to the frequency of follicles have indicated to us that cleaved FCC are related to follicle formation, but when transformation occurs so that the noncleaved cells with a high proliferative rate predominate, the proliferation rapidly "breaks through" the follicular confinement and quickly becomes a diffuse process. Whether the follicular confinement is provided by the perifollicular stroma of cells is unknown. An interesting case could be made for a T-cell role in limiting FCC lymphomas to follicles.

ROBERT J. LUKES AND
JOHN W. PARKER

3.2.4. Immunoblastic Sarcoma of B Cells

This lymphoma of transformed B cells [see Figure 4(6)] resembles the large noncleaved FCC, but has more deeply staining amphophilic and pyroninophilic cytoplasm, often with plasmacytoid features. It lacks the typical features of the FCC types, specifically the cleaved FCC component and the follicular pattern. The process is frequently observed initially as partial involvement of a lymph node in abnormal immune states. It presents as monomorphous collections (clones) of large abnormal immunoblasts in a background of severe and abnormal immunoblastic reaction. Later in the process, the proliferation may totally involve and replace the lymph node or present as a tumor mass. The immunoblasts of B-cell type are differentiated from T immunoblasts on the basis of their deeply staining and pyroninophilic cytoplasm and their frequent plasmacytoid character. The size, number, and distribution of nucleoli may be distinctive, but the reliability of this criterion is not yet established. The demonstration of the cytoplasmic Ig by the immunoperoxidase technique (Taylor, 1976a) further indicates their B-cell nature, particularly if the Ig is monoclonal in character.

3.2.5. Hairy-Cell Leukemia (Leukemic Reticuloendotheliosis)

This cellular proliferation [see Figure 4(8)] in tissue sections consists of medium-size cells with abundant pale cytoplasm and round-to-oval nuclei with finely dispersed chromatin. At times, the nuclei have a deep central indentation and appear to be binucleated. The cytoplasm is pale-staining and occasionally almost inapparent, depending on the fixation and processing. In ideally prepared tissue, the cellular borders are sharply demarcated and interlocking with a prominent acidophilic intercellular zone. In smears of peripheral blood and bone marrow or tissue imprints, the cytoplasm is generally abundant and finely granular and the cellular margin ill defined, with hairlike processes. Often, however, the cellular borders are simply irregular without hairy processes. The nuclei are oval or binucleated, with finely dispersed chromatin. The cytoplasm contains a variable number of tartrate-resistant acid phosphatase granules (Yam *et al.*, 1971b), but shows no NSE activity (α-naphthyl butyrate substrate). The precise origin of the cell is still debated. In our studies and those of Dr. Collins' group at Vanderbilt University, the majority of 17 cases exhibited monoclonal SIg. The cells in three cases studied by Collins' group resynthesized SIg after the original SIg was removed with trypsin, indicating that it was not passively absorbed cytophilic antibody. In our opinion, these findings leave little doubt that the cells are B lymphocytes, although atypical. The demonstration of phagocytosis of latex and zymosan particles by the hairy cells has been offered, however, as evidence of their monocyte–histiocyte nature. A recent study by Boldt *et al.* (1977) demonstrated that hairy cells possessed an unusual combination of both lymphocytic and histiocytic functional capabilities and structural features. These confusing results may indicate origin of this very interesting cell from an as yet unidentified normal counterpart in lymphoid tissue or simply the aberrant expression of features not normally expressed.

3.3. Histiocytic Type

The true histiocytic lymphoma seems to exist as an interrelated histiocyte–monocyte proliferation, and from our experience is the least common cytological type of malignant lymphoma. The number of proved cases with functional studies is too small at present to establish an accurate description of the variations in morphological expression. To identify a lymphoma as a true histiocytic type, the demonstration of macrophage–monocyte enzymes such as α-naphthyl butyrase or muramidase is required, and ideally, there should be no T or B surface markers. The small number of proved cases we have had the opportunity to study have been variable in their histological appearance, but have had an identifiable histiocyte component, the macrophage, as well as a monocyte component. Several of these cases terminated in a leukemic process resembling a poorly differentiated monocytic leukemia (Lukes and Collins, 1977).

3.4. Hodgkin's Disease

The basic process in Hodgkin's disease and the precise nature of the Reed–Sternberg cell remain controversial. The histological types of the Rye classification (Lukes *et al.*, 1966a) adapted from the original Lukes–Butler types (Lukes *et al.*, 1966b), however, have long been accepted. In both classifications, the histological types are designed to classify the host response and are based on our concept that the basic process in Hodgkin's disease is a struggle between the host and the factors involved in the induction of Reed–Sternberg cells. The lymphocyte-predominance type of the Rye classification is interpreted as an expression of a fairly effective host response, characterized morphologically by a prominence of lymphocytes with a variable component of reactive histiocytes, a rarity of diagnostic Reed–Sternberg cells, and, clinically, by disease of limited extent. In contrast, the lymphocyte-depletion type is regarded as an ineffective host response represented morphologically by decreased numbers of lymphocytes accompanied by either a distinctive type of diffuse fibrosis or numerous diagnostic Reed–Sternberg cells and clinically by widespread stage III or IV disease with rapid progression. The mixed-cellularity type occupies an intermediate position between lymphocyte predominance and lymphocyte depletion, and indicates a failing host response expressed clinically by changing disease. These three types—lymphocyte predominance, mixed cellularity, and lymphocyte depletion—appear to represent morphological expressions of stages in the evolution of the process. We regard nodular sclerosis separately, with its dominant association with the anterior superior mediastinum and adjacent cervical, hilar, and axillary lymph nodes, since it seems to represent a regional expression of Hodgkin's disease. It includes cases with both quiescent and aggressive disease. The spread of nodular sclerosis appears to be contiguous and predictable, while in the other types, the process usually skips the mediastinum and is noncontiguous in its spread.

Reed–Sternberg cells have long been regarded as modified reticulum cells or histiocytes because of their large size. From our experience with the morphological expressions of transformed lymphocytes and our observation of diagnostic Reed–Sternberg cells in infectious mononucleosis, we proposed that Reed–Sternberg cells may be polyploid transformed lymphocytes (Lukes *et al.*, 1969; Tindle *et al.*, 1972). The lacunar cells and L & H cells, the biological Reed–Sternberg cell variants according to this view, represent partially developed or modified Reed–Sternberg cells (Lukes, 1971; Anagnostou *et al.*, 1977). The Order and Hellman (1972) hypothesis of the development of Hodgkin's disease is based on a defective T-cell surveillance that allows Reed–Sternberg cells to develop from *reticulum cells.* In our view, the T cells are defective in Hodgkin's disease, though the precise abnormality is unknown. Defective T cells permit abnormal lymphocyte transformation to occur, leading to the formation of Reed–Sternberg cells as polyploid transformed lymphocytes (Figure 10). The lymphocyte abnormality may be acquired through a viral infection, or it may be the result of a genetic predisposition related to a specific (?aberrant) immune response gene *(HLA-D)*. If the T cells were unaltered or normal, any defective transformed lymphocytes would be eliminated by T cells. When the host reponse is more effective, though not normal, many partially developed Reed–Sternberg variants such as lacunar cells are formed. The abundant pale cytoplasm of the lacunar cell may be the result of host lymphocyte damage (Anagnostou *et al.*, 1977). This hypothesis fits with our original proposal that the Hodgkin's disease process represents a struggle between the host and the attempted formation of Reed–Sternberg cells, with the diverse morphological types and clinical expressions being the result of differences in host responsiveness (Lukes *et al.*, 1966b).

In the following sections, each histological type of the Rye classification is briefly defined.

3.4.1. Lymphocyte Predominance

Included within this type are the lymphocytic and histiocytic types, both nodular and diffuse, of our original classification (Lukes *et al.*, 1966b). The term *lymphocyte predominance* is misleading at times, since the process may be composed primarily of lymphocytes or histiocytes in varying proportions, although a predominance of lymphocytes is most commonly observed. The proliferation in approximately half the cases is aggregated into large, poorly defined nodules and is usually manifested clinically by stage I disease. Both the lymphocytic and histiocytic components are believed to represent attempted host responses. The lymphocytes are small and have round to irregular nuclei and scanty cytoplasm. The

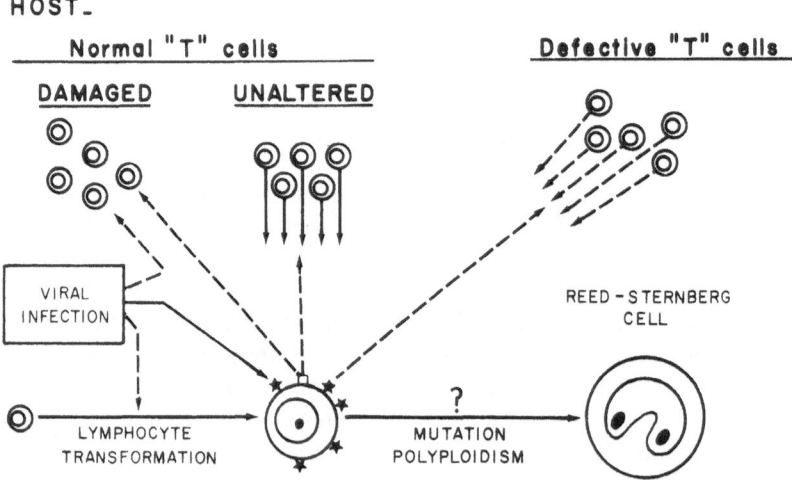

Figure 10. Schematic representation of proposed interaction between host T cells and transformed lymphocytes. It is hypothesized that Reed–Sternberg cells are polyploid transformed lymphocytes resulting from abnormal control of transformation by defective T cells.

histiocytes occur singly or in small clusters and are grouped, on occasion, as small epithelioid "sarcoidlike" aggregations. Throughout the lymphocytic and histiocytic proliferation, in varying frequency, there is a prominent component of large cells with lobated, folded, and overlapping large nuclei with finely dispersed chromatin and small or inconspicuous nucleoli. The cytoplasm is pale-staining and usually limited in amount. We have referred to these cells as the *L & H variants* of the Reed–Sternberg cell, because of the consistent association with this histological type and their usefulness in recognizing it (Lukes, 1971). In contrast, the diagnostic Reed–Sternberg cell, with huge nucleoli and amphophilic cytoplasm, is typically extremely rare in this histological type, and therefore difficult to find.

3.4.2. Mixed Cellularity

In this type, a variety of cellular components are found in differing proportions in each case. Diagnostic bi- or multinucleated Reed–Sternberg cells with large nucleoli are conspicuous, while histiocytes, eosinophils, and fibrosis are prominent. In addition, the mixed type provides a category for cases in which the morphological findings do not fulfill the criteria for any of the other histological types.

3.4.3. Lymphocyte Depletion

Included in this type are the diffuse fibrosis and reticular types of our original classification (Lukes *et al.*, 1966b). Diffuse fibrosis is characterized by a marked reduction in cellularity, particularly of lymphocytes, associated with a distinctive type of disorderly fibrosis characterized by loose, amorphous, and poorly formed nonbirefringent connective tissue that extends throughout most of the lymph node. Diagnostic Reed–Sternberg cells are generally infrequent in the hypocellular nodes. In the reticular variant, diagnostic Reed–Sternberg cells are extremely numerous, and on rare occasions are pleomorphic and appear sarcomatous. At times, both the reticular and diffuse fibrosing types are found in the same biopsy or in an individual case at autopsy, in different tissues, indicating different expressions of the failing host response.

3.4.4. Nodular Sclerosis

This histological type has two distinctive features essential for diagnosis: (1) thick birefringent collagen bands and (2) lacunar-cell variants of the Reed–Sternberg cell. The nodular sclerosing type, however, exhibits wide variations in expression, from total sclerosis to almost complete cellularity with only a single demonstrable thick collagen band. The cellularity is similarly variable. It may be predominantly lymphocytic with varying numbers of lacunar cells, mixed in cellularity, or predominantly composed of lacunar cells. This distinct Reed–Sternberg cell variant of nodular sclerosis, the lacunar cell, has, in formalin-fixed tissue, abundant water-clear cytoplasm, which often retracts from its cell borders. The nucleus is hyperlobated with small nucleoli. Lacunar cells often occur in cohesive clusters, which commonly exhibit central necrosis associated with granulocyte infiltration. In the aggressive infiltrative form of nodular sclerosis, the process may be primarily composed of lacunar cells with large nucleoli and little collagen formation.

262

3.5. Comparison of Lymphoma Classifications

ROBERT J. LUKES AND
JOHN W. PARKER

The cytological types in traditional lymphoma classification—reticulum-cell sarcoma, lymphosarcoma, and follicular lymphoma—were all proposed three decades before the modern developments in immunology. In addition, they have been demonstrated to be meaningless terms because of the extraordinary variation in their application (Gall, 1958; Lukes, 1968). Nevertheless, these terms remain in use in a limited number of laboratories and still appear occasionally in the literature, even though their value has been questioned and they bear no relationship to modern immunology.

The approach of Rappaport, also proposed before the dramatic progress in immunology of the past decade, is based on the concept that each of the cytological types of the classification may proliferate in a nodular or diffuse histological fashion, and when the proliferation exhibits a nodular pattern, it is less aggressive than when the same cytological types has a diffuse pattern. Recent clinical studies have supported this contention, with significantly longer median survivals for those patients with nodular than for those with diffuse histological patterns (Jones *et al.*, 1973). The cytological types of Rappaport are based primarily on size, and as a result are limited in specificity. When they are compared with the cytological types of Lukes and Collins (Table 2), three major points are apparent: (1) each of the cytological types of Rappaport is considered to have a nodular and diffuse expression, and each includes both T- and B-cell types and is thus heterogeneous; (2) in the Rappaport classification, a relationship to follicles is avoided; and (3) a practical and conceptual basis for the investigation of lymphomas is provided by our immunological approach. The criss-cross pattern of arrows dramatically demonstrates the heterogeneity of each of the cytological types of Rappaport. The histiocytic

TABLE 2. Comparison of Lymphoma Classifications of Rappaport and Lukes and Collins

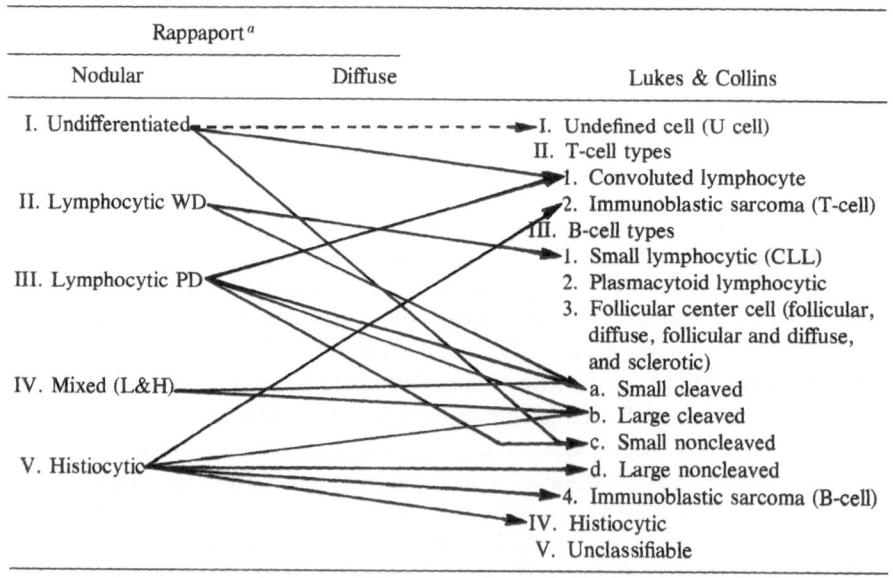

*(WD) Well-differentiated; (PD) poorly differentiated; (L&H) lymphocytic and histiocytic.

lymphoma of Rappaport includes IBSs of both T- and B-cell types, the large cleaved and the large noncleaved FCC types, and the true histiocytic type. As an intermediate-size cell, the poorly differentiated lymphocytic lymphoma of Rappaport includes the convoluted T lymphocyte, the small noncleaved FCC, the small cleaved FCC, and the large cleaved FCC, depending on its size. The well-differentiated lymphocytic type (small cell) and the undifferentiated cell are similarly heterogeneous and also contain several cell types in our classification. The mixed type of Rappaport is difficult to illustrate as a result of the variability in application and since a number of cytological types of lymphoma may have varying degrees of cell mixture, although one cell type predominates.

In the time since our proposal of a new functional classification, a number of other classifications have appeared (Bennett *et al.*, 1974; Dorfman, 1974; Gerard-Marchant *et al.*, 1974; Lennert *et al.*, 1975). The Kiel classification (Gerard-Marchant *et al.*, 1974)—a modification of the proposal of Lennert *et al.* (1975)—has a conceptual and immunological basis similar to that of ours, but it is uncertain how closely related the cytological types are. The remaining classifications are essentially modifications of the Rappaport classifications, with the exception that several of our terms are included in the working classification of Dorfman (1974).

4. Immunological and Cytochemical Marker Studies

The application of immunological methods to the study of lymphomas has added a new dimension to our understanding of this complex field. We began our studies with the point of view that cytomorphological differences among lymphomas indicated their origin from T or B lymphocytes or U cells, and that this relationship would be confirmed with the appropriate immunological surface-marker and cytochemical techniques as they became available and were applied.

4.1. Techniques

A variety of methods are now available for distinguishing T and B lymphocytes and monocytes, and a number of these methods have found wide application. Others have been used by only a few investigators. None of the methods provides absolute criteria for distinguishing the cell types. For this reason, many laboratories, including our own, use a panel of several methods for the assessment of cell populations for the presence of T and B cells and histiocytes (monocytes). Table 3 lists the most commonly used techniques, including cytochemistry. Particular emphasis will be placed on spontaneous sheep erythrocyte (SRBC) rosette formation (E rosettes) for T cells and SIg for B cells, since these are the most widely employed and reliable procedures. The pitfalls and factors that influence these various tests were reviewed recently by Taylor (1976b) and others (Braylan *et al.*, 1975; Green *et al.*, 1975; Kunkel, 1975), and are discussed in some detail in Chapter 10.

Our approach to the study of lymphomas and leukemias has been to relate morphology, cytochemistry, electron microscopy, and immunological surface markers in an attempt to characterize various types of proliferations. Where possible, other techniques such as measurement of Ig synthesis by lymphoma cells and cell kinetics are used to further characterize the cells. The immunological

ROBERT J. LUKES AND
JOHN W. PARKER

TABLE 3. Techniques Most Commonly Used for Identification of T and B Cells and Histiocytes

Technique	T cells[a]	B cells[a]	Histiocytes, monocytes[a]	Comments
SRBC rosettes[b]				Cytocentrifuge preparations essential in evaluating lymphomas.
E	+	−	−	Currently most useful T-cell marker.
EAC (IgM) (Complement)	(+)	+	+	Some T cells. Convoluted T-cell lymphomas observed with complement receptors.
EA (IgG) (Fc receptor)	−	+	+	Limited usefulness.
Surface Ig[c]	−	+	(+)	By immunofluorescence. Monocytes mark because of Fc receptors.
Cytoplasmic Ig	−	+	−	Immunoperoxidase more useful than immunofluorescence in lymphomas because it can be used on paraffin sections.
Antisera[d]				
HTLA	+	−	−	Antigen source: thymus, brain. Specificity a problem.
HBLA	−	+	−	Antigen source: CLL cells, B-lymphoblastoid cell lines. Specificity a problem.
Cytochemistry				
α-Naphthyl butyrase (NSE)	(+)	−	+	Globules reported in T cells. Specificity for T cells doubtful.
Acid phosphatase	(+)	−	−	Reported in convoluted T-cell and T-cell ALL.
Tartrate-resistant acid phosphatase	−	(+)	−	Hairy-cell leukemia.
Muramidase (lysozyme)	−	−	+	Immunoperoxidase method on paraffin sections.

[a] (+) Lacks specificity, is controversial, or is seen only with certain types of lymphoma–leukemia.
[b] (EAC) Erythrocyte–antibody–complement complex; (EA) erythrocyte–antibody complex.
[c] T cells have a small amount of SIg that is not detected by immunofluorescent methods.
[d] (HTLA) Human T-lymphocyte antigen; (HBLA) human B-lymphocyte antigen.

surface-marker techniques have been helpful in the study of immune deficiencies, and more recently have proved of value in the study of malignant lymphomas and their leukemic expressions. The results of these studies from our laboratory and from those of others support our initial proposal that most of these neoplasms mark as T or B cells, and only rarely as histiocytes. The morphological features of the cell types in the Lukes and Collins classification of lymphomas predict the T- or B-cell nature of the cells in a high proportion of cases (Lukes and Collins, 1977).

Pretherapy lymphoid material for our studies has been collected from lymph node biopsies, spleens, bone marrow, and peripheral blood. Frequently, additional specimens from patients in relapse have been obtained as well. Cells from spinal, pleural, and peritoneal fluids have also been studied. The specimens were obtained from the patients at the Los Angeles County–University of Southern California Medical Center, the Children's Hospital of Los Angeles, and participating hospitals of the Southern California Lymphoma Group, which includes 20 major hospitals. Cell suspensions of lymphoid tissues are prepared in our institution by gently teasing the specimen through stainless steel wire mesh in RPMI 1640. Pathologists or technologists who have been instructed in our laboratory similarly prepare suspensions in the other hospitals, and messengers deliver the cell suspensions to our laboratory. Mononuclear cells from peripheral blood are separated on Ficoll–Hypaque.

Spontaneous SRBC rosette formation as well as SRBC-rosetting techniques for detecting complement (EAC) and Fc receptors (EA) are performed on cell suspensions using the methods of Jondal *et al.* (1972) with minor modifications. Surface Ig's are detected with fluorescein–isothiocyanate-labeled monospecific antiglobulins. Whenever sufficient cells are available, the cells are examined for the presence of the heavy (H) chains α, γ, δ, μ, and occasionally ϵ, and the light (L) chains κ and λ. In our early studies, commercial antisera that we characterized for specificity by immunoprecipitation techniques were used, but more recently, specific antisera raised in rabbits and goats have been prepared and characterized in our own laboratory.

Shandon cytocentrifuge preparations are prepared from the cell suspensions for cytochemical determinations, as are touch imprints of the cut surfaces of the lymphoid tissues. The cytochemical procedures routinely applied include Wright's stain, PAS, MGP, granulocyte stains (peroxidase, Sudan black, and chloroacetate esterase), and NSE (α-naphthyl butyrase) for histiocytes (see Table 3). From the same specimen from which the suspensions are prepared, slices 2–4 mm thick are fixed in Zenker's or B-5 fixative (Lillie and Fullmer, 1976) for paraffin embedding and 2×2 mm fragments are fixed in Karnovsky's fixative (Graham and Karnovsky, 1966) for transmission electron microscopy. Paraffin sections are examined for the presence of cytoplasmic Ig's and muramidase by the immunoperoxidase technique (Taylor and Mason, 1974).

4.2. General Results of Immunological and Cytochemical Studies

A number of studies of malignant lymphomas and leukemias have been reported using surface-marker techniques (Aisenberg and Long, 1975; Berard *et al.*, 1976; Braylan *et al.*, 1975; Brouet *et al.*, 1975; Davey *et al.*, 1976; Gajl-Peczalska *et al.*, 1975; Leech *et al.*, 1975). These studies and our own results, which are described below, support our original proposal that malignant lymphomas are neoplasms of the immune system, and that for the most part, these proliferations mark as T- and B-cell types, whereas lymphomas of histiocytes are quite rare (Lukes and Collins, 1977). It is clear from these reports and from our own experience that we have much to learn about the techniques used and their interpretation. Taylor (1976b) pointed out many potential sources of error and confusion. Refinement and standardization of these techniques and the development of other methods, however, will add greater precision and reproducibility to these studies.

As indicated in Table 3, E-rosette formation is the marker of T lymphocytes that we have found most reliable in studying lymphomas. The EAC rosettes, which

ROBERT J. LUKES AND
JOHN W. PARKER

detect complement-receptor-bearing cells, form with some B-lymphoma cells, but the correlation with SIg's on these same cells is not high. Generally, the percentage of EAC-rosette-forming cells is less than the percentage of SIg-bearing cells. In addition, some T-cell lymphomas, particularly the convoluted T cell, form EAC rosettes, as do some normal histiocytes. The EA-rosette technique apparently detects Fc receptors, and has been used by some workers (Green et al., 1975) as a marker for histiocytes. In our hands, in cell suspensions, it has not been a reliable identifier of histiocytes, and other methods for detecting Fc receptors promise to be better (Gordon et al., 1977; Taylor et al., 1977). SIg's appear to be the most reliable markers for lymphomatous B cells. In most instances, the cells from different types of B-cell lymphomas have shown evidence that they belong, in each instance, to a single clone, since only one H chain (occasionally two) and one L chain have been present on the surface of cells from a given lymphoma. A significant number have shown a polyclonal pattern of staining, however, with more than one H and L chain being present in the population. As Taylor (1976b) discussed, this result may be due to technical factors such as lack of specificity of antisera or use of a nonoptimal titer of antiserum, or to biological factors such as the presence of Fc receptors, which results in adsorbtion of serum IgG or IgG antisera or both, the latter emphasizing the need for the use of Fab antisera. Unfortunately, these antisera have not been readily available in quantity. Preud'homme and Seligmann (1974) also discussed the variety of ways in which adsorption of fluorescent antisera to cells may occur; e.g., anti-lymphoma cell antibodies produced by the patient may attach to the lymphoma cells and be detected as SIg. Despite these problems, it is readily apparent that the bulk of B-cell lymphomas show a monoclonal staining pattern, particularly when cells are incubated at 37°C prior to immunofluorescence staining to allow loss of Ig adsorbed to Fc receptors.

The immunoperoxidase method for detecting intracytoplasmic antigens, specifically Ig's in B cells and muramidase in histiocytes or monocytes, has proved to be quite useful in identifying lymphomas in paraffin sections. We have not used anti-HTLA or HBLA sera, although in principle these antisera should be valuable additions to the marker panel, because specific antisera have not been readily available.

Among the cytochemical determinations that we have used, the NSE, using an α-naphthyl butyrate substrate, is a good identifier of histiocytes and monocytes. Some workers have reported focal cytoplasmic NSE activity in T cells, but we have not been able to confirm this observation. Localized acid phosphatase activity has been reported to identify the cells of convoluted T-cell lymphomas (Stein et al., 1976) and T cells from ALL (Catovsky et al., 1974), but this identification has not been a consistent finding in our hands. Tartrate-resistant acid phosphatase is used as a marker for the cells of hairy-cell leukemia (leukemic reticuloendotheliosis), and we have found it generally reliable. Terminal deoxyribonucleotidyl transferase activity reported in thymocytes and ALL (McCaffrey et al., 1973) may prove useful in the study of lymphomas, but the methodology is not easily applied to the clinical situation, and there is some question as to specificity for human T cells (Hutton and Coleman, 1975; Bhattacharyza, 1975). Some workers have reported B-glucuronidase activity in T cells (Catovsky et al., 1974), but again our experience has not indicated specificity.

To date, we have studied over 300 cases of non-Hodgkin's lymphomas and related leukemias. The detailed results are being reported elsewhere. In summary, however, approximately two thirds of all the lymphomas studied have marked as B cells and 20% as T cells. There have been approximately 15% that have not marked as either T or B cells with the techniques used, and only one histiocytic lymphoma has been encountered. The majority of T-cell lymphomas have possessed convoluted nuclei and have developed largely in patients under 20 years of age. The other T-cell proliferations have been classified as T-cell IBS, mycosis fungoides, Sézary's syndrome, or ALL. The great majority (approximately 65%) of the B-cell lymphomas have been FCC lymphomas. The rest have been classified as small lymphocyte, plasmacytoid lymphocyte, or B-type IBS.

The monoclonicity of the SIg's present on lymphoma cells remains the most important indicator of the neoplastic nature of a B-cell proliferation, but is subject to the vagaries discussed above. In the case of the T-cell lymphomas, we have encountered a wide range of percentages of E-rosette-forming lymphoma cells as counted in wet mounts. A most important observation is that in a significant number of T-cell proliferations, only a small percentage of the cells form E rosettes, but stained cytocentrifuge preparations convincingly demonstrate rosette formation by some of the lymphoma cells. Thus, there have been a number of low-marking convoluted T-cell lymphomas.

Since every cell suspension prepared from lymphoid tissue, whether reactive or neoplastic, contains a mixture of both neoplastic cells and reactive lymphocytes, the percentages of T and B cells will inevitably be colored by this admixture. In the case of the relatively homogeneous population obtained from completely replaced lymph nodes, the problem is less severe, but even then, varying numbers of residual reactive T lymphocytes will be present in a B-cell lymphoma and vice versa. For that reason, the importance of identifying the cells that are marking is important. As mentioned, this can be achieved relatively easily with the E rosettes, but very poorly using immunofluorescent techniques for SIg's. The immunoperoxidase technique for detecting SIg's is not as satisfactory as it is in identifying intracytoplasmic Ig's, but we have developed a new method for identifying SIg-bearing B cells by using polymeric microspheres conjugated to anti-human Ig's (Gordon *et al.*, 1977). This technique, like that employing E rosettes, provides a permanent specimen with acceptably discernible morphological details.

5. Illustrative Cases

The clinical importance and reliability of using the classification and markers we have discussed above are probably best illustrated by specific case examples. In the remainder of this chapter, therefore, we will describe cases that we have studied and that are representative of the various cytological types.

Case 1: Small Lymphocytic Lymphoma (B-Cell, CLL) Progressing to IBS. The patient was a 71-year-old male with an 8-year history of relatively asymptomatic CLL. Lymphocytosis ranged from 20,000 to 50,000 and was associated with only mild anemia. There was a dramatic terminal change in symptomatology associated with a prominent increase in the size of lymph nodes. Biopsy revealed most of the lymph node to be composed of small, round lymphocytes of B-

ROBERT J. LUKES AND
JOHN W. PARKER

cell type [see Figure 4(1)] with monomorphous areas of large transformed lymphocytes or immunoblasts. These areas were interpreted as IBS, B-cell type [see Figure
4(6)]. The patient died 2 weeks later. The results of immunological surface-marker
studies on three specimens were as follows:

Study	Rosettes*			Ig*						
	E	EAC	EA	PV†	μ	γ	α	Δ	κ	λ
PB† 1973	0	10	—	87	20	77	0	—	—	—
LN† 1976	12	12	13	83	0	79	0	0	0	76
PB 1976	4	21	6	91	0	89	0	0	0	84

There were insufficient numbers of cells to complete the studies on the 1973
specimen. Nevertheless, the general features, with a high proportion of cells
staining with a polyvalent anti-Ig serum (PV) and anti-IgG, were similar to the latter
two specimens, which marked in a monoclonal fashion (IgG λ). In the latter
specimens, few cells formed E rosettes (spontaneous SRBC rosettes—T cells) and
only a limited number EAC or EA rosettes. Thus, the markers were maintained
even with the evolution of the process to an IBS. In the past, this change from a
small lymphocyte to a large cell associated with a change in aggressiveness was
known as CLL developing into reticulum-cell sarcoma or Richter's syndrome
(Richter, 1928; Long and Aisenberg, 1975). This case illustrates the "switch on" or
derepression of the lymphocyte-transformation mechanism with maintenance of the
same monoclonicity, rather than an inexplicable change in cell type from a lymphocyte to a reticulum cell.

Case 2: Plasmacytoid Lymphocytic Type. This 76-year-old female presented with generalized asymptomatic lymphadenopathy. The spleen and liver were
not palpably enlarged. The WBC was 64,000, with 87% small and plasmacytoid
lymphocytes. A lymph node biopsy revealed diffuse involvement by a cellular
proliferation that varied from small lymphocytes with round nuclei, compact chromatin, and a moderate amount of cytoplasm to plasmacytoid lymphocytes that had
eccentric lymphocyte nuclei and varying amounts of plasmacytoid pyroninophilic
cytoplasm [see Figure 4(7)]. Serum immunoelectrophoresis revealed an IgG κ
monoclonal pattern. The immunological surface-marker study results were as
follows:

Study	Rosettes			Ig						
	E	EAC	EA	PV	μ	γ	α	Δ	κ	λ
PB	5	0	0	84	0	81	0	0	83	0
PB	4	4	2	80	0	78	0	0	82	0

Here and throughout this section:
*Results are expressed as percentages of mononuclear cells marking.
†(PB) Peripheral blood; (LN) lymph node; (PV) polyvalent anti-Ig serum.

Three other studies of peripheral blood for immunological surface markers gave similar results. All showed a monoclonal, IgG κ, pattern, with few E rosettes. The serum Ig abnormality was apparently related to the Ig produced by the lymphoma cells. The lymph node biopsy obtained 1 year after the peripheral blood yielded too few cells for a complete study. Only 3% of the cells marked as T cells, 41% possessed SIg, and the remainder were unmarked. The latter may be attributed to the absence of SIg on plasma cells. The disparity in the number of marking cells between the peripheral blood and lymph node appears to relate to the prominent proportion of plasmacytoid lymphocytes that may have reached a functional state in which the SIg is lost. The majority of plasmacytoid lymphomas are associated with monoclonal serum spikes (IgM) and a predominance of SIgM, and at times are expressed as the Waldenström syndrome.

In our series of these cases, a small group has exhibited a serum monoclonal IgG spike and SIgG similar to this case. In the past, such cases have been included with CLL or the diffuse well-differentiated lymphocytic type of lymphoma of Rappaport, both of which fail to acknowledge the plasmacytoid features of the lymphocyte.

Case 3: Small Cleaved FCC, Infiltrative Follicular Type. This 39-year-old asymptomatic female had noted painless enlargement of right inguinal lymph nodes. Enlarged left axillary lymph nodes were the only other abnormality on physical examination. There were no abnormal laboratory findings. A lymphangiogram revealed enlarged abnormal periaortic lymph nodes. Biopsy of the inguinal and axillary lymph nodes showed an infiltrative follicular (nodular) pattern of involvement by a small cleaved FCC [see Figures 4(2) and 5A,C] that extended throughout the follicular and interfollicular tissue and into the lymph node capsule. In the sections of the marrow biopsy, a similar small cleaved FCC proliferation was found in peritrabecular areas. The immunological surface-marker studies of cells from the axillary lymph node revealed monoclonal surface staining (IgM κ):

Study	E	EAC	EA	PV	μ	γ	α	Δ	κ	λ
LN	29	11	0	75	72	0	1	5	74	6

This case illustrates the monoclonal surface marking we have observed in the majority of this cytological type of B cell proliferation. Clinically, it illustrates the common widespread distribution of this low-turnover-rate proliferation and its asymptomatic presentation. From our experience, the marrow is involved at initial presentation in over 70% of cases. This cytological type in kinetic studies is diploid or slightly hyperdiploid, has a low-turnover proliferative rate (Riccardi *et al.*, 1976), and paradoxically has a widespread distribution, but prolonged median survival (Lukes and Peckham, unpublished).

Case 4: Large Cleaved FCC, Minimally Follicular, with Sclerosis. This 63-year-old male noticed abdominal fullness and was discovered to have a large abdominal mass. There was no peripheral lymphadenopathy or hepatosplenomegaly. Surgical exploration of the abdomen revealed a large mass in the base of the mesentery. There was only mild anemia, and no other significant laboratory find-

ROBERT J. LUKES AND
JOHN W. PARKER

ings. There was no evidence of marrow involvement. A biopsy of a small satellite mass in the mesentery showed some areas with follicle (nodule) formation, a region of sclerosis, and the remainder involved by a diffuse proliferation of large cleaved cells, some of which contained large, single, acidophilic globular structures in the cytoplasm [see Figure 4(3)a]. Immunoperoxidase staining for Ig showed this material to be IgA λ. Immunological surface-marker studies on the cell suspensions prepared from the mass yielded the following results:

Study	E	EAC	EA	PV	μ	γ	α	Δ	κ	λ
LN	34	30	0	39	0	2	57	2	2	53

SIg on the lymphoma cells was also IgA λ, a monoclonal pattern.

Our large series of sclerosing lymphomas (to be published) have all been composed of FCC, and are predominantly of the small or large cleaved types. They were originally reported by Bennett and Millet (1969) as nodular sclerosing retroperitoneal lymphomas. Approximately two thirds of the cases in our large series have presented in the mesentery, retroperitoneum, or inguinal region. They are also found in the salivary gland region and in a wide variety of sites, often in unusual extranodal locations, such as the scalp. The reason for the common association of the cleaved FCC with sclerosis and the frequent regional distribution in the retroperitoneum or mesentery is unclear.

Case 5: Small Noncleaved (Transformed) FCC, Diffuse. This 5-year-old male was well until 10 days before admission, when constipation, nausea, vomiting, and abdominal pain developed. On physical examination, a large abdominal mass was found and was confirmed at laparatomy. A biopsy revealed a diffuse proliferation of medium-size cells with moderate amounts of pyroninophilic cytoplasm, cohesive cellular borders, and variably sized round to oval nuclei with finely dispersed chromatin and one to three small nucleoli [see Figure 4(4)]. Mitoses were numerous. The frequently interspersed reactive phagocytes imparted a resemblance to Burkitt's lymphoma, but the lymphoma cells and their nuclei were more variable in size and the nucleoli larger than are seen in the typical African Burkitt's lymphoma, according to the criteria of the W.H.O. Conference (Berard *et al.*, 1969). The patient survived only 4 months on combination chemotherapy. The immunological surface-marker study results on the lymph node suspension were as follows:

Study	E	EAC	EA	PV	μ	γ	α	Δ	κ	λ
LN	6	43	13	88	74	0	0	0	0	61

Almost all the cells showed a monoclonal pattern of SIg staining (IgM λ), supporting their proposed B-cell nature. Less than half these cells, however, possessed complement receptors (EAC).

Clinically, the abdominal presentation is characteristic of this lymphoma in American children, and was observed in over 70% of similar cases in our recent study (Schneider *et al.*, 1978). This lymphoma commonly presents as an obstructive ileocecal wall mass, and apparently arises in the lymphoid tissue of the lamina propria of the region.

Case 6: Large Noncleaved (Transformed) FCC, Minimally Follicular. This 75-year-old male complained of difficulty in swallowing, and was found to have massive unilateral tonsillar enlargement and large ipsilateral, submandibular lymph nodes. The tonsillar surface was ulcerated and replaced by a predominantly diffuse proliferation of large noncleaved cells resembling *in vitro* transformed lymphocytes [see Figure 4(5)]. In one area, several lymphomatous follicles composed of the large noncleaved FCC were identified. The patient was treated with radiation of the tonsillar bed and regional lymph nodes and combination chemotherapy. Six months later, multiple cutaneous nodules and hepatosplenomegaly developed. A biopsy of a cutaneous nodule showed a lymphomatous infiltrate essentially identical to that of the tonsil. The patient died 13 months after the initial diagnosis. The results of immunological surface-marker studies were as follows:

Study	E	EAC	EA	PV	μ	γ	α	Δ	κ	λ
Tonsil	39	—	—	34	31	1	1	—	16	0
Skin nodule	17	22	29	14	12	0	1	0	7	0

The aggressiveness of this high-turnover-rate proliferation of large noncleaved FCC is apparent in this case. The cells in both specimens showed a similar monoclonal pattern of SIg staining (IgM κ), though the number of cells with SIg was low, particularly in the cutaneous nodule. The number of unmarked cells was high.

This case demonstrates that specimens from different sites possess the same monoclonal pattern of SIg and the rapid clinical progression and dissemination of this high-turnover-rate proliferation. Kinetic studies have characterized this type of proliferation as hypertetraploid with frequent aneuploidy (Riccardi *et al.*, 1976).

Case 7: IBS, B-Cell Type (IBS-B), Developing in Immunoblastic Lymphadenopathy. A 51-year-old male developed generalized severe pruritus, fever, and moderate lymphadenopathy. A lymph node biopsy was interpreted as immunoblastic lymphadenopathy (IBL). Lymphocytopenia and a serum lymphocytotoxic factor were demonstrated along with mild polyclonic hyperglobulinemia. His symptoms and signs gradually subsided without therapy, only to reappear dramatically in 15 months. A lymph node biopsy at that time revealed a lymphoma of transformed lymphocytes with plasmacytoid features, i.e., an IBS of B-cell type [see Figures 2D and 4(6)]. Clinical progression was rapid despite combination chemotherapy, and death occurred 3 months later, with generalized IBS confirmed at autopsy.

IBL was reported by Lukes and Tindle (1975) as an abnormal hyperimmune B-cell disorder that is commonly associated (35%) with hypersensitivity reactions to therapeutic agents as the initial clinical manifestation, and with the development of IBS in approximately 10% of our cases. The process is usually associated with polyclonal hyperglobulinemia and commonly with Coomb's-positive hemolytic anemia, both evidence of the hyperimmune B-cell response. The initial hypersensitivity phenomenon is interpreted as a triggering of an abnormal immune system. The progression to IBS seems to represent the neoplastic "switch on" or derepression of lymphocyte transformation in an abnormal immune state, parallel to that observed in a variety of abnormal immune states—immunosuppressed transplant patients, α-chain disease, SLE, Sjögren's syndrome, and others (Lukes and Collins, 1974a).

Case 8: Small Lymphocytic Lymphoma, T-Cell Type. An 81-year-old male was discovered to have an absolute lymphocytosis during an admission for insertion of a cardiac pacemaker. At 1 year later, there was hepatosplenomegaly with mild axillary and inguinal lymphadenopathy. The leukocyte count was 23,000, with 88% small lymphocytes that exhibited irregularly shaped nuclei. Following institution of chemotherapy, the patient abruptly expired. An autopsy revealed widespread involvement of lymph nodes, spleen, liver, and bone marrow by a proliferation of small- to medium-size lymphocytes with compact nuclear chromatin and irregular nuclear configuration [see Figure 3(1)], and a small amount of acidophilic cytoplasm. Mitoses were rare. Immunological surface-marker studies on the pretreatment peripheral blood yielded the following results:

Study	E	EAC	EA	PV	μ	γ	α	Δ	κ	λ
PB	53	—	—	0	0	0	0	0	0	0

The abnormal lymphocytes formed E rosettes in cytocentrifuge preparations.

Only a small group of cases of lymphomas of small T lymphocytes, including CLL of T cells, have been reported. These cases in general have dramatic splenomegaly and commonly show skin involvement. The number of cases is insufficient, however, to establish a distinctive clinical entity.

Case 9: Malignant Lymphoma, Convoluted T-Cell Type. A 13-year-old male was admitted with a sore throat, bleeding gums, lymphadenopathy, and groin pain. He was febrile and exhibited a generalized rash. The leukocyte count was 243,000, with 60% blasts. Hemoglobin was 12g/dl, and platelets, 4000/mm³. The marrow was diffusely involved by a proliferation of primitive-appearing "convoluted" lymphocytes [see Figure 3(2)]. Surface markers were as follows:

Study	E	EAC	EA	PV	μ	γ	α	Δ	κ	λ
PB Day 1	84	44	0	0	0	0	0	0	0	0
PB Day 2	97	65	0	0	0	0	0	0	0	0

C_3-receptor-bearing cells with fluoresceinated anti-C_3: patient, 93%; control, 16%.

The abnormal lymphocytes in both specimens formed E rosettes as seen in cytocentrifuge preparations. The cytoplasm contained PAS-positive globules and focal acid phosphatase activity.

The patient was treated initially with vincristine and prednisone for 2 months, but developed increasing lymphadenopathy without a mediastinal mass. Therapy was switched to the L_2 protocol of Wolner (Wolner et al., 1975), including prophylactic radiation to the central nervous system and mediastinum. Relapse in the CNS nevertheless occurred 8 months after onset of disease, and convoluted T cells (E-rosette-forming) were observed in the spinal fluid in cytocentrifuge preparations. Involvement of the spinal fluid persisted, despite therapy, until death 14 months after onset of the disease.

The lymphoma of convoluted T lymphocytes is a lymphoma–leukemia process that develops predominantly in children (Barcos and Lukes, 1975). It appears initially outside the bone marrow in lymph nodes or mediastinum, and subsequently involves the bone marrow diffusely, as in a leukemia. The cells form E rosettes in varying degrees. EAC rosettes are also common, and a distinctive acid phosphatase area in the Golgi region may be present. Both these features were also observed by Stein *et al.* (1976) and Catovsky *et al.* (1974). This process occurs predominantly in children or young adults, often with a male predominance. There is frequently a large mediastinal mass, and in our experience, CNS relapses are common. In the past, this entity has been included in the ALL group, though it appears that the median survival in two of our case series (Barcos and Lukes, 1975; Schneider *et al.*, 1978) is 10 months, which differs considerably from the prolonged survival in ALL. In our view, the convoluted lymphocyte of T cells interrelates with ALL of T-cell type in both children and adults. Its poor response to conventional therapy for ALL and short survival dramatically demonstrate the importance of initial recognition and separation of this cytological type from ALL and the need for development of effective therapy for this distinctive lymphoma. The recent demonstration of the dependence of T-cell-type ALL on L-asparagine (Ohnuma *et al.*, 1976) further illustrates its biological distinctiveness.

Case 10: Malignant Lymphoma, Cerebriform T Cells with Mycosis Fungoides. A 48-year-old female was in good health until she noted dry skin on her arms and breasts. The dryness became progressively worse over a 2-year period until she became aware of pruritic lumps on the skin of her face. The lumps rapidly became numerous on her forehead and cheeks, and several were noted on the areolae of her breasts.

On physical examination, enlarged cervical and axillary lymph nodes were also observed. There were no laboratory abnormalities. The skin and an axillary lymph node were biopsied. An abnormal mononuclear lymphoid infiltrate [see Figure 3(4)] extended about the dermal appendages and into the epidermis, forming Pautrier's abscesses. Mitoses were numerous. In the lymph node biopsy, a similar infiltrate extended throughout the paracortical (T-cell) region. Multiparameter studies were obtained only from the lymph node. The results on peripheral blood and lymph node were as follows:

Study	E	EAC	EA	PV	μ	γ	α	Δ	κ	λ
LN	47	2	0	32	16	7	3	14	22	17

SIg staining showed a polyclonal pattern. E-rosette-forming cells, observed in cytocentrifuge preparations, were abnormal, but resembled transformed lymphocytes. Ultrastructural studies revealed the typical cerebriform cells of mycosis fungoides and Sézary's syndrome. This initial presentation as the tumor phase of mycosis fungoides is unusual, but occurs in so-called "mycosis fungoides d'Amblé."

ROBERT J. LUKES AND
JOHN W. PARKER

Mycosis fungoides and Sézary's syndrome, the latter a chronic generalized erythroderma associated with lymphocytosis, are closely related and possibly interrelated expressions of a lymphoma–leukemia of cerebriform T cells, as suggested by Lutzner (Lutzner *et al.*, 1975). The development of this T-cell process in the skin with subsequent dissemination to lymph nodes, spleen, and other organs only late in the process demonstrates the known affinity of T cells for the skin. The recent proposal of the helper-T-cell nature of Sézary cells by Broder *et al.* (1976) suggests that the process involves an alteration of regulation of inflammatory processes in the skin.

6. Conclusions and Summary

I. The malignant lymphomas have been for decades the subject of dispute and controversy over terminology and concept as the result of the imprecision of cytological techniques and the limited understanding of basic immunology.

II. Recently, we proposed a new approach to the understanding of the malignant lymphomas, emphasizing that they are neoplasms of the immune system and relating these disorders to the T- and B-lymphocyte systems and alterations in lymphocyte transformation. A new classification was also put forth with five major groups: (1) U cell (undefined); (2) T cell; (3) B cell; (4) histiocytic; and (5) Hodgkin's disease (cell of uncertain origin).

III. A multiparameter investigative approach to the redefinition of these disorders as related to the T- and B-cell systems was outlined. These techniques include special morphology, cytochemistry, electron microscopy, immunological surface-marker techniques, *in vitro* lymphocyte transformation, and immunoperoxidase techniques for cytoplasmic Ig and muramidase localization. Our studies on over 300 cases of non-Hodgkin's lymphomas and related leukemias reveal that the majority mark as T or B cells, with the exception of a portion of ALLs and a rare case of apparently true histiocytic neoplasm. The cytomorphology of the various types is predictive of their T- and B-cell nature, but their reliability is dependent on carefully collected and prepared histological sections and an experienced observer. Of major importance is the demonstrated heterogeneity of the histological types of lymphoma in traditional classifications, particularly the diffuse lymphomas of Rappaport and ALL of childhood. In contrast, our results and those of others permit the identification of a number of new homogeneous cytological types that are emerging as clinical–morphological–immunological entities, such as the convoluted T-cell lymphoma–leukemia that interrelates with T-cell ALL, the plasmacytoid lymphocytic lymphoma that is commonly associated with monoclonal gammopathies, the cerebriform T-cell lymphoma associated with Sézary's syndrome and mycosis fungoides, the FCC lymphomas, and the IBS of B cells that commonly develops in abnormal immune disorders.

IV. The functional approach has a number of immediate and future implications. Application of the new approach by pathologists will require a change in the collection and processing of biopsy material to provide the excellent cytological detail necessary for morphological evaluation. Since the morphological features are predictive for the most part, the only new histological technique necessary for paraffin sections will be the immunoperoxidase technique for detection of cytoplasmic Ig in B cells, muramidase in histiocytes and monocytes, and other antigenic cell components that may ultimately be identified as specific markers for a particular type of lymphoma. α-Naphthyl butyrase (NSE) activity, which requires tissue imprints or frozen fresh tissue, remains the most effective method for identifying histiocytes and monocytes, and will be useful in the redefinition of the varied expressions of the histiocyte-monocyte neoplasms. At present, E rosettes remain essential for identifying the T-cell type of ALL, though the acid phosphatase may prove helpful. It seems likely that in the future, precise identification of T and B cells will be achieved most effectively with specific antisera. It also appears likely that subtypes of T- and B-cell lymphomas will be identified by virtue of certain retained differentiated functions such as suppressor- or helper-T-cell activity, cytotoxic activity, or lymphokine production. Recognition of these subtypes will allow understanding of their clinical expression and development of meaningful therapy.

V. Identification of homogeneous cytological types of T- and B-cell lymphomas and clinical–morphological entities permits investigation of the basic biological mechanisms, and ultimately it will lead to the design of more fundamental biological approaches to therapy.

References

Aisenberg, A. C., and Long, J. C., 1975, Lymphocyte surface characteristics in malignant lymphoma, *Am. J. Med.* **58**:300–306.

Anagnostou, D., Parker, J. W., Taylor, C. R., Tindle, B. H., and Lukes, R. J., 1977, Lacunar cells of nodular sclerosing Hodgkin's disease: An ultrastructural and immunohistologic study, *Cancer* **39**:1032–1043.

Bain, B., Vas, M. R., and Lowenstein, L., 1964, The development of large immature mononuclear cells in mixed lymphocyte cultures, *Blood* **23**:108–116.

Barcos, M. P., and Lukes, R. J., 1975, Malignant lymphoma of convoluted lymphocytes: A new entity of possible T-cell type, in: *Conflicts in Childhood Cancer* (L. F. Sinks, and J. O. Godden, eds.), pp. 147–178, Alan R. Liss, New York.

Bennett, M. H., and Millet, Y. L., 1969, Nodular sclerotic lymphosarcoma: A possible new clinicopathological entity, *Clin. Radiol.* **20**:339–343.

Bennett, M. H., Farrer-Brown, G., Henry, K., and Jelliffe, A. M., 1974, Classification of non-Hodgkin's lymphomas, *Lancet* **2**:405.

Berard, C., O'Connor, G. T., Thomas, L. B., and Torloni, H., 1969, Histopathologic definition of Burkitt's tumour, *Bull. W. H. O.* **40**:601–607.

Berard, C. W., Gallo, R. C., Jaffe, E., Green, I., and Devita, V. T., 1976, Current concepts of leukemia and lymphoma: Etiology, pathogenesis and therapy, *Ann. Intern. Med.* **85**:351–366.

Berger, N. A., and Skinner, A. M., 1974, Characterization of lymphocyte transformation induced by zinc ions, *J. Cell Biol.* **61**:45–55.

Bhattacharyza, J. R., 1975, Terminal deoxyribonucleotidyl transferase in human leukemia, *Biochem. Biophys. Res. Commun.* **62**:367.

Boldt, D. H., Speckart, S. R., MacDermott, R. P., Nash, G. S., and Valeski, J. E., 1977, Leukemic reticuloendotheliosis: "Hairy cell leukemia," functional and structural features of the abnormal cell in a patient with profound leukocytosis, *Blood* **49**:745–757.

Braylan, R. C., Jaffe, E. S., and Berard, C. W., 1975, Malignant lymphomas: Current classifications and new observations, in: *Pathology Annual*, Vol. 10 (S. C. Sommers, ed.), pp. 213–270, Appleton-Century-Crofts, New York.

Brochier, J., Bona, C., Ciorbaru, R., Revillard, J. P., and Chedid, L., 1976, A human T-independent B lymphocyte mitogen extracted from *Nocardia opaca*, *J. Immunol.* **117**:1434–1439.

Broder, S., Edelson, R. L., Lutzner, M. A., Nelson, D. L., MacDermott, R. P., Durm, M. E., Goldman,

C. K., Meade, B. D., and Waldmann, T. A., 1976, The Sézary syndrome—A malignant proliferation of helper T cells, *J. Clin. Invest.* **58**:1297–1306.

Brouet, J., LaBaume, S., and Seligmann, M., 1975, Evaluation of T and B lymphocyte membrane markers in human non-Hodgkin's malignant lymphomas, *Br. J. Cancer* **31**(Suppl. 2):121–127.

Caron, G. A., Poutala, S., and Provost, T. T., 1970, Lymphocyte transformation induced by inorganic and organic mercury, *Int. Arch. Allergy Appl. Immunol.* **37**:76–87.

Catovsky, D., Galetto, J., Okos, A., Milliani, E., and Galton, D. A. G., 1974, Cytochemical profile of B and T leukaemic lymphocytes with special reference to acute lymphoblastic leukaemia, *J. Clin. Pathol.* **27**:767–771.

Collins, R. D., and Lukes, R. J., 1971, Studies on possible derivation of some malignant lymphomas from follicular center cells, *Am. J. Pathol.* **62**:63a.

Davey, F. R., Goldberg, J., Stockman, J., and Gottlieb, A. J., 1976, Immunologic and cytochemical cell markers in non-Hodgkin's lymphomas, *Lab. Invest.* **35**:430–438.

Dorfman, R. F., 1974, Classification of non-Hodgkin's lymphomas, *Lancet* **1**:1295.

Dutcher, T. F., and Fahey, J. L., 1959, The histopathology of the macroglobulinemia of Waldenström, *J. Natl. Cancer Inst.* **22**:887–916.

Gajl-Peczalska, K. J., Bloomfield, C. D., Coccia, P. F., Sosin, H., Brunning, R. D., and Kersey, J. H., 1975, B and T cell lymphomas, *Am. J. Med.* **59**:674–685.

Gall, E. A., 1958, The reticulum cell: The cytological identity and interrelation of mesenchymal cells of lymphoid tissue, *Ann. N.Y. Acad. Sci.* **73**:120–130.

Gerard-Merchant, R., Hamlin, I., Lennert, K., Rilke, F., Stansfeld, A. G., and Van Unnik, J. A. M., 1974, Classification of non-Hodgkin's lymphomas, *Lancet* **2**:406.

Good, R. A., and Finstad, J., 1968, The association of lymphoid malignancy and immunologic functions, in: *Proceedings of the International Conference on Leukemia–Lymphoma* (C. J. D. Zarafonetis, ed.), pp. 175–197, Lea & Febiger, Philadelphia.

Gordon, I. L., Lukes, R. J., O'Brien, R. L., Parker, J. W., Rembaum, A., Russell, R., and Taylor, C. R., 1977, Visualization of surface immunoglobulin of human B lymphocytes using microsphere-immunoglobulin conjugates in Giemsa stained preparations, *Clin. Immunol. Immunopathol.* **8**:51–63.

Graham, R. C., Jr., and Karnovsky, M. J., 1966, The early stages of absorption of injected horseradish peroxidase in the proximal tubules of mouse kidney: Ultrastructural cytochemistry by a new technique, *J. Histochem. Cytochem.* **14**:291–302.

Green, I., Jaffe, E., Shevach, E. M., Edelson, R. L., Frank, M. M., and Berard, C. W., 1975, Determination of the origin of malignant reticular cells by the use of surface membrane markers, in: *The Reticuloendothelial System*, International Academy of Pathology Monograph No. 16 (J. W. Rebuck, C. W. Berard, and M. R. Abell, eds.), pp. 282–300, Williams and Wilkins Co., Baltimore.

Hansen, J. A., and Good, R. A., 1974, Malignant disease of the lymphoid system in immunologic perspective, *Hum. Pathol.* **5**:567–599.

Hovi, T., Allison, A. C., and Williams, S. C., 1976, Proliferation of human peripheral blood lymphocytes induced by A23187, a *Streptomyces* antibiotic, *Exp. Cell Res.* **97**:92–100.

Hungerford, D. A., Donnelly, A. J., Nowell, P. C., and Beck, S., 1959, The chromosome constitution of a human phenotypic intersex, *Am. J. Hum. Genet.* **11**:215–236.

Hutton, J. J., and Coleman, M. S., 1975, Terminal deoxyribonucleotidyl transferase in adult leukemia, *Blood* **46**:1043.

Jondal, M., Holm, G., and Wigzell, H., 1972, Surface markers on human T and B lymphocytes, *J. Exp. Med.* **136**:207–215.

Jones, S. E., Fuks, Z., Bull, M., Kadin, M., Dorfman, R. F., Kaplan, H. S., Rosenberg, S. A., and Kim, H., 1973, Non-Hodgkin's lymphomas. IV. Clinico–pathologic correlation in 405 cases, *Cancer* **32**:682–691.

Kaplan, J. G., and Bona, C., 1974, Proteases as mitogens: The effect of trypsin and pronase on mouse and human lymphocytes, *Exp. Cell Res.* **88**:388–394.

Kaplan, J., Ravindranath, Y., and Peterson, W. D., 1977, Lymphocyte antigen-positive null cell leukemias, *Blood* **49**:371–378.

Kojima, M., and Tsunoda, R., 1976, Localization of immunoglobulins in germinal centers of human tonsils, in: *The Reticuloendothelial System in Health and Disease: Immunologic and Pathologic Aspects* (H. Friedman, ed.), pp. 77–86, Plenum Publishing Corp., New York.

Kunkel, H. G., 1975, Surface markers of human lymphocytes, *Johns Hopkins Med. J.* **137**:216–223.

Leech, J., Glick, A., Horn, R., and Collins, R., 1975, Immunologic, histochemical and ultrastructural studies of malignant lymphomas presumed to be of follicular center cell origin, *J. Natl. Cancer Inst.* **54**:11–21.

Lennert, K., and Mestdagh, J., 1968, Lymphogranulomatosen mit konstant hohem Epitheloidzellgehalt, *Virchows Arch. Pathol. Anat. Physiol.* **344**:1–20.

Lennert, K., Mohri, N., Stein, H., and Kaiserling, E., 1975, The histopathology of malignant lymphomas, *Br. J. Haematol.* **31**(Suppl. 2):193–203.

Lillie, R. D., and Fullmer, H. M., 1976, *Histopathologic Technic and Practical Histochemistry*, 4th Ed., pp. 52–53, McGraw-Hill, New York.

Long, J. C., and Aisenberg, A. C., 1975, Richter's syndrome: A terminal complication of chronic lymphocytic leukemia with distinct clinicopathologic features, *Am. J. Clin. Pathol.* **63**:786–795.

Lukes, R. J., 1968, The pathological picture of the malignant lymphomas, in: *Proceedings of the International Conference on Leukemia–Lymphoma* (C. J. D. Zarafonetis, ed.), pp. 333–356, Lea & Febiger, Philadelphia.

Lukes, R. J., 1971, Criteria for involvement of lymph node, bone marrow, spleen and liver in Hodgkin's disease, *Cancer Res.* **31**:1755–1767.

Lukes, R. J., and Collins, R. D., 1973, New observations on follicular lymphoma, in: *Gann Monogr. Cancer Res. 15: Malignant Diseases of the Hematopoietic System* (K. Akazaki *et al.*, eds.), pp. 209–215, University Park Press, Baltimore—London—Tokyo.

Lukes, R. J., and Collins, R. D., 1974a, Immunologic characterization of human malignant lymphomas, *Cancer* **34**:1488–1503.

Lukes, R. J., and Collins, R. D., 1974b, A functional approach to the classification of malignant lymphoma, *Recent Results Cancer Res.* **46**:18–30.

Lukes, R. J., and Collins, R. D., 1975, New approaches to the classification of the lymphomata, *Br. J. Cancer* **31**(Suppl. 2):1–28.

Lukes, R. J., and Collins, R. D., 1977, The Lukes–Collins classification and its significance, Conference on the Non-Hodgkin's Lymphomas, San Francisco, September 30–October 2, 1976, in: *Cancer Treatment Rep.* **61**:971–979.

Lukes, R. J., and Tindle, B. H., 1975, Immunoblastic lymphadenopathy: A hyperimmune entity resembling Hodgkin's disease, *N. Engl. J. Med.* **292**:1–8.

Lukes, R. J., Craver, L. L., Hall, T. C., Rappaport, H., and Ruben, P., 1966a, Hodgkin's disease: Report of Nomenclature Committee, *Cancer Res.* **26**:1311.

Lukes, R. J., Butler, J. J., and Hicks, E. B., 1966b, Natural history of Hodgkin's disease as related to its pathologic picture, *Cancer* **19**:317–344.

Lukes, R. J., Tindle, B. H., and Parker, J. W., 1969, Reed–Sternberg-like cells in infectious mononucleosis, *Lancet* **2**:1003–1004.

Lutzner, M., Edelson, R., Schein, P., Green, I., Kirkpatrick, C., and Ahmed, A., 1975, Cutaneous T cell lymphoma: The Sézary syndrome, mycosis fungoides and related disorders, *Ann. Intern. Med.* **85**:534–552.

Maino, V. C., Green, N. M., and Crumpton, M. J., 1974, The role of calcium ions in initiating transformation of lymphocytes, *Nature (London)* **251**:324–327.

Mann, R. B., Jaffe, E. S., Braylan, R. C., Nanba, K., Frank, M. M., Ziegler, J. L., and Berard, C. W., 1976, Non-endemic Burkitt's lymphoma: A B-cell tumor related to germinal centers, *N. Engl. J. Med.* **295**:685–691.

Mason, D. Y., and Taylor, C. R., 1975, The distribution of muramidase (lysozyme) in human tissues, *J. Clin. Pathol.* **28**:124.

McCaffrey, A., Smoler, D. F., and Baltimore, D., 1973, Terminal deoxynucleotidyl transferases in a case of childhood acute lymphoblastic leukaemia, *Proc. Natl. Acad. Sci. U.S.A.* **70**:521–525.

Nossal, G. J. V., Abbot, A., Mitchell, J., and Lummus, Z., 1968, Antigens in immunity. XV. Ultrastructural features of antigen capture in primary and secondary lymphoid follicles, *J. Exp. Med.* **127**:277–289.

Nowell, P. C., 1960, Phytohemagglutinin: An initiator of mitosis in cultures of normal human leukocytes, *Cancer Res.* **20**:462–466.

O'Brien, R. L., and Parker, J. W., 1976, Oxidation-induced lymphocyte transformation: A review, *Cell* **7**:13–20.

O'Brien, R. L., Parker, J. W., and Dixon, J. F. P., 1978, Mechanisms of lymphocyte transformation, in: *Progress in Molecular and Subcellular Biology*, Vol. 6 (F. Hahn, ed.), Springer-Verlag, Berlin—Heidelberg—New York (in press).

Ohnuma, T., Orlowski, M., Minowada, J., and Holland, J. F., 1976, Differences in amino acid metabolism of human T- and B-cells in culture, presented at the Proceedings of the 16th International Congress of Hematology, Kyoto, Japan, September 5–11, 1976.

Oppenheim, J. J., and Rosenstreich, D. L., 1976, Signals regulating *in vitro* activation of lymphocytes, *Prog. Allergy* **20**:65–194.

Order, S. E., and Hellman, S., 1972, Pathogenesis of Hodgkin's disease, *Lancet* **1**;571–573.

Parker, J. W., Steiner, J., Coffin, A., Lukes, R. J., Burr, K., and Brilliantine, L., 1969, Blastomitogenic agents in Leguminosae and other families, *Experientia* **25**:187–188.

Parker, J. W., Royston, A. I., Pattengale, P., Taylor, C. R., Tindle, B. H., Cain, M. J., and Lukes, R. J., 1978, Morphological differences between cultured human B and T lymphoblastoid cell lines: A light and electron microscopic and cytochemical study, *J. Natl. Cancer Inst.* **60**(in press).

Pearmain, G., Lycette, R. R., and Fitzgerald, P. H., 1963, Tuberculin-induced mitosis in peripheral blood leucocytes, *Lancet* **1**:637–638.

Preud'homme, J. L., and Seligmann, M., 1974, Surface immunoglobulins on human lymphoid cells, *Prog. Clin. Immunol.* **2**:121–174.

Rappaport, R., Winter, W. J., and Hicks, E. B., 1956, Follicular lymphoma: Re-evaluation of its position in the scheme of malignant lymphoma, based on survey of 253 cases, *Cancer* **9**:792–821.

Riccardi, A., Piazza, R., and Perugini, S., 1976, Deoxyribonucleic acid content of cleaved and non-cleaved cells in follicular center cell lymphomas: A cytofluorometric study, *Haematologica* **61**:170–183.

Richter, M. N., 1928, Generalized reticular cell sarcoma of lymph nodes associated with lymphatic leukemia, *Am. J. Pathol.* **4**:285–292.

Rosen, P. J., Feinstein, D. I., Bonorris, J. M., Parker, J. W., Pattengale, P. K., Tindle, B. H., and Lukes, R. J., 1975, Convoluted lymphocytic (T-cell) lymphoma: A distinct clinical–pathologic entity, Annual Meeting of the American Society of Hematology, Dallas, Texas, Dec. 8, 1975 (abstract).

Schlossman, S. F., Chess, L., Humphreys, R. E., and Strominger, J. L., 1976, Distribution of Ia-like molecules on the surface of normal and leukemic human cells, *Proc. Natl. Acad. Sci. U.S.A.* **73**:1288–1292.

Schneider, B. K., Higgins, G. R., Swanson, V., Isaacs, H., Tindle, B. H., and Lukes, R. J., 1978, Malignant lymphomas of childhood (submitted).

Schöpf, E., Schulz, K. H., and Grom, M., 1967, Transformationen und Mitosen von Lymphocyten *in vitro* durch Quecksilber (II)-chlorid, *Naturwissenschaften* **54**:568–569.

Stein, H., Peterson, N., Gaedicke, G., Lennert, K., and Landberg, C., 1976, Lymphoblastic lymphoma of convoluted or acid phosphatase type—A tumor of T precursor cells, *Int. J. Cancer* **17**:292–295.

Taylor, C. R., 1976a, An immunohistological study of follicular lymphoma, reticulum cell sarcoma and Hodgkin's disease, *Eur. J. Cancer* **12**:61–75.

Taylor, C. R., 1976b, *Hodgkin's Disease and the Lymphomas, Annual Research Reviews* (D. F. Horrobin, ed.), Eden Press, Montreal.

Taylor, C. R., and Mason, D. Y., 1974, The immunohistological detection of intracellular immunoglobulin in formalin–paraffin sections from multiple myeloma and related conditions using the immunoperoxidase technique, *Clin. Exp. Immunol.* **18**:417–429.

Taylor, C. R., Gordon, I. L., Rembaum, A., Russell, R., Parker, J. W., O'Brien, R. L., and Lukes, R. J., 1977, Human B lymphocytes in Giemsa stained preparations, *J. Immunol. Methods* **17**:81–89.

Tindle, B. H., Parker, J. W., and Lukes, R. J., 1972, "Reed–Sternberg cells" in infectious mononucleosis?, *Am. J. Clin. Pathol.* **58**:607–617.

Toyoshima, S., Osawa, T., and Tonomura, A., 1970, Some properties of purified phytohemagglutinin from *Lens culinaris* seeds, *Biochim. Biophys. Acta* **21**:514–521.

Vischer, T. L., 1974, Stimulation of mouse B lymphocytes by trypsin, *J. Immunol.* **113**:58–62.

Waxdal, M. J., and Basham, T. Y., 1974, B and T-cell stimulatory activities of multiple mitogens from pokeweed, *Nature (London)* **251**:163–164.

Weinstein, Y., Chambers, D. A., Bourne, H. R., and Melmon, K. L., 1974, Cyclic GMP stimulates lymphocyte nucleic acid synthesis, *Nature (London)* **251**:352–353.

Weinstein, Y., Segal, S., and Melmon, K. L., 1975, Specific mitogenic activity of 8-Br-guanosine 3′,5′-monophosphate (Br-cyclic GMP) on B lymphocytes, *J. Immunol.* **115**:112–117.

Wolner, N., Lieberman, P., Exelby, P., Dongio, G., Burcheval, J., Fang, S., and Murphy, M. L., 1975, Non-Hodgkin's lymphoma in children: Results of treatment with LSA-L protocol, *Br. J. Cancer* **31**(Suppl. 2):337.

Yam, L. T., Li, C. Y., and Crosby, W. H., 1971a, Cytochemical identification of monocytes and granulocytes, *Am. J. Clin. Pathol.* **55**:283–290.

Yam, L. T., Li, C. Y., and Lam, K. W., 1971b, Tartrate resistant acid phosphatase isoenzyme in the reticulum cells of leukemic reticuloendotheliosis, *N. Engl. J. Med.* **284**:357–360.

Yeckley, J. A., Weston, W. L., Thorne, G., and Kruger, G. G., 1975, Production of Sézary-like cells from normal human lymphocytes, *Arch. Dermatol.* **111**:29–32.

Yoshida, T., Edelson, R., Cohen, S., and Green, I., 1975, Migration inhibitory activity in serum and cell supernatants in patients with Sézary syndrome, *J. Immunol.* **114**:915–918.

10

Cytoidentity of the Lymphoreticular Neoplasms

FREDERICK P. SIEGAL

1. Introduction*

The motile mononuclear cells present in the tissues of man are functionally, morphologically, and developmentally heterogeneous. Despite this variety, it had not been possible to discriminate among normal or malignant mononuclear cells via conventional morphological and cytochemical approaches, and thus there is a continuing controversy over classification of the lymphomas (Dorfman, 1974). Schemes for the reclassification of neoplasms of these cells as proposed by Lukes and Collins (1974) and by Lennert *et al.* (1975) have depended on the recognition, based largely on morphological considerations, that cells participating in the lymphoproliferative diseases are counterparts of normal cells found in certain areas of normal lymph nodes. This recognition, in turn, depended heavily on certain developments of modern immunology, which demonstrated that normal lymphocytes were functionally divisible into several groups, and that these groups could be identified on the basis of characteristic markers of differentiation.

*Abbreviations used in this chapter: (ALL) Acute lymphoblastic leukemia; (CLL) chronic lymphocytic leukemia; (Con A) concanavalin A; (DPDL) diffuse, poorly differentiated lymphocytic lymphoma; (DWDL) diffuse, well-differentiated lymphocytic lymphoma; (EA) erythrocyte–antibody complex; (EAC) antibody- and complement-coated erythrocytes (utilized in rosetting assays); (EBV) Epstein–Barr virus; (EM) electron microscopy; (FCC) follicular center cell; (FcR) Fc receptor; (Ig) immunoglobulin; (IgGEA) IgG-coated erythrocytes; (IgMEAC) IgM- and complement-coated erythrocytes (=EAC); (MRFC) mouse rosette-forming cells; (NH) nodular histiocytic lymphoma; (PBL) peripheral blood lymphocytes; (PHA) phytohemagglutinin; (PWM) pokeweed mitogen; (RFC) rosette-forming cells; (SEM) scanning electron microscopy; (SIg) surface immunoglobulin; (SRBC) sheep erythrocytes; (TdT) terminal deoxynucleotidyltransferase; (TEM) transmission electron microscopy.

FREDERICK P. SIEGAL • Memorial Sloan-Kettering Cancer Center, New York, New York 10021.

Reif and Allen (1964) recognized an antigen present on murine thymocytes, some peripheral blood splenic and lymph node lymphocytes, in nervous system tissue, and in some murine leukemias. Boyse, Old, and their colleagues (for a review, see Boyse and Bennett, 1974) termed these and several other cell-surface antigens *differentiation antigens*, since they appeared to discriminate among developmental stages of cells that were morphologically indistinguishable. For example, the antigen described by Reif and Allen, now known as *Thy-1* (formerly theta), is absent from certain lymphoid cells that, on gaining entry to the thymus, express large amounts of the antigen. As these cells pass out of the thymus following one or several differentiative steps, the density of that antigen on the cell surface decreases. The peripheral thymus-derived cell retains the lesser amount for its life span. Thy-1 is consequently a T-cell differentiation marker, one of the several described in the mouse (Boyse and Bennett, 1974). Two subgroups of murine lymphoid cells, one carrying Thy-1 and the other surface immunoglobulin and a receptor for complement, have been recognized (Raff, 1970; Bianco and Nussenzweig, 1971).

Meanwhile, developments in human immunobiology and in extensive experimental work on lymphoid differentiation, particularly in the chicken (see Chapter 1), led to the beginnings of an understanding of the cellular basis of the older terms *delayed-type hypersensitivity* and *humoral immunity*. The former term was associated with cells passing through the thymus, and localized in the deep cortical areas of lymph nodes (see Chapter 11), now known as *T lymphocytes*. On the other hand, the plasma cells, producing antibodies, were recognized as originating as lymphoid cells in the yolk sac and fetal liver and differentiating through an inducing environment. In avian species, this milieu is provided by the bursa of Fabricius, but in mammals, it remains undefined. These lymphocytes, which are capable of differentiating into plasma cells on appropriate antigenic stimulation, have been termed *B cells* because of their apparent derivation in bone marrow in mammals. They too have a characteristic localization, particularly in the germinal centers of lymph nodes.

The convergence of functional and cell-surface analyses has culminated in the last five years in the development of differentiation markers for lymphoid and other mononuclear cells in man, as well as in many experimental animals. These markers, and their application to the classification of the lymphoreticular malignancies, are the subject of this chapter.

2. Identification of Mononuclear Cell Populations

2.1. Cell-Surface Markers

The definition of mononuclear cells can be accomplished in a number of ways. Because of the rapid recent proliferation of cell-surface-marker techniques, these methods have tended to take precedence over some of the more traditional approaches to classification, such as "functional" characterizations (e.g., responses to mitogens, phagocytic ability, capacity to act in cell-mediated cytotoxic reactions). Since the earliest applications of lymphocyte cell-surface markers in humans (Klein *et al.*, 1968; Pernis *et al.*, 1971; Papamichail *et al.*, 1971; Cooper, M. D., *et al.*, 1971; Siegal *et al.*, 1971; Grey *et al.*, 1971; Wilson and Nossal, 1971; Frøland *et al.*, 1971), considerable advances have been made, particularly in the range of techniques available and the sophistication with which they are applied. Several excellent reviews on cell-surface markers in man and in experimental animals (Preud'homme and Seligmann, 1974; Greaves *et al.*, 1973; Möller, 1973) and a symposium (Seligmann *et al.*, 1975) have been published.

2.1.1. Cell-Surface Immunoglobulin

Immunoglobulins (Ig) on lymphoid cells have been convincingly shown to provide the receptor for antigen, conferring on a particular lymphocyte its specificity for particular antigenic determinants (reviewed by Vitetta and Uhr, 1975). Although Ig's are readily detected on B lymphocytes as indeed the hallmark of those cells (Pernis *et al.*, 1971), considerable debate has raged concerning their presence on T cells (Uhr and Vitetta, 1973). While the question is still incompletely resolved, evidence has accumulated from several laboratories (Binz and Wigzell, 1975; Eichmann and Rajewsky, 1975) that T-cell antigen receptors are quire similar to those on B cells, at least in the area of the combining site. The chief evidence that they are is the finding of idiotypic antigenic determinants present on both B and T cells in appropriately immunized animals. Idiotypic antigens are those peculiar to the regions of Ig molecules that comprise the combining site. They are unique to a particular antibody, or to the Ig products of a single clone. Despite the debate, the detection of intrinsic surface immunoglobulin (SIg) in man has, as a rule, been limited to cells of the B-lymphocyte line. except in certain complex situations discussed below. Consequently, malignant lymphoid cells that bear SIg have generally been regarded as B cells. For the most part, this conclusion has been justified.

Lymphocyte SIg has most commonly been detected by immunofluorescence (Pernis *et al.*, 1970; Siegal *et al.*, 1971; Grey *et al.*, 1971; Cooper, M. D., *et al.*, 1971; Papamichail *et al.*, 1971; Preud'homme and Seligmann, 1972a–c; Klein *et al.*, 1968; Aisenberg and Bloch, 1972), and generally by direct immunofluorescence, whereby a fluorochrome-conjugated antiserum is reacted directly with living cells. Mixed cell agglutination has also been used to detect SIg: erythrocytes coated with the Ig to be detected are mixed with lymphocytes and with an antiserum specific for the Ig in question; lymphoid cells bearing the relevant Ig determinants are coagglutinated with the coated erythrocytes and form rosettes (Hallberg *et al.*, 1973a). This methodology has certain advantages over immunofluorescence, in that it does not require a fluorescence microscope. Both cytotoxicity (Wernet *et al.*, 1972) and radioautography (Wilson and Nossal, 1971) have been employed on occasion to detect SIg. Additionally, immunoperoxidase techniques lend themselves to demonstration of SIg, especially since they can be applied to both light and electron microscopy; while sharing certain of the advantages of immunofluorescence, particularly sensitivity, they too avoid the necessity for highly specialized equipment.

Because immunofluorescence has been the mainstay of detection of cell-surface Ig in most clinical studies, the problems associated with it will be discussed in some depth. They deserve emphasis inasmuch as the literature on cell-surface markers has been greatly complicated by a lack of general appreciation of the pitfalls of immunofluorescence. These difficulties center mostly around specificity of reagents and the nature of the SIg detected by the reagents. The variety of difficulties encountered in the use of immunofluorescence of the detection of cell-surface antigens, especially of Ig's, was recently reviewed by Aiuti *et al.* (1974) and Preud'homme and Labaume (1975).

Questions of specificity of reagents present a major problem. Commercially available fluorescent antisera are often not truly specific; all need careful specificity testing, both at the cell surface and by cytoplasmic staining, through the use of plasma cells of known Ig heavy chain and light chain, or by staining purified Ig covalently bound to agarose beads. Screening of an antiserum for specificity by using gel precipitation methods is insufficiently sensitive if the antiserum is ultimately to be used in immunofluorescence. One problem that occasionally arises is that truly specific antisera behave as if they were nonspecific when used to detect Ig on the surface of cells that carry Fc receptors (FcRs).

Since B cells and most other non-T mononuclear cells have such receptors (Dickler and Kunkel, 1972; Dickler, 1974; Huber et al., 1969; Frøland and Natvig, 1973), this lack of specificity has been a significant problem. The fault appears to lie, in part, in the common tendency of fluoresceinated antisera to aggregate; the aggregated γ-globulins in the reagents adhere nonspecifically to cells with FcRs. Two methods can be used to overcome this difficulty: (1) antisera can be deaggregated by centrifugation or by filtration or (2) they can be rendered nonadherent by pepsin digestion and use of only the F(ab')₂ fragments (Winchester et al., 1974). The latter procedure is the only sure way to eliminate the adherence to FcRs of immune complexes formed at the cell surface between the reagent and loosely associated (adherent rather than intrinsic?) Ig (see below). Additional sources of error include immune complexes present in the antisera as a result of absorption with soluble antigens to achieve specificity. Sera used in immunofluorescence must consequently be absorbed on insolubilized antigens (Cuatrecasas, 1970).

There are certain situations in which cell-surface Ig is not intrinsic to the cell on which it is found. This can occur if antilymphocyte antibodies, immune complexes, or rheumatoid factors are present in the serum of the cell donor (Winchester et al., 1974; Winfield et al., 1975; Grifoni et al., 1975). In this case, unlike that in which the reagents are aggregated or complexed, the Ig is really present on the cells, as SIg, but its presence does not signify that the cell is a B lymphocyte. Such cell-bound Ig can lead to inappropriate conclusions in terms of the proportion of B or T cells, or of the class of SIg found. Elimination of this passively bound anti-cell Ig is relatively easy, requiring brief incubation at 37°C in the absence of serum, often for a few hours or overnight. Trypsinization and resynthesis of SIg (Osunkoya et al., 1969; Preud'homme and Seligmann, 1972c; Siegal et al., 1975) is another approach that has been employed to prove the intrinsic nature of the cell-surface Ig. This is especially important when lymphoproliferative disorders are characterized by the presence of several SIg classes (e.g., Papamichail et al., 1971; Piessens et al., 1973), since most careful studies that have employed short-term culture or trypsinization–resynthesis (Preud'homme and Seligmann, 1972c; Leech et al., 1975) have concluded that the vast majority of B-cell lymphoproliferative states are characterized by a single (monoclonal) heavy- and light-chain SIg. The presence of antibodies directed against the malignant cells may be suspected when a polyclonal staining pattern is observed (Preud'homme and Seligmann, 1974; Winfield et al., 1975), although a few apparently bona fide polyclonal cell-surface Ig patterns have survived the rigors of trypsinization and long-term culture (Preud'homme and Seligmann, 1972c; Leech et al., 1975). The explanation for such findings is not known.

Still another source of nonintrinsic SIg, which has been less of a problem with the lymphoproliferative states than with polyclonal lymphoid abnormal states and with normals, is the binding by lymphoid cells of serum IgG, through their Fc receptors. Originally, SIg on normal human cells was reported on a large proportion of cells from peripheral blood, with averages sometimes as high as 35%. As soon as it was recognized that monocytes, with their receptors for IgG Fc (Huber *et al.,* 1969), were included because of adherent IgG, the proportion of Ig-bearing "lymphocytes" reported fell (Aiuti *et al.,* 1974). There nevertheless remained a significant proportion of IgG-bearing lymphocytes in the peripheral blood, although the proportion reported varied markedly from laboratory to laboratory. The IgG-positive lymphocytes tended to have a more "clumpy" SIg (Kumagai *et al.,* 1975) than did cells bearing SIgM. In contrast to human cells, most rabbit B lymphocytes bore SIgM (Pernis *et al.,* 1970). Similarly, Vitetta and Uhr (1975) were unable to detect SIgG on mouse lymphoid cells. The large proportion of IgG-positive cells in normal human peripheral blood lymphocytes (PBL) was also in sharp contrast to the rarity of IgG-bearing chronic lymphocytic leukemia cells (Preud'homme and Seligmann, 1972c, 1974). Winchester *et al.* (1975a), Horwitz and Lobo (1975), and Kumagai *et al.* (1975) showed that the SIgG on most or many IgG-positive non-T lymphocytes was adherent through their FcRs. The cells bearing labile, or FcR-dependent, SIgG have been shown to coincide generally with non-B, non-T, lymphoid-appearing, nonphagocytic cells described as the *third population* by Frøland and Natvig (1973) and as *null cells* by Schlossman and his collaborators (Chess *et al.,* 1975). These lymphoid cells, which do not carry intrinsic SIg but may have other characteristics of B cells (FcRs or complement receptors or both), are probably a heterogeneous group, including cells participating in antibody-dependent cell-mediated cytotoxicity (*K cells*) (Revillard *et al.,* 1975; Perlmann *et al.,* 1972), precursors of B cells (Siegal *et al.,* 1975), some T cells (Moretta *et al.,* 1975), and nonphagocytic monocytes (Hayward and Greaves, 1975; Greaves *et al.,* 1975a; Greenberg *et al.,* 1973). The existence of such cells has provoked considerable interest, since they constitute about 10% of human PBL; it is of some note that so far no lymphoproliferative state has been clearly identified as their counterpart.

SIgG is often detected as a membrane component of these non-B, non-T cells, apparently because their FcRs are more effective in binding IgG than are those of the B cells (Kurnick and Grey, 1975). Under certain circumstances, notably in the blood of infants (Siegal, 1976), B-cell FcRs also appear to be capable of binding IgG avidly, which can complicate the analysis of SIg on B cells. Additionally, if the IgM present on the B-cell surface has measurable antibody activity against IgG, as in certain cases of mixed cryoglobulinemia (Preud'homme and Seligmann, 1972b; Siegal and Winchester, 1972), both IgG and IgM may appear on the same malignant clone, the IgG being bound not by the FcRs but by the IgM antigen receptors on the malignant cells.

SIg may be quantitated by radioimmunoassay (Grey *et al.,* 1972), by hemagglutination-inhibition (Cooper, A. G., *et al.,* 1973), or by fluorescence intensity (Aisenberg and Bloch, 1972). Membrane Ig quantitation is complicated by the fact that certain antisera may recognize primarily Ig determinants that are ordinarily submerged in the lipid membrane, and thus give relatively little fluorescence on cells having those determinants "buried." Differences in fluorescence intensity may nevertheless really reflect the amount of SIg on or in the membrane. The loss of Thy-1 fluorescence intensity in T cell maturation (Raff, 1970) provides a precedent for this. Staining brightness may prove to be an important discriminant of different groups of B-cell proliferations (Aisenberg and Bloch, 1972).

The detection of SIg and its careful delineation has provided an important tool for the study of lymphoproliferative disease, which in turn has become a crucial model for the understanding of normal lymphocyte function, much as the study of myeloma proteins led the way to an understanding of Ig structure. For example, the formal proof that the IgM and IgD found on individual cells share the same Fab rests on the observation that both moieties shared identical idiotypes (Fu *et al.*, 1974) and antibody activity (Pernis *et al.*, 1974) when present on monoclonal lymphoid proliferations. Similarly, the demonstration that shared idiotypy between the monoclonal proteins in a diclonal gammopathy was reflected on the cell surfaces in that disease (Rudders and Ross, 1975) has provided further evidence for the "switch" (Pernis *et al.*, 1971) from production of one to another Ig constant-region gene in human lymphoid cells. Such studies have confirmed that Ig synthesis in a single cell is capable of switching between heavy-chain constant-region genes while maintaining the same heavy- and light-chain variable-region genes.

Current evidence appears to indicate that, as in the mouse and rabbit, human B cells (plasma-cell precursors) carry intrinsic Ig that is largely IgM and IgD. Usually, both these classes appear on the same cells (Rowe *et al.*, 1973; Ferrarini *et al.*, 1975; Vossen and Hijmans, 1975; Siegal, 1976; Kubo *et al.*, 1974), although some B cells apparently express only one of the two classes. The functional significance of this double expression is not yet apparent, although several hypotheses have been advanced (Vitetta and Uhr, 1975). IgM is now thought to be the primordial Ig, appearing first in ontogeny in both mouse and man (Vitetta and Uhr, 1975; Gupta *et al.*, 1976a; Gathings *et al.*, 1976; Vossen and Hijmans, 1975). There is some indication that a few IgG-bearing cells are included in the "true B" populations, as defined by stable IgG (Horwitz and Lobo, 1975; Kumagai *et al.*, 1975) or by the ability to be stained by F(ab')$_2$ reagents (Winchester *et al.*, 1975a). These IgG B cells may account for only 1% or fewer of the PBL. Since an F(ab')$_2$ reagent might be expected to complex with and remove loosely bound membrane Ig, the significance of results obtained with short-term incubation prior to staining and those using pepsin-digested antisera may be the same. There is some additional evidence (Siegal, 1976; Winchester *et al.*, 1975a) that short-term incubation or use of F(ab')$_2$ reagents can also reduce SIgM and SIgA staining to a certain extent. The role of IgA-bearing cells is not yet clear, although gut-associated lymphoid tissue has many IgA-bearing cells (Vitetta and Uhr, 1975). The recent demonstration of a receptor for secretory component on porcine lymphocytes may add to current suspicion about IgA-bearing cells (Setcavage *et al.*, 1976).

Additional problems with FcRs of various types that appear on various hematopoietic and lymphoid cells are discussed in the next section.

2.1.2. Fc Receptors

Cells of several types have sites that can react to varying degrees with the Fc portions of Ig molecules. Huber *et al.* (1969) showed that monocytes can form rosettes with IgG-coated erythrocytes. Other cells capable of binding IgG Fc include granulocytes, eosinophils (Gupta *et al.*, 1976b), and some tumor cells (Tönder *et al.*, 1974). Certain lymphoid cells can bind Fc of IgG (Dickler and Kunkel, 1972; Frøland and Natvig, 1973; Frøland *et al.*, 1974). Originally, such cells were generally regarded as B cells, although the proof of this was not rigorous. Recent work, which was discussed in the preceding section, has indicated that at least two major groups of human PBL have FcRs of varying apparent avidity. There is some evidence that activated murine T cells and human T cells can also express FcRs for IgG (Dickler, 1974). More recent work indicates that certain T cells can bind IgM as well (Webb and Cooper, 1973; Moretta et al., 1975), and that these T cells may be functionally discrete from those that can bind IgG (Moretta et al., 1976). The IgM reported to be present on human T cells after incubation in AB serum (Whiteside and Rabin, 1976) may be a reflection of this phenomenon.

FcRs have been detected in several ways. Rosette formation (mixed agglutination) was effectively employed by Haegert et al. (1974), who used ox cells coated with IgG antibody to bovine erythrocytes as the indicator (Hallberg et al., 1973b). This indicator labeled most of the FcR-positive mononuclear cells. Such antierythrocyte antibodies presumably recognize multiple antigenic determinants on erythrocytes and provide a relatively heavy coat of poorly agglutinating antibody, and a densely packed array of Fc pieces to react with nucleated-cell FcRs. Similar results were obtained by Dickler and Kunkel (1972), using heat-aggregated human IgG conjugated to fluorochromes as the detection system. This immune-complex-like aggregate provides concentrations of Fc pieces apparently similar to those achieved by the ox cell system, since, under optimal conditions of size and pH, such aggregates are bound by essentially all cells having FcRs (as determined by the attainment of a plateau). In general practice, the direct fluorescence method described by Dickler has been difficult to use because of the necessity for optimal aggregate size, and other less well defined factors. Methods of preparing aggregates of the proper characteristics other than centrifugation have been employed, e.g., gel filtration (Hayward and Greaves, 1975). One problem has been that the conjugation of IgG to fluorescein appears to block some of the sites necessary for efficient binding to the cell-surface receptors (Thrasher et al., 1975). Others (Forni and Pernis, 1975; Winchester and Ross, 1976) have employed antigen–antibody complexes in which one member of the complex was conjugated to fluorescein. Still another approach is the indirect aggregate-binding assay, in which heated IgG is purified by centrifugation and reacted with cells. After several washes, the cells are stained with an anti-IgG. Given the knowledge that blood lymphocytes with intrinsic IgG are rare in man, it is possible to enumerate cells with FcRs with fair certainty. This quite simple method has particular application in the study of patients with lymphoproliferative or immunodeficiency diseases, in whom cells having FcRs but little or no SIg are often encountered. It has the theoretical disadvantage of failing to detect cells bearing intrinsic IgG without FcRs; such cells are probably very rare, since essentially all cells with SIg also have FcRs (Dickler and Kunkel, 1972).

J. F. Bach and his colleagues (Bach et al., 1970) described a rosette test that employed a human anti-Rh serum (Ripley) to coat human Rh-positive (CDe) red cells; the IgG-coated cells [erythrocyte–antibody complex (EA)] were used to detect lymphocytes presumed to have rheumatoid factor on their surface. Frøland and Natvig (1973) later employed the same reagent to define a lymphoid population of non-T, non-B cells (discussed in the preceding section). Others (Kurnick and Grey, 1975; Gupta et al., 1976c; Siegal, 1976) have in general confirmed that cells with FcRs of sufficient binding avidity to react with the Ripley-coated erythrocytes are distinct, for the most part, from B cells. The FcRs of normal monocytes have similar binding characteristics. The exact nature of the difference between B-cell and "third-population" FcRs is not known, although some differences in specificity or avidity of binding of the IgG of different subclasses (Spiegelberg *et al.*, 1976) or of species (Ross, 1977) have been suggested. Alternatively, the FcRs may be similar in specificity but different in their display on the cell surface. This author (Siegal, 1976) has suggested that FcR avidity may change with the functional state of the cell over time, so that increased amounts of IgG may bind to B cells under certain circumstances.

In the study of lymphoreticular malignancy, FcR assays have found their most useful application in identifying cells that have relatively little SIg, but lack cytochemical or functional characteristics of myeloid or monocytoid cells, such as phagocytosis. For example, certain chronic lymphocytic leukemia (CLL) proliferations are Ig-negative but still express FcRs detectable by binding of aggregated IgG (Dickler *et al.*, 1973; Augener *et al.*, 1974). The anti-Rh (Ripley) EA rosette assay has been especially useful in the study of some diffuse histiocytic lymphomas that, like normal monocytes, are capable of binding EA as well as aggregated IgG, but fail to ingest latex or carry intrinsic SIg. These proliferations (Koziner *et al.*, 1977b) possess some of the characteristics of monocytes, but do not have the morphology of myelomonocytic or monocytic leukemias. They may be considered true histiocytic proliferations or perhaps even a malignant counterpart of cells included in the "third population."

2.1.3. Complement Receptors

Cells that bear complement receptors include B lymphocytes (Bianco and Nussenzweig, 1971), monocytes and granulocytes (Ross and Polley, 1975), some "third-population" cells (Perlmann *et al.*, 1972; Ross, 1977), certain cells that otherwise might be considered T cells (Shevach *et al.*, 1974; Chiao *et al.*, 1974), and glomerular epithelial cells (Gelfand *et al.*, 1976). Since essentially all the cell types under consideration as participants in the lymphoreticular malignancies have been associated with complement receptors, this marker may be less useful than some of the others as a discriminant among them.

Complement receptors are commonly detected by rosetting assays utilizing erythrocytes (E) coated with antibody (A) (usually IgM, to avoid reaction with the FcRs of the non-T cells) and complement (C) (often from a C5-deficient mouse source such as AKR) (Bianco *et al.*, 1970; Winchester and Ross, 1976); hence the tern *EAC rosettes*. Human, ox, avian, and sheep erythrocytes have been used as substrates for the EAC. Human E have the largely theoretical disadvantage of carrying a C3 (immune adherence) receptor of their own (Aiuti *et al.*, 1974), and might tend to clump following C sensitization, although human E have been successfully used in EAC assays (Siegal *et al.*, 1976b). Both sheep and, to a lesser extent, human E form spontaneous rosettes with human T lymphocytes (Branganza *et al.*, 1975), which also constitutes a difficulty in the use of these cells in EAC. To obviate this, EAC rosettes are best formed with constant shaking at 37°C (a temperature at which spontaneous E rosetting is minimized when applied to normal PBL) in the presence of 0.2% sodium azide (Winchester and Ross, 1976). However, since sheep rosettes formed with normal thymic lymphocytes and malignant T cells (Galili and Schlesinger, 1975) do not dissociate at 37°C, being more stable than most normal peripheral-T-cell rosettes, even these conditions may not always be sufficient to prevent some spontaneous rosetting. For example, even with other precautions, thymoma lymphocytes form stable E rosettes at 37°C (Filippa and Siegal, 1975), and accordingly form sheep EAC rosettes as well. Consequently, if sheep E are used in EAC assays, E and EA controls must be run to assess the significance of the C coat.

Other systems have been utilized to detect C receptors. Ross and Polley (1975) used indirect immunofluorescence with fluid-phase C components to demonstrate receptors and their membrane redistribution. Mendes *et al.* (1974) introduced the use of zymosan (Z) particles as a substrate for C3 activation via the alternate complement pathway, with the formation of ZC complexes. These complexes do not depend on the presence of antibody, and can be frozen and stored far longer than can conventional EAC reagents. ZC complexes have the additional advantage of providing an indicator distinct from E for rosette formation, which both avoids the problem of spontaneous rosetting and facilitates the demonstration of "double" rosettes, i.e., rosettes around cells capable of spontaneously binding sheep or mouse E and having a C receptor (Mendes *et al.*, 1974; Lin and Hsu, 1976). Others have used nucleated avian E (Chiao *et al.*, 1974), E of differing sizes (Siegal *et al.*, 1976b), or fluorochrome-labeled E (Pellegrino *et al.*, 1975) in the formation of identifiable mixed rosettes.

One major source of confusion in the interpretation of C receptors on mononuclear cells is that there are two distinct C receptors, which are antigenically and functionally distinct and occur on separate cell-surface macromolecules (Ross and Polley, 1975) and to some extent on different cells. The detection of these two receptors depends heavily on the C coat present on the particular EAC employed. EAC prepared by whole serum have on their surface a mixture of C3b and C3d, with the relative amounts of each depending on the level of activity of C3b inactivator present in normal serum. The inactivator cleaves C3b into C3c and C3d, leaving C3d at the E surface and releasing C3c into the medium. C3c contains structures that interact with a "C3b" receptor, while C3d carries a structure that interacts with C3d receptor. The "C3b" receptor is functionally and antigenically identical to the immune adherence receptor found on primate E, and appears to be the same receptor described by Bokisch and Sobel (1974) for C4. The C4 molecule lacks the structures found in the C3d part of C3b, so it does not bind to C3d receptor sites. Fluid-phase C3c and C4b inhibit the C3b receptor, while C3d inhibits only its own receptor, without significant cross-inhibition. Intact C3b binds to both types of C receptors. Workers in the field—Ross, Polley, Bianco, and Nussenzweig—have informally agreed to simplify this confusing nomenclature by referring to the immune adherence (Primate RBC, C3b, C4, C4b) receptors as CR_1, and to C3d receptor as CR_2. The observation of Ross *et al.* (1973) that EAC made with mouse serum reacted better with CLL lymphocytes than did EAC prepared with human complement components, while normal PBL formed C rosettes equally well with both kinds of EAC, is now explained by the predominance of C3d (CR_2) receptors on CLL cells; mouse serum contains C3b inactivator, which cleaves C3b to C3c and C3d, and produces C3d sites on EAC mouse. Purified C components lack that inactivator, so EAC made with mouse components have predominantly C3b sites (Ross and Polley, 1975). The CLL receptor profile (C3d predominant) is also found among normal tonsillar cells.

Monocytes have CR_1 and CR_2 similar in relative proportion to those on lymphocytes. Jaffe *et al.* (1975) reported that splenic histiocytes in the cords of Billroth do not bind EAC reagents, while lymph node histiocytes do so when studied on frozen section material and in suspension. This may reflect differences in specific C-receptor display in different organs; Jaffe and colleagues utilized EAC prepared from fresh mouse serum in their studies.

At the time of review, the nature of cells that form C rosettes is a point of some disagreement. Ehlenberger *et al.* (1976) and Horwitz (1976) presented evidence that C-rosetting cells are all B lymphocytes, i.e., that they have stable membrane Ig, and that the C3 rosette is definitive for B lymphocytes. On the other hand, patients without B lymphocytes (thymoma and agammaglobulinemia; X-linked agammaglobulinemia) have lymphoid cells that do bind EAC (Schiff *et al.*, 1974; Yata and Tsukimoto, 1972). The nature of these mononuclear cells is in turn controversial [Hayward and Greaves (1975) reported that they are monocytes], but many of them are nonphagocytic, peroxidase- and α-naphthyl-esterase-negative, and nonadherent (Siegal *et al.*, 1976c) and EAC-positive. Ross and Winchester did extensive double-marker analyses with F(ab')$_2$ antisera and directly demonstrated normal cells that do not have instrinsic SIg but that form EAC rosettes (Ross, 1977). Finally, the observations that small numbers of normal PBL, several malignant clones (Siegal *et al.*, 1976b; Lin and Hsu, 1976; Shevach *et al.*, 1974), and the T-cell line MOLT-4 (West and Herberman, 1974) simultaneously form spontaneous sheep rosettes and EAC rosettes, but lack SIg and FcRs, have made it difficult to conclude that C receptors are exclusively on B cells. In practice, the EAC rosette has nevertheless been a relatively simple marker to use, and has been widely employed in the study of lymphoreticular malignancy. Insofar as the receptor can appear on a variety of cell types, EAC rosetting should be utilized as a marker of lymphoproliferative states only as part of a battery of other confirmatory reagents.

2.1.4. Spontaneous Mouse Erythrocyte Rosette Formation

Mouse erythrocytes (MRBC) were recently shown to form clusters around certain human lymphocytes, which have surface characteristics of B cells (Stathopoulos and Elliott, 1974; Gupta and Grieco, 1975). The method of making the rosettes appears to bear heavily on the types of cells labeled by the MRBC. In our own laboratory, the mouse rosette-forming cells (MRFC) appear to detect a subpopulation of true B cells, since essentially all the MRFC have SIgM or SIgD. When the lymphocytes are treated with neuraminidase, a larger proportion form rosettes. This population appears to include all the cells that do not form spontaneous sheep E rosettes, i.e., the B cells and the "third population" (Gupta *et al.*, 1976c). Thus, the MRFC are an excellent rosetting marker for B cells: they do not appear to form around monocytes or granulocytes, and can be used in conjunction with the Ripley EA (discussed in Section 2.1.2) and the spontaneous sheep RFC (see Section 2.1.6) to give a reasonable indication of the lymphoid populations present among human mononuclear cells. At least in our hands (Gupta *et al.*, 1976c), these three populations appear to be generally exclusive of one another.

Apparently for technical reasons, the MRFC have either been extremely difficult to reproduce (Greaves, 1974), or have detected all the non-T cells without the use of neuraminidase (Dobozy *et al.*, 1976). Under standard conditions of centrifugation, temperature of incubation, and resuspension, most true B cells can form MRFC, and a plateau value can be obtained (Gupta *et al.*, 1976c). In routine practice, however, the proportion of MRFC is highly dependent on technique; we have found fewer MRFC than IgM-bearing cells over an extended number of normal controls, and have frequently detected so few in normals that the usefulness of the MRFC is mainly in the investigation of situations in which there is a monoclonal expansion of B cells of certain types: CLL B cells appear to be MRFC, while interestingly enough, the B cells of certain lymphosarcoma cell leukemias do not (see Section 3.1). Coupling these observations with our finding of MRFC as a very early marker for B cells in ontogeny (Gupta *et al.*, 1976a), it seems possible that this rosette functions as a differentiation marker similar to the thymus-leukemia antigen (TL) in the mouse, which is expressed on thymocytes but not on peripheralized T cells (Boyse and Bennett, 1974); as in the mouse, some markers can be transiently expressed on cells during one phase of differentiation only. The MRBC receptor is independent of SIg, Fc, and C3 receptors on the cells recognized (Gupta *et al.*, 1976c,d).

2.1.5. Spontaneous Monkey Erythrocyte Rosette Formation

Simian RBC also bind spontaneously to certain human lymphocytes; the species used seems to determine the specificity of the rosette. Pellegrino *et al.* (1975) showed that RBC of the Japanese ape, *Macaca speciosa*, form rosettes with B lymphocytes, in that they formed double rosettes with EAC and reacted with Ig-bearing cells. The majority of non-sheep-rosetting cells (non-T cells; see Section 2.1.6) were found to bind these monkey RBC, suggesting that not only B but also "third-population" cells were capable of reacting; the proportions of RFC were somewhat less than the proportion of cells with FcRs in their study. Brain *et al.* (1970) observed apparent rosette formation of RBC from vervet monkeys and baboons with some human leukocytes.

In contrast, RBC of the rhesus monkey form rosettes with a larger group of cells, which appear to be primarily T lymphocytes (Lohrmann and Novikovs, 1974), and with neuraminidase-treated non-T cells. Simian RBC have not been used extensively as markers for lymphoreticular malignancies, but cells from some patients with CLL, probably B cells, were (somewhat paradoxically) positive for rhesus rosettes, as though they had been treated with neuraminidase (Lohrmann and Novikovs, 1974).

2.1.6. Spontaneous Sheep Erythrocyte Rosette Formation

Brain *et al.* (1970), Coombs *et al.* (1970), and Lay *et al.* (1971) observed a large population of PBL that formed rosettes with sheep RBC (SRBC). The aggregation was independent of SIg or of serum antibody to sheep cells. There followed quickly the recognition that such cells were thymus-derived (Wybran and Fudenberg, 1971). A method for obtaining a plateau value detecting essentially all thymus-derived cells (and some other less well defined cells) was reported (Jondal *et al.*, 1972) and expanded on (Bentwich *et al.*, 1973a). Both because of its simplicity and reproducibility and because of its capacity to detect T cells, this type of rosette formation has been widely used in the study of lymphoproliferative states. One of its major advantages is that sheep cells do not form rosettes with nonlymphoid cells [excepting one report of sheep cells rosetting with granulocytes from some normal persons and from a patient with X-linked agammaglobulinemia (Hsu and Fell, 1974)].

Technical matters are highly important in the formation of SRBC rosettes, as in most other rosette assays. Optimal ("total") rosetting, which detects about 80% of normal PBL, depends on adequate cell viability, the sheep (some sheep provide especially good rosette-forming cells), the age of the RBC, the presence of serum, adequate centrifugation, incubation temperatures and times, and especially, gentleness of resuspension. These details may be found in the literature (Aiuti *et al.*, 1974; Bentwich *et al.*, 1973a; Jondal *et al.*, 1972; Winchester and Ross, 1976). A number of methodological alterations, such as pretreatment of the SRBC with neuraminidase or with 2-amino-ethylisothiouronium bromide hydrobromide (Pellegrino *et al.*, 1975), stabilize the rosettes and allow more rapid attainment of a plateau. Cold overnight incubation appears to have a similar effect, although this prolongs the assay time. Maximum numbers of RFC are attained if, in addition to strict attention to the aforementioned factors, lymphocytes that form rosettes with only one or two sheep cells are included in the counts (Bentwich *et al.*, 1973a), since in double-marker experiments with aggregated IgG, the few cells that are double-marked have large numbers of adherent SRBC, while the "small" rosettes do not have that marker. Most thymocytes bind very many SRBC ("morula formation"), and tend to form larger rosettes than do the PBL.

The "active" rosette of Wybran and Fudenberg (1973) is formed after preincubation of only the lymphocytes with high concentrations of fetal calf serum, followed by the addition of SRBC, a brief centrifugation, and immediate resuspension at room temperature. Only about 25–30% of human PBL form rosettes under these conditions (Wybran and Fudenberg, 1973; Taniguchi *et al.*, 1976). Taniguchi demonstrated that it is only these rosettes that are preferentially inhibited by SRBC fragments, indicating differences in the lymphocyte surfaces between cells that form "active" rosettes and the cells that eventually form rosettes under optimal conditions ("total" rosettes). By a similar definition, the "active" RFC are a subset of cells with more "avid" binding of SRBC, possibly because the rate of rosette formation is more rapid than it is with the later-forming rosettes. Similar conclusions were drawn by Yu (1975) and by West *et al.* (1976), who used a high-temperature incubation after centrifugation to discriminate between high and low avidity (early–late, active–total) rosetting lymphocytes.

Many laboratories have reported proportions of positive cells intermediate between "total" and "active" rosette values for normal cells. This reflects technical factors that give less than plateau values.

Various sheep-rosetting assays differ in their ability to be inhibited by anti-cell antibodies, serum "factors," and drugs. Optimal assays for "total" rosettes tend not to reveal such inhibitors (West *et al.*, 1976). These assay differences account for certain discrepancies in the literature of Hodgkin's disease and perhaps other lymphomas (see Section 3.6).

In certain hands, the SRBC rosettes also detect a proportion of cells of the "third population," both with neuraminidase (Bentwich *et al.*, 1973b; Lohrmann and Novikovs, 1974) and without (Winchester *et al.*, 1975a).

Thymocytes have special characteristics in the sheep rosette assay in that in addition to the size of the rosettes formed, most are generally quite stable (Galili and Schlesinger, 1975; Borella and Sen, 1975; Yu, 1975), and do not, as do the majority of peripheral T cells, dissociate at 37°C. Neuraminidase-treated peripheral T cells are similarly stable. It is of some interest that the stability of thymocyte rosettes seems to be mimicked by certain acute lymphoblastic leukemia cells (Borella and

"active" PBL rosettes is not known, but most thymocytes are poor responders in
lymphocyte transformation assays [e.g., phytohemagglutinin (PHA)], while it may
be the "active" rosettes that respond best to mitogens (Wybran and Fudenberg,
1973).

Because of its simplicity, the sheep rosette is perhaps the most widely used
discriminant of human lymphoid cells in use today.

2.1.7. Spontaneous Human Erythrocyte Rosette Formation

Human erythrocytes were found to spontaneously form aggregates with a large
proportion of human thymocytes (Baxley *et al.*, 1973); following neuraminidase
treatment of the erythrocytes, almost all thymocytes formed rosettes, and approximately 25% of PBL did so. Baxley and colleagues further showed that essentially all
the positive lymphocytes also formed rosettes with SRBC. Although they did not
find spontaneous rosetting of human erythrocytes with PBL, others (Gluckman and
Montambault, 1975; Kaplan, J., 1975) observed a small proportion ($\approx 3-8\%$) of human
PBL forming spontaneous "autorosettes" in the absence of neuraminidase treatment. Autorosette formation appears to be a property of a subpopulation of T cells,
since the experience of Gluckman and Montambault and J. Kaplan indicates that the
autorosette-forming cells do not have SIg, form mixed rosettes with SRBC (see
Section 2.1.6), and are sensitive to antithymocyte globulin. Insofar as thymocytes,
PBL, and tonsillar lymphocytes have receptors for human RBC, but to a more
concealed or lesser degree on PBL and tonsillar cells, it is possible that the
autorosette represents a relatively thymus-specific marker like Thy-1, which is less
apparent on peripheralized T cells than it is on cells in the thymus. Similar findings
have been reported for human lymphocyte–sheep erythrocyte interactions (see
Section 2.1.6). Human rosette formation has not been commonly used in the
analysis of lymphoreticular malignancy.

2.1.8. Differentiation Antigens on Human Mononuclear Cells

The use of differentiation antigens (as opposed to "receptors" specific for
various cell types) has been of great importance in the definition of lymphoid cells in
both man and experimental animals (for discussion of the latter, see Section 1). A
variety of antisera have been employed for the study of cell-surface antigens as
differentiation markers of mononuclear cells in man. The problem of specificity for
one or another cell type has been considerable, and certain antisera regarded as
definitive of one or another subpopulation must be viewed with some suspicion in
reviewing the literature on the subject. Malignant cells may be useful models for
their normal counterparts, but their surface antigens (as well as other markers) may
reflect derepression of genes that are not active on normal cells. The antigen
detected may not be truly specific for a particular cell type, but may appear to be
definitive if it is sought on only a few other cells and found lacking, since a surface
component of an infrequent stem cell in blood or marrow might not be recognized.
The use of a fluorescence-activated cell sorter (Herzenberg *et al.*, 1976) may
facilitate analysis of infrequent but reactive cells (Brown *et al.*, 1975).

Technically, an antiserum may be specific by cytotoxicity, but not by immunofluorescence; it may be specific at one dilution, but not if more concentrated. The

activity of particular reagents may depend on secondary effectors, such as complement or even cell-mediated cytotoxicity. Many heteroantisera contain natural antibodies to human antigens present at the cell surface; normal rabbit serum frequently contains anti-human cell antibodies. Specificity is achieved by multiple absorptions with (usually living) cells thought not to present the antigens in question; absorbing cells have included monoclonal lymphocytes, platelets, granulocytes, erythrocytes, lymphoid cell lines (both T and B), and cells from patients lacking certain cells (e.g., from patients with Bruton-type agammaglobulinemia, who lack fully formed B cells).

Specificity is checked during the absorptions on defined cell populations, and multiple criteria are generally utilized for adequate definition. The process is outlined in Aiuti *et al.* (1974).

a. **Differentiation Isoantigens.**   Isoantigens, or alloantigens, have not been extensively utilized as differentiation markers in man, although in the mouse (see Section 1), they have been exceedingly useful. Several systems of human antilymphocyte antibodies have been described, but only one has been applied in the study of lymphoproliferative states. Winchester *et al.* (1975b) collected a panel of several pregnancy sera capable of recognizing antigens on mononuclear cells. Absorption with platelets of appropriate HLA type removed HLA-A and HLA-B specificities, leaving reactivity with an alloantigen limited to non-T mononuclear cells, including monocytes. The presence of these antigens, considered characteristic of B but not T cells, on the blasts of certain cases of acute lymphoblastic leukemia has been considered as evidence that these are proliferations of cells other than T lymphocytes (Fu *et al.*, 1975a). Subsequent analysis by this group and others has revealed that the antigens are characteristic of various hematopoietic cells, apparently lost during differentiation along the T-cell pathway. Some of these "B-cell antigens," also employed by Billing *et al.* (1976), may be analogous to the Ia antigens of the mouse, which are present on B cells and monocytes, and are closely associated on the cell surface with FcRs.

b. **Autoantibodies That Detect Cell-Surface Differentiation Antigens.** Sera of certain patients with systemic lupus erythematosus (SLE) (Winchester *et al.*, 1974; Winfield *et al.*, 1975; Glinski *et al.*, 1976; Korsmeyer *et al.*, 1976) contain antibodies reactive with lymphocytes. Certain of these antibodies recognize differentiation antigens insofar as they do not detect all PBL. Winfield *et al.* (1975) recognized antibodies of the IgM class that were cold-reactive and tended to react with both B and T cells. Glinski *et al.* (1976) showed the presence of IgG antibodies that could be detected by cell-mediated cytotoxic reactions, which appeared specific for a T-cell subset. Thomas (1973) observed antilymphocyte antibodies in infectious mononucleosis and several other human diseases that were reactive with T cells. The applicability of such reagents to the study of the lymphoproliferative diseases depends on the demonstration that they specifically detect a functionally defined subpopulation. Definitive information of this sort is not yet available, although one study (Korsmeyer *et al.*, 1976) unsuccessfully attempted to demonstrate antibodies to suppressor T cells in SLE sera.

c. **Heteroantibodies That Detect Cell-Surface Differentiation Antigens.** SIg's are, of course, differentiation antigens identified in this way (see Section 2.1.1). To detect other surface antigens, antisera have been prepared in horses, goats, rabbits, and other species by immunization with whole cells or with cell extracts. Unfortunately, the determinants recognized by these reagents have often been given similar names (e.g., "HTLA" for human T-lymphocyte antigen), although there is no evidence that the specificities recognized are identical (Touraine *et al.*, 1974). Because these reagents are difficult to prepare and the absorbing cells are sometimes hard to obtain in sufficient amounts to prepare large volumes of sera, antisera have rarely (if ever) been checked for specificity in more than one laboratory, making comparison of the different sera difficult and greatly dependent on the specificity testing described in the published work.

Immunizing cells have included a variety of hematopoietic cell types, as well as brain (by analogy with the murine antigen, Thy-1, found on T cells, thymocytes and brain).

Several laboratories have reported antisera to T cells, some of which appear to recognize subsets of T cells (Brouet *et al.*, 1975c; Kersey *et al.*, 1975; Chin *et al.*, 1973; Touraine *et al.*, 1974; Brown and Greaves, 1974).

Various antisera have been regarded as specific for B cells, T cells, thymocytes, and T and B lymphoblasts, and against monocytes (see Section 2.1.10). These reagents have been useful, but for reasons expressed previously, strong interpretations based solely on their use must be tempered with the realization of their limitations; ideally, cell-specific antisera will be used in conjunction with other marker systems.

2.1.9. Other Cell-Surface Markers

Harris (1974) described an antiserum raised against cultured human plasmacytoma cells which detected surface antigens on approximately 12% of human peripheral blood mononuclear cells and on an increased proportion of pokeweed-mitogen (PWM)-stimulated PBL. Cells with the "plasma cell antigen" did not bear SIg in double-marker analysis. Cytoplasmic Ig (see below) was not sought in these cells. It is not possible at this time to identify the reactive population in the framework of multiple-marker analysis using more conventional markers, since Harris found 25% of the normal PBL to have SIg, and an additional 12% would already account for 37% of the lymphoid cells as belonging to the B or third population series, a number in considerable excess of that usually considered non-T in many other studies.

Jondal and Klein (1973) described the adhesion of Epstein–Barr virus (EBV)-coated cells to B cells, but not T cells, and reported this as a marker of B lymphocytes. Greaves *et al.* (1975b) utilized the binding of virus-containing cell extracts, followed by a fluorescent anti-EBV serum, to detect EBV receptors on peripheral blood cells. Their system recognized approximately 16% of normal PBL, a proportion that, judging from their other parallel marker studies, almost certainly includes some "third-population" cells. Of some interest is the total lack of EBV-reactive cells in patients with Bruton-type agammaglobulinemia (Hayward and Greaves, 1975).

Hammarström *et al.* (1973) isolated a lectinlike molecule from the snail, *Helix pomatia*, that may have some value as a T-cell marker, but it has so far found only limited application to lymphoreticular malignancies.

2.1.10. Identification of Monocytes

Mononuclear cells from normal peripheral blood, isolated on Ficoll–Hypaque gradients, may abound in monocytes (Zucker-Franklin, 1974). Monocytes can be exceedingly difficult to differentiate from lymphoid cells, both in conventional light microscopy on fixed, stained smears and in the cell suspensions commonly used for rosette and immunofluorescence testing, and they can complicate the interpretation of such assays unless rigorously controlled for. It is essential in the analysis of surface markers to exclude or identify these nonlymphoid cells. One extremely useful marker is the ability of these cells to effectively ingest small polystyrene (latex) particles in the presence of serum or plasma. The usual latex-ingestion procedures are better than 90% efficient in obviously labeling nonlymphoid cells, insofar as following latex ingestion, only a small proportion of the remaining latex-negative cells can be found to stain for cytochemical markers of monocytes (see below). Additionally, this marker has been quite valuable in the identification of monocytic and myelomonocytic leukemias (Koziner *et al.*, 1977a) and in the recognition of some morphologically less well defined proliferations that appear by other criteria to be true histiocytic "lymphomas" (Koziner *et al.*, 1977b). Unfortunately, monoclonal proliferations of certain cells may be functionally unable to ingest latex particles despite their monocytic–histiocytic origins. Nevertheless, combined assays with other markers may confirm the tendency to latex ingestion in cells with high-avidity FcRs and adherent polyclonal IgG, a pattern that is certainly consistent with monocytoid rather than lymphoid cells.

Latex ingestion has been noted among cells characterized by morphological or histochemical criteria as hairy cells (leukemic reticuloendotheliosis, hairy-cell leukemia) (Koziner *et al.*, 1976; Fu *et al.*, 1974). These cells have been shown to ingest (adhere to?) the latex particles. By other criteria (see below), however, they appear to be B cells of an unusual type, so the latex-ingestion criterion must be evaluated in the context of other markers when studying lymphoreticular malignancy.

Certain enzymes in monocytes or lymphocytes can serve as cytochemical differentiation markers, although they are useful only on fixed smears. Peroxidase (myeloperoxidase) has been widely used as a marker of granulocytes and monocytes, but has the disadvantage that its detection system includes benzidine, which is now difficult to obtain and is thought to be carcinogenic. Peroxidase staining is most intense in the cells of the granulocytic series, finer granules appearing in monocytes, which may be negatively or very weakly stained (Zucker-Franklin, 1975). Cells that have ingested latex or other particles are usually negatively stained for peroxidase, because of lysosomal discharge during phagocytosis. More useful for monocytes is the α-naphthylacetate esterase stain. The enzyme, which is stable after treatment with sodium fluoride, is regarded as specific for the monocyte-macrophage system. Small amounts of α-naphthylacetate esterase have been observed in lymphoid cells. The enzyme appears to be limited to T cells, and may prove an important differentiation marker (Ranki *et al.*, 1976). These histochemical stains are most useful in defining a population of indeterminate morphology that has been marked by one or another of the surface markers, in a double-label system (Preud'homme and Labaume, 1975) (see Section 2.1.11).

Greaves *et al.* (1975a) described an antiserum raised against human peritoneal macrophages that appears to identify human blood monocytes. Interestingly enough, a significant proportion of the non-T, non-B, nonphagocytic small lymphoid cells of peripheral blood (the third population of Frøland and Natvig, 1973) was reactive with this reagent, which Baker *et al.* (1976) applied to leukemic proliferations. They found reactivity with cells from patients with acute myelomon-ocytic leukemia, but not from patients with lymphocytic leukemias or from most patients with acute myelocytic leukemia.

The importance of monocyte identification cannot be overemphasized. It is not only essential in the correct definition of lymphoreticular malignancies, but also is crucial for the adequate interpretation of "lymphocyte"-surface-marker counting in uninvolved peripheral blood, since some markers interact with monocytes (IgG Fc, EAC3d, and EAC3b), while others (SRBC, MRBC) do not. Monocyte identification is complicated further by the almost inevitable inconsistency of morphological criteria when employing these various markers.

2.1.11. Studies Utilizing Combinations of Markers

Uncertainties concerning the coexistence of particular surface markers on malignant lymphoid cells may be resolved by combining marker studies on the same sample of cells. Fluorescent and rosette analyses (Siegal, 1976; Bentwich *et al.*, 1973b; Dickler *et al.*, 1973), or two different rosette analyses (Siegal *et al.*, 1976b; Chiao *et al.*, 1974; Pellegrino *et al.*, 1975), have been simultaneously employed. Indeed, the combined use of three or more markers is possible, particularly when histochemical methods are coupled with the surface-marker methodologies (Ross, 1977). For example, we have developed a simple method of safely identifying rosette-forming cells morphologically by isolating the rosetting cells on a one-step gradient (e.g., Bentwich *et al.*, 1973a; Wybran *et al.*, 1973) and making cytocentri-fuge smears of the resulting rosetted cells, which can then be stained for a specific enzyme or for cytoplasmic Ig (see Section 2.2.1). Both SIg and cytoplasmic Ig can be identified in single cells by first staining the cell surface while the cell is alive, then the cytoplasm following appropriate fixation (Pernis *et al.*, 1971; Rudders and Ross, 1975). Almost any set of markers can be used together, provided the conditions of temperature, incubation, and resuspension, and the types of cells involved in mixed agglutination, can be made compatible. Sometimes a compromise away from the conditions optimal to each pair of markers is necessary to demon-strate coincidence of two markers. When markers are used conjointly, it is impor-tant to show a lack of mutual interference; consequently, double-marker analyses should be done in parallel with studies in which each of the markers is used alone on other aliquots of the same cells. Inhibition by one marker system of another is usually easily recognized under these circumstances.

2.1.12. Application of Surface Markers to Tissue Section

Certain lymphoid malignancies, such as the nodular lymphomas, are character-ized by architectural features that require specialized evaluation. Cell suspensions from such nodes may contain a mixture of malignant and normal, possibly reactive, lymphoid cells. Localization of a particular marker system in the areas of lympho-matous involvement may facilitate the identification of the malignant cell type. Dukor *et al.* (1970) first applied this kind of technique to localize B cells in germinal centers through binding of C3-coated erythrocytes to lymphoid cells in frozen sections. Jaffe *et al.* (1975) and Gajl-Peczalska *et al.* (1975) employed these elegant techniques in the analysis of lymphoreticular malignancies (see Section 3.4). The indicator systems used have been IgG-coated erythrocytes (IgGEA) for the detection of high-avidity (monocyte-type) FcRs, and IgM- and complement-coated erythrocytes (IgMEAC = EAC; see Section 2.1.3) for CR_1 or CR_2. Although most groups working with this kind of assay did not employ SRBC rosette formation on frozen tissue because of the apparent requirement for viable cells, Mendes et al. (1974) reported the successful use of this rosette, in conjunction with Zymosan-C, on fixed tissue.

2.2. Cytoplasmic and Nuclear Differentiation Markers

2.2.1. Antigens

Cytoplasmic Ig detected by immunofluorescence appears to be a good marker for terminally differentiated B cells (Wu et al., 1973; Pernis et al., 1971; Andersson and Melchers, 1974; Siegal et al., 1976a), and is a classic tool for the identification of Ig classes in fully formed plasma cells (Coons et al., 1955; Taylor, 1974), in tissue (Broom et al., 1975), and in cell suspensions from peripheral blood and tissues (Preud'homme and Seligmann, 1972a,c). Crystalloids containing monoclonal Ig were demonstrated in the cytoplasm of a proportion of cells from some patients with CLL or lymphoma, particularly those with IgMλ SIg by Clark et al. (1973) and Mennemeyer et al. (1974). More recently, Raff et al. (1976) showed cytoplasmic Ig to be also a marker of B cells very early in ontogeny, in precursors of Ig-bearing cells.

J chain, a component of most polymeric Ig's, may be a marker for plasma cells, since it appears in essentially all Ig-containing cells, as detected by immunofluorescence (Mestecky, 1976). Some tissue plasma cells involved in chronic inflammation, but not in the production of secretory Ig, may lack J chain (Brandtzaeg, 1974).

Certain enzymes can be detected as antigens by immunofluorescence, and can function as differentiation antigens. Terminal deoxynucleotidyltransferase (TdT), which is discussed more fully in the next section, can be detected as a nuclear component of T-cell precursors by immunofluorescence (Baltimore et al., 1976). Fluorescent antisera against TdT and other enzymes specific for particular cell types may eventually be extremely useful probes for differentiation.

Fagraeus et al. (1973, 1974) observed that smooth muscle antibodies (SMA) from patients with chronic active hepatitis react with peripheral antigens within lymphoid cells, which are not available to surface staining but are apparently membrane-associated. These antigens, presumed to be determinants of contractile proteins, are associated with microvilli on the membranes of various cells. While they are apparently not true differentiation antigens, the SMA do seem to reflect differences among cells, insofar as the villous B-cell lines tested had significant reactivity with SMA, while the MOLT-4 line, with short, stubby microvilli, has considerably less. Medullary, cortisone-resistant thymocytes, as well as about 70% of human PBL, were reactive with the antisera used (Fagraeus et al., 1973).

2.2.2. Enzymes

Certain enzymatic markers have been associated with lymphoid cells, but only a few seem to have relative specificity for T or B cells. Acid phosphatase appears to have some specificity for thymus-related cells, found in a patchy paranuclear

(Golgi) distribution (Schwarze, 1975). This enzyme has been described in association with T-cell leukemias (Catovsky *et al.*, 1975; Brouet *et al.*, 1975b; Nathwani *et al.*, 1976), but its usefulness as a specific marker needs further evaluation. Tartrate-resistant acid phosphatase appears to be a marker unique to the cells of leukemic reticuloendotheliosis (hairy-cell leukemia) (Catovsky *et al.*, 1974a). This disease, the exact nature of which is still uncertain, is discussed in Section 3.4.

The enzyme that has received the greatest recent interest as a lymphoid cell marker, TdT (terminal deoxynucleotidyltransferase), was initially isolated and characterized by Bollum and his associates as capable of polymerization of deoxynucleotides onto a primer in the absence of a template. Chang and Bollum (1971) recognized the organ distribution of the enzyme to be restricted to thymic tissue, and observed its presence in a number of species. Subsequently, its activity in much smaller amounts in bone marrow was appreciated. McCaffrey *et al.* (1975) soon demonstrated TdT in the cells of patients with acute lymphatic leukemia. More recent investigations, summarized by McCaffrey *et al.* (1976) and Baltimore *et al.* (1976), showed the enzyme to be a marker for lymphoid cells destined to differentiate into thymocytes and T cells, i.e., prothymocytes. Such precommitted (Boyse and Bennett, 1974) cells are found in the marrow as well as in the thymus. Of considerable interest is the demonstration that cells from certain cases of blast crisis of chronic myelogenous leukemia, acute undifferentiated and "myelomonocytic" leukemias (McCaffrey *et al.*, 1976; Marcus *et al.*, 1976), and leukemic lymphosarcoma (Koziner *et al.*, 1977b) also contained the enzyme. The possibility that these findings indicate a common pre-T lymphoid cell origin for the various morphological forms of leukemia must be balanced by the other alternatives: (1) that the enzyme is not truly a lymphoid marker or (2) that lymphoid "transformation" of other leukemias is the result of a second independent leukemia developing in certain patients, perhaps as the result of chronic antigenic stimulation by leukemia-associated antigens or of antileukemia chemotherapy. The weight of the evidence so far is in favor of the enzymes being restricted to cells early in the differentiation pathway of T lymphocytes. Baltimore *et al.* (1976) raised the appealing but unproved hypothesis that enzymes with activities like those of TdT could provide a mechanism of base insertion into genes encoding for the hypervariable regions of antibody-combining sites. In view of the increasing evidence for similar or identical sites on T cells (Eichmann and Rajewsky, 1975; Binz and Wigzell, 1975), the absence of this particular enzyme from B cells seems less disturbing than when the hypothesis was initially proposed. A similar enzymatic activity recently demonstrated in avian bursal cells (Baltimore *et al.*, 1976) might serve an analogous function in B lymphocytes. Kung *et al.* (1976) and Bollum (1975) prepared antisera against TdT, and Baltimore's group used their reagent in a fluorescent assay (see Section 2.2.1) that may prove to be an important differentiation marker for human prothymocytes.

Adenosine deaminase (ADA) is an enzyme of great importance in the intact differentiation of lymphoid cells. Its absence is associated with certain cases of severe combined immunodeficiency, and excess adenosine has been shown to be toxic to lymphoid cells (Ballet *et al.*, 1976; Hirschhorn *et al.*, 1976; Meuwissen *et al.*, 1975). Tung *et al.* (1976) investigated the distribution of ADA and of its isozyme in B and T chronic lymphocytic leukemia cells and in enriched populations of normal B and T cells. They found somewhat higher levels of ADA in T cells than in B cells, but the differences do not appear sufficient to make that enzyme useful as a differentiation marker. Lactic dehydrogenase isoenzyme patterns differ between B and T cells, the latter having a significantly higher amount of the LDH-1 isoenzyme than do B cells (Plum and Ringoir, 1975).

5'-Nucleotidase, which is detectable by either enzymatic activity (Quagliata *et al.*, 1974) or immunofluorescence (LaMantia *et al.*, 1976) on a proportion (15–43%) of normal lymphoid cells, is missing from the cells of most patients with CLL. The enzyme is not specific to either B or T cells. α-Naphthylacetate esterase appears to be present in small amounts in T, but not B, cells (Ränki *et al.*, 1976).

2.3. Morphology

2.3.1. Light Microscopy

In less sophisticated times, all lymphocytes were regarded as large, medium, or small, and the larger ones were thought to be "less mature." Grundmann, in 1961, described two types of PBL on the basis of special stains revealing nucleolar and nuclear morphology [macronucleolar (follicle) and polynucleolar (sinus, micronucleolar)] and indicated that the micro- or polynucleolar type accounted for perhaps 25% of the PBL (Millikin, 1974). Such differences, not readily appreciated by most observers, might now strike one's fancy were it not that in CLL, the macronucleolar forms predominate. Thus, this morphological approach to discrimination between B and T cells does not seem to be useful. On the other hand, Lennert *et al.* (1975) and Lukes and Collins (1974) discerned similarities between the morphology of cells in normal germinal centers and the cells of certain lymphomas. They termed these cells *germinocytes, germinoblasts* (Lennert), and *follicular center cells* (FCC) (Lukes). Since the far cortical region of lymph nodes, particularly the germinal centers (see Chapters 9 and 11), contain B cells, it would seem reasonable that such cells are B cells. It may therefore be possible to draw certain distinctions in the light microscope between germinal center cells and other lymphoid cells; the non-FCC (which include the cells of CLL, also B cells) cannot be divided morphologically into B and T types. Lukes and Collins (1974) noted, however, the marked nuclear convolutions of certain T-leukemic proliferations associated with thymic tumors in children and young adults (leukemic lymphosarcoma) and older children; further, the nuclear convolutions found in Sézary cells, both large and small (see Chapter 16), appear to indicate that cells with bizarre nuclear shapes tend to be T-cell-related. Brouet *et al.* (1975c) also observed bizarre nuclear morphology "clearly distinct from . . . [that] of Sézary cells" in lymphocytes from patients with T-cell CLL.

Stimulated primarily by the reports of surface morphological differences between B and T cells by Polliack *et al.* (1973) and Lin *et al.* (1973) by scanning electron microscopy, a number of investigators observed differences between these types by phase-contrast light microscopy. These differences are considered in the next section.

2.3.2. Electron Microscopy

Although significant differences between lymphocytes and plasma cells are apparent in transmission electron microscopy (TEM) (Douglas, 1971), B and T cells had not been regarded as distinguishable by EM until the observations of Polliack *et al.* (1973) and Lin *et al.* (1973). Their pictures by scanning electron microscopy (SEM) revealed differences in the size, number, and distribution of surface microvilli, B cells tending to have more and larger microvilli than T cells. Alexander and Wetzel (1975) and M. M. Kay *et al.* (1974) used different techniques of fixation and challenged the earlier studies, concluding that there was no difference in surface morphology between the two lymphoid cell types. The various technical considerations were reviewed by Polliack and de Harven (1975). The subsequent observations on living cells by Sullivan *et al.* (1974), Padnos (1976), Fogh (1974), and Vila and Taub (1975) indicated, however, that significant surface morphological differences probably do exist, although not in direct correlation with the markers. Furthermore, the recent publication of Lipscomb *et al.* (1975), utilizing the hybrid antibody technique, and our own unpublished experiences with T lymphocytic leukemic proliferations using the methods advocated by Alexander and Wetzel, appear to favor the return to a concept of real differences between B and T cells. The difficulty of the surface morphological approach with malignant proliferations, however, is that correlations with immunological markers are poor, and bizarre surface shapes occur. In our later study of 84 leukemic proliferations (Polliack *et al.*, 1975), TEM seems to have pointed up the possibility of recognizing surface structures that were not previously appreciated as being of any significance. Correlations among smooth, villous, and blebbed surfaces in SEM and TEM were observed in both independent techniques. The usefulness of surface morphological differences among lymphoid cells in discriminating B and T cells is limited by the large number of "intermediate" forms, which may be either B or T, if the original reports are to be believed. It is possible that the smooth muscle antibodies described by Fagraeus (see Section 2.2.1) will add to the study of surface morphology and point up differences when used in combined assays. The identification of monocytes, which is regarded as the simplest discrimination in SEM morphology (the characteristic "ridged and ruffled" membrane), is complicated somewhat by the observation of Golomb *et al.* (1975) on hairy-cell leukemia, in which the leukemic cells had the aspect of monocytes. Some of these same cells were studied by the author and found to have monoclonal IgM or IgD on their surfaces, and thus to have the immunological characteristics of B cells.

2.4. Functional Cell Markers

Most of the markers discussed already can be regarded as "functional" in evolutionary terms. Phagocytosis as a marker of nonlymphoid cells was discussed in Section 2.1.10. Most of the *in vitro* "functional" characterizations of mononuclear cells in use today are only relatively specific for B and T cells, although differences certainly exist. For the most part, they seem somewhat less useful than the surface markers in discriminating among mononuclear cells. The ability to form colonies in soft agar culture is characteristic of a few "lymphoid" mononuclear cells in peripheral blood (Barr *et al.*, 1975); these cells have the morphological appearance of large lymphocytes that carry none of the conventional markers of B and T cells, and therefore fall into the "null" category. The ability to adhere to glass and nylon surfaces is a property particularly of monocytes, but B cells will adhere to surfaces under appropriate conditions (Aiuti *et al.*, 1974; Aisenberg *et al.*, 1974), and can be removed along with monocytes by column chromatographic procedures. "Third-population" cells, K cells, and T cells do not usually adhere (Frøland *et al.*, 1974). The ability of certain cell types to function in various cytotoxicity systems may differentiate among them. PHA-induced cytotoxicity, for instance, may be specific for T cells; antibody-dependent cytotoxicity, for cells with certain types of FcRs (Perlmann *et al.*, 1972; Revillard *et al.*, 1975), particularly monocytes and some "third-population" lymphoid cells (K cells).

Secretion of Ig (by definition a functional B-cell-line marker) was used by Kaiserling *et al.* (1973) and others to define B-cell populations, and is roughly equivalent in its significance to demonstration of cytoplasmic or intrinsic SIg. This is also true of the demonstration of monoclonal Ig secretory activity after stimulation of leukemic proliferations by PWM (Litwin, 1976).

Responses to a variety of plant lectins, or mitogens, have been useful in the study of lymphoproliferative states, as they have been with normal and immunodeficient lymphocytes. Concanavalin A (Con A) appears to be the lectin most specific for human T cells, giving no or minimal stimulation of cells definable as B cells. A small proportion of the blasts resulting from PHA have had B-cell markers, although it is not known whether these cells are directly stimulated by PHA or are the result of B-cell mitogenic factors released by stimulated T cells (Greaves and Janossy, 1972). PWM has the capacity to stimulate both B and T cells, though the dependence on T cells may indicate considerations similar to those mentioned for PHA. These mitogens, particularly PWM, have the additional function of pushing B cells to terminally differentiate into plasmacytoid cells, as defined by the presence of cytoplasmic Ig (Janossy and Greaves, 1975). This is a function that should be discriminated from induction of blast transformation and mitosis. The EM morphology of these transformed cells was reviewed by Douglas (1971). The chief usefulness of the evaluation of mitogen responses by cells from lymphoproliferative states is to evaluate the question whether the cells, once defined by surface markers, behave in a normal fashion for the particular subpopulation identified. For example, if a patient has an absolute T lymphocytosis, absent or depressed mitogen responses to PHA and Con A would be markedly abnormal. In the absence of another marker of malignancy, such a finding would be quite significant.

There are several problems with mitogen responses that must be recognized. An observed response may be attributed to the malignant clone when it is, in fact, a small population of normal cells that accounts for the observed transformation. This appears to be the case with most CLL proliferations, which were long regarded as very weak responders to PHA. Havemann and Rubin (1968) noted a delayed response to PHA, and attributed it to the leukemic cells. The observed PHA response in CLL is probably made by normal T cells present in relatively low numbers among the leukemic lymphocytes (Wybran *et al.*, 1973; Aisenberg *et al.*, 1974). Given the stimulus of PHA, the normal T cells overgrow the culture and eventually give a detectable response. A more recent report (Schultz *et al.*, 1976), however, would seem to indicate T cell abnormalities in CLL that are not attributable merely to dilution.

Another problem is the possible lack of sufficient numbers of cooperating cells necessary for a mitotic response. For instance, a few monocytes (on the order of 1%) are necessary for optimal transformation to Con A, or to allogeneic cells in the mixed leukocyte culture (MLC) and probably to a lesser extent to PHA and PWM.

T cells are important in the transformation of B cells to PWM (Janossy and Greaves, 1975). Extreme dilution of these cooperating cells by a malignant clone may alter the apparent response, even when the leukemic cells themselves might have made a response, provided with cooperating factors. Mercaptoethanol has been shown to at least partially restore MLC responsiveness diminished by the removal of monocytes by adherence columns (Chen, C., and Hirsch, 1972; Berlinger *et al.*, 1976).

3. Application of Differentiation Markers to the Lymphoreticular Malignancies

The taxonomy of the various malignancies of the lymphoid and monocyte–macrophage systems has undergone almost constant revision in recent years because of growing recognition of functional cellular heterogeneity among cases grouped together on strictly morphological grounds.

Markers of cellular differentiation, particularly when employed in concert with morphological and clinical data, have improved our ability to classify these disease states, and may aid the rational development of specific therapy. Some fairly clear-cut distinctions can already be drawn among certain diseases that previously could not be reliably separated on the basis of morphological criteria alone. Along with this has come an improved ability to arrive at prognoses (Berard *et al.*, 1976).

These malignancies may reasonably be thought of as representing certain stages in the normal differentiation of lymphoid and monocytic cells. In some, e.g., in chronic lymphocytic leukemia (CLL), a block in normal differentiation might be viewed as the primary problem. The CLL cells remain in their partially differentiated state, while others of their own afflicted kind continue to accumulate. In contrast, normal cells are produced and differentiate, cycle, and die. The concept of a differentiative block is perhaps less attractive in states characterized by high labeling indices, such as acute leukemia. Perhaps here, too, the failure to differentiate even under ''good'' environmental conditions (development within the thymic epithelium in some cases of acute lymphoblastic leukemia (ALL) or childhood lymphoblastic lymphoma) may be a contributing factor in the malignant quality of such cellular proliferations. It is relatively easy to assign ''stages'' to the various B-cell proliferations, recognizing a spectrum of diseases from CLL to multiple myeloma, which were analyzed by Davis (1975) and Salmon and Seligmann (1974). A similar conceptual organization of human T-cell malignancies has been limited by the paucity of clear-cut differentiation markers for these cells.

No formal attempts at classification of lymphoreticular malignancy will be attempted in this chapter. Diseases described in more traditional terms will be related to the surface markers discussed previously.

3.1. Chronic Lymphocytic Leukemia

In its most common state, CLL is characterized by the initially asymptomatic accumulation of small or medium-sized lymphoid cells, but there are many variations on this theme. Some proliferations are associated with an obvious monoclonal ''M component''; with sensitive methods, Eipe *et al.* (1976) detected monoclonal serum Ig in 22 of 29 CLL sera. Some cases blend into the diesease known as

Waldenström's macroglobulinemia. The vast majority of CLL proliferations consist of B cells having among them a fairly consistent pattern of monoclonal SIg (Preud'homme and Seligmann, 1972c; Pernis *et al.*, 1971; Aisenberg and Bloch, 1972; Möller, 1973; Schroer *et al.*, 1974), FcRs (Dickler *et al.*, 1973; Augener *et al.*, 1974), C3 receptors (Ross *et al.*, 1973), and mouse erythrocyte rosetting (Stathopoulos and Elliott, 1974; Stathopoulos and Davies, 1976; Gupta and Grieco, 1975; Gupta *et al.*, 1976d; Koziner *et al.*, 1977b), but lacking the ability to form sheep rosettes (Dickler *et al.*, 1973; Jondal *et al.*, 1972; Wybran *et al.*, 1973). The SIg staining is often quite faint compared with that of the majority of normal lymphocytes, as detected by immunofluorescence (Aisenberg and Bloch, 1972), and this appears to correlate with decreased amounts of cell-membrane-associated Ig as detected by radioautography (Wilson and Nossal, 1971) or hemagglutination-inhibition (Cooper, A. G., *et al.*, 1973). The Ig class most regularly associated with CLL proliferations has been IgM, although since IgD was recognized as a major component of B-cell surfaces, it has been detected with considerable frequency on CLL cells, often but not always in association with IgM (Kubo *et al.*, 1974; Pernis *et al.*, 1974; Fu *et al.*, 1975b; Koziner *et al.*, 1977b). Occasional monoclonal proliferations bearing Ig of classes other than IgM-D have been observed (Preud'homme and Seligmann, 1972c; Rudders, 1976), but the presence of multiple heavy chains other than IgM and IgD on the surface of these proliferations is heavily suspect, as was discussed in Section 2.1.1. Cases associated with a monoclonal serum Ig almost always carry the same Ig on the cell surface. Some CLL proliferations contain cytoplasmic Ig in crystallinelike inclusions (Clark *et al.*, 1973) found in variable proportions of the cells of the proliferation. These inclusions may be recognized by their typical appearance on standard blood smears and confirmed by anti-Ig immunofluorescence. We have studied (Siegal and Litwin, 1976) one CLL proliferation containing such inclusions, which appeared to secrete unusually large amounts of λ light chains when cultured with PWM. Occasional diclonal proliferations of CLL have been noted (Preud'homme and Seligmann, 1972c).

The complement receptors, particularly CR_2 (Ross *et al.*, 1973), are present on CLL cells. Ross (1976) believes the CR_2 receptor may be associated with early stages of differentiation, the CR_1 receptors appearing later. Mouse erythrocyte rosette formation also seems to occur with typical CLL proliferations, but not on the cells of B-cell lymphomas in leukemic phase (CLSL) (Stathopoulos and Davies, 1976; Koziner *et al.*, 1977b). Because of this distinction, as well as the brighter SIg staining of CLSL cells emphasized by Aisenberg *et al.* (1973), and Aisenberg and Long (1975), it may be possible to separate CLSL and CLL reliably. These findings indicate that not all leukemic B-cell proliferations are the same, and suggest that different stages of B-cell differentiation may be involved. Also of interest is the early appearance of the mouse rosette in the normal ontogeny of B cells, suggesting that this rosette may be a marker of B cells early in their differentiation (Gupta *et al.*, 1976a), and that the CLL cells (which react with MRBC) are representative of early steps in B-cell development. Such an idea would be strengthened if CLL cells showing some plasmacytoid differentiation or cells of Waldenström's macroglobulinemia (see the next section) did not form MRBC rosettes.

A few cases of T-cell proliferations have originally been diagnosed as CLL. In the author's personal series, such cases are rare, on the order of 1% of all examples of CLL. Brouet *et al.* (1975) recorded a somewhat higher frequency (2.9%), and described a clinical syndrome suggestive of T-cell CLL, in which the cells have azurophilic granules, stain for acid phosphatase and β-glucuronidase and form sheep rosettes, but fail to carry markers of B cells. Whether this "syndrome" is characteristic of all the other cases of apparent T-cell CLL so far described (Yodoi et al., 1974; Dickler et al., 1973; Sumiya et al., 1973) is not known. Also complicating these findings is the presence in the literature of several cases of apparent T-cell proliferations that were CLL or leukemic lymphomas [some indeed apparently related to Sézary syndrome (see Section 3.4)] in which the cells carried both the sheep erythrocyte receptor and markers usually associated with B cells (most commonly C3 receptors, but also FcRs and SIg). The classification of such cases is still undetermined.

Associated with some cases of CLL is a variable lymphadenopathy in which the histology is most usually that of diffuse, well-differentiated lymphocytic lymphoma (DWDL). When such tissue has been investigated, the results have been conflicting. Thus, Aisenberg and Long (1975) and Braylan et al. (1976) found faint staining to be the rule on the DWDL cases, while they observed diffuse, poorly differentiated lymphocytic lymphoma (DPDL) to generally have bright staining for SIg. On the other hand, Klein and her collaborators (Johansson et al., 1976) found the reverse situation, the poorly differentiated cases having the least SIg. Whether this can be attributed to discrepancies in terminology, to some technical factor (such as FcRs), or to a true difference cannot be assessed at present. Study of CLL cases by SEM, which was initially thought to be helpful (Polliack et al., 1973) has proved, on further analysis, to be unreliable (Polliack et al., 1975) as a way of distinguishing B- and T-cell types.

Galton et al. (1974) described a type of lymphocytic leukemia having a subacute course, associated with massive splenomegaly, extremely high lymphocyte counts, and a characteristic cellular morphology, which they have termed prolymphocytic. Although this may be a clinical entity, the finding of both B- and T-cell proliferations that could be included in this group (Brouet et al., 1975b; Catovsky et al., 1975) must raise serious doubts as to its significance.

3.2. Waldenström's Macroglobulinemia and Heavy-Chain Disease

These diseases, by definition proliferations of B cells and their progeny, may be thought of as CLL-like proliferations that have the capability for partial terminal differentiation. Preud'homme and Seligmann (1972a) clearly showed an increase in the proportion of IgM-bearing PBL in macroglobulinemia and cytoplasmic Ig in a variable proportion of these cells. In contrast to CLL cells, a spectrum of marker-defined B-cell differentiation is present, associated with the usual morphological characterization of Waldenström's macroglobulinemia cells as plasmacytoid lymphocytes. The cytology and cell markers in heavy-chain diseases are often similar to those found in Waldenström's macroglobulinemia (Salmon and Seligmann, 1974) (see also Chapter 14).

3.3. Multiple Myeloma

In myeloma, the terminal differentiation of the B-cell lineage is represented. It is not known, however, at which stage of B-cell differentiation the malignant cells arise. The PBL in untreated myeloma are characterized in some studies by an increased proportion of SIg- and complement-receptor bearers and a reciprocally decreased sheep-rosetting population (Mellstedt *et al.*, 1973, 1974, 1976). Mellstedt found these cells to have a supranormal ability to function in antibody-dependent killing, which correlated with the proportion of non-T cells in the population. This was in contrast to B cells in CLL, which did not seem to function in antibody-dependent killing. Some other reports have indicated, however, that SIg-bearing cells are decreased, suggesting in myeloma an increased proportion of lymphocytes having complement receptors but no SIg (Lindstrom *et al.*, 1973; Jones and McFarlane, 1975). This, too, is in interesting contrast to the finding that the proportion of cells carrying the idiotypic determinants of the M component is elevated, often above the proportion of those cells that have detectable Ig classes using conventional, nonidiotypic antisera (Chen, Y., *et al.*, 1975; Abdou and Abdou, 1975). Relevant to this is the recent report (Mills, R. J., *et al.*, 1976) of a case of IgE myeloma in which a large proportion of the PBL carried monoclonal IgE. Unfortunately, overnight culture or enzymatic stripping of these cells to prove that the IgE was intrinsic was not carried out. The significance of these apparently conflicting data remains to be elucidated. Absolutely rigorous exclusion of the adherence of serum myeloma proteins to the cells using trypsinization and resynthesis seems essential, and has already been done in some studies (Chen, Y., *et al.*, 1975; Abdou and Abdou, 1975). Since the blood B lymphoid cells in at least some cases of myeloma (Mellstedt *et al.*, 1976), like those in macroglobulinemia, make the idiotype produced by plasma cells, the disease may be said to arise in B cells that are capable of full differentiation. Still another possibility raised by the studies of Y. Chen *et al.* (1975) is that idiotype-specific messenger RNA in myeloma serum recruits cells, altering their phenotypic expression of SIg to conform to that of the malignant clone. Although final conclusions cannot yet be reached, it seems possible that multiple myeloma plasma-cell proliferations in different patients may arise at different points in the B-cell scheme of differentiation.

The polyclonal hypogammaglobulinemia observed in myeloma has been attributed to several mechanisms. Salmon (1973) presented evidence of antimitotic chalones produced by the tumor. More recently, Broder *et al.* (1975) demonstrated in the blood of myeloma patients suppressor leukocytes that inhibit synthesis and secretion of Ig by normal lymphocytes. These cells may be phagocytic, which seems to differentiate them from the T suppressor cells detected in several forms of hypogammaglobulinemia (Siegal *et al.*, 1976a). Alternatively, the "infectious" RNA may alter the antigen receptors on normal B lymphocytes so that they are unable to respond normally to antigen (Chen, Y., *et al.*, 1975; Giacomoni *et al.*, 1974).

3.4. Solid-Tissue (Non-Hodgkin's) Lymphomas

Fewer data are available concerning malignant cells from lymph nodes than from the peripheral blood manifestations of the lymphomas. Lymphomatous involvement of the blood and bone marrow is not uncommon, as manifested by surface markers, even in the absence of morphologically abnormal blood lymphocytes, occuring in 13% of adult cases in one series (Gajl-Peczalska *et al.*, 1975).

Analysis of lymph node lymphocytes in suspension is complicated by the frequent occurrence of apparently normal cells admixed with the malignant ones in partially involved nodes or nodes containing reactive cells. In the evaluation of malignant nodes, it is necessary to assess the cells labeled by the various markers by cytocentrifuge smears or on Millipore filters (Jaffe *et al.*, 1975; Leech *et al.*, 1975). Additional help has come from the use of the markers on frozen section, so as to preserve the pathological architecture.

When these techniques have been carefully applied, proliferations originally classified as having a nodular architecture have been found to be composed of B cells, generally having monoclonal membrane IgM (+IgD) or, less often, IgG (Leech *et al.*, 1975; Gajl-Peczalska *et al.*, 1975) or complement receptors (Jaffe *et al.*, 1975). There are a few discordant cases of nodular histology among those of Aisenberg and Long (1975) and Peter *et al.* (1974), which were not, however, evaluated by tissue-sectional analysis. These were found to have a predominance of T cells, either by anti-T-cell sera (Aisenberg) or by sheep rosettes (Peter), and might be interpreted as showing that at least some nodular lymphomas are of T-cell origin. The author believes that great caution must be exercised in the present interpretation of these data, for the reasons elaborated in Section 2. A proportion of the nodular lymphomas in all reports could not be positively identified as monoclonal. When studied, FcRs by the aggregated IgG method were detected on a similar proportion of cells found to carry membrane Ig; a few cases, as in CLL, showed discordance of these two markers.

The findings in nodular lymphoma would appear at least tentatively to support the concept of follicular center cell neoplasia of Lukes and Collins (1974) and Lennert *et al.* (1975) (see Section 2.3.1), since nodular disease would be expected to be composed of B cells.

The situation in the case of the lymphocytic lymphomas of diffuse architecture is more complex. Those identified by Leech *et al.* (1975) as FCC tumors, having cleaved nuclear morphology, were B cells by marker criteria as well. This finding confirms the usefulness of nuclear cleavage as a criterion for FCC origin, even in the diffuse lymphomas. Peter *et al.* (1974) reported a nodular lymphoma of small cleaved cells that consisted primarily of sheep-rosette-forming cells, the only marker used (see above). Overall, the study of Leech and colleagues concluded that of 45 consecutively studied patients with non-Hodgkin's lymphoma, 60% were morphologically of FCC type. All these patients could be shown to have surface markers consistent with B cells. Among the remaining 40% uncleaved, diffuse types, Leech, Waldron, and their colleagues detected some with B, some with T, and some without markers of either type of cell. Others, who have not used the same morphological classification (Gajl-Peczalska *et al.*, 1975; Aisenberg and Long, 1975; Johansson *et al.*, 1976; Brouet *et al.*, 1975a), found most diffuse, poorly differentiated lymphocytic lymphomas to be of monoclonal B-cell origin. Jaffe *et al.* (1975), on the other hand, found 3 of 3 cases studied to form sheep rosettes, indicating a probable T-cell origin. Patient age is an important factor in the cell type participating in DPDL. The disease in adults is most often of B cells, while in childhood it is commonly of T-cell or indeterminate type (Gajl-Peczalska *et al.*, 1975; Mann *et al.*, 1975).

Cytoplasmic immunofluorescence for detection of plasmacytoid cells in non-Hodgkin's lymphoma was carried out in a few studies in conjunction with surface markers, and was positive in only occasional cases (Gajl-Peczalska *et al.*, 1975; Johansson *et al.*, 1976), although Taylor (1974), using a sensitive immunoperoxidase technique (which may have detected SIg), found a high proportion of positive cells.

Leech *et al.* (1975) made the interesting observation that λ-bearing proliferations appeared to occur almost exclusively in diffuse lymphomas. Considering both leukemic and nodal cellular analyses, of the λ proliferations so far reported in this way (Leech *et al.*, 1975; Gajl-Peczalska *et al.*, 1975; Aisenberg and Long, 1975; Peter *et al.*, 1974), 20 have been associated with diffuse, and only 5 with nodular, lymphomas; κ-bearing lymphomas were nodular in 18 and diffuse in 11 cases. Leech *et al.* (1975) also noted that IgA- and IgG-bearing cells appeared to be associated with the noncleaved varieties of B-cell lymphomas, which may reflect different stages in B-cell differentiation between noncleaved and cleaved cells.

When the larger number of cases analyzed in blood or marrow as leukemic manifestations are considered, similar relationships appear to be maintained. Nodular lymphomas in leukemic phase consist of B cells (Aisenberg and Long, 1975; Koziner *et al.*, 1977b; Brouet *et al.*, 1975a; Cohnen *et al.*, 1974; Mathé *et al.*, 1975; Gajl-Peczalska *et al.*, 1973), and diffuse lymphomas of either T, B, or undefined cells. In our series of adult leukemic DPDL, however, there seemed to be an unusual frequency of T-cell proliferations (4 of 12 cases) or unidentifiable cells (7 of 12), and only 1 that appeared to be of monoclonal B-cell type (Koziner *et al.*, 1976). These cases appeared both by marker criteria and clinically to resemble acute lymphoblastic leukemia. Since a large proportion of cases of adult DPDL in solid tissue are of B-cell origin, it may be that T- and null-cell varieties have a greater tendency to become leukemic or, alternatively, that they arise from tumors bearing B-cell markers. The latter seems unlikely, since all these leukemias tested (six) had TdT activity, a marker of the T-cell mode of differentiation. Those adults with leukemic DPDL may therefore most resemble cases of childhood lymphoma (see Section 3.5).

Chin *et al.* (1973) found only 1 leukemic proliferation in their series of peripheral blood samples from 17 patients with NHL, but did observe excess amounts of reactivity with an antithymocyte antiserum and antiimmunoglobulins, since many cells from those patients appeared to show both types of markers. This observation remains to be explained, as do the findings of Schedel *et al.* (1976) that the predominant Ig on 6 lymphosarcoma patients was IgG, which was shown by trypsinization to be intrinsic, and was associated with anti-IgG activity. It is possible that the demonstrated anti-IgG activity was not a property of the SIg but rather of isolated FcRs.

Proliferations characterized as "histiocytic" by the Rappaport scheme, and as reticulum-cell sarcomas in older terminologies, have been found to be heterogeneous, as recently reviewed by Brouet *et al.* (1976). They collected 38 cases from their own series and from the literature. Of this total, 16 were of B-cell origin (6 of these "supervening on previous B cell neoplasms"), 4 of T-cell, and 3 apparently of bona fide monocytic origins. The rest were unclassifiable by the markers utilized. In our more recent series, 4 patients with leukemic histiocytic lymphoma were studied: 2 were monoclonal IgMκ proliferations, while 2 had FcRs characteristic of monocytes or "third-population" lymphoid cells (Koziner *et al.*, 1977b).

In proliferations of mixed type, consisting of small and large cells (mixed histiocytic–lymphocytic), both types of cells appear to share the same membrane markers, being either "null" or of B-cell origin (Brouet *et al.*, 1976; Jaffe *et al.*, 1975). Nodularity again favors a B lineage (Jaffe *et al.*, 1975). Since many or most of these proliferations would also be included in the group of "immunoblastic" sarcomas or of large, uncleaved lymphocytic proliferations in the system of Lukes and Collins (1974), the heterogeneity of these cellular types from a marker point of view would again indicate the need for caution in classification by morphology alone.

Leukemic reticuloendotheliosis is an entity that may now be properly classified as a lymphoma. It is characterized by subacute course splenomegaly, grossly normal immune function, and the presence, in blood and spleen, of large mononuclear cells with an extremely villous or "hairy" membrane. This has led to its designation as *hairy-cell leukemia*. A variety of markers have been associated with these cells, and their origin is still somewhat controversial, particularly since no normal counterpart has been recognized. Jaffe *et al.* (1975) regarded them as monocytic or histiocytic on the grounds that they bound IgGEA, but not IgMEAC, in tissue section and in suspension, as is characteristic of most normal splenic histiocytes. Lennert (1975), on the other hand, concluded on the basis of primary tissue localization to the B-cell areas that these cells were in the B-cell lineage. Studies with other markers (Rubin *et al.*, 1969; Aisenberg and Bloch, 1972; Catovsky *et al.*, 1974b; Fu *et al.*, 1974; Siegal and Koziner, 1976; Leech *et al.*, 1976) also favored their positioning among the B cells, since they bear usually intrinsic (Leech *et al.*, 1976) monoclonal SIg (often IgM, IgD, or both) and have FcRs, but do not form sheep rosettes. A few proliferations have formed mouse rosettes as well. The cells do tend to associate with (?phagocytize) latex particles (Siegal and Koziner, 1976; Fu *et al.*, 1974), but do not seem to phagocytize other types of particles or contain enzymes characteristic of the monocyte–macrophage axis (Stein and Kaiserling, 1974). Golomb *et al.* (1975) studied the cells by SEM and found their membrane morphology to resemble that of monocytes; on some of these same cells, the author has found markers characteristic of B lymphocytes. The weight of the evidence so far favors their inclusion as B cells, but their place in the immunological scheme is not totally secure.

Burkitt's lymphoma was the first lymphoid tumor to be studied for SIg, before the significance of SIg as a marker of B cells was even recognized (Klein *et al.*, 1968). Both the African and American variants of this distinctive tumor have been characterized as B-cell proliferations (Binder *et al.*, 1975). Interestingly enough, they do not all share exactly the same pattern of surface markers, including EBV receptors, which are apparently lacking (or are relatively few) in certain Burkitt tumors and cell lines (Epstein *et al.*, 1976).

Sézary syndrome and mycosis fungoides have been grouped together by several investigators by virtue of their dermal involvement and common cellular morphology, frequent aneuploidy, and the presence of T, but not B, markers in most cases (Braylan *et al.*, 1973; Broome *et al.*, 1973; Brouet *et al.*, 1973) [a few have shown both B and T cell markers (e.g., Shevach *et al.*, 1974)]. These cells are variable in their response to mitogens, but unlike most B-cell proliferations, a substantial proportion do respond to PHA, which is regarded as a T-cell lectin. Surface markers of these cells have not yet provided clear evidence of monoclonality. Cells of certain cases of Sézary syndrone have been shown to be capable of increasing B-cell differentiation and are thus classifiable as "helper" T cells (Broder *et al.*, 1976).

3.5. Acute Lymphoblastic Leukemia

Acute lymphocytic leukemia appears to occur in two fairly distinctive forms, as defined by surface-marker analysis. A substantial proportion of such cases have surface markers of T cells (either T-cell-related antigens or sheep-rosette-forming ability), but the majority are "null" types without detectable conventional markers (Kaplan, J., et al., 1974; Kersey et al., 1975; Sen and Borella, 1975; Brouet et al., 1975b; Mills, B., et al., 1975). In about 25% of the cases, the leukemic cells form sheep rosettes, some additional cases having T-cell antigens (Kersey et al., 1975). Sen and Borella (1975) pointed out that the cases associated with rosetting ability form a clinically distinctive group of older children, who have a mediastinal (thymic) mass and higher peripheral blast counts than do the children with "null"-cell ALL. There appears to be a strong relationship of the rosette-forming group to the cells of patients with "convoluted-cell" leukemia (Lukes and Collins, 1974), Sternberg sarcoma (lymphoblastic lymphosarcoma) (Nathwani et al., 1976), and perhaps to the forms of DPDL that in adults tend to become leukemic (Koziner et al., 1977b), all of which perhaps will ultimately be grouped together. Cells of this type often give a positive acid phosphatase stain (Nathwani et al., 1976). In early childhood, ALL tends to be a disease of "null" cells, as it does in adulthood. Jaffe et al. (1976) and Coccia et al. (1976) studied patients with childhood lymphoblastic lymphoma or DPDL and found a heterogeneous marker pattern. Some cases displayed complement receptors, some sheep-rosetting, some both of these markers, and some, neither. As discussed elsewhere in Section 2.1.3, the complement marker may not be specific for B cells. None of these proliferations carried SIg, FcRs, or other B-cell markers.

Those cases of ALL in which the cells do not carry sheep-rosetting ability do seem to be characterized by surface alloantigens, initially associated with myeloid and B cells, the Ia-like, "HL-B" or "B-cell" antigens (Fu et al., 1975a; Billing et al., 1976). Brown et al. (1975), moreover, developed a heteroantiserum that also detects the "null" ALL cells, but not antigens of normal B cells or of the sheep-rosetting type of ALL, further drawing the distinction between these two types of ALL. Perhaps linking these two apparently disparate groups of cases, however, is the observation that both cell types contain the enzyme TdT, which seems to be a useful marker of prethymic cells (McCaffrey et al., 1976). This seeming contradiction might be resolved if the "HL-B" and "leukemia-associated" antigens, which are also known to occur on nonlymphoid hematopoietic cells, are actually stem-cell antigens lost during the early differentiation of T, but not of B, cells. In this case, the sheep-rosette-negative ALL cases would represent a very early stage in lymphoid development along the T-cell pathway. In this regard, the "null" leukemic cells do not develop sheep-rosetting ability when incubated with thymic extracts (Tsukimoto and Lampkin, 1975).

A few cases of ALL carrying conventional B-cell markers have also been observed, all of which appear to have developed out of a substrate of chronic B-cell malignancy (CLL or Burkitt's lymphoma) (Brouet et al., 1975b). A case of apparently simultaneous acute leukemia by independent B- and T-cell clones was observed by Haegert et al. (1974). Very recently, several cases of non-rosette-forming SIg-negative ALL have been described which have cytoplasmic IgM and are TdT-negative. They have been regarded as "pre-B" ALL (Balch et al., 1978).

A variety of uncommon leukemias and lymphomas of morphologically diverse types that have been reported in the literature will not be discussed here. Certain anomalous cases of leukemic lymphoma that have had markers of both B and T cells (Siegal et al., 1976b; Lin and Hsu, 1976; Shevach et al., 1974; Hsu et al., 1975) have not been morphologically or histologically classified as a specific group, and in any event probably do not qualify as a specific "disease."

The polymorphous cellular infiltrates in involved nodal and some splenic tissue in this disease cannot be clearly distinguished from those of hyperplastic lymphoid tissue by cell-surface markers (Aisenberg and Long, 1975; Payne et al., 1976; Gajl-Peczalska et al., 1973), although they tend to have somewhat increased T-cell proportions (Aisenberg and Long, 1975; Payne et al., 1976; Braylan et al., 1974). Peripheral blood B and T values have been reported by various groups (reviewed by Gajl-Peczalska et al., 1976), but either have been normal or have shown an increase in the proportion of cells coated with IgG (Grifoni et al., 1975; Chin et al., 1973) (possibly antilymphocyte antibodies) and decreased T-cell rosettes. Serum factors blocking sheep-rosette formation were reported by Fuks et al. (1976). Excess Ig staining (of T cells) was observed in HD nodes (Payne et al., 1976). Such interfering factors, which are similar to those found in systemic lupus erythematosus sera (see Section 2.1.8b), may finally explain the variety of conflicting results reported earlier in this disease.

Although the exact nature of the Hodgkin's infiltrate is not known, the component presumed to be neoplastic includes the classic large multinucleated Reed–Sternberg (R-S) cells, the large mononuclear "Hodgkin's cells," and possibly the lymphoblasts (the last of which are mostly T cells). The nature of the R-S cells has not yet clearly been defined. SIg (Leech, 1973), sparse FcR activity (ox cell reagent) (Payne et al., 1976), and a general absence of sheep-rosette formation were observed on both R-S and HD cells. Payne et al. (1976) observed occasional Hodgkin's cells forming sheep rosettes, possibly indicating their heterogeneity, but the presence of cytophilic antibody reactive with sheep-cell antigens has not been excluded. The presence of intracellular IgG (but not IgM) was noted (Payne et al., 1976; Taylor, 1974; Garvin et al., 1974), but interestingly, the cytoplasmic fluorescence was described as less intense than that of normal plasma cells found in the same biopsy specimen and was not found consistently in all R-S or HD cells (Payne et al., 1976). Taylor (1974) reported that "in some cases both kappa and lambda light chains were clearly present in the same cell, as confirmed by dilution and blocking studies," detected by an immunoperoxidase technique. Leech's study with several monospecific antiglobulin sera (not including anti-λ) showed only IgG and κ surface and cytoplasmic staining. Staining of R-S and HD cells with Schiff–methylene blue showed considerable cytoplasmic RNA, and EM demonstrated a large number of free ribosomes, usually not membrane-bound, suggesting to the observers that the cytoplasmic IgG was synthesized by unbound ribosomes and not exported (Garvin et al., 1974). The accumulated data have indicated to some the B-cell origins of these cells. In the light of knowledge, however, particularly of the observations both of Winchester et al. (1975a) and of Grifoni et al. (1975), the findings to date are perfectly consistent with non-B cells coated with IgG antibody, perhaps chronically endocytosed through a capping mechanism to account for the cytoplasmic staining. While first described in lymphoid cells, capping is now known to occur in nonlymphoid cells as well (Raff, 1976). Histiocytic and other cell types should be excellent alternatives to cells of the B series as the source of these peculiar cells. Data from several laboratories now appear to support the monocyte–macrophage lineage of the R-S cell. The evidence has been derived from both combined cell-culture and marker analysis (Long et al., 1977; Kaplan, H. S., and Gartner, 1977) and histochemical staining (Curran and Jones, 1977). Nevertheless, the nature of the malignant cells in Hodgkin's disease is still uncertain, requiring further and more definitive study.

3.7. Histiocytic Medullary Reticulosis

Unlike leukemic reticuloendotheliosis, this unusual malignant disorder has not been widely studied. Jaffe *et al.* (1975) investigated a case as a way of validating their IgGEA reagent for the detection of FcRs on monocytes. The disease is characterized by a histiocytic proliferation marked by erythrophagocytosis. Because of the phagocytic activity of the cells, as well as their reactivity with the Fc reagent, this is the prototype of a true histiocytic malignancy.

References

Abdou, N. I., and Abou, N. L., 1975, The monoclonal nature of lymphocytes in multiple myeloma: Effects of therapy, *Ann. Intern. Med.* **83**:42–45.

Aisenberg, A. C., and Bloch, K. J., 1972, Immunoglobulins on the surface of neoplastic lymphocytes, *N. Engl. J. Med.* **287**:272–276.

Aisenberg, C., and Long, C., 1975, Lymphocyte surface characteristics in malignant lymphoma, *Am. J. Med.* **58**:300–306.

Aisenberg, A. C., Bloch, K. J., and Long, J., 1973, Cell-surface immunoglobulin in chronic lymphocytic leukemia and allied disorders, *Am. J. Med.* **55**:184–191.

Aisenberg, A. C., Long, J. C., and Wilkes, B., 1974, Chronic lymphocytic leukemia cells; Rosette formation and adherence to nylon fiber columns, *J. Natl. Cancer Inst.* **52**:13–17.

Aiuti, F., Cerottini, J.-C., Coombs, R. R. A., Cooper, M., Dickler, H. B., Frøland, S., Fudenberg, H. H., Greaves, M. F., Grey, H. M., Kunkel, H. G., Natvig, J., Preud'homme, J.-L., Rabellino, E., Ritts, R. E., Rowe, D. S., Seligmann, M., Siegal, F. P., Stjernsward, J., Terry, W. D., and Wybran, J., 1974, Identification, enumeration and isolation of B and T lymphocytes from human peripheral blood; Report of a WHO/IARC-sponsored workshop on human B and T cells, London, 15–17 July 1974 (special technical report), *Scand. J. Immunol.* **3**:521–532.

Alexander, E. L., and Wetzel, B., 1975, Human Lymphocytes: Similarity of B and T cell surface morphology, *Science* **188**:732–734.

Andersson, J., and Melchers, F., 1974, Maturation of mitogen-activated bone marrow-derived lymphocytes in the absence of proliferation, *Eur. J. Immunol.* **4**:533–538.

Augener, W., Cohnen, G., and Brittinger, G., 1974, Binding of aggregated IgG by lymphocytes in chronic lymphocytic leukemia, *Biomedicine* **21**:6–8.

Bach, J.-F., Delrieu, F., and Delbarre, F., 1970, The rheumatoid rosette; A diagnostic test unifying seropositive and seronegative rheumatoid arthritis, *Am. J. Med.* **49**:213–222.

Baker, M. A., Falk, R. E., Falk, J., and Greaves, M. F., 1976, Detection of monocyte specific antigen on human acute leukaemia cells, *Br. J. Haematol.* **32**:13–19.

Balch, C. M., Vogler, L. B., and Dougherty, P. A., 1978, Distribution and immunochemical properties of a unique B-cell differentiation antigen on human leukemic lymphocytes, American Association for Cancer Research, Washington, D.C. (abstract).

Ballet, J.-J., Insel, R., Merler, E., and Rosen, F. S., 1976, Inhibition of maturation of human precursor lymphocytes by coformycin, an inhibitor of the enzyme adenosine deaminase, *J. Exp. Med.* **143**:1271–1276.

Baltimore, D., Kung, P., Silverstone, A., Harrison, T., and McCaffrey, R., 1976, Specialized DNA polymerases in lymphoid cells, *Cold Spring Harbor Symp. Quant. Biol.* **41**:63–72.

Barr, R. E., Whang-Peng, J., and Perry, S., 1975, Hemopoietic stem cells in human peripheral blood, *Science* **190**:284–285.

Baxley, G., Bishop, G. B., Cooper, A. G., and Wortis, H. H., 1973, Rosetting of human red blood cells to thymocytes and thymus-derived cells, *Clin. Exp. Immunol.* **15**:385–392.

Bentwich, Z., Douglas, S. D., Siegal, F. P., and Kunkel, H. G., 1973a, Human lymphocyte–sheep erythrocyte rosette formation: Some characteristics of the interaction, *Clin. Immunol. Immunopathol.* **1**:511–522.

Bentwich, Z., Douglas, S. D., Skutelsky, E., and Kunkel, H. G., 1973b, Sheep red blood cell binding to human lymphocytes treated with neuraminidase: enhancement of T cell binding and identification of a subpopulation of B cells, *J. Exp. Med.* **137**:1532–1537.

Berard, C. W., Gallo, R. C., Jaffe, E. S., Green, I., and Devita, V. T., Jr., 1976, Current concepts of leukemia and lymphoma: Etiology, pathogenesis and therapy, *Ann. Intern. Med.* **85**:351–366.

Berlinger, N. T., Lopez, C., and Good, R. A., 1976, Facilitation or attenuation of mixed leukocyte culture responsiveness by adherent cells, *Nature (London)* **260**:145–146.

Bianco, C., and Nussenzweig, V., 1971, Theta-bearing and complement-receptor lymphocytes are distinct populations of cells, *Science* **173**:154–156.

Bianco, C., Patrick, R., and Nussenzweig, V., 1970, A population of lymphocytes bearing a membrane receptor for antigen–antibody–complement complexes. I. Separation and characterization, *J. Exp. Med.* **132**:702–720.

Billing, J., Terasaki, P., Honig, R., and Peterson, P., 1976, The absence of B-cell antigen B2 from leukaemia cells and lymphoblastoid cell lines, *Lancet* **1**:1365–1367.

Binder, R. A., Jencks, J. A., Chun, B., and Rath, C. E., 1975, "B" cell origin of malignant cells in a case of American Burkitt's lymphoma, *Cancer* **36**:161–168.

Binz, H., and Wigzell, H., 1975, Shared idiotypic determinants on B and T lymphocytes reactive against the same antigenic determinants. II. Determination of frequency and characteristics of idiotypic T and B lymphocytes in normal rats using direct visualization, *J. Exp. Med.* **142**:1218–1230.

Bokisch, V. A., and Sobel, A. T., 1974, Receptor for the fourth component of complement on human B lymphocytes and cultured human lymphoblastoid cells, *J. Exp. Med.* **140**:1336–1347.

Bollum, F. J., 1975, Antibody to terminal deoxynucleotidyl transferase, *Proc. Natl. Acad. Sci. U.S.A.* **72**:4119–4122.

Borella, L., and Sen, L., 1975, E receptors on blasts from untreated acute lymphocytic leukemia (ALL): Comparison of temperature dependence of E rosettes formed by normal and leukemic lymphoid cells, *J. Immunol.* **114**:187–190.

Boyse, E. A., and Bennett, D., 1974, Differentiation and the cell surface: Illustrations from work with T cells and sperm, in: *Cellular Selection and Regulation in the Immune Response* (G. M. Edelman, ed.), pp. 155–176, Raven Press, New York.

Brain, P., Gordon, J., and Willetts, W. A., 1970, Rosette formation by peripheral lymphocytes, *Clin. Exp. Immunol.* **6**:681–688.

Brandtzaeg, P., 1974, Presence of J chain in human immunocytes containing various immunoglobulin classes, *Nature (London)* **252**:418–419.

Branganza, C. M., Stathopoulos, G., Davies, A. J. S., Elliott, E. V., Kerbel, R. S., Papamichael, M., and Holborow, E. J., 1975, Lymphocyte:erythrocyte (L.E.) rosettes as indicators of the heterogeneity of lymphocytes in a variety of mammalian species, *Cell* **4**:103–106.

Braylan, R. C., Jaffe, E. S., and Berard, C. W., 1974, Surface characteristics of Hodgkin's lymphoma cells, *Lancet* **2**:1328–1329.

Braylan, R. C., Variakojis, and Yachnin, S., 1975, The Sézary syndrome lymphoid cell: Abnormal surface properties and mitogen responsiveness, *Br. J. Haematol.* **31**:553–564.

Braylan, R. C., Jaffe, E. S., Burbach, J. W., Frank, M. M., and Berard, C. W., 1976, Surface characteristics of malignant well differentiated lymphocytes, *Blood* **46**:1036.

Broder, S., Humphrey, R., Durm, M., Blackman, M., Meade, B., Goldman, C., Strober, W., and Waldmann, T., 1975, Impaired synthesis of polyclonal (non-paraprotein) immunoglobulins by circulating lymphocytes from patients with multiple myeloma (role of suppressor cells), *N. Engl. J. Med.* **203**:887–892.

Broder S., Edelson, R. L., Lutzner, M. A., Nelson, D. L., MacDermott, R. P., Durm, M. E., Goldman, C. K., Meade, B. D., and Waldman, T. A., 1976, The Sézary syndrome. A malignant proliferation of helper T cells, *J. Clin. Invest.* **58**:1297–1306.

Broom, B. C., Webster, A. D. B., de la Concha, E. G., Loewi, G., and Asherson, G. L., 1975, Dichotomy between immunoglobulin synthesis by cells in gut and blood of patients with hypogammaglobulinemia, *Lancet* **2**:253–256.

Broome, J. D., Zucker-Franklin, D., Weiner, M. S., Bianco, C., and Nussenzweig, V., 1973, leukemic cells with membrane properties of thymus-derived (T) lymphocytes in a case of Sézary's syndrome: Morphologic and immunologic studies, *Clin. Immunol. Immunopathol.* **1**:319–329.

Brouet, J.-C., Flandrin, G., and Seligmann, M., 1973, Indications of the thymus-derived nature of the proliferating cells in six patients with Sézary's syndrome, *N. Engl. J. Med.* **289**:341–344.

Brouet, J.-C., Preud'homme, J.-L., Flandrin, G., Chelloul, N., and Seligmann, M., 1976, Membrane markers in "histiocytic" lymphomas (reticulum cell sarcomas), *J. Natl. Cancer Inst.* **56**:631–633.

Brouet, J.-C., Preud'homme, J.-L., and Seligmann, M., 1975b, The use of B and T membrane markers in

314

FREDERICK P. SIEGAL

the classification of human leukemias, with special reference to acute lymphoblastic leukemia, *Blood Cells* 1:81–90.

Brouet, J.-C., Flandrin, G., Sasportes, M., Preud'homme, J.-L., and Seligmann, M., 1975c, Chronic lymphocytic leukaemia of T-cell origin; Immunological and clinical evaluation in eleven patients, *Lancet* 2:890–893.

Brouet, J.-C., Preud'homme, J.-L., Flandrin, G., Chelloul, N., and Seligmann, M., 1976, Membrane markers in "histiocytic" lymphomas (reticulum cell sarcomas), *J. Natl. Cancer Inst.* 56:631–633.

Brown, G., and Greaves, M. F., 1974, Cell surface markers for human T and B lymphocytes, *Eur. J. Immunol.* 4:302–310.

Brown, G., Capellaro, D., and Greaves, M., 1975, Leukemia-associated antigens in man, *J. Natl. Cancer Inst.* 55:1281–1289.

Catovsky, D., Pettit, J. E., Galton, D. G. A., Spiers, A. S. D., and Harrison, C. V., 1974a, Leukaemic reticuloendotheliosis ("hairy" cell leukaemia): A distinct clinico-pathological entity, *Br. J. Haematol.* 26:9–21.

Catovsky, D., Pettit, J. E., Galetto, J., Ikos, A., and Galton, D. A. G., 1974b, The B-lymphocyte nature of the hairy cell of leukaemic reticuloendotheliosis, *Br. J. Haematol.* 26:29–37.

Catovsky, D., Frisch, B., and Van Noorden, S., 1975, B, T, and "null" cell leukaemias: Electron cytochemistry and surface morphology, *Blood Cells* 1:115–124.

Chang, L. M. S., and Bollum, F. J., 1971, Deoxynucleotide-polymerizing enzymes of calf thymus gland. V. Homogeneous terminal deoxynucleotidyl transferase, *J. Biol. Chem.* 246:909–916.

Chen, C., and Hirsch, J. G., 1972, The effects of mercaptoethanol and of peritoneal macrophages on the antibody-forming capacity of nonadherent spleen cells *in vitro, J. Exp. Med.* 136:604–617.

Chen, Y., Bhoopalam, N., Yakulis, V., and Heller, P., 1975, Changes in lymphocyte surface immunoglobulins in myeloma and the effect of an RNA-containing plasma factor, *Ann. Intern. Med.* 83:625–631.

Chess, L., Levine, H., MacDermott, R. P., and Schlossman, S. F., 1975, Immunologic functions of isolated human lymphocyte subpopulations. VI. Further characterization of the surface Ig-negative, E rosette negative (null cell) subset, *J. Immunol.* 115:1483–1487.

Chiao, J. W., Pantic, V. S., and Good, R. A., 1974, Human peripheral lymphocytes bearing both B-cell complement receptors and T-cell characteristics for sheep erythrocytes detected by a mixed rosette method, *Clin. Exp. Immunol.* 18:483–490.

Chin, A. H., Saiki, J. H., Trujillo, J. M., and Williams, R. C., Jr., 1973, Peripheral blood T and B lymphocytes in patients with lymphoma and acute leukemia, *Clin. Immunol. Immunopathol.* 1:499–510.

Clark, C., Rydell, R. E., and Kaplan, M. E., 1973, Frequent association of IgMλ with crystalline inclusions in chronic lymphatic leukemic lymphocytes, *N. Engl. J. Med.* 289:113–117.

Coccia, P. F., Kersey, J. H., Corte, J., Chartrand, S., Gajl-Peczalska, K., Krivit, W., and Nesbit, M. E., 1976, Lymphoblasts with receptors for both sheep erythrocytes and complement in childhood diffuse poorly differentiated lymphocytic lymphoma (dPDLL), *Blood* 46:1036.

Cohnen, G., Augener, W., Buka, A., and Brittinger, G., 1974, Rosette-forming lymphocytes in normals and patients with malignant lymphomas, *Acta Haematol.* 51:65–75.

Coombs, R. R. A., Gurner, B. W., Wilson, A. B., Holm, G., and Lindgren, B., 1970, Rosette-formation between human lymphocytes and sheep red cells not involving immunoglobulin receptors, *Int. Arch. Allergy Appl. Immunol.* 39:658–663.

Coons, A. H., Leduc, E. H., and Connolly, E., 1955, Study on antibody production. I. A method for the histochemical demonstration of specific antibody and its application to a study of the hyperimmune rabbit, *J. Exp. Med.* 102:49–54.

Cooper, A. G., Brown, M. C., Derby, H. A. and Wortis, H. H., 1973, Quantitation of surface-membrane and intracellular gamma, mu and kappa chains of normal and neoplastic human lymphocytes, *Clin. Exp. Immunol.* 13:487–496.

Cooper, M. D., Lawton, A. R., and Bockman, D. E., 1971, Agammaglobulinemia with B lymphocytes: Specific defect of plasma cell differentiation, *Lancet* 2:791–794.

Cuatrecasas, P., 1970, Protein purification by affinity chromatography: Derivations of agarose and polyacrylamide beads, *J. Biol. Chem.* 245:3059–3065.

Curran, R. C., and Jones, E. L., 1977, Dendritic cells and B lymphocytes in Hodgkin's disease, *Lancet* 2:349 (letter).

Davis, S., 1975, Hypothesis: Differentiation of the human lymphoid system based on cell surface markers, *Blood* 45:870–880.

Dickler, H. B., 1974, Studies of the human lymphocyte receptor for heat-aggregated or antigen complexed immunoglobulin, *J. Exp. Med.* **140**:508–522.

Dickler, H. B., and Kunkel, H. G., 1972, Interaction of aggregated gammaglobulin with B lymphocytes, *J. Exp. Med.* **136**:191–196.

Dickler, H. B., Siegal, F. P., Bentwich, Z., and Kunkel, H. G., 1973, Lymphocyte binding of aggregated IgG and surface Ig staining in chronic lymphocytic leukemia, *Clin. Exp. Immunol.* **14**:97–107.

Dobozy, A., Husz, S., Hunyadi, J., and Simon, N., 1976, Formation of mouse erythrocyte rosettes by human lymphocytes, a B-cell marker, *Clin. Exp. Immunol.* **23**:382–384.

Dorfman, R. F., 1974, Classification of non-Hodgkin's lymphomas, *Lancet* **1**:1295–1296.

Douglas, S. D., 1971, Human lymphocyte growth in vitro: morphologic, biochemical and immunologic significance. *Int. Rev. Exp. Pathol.* **10**:41–114.

Dukor, P., Bianco, C., and Nussenzweig, V., 1970, Tissue localization of lymphocytes bearing a membrane receptor for antigen–antibody–complement complexes, *Proc. Natl. Acad. Sci. U.S.A.* **67**:991–997.

Ehlenberger, A. G., McWilliams, M., Phillips-Quagliata, J. M., Lamm, M. E., and Nussenzweig, V., 1976, Immunoglobulin-bearing and complement-receptor lymphocytes constitute the same population in human peripheral blood, *J. Clin. Invest.* **57**:53–56.

Eichmann, K., and Rajewsky, K., 1975, Induction of T and B cell immunity by anti-idiotypic antibody, *Eur. J. Immunol.* **5**:661–666.

Eipe, J., Yakulis, V., and Costea, N., 1976, Idiotypic specificity of lymphocyte surface Ig (SIg) and serum monoclonal IgM in patients with malignant lymphoproliferative disorders, *Blood* **46**:1036.

Epstein, A. L., Henle, W., Henle, G., Hewetson, J. F., and Kaplan, H., 1976, Surface marker characteristics and Epstein–Barr virus studies of two established North American Burkitt's lymphoma cell lines, *Proc. Natl. Acad. Sci. U.S.A.* **73**:228–232.

Fagraeus, A., The, H., and Biberfield, G., 1973, Reaction of human smooth muscle antibody with thymus medullary cells, *Nature (London) New Biol.* **246**:113–115.

Fagraeus, A., Lidman, K. and Biberfeld, G., 1974, Reaction of human smooth muscle antibodies with human blood lymphocytes and lymphoid cell lines, *Nature (London)* **252**:246–247.

Ferrarini, M., Bargellesi, A., Corte, G., Viale, F., and Pernis, B., 1975, Comparative study of membrane and intracytoplasmic immunoglobulin classes in human lymphoid cells, *Ann. N.Y. Acad. Sci.* **254**:243–253.

Filippa, D. A., and Siegal, F. P., 1975 (unpublished).

Fogh, J. 1974 (personal communication).

Forni, L., and Pernis, B., 1975, Interactions between Fc receptors and membrane immunoglobulins on B lymphocytes, in: *Membrane Receptors of Lymphocytes,* INSERM Symposium I (M. Seligmann, J.-L. Preud'homme, and F. M. Kourilsky, eds.), pp. 193–201, American-Elsevier, New York.

Frøland, S., and Natvig, J. B., 1973, Identification of three different human lymphocyte populations by surface markers, *Transplant. Rev.* **16**:114–162.

Frøland, S., Natvig, J. B., and Berdal, P., 1971, Surface-bound immunoglobulin as a marker of B lymphocytes in man, *Nature (London) New Biol.* **234**:251–252.

Frøland, S. S., Wisloff, F., and Michaelsen, T. E., 1974, Human lymphocytes with receptors for IgG, a population of cells distinct from T- and B-lymphocytes, *Int. Arch. Allergy Appl. Immunol.* **47**:124–138.

Fu, S. M., Winchester, R. J., Rai, K. R., and Kunkel, H. G., 1974, Hairy cell leukemia: Proliferation of a cell with phagocytic and B lymphocyte properties, *Scand. J. Immunol.* **3**:847–851.

Fu, S. M., Winchester, R. J., and Kunkel, H. G., 1975a, The occurrence of the *HL-B* alloantigens on the cells of unclassified acute lymphoblastic leukemias, *J. Exp. Med.* **142**:1334–1338.

Fu, S. M., Winchester, R. J., and Kunkel, H. G., 1975b, Similar idiotypic specificity of the membrane IgD and IgM of human B lymphocytes, *J. Immunol.* **114**:250–252.

Fuks, Z., Strober, S., and Kaplan, H. S., 1976, Interaction between serum factors and T lymphocytes in Hodgkin's disease: Use as a diagnostic test, *N. Engl. J. Med.* **295**:1275–1278.

Gajl-Peczalska, K. J., Hansen, J. A., Bloomfield, C. D., and Good, R. A., 1973, B lymphocytes in untreated patients with malignant lymphoma and Hodgkin's disease, *J. Clin. Invest.* **52**:3064–3073.

Gajl-Peczalska, K. J., Bloomfield, C. D., Coccia, P. F., Sosin, H., Brunning, R. D., and Kersey, J. H., 1975, B and T cell lymphomas: Analysis of blood and lymph nodes in 87 patients, *Am. J. Med.* **59**:674–685.

Gajl-Peczalska, K. J., Bloomfield, C. D., Sosin, H., and Kersey, J. H., 1976, B and T lymphocytes in Hodgkin's disease: Analysis at diagnosis and following therapy, *Clin. Exp. Immunol.* **23**:47–55.

Galili, U., and Schlesinger, M., 1975, Subpopulations of human thymus cells differing in their capacity to form stable E-rosettes and in their immunologic reactivity, *J. Immunol.* **115**:827–833.

Galton, D. A. G., Goldman, J. M., Witshaw, E., Catovsky, D., Henry, D., and Goldenberg, G. J., 1974, Prolymphocytic leukaemia, *Br. J. Haematol.* **27**:7–23.

Garvin, A. J., Spicer, S. S., Parmley, R. T., and Munster, A. M., 1974, Immunohistochemical demonstration of IgG in Reed–Sternberg and other cells in Hodgkin's desease, *J. Exp. Med.* **139**:1077–1083.

Gathings, W. E., Cooper, M. D., Lawton, A. R., and Alford, C. A., Jr., 1976, B cell ontogeny in humans, *Fed. Proc. Fed. Am. Soc. Exp. Biol.* **35**:276.

Gelfand, M. C., Shin, M. L., Nagle, R. B., Green, I., and Frank, M. M., 1976, The glomerular complement receptor in immunologically mediated renal glomerular injury, *N. Engl. J. Med.* **295**:10–14.

Giacomoni, D., Yakulis, V., Wang, S. R., Cooke, A., Dray, S., and Heller, P., 1975, *In vitro* conversion of normal mouse lymphocytes by plasmacytoma RNA to express idiotypic specificities on their surface characteristic of the plasmacytoma immunoglobulin, *Cell. Immunol.* **11**:389–400.

Glinski, W., Gershwin, M. E., and Steinberg, A. D., 1976, Fractionation of lymphoid cells on a discontinuous Ficoll gradient—Study of subpopulations of human T-cells using anti-T-cell antibodies from patients with systemic lupus erythematosus, *J. Clin. Invest.* **57**:604–614.

Gluckman, J. C., and Montambault, P., 1974, Spontaneous autorosette-forming cells in man: A marker for a subset population of T lymphocytes?, *Clin. Exp. Immunol.* **22**:302–310.

Golomb, H., Braylan, R., and Polliack, A., 1975, "Hairy cell leukemia" (Leukemic reticuloendotheliosis): A scanning electron microscopy study of eight cases, *Br. J. Haematol.* **29**:455–460.

Greaves, M. F., 1974 (personal communication).

Greaves, M., and Janossy, G., 1972, Elicitation of selective T and B lymphocyte responses by cell surface binding ligands, *Transplant. Rev.* **11**:87–130.

Greaves, M. F., Owen, J. J. T., and Raff, M. C., 1973, *T and B Lymphocytes: Origins, Properties and Roles in Immune Responses*, American Elsevier, New York.

Greaves, M. F., Falk, J. A., and Falk, R. E., 1975a, A surface antigen marker for human monocytes, *Scand. J. Immunol.* **4**:555–562.

Greaves, M. F., Brown, G., and Rickinson, A. B., 1975b, Epstein–Barr virus binding sites on lymphocyte subpopulations and the origin of lymphoblasts in cyltured lymphoid cell lines and in the blood of patients with infectious mononucleosis, *Clin. Immunol. Immunopathol.* **3**:514–524.

Greenberg, A. H., Shen, L., and Roitt, I. M., 1973, Characterization of the antibody-dependent cytotoxic cell: A non-phagocytic monocyte?, *Clin. Exp. Immunol.* **15**:251–259.

Grey, H. M., Rabellino, E., and Pirofsky, B., 1971, Immunoglobulins on the surface of lymphocytes. IV. Distribution in hypogammaglobulinemia, cellular immune deficiency, and chronic lymphatic leukemia, *J. Clin. Invest.* **50**:2368–2375.

Grey, H. M., Colon, S. M., Campbell, P., and Rabellino, E., 1972, Immunoglobulins on surface of lymphocytes. 5. Quantitative studies on question of whether immunoglobulins are associated with T cells in mouse, *J. Immunol.* **109**:776–778.

Grifoni, V., Del Giacco, G. S., Manconi, P. E., Tognella, S., and Mantovani, G., 1975, Lymphocytes in the spleen in Hodgkin's disease, *Lancet* **1**:332–333.

Gupta, S., and Grieco, M. H., 1975, Rosette-formation with mouse erythrocytes: Probable marker for human B lymphocytes, *Int. Arch. Allergy Appl. Immunol.* **49**:734–742.

Gupta, S., Pahwa, R., O'Reilly, R., Good, R. A., and Siegal, F. P., 1976a, Ontogeny of lymphocyte subpopulations in human fetal liver, *Proc. Natl. Acad. Sci. U.S.A.* **73**:919.

Gupta, S., Ross, G., Good, R. A., and Siegal, F. P., 1976b, Surface markers on human eosinophils, *Blood* **48**:755–763.

Gupta, S., Good, R. A., and Siegal, F. P., 1976c, Rosette-formation with mouse erythrocytes. II. A marker for human B and non-T lymphocytes, *Clin. Exp. Immunol.* **25**:319–327.

Gupta, S., Good, R. A., and Siegal, F. P., 1976d, Rosette-formation with mouse erythrocytes. III. Studies in patients with primary immunodeficiency and lymphoproliferative disorders, *Clin. Exp. Immunol.* **26**:204–213.

Haegert, D. G., Cawley, J. C., Karpas, A., and Goldstone, A. H., 1974, Combined T and B cell acute lymphoblastic leukaemia, *Br. Med. J.* **4**:79–82.

Hallberg, T., Haegert, D., Clein, G. P., Coombs, R. R. A., Feinstein, A., and Gurner, B. W., 1973a, Observations on the mixed antiglobulin reaction as a test for immunogloublin-bearing lymphocytes in normal persons and in patients with chronic lymphatic leukaemia, *J. Immunol. Methods* **4**:317–332.

Hallberg, T., Gurner, B. W., and Coombs, R. R. A., 1973b, Opsonic adherence of sensitized ox red cells to human lymphocytes as measured by rosette formation, *Int. Arch. Allergy Appl. Immunol.* **44**:500–513.

Hammarström, S., Hellström, U., Perlmann, P., and Dillner, M.-L., 1973, A new surface marker on T lymphocytes of human peripheral blood, *J. Exp. Med.* **138**:1270–1275.

Harris, N. S., 1974, Plasma cell surface antigen on human blood lymphocytes, *Nature (London)* **250**:507–509.

Havemann, K., and Rubin, A. D., 1968, The delayed response of chronic lymphocytic leukemia lymphocytes to phytohemagglutinin *in vitro, Proc. Soc. Exp. Biol. Med.* **127**:668–671.

Hayward, A. R., and Greaves, M. F., 1975, Identification of cells with monocyte markers in panhypogammaglobulinaemia, *Scand. J. Immunol.* **4**:563–570.

Herzenberg, L. S., Sweet, R. G., and Herzenberg, S. A., 1976, Fluorescence-activated cell sorting, *Sci. Am.* **234**:108–117.

Hirschhorn, R., Beratis, N., and Rosen, F. S., 1976, Characterization of residual enzyme activity in fibroblasts from patients with adenosine deaminase deficiency and combined immunodeficiency: Evidence for a mutant enzyme, *Proc. Natl. Acad. Sci. U.S.A.* **73**:213–217.

Horwitz, D. A., 1976, Functional characterization of human peripheral blood lymphocytes, *Fed. Proc. Fed. Am. Soc. Exp. Biol.* **35**:473.

Horwitz, D. A., and Lobo, P. I., 1975, Characterization of two populations of human lymphocytes bearing easily detectable surface immunoglobulin, *J. Clin. Invest.* **56**:1464–1472.

Hsu, C. C. S., and Fell, A., 1974, Polymorphonuclear cells form E rosettes, *N. Engl. J. Med.* **290**:402–403.

Hsu, C. C. S., Marti, G. E., Schrek, R., and Williams, R. C., Jr., 1975, Lymphocytes bearing B- and T-cell markers in patient with lymphosarcoma cell leukemia, *Clin. Immunol. Immunopathol.* **3**:385–395.

Huber, H., Douglas, S. D., and Fudenberg, H. H., 1969, The IgG receptor: An immunological marker for the characterization of mononuclear cells, *Immunology* **17**:7–21.

Jaffe, E. S., Shevach, E. M., Sussman, E. H., Frank, M., Green, I., and Berard, C. W., 1975, Membrane receptor sites for the identification of lymphoreticular cells in benign and malignant conditions, *Br. J. Cancer* **31**(*Suppl. 2*):107–120.

Jaffe, E. S., Braylan, R., Frank, M. M., Green, I., and Berard, C., 1976, Heterogeneity of immunologic markers and surface morphology in "childhood lymphoblastic lymphoma," *Blood* **48**:213–222.

Janossy, G., and Greaves, M. F., 1975, Functional analysis of murine and human B. lymphocyte subsets, *Transplant. Rev.* **24**:177–236.

Johansson, B., Klein, E., and Haglund, S., 1976, Correlation between the presence of surface localized immunoglobulin (Ig) and the histological type of human malignant lymphomas, *Clin. Immunol. Immunopathol.* **5**:119–132.

Jondal, M., and Klein, G., 1973, Surface markers on human B and T lymphocytes II. Presence of Epstein–Barr virus receptors on B lymphocytes, *J. Exp. Med.* **138**:1365–1378.

Jondal, M., Holm, G., and Wigzell, H., 1972, Surface markers on human B and T lymphocytes. I. A large population of lymphocytes forming nonimmune rosettes with sheep red blood cells, *J. Exp. Med.* **136**:207–215.

Jones, S. V., and McFarlane, H., 1975, T and B cells in myelomatosis, *Br. J. Haematol.* **31**:545–552.

Kaiserling, E., Stein, H., and Lennert, K., 1973, IgM-producing malignant lymphomas without macroglobulinemia—Morphological and immunochemical findings, *Virchows Arch. B* **14**:1–18.

Kaplan, H. S., and Gartner, S. 1977, "Sternberg–Reed" giant cells of Hodgkin's disease: Cultivation *in vitro*, heterotransplantation, and characterization as neoplastic macrophages, *Int. J. Cancer* **19**:511–525.

Kaplan, J., 1975, Human T lymphocytes form rosettes with autologous and allogeneic human red blood cells, *Clin. Immunol. Immunopathol.* **3**:471–475.

Kaplan, J., Mastrangelo, R., and Peterson, W. D., Jr., 1974, Childhood lymphoblastic lymphoma, a cancer of thymus-derived lymphocytes, *Cancer Res.* **34**:521–525.

Kay, M. M., Belohradsky, B., Yee, K., Vogel, J., Butcher, D., Wybran, J., and Fudenberg, H. H., 1974, Cellular interactions: Scanning electron microscopy of human thymus-derived rosette-forming lymphocytes, *Clin. Immunol. Immunopathol.* **2**:301–309.

Kersey, J., Nesbit, M., Hallgren, H., Sabad, A., Yunis, E., and Gajl-Peczalska, K., 1975, Evidence for origin of certain childhood acute lymphoblastic leukemias and lymphomas in thymus-derived lymphocytes, *Cancer* **36**:1348–1352.

Klein, E., Klein, G., Nadkarni, J. S., Nadkarni, J. J., Wigzell, H., and Clifford, P., 1968, Surface IgM-kappa specificity on a Burkitt lymphoma cell *in vivo* and in derived culture lines, *Cancer Res.* **28**:1300–1310.

Korsmeyer, S. J., Strickland, R. G., Ammann, A. J., Waldmann, T. A., and Williams, R. C., Jr.,.1976, Differential specificity of lymphocytotoxins from patients with systemic lupus erythematosus and inflammatory bowel disease, *Clin. Immunol. Immunopathol.* **5**:67–73.

Koziner, B., McKenzie, S., Straus, D., Clarkson, B., Good, R. A., and Siegal, F. P., 1977a, Cell marker analysis in acute monocytic leukemias, *Blood* **49**:895–901.

Koziner, B., Filippa, D. A., Mertelsmann, R., Gupta, S., Clarkson, B., Good, R. A., and Siegal, F. P., 1977b, Characterization of lymphomas in a leukemic phase by multiple differentiation markers of mononuclear cells: Correlation with clinical features and conventional morphology, *Amer. J. Med.* **63**:556–567.

Kubo, R. T., Grey, H. M., and Pirofsky, B., 1974, IgD: A major immunoglobulin on the surface of lymphocytes from patients with chronic lymphatic leukemia, *J. Immunol.* **112**:1952–1954.

Kumagai, K., Abo, R., Sekizawa, T., and Sasaki, M., 1975, Studies of surface immunoglobulins on human B lymphocytes. I. Dissociation of cell-bound immunoglobulins with acid pH or at 37 °C, *J. Immunol.* **115**:982–987.

Kung, P. C., Gottlieb, P. D., and Baltimore, D., 1976, Terminal deoxynucleotidyl transferase: Serological studies and radioimmunoassay, *J. Biol. Chem.* **251**:2399–2404.

Kurnick, J. T., and Grey, H. M., 1975, Relationship between immunoglobulin-bearing lymphocytes and cells reactive with sensitized human erythrocytes, *J. Immunol.* **115**:305–307.

LaMantia, K., Conklyn, M., Quagliata, F., and Silber, R., 1976, Immunologic studies of 5'-nucleotidase in normal and chronic lymphocytic leukemia lymphocytes, *Blood* **46**:1042.

Lay, W. H., Mendes, H. F., Bianco, C., and Nussenzweig, V., 1971, Binding of sheep red blood cells to a large population of human lymphocytes, *Nature (London)* **230**:531–532.

Leech, J., 1973, Immunoglobulin-positive Reed–Sternberg cells in Hodgkin's disease, *Lancet* **2**:265–266.

Leech, J. H., Glick, A. D., Waldron, J. A., Flexner, J. M., Horn, R. G., and Collins, R. D., 1975, Malignant lymphomas of follicular center cell origin in man. I. Immunologic studies, *J. Natl. Cancer Inst.* **54**:11–21.

Leech, J., Roy, R. M., Flexner, J. M., Glick, A. D., Waldron, J. A., and Collins, R. D., 1976, Evidence for synthesis of surface immunoglobulin in leukemic reticuloendotheliosis, *Blood* **46**:1037.

Lennert, K., Stein, H., and Kaiserling, E., 1975, Cytological and functional criteria for the classification of malignant lymphoma, *Br. J. Cancer* **31**(*Suppl. 2*):29–43.

Lin, P. S., and Hsu, C. C. S., 1976, Human leukaemic T cells with complement receptors, *Clin. Exp. Immunol.* **23**:209–213.

Lin, P. S., Cooper, A. G., and Wortis, H. H., 1973, Scanning electron microscopy of human T-cell and B-cell rosettes, *N. Engl. J. Med.* **289**:548–551.

Lindstrom, F. D., Hardy, W. R., Eberle, B. J., and Williams, R. C., 1973, Multiple myeloma and benign monoclonal gammapathy: Differentiation by immunofluorescence of lymphocytes, *Ann. Intern. Med.* **78**:837–844.

Lipscomb, M. F., Holmes, K. V., Vitetta, E. S., Hammerling, U., and Uhr, J. W., 1975, Cell-surface immunoglobulin 12: Localization of immunoglobulin on murine lymphocytes by scanning immunoelectron microscopy, *Eur. J. Immunol.* **5**:255–259.

Litwin, S., 1976, Pokeweed mitogen induced terminal differentiation to monoclonal Ig production in human leukemic lymphocytes, *Clin. Res.* **24**:448A.

Lohrmann, H.-P., and Novikovs, L., 1974, Rosette formation between human T-lymphocytes and unsensitized rhesus monkey erythrocytes, *Clin. Immunol. Immunopathol.* **3**:99–111.

Long, J. C., Zamecnik, P. C., Aisenberg, A. C., and Atkins, L., 1977, Tissue culture studies in Hodgkin's disease, *J. Exp. Med.* **145**:1484–1500.

Lukes, J. R., and Collins, R. D., 1974, Immunologic characterization of human malignant lymphomas, *Cancer* **34**:1388–1503.

Lutzner, A., Emerit, I., Durepaire, R., Flandrin, G., Grupper, C., and Prunieras, M., 1973, Cytogenetic, cytophotometric, and ultrastructural study of large cerebriform cells of the Sézary syndrome and description of a small-cell variant, *J. Natl. Cancer Inst.* **50**:1145–1162.

Mann, R. B., Jaffe, E. S., Braylan, R. C., Eggleston, J. C., Ransom, L., Kaizer, H., and Berard, C., 1975, Immunologic and morphologic studies of T cell lymphoma, *Am. J. Med.* **58**:307–313.

Marcus, S. L., Smith, S. W., Jarowski, C. I., and Modak, M., 1976, Terminal deoxynucleotidyl transferase activity in acute undifferentiated leukemia, *Biochem. Biophys. Res. Commun.* **70**:37–44.

Mathé, G., Belpomme, D., Dantchev, D., Pouillart, P., Schlumberger, J. R., and Lafleur, M., 1975,

Leukaemic lymphosarcomas: Respective prognosis of the three types: prolymphocytic, lympho-blastic (or lymphoblastoid) and immunoblastic, *Blood Cells* 1:25–36.

McCaffrey, R., Harrison, R. A., Parkman, R., and Baltimore, D., 1975, Terminal deoxynucleotidyl transferase activity in human leukemic cells and in normal human thymocytes, *N. Engl. J. Med.* 292:775–780.

McCaffrey, R., Harrison, T. A., Kung, P. C., Parkman, R., Silverstone, A. E., and Baltimore, D., 1976, Terminal deoxynucleotidyl transferase in normal and neoplastic hematopoietic cells, in: *Modern Trends in Human Leukemia* (R. Neth, ed.), pp. 503–513, J. F. Lehmanns, Munich.

Mellstedt, H., Jondal, M., and Holm, G., 1973, *In vitro* studies of lymphocytes from patients with plasma cell myeloma. II. Characterization by cell surface markers, *Clin. Exp. Immunol.* 15:321–330.

Mellstedt, H., Hammarström, S., and Holm, G., 1974, Monoclonal lymphocyte population in human plasma cell myeloma, *Clin. Exp. Immunol.* 17:371–384.

Mellstedt, H., Pettersson, D., and Holm, G., 1976, Monoclonal B lymphocytes in peripheral blood of patients with plasma cell myeloma: Relation to activity of the disease, *Scand. J. Hematol.* 16:112–120.

Mendes, N. F., Miki, S. S., and Peixinho, F., 1974, Combined detection of human T and B lymphocytes by rosette formation with sheep erythrocytes and zymosan–C3 complexes, *J. Immunol.* 113:531–536.

Mennemeyer, R., Hammar, S. P., and Cathey, J., 1974, Malignant lymphoma with intracytoplasmic IgM crystalline inclusions, *N. Engl. J. Med.* 291:960–963.

Mestecky, J., 1976 (personal communication).

Meuwissen, H. J., Pollara, B., and Pickering, R. J., 1975, Combined immunodeficiency disease associ-ated with adenosine deaminase deficiency (special article), *J. Pediatr.* 86:169–181.

Millikin, P. D., 1974, A supravital stain for nucleoli in human lymphocytes, *Amer. J. Clin. Path.* 62:520–524.

Mills, B., Sen, L., and Borella, L., 1974, Reactivity of antihuman thymocyte serum with acute leukemic blasts, *J. Immunol.* 115:1038–1044.

Mills, R. J., Fahie-Wilson, M. N., Carter, P. M., and Hobbs, J. R., 1976, IgE myelomatosis, *Clin. Exp. Immunol.* 23:228–232.

Möller, G. (ed.), 1973, T and B lymphocytes in humans, *Transplant. Rev.* 16:1–217.

Moretta, L., Ferrarini, M., Durante, M. L., and Minari, M. C., 1975, Expression of a receptor for IgM by human T-cells *in vitro*, *Eur. J. Immunol.* 5:565–569.

Moretta, L., Webb, S. R., Grossi, C. E., Lydyard, P. M., and Cooper, M. D., 1976, Functional analysis of two subpopulations of human T cells and their distribution in immunodeficient patients, *Clin. Res.* 24:448A.

Nathwani, B. N., Kim, H., and Rappaport, H., 1976, Malignant lymphoma, lymphoblastic, *Cancer* 38:964–983.

Osunkoya, B. O., Mottram, F. C., and Isoun, M. J., 1969, Synthesis and fate of immunological surface receptors on cultured Burkitt lymphoma cells, *Int. J. Cancer* 4:159–165.

Padnos, M., 1976, Differentiation of B and T mouse lymphocytes in cell suspension and smears, *Nature (London)* 259:218–220.

Papamichail, M., Brown, J. C., and Holborow, E. J., 1971, Immunoglobulins on the surface of human lymphocytes, *Lancet* 2:850–852.

Payne, S. V., Jones, D. B., Haegert, D. G., Smith, J. L., and Wright, D. H., 1976, T and B lymphocytes and Reed–Sternberg cells in Hodgkin's disease lymph nodes and spleens, *Clin. Exp. Immunol.* 24:280–286.

Pellegrino, M. A., Ferrone, S., and Theofilopoulos, A. N., 1975, Rosette formation of human lymphoid cells with monkey red blood cells, *J. Immunol.* 115:1065–1071.

Perlmann, P., Perlmann, H., and Wigzell, H., 1972, Lymphocyte mediated cytotoxicity *in vitro*: Induction and inhibition by humoral antibody and nature of effector cells, *Transplant. Rev.* 13:91–114.

Pernis, B., Forni, L., and Amante, L., 1970, Immunoglobulin spots on the surface of rabbit lymphocytes, *J. Exp. Med.* 132:1001–1018.

Pernis, B., Forni, L., and Amante, L., 1971, Immunoglobulins as cell receptors, *Ann. N.Y. Acad. Sci.* 190:420–431.

Pernis, B., Brouet, J. C., and Seligmann, M., 1974, IgD and IgM on the membrane of lymphoid cells in macroglobulinemia: Evidence for identity of membrane IgD and IgM antibody activity in a case with anti-IgG receptors, *Eur. J. Immunol.* 4:776–778.

Peter, C. R., MacKenzie, M. R., and Glassy, F. J., 1974, T or B cell origin of some non-Hodgkin's lymphomas, *Lancet* **2**:686–689.

Piessens, W. F., Schur, P. H., Moloney, W. C., and Churchill, W. H., 1973, Lymphocyte surface immunoglobulins: Distribution and frequency in lymphoproliferative diseases, *N. Engl. J. Med.* **288**:176–180.

Plum, J., and Ringoir, S., 1975, A characterization of human B and T lymphocytes by their lactate dehydrogenase isoenzyme pattern, *Eur. J. Immunol.* **5**:871–874.

Polliack, A., and de Harven, E., 1975, Surface features of normal and leukemic lymphocytes as seen by scanning electron microscopy: An interpretative review, *Clin. Immunol. Immunopathol.* **3**:412–430.

Polliack, A., Lampen, N., Clarkson, B. D., De Harven, E., Bentwich, A., Siegal, F. P., and Kunkel, H. G., 1973, Identification of human B and T lymphocytes by scanning electron microscopy, *J. Exp. Med.* **138**:607.

Polliack, A., Siegal, F. P., Clarkson, B. D., Fu, S. M., Winchester, R. J., Lampen, N., Siegal, M., and de Harven, E., 1975, A scanning electron microscopy and immunological study of 84 cases of lymphocytic leukaemia and related lymphoproliferative disorders, *Scand. J. Haematol.* **15**:359–376.

Preud'homme, J.-L., and Labaume, S., 1975, Immunofluorescent staining of human lymphocytes for the detection of surface immunoglobulins, *Ann. N. Y. Acad. Sci.* **254**:254–261.

Preud'homme, J.-L., and Seligmann, M., 1972a, Immunoglobulins on the surface of lymphoid cells in Waldenström's macroglobulinemia, *J. Clin. Invest.* **51**:701–705.

Preud'homme, J.-L., and Seligmann, M., 1972b, Anti-human immunoglobulin G activity of membrane-bound monoclonal immunoglobulin M in lymphoproliferative disorders, *Proc. Natl. Acad. Sci. U.S.A.* **69**:2132–2135.

Preud'homme, J.-L., and Seligmann, M., 1972c, Surface bound immunoglobulins as a cell marker in human lymphoproliferative diseases, *Blood* **40**:777–794.

Preud'homme, J.-L., and Seligmann, M., 1974, Surface immunoglobulins on human lymphoid cells, in: *Progress in Clinical Immunology* (R. S. Schwartz, ed.), pp. 121–174, Grune & Stratton, New York.

Quagliata, F., Faig, D., Conklyn, M., and Silber, R., 1974, Studies on the lymphocyte 5'-nucleotidase in chronic lymphocytic leukemia, infectious mononucleosis, normal subpopulations, and phytohemagglutinin-stimulated cells, *Cancer Res.* **34**:3197–3202.

Raff, M. C., 1970, Two distinct populations of peripheral lymphocytes in mice distinguishable by immunofluorescence, *Immunology* **19**:637–650.

Raff, M., 1976, Cell surface immunology, *Sci. Am.* **234**:30–39.

Raff, M. C., Megson, M., Owen, J. J. T., and Cooper, M. D., 1976, Early production of intracellular IgM by B-lymphocyte precursors in mouse, *Nature (London)* **259**:224–226.

Ranki, A., Tötterman, T. H., and Häyry, P., 1976, Identification of resting human T and B lymphocytes by acid α-naphthylacetate esterase staining combined with rosette formation with *Staphylococcus aureus* strain Cowan 1, *Scand. J. Immunol.* **5**:1129–1138.

Reif, A. E., and Allen, J. M. V., 1964, The AKR thymic antigen and its distribution in leukemias and nervous tissues, *J. Exp. Med.* **120**:413–433.

Revillard, J. P., Samarut, C., Cordier, G., and Brochier, J., 1975, Characterization of human lymphocytes bearing Ig receptors with special reference to cytotoxic (K) cells, in: *Membrane Receptors of Lymphocytes*, INSERM Symposium I (M. Seligmann, J.-L. Preud'homme, and F. M. Kourilsky, eds.), pp. 171–184, American-Elsevier, New York.

Ross, G. D., 1976 (personal communication).

Ross, G. D., 1977, Surface markers of B and T cells, *Arch. Pathol. Lab. Med.* **101**:337–341.

Ross, G. D., and Polley, M. J., 1975, Specificity of human lymphocyte complement receptors, *J. Exp. Med.* **141**:1163–1180.

Ross, G. D., Rabellino, E. M., Polley, M. J., and Grey, H. M., 1973, Combined studies of complement receptor and surface immunoglobulin-bearing cells and sheep erythrocyte rosette-forming cells in normal and leukemic human lymphocytes, *J. Clin. Invest.* **52**:377–385.

Rowe, D., Hug, K., Forni, L., and Pernis, B., 1973, Immunoglobulin D as a lymphocyte receptor, *J. Exp. Med.* **138**:965–972.

Rubin, A. D., Douglas, S. D., Chessin, J. N., Glade, P. R., and Dameshek, W., 1969, Chronic reticulolymphocytic leukemia: Reclassification of "leukemic reticuloendotheliosis" through functional characterization of the circulating mononuclear cells, *Am. J. Med.* **47**:149–162.

Rudders, R. A., 1976, B lymphocyte subpopulations in chronic lymphocytic leukemia, *Blood* **47**:229–235.

Rudders, A., and Ross, R., 1975, Partial characterization of the shift from IgG to IgA synthesis in the clonal differentiation of human leukemia bone marrow-derived lymphocytes, *J. Exp. Med.* **142**:549–559.

Salmon, S. E., 1973, Immunoglobulin synthesis and tumor kinetics of multiple myeloma, *Semin. Hematol.* **10**:135–147.

Salmon, S. E., and Seligmann, M., 1974, B-cell neoplasia in man, *Lancet* **2**:1230–1233.

Schedel, I., Fink, P. C., Bodenberger, M., and Deicher, H., 1976, Monoclonal lymphoid cell surface immunoglobulins with tumor-specific determinants in lymphosarcoma, *Clin. Immunol. Immunopathol.* **5**:74–83.

Schiff, R. I., Buckley, R. H., Gilbertsen, R. B., and Metzgar, R. S., 1974, Membrane receptors and *in vitro* responsiveness of lymphocytes in human immunodeficiency, *J. Immunol.* **112**:376–385.

Schroer, K. R., Briles, D. E., Van Boxel, J. A., and Davie, J. M., 1974, Idiotypic uniformity of cell surface immunoglobulin in chronic lymphocytic leukemia, *J. Exp. Med.* **140**:1416–1420.

Schultz, E. F., Davis, S., and Rubin, A. D., 1976, Further characterization of the circulating cell in chronic lymphocytic leukemia, *Blood* **48**:223–234.

Schwarze, W.-W., 1975, T-cell origin of acid-phosphatase-positive lymphoblasts, *Lancet* **2**:1264.

Seligmann, M., Preud'homme, J.-L., and Kourilsky, F. M., (eds.), 1975, *Membrane Receptors of Lymphocytes,* Proceedings of an International Symposium, Paris, 1974, INSERM Symposium I, American-Elsevier, New York.

Sen, L., and Borella, L., 1975, Clinical importance of lymphoblasts with T markers in childhood acute leukemia, *N. Engl. J. Med.* **292**:828–832.

Setcavage, T. M., Rothlein, R., Muscoplat, C. C., and Kim, Y. B., 1976, A novel receptor for secretory component on porcine mononuclear cells, *Fed. Proc. Fed. Am. Soc. Exp. Biol.* **35**:857.

Shevach, E., Edelson, R., Frank, M., Lutzner, M., and Green, I., 1974, A human leukemia cell with both B and T cell surface markers, *Proc. Natl. Acad. Sci. U.S.A.* **71**:863–866.

Siegal, F. P., 1976, IgG on infants' B lymphocytes: Enhanced binding of IgG by IgM bearing lymphoid cells in early childhood, *Scand. J. Immunol.* **5**:721–729.

Siegal, F. P., and Koziner, B., 1976 (unpublished).

Siegal, F. P., and Litwin, S., 1976 (unpublished).

Siegal, F. P., and Winchester, R. J., 1972 (unpublished).

Siegal, F. P., Pernis, B., and Kunkel, H. G., 1971, Lymphocytes in human immunodeficiency states: A study of membrane-associated immunoglobulins, *Eur. J. Immunol.* **1**:482–486.

Siegal, F. P., Wernet, P., Dickler, H. B., Fu, S. M., and Kunkel, H. G., 1975, B lymphocytes lacking surface Ig in patients with immune deficiency: Initiation of Ig synthesis in culture in cells of a patient with thymoma, in: *Immunodeficiency in Man and Animals: Birth Defects Orig Artic. Ser.,* Vol. XI, No. 1, pp. 40–44.

Siegal, F. P., Siegal, M., and Good, R. A., 1976a, Suppression of plasma cell formation by leukocytes from hypogammaglobulinemic patients, *J. Clin. Invest.* **58**:109.

Siegal, F. P., Voss, R., Al-Mondhiry, H., Polliack, A., Hansen, J. A., Siegal, M., and Good, R. A., 1976b, Association of a chromosomal abnormality with lymphocytes having both T and B markers in a patient with lymphoproliferative disease, *Am. J. Med.* **60**:157–166.

Siegal, F. P., Berlinger, N. T., McKenzie, S., and Czeczotka, V., 1976c (unpublished).

Spiegelberg, H. L., Perlmann, H., and Perlmann, P., 1976, Interaction of IgG subclasses with K lymphocytes, *Fed. Proc. Fed. Am. Soc. Exp. Biol.* **35**:473.

Stathopoulos, G., and Davies, A. J. S., 1976, Human lymphocytes and mouse red cells, *Lancet* **1**:1078.

Stathopoulos, G., and Elliot, E. V., 1974, Formation of mouse or sheep red-blood cell rosettes by lymphocytes from normal and leukaemic individuals, *Lancet* **2**:600–601.

Stein, H., and Kaiserling, E., 1974, Surface immunoglobulins and lymphocyte-specific surface antigens on leukaemic reticuloendotheliosis cells, *Clin. Exp. Immunol.* **18**:63–71.

Sullivan, A. K., Adams, L. S., Silke, I., and Jerry, L. M., 1974, Hairy B-cells and smooth T cells, *N. Engl. J. Med.* **290**:689–690.

Sumiya, M., Mizoguchi, H., Kosaka, K., Miuri, Y., Takaku, F., and Yata, J., 1973, Chronic lymphocytic leukemia of T-cell origin?, *Lancet* **2**:910.

Taniguchi, N., Okuda, N., Moriya, N., Miyawaki, T., and Nagaoki, T., 1976, Inhibitory effect of sheep erythrocyte fragments on rosette formation of human T lymphocytes with sheep red blood cells, *Clin. Exp. Immunol.* **24**:370–373.

Taylor, C. R., 1974, The nature of Reed–Sternberg cells and other malignant "reticulum" cells, *Lancet* **2**:802–807.

Thomas, D. B., 1973, Antibodies specific for T lymphocytes in cold agglutinin and lymphocytotoxic sera, *Eur. J. Immunol.* **3**:824–828.

Thrasher, S. G., Bigazzi, P. E., Yoshida, T., and Cohen, S., 1974, The effect of fluorescein conjugation on Fc-dependent properties of rabbit antibody, *J. Immunol.* **114**:762–764.

Tönder, O., Morse, P. A., and Humphrey, L. J., 1974, Similarities of Fc receptors in human malignant tissue and normal lymphoid tissue, *J. Immunol.* **113**:1162–1169.

Touraine, J.-L., Touraine, F., Kiszkiss, D. F., Choi, Y. S., and Good, R. A., 1974, Heterologous specific antiserum for identification of human T lymphocytes, *Clin. Exp. Immunol.* **16**:503–520.

Tsukimoto, I., and Lampkin, B., 1975, Effects of thymosin on lymphoblasts, *N. Engl. J. Med.* **293**:455–456.

Tung, R., Silber, R., Quagliata, F., Conklyn, M., Gottesman, J., and Hirschhorn, R., 1976, Adenosine deaminase activity in chronic lymphocytic leukemia: relationship to B- and T-cell subpopulations, *J. Clin. Invest.* **57**:756–761.

Uhr, J. W., and Vitetta, E. S., 1973, Synthesis, biochemistry and dynamics of cell surface immunoglobulin on lymphocytes, *Fed. Proc. Fed. Am. Soc. Exp. Biol.* **32**:35–40.

Vila, J. N., and Taub, R. N., 1975, Nomarski optics and T and B markers, *Lancet* **1**:977.

Vitetta, E. S., and Uhr, J. W., 1975, Immunoglobulin-receptors revisited: A model for the differentiation of bone marrow-derived lymphocytes is described, *Science* **189**:964–969.

Vossen, J. M., and Hijmans, W., 1975, Membrane-associated immunoglobulin determinants on bone marrow and blood lymphocytes in the pediatric age group and on fetal tissues, *Ann. N. Y. Acad. Sci.* **254**:262–279.

Webb, S. R., and Cooper, M. D., 1973, T cells can bind antigen via cytophilic IgM antibody made by B cells, *J. Immunol.* **111**:275–277.

Wernet, P., Feizi, T., and Kunkel, H. G., 1972, Idiotypic determinants of immunoglobulin M detected on the surface of human lymphocytes by cytotoxic assay, *J. Exp. Med.* **136**:650–655.

West, W., and Herberman, R. B., 1974, A human lymphoid cell line with receptors for both sheep red blood cells and complement, *Cell. Immunol.* **14**:139–145.

West, W. H., Sienknecht, C. W., Townes, A. S., and Herberman, R. B., 1976, Performance of a rosette assay between lymphocytes and sheep erythrocytes at elevated temperatures to study patients with cancer and other diseases, *Clin. Immunol. Immunopathol.* **5**:60–66.

Whiteside, T. L., and Rabin, B. S., 1976, Surface immunoglobulin on activated human peripheral blood thymus-derived cells, *J. Clin. Invest.* **57**:762–771.

Wilson, J. D., and Nossal, G. J. V., 1971, Identification of human T and B lymphocytes in normal peripheral blood and in chronic lymphocytic leukaemia, *Lancet* **2**:788–791.

Winchester, R. J., and Ross, G., 1976, Methods for enumerating lymphocyte populations, in: *Manual of Clinical Immunology* (N. R. Rose and H. Friedman, eds.), pp. 64–76, American Society for Microbiology, Washington, D.C.

Winchester, R. J., Winfield, J. B., Siegal, F. P., Wernet, P., Bentwich, Z., and Kunkel, H. G., 1974, Analyses of lymphocytes from patients with rheumatoid arthritis and systemic lupus erythematosus, *J. Clin. Invest.* **54**:1082–1092.

Winchester, R. J., Fu, S. M., Hoffman, T., and Kunkel, H. G., 1975a, IgG on lymphocyte surfaces: Technical problems and the significance of a third cell population, *J. Immunol.* **114**:1210–1212.

Winchester, R. J., Fu, S. M., Wernet, P., Kunkel, H. G., Dupont, B., and Jersild, C., 1975b, Recognition by pregnancy serums of non-*HL-A* alloantigens selectively expressed on B lymphocytes, *J. Exp. Med.* **141**:924–929.

Winfield, J. B., Winchester, R. J., Wernet, P., Fu, S. M., and Kunkel, H. G., 1974, Nature of cold-reactive antibodies to lymphocyte surface determinants in systemic lupus erythematosus, *Arthritis Rheum.* **18**:1–8.

Wu, L. Y. T., Lawton, A. R., and Cooper, M. D., 1973, Differentiation capacity of cultured B lymphocytes from immunodeficient patients, *J. Clin. Invest.* **52**:3180–3189.

Wybran, J., and Fudenberg, H. H., 1971, Rosette-formation, a test for cellular immunity, *Trans. Assoc. Am. Physicians* **84**:239–244.

Wybran, J., and Fudenberg, H. H., 1973, Thymus-derived rosette-forming cells in various human disease states: cancer, lymphoma, bacterial and viral infections, and other diseases, *J. Clin. Invest.* **52**:1026–1032.

Wybran, J., Chantler, S., and Fudenberg, H. H., 1973, Isolation of normal T cells in chronic lymphocytic leukemia, *Lancet* **1**:126–129.

Yata, J., and Tsukimoto, I., 1972, Maturation of cell-surface structure of human B lymphocytes, *Lancet* **2**:1425.

Yodoi, J., Takatsuki, K., and Masuda, T., 1974, Two cases of T-cell chronic lymphocytic leukemia in Japan, *N. Engl. J. Med.* **290**:572–573.

Yu, D. T. Y., 1975, Human lymphocyte subpopulations: early and late rosettes, *J. Immunol.* **115**:91–93.

Zucker-Franklin, D., 1974, The percentage of monocytes among "mononuclear" cell fractions obtained from normal human blood, *J. Immunol.* **112**:236–240.

Zucker-Franklin, D., 1975, Physiological and pathological variations in the ultrastructure of neutrophils and granulocytes, *Clin. Haematol.* **4**:485–508.

11

Ecotaxis, Ecotaxopathy, and Lymphoid Malignancy: Terms, Facts, and Predictions

1. Ecotaxis

1.1. Definition of the Term and Introduction

The term *ecotaxis* was designed originally to define the capacity of mature cells within the lymphomyeloid system to migrate and arrange themselves in clear-cut microenvironments of the peripheral lymphoid organs (de Sousa, 1971, 1973). Each of the mammalian peripheral lymphoid organs—the spleen, the lymph node, and the Peyer's patch—can be divided into a number of clearly defined areas that can be represented diagramatically as in Figure 1. The spleen, in addition to containing the lymphoid component originally described by Malpighi (1686) as the follicular white pulp, contains a mixed white- and red-cell component, the red pulp; in the mouse, the red pulp is also a site of hemopoiesis (see Section 1.2.1). The splenic red pulp consists of cords and sinuses that are features of importance for the subsequent fate of circulating cells (see Sections 1.2.2 and 1.2.3). The white pulp, the lymph nodes, and the cortical areas of Peyer's patches can be divided into thymus-dependent (T) and thymus-independent (B) zones, which contain a predominance of thymus-derived (T) and thymus-independent (B) cells, respectively (Parrott and de Sousa, 1971; de Sousa, 1973; de Sousa and Anderson, 1969). Ultrastructural studies (Veldman, 1970; Hoefschmit, 1974) and studies of the reticulum framework of the spleen and lymph nodes (Veerman, 1974; de Sousa, 1969) have revealed cellular

---

MARIA DE SOUSA • Sloan-Kettering Institute for Cancer Research, New York, New York 10021.

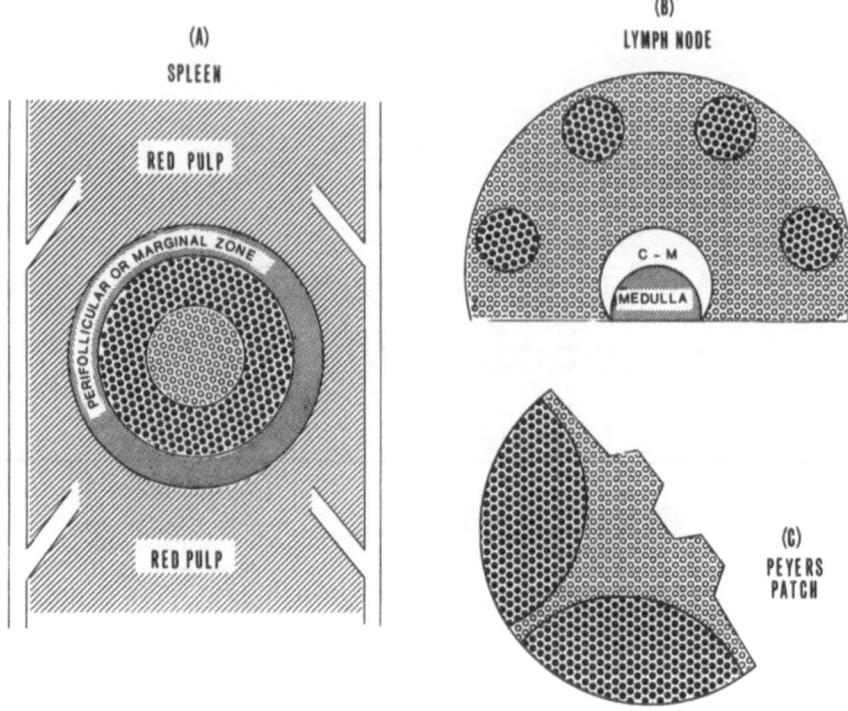

Figure 1. Diagrammatic representation of the main microenvironments of the spleen (A), the lymph node (B), and the Peyer's patch (C) in the mammal. (○) Thymus-dependent areas; (●) thymus-independent areas; (C − M) corticomedullary junction.

features peculiar to the two areas. The reticulin framework of the thymus and thymus-dependent areas differs from that of other lymphoid tissues: an interdigitating cell with dendritic processes (Veldman, 1970) is unique to these thymic (Hoefschmit and Gerver, 1975) and thymus-dependent areas (TDAs) (Figure 2), which are also characterized by their "open" structural pattern (de Sousa, 1969) (Figure 3A). The medulla in the lymph nodes, the equivalent medullary region in Peyer's patches, and the peritrabecular areas in the splenic red pulp contain most antibody-producing cell populations. The reticulin framework in the lymph node medulla has a characteristic "closed" pattern, containing single cells (Figure 3B). The nodular peripheral areas in splenic follicles and in the outer cortex of the lymph nodes or Peyer's patches contain little reticulin and have a different type of dendritic cell that is indentified with the macrophage series (Veldman, 1970).

Individual lymphocyte populations enter the bloodstream through common routes and are subsequently distributed in anatomical locations that are specific to each population. Circulating cells can also discriminate between lymphoid and nonlymphoid tissue macroenvironments. For instance, 70–80% of thoracic duct or lymph node lymphocytes migrate to T and B areas of the peripheral lymphoid organs soon after intravenous injection (Ford, 1975), despite the natural circulating "advantage" of passing first the pulmonary, hepatic, and red pulp capillary networks. The acquisition of "environmental discrimination" may be an important

327

ECOTAXIS,
ECOTAXOPATHY,
AND LYMPHOID
MALIGNANCY:
TERMS, FACTS AND
PREDICTIONS

facet of the physiological process of lymphoid cell maturation (de Sousa, 1971, 1973).

In its wider sense, ecotaxis cannot be restricted to lymphoid cells. Other circulating cells (e.g., erythrocytes and granulocytes) are predominantly confined to well-defined compartments of the blood circulation (de Sousa, 1976a). Removal or dislodgment of a circulating cell population from its normal environment may have severe functional consequences, e.g., in autoimmune hemolytic anemia (see Section 1.2.2).

This section of this chapter discusses examples of ecotaxis in this broad context, the possible underlying control mechanisms of ecotaxis, and potential implications of their failure. Section 2 analyzes the question how failure of ecotaxis may be related to the pathophysiology of certain lymphoid neoplasms.

1.2. Factual Basis for Definition of the Term

1.2.1. Experiments on Bone Marrow Cell Distribution

An elegant demonstration of the multiple, well-defined microenvironments that exist within the lymphomyeloid system is provided by events that follow colonization of bone marrow stem cells in marrow and spleen in mice (Trentin *et al.*, 1971). At 9 days after intravenous injection of small numbers of bone marrow cells into irradiated syngeneic mice, colonies that can be counted macroscopically develop in the spleen. Each colony is derived from a single multipotential stem cell maturing along specific erythroid, neutrophilic, eosinophilic, or megakaryocytic cell lines; this maturation appears to be determined by the stroma with which the stem cell interacts (Wolf and Trentin, 1968). Thus, hematopoietic stem cells in bone marrow stroma that is implanted in the spleen differentiate along granulocytic lines (which predominate in normal bone marrow), while similar multipotential cells placed directly in spleen stroma give rise mostly to erythroid colonies (Table 1).

Stem cells are not the only bone marrow cells that migrate to and settle in the red pulp of the spleen. The fate of mouse bone marrow cells labeled *in vitro* with [³H]adenosine has been observed after infusion into intact recipients. Labeled cells are found in the perifollicular areas and red pulp sinuses shortly after infusion. At

TABLE 1. Types of Bone-Marrow-Cell-Derived[a] Spleen Colonies That Develop When Placed in Contact with Marrow Stroma[b] or with Spleen Stroma[c]

Number of mice	Colony-forming unit route of entry	Colony type (erythroid granuloid ratio)
28	Trocar-implanted	0.1 : 1
30	Intravenous	2–8 : 1

[a]Data from Wolf and Trentin (1968). Primary recipients irradiated with 1000 rads received an intravenous injection of $2.5–3 \times 10^7$ viable bone marrow cells; 18–24 hr later, the content of their femoral cavities was used to repopulate similarly irradiated secondary recipients as described in footnotes *b* and *c*.
[b]As much marrow stroma as possible from a single femur was implanted into the spleen by trocar.
[c]A suspension of marrow cells from the supralateral femur was injected intravenously.

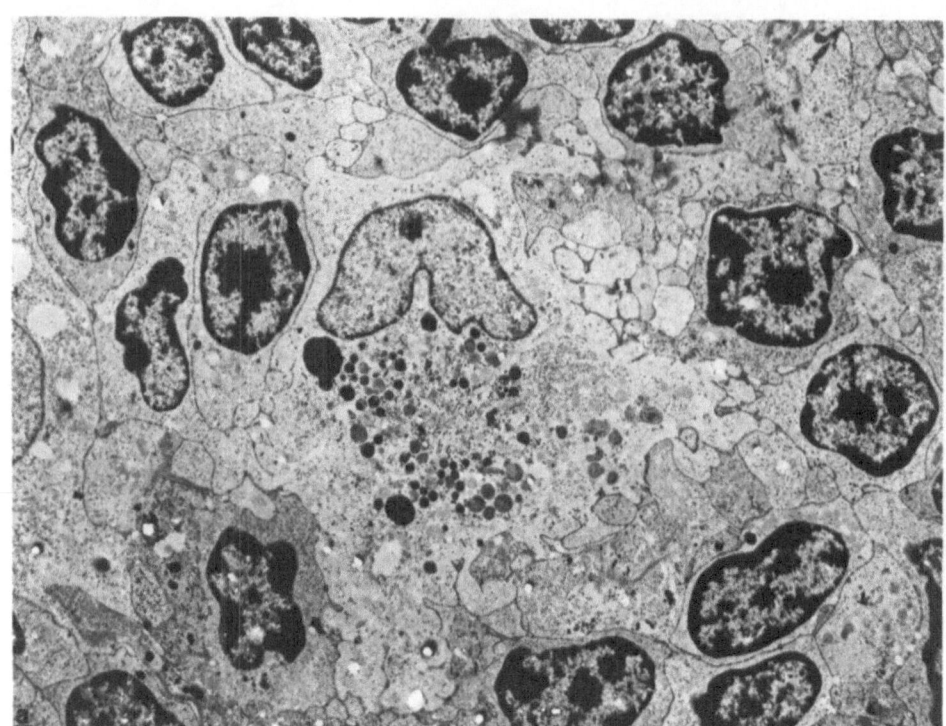

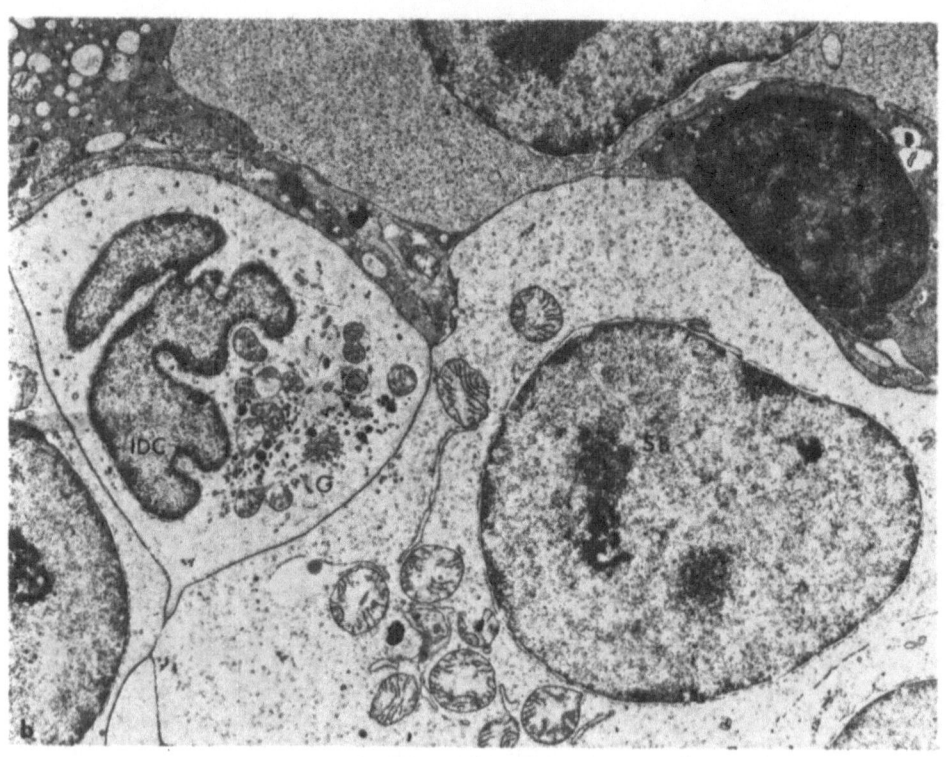

329

ECOTAXIS,
ECOTAXOPATHY,
AND LYMPHOID
MALIGNANCY:
TERMS, FACTS AND
PREDICTIONS

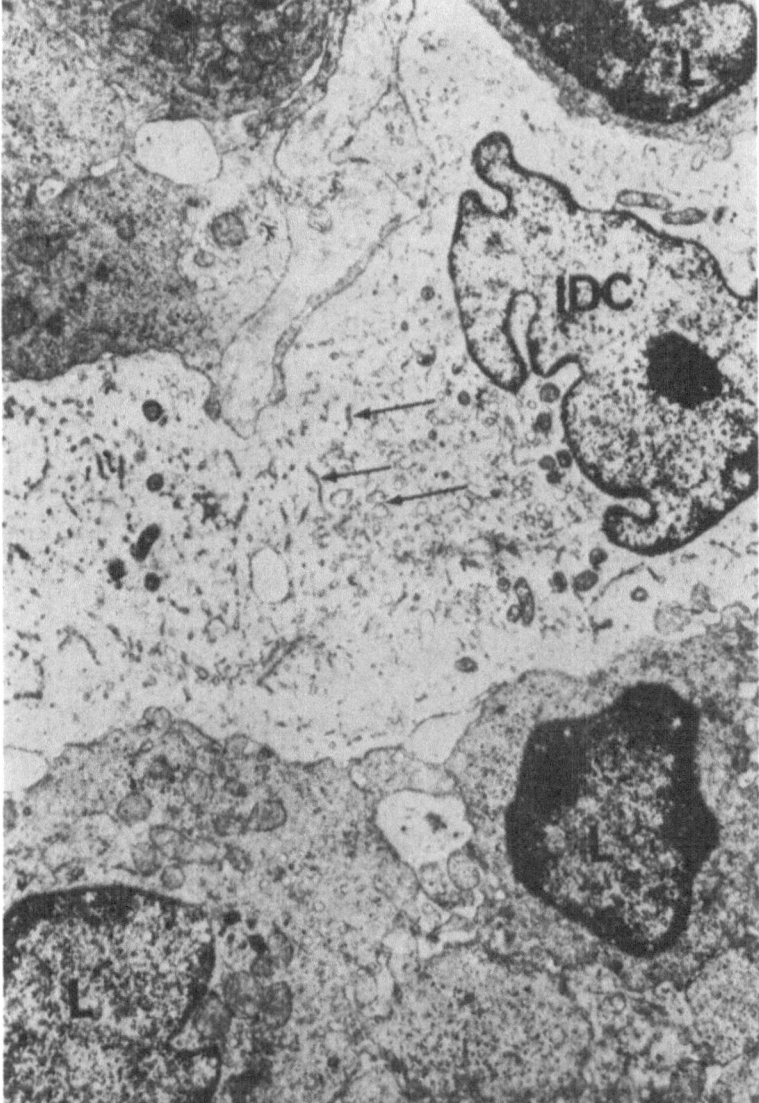

Figure 2. Interdigitating cell (IDC), which is seemingly confined to the thymus (a) and thymus-dependent areas (b) and to the skin of patients with mycosis fungoides (c). The silver metheneamine reaction shows positive Golgi stacks (G), small vesicles, and tubules. Figures courtesy of Drs. Hoefschmit and Gerver (a), Veldman (b), and Goos (c). (L) Lymphatic tumor cells.

24–72 hr, the majority of labeled hematopoietic cells remain in the trabecular areas of the red pulp and in the cords. In contrast, lymphoid populations migrate predominantly into the white pulp (see Section 1.2.3). Bone marrow cells transfused into nonirradiated recipients (although they ecotax to environments that are capable of inducing differentiation and rapid cell division) do not produce large colonies. That they do not indicates that the fate of a cell population depends on interaction

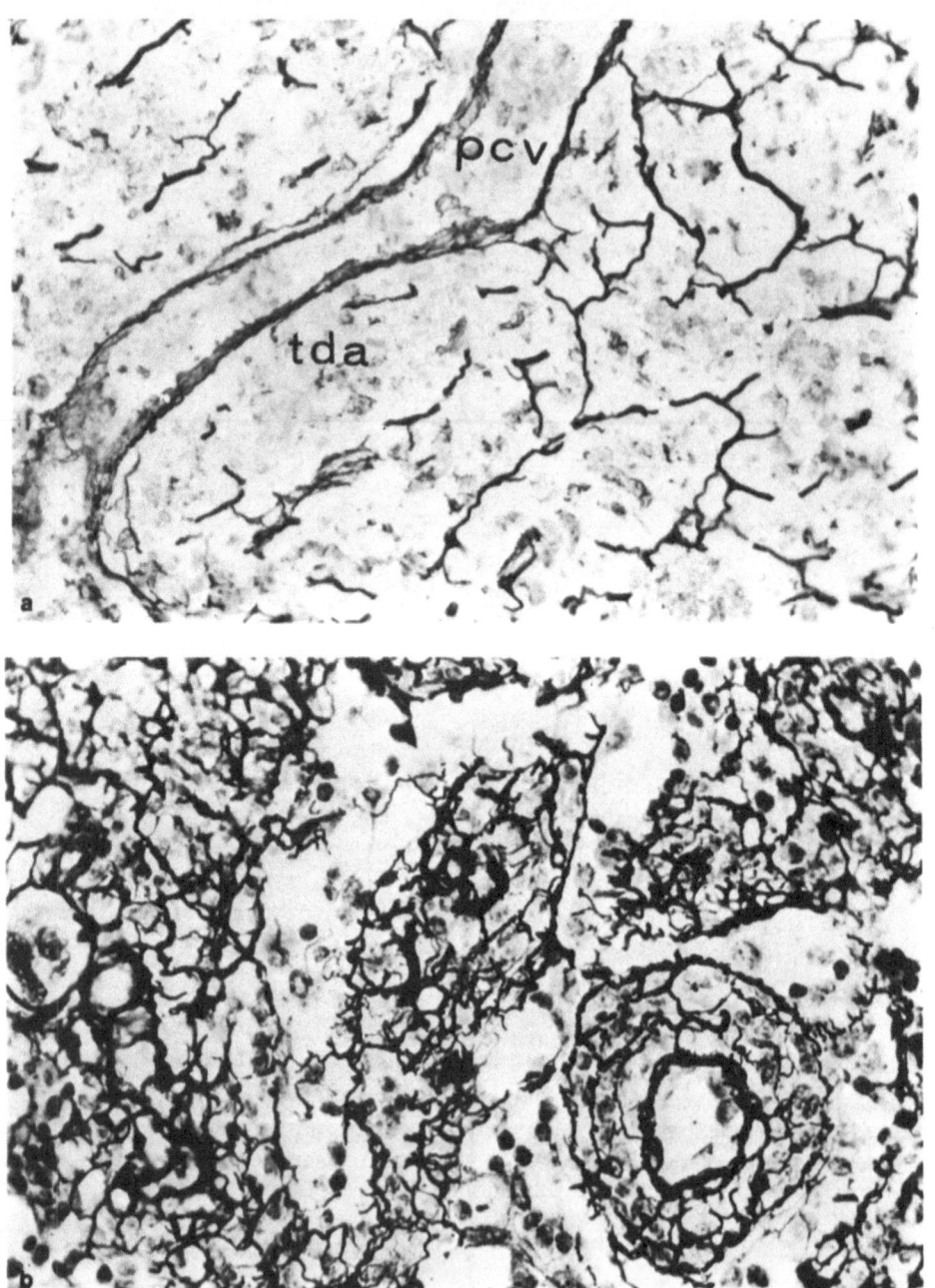

Figure 3. Sections of lymph nodes from neonatally thymectomized (a) and intact (b) mice (Gordon–Sweets staining method for reticulin). The two distinct reticular patterns of thymus-dependent areas (tda in a) and of medullary areas (b) are illustrated. Note the delineation of the basement membrane of a postcapillary venule (pcv) in the tda. Reproduced from de Sousa (1969).

not only with other neighboring cells, but also with local stroma. This point will be the *leitmotiv* of this chapter.

331

ECOTAXIS,
ECOTAXOPATHY,
AND LYMPHOID
MALIGNANCY:
TERMS, FACTS AND
PREDICTIONS

There is extensive evidence that a subpopulation in the bone marrow cells enters the thymus and therein differentiates along a lymphoid line (Greaves *et al.*, 1974). The actual microenvironment within the thymus in which this process takes place is not known. The epithelial framework of the thymus comprises its "constant region" and may influence differentiation of lymphoid cells, which may, in turn, build up the "variable region" of the thymus (de Sousa and Incefy, 1975).

Sequential autoradiographic studies were performed using [^{3}H]thymidine-labeled newborn thymuses grafted into intact and neonatally thymectomized recipients (Parrott and de Sousa, 1967). Large, long-lived cells located between the cortex and medulla (Figure 4) were observed to remain labeled for longer than 40 days. The significance of these long-lived cells is not known. This observation and the results of electron-microscopic studies of thymic structure (Clark, 1966) suggest that the cells that are likely to influence differentiation of incoming bone marrow cells are located in the medulla or adjacent areas. Difficulty in obtaining relatively pure suspensions of thymus precursor cells hampers studies of this nature.

1.2.2. Experiments on Red Cell Distribution

Interest in the distribution of red cells has been closely associated with the study of hemolytic anemia. Attention has focused largely on the fate of ^{51}Cr-labeled

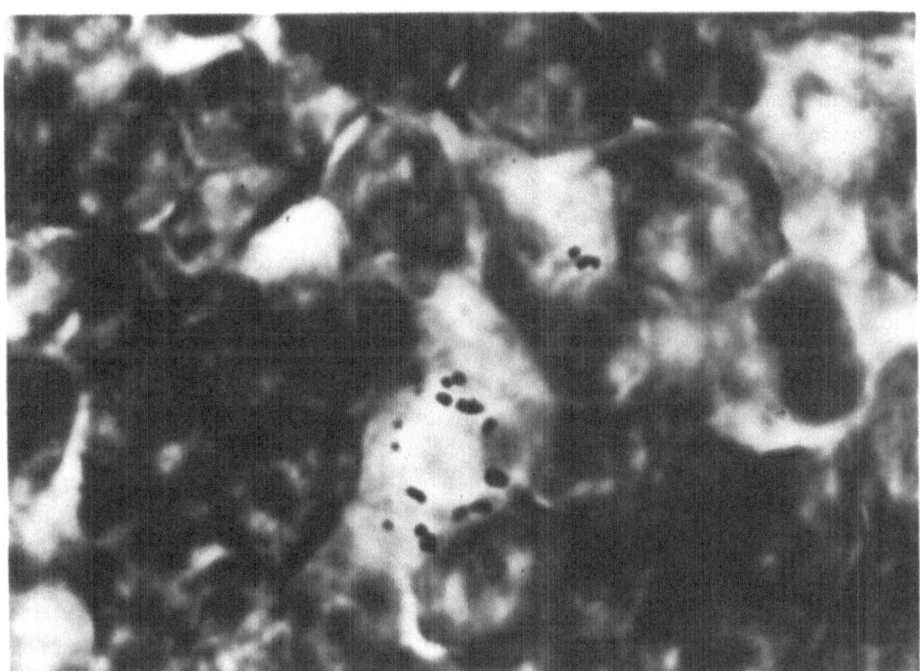

Figure 4. A persisting labeled epithelial reticular cell in the medulla of thymus that had been implanted under the kidney capsule 41 days earlier. The thymus donor had been injected with four 2-μCi doses of [^{3}H]thymidine over 3 days immediately after birth and before thymic tissue implantation. Reproduced from Parrott and de Sousa (1967).

TABLE 2.   Distribution of ^{51}Cr-Labeled Mouse Erythrocytes in Syngeneic Intact or Splenectomized Recipients

Red cell treatment	Recipient	Percentage of injected radioactivity[a]			
		Blood	Lung	Liver	Spleen
None	Intact	32	2	6	3
	Splenectomized	30	2	6	—
Neuraminidase	Intact	21	2	33	2
Trypsin	Intact	22	2	34	16
	Splenectomized	28	3	16	—
Con A	Intact	18	2	8	18

[a]At 1 hr after intravenous injection of 0.2 ml of a 10% cell suspension. Each value is the mean of 4–12 mice. (Previously unpublished data from Freitas and de Sousa, 1976.)

red cells (Jandl *et al.*, 1957) modified by antibody and complement or by other procedures that induce the formation of spherocytes (i.e., heat damage) (Kimber and Lander, 1964; Crome and Mollison, 1964; Marsh *et al.*, 1966; Schreiber and Frank, 1972; Brown, 1973; Brown *et al.*, 1970). After intravenous injection of normal autologous red cells, 80–90% of the injected radioactivity is recovered from the blood. Pretreatment of the red cells with antibody and complement or with heat substantially modifies this pattern. Under these circumstances, the altered red cells are found mostly in the spleen or liver, and their distribution is influenced by the nature of the *in vitro* treatment, e.g., class of antibody (Atkinson *et al.*, 1973), source of complement employed (Brown *et al.*, 1970), or degree of heat damage (Kimber and Lander, 1964; see de Sousa, 1976a). Brown *et al.* (1970) reported that large numbers of complement-pretreated erythrocytes became attached to the Kupffer cells, reflecting the abnormal interaction between the altered red blood cells and the cells lining the liver sinusoids. We analyzed the question of the effect of pretreatment of mouse red cells *in vitro* with enzymes or concanavalin A (Con A) (Table 2) and found that these manipulations induce liver or spleen sequestration of red blood cells. Such techniques are also used to study the distribution of lymphocytes *in vivo* (see Section 1.2.3).

Experiments on the effect of neuraminidase on the distribution and morphology of rat platelets were performed by Choi *et al.* (1972). These studies showed that the platelet counts drop after the intravenous injection of bacterial and viral neuraminidase. This thrombocytopenia could be related to the redistribution of structurally altered platelets to the splenic sinusoids and their macrophages. Thus, the large numbers of erythrocytes and platelets in the normal blood compartment reflect "negative" interactions between these formed elements and macrophages in organs with sinusoidal capillary beds, such as the liver and spleen. Minor membrane modifications of these circulating cells are "detected" by cells that reside in the sinusoids. The result is progressive removal of the abnormal cells from the circulation. It is therefore not unexpected that splenectomy prolongs the survival of abnormal red cells and platelets in the circulation both in man (Marsh *et al.*, 1966) and in experimental animals (Atkinson *et al.*, 1973; Choi *et al.*, 1972; de Sousa, 1976a).

1.2.3.   Experiments on Lymphocyte Distribution

a. Tempo and Patterns of Normal Lymphocyte Circulation.   The normal environment for erythrocytes is within the circulation and communicating vascular

333

ECOTAXIS,
ECOTAXOPATHY,
AND LYMPHOID
MALIGNANCY:
TERMS, FACTS AND
PREDICTIONS

spaces. Lymphocytes are present in the blood in relatively small numbers, and also freely leave the blood circuit and enter the lymph circuit. The existence of a physiological circulation of lymphocytes between blood and lymph has been demonstrated in fish (Ellis and de Sousa, 1974), birds (Bell, R. G., and Lafferty, 1972), and mammals (Gowans, 1966; Ford and Gowans, 1969; Ford, 1975; Frost, H., *et al.*, 1975). Pearson *et al.* (1976) showed elegantly in the fetal lamb that this blood–lymph circulation of lymphocytes develops during fetal life, independently of encounter with external antigen. Labeled lymphocytes injected intravenously reach the lymph most slowly in mammals (15–20 hr in the rat, 12–18 hr in the fetal lamb, 27–36 hr in the adult sheep, 18–24 hr in the young lamb) and most rapidly in fish (0.5 hr). The tempo of circulation from blood to lymph is different for T and B cells in mammals. Labeled B thoracic duct cells from mice (Sprent, 1974) or rats (Howard, 1972) have a slower tempo of circulation than do normal thoracic duct cells. This difference has been interpreted as reflecting a relatively long sojourn of B cells in the major capillary networks after intravenous injection, and may be due to intrinsic differences of lymphocyte subpopulations. The distribution of pure suspensions of ^{51}Cr-labeled T or B lymph node cells from mice is summarized in Table 3 (Freitas and de Sousa, 1975). At 1 hr after injection, 47% of the labeled T cells are found in the spleen (41%) and lymph nodes (6%) and 22% in the lungs (12%) and liver (10%). In contrast, only 17% of B-cell label is found in the spleen and lymph nodes, while 58% is present in the lungs and liver. T and B cells also circulate through different routes within lymphoid organs (Parrott and de Sousa, 1971; de Sousa, 1973; de Sousa *et al.*, 1973; Howard, 1972; Sprent, 1974). T cells that enter postcapillary venules in the midcortex of lymph nodes and the perifollicular and red pulp areas in the spleen localize in TDAs. These TDAs include the midcortex in lymph nodes and the periarteriolar sheath in the spleen. B cells are found in the primary nodules of the outer cortex of the lymph nodes and in the periphery of Malpighian follicles in the spleen (Figure 5). In Peyer's patches, T cells localize in the dome and interfollicular areas, while the distribution of B cells is similar to that in lymph nodes.

The sections of the postcapillary venules of lymph nodes through which there is considerable lymphocyte traffic are lined with high cuboidal endothelial cells (Gowans and Knight, 1964; Parrott *et al.*, 1966; Godschneider and McGregor, 1968; Herman *et al.*, 1972). In animals with reduced cell traffic induced by T-cell depletion, these venules are difficult to discern because their endothelium assumes a flattened morphology (Parrott *et al.*, 1966; de Sousa, 1969). The interaction between circulating lymphocytes and endothelial cells of postcapillary venules has been the subject of considerable attention (Gowans and Knight, 1964; Marchesi and

TABLE 3. Illustration of the Slower Traffic of ^{51}Cr-Labeled B Cells in the Mouse

Time after injection	Cell type	Distribution[a]		
		Lungs and liver	Spleen	Lymph node
1 hr	T	22	41	6
	B	58	16	1
24 hr	T	9	24	16
	B	26	23	4

[a]Expressed as the percentage of injected radioactivity. Each value is the mean of 2–6 mice.

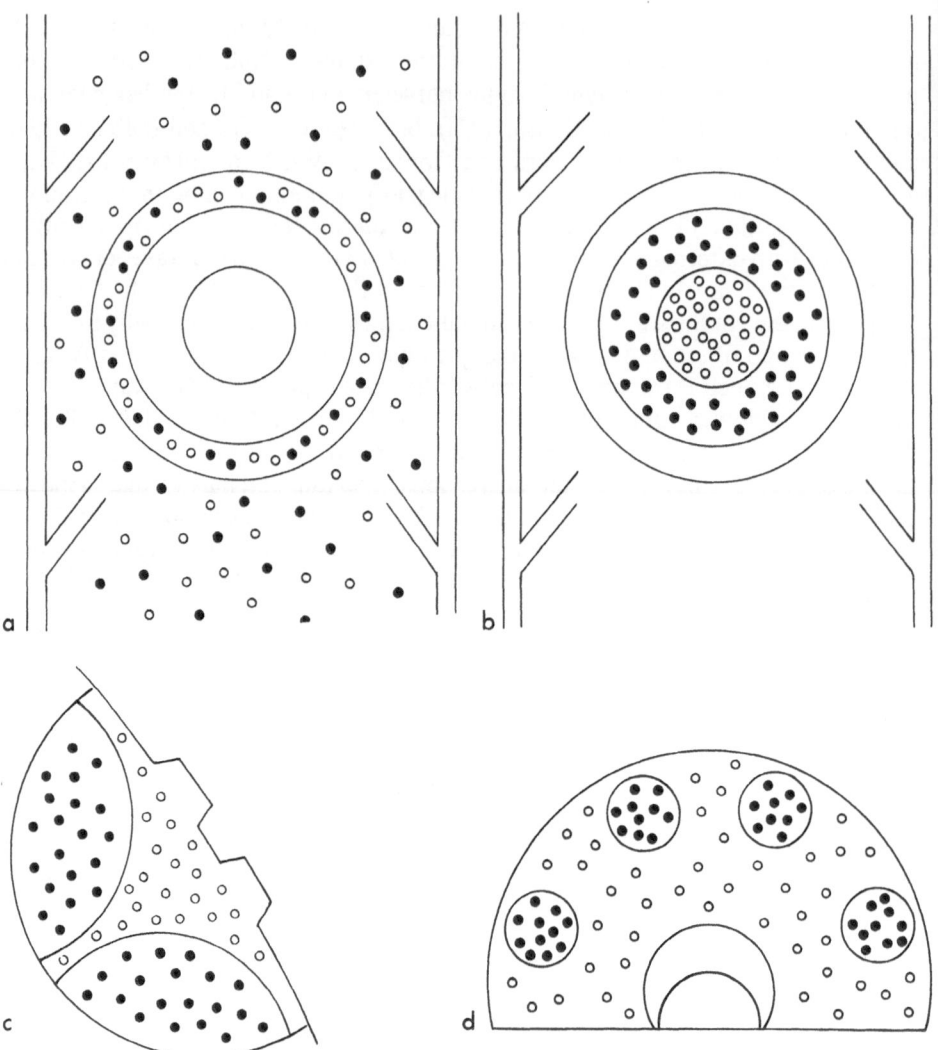

Figure 5. Diagrams representing the distribution patterns of T (○) and B (●) cells in the spleen (a, b), lymph nodes (c), and Peyer's patches (d). After utilizing common routes of entry (represented here only for the spleen), T and B cells ultimately ecotax to T and B microenvironments (see Figure 1).

Gowans, 1964; Mikata and Niki, 1971; Schoefl and Miles, 1972; van Ewijk *et al.*, 1975). It was suggested by Gesner and Ginsburg (1964) that carbohydrate receptors on lymphocytes might interact with receptors on endothelial cells of postcapillary venules, and thereby contribute to lymphocyte entry into the lymph node cortex.

b. Modified Lymphocyte Circulation. *1. Circulation of Modified Lymphocytes in Intact Hosts.* Most experiments on the modulation of lymphocyte traffic are based on the aforementioned suggestion that carbohydrates on lymphocyte membranes contribute to recognition processes associated with the entry of the lymphocytes into lymph nodes (Gesner and Ginsburg, 1967; Woodruff and Gesner, 1969; Woodruff, 1974; Gillette *et al.*, 1973; Schlesinger and Israel, 1974; Freitas and de

Sousa, 1975). In these studies, ^{51}Cr-labeled lymphocytes were first treated with enzymes and lectins that cleave or bind to surface carbohydrates *in vitro* and the fate and distribution of the lymphocytes were then followed *in vivo*.

Neuraminidase treatment results in a transient increase in the number of lymphocytes that lodge in the liver (Gesner and Ginsburg, 1964; Woodruff and Gesner, 1969; Freitas and de Sousa, 1976a); this effect is lost within 24 hr. Lymphocytes pretreated with trypsin also accumulate in the liver and spleen for a period of less than 24 hr. (Woodruff and Gesner, 1968; Freitas and de Sousa, 1975) Pretreatment with Con A causes an inconsistent inital increased localization in the spleen (Gillette *et al.*, 1973; Freitas and de Sousa, 1975; Schlesinger and Israel, 1974). There is a concomitant reduced entry of these manipulated lymphocytes into lymph nodes.

We examined the fate of untreated lymph node cells and cells treated with Con A and with lipopolysaccharide (LPS) in intact and in splenectomized recipients (Freitas and de Sousa, 1975). These studies are somewhat analogous to those on splenectomized animals in which modified red cells or platelets were studied. Cells pretreated with Con A and untreated cells were recovered in equal numbers from the lymph nodes of splenectomized recipients (Table 4). Ford *et al.* (1976) performed direct studies on entry of neuraminidase-treated rat thoracic duct lymphocytes into perfused mesenteric lymph nodes. The number of neuraminidase-treated cells that entered lymph nodes under these experimental conditions was similar to the number of untreated cells that entered lymph nodes when presented "directly" to the nodes.

The distribution of [^{3}H]adenosine-labeled lymph node cells, however, was shown by autoradiography to be modified after Con A treatment; a greater number of treated than of untreated cells were present in the lumen of venules 1 hr after intravenous injection (Freitas *et al.*, 1978).

Surface carbohydrates are probably not the only membrane components involved in the control of lymphocyte circulation. LPS (Freitas and de Sousa, 1976b) and phospholipases (Freitas and de Sousa, 1976a) also cause reduced entry of lymph node cells into lymph nodes from mice. After LPS treatment, radioactivity was increased in the spleen, while after phospholipase A treatment, the cell traffic

335

ECOTAXIS,
ECOTAXOPATHY,
AND LYMPHOID
MALIGNANCY:
TERMS, FACTS AND
PREDICTIONS

TABLE 4. Effect of Splenectomy on Entry of Modified
^{51}Cr-Labeled Lymphocytes into Lymph Nodes

Lymphocyte treatment	Recipient	Percentage of injected radioactivity in lymph node
—	Intact	12
Con A	Intact	4
Con A	Splenectomized	15
—	Splenectomized	15
—	Intact	13
LPS	Intact	9
LPS	Splenectomized	22
—	Splenectomized	21

to lymph nodes was delayed as a consequence of a considerable holdup in the lungs. Other substances that modify the lymphocyte surface and alter lymphocyte distribution include a factor present in the supernatants of cultures of *Bordetella pertussis* (Taub *et al.*, 1972) and antilymphocyte antiserum (Martin, 1969).

2. Circulation of Intact Lymphocytes in Modified Hosts. The circulation of lymphocytes from blood to lymph can be visualized as a journey through a series of different territories. The tempo of this journey is determined by the interactions between the circulating cells and the territory crossed by these cells (de Sousa, 1976a,b; Freitas and de Sousa, 1975, 1976a). Alterations of the territory, as well as of the traveling cells, should alter the normal pattern of circulation. In the preceding section, we saw that, on the whole, *any* modification of the lymphocyte surface results in reduced entry into lymph nodes and a concomitant increase in the number of cells that enter other compartments. In this section, a number of situations will be described in which modulation of territory alters lymphocyte circulation. This work with modified hosts is pertinent to the development of immunological reactivity.

Hall and Morris (1965) showed that local administration of antigen was followed by a transient reduction or "shutdown" in the numbers of lymphocytes leaving the draining lymph node via the efferent lymphatic. Later, it was demonstrated (Dresser *et al.*, 1970; Zatz and Lance, 1971) that either adjuvant or antigen causes a temporary sequestration of circulating cells in the lymphoid organ that drains the site of injection. Labeled circulating cells accumulate transiently in the node that drains the site of a subcutaneous injection (Dresser *et al.*, 1970; Zatz and Lance, 1971; Lance and Frost, 1974). If the injection is given intravenously or intraperitoneally, sequestration occurs in the spleen (Lance and Frost, 1974). *Bordetella pertussis* is one adjuvant that causes both sequestration and redistribution of lymphocytes (Taub *et al.*, 1972). *Bordetella pertussis* causes a dramatic lymphocytosis in mice (Morse, 1964); this lymphocytosis is due to failure of long-lived cells to circulate from the blood compartment into the lymphatics (Morse and Riester, 1967), and is not significantly influenced by increased lymphopoiesis. When the whole organism is administered intravenously, simultaneously injected labeled lymphocytes are "trapped" in the spleen. When a purified "lymphocytosis-promoter factor" obtained from *B. pertussis* culture supernatants is injected, no organ trapping is observed, and the labeled cells remain in the blood compartment (Taub *et al.*, 1972).

The cellular basis of antigen-induced lymphocyte trapping is not understood. The evidence suggests that this phenomenon is another example of a modified interaction between "neighbors" within a lymphoid organ. The macrophage may be the resident cell responsible for the delay of lymphocytes in the area local to antigen injection (Frost, P., 1974; Mongini and Rosenberg, 1976).

Other delays in lymphocyte circulation have been reported after stress (Spry, 1972), after injection of Newcastle disease virus (NDV) (Woodruff and Woodruff, 1974), and after whole-body irradiation (Bell, E. B., and Shand, 1975). Data are available from the experiments on the effect of NDV and of whole-body irradiation on organ distribution of labeled cells after injection. In the NDV experiments, recovery of labeled cells from the spleen was increased 85%. When the virus was injected shortly before injection of labeled cells, neither reduced entry into lymph nodes (72% of control) nor the simultaneous increased localization in the spleen (131% of control) was so striking. One possible interpretation of these experiments

337

ECOTAXIS,
ECOTAXOPATHY,
AND LYMPHOID
MALIGNANCY:
TERMS, FACTS AND
PREDICTIONS

is that they offer another illustration of lymphocyte trapping in the spleen resulting from the intravenous injection of the virus.

Finally, experiments were conducted by E. B. Bell and Shand (1975) on the fate of labeled rat thoracic duct lymphocytes (TDL) from immunized donors after injection into irradiated hosts. These experiments are particularly important, since modified lymphocyte circulation was related to modified immunological function. The experiments were based on the Dresser (1961) and Celada (1966) models of adoptive transfer of immunity in irradiated recipients. TDL from animals immunized with human serum albumin were shown to transfer immunity successfully to irradiated but not to intact recipients. Both the magnitude and the affinity of antibody were greater in irradiated recipients, correlated with impaired blood–lymph circulation of labeled cells. Reduction in recovered radioactivity from the recipients' thoracic duct lymph coincided with increased recovery of radioactivity in lymphoid organs (Table 5). Moreover, administration of unlabeled nonimmune TDL before the injection of the labeled cells corrected the impairment in lymphocyte circulation. This prior administration of nonimmune cells also suppressed the adoptive transfer of the immune response.

1.3. Predictions

1.3.1. Role of Cell Interactions in Control of Ecotaxis

For both T and B lymphocytes, ecotaxis involves circulation from blood to lymph and includes passage through large nonlymphoid capillary filters in the lungs and liver and slow penetration through distinct territories of the peripheral lymphoid organs. Situations that deviate from the normal pattern have been analyzed. Minor modifications of the lymphocyte surface can cause their delay in nonlymphoid organs and delay their arrival in lymph nodes by prolonging the time spent in the spleen. Modifications of the lymphoid organs themselves by irradiation, stress, or the injection of viruses, antigens, or adjuvants can also delay the overall tempo of lymphocyte circulation.

What interaction or interactions actually control the tempo of blood-to-lymph circulation of T and B lymphocytes and determine the distinct positioning of these cells in peripheral lymphoid organs? Greatest attention has been directed to the

TABLE 5. Effect of Unlabeled Rat TDL on the Circulation of Labeled TDL from Blood to Lymph in Irradiated Recipients[a]

Interval before lymph collection (hr)	Percentage of input	
	Irradiated recipients	Irradiated + normal TDL
0–5	0.03	0.27
17	0.49	1.71
29	0.29	1.76
41	0.12	0.61
53	0.09	0.11
65	0.12	0.09

[a] Data from E. B. Bell and Shand (1975). Unlabeled TDL (6×10^8) were injected 1.5 hr before labeled TDL.

interaction between circulating lymphocytes and endothelial cells of postcapillary venules in lymph nodes. Whether lymphocytes cross venules *through* or *between* endothelial cells (Marchesi and Gowans, 1964; Mikata and Niki, 1971; Schoefl and Miles, 1972; van Ewijk *et al.*, 1975) and whether membrane carbohydrates are responsible for preserving this interaction (Gesner and Ginsburg, 1964; Woodruff, 1974) has also been of considerable interest. It is important to clarify the molecular basis of interactions that involve the departure of lymphocytes from the circulation. Lymphocytes enter the white pulp in the mammalian spleen and migrate from blood to lymph in species that lack lymph nodes (Ellis and de Sousa, 1974; Bell, R. G., and Lafferty, 1972). The interaction between lymphocytes and postcapillary venules is particularly sensitive to pretreatment of the lymphocytes with trypsin (Ford *et al.*, 1976; Woodruff, 1974; Freitas and de Sousa, 1976a). For example, trypsin-treated cells fail to leave the blood circuit even in splenectomized recipients (Freitas and de Sousa, 1976a). This result may reflect the relatively generalized action of trypsin on processes such as cell adhesion (Curtis, 1973), rather than the tryptic removal of a lymphocyte receptor for a surface component in the cells of postcapillary venules.

Other interactions must also be considered. In theory, interactions that potentially control the circulation and positioning of lymphoid cells fall into three major groups: (1) those that occur at the site of entry; (2) those that occur within organs traversed by cells en route to the lymph; and (3) those that occur at the exit point.

Cells that penetrate a lymph node enter a pathway that leads them into the efferent lymphatics. Obstruction of the exit route will lead to the accumulation of fluid and cells within the lymphoid organ. Exit of lymphoid cells from nonlymphoid organs is more difficult to envisage. For example, normal lymphoid cells that have extravasated into the skin may be more likely to reenter and circulate in the lymphatics.

The most sensitive anatomical site for altered interactions between lymphocytes and postcapillary venules is located in the midcortex of lymph nodes. The effects of lymphocyte membrane manipulations on lymphocyte traffic in these areas are masked in large part, however, because lymphocytes are "held up" elsewhere. A number of questions are therefore raised: Why does removal of terminal sialic acid from cell membranes by neuraminidase treatment modify the interaction between circulating lymphocytes and liver sinusoidal cells? Why does membrane binding of Con A result first in a modified interaction with the pulmonary capillary wall and later in cell accumulation within the splenic white pulp? Why does phospholipase A modify the interaction between lymphocytes and the alveolar capillary network and delay traffic of lymphocytes through the splenic red pulp (Freitas and de Sousa, 1975, 1976c)? The question with the most clear-cut answer relates to neuraminidase treatment. It is known that asialated glycoproteins are rapidly removed from the blood into the liver (Morell *et al.*, 1971). Thus, the temporary sequestration of the neuraminidase-treated lymphocytes in the liver may simply reflect the expected fate of their surface glycoproteins.

Finally, the interactions that determine the traffic and positioning of lymphocytes that have penetrated into lymphoid organs must be considered. It is indeed intriguing how T and B cells find their separate ways and anatomical locations within an organ after reaching it through a common entry route.

339

ECOTAXIS,
ECOTAXOPATHY,
AND LYMPHOID
MALIGNANCY:
TERMS, FACTS AND
PREDICTIONS

Lymphocytes within a lymphoid organ have basically two kinds of "neighbors"—the "obvious" neighbors and the "underlying" neighbors (de Sousa, 1976b). The obvious neighbor to a lymphocyte is another lymphocyte of the same or a different subpopulation. The underlying neighbors are those permanent elements in the stroma that are easily overlooked on histological examination of normal tissues and are revealed only when T or B lymphocytes have been depleted or have failed to develop. The combined use of lymphocyte depletion and careful ultrastructural analytical techniques permitted Veldman (1970) to define distinct types of dendritic cells peculiar to the stroma of T or B areas (see Figure 2B). Thus, it is conceivable (de Sousa *et al.*, 1973) that localization of T lymphocytes in TDAs is influenced by interactions between these T cells after they leave the postcapillary venules and particular underlying interdigitating dendritic cells (Figure 2B). A distinct set of interactions between lymphocytes and dentritic cells may be responsible for B-cell ecotaxis to the outer cortex.

Recently, it was suggested (Curtis and de Sousa, 1975; de Sousa, 1976b) that modulation of adhesive interactions between "obvious" neighbors (i.e., T and B lymphocytes) within lymphoid organs plays an important role in the control of lymphocyte positioning and the tempo of their circulation. It was found that T and B lymphocytes differ in their adhesiveness *in vitro;* each type of lymphocyte releases a low-molecular-weight factor capable of diminishing the adhesiveness of the other population of lymphocytes without altering the adhesiveness of its own population. Factors that are released by cells and are responsible for their positioning have been termed *morphogens* (Edelstein, 1970; Curtis and van de Wyver, 1971; Curtis, 1974). We prefer the term *interaction-modulation factor* (IMF) for this activity because it provides a more accurate description of function.

The rate at which a cell travels in a given environment may depend on the local concentration of factors produced by other cells in that environment that alter its propensity for adhesion. Evidence for a direct influence of IMF on the rate of lymphocyte traffic stems from a single observation of Curtis and de Sousa (1975). This study showed that ^{51}Cr-labeled *nu/nu* lymphoid cells had an increased entry rate into lymph nodes when injected into *nu/nu* recipients together with T-cell factor. There is considerable indirect evidence, however, to suggest that the rate of lymphocyte traffic is influenced by the host's lymphocyte makeup. Sprent (1974) compared the distribution of ^{51}Cr-labeled *nu/nu* TDL in outbred *nu/nu* or histoincompatible, intact CBA recipients. These studies showed that the ratio of radioactivity recovered from the spleen and mesenteric lymph nodes after injection was higher in *nu/nu* recipients than in intact CBA recipients. This observation indicates that unlabeled host cells facilitated the migration to the lymph nodes of labeled B cells from the athymic mice. These observations are supported by the studies of Spry (1972) on lymphocyte circulation in rats submitted to stress or treatment with corticosteroids and by the studies of E. B. Bell and Shand (1975) on factors that influence the circulation of rat TDL adoptively transferred into syngeneic irradiated hosts. Recirculation of labeled TDL from blood to lymph was reduced after both stress and irradiation. One would expect that if lymphocyte recirculation in a normal host is influenced by the release of factors that modulate the adhesion of T or B cells, a reduction in the circulation of one lymphocyte population will also reduce the rate at which the second population recirculates. Moreover, replacement in animals depleted of lymphoid cells with normal IMF-releasing cells should normalize the tempo of lymphocyte circulation. This indeed proved to be the case. E. B. Bell and Shand (1975) measured radioactivity in thoracic lymph of irradiated recipients of [^{14}C]leucine-labeled immune TDL and found that after these recipients had been administered nonimmune and unlabeled TDL, the recovery rate of radioactivity was normalized (Table 5).

One of the most interesting aspects of Bell and Shand's study is the correlation observed between the rate of traffic of adoptively transferred lymphocytes in irradiated and unirradiated hosts and the magnitude of the secondary response in both animal models. Responses were two orders of magnitude higher in irradiated than in unirradiated animals. The obligatory requirement of host irradiation for the effective adoptive transfer of an immune response has been realized for some time (Dresser, 1961; Celada, 1966). The nature of the functional "barrier" faced by adoptively transferred cells in intact hosts is not known, but may be influenced by the control mechanism of lymphoid cell interactions proposed at present.

We recently reported (de Sousa and Haston, 1976) that partial reduction of a T-cell population by treatment with antilymphocyte serum (ALS) significantly increases the frequency of heterologous and B–B cell interactions in lymph node cell suspensions (Table 6). In an intact host, production of IMF by both T and B cells must be high, thereby hindering interaction between adoptively transferred cells. Partial reduction of the host's lymphoid cell population by sublethal irradiation (500 rads in the mouse, 900 rads in the rat) creates the physical conditions conducive to interactions that favor clonal expansion of adoptively transferred cells. Conversely, administration of nonimmune cells increases IMF concentrations in lymphoid organs of the recipients, which would diminish interactions between the transferred cells and thereby reduce the adoptive response (Bell, E. B., and Shand, 1975).

Such a mechanism would explain why a small dose of ALS enhances background IgM plaque formation by spleen cells from *nonimmunized* mice (Anderson *et al.*, 1972). This mechanism would also explain the observations of Baker *et al.* (1974) that partial depletion of T cells with ALS "enhances" the production of antibodies to thymus-independent antigens; this effect can be reversed by administering thymocytes. We found (de Sousa and Haston, 1976) that administration of thymocytes to mice pretreated with ALS considerably reduces the frequency of direct B–B cell interactions. This observation must constitute the basis, at least in large part, for most nonspecific suppressor effects of thymocytes (Gershon, 1974).

TABLE 6. Nature of Cell Pairs Found in Lymph Node Suspension[a] of ALS-Treated Mice, Normal Mice, and ALS-Treated Mice Reconstituted with Thymocytes

Group	Pairs (%)	Cell pairs[b]		
		−/−	−/+	+/+
Control	2.44 ± 1.02	1.71 ± 0.81	0.3 ± 0.35	0.57 ± 0.48
ALS	9.44 ± 2.02	1.07 ± 0.90	3.74 ± 1.83	4.74 ± 0.95
ALS + thymocytes	2.97 ± 0.34	1.33 ± 0.84	0.94 ± 0.04	0.71 ± 0.54

[a]Suspensions were stained with a fluorescein-isothiocyanate-labeled rabbit anti-mouse IgG antiserum.
[b](−/−) Homologous, surface-IgG-negative; (−/+) heterologous, consisting of 1 labeled and 1 unlabeled cell; (+/+) homologous, surface-IgG-positive.

341

ECOTAXIS,
ECOTAXOPATHY,
AND LYMPHOID
MALIGNANCY:
TERMS, FACTS AND
PREDICTIONS

A physiological situation in which partial T-cell depletion occurs is during the early stages of primary responses to a number of thymus-dependent antigens (de Sousa and Parrott, 1967). Within the first 24 hr after antigenic challenge, a transient depletion of TDAs in the spleen is observed. This partial T-cell depletion has considerable potential importance for the subsequent development of a normal immune response to an administered antigen because it increases the frequency of direct cell interactions in the organ containing the highest concentration of antigen.

1.3.2. Abnormal Lymphocyte Traffic and Disease

Most experimental models of abnormal cell traffic have a transient duration. For example, most of the changes observed as a result of enzyme, lectin, or viral pretreatment last for less than 24 or 48 hr. The value of an experimental model, however, is to prove that a certain event *can* happen. That it can happen should alert us to the possibility that it can also occur in nature. Thus, it is possible to predict the existence of clinical situations in which a permanent lesion of the lymphocyte surface will result in its progressive sequestration in the spleen or liver, and slow its removal from the blood (see Section 2.2).

More recently, in an autoradiographic study of the fate of [³H]adenosine-labeled lymph node cells in recipients pretreated with dextran sulfate or pentosan sulfate (Freitas and de Sousa, 1977), it was demonstrated that modification of the host also results in slower circulation of lymphocytes through the lung, and red pulp and marginal zone in the spleen. Thus, in disease, progressive sequestration of a cell may reflect a progressive lesion of the environment through which the cell is circulating (see also Section 2.2.3, p. 347).

Interest in problems of lymphocyte traffic has evolved separately from interest in the mechanism of red cell traffic. Antibody, however, is instrumental in removal of erythrocytes *as well as* lymphocytes from the blood (Martin, 1969). The consequences for immunological function of a slowed circulation of lymphocytes and the resulting abnormal interactions occurring within lymphoid organs partially depleted of one cell population were well illustrated by the experiments discussed above. These observations (Bell, E. B., and Shand, 1975; de Sousa and Haston, 1976) are relevant to understanding the association of autoimmune hemolytic anemia, macroglobulinemia, and lymphoid malignancy in the New Zealand Black (NZB) mouse (East *et al.,* 1965; Talal and Steinberg, 1974).

The position occupied by a cell in a lymphoid organ reflects a series of interactions with both obvious and underlying neighbor cells. It is therefore predictable that the accumulation or proliferation of one malignant cell type exemplifies a defect in those interactions as well as a defect of the malignant population itself.

Finally, if the spleen, by virtue of its structure and position in the blood circuit, is one of the major sequestration sites of abnormal circulating cells, splenectomy will predictably help improve cell maldistribution.

2. Ecotaxopathy

2.1. Definition of the Term and Introduction

Ecotaxopathy refers to abnormal ecotaxis and is due to failure of circulating cells to migrate and occupy their normal environment. Ecotaxis results from a series of interactions of the circulating cells with resident or other circulating cells in the organs through which they travel in blood, blood-to-lymph, or lymph circulations. Excessive proliferation or accumulation of one cell type in one compartment of the lymphoid system occurs with lymphoid malignancy. This may be the result of abnormal function of normal neighboring cells, rather than of the primary neoplastic cells themselves.

A number of experimental and human lymphoid malignancies will now be discussed to illustrate how progressive depletion of one lymphoid cell population in its normal environment could lead to the development of malignancy among its usual neighbors. These modified cell interactions may offer an explanation for some anomalies of immunological function that are often associated with lymphoid malignancy.

2.2. Experimental and Clinical Basis for Definition of the Term

2.2.1. Autoimmunity and Malignancy in the New Zealand Black Mouse

In 1959, it was discovered that NZB mice developed hemolytic anemia (Bielschowsky et al., 1959). The interpretation of this discovery illustrates how interpretation of facts tends to reflect prevailing theoretical views (Burnet, 1962; Gershon, 1974) and also influences clinical decisions on therapy and management of human disease.

The abnormalities found in NZB mice include (1) autoimmune hemolytic anemia; (2) the appearance of germinal centers in the thymus; (3) immune complex renal disease (East, 1970); (4) immunological hyperresponsiveness during early life (Playfair, 1968; Evans et al., 1968; Staples and Talal, 1969; Cantor et al., 1970; Talal and Steinberg, 1974; Palmer et al., 1976); (5) depressed cell-mediated immunity (CMI) later in life (Gazdar et al., 1971; Gelfland and Steinberg, 1973); (6) depletion of recirculating and long-lived lymphocytes (Zatz et al., 1971; Denman and Denman, 1970); (7) lymphoid hyperplasia; and (8) malignancy (East et al., 1965; East and de Sousa, 1966; Mellors, 1966a,b) and macroglobulinemia (East et al., 1965; East and de Sousa, 1966).

The appearance of germinal centers in the thymus was interpreted as the expression of uncontrolled proliferation of forbidden clones of cells producing autoantibodies in the thymus (Burnet and Holmes, 1962). This hypothesis suggested that thymectomy might be clinically beneficial for patients with various autoimmune diseases (MacKay and Smalley, 1966; Alarcón-Segovia et al., 1963). This hypothesis, however, was shown not to be valid; experimental thymectomy did not prove to be beneficial. In fact, thymectomy may precipitate the development of the hemolytic anemia and the kidney lesions in NZB mice (East et al., 1967a).

An alternative explanation was that the thymus normally exercises regulatory control over populations of immune reactive cells, and that this regulatory mechanism is defective in NZB mice (East and de Sousa, 1966; Gershon, 1974; Barthold et al., 1974; Talal and Steinberg, 1974). From the study of thymus-dependent responses, it has become apparent that older NZB mice develop a defect of thymus-controlled functions that precedes the onset of autoimmune phenomena (Talal and Steinberg, 1974). This defect develops with advancing age and is reflected both in depressed CMI responses and in abnormally high responsiveness to thymus-independent antigens (Barthold et al., 1974).

The peripheral lymphoid organs (particularly the peripheral lymph nodes and spleen) of NZB mice are considerably enlarged. This enlargement of lymphoid tissues is due to overt proliferation of the cells in the B areas, large primary nodules, and germinal centers. Sheets of plasma cells, early plasma cell precursors, and reticulum cells make their appearance in the red pulp of the spleen and in the medullary cords of lymph nodes (Figure 6). These cells have malignant properties that can be demonstrated in transfer experiments (Mellors, 1966a; East and de Sousa, 1966; East *et al.*, 1967b). In fact, the pathological changes in lymphoid organs of these mice are similar to those in the organs of patients with macroglobuli-nemia (Dutcher and Fahey, 1959). At the same time, lymphoid cells accumulate in nonlymphoid organs such as the lungs and liver, while relatively fewer lymphocytes circulate in the blood than in other inbred strains of mice (East *et al.*, 1965). The distribution of ^{51}Cr-labeled spleen and lymph node cells (Zatz *et al.*, 1971) from NZB mice showed a sharp increase in the numbers of nonrecirculating cells in the spleen by age 3 months, while there was an absolute decrease in recirculating cells. The predominant localization of cells that did not recirculate shifted from lymph nodes to the liver. These changes precede detection of Coombs positivity by about 1 month and coincide with the appearance of soluble type-specific Gross virus antigen in the circulation at 3–4 months (Mellors *et al.*, 1969).

Are these different facts interrelated? The answer is yes. These phenomena are interrelated through the absence in peripheral lymphoid organs of older NZB mice of a thymus-derived population of lymphocytes that normally control B-cell interactions. This T-cell deficit could be due to (1) a central deficit of the thymus or (2) ecotaxopathy of a modified population (perhaps due to greater susceptibility to

343

ECOTAXIS,
ECOTAXOPATHY,
AND LYMPHOID
MALIGNANCY:
TERMS, FACTS AND
PREDICTIONS

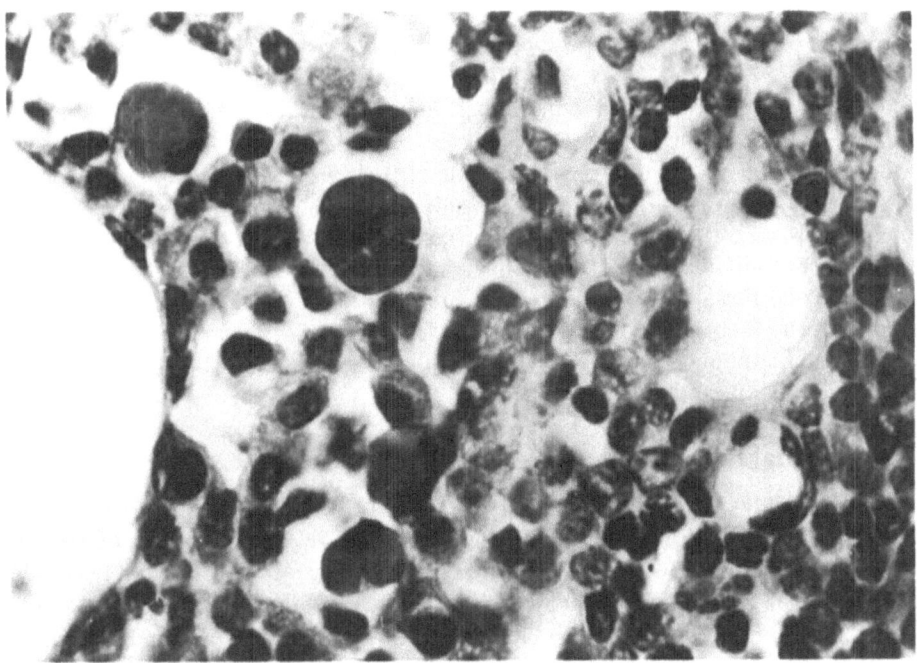

Figure 6. A peripheral lymph node from a Coombs-positive NZB mouse. Note the large periodic-acid–Schiff-positive Russell bodies and the numerous plasma cells and plasmablasts.

virus infection) sequestered from blood and peripheral lymphoid organs into non-lymphoid sites, especially the liver.

If the release of IMF by T cells controls the frequency and nature of B-cell interactions (see Section 1.3.1), these factors are likely to influence B-cell proliferation and function. Lack of the controlling cell population would then explain increased IgM production and the appearance of circulating autoantibodies, which perhaps lead to the eventual development of B-cell malignancy.

It is of interest to recall at this point the numerous IgG antibodies, including autoantibodies, that occur with infectious mononucleosis (Carter, 1966) (see also Chapter 13). Infectious mononucleosis is a human disease in which a modified population of circulating lymphocytes suddenly appears in the blood for a transient period of time. This clinical event probably reflects alteration of interactions within peripheral lymphoid organs. Continuous production of autoantibodies such as occurs in NZB mice is likely to give rise to further ecotaxopathies such as red cell sequestration in the spleen and lymphocyte maldistribution related to the production of antilymphocyte antibodies.

The logical therapy for abnormalities that occur with autoimmune conditions may be replacement of thymus-derived cells, not thymectomy. This form of therapeutic manipulation has been achieved with transfer of thymus cells from young into older NZB mice. This procedure corrects the abnormal responses to thymus-independent antigens of the older animals (Barthold *et al.*, 1974). In addition, Denman *et al.* (1971) reported that rat spleen cells that are first passed through glass wool columns (a maneuver that is likely to cause T-cell enrichment) had a dramatic therapeutic effect on the hemolytic anemia when administered to thymectomized and ALS-treated NZB mice. Complete remission of macroglobulinemia also took place.

2.2.2. B-Cell Lymphomas

Most studies on B-cell lymphomas have focused on the identification and characterization of the abnormal cell clones (see Chapter 10). The possibility that a situation similar to the one postulated for NZB murine neoplasms also occurs in man with lymphoma is deserving of consideration. The appearance of a neoplastic B-cell lymphoma may represent local or generalized derangement of B-cell traffic, which is normally controlled by T cells. Alternatively, an unrecognized abnormality of the "underlying" stroma cell neighbors may occur in these patients. Further studies of the function of T cells separated from lymph nodes and blood of patients with B-cell lymphomas should provide useful new information about the pathophysiology of these lymphomas.

2.2.3. Hodgkin's Disease

Why Hodgkin's disease?

How can the concept of ecotaxopathy be of relevance to one of the most extensively studied and best documented primary diseases of lymphoid tissues?

Hodgkin's disease is a progressive disorder of the lymphoid system often accompanied by lymphopenia and deficits of CMI (Hansen, J. A., and Good, 1974) (see also Chapter 19). This lymphopenia could result from an absolute deficit of circulating lymphocytes or from displacement of cells from one compartment, resulting in their accumulation in another compartment (de Sousa, 1976c; de Sousa et al., 1976). Lymphocyte ecotaxopathy may have fundamental relevance to understanding the basic pathogenesis of Hodgkin's disease.

345

ECOTAXIS,
ECOTAXOPATHY,
AND LYMPHOID
MALIGNANCY:
TERMS, FACTS AND
PREDICTIONS

Recent studies on the distribution of T and B lymphocytes in the blood and spleen of patients with Hodgkin's disease (Matchett et al., 1973; Kaur et al., 1974; Payne et al., 1976; de Sousa et al., 1977) indicate that depletion of T lymphocytes from the blood may not be a reflection of an overall T-cell deficit, but instead could be related to an accumulation of T cells in the spleen. There is some controversy as to whether splenic sequestration of T cells occurs primarily at sites that are involved with the disease. That a similar maldistribution of lymphocytes occurs in splenectomized patients with stage I Hodgkin's disease indicates that the spleen, with or without tumor involvement, need not be present for T-cell sequestration to occur with Hodgkin's disease. One is therefore tempted to speculate that patients with Hodgkin's disease have an anomaly of the lymphocyte surface similar to that induced under experimental conditions. An anomaly of this nature would result in the progressive sequestration of affected cells in the spleen or other reticuloendothelial tissues. Evidence derived from a number of in vitro abnormalities of lymphocyte function (even with stage I disease) (Matchett et al., 1973; Levy and Kaplan, 1974) suggests that these patients may have a basic defect of their lymphocyte membranes. We studied responses to various mitogens by spleen and blood lymphocytes (de Sousa et al., 1976) from children with Hodgkin's disease. While peripheral blood cells failed to respond normally to lower doses of phytohemagglutinin (PHA), normal or increased responses by cells from the spleen and uninvolved lymph nodes from the same patients were observed. Similar observations were made by Twomey et al. (Chapter 20), using cells from tissues that were involved with tumor. Furthermore, responses by cultured blood lymphocytes to T-cell mitogens increased following splenectomy (Figure 7).

These findings could probably be related to the currently attractive concept that a viral infection underlies Hodgkin's disease (see Chapter 6). Perhaps the membrane defect detected by PHA stimulation and by the possible failure of the lymphocytes to ecotax is due to the binding of a virus or viral component to receptors on the T-cell surface that are needed for proliferative responses to lectins (Hughes and Mautner, 1973) and for normal lymphocyte traffic (Woodruff and Woodruff, 1974) (see Section 1.2.3b). Alternatively, proliferative hyporesponsiveness by peripheral blood lymphocytes, despite unimpaired responses by lymphocytes from uninvolved lymphoid organs, may indicate a lack of membrane receptors on circulating cells, which is corrected by compensatory synthesis of the receptor while the cells reside in the lymphoid organs. This would render these cells vulnerable to infection by viruses that utilize similar binding sites.

Recent studies of the mechanism of the hyporesponsiveness of peripheral blood T lymphocytes in Hodgkin's disease (Fuks et al., 1976) have revealed the presence in the serum of these patients of blocking factors of sheep erythrocyte rosette formation and of the PHA response. The nature of the factors is not clear. The finding of Moroz et al. (1977) that a population of lymphocytes with ferritin on the surface appears in the peripheral blood of Hodgkin's disease patients indicates that ferritin is responsible for the blocking effect. However, the reason why T lymphocytes in the blood are unresponsive to PHA while T lymphocytes in the spleen respond normally to stimulation by the same mitogen is not understood.

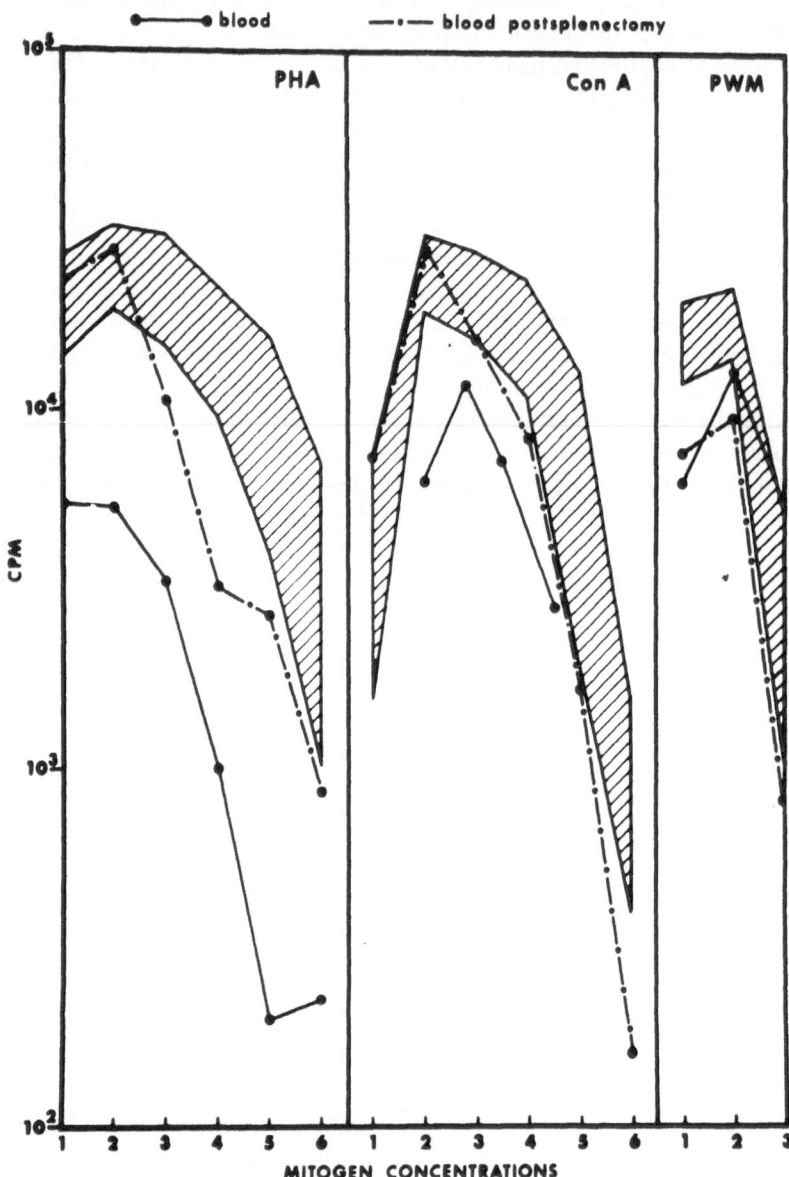

Figure 7. Comparison of mitogen response by cultured blood lymphocytes from a 5-year-old patient with stage IA Hodgkin's disease before (•———•) and 3 months after splenectomy (• · · · · · · •). The percentage of T cells was 23.5% in peripheral blood and 61% in splenic tissue. The percentage of T cells in the peripheral blood increased to 43.5% after splenectomy. Total lymphocyte counts before were 1072/mm³ of blood before splenectomy and 2550/mm³ after. The hatched areas represent standard deviations of values obtained with normal blood. Mitogen concentrations (μg/ml): Phytohemagglutinin (PHA): 1 : 50, 2 : 12.5, 3 : 4.2, 4 : 21, 5 :1.0, 6 : 0.5; concanavalin A (Con A): 1 : 50, 2 : 25, 3 : 6, 4 : 1.6, 5 : 0.4, 6 : 0.1; pokeweed mitogen (PWM): 1 : 1/10, 2 : 1/50, 3 : 1/250.

347

ECOTAXIS,
ECOTAXOPATHY,
AND LYMPHOID
MALIGNANCY:
TERMS, FACTS AND
PREDICTIONS

Recently we have been exploring the possibility that the finding of high numbers of T lymphocytes in the spleen is associated with an abnormality of the spleen environment. Following the early observation of Bieber and Bieber (1973), who found abnormally high amounts of ferritin in tissues involved by the disease, we have been studying the distribution of the three major iron-binding proteins—ferritin, lactoferrin, and transferrin—in the spleen and other tissues from Hodgkin's disease patients. We confirm the finding of excessive amounts of ferritin; in addition, excessive amounts of the other two iron-binding proteins were also observed. These findings and the reported observations of siderosis of the lymph nodes (Dumont *et al.*, 1976) and of other abnormalities of iron metabolism in Hodgkin's disease (Beamish *et al.*, 1972) have led us to postulate that the central defect in the disease is an iron-handling defect of spleen and lymph node macrophages (de Sousa *et al.*, 1978). The recent demonstrations that lymphocytes have receptors for lactoferrin (van Snick and Masson, 1976) and for transferrin (Phillips, 1976) offer a plausible mechanism for the ecotaxopathy of lymphocytes in environments rich in these proteins.

2.2.4. Mycosis Fungoides

The association of a deficit of immunological function with Hodgkin's disease has been known for some time (Parker *et al.*, 1932; Steiner, 1934). Interest has recently focused on the immunopathology of mycosis fungoides, in which there is an accumulation of lymphoid cells in the skin (see Chapter 16) (Tan *et al.*, 1974; Zacharie *et al.*, 1975; Lutzner *et al.*, 1975; Mackie *et al.*, 1976; Goos *et al.*, 1976). One consequence of the accumulation of circulating cells in the "wrong" environment is their depletion elsewhere. This point is most dramatically illustrated by one patient (Lutzner *et al.*, 1975) with Sézary syndrome who had a form of the disease in which skin infiltration and blood lymphocyte counts varied reciprocally (Figure 8).

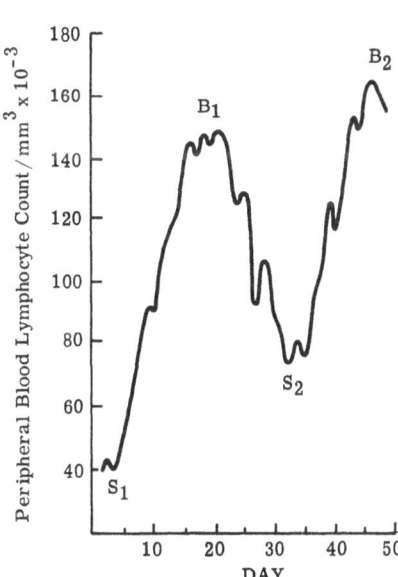

Figure 8. Spontaneous cyclic pattern of peripheral blood lymphocyte counts in a patient with mycosis fungoides. At points B_1 and B_2, skin involvement was improved, while cutaneous infiltration was most marked at points S_1 and S_2. Reproduced with modifications from Lutzner *et al.* (1975).

We and others have recently shown (MacKie *et al.*, 1976; Tan *et al.*, 1974; Zacharie *et al.*, 1975) that the portion of total body T cells in the peripheral blood of patients with mycosis fungoides is considerably lower than that in normal persons (Figure 9). Moreover, it is apparent from absolute cell counts on blood that there is a depletion of both T and B cells, with a simultaneous increase in cells that form neither sheep erythrocyte (E) nor erythrocyte–antibody–complement (EAC) rosettes. The discovery of lymphoid ecotaxopathy in mycosis fungoides is important because it permits analysis of possible pathophysiological mechanisms of the disease.

Lymphocyte emigration from the blood into the skin could be due to an abnormality of the skin environment, abnormal capillary permeability, or an abnormality of circulating cells themselves. These possibilities are discussed below.

a. An Abnormality of the Skin Environment. One mechanism for experimental lymphocyte sequestration is the administration of antigen (see Section 1.2.3b). It is possible that an unidentified antigenic stimulus in the skin of patients with mycosis fungoides causes cells to accumulate in the skin. Recently, however, Goos *et al.* (1976) discovered the presence in the skin of one such patient of "interdigitating dendritic" cells (see Figure 2C). Hitherto, this morphological type of cell had been associated only with the thymus and TDAs within lymphoid tissues (Veldman, 1970; Hoefschmit, 1974). This observation, if confirmed, could greatly enhance understanding of the pathogenesis of mycosis fungoides. It would also confirm the prediction of Goudie *et al.* (1974) that situations in which abnormal lymphocyte accumulations occur in nonlymphoid sites represent examples of "ecotaxis." Skin involvement with mycosis fungoides may be related to the existence of certain characteristic structural similarities between cutaneous and thymic tissues.

b. Abnormal Capillary Permeability. Patients with mycosis fungoides often demonstrate an abnormal Hess test, indicating some degree of increased capillary permeability (MacKie, personal observations). This could result in increased cell traffic through capillary membranes. Sézary syndrome has been considered a "malignant caricature" of mycosis fungoides. That leukopheresis has been used successfully to deplete skin lymphocytes in Sézary syndrome (Edelson *et*

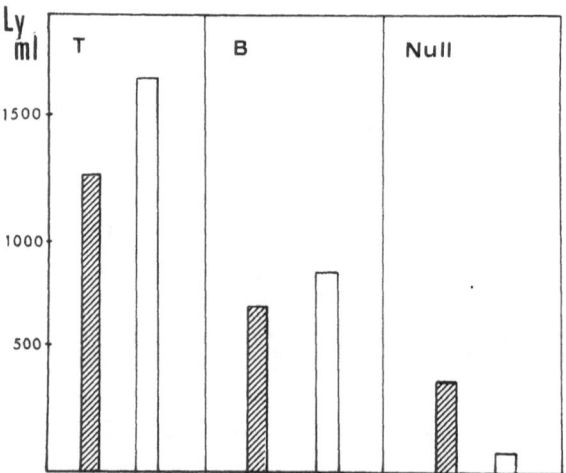

Figure 9. Peripheral blood counts of E-rosette-forming cells (T), EAC-rosette-forming cells (B), and lymphoid cells that failed to form rosettes (Null) in 28 patients with mycosis fungoides (hatched bars) and 20 age-matched healthy subjects (open bars). (Unpublished data from MacKie *et al.*, 1976.)

349

ECOTAXIS,
ECOTAXOPATHY,
AND LYMPHOID
MALIGNANCY:
TERMS, FACTS AND
PREDICTIONS

al., 1974a) also points to an unusually easy reentry into the blood of cells that accumulate in the skin.

That polymorphonuclear leukocytes are seldom found in the skin infiltrates of mycosis fungoides is not surprising. Hurley (1963) demonstrated clearly that granulocyte emigration is related, not to increased vascular permeability, but instead to the presence of chemotaxis-inducing factors.

c. An Abnormality of the Circulating Cells Themselves. Experimental maneuvers that lead to lymphocyte maldistribution are not limited to the administration of antigens. Pretreatment of labeled lymphocytes *in vitro* with a number of substances that modify the lymphocyte membrane also results in lymphocyte maldistribution (see Section 1.2.3a). Lymphocyte sequestration occurs more frequently in organs with sinusoids, such as the spleen and liver. If, however, there were a slight abnormality of the skin capillaries plus a minor defect of lymphocyte membranes (that would modify interactions between circulating lymphocytes and the dermal cells), lymphocyte immigration and accumulation in the dermis would follow, as they do in mycosis fungoides.

d. High IgE Levels: A Functional Consequence of Lymphocyte Ecotaxopathy? Three separate groups of workers have now reported a high level of circulating IgE in a subpopulation of patients with mycosis fungoides who have no history of atopy (MacKie *et al.*, 1976; Tan *et al.*, 1974; Zacharie *et al.*, 1975). Elevated IgE levels are also found in bullous pemphigoides (Arbesman *et al.*, 1974). These observations suggest indirectly that elevated serum IgE levels may not be associated exclusively with atopy. The common factor in these three conditions may well be a maldistribution of lymphocytes. The possibility that the subpopulation of lymphocytes that accumulate in the dermis is related to control of IgE production merits serious consideration. Experimental work on the regulation of IgE antibody responses in rats (Tada *et al.*, 1973) established the importance of a T-cell population in controlling IgE antibody levels.

2.3. Beneficial Effect of Splenectomy

Recent studies of the effect of splenectomy on hematological cytopenias complicating malignant lymphomas have stressed the clinical benefits often derived from this operation, even in cases with no demonstrable increase in splenic sequestration of ^{51}Cr-labeled erythrocytes (Adler *et al.*, 1975; Morris, 1975). The value of these observations to the understanding of the pathogenesis of diseases such as Hodgkin's disease, chronic lymphocytic leukemia (CLL), and nodular (but not diffuse) histiocytic lymphomas (Morris, 1975) can be appreciated only in the context of understanding splenic structure and its role in the control of ecotaxis.

Until now, the cytopenias with splenomegaly in patients with lymphoproliferative disorders have been attributed to "hypersplenism." When considered in the context of cell traffic, however, the spleen is simply a passive, if unique, part of the blood circuit that sequesters modified lymphocytes, erythrocytes, and platelets by virtue of its anatomical position and the structure of its capillary network (see Section 1.2). Removal of the spleen even from healthy subjects results in increased numbers of leukocytes elsewhere in the blood circulation.

Sequestration of lymphoid cells occurs when the spleen environment is modified (e.g., following experimental intravenous administration of antigen) (see Section 1.2.3b). Partial depletion of T cells with ALS results in a marked increase in spleen cells capable of spontaneous IgM plaque formation with sheep erythrocytes (Anderson *et al.*, 1972). Thus, the spleen has to be visualized as a special part of the blood circuit, where minor qualitative or quantitative modifications of one cell population may alter the function of another cell population, such as the production of antibody. Autoantibodies may be part of this spontaneous change in antibody production (see Section 2.2.1), which, in turn, has the potential to modify other circulating cells. On subsequent splenic passage, these other circulating cells will be recognized and removed by the pericapillary macrophages.

Things can therefore "go wrong" in the spleen at at least two interrelated points—(1) at the point of antibody production and (2) at the point of cell traffic control—because, in part, the spleen evolved as the peripheral lymphoid organ in which circulating cells are most freely mixed and the chances of direct interactions between antigen, macrophages, T cells, B cells, erythrocytes, platelets, and other cell types are highest.

Removal of the spleen should, on the whole, improve clinical situations in which circulating cells are abnormal and at risk of sequestration. In the case of Hodgkin's disease, this latter risk is greater because there seems to be an additional abnormality of the splenic biochemical makeup. Originally, this was thought to be a tumor-associated antigen (Order *et al.*, 1971), but more recently it was found to be a high concentration of normal ferritin (Eshhar *et al.*, 1974). Whatever the nature of the splenic abnormality, it could constitute an additional reason for the local accumulation of circulating T cells. This possibility, though it is attractive and is borne out to some extent by the short-term improvement in peripheral blood lymphocyte counts in splenectomized patients with Hodgkin's disease, does not persist over a longer period. Eventually (by 10 months), the lymphocyte count starts to decline, and it has been suggested that the liver then takes over from the spleen as the abnormal lodging site of the circulating cells (de Sousa *et al.*, 1977).

2.4. Lymphocyte Ecotaxopathy: Some Conclusions

In conclusion, I wish to stress that diseases in which T- or B-lymphocyte depletion is observed in one compartment of the circulatory pathway should be analyzed in the light of the principle of ecotaxis—that lymphocytes normally have the capacity to discriminate between lymphoid and nonlymphoid environments and among separate microenvironments within the lymphoid organs. If accumulation or depletion is observed in one compartment (the compartment most frequently studied being the peripheral blood) with concurrent depletion or accumulation in others, reasons for this lymphocyte maldistribution should be sought.

Lymphocyte ecotaxopathy may in some cases reflect an abnormality of the cell itself, but more likely it may act as a pointer of diagnostic and prognostic value in the detection of other generalized abnormalities occurring at control points of lymphoid cell traffic (see Section 1.3.1).

3. Predictions

3.1. Reading New Diagnostic Meanings

The merit of an experimental or conceptual model in biology ultimately resides in its application to the understanding of disease. The finding of the specific

351

ECOTAXIS,
ECOTAXOPATHY,
AND LYMPHOID
MALIGNANCY:
TERMS, FACTS AND
PREDICTIONS

positioning of the two major lymphoid cell populations that occurs in experimental animals is now also firmly established in man. Knowledge concerning the position of lymphoid cells in lymphoid tissues, their changes in response to various immunological stimuli, and the functional implications of these changes has provided new insight into pathological changes of the lymphoid system in man (Hansen, J. A., and Good, 1974; Green *et al.*, 1975). What contribution can knowledge of ecotaxis and the concept of "neighbor control" make to the understanding of lymphoid malignancy? What new diagnostic meaning can be inferred, for instance, from the knowledge that after intravenous injection, labeled mouse bone marrow cells are found in larger numbers in the recipient's bone marrow and splenic red pulp than a similar inoculum of thymus cells?

One answer is to be found in Edelson's perspective on T-cell lymphomas (Lutzner *et al.*, 1975):

> It is of major interest that the abnormal T cells, like their normal counterparts, tend to localize in specific regions of soft tissues. Besides preferential infiltration of the skin and T cell zones of lymphoid tissues, they initially spare the bone marrow to a remarkable extent (Edelson *et al.*, 1974b). Leukemias of B (bone marrow derived) cells significantly involve the bone marrow, replacing normal marrow elements (Hansen, M. M., 1973). Therefore, despite extreme peripheral blood lymphocytosis in individual cases, severe anemia, granulocytopenia and thrombocytopenia are not prominent features of these T-cell leukemias. Indeed, like widespread cutaneous infiltration, surprising marrow sparing in patients suspected to have chronic lymphocytic leukemia should alert the physician to the possibility of a T-cell leukemia.

The physician must become alerted to the new anatomical and functional meanings of depletion or accumulation of lymphocytes in soft tissue or fluid compartments of the cells' circuit, such as the blood and lymph. The blood has been the compartment most extensively studied for cell content and immunological function. Lymph node biopsies, however, are frequently done *without* a simultaneous analysis of the blood compartment. Any attempt to investigate a disease of the lymphoid system is incomplete if only one compartment is analyzed. Except for congenital thymus or marrow aplasias, no single compartment is representative of the whole system. Lymphocyte depletion in one compartment may mean that cells are accumulating elsewhere, and it is the accumulation, not the depletion, that is of relevance to the primary disease pathology. Figure 10 illustrates the application of this reasoning to Hodgkin's disease. On the other hand, accumulation of a cell clone, i.e., B cells in the blood in CLL or in a lymph node with a nodular lymphoma, may mean that the cells are failing to circulate normally. This failure to circulate, rather than excessive accumulation of cells, may hold clues to pathogenesis of these neoplasms.

Then there is the question of the *functional* repercussions of partial depletion or accumulation of one lymphoid cell type. Interactions that control positioning and traffic of lymphocyte populations may be important to the same controlling immunological function, especially of B cells. For example, partial T-cell depletion in the spleen may result in increased IgM production. On the other hand, progressive T-cell accumulation in the same organ may stimulate IgG production by B cells (Longmire *et al.*, 1973). Depletion of T-cell subpopulations, through their extravasation into the skin, may result in uncontrolled production of IgE in mycosis fungoides and, perhaps, atopy. Disease processes cannot be attributed, however, to altered T–B cell interactions alone. Knowledge that T and B cells circulate and interact continuously and that these processes are subject to derangement adds a

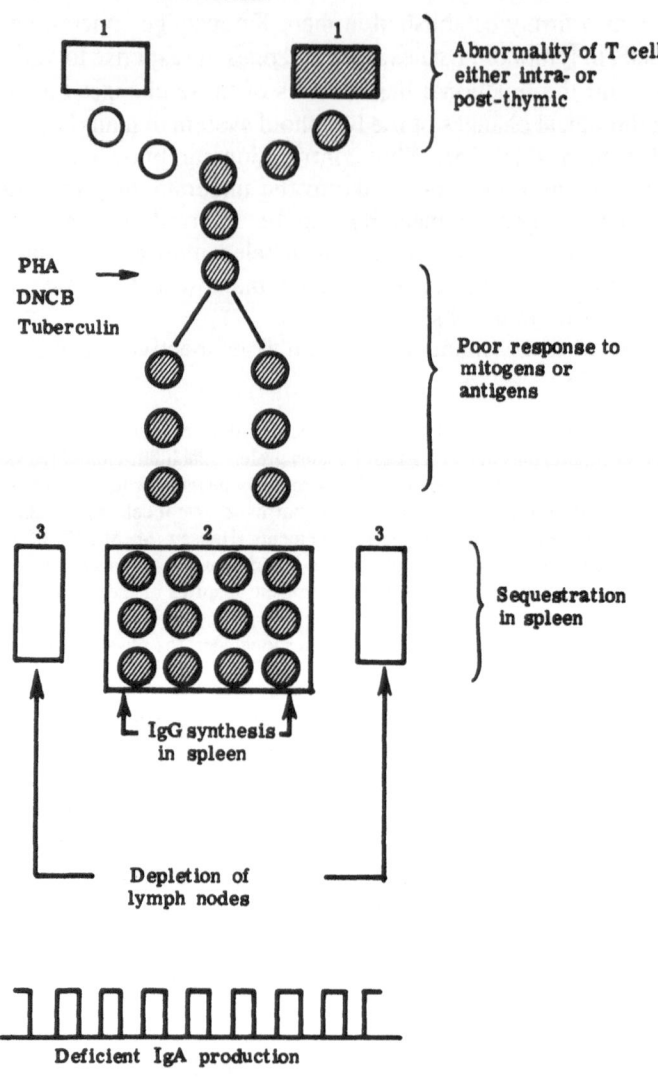

Figure 10. A hypothesis for the redistribution of abnormal T cells with Hodgkin's disease. The basic abnormality may occur before or after cells leave the thymus (1), and is reflected by hyporesponsiveness by circulating lymphocytes to mitogens and antigens. Sequestration of the cells occurs in the spleen (2), thereby causing progressive depletion of lymphocytes from other peripheral lymphoid sites such as lymph nodes (3) and gut (⊓⊓⊓). This maldistribution could explain increased splenic IgG synthesis and deficient IgA production.

new dimension to our understanding of the pathogenesis of certain diseases. These derangements include anomalies of lymphocyte positioning and of immunological function.

3.2. Finding New Therapeutic Tools

The quality of therapy reflects understanding of disease pathogenesis. If the pathogenesis of lymphoid malignancy is associated with the failure of neighboring

353

ECOTAXIS,
ECOTAXOPATHY,
AND LYMPHOID
MALIGNANCY:
TERMS, FACTS AND
PREDICTIONS

cells to control the traffic and proliferation of malignant cells, therapy designed to eliminate the accumulating cells may be only temporarily beneficial.

What manipulations other than radiotherapy and chemotherapy for the lymphomas (see Chapter 22) can be foreseen as possible viable future forms of therapy? Mechanical manipulation and drainage of accumulated malignant cells has been attempted. Extensive leukopheresis with Sézary syndrome was reported to lower cellular infiltration in the skin (Edelson *et al.*, 1974a). Success with prolonged thoracic duct drainage was reported in the management of rheumatoid arthritis (Paulus *et al.*, 1973). This report is of particular interest because the lymphocyte drainage was accompanied by reinfusion into the bloodstream of the cell-free lymph without untoward effect. Conversely, reinfusion of cell-free lymph into patients with myasthenia gravis after prolonged thoracic duct drainage aggravates clinical manifestations of the disease (Bergström *et al.*, 1973). These seemingly unrelated observations may be relevant to future management of lymphoid malignancy because they suggest the presence in lymph of products capable of modulating disease. There is evidence that immunochemical differences (perhaps including low-molecular-weight substances) do exist between blood and lymph (Nash and Heremans, 1972; Vaerman *et al.*, 1973; Kaartinen *et al.*, 1973). IMFs (mol. wt. <10,000) fall in this low-molecular-weight category. We have evidence that these substances are present in serum (Curtis and de Sousa, 1975) and should be present in higher concentrations in lymph.

In some forms of lymphoid malignancy, especially Waldenström's macroglobulinemia, a generalized deficit of IMF production by T cells may exist. Such deficits should lead to the accumulation and slow expansion of B-cell clones, and contribute to the unusually high viscosity of blood related to the high concentrations of IgM in these patients. Transfusions of normal, cell-free lymph may become beneficial in management of NZB mice instead of thymus-cell transfer (see Section 2.2.1). Similarly, the local infusion of normal lymph (or T-cell IMF) could be considered in cases of nodular B-cell lymphomas.

Corrections of abnormal interactions with "underlying neighbors" are at present more difficult to visualize, although the reported success of β-irradiation of skin involved with mycosis fungoides (see Chapter 16) may be due to the action of irradiation on the abnormal skin environment (Goos *et al.*, 1976), rather than on the infiltrating cells.

4. Conclusion

To conclude, if the central notion of microenvironment to a cell is interaction with its neighbors, the central intention of this chapter and its strange new words is to focus attention on that notion.

Time may permit the words to be forgotten once their purpose has been served, but let us remember the facts and challenge the predictions.

5. Note Added in Proof

During the time since completion of this chapter, a number of papers have appeared of direct relevance to many of the points raised. In addition, further work from our group substantiated some of the ideas first raised here as possibilities. A short list of some of the most significant references not included in the text is reviewed below.

Recent work from Judith Woodruff's laboratory (1977, *J. Immunol.* **119**:1603–1610) demonstrated that treatment of lymphocytes with neuraminidase does not alter their adhesion to the endothelium of postcapillary venules *in vitro,* thus confirming the view discussed in Section 1.3.1 that the maldistribution of ^{51}Cr-labeled neuraminidase-treated lymphocytes *in vivo* is due to the modified interaction of the treated cells with liver cells.

Further work from Kaplan's (1977, *Int. J. Cancer* **19**:511–525) and Aisenberg's (1977, *J. Exp. Med.* **145**:1484–1500) groups suggests that the malignant cell in Hodgkin's disease is a monocyte. Further suppressor effects of the E-rosette formation were reported by Bieber *et al.* with spleen extracts from HD patients (1977, *Clin. Exp. Immunol.* **29**:369–375) and attributed by Goodwin *et al.* to the manufacture of prostaglandins by an adherent cell in HD peripheral blood (1977, *N. Engl. J. Med.* **297**:963–968). We have suggested that the presence of a defective monocyte population, excessively avid for iron in HD, may be the linking factor of the multiple immunological, hematological, pathological, and epidemiological aspects of the disease (de Sousa *et al.* 1978, *Am. J. Pathol.* **90**:497).

References

Adler, S., Stutzman, L., Sokal, J. E., and Mittelman, A., 1975, Splenectomy for hematologic depression in lymphocytic lymphoma and leukemia, *Cancer* **35**:521.

Alarcón-Segovia, D., Galbraith, R. F., Maldonado, J. E., and Howard, F. M., 1963, Systemic lupus erythematosus following thymectomy for myasthenia gravis, *Lancet* **2**:662.

Anderson, H. R., Dresser, D. W., Iverson, G. M., Lance, E. M., Wortis, H. H., and Zebra, J., 1972, The effects of ALG on the murine immune response to sheep erythrocytes, *Immunology* **22**:277.

Arbesman, C. E., Wypych, J. L., Reisman, R. E., and Peutner, E. M., 1974, IgE levels in sera of patients with permiphigus or bullous permiphigoid, *Arch. Dermatol.* **110**:378.

Atkinson, J. P., Schreiber, A. D., and Frank M. M., 1973, Effects of cortico steroids and splenectomy on the immune clearance and destruction of erythrocytes, *J. Clin. Invest.* **52**:1509.

Baker, P. J., Prescott, B., Stashak, P. W., and Ausbaugh, D. F., 1974, Regulation of the antibody response to type III pneumococcal polysaccharide by thymic derived cells, in: *The Immune System—Genes, Receptors, Signals* (E. E. Sercaz, A. R. Williamson, and C. F. Fox, eds.), p. 415, Academic Press, New York.

Barthold, D. R., Kysela, S., and Steinberg, A. D., 1974, Decline in suppressor T cell function with age in female NZB mice, *J. Immunol.* **112**:9.

Beamish, M. R., Ashley Jones, P., Trevett, D., Evans, H. and Jacobs, A., 1972, Iron metabolism in Hodgkin's disease, *Brit. J. Cancer* **26**:444.

Bell, E. B., and Shand, F. L., 1975, Changes in lymphocyte recirculation and liberation of the adoptive memory response from cellular recognition in irradiated recipients, *Eur. J. Immunol.* **5**:4.

Bell, R. G., and Lafferty, K. J., 1972, The flow and cellular characteristics of cervical lymph from unanaesthetized ducks, *Aust. J. Exp. Biol. Med.* **50**:611.

Bergström, K., Franksson, C., Matell, G., and von Reis, G., 1973, The effect of thoracic duct lymph drainage in myasthenia gravis, *Eur. Neurol.* **9**:157.

Bieber, C. P. and Bieber, M. M., 1973, Detection of ferritin as a circulating tumour associated antigen in Hodgkin's disease, *Nat. Canc. Inst. Monograph* **36**:147.

Bielschowsky, M., Helyer, B. J. and Howie, J. B., 1959, Spontaneous hemolytic anemia in NZB/Bl mice. *Proc. Univ. Otago Med. Sch.,* **37**:9

Brown, D. L., 1973, The immune interaction between red cells and leukocytes and the pathogenesis of spherocytosis, *Annotation Brit. J. Haematol.* **25**:691.

Brown, D. L., Lachman, P. J., and Dacie, J. V., 1970, The *in vivo* behaviour of complement coated red cells: Studies in C6-deficient, C3-depleted and normal rabbits, *Clin. Exp. Immunol.* **7**:401.

Burnet, F. M., 1962, Role of the thymus and related organs in immunity, *Br. Med. J.* **2**:807.

Burnet, F. M., and Holmes, M., 1962, Thymus lesions in an autoimmune disease of mice, *Nature* (London) **194**:146.

355

ECOTAXIS,
ECOTAXOPATHY,
AND LYMPHOID
MALIGNANCY:
TERMS, FACTS AND
PREDICTIONS

Cantor, H., Asofsky, R., and Talal, N., 1970, Synergy among lymphoid cells mediating the graft versus host response. I. Syngergy in graft versus host reactions produced by cells from NZB/B1 mice, *J. Exp. Med.* **131**:223.

Carter, R. L., 1966, Antibody formation in infectious mononucleosis. II. Other IgS antibodies and false positive serology, *Br. J. Haematol.* **12**:268.

Celada, F., 1966, Quantitative studies of the adoptive immunological memory in mice. I. An age-dependent barrier to syngeneic transplantation, *J. Exp. Med.* **124**:1.

Choi, S. -I., Simone, J. V., and Journey, L. J., 1972, Neuraminidase-induced thrombocytopenia in rats, *Br. J. Haematol.* **22**:93.

Clark, S. L., 1966, Cytological evidence of secretion in the thymus, in: *Ciba Found. Symp. The Thymus: Experimental and Clinical Studies* (G. E. W. Wolstenholme and R. Porter, eds.), p. 3, Churchill, London.

Crome, P., and Mollison, P. L., 1964, Splenic destruction of Rh-sensitized and of heated red cells, *Br. J. Haematol.* **10**:137.

Curtis, A. S. G., 1973, Cell adhesion, *Prog. Biophys. Mol. Biol.* **27**:317.

Curtis, A. S. G., 1974, The specific control of cell positioning, *Arch. Biol.* **85**:105.

Curtis, A. S. G., and van de Wyver, G., 1971, The control of cell adhesion in a morphogenetic system, *J. Embryol. Exp. Morphol.* **26**:295.

Curtis, A. S. G., and de Sousa, M., 1975, Lymphocyte interactions and positioning. I. Adhesive interactions, *Cell. Immunol.* **19**:282.

Denman, A. M., and Denman, E. J., 1970, Depletion of long lived lymphocytes in old New Zealand Black mice, *Clin. Exp. Immunol.* **6**:457.

Denman, A. M., Russel, A. S., Loewi, G., and Denman, E. J., 1971, Immunopathology of New Zealand Black mice treated with antilymphocyte globulin, *Immunology* **20**:973.

de Sousa, M. A. B., 1969, Reticulum arrangement related to the behaviour of cell populations in the mouse lymph node, *Adv. Exp. Med. Biol.* **5**:49.

de Sousa, M., 1971, Kinetics of the distribution of thymus and marrow cells in the peripheral lymphoid organs of the mouse: Ecotaxis, *Clin. Exp. Immunol.* **9**:371.

de Sousa, M., 1973, The ecology of thymus-dependency, in: *Contemporary Topics in Immunobiology* (A. J. S. Davies and R. L. Carter, eds.), Vol. 2, p. 119, Plenum Press, New York.

de Sousa, M., 1976a, Cell traffic, in: *Receptors and Recognition*, Vol. 2 (P. Cuatrecasas and M. F. Greaves, eds.), p. 105, Chapman and Hall, London.

de Sousa, M., 1976b, Microenvironment to a lymphoid cell is nothing more than interaction with its neighbours, *Adv. Exp. Med. Biol.* **66**:165.

de Sousa, M. A. B., and Anderson, J. M., 1969, A study of human lymph node biopsies, in: *The Biology and Surgery of Tissue Transplantation* (J. M. Anderson, ed.), p. 175, Blackwell Scientific Publications, Oxford.

de Sousa, M., and Haston, W., 1976, Modulation of B cell interactions by T cells, *Nature (London)* **260**:429.

de Sousa, M., and Incefy, G., 1975, The possible contribution of the thymus lymphocyte to thymus humoral function, in: *The Biological Activity of Thymic Hormones* (D. W. van Bekkum, ed.), p. 49, Kooyker Scientific Publications, Rotterdam.

de Sousa, M. A. B., and Parrott, D. M. V., 1967, The definition of a germinal centre area as distinct from the thymus-dependent area in the lymphoid tissue of the mouse, in: *Germinal Centers in Immune Responses* (H. Cottier and Odarchenko, eds.), p. 361, Springer-Verlag, New York.

de Sousa, M., Ferguson, A., and Parrott, D. M. V., 1973, Ecotaxis of B cells in the mouse, *Adv. Exp. Med. Biol.* **29**:55.

de Sousa, M., Smithyman, A. E., and Tan, C. T. C., 1978, Suggested models of ecotaxopathy in lymphoreticular malignancy: A role for iron and iron binding proteins in the control of lymphoid cell migration, *Am. J. Pathol.* **90**:497.

de Sousa, M., Yang, M., Lopes-Corrales, E., Tan, C., Dupont, B., and Good, R. A., 1977, Ecotaxis: The principle and its application to the study of Hodgkin's disease, *Clin. Exp. Immunol.* **27**:143.

Dresser, D. W. A., 1961, A study of the adoptive secondary response to a protein antigen in mice, *Proc. R. Soc. London Ser. B* **154**:398.

Dresser, D. W. A., Taub, R. N., and Krantz, A. R., 1970, The effect of localized injection of adjuvant material on the draining lymph node, *Immunology* **18**:663.

Dumont, A. E., Ford, R. J. and Becker, F. F., 1976, Siderosis of lymph nodes in patients with Hodgkin's disease, *Cancer* **38**:1247.

Dutcher, T. F., and Fahey, J. L., 1959, The histopathology of macroglobulinemia of Waldenström, *J. Natl. Cancer Inst.* **22**:887.

East, J., 1970, Immunopathology and neoplasms in New Zealand Black (NZB) and SJL/J mice, *Prog. Exp. Tumor Res.* **13**:84.

East, J., and de Sousa, M. A. B., 1966, The thymus, autoimmunity and malignancy in New Zealand Black mice, *Natl. Cancer Inst. Monogr.* **22**:605.

East, J., de Sousa, M. A. B., and Parrott, D. M. V., 1965, Immunopathology of New Zealand Black (NZB/B1) mice, *Transplantation* **3**:711.

East, J., de Sousa, M. A. B., Parrott, D. M. V., and Jaquet, H., 1967a, Consequences of neonatal thymectomy in New Zealand Black mice, *Clin. Exp. Immunol.* **2**:203.

East, J., de Sousa, M. A. B., Prosser, P. R., and Jaquet, H., 1967b, Malignant changes in New Zealand Black mice, *Clin. Exp. Immunol.* **2**:427.

Edelson, R. L., Fackton, M., Andrews, A., Lutzner, M., and Schein, P., 1974a, Successful management of the Sézary syndrome: Mobilization and removal of extravascular neoplastic T cells by leukopheresis, *N. Engl. J. Med.* **291**:293.

Edelson, R. L., Kirkpatrick, C. H., Shevach, E. M., Schein, P. S., Smith, R. W., Green, I., and Lutzner, M., 1974b, Preferential cutaneous infiltration by neoplastic thymus-derived lymphocytes: Morphological and functional studies, *Ann. Intern. Med.* **80**:685; cited in Lutzner *et al.* (1975).

Edelstein, B. B., 1970, Cell specific diffusion model of morphogens, *J. Theor. Biol.* **30**:515.

Ellis, A. E., and de Sousa, M., 1974, Phylogeny of the lymphoid system: A study of the fate of circulating lymphocytes in plaice, *Eur. J. Immunol.* **4**:338.

Eshhar, Z., Order, S. E., and Katz, D. H., 1974, Ferritin: A Hodgkin's disease associated antigen, *Proc. Natl. Acad. Sci. U.S.A.* **71**:3956.

Evans, M. M., Williamson, W. G., and Irvine, W. J., 1968, The appearance of immunological competence at an early age in New Zealand Black mice, *Clin. Exp. Immunol.* **3**:375.

Ford, W. L., 1975, Lymphocyte migration and immune responses, *Prog. Allergy* **19**:1.

Ford, W. L., and Gowans, J. L., 1969, The traffic of lymphocytes, *Semin. Hematol.* **6**:67.

Ford, W. L., Sedgley, M., Sparshott, S. M., and Smith, M. E., 1976, The migration of lymphocytes across specialised endothelium. 2. The contrasting consequences of treating lymphocytes with trypsin or neuraminidase, *Cell Tissue Kinet.* **9**:351.

Freitas, A. A., and de Sousa, M., 1975, Control mechanisms of lymphocyte traffic: Modification of the traffic of ^{51}Cr labelled mouse lymph node cells by treatment with plant lectins, *Eur. J. Immunol.* **5**:831.

Freitas, A. A., and de Sousa, M., 1976a, The role of cell interactions in the control of lymphocyte traffic, *Cell. Immunol.* **22**:435.

Freitas, A. A., and de Sousa, M., 1976b, Control mechanism of lymphocyte traffic: Altered distribution of ^{51}Cr labelled mouse lymph node cells pretreated *in vitro* with lipopolysaccharide, *Eur. J. Immunol.* **6**:269.

Freitas, A. A., and de Sousa, M., 1976c, Control mechanism of lymphocyte traffic. Altered migration of ^{51}Cr-labeled mouse lymph node cells pretreated *in vitro* with phospholipases, *Eur. J. Immunol* **10**:703.

Freitas, A. A., and de Sousa, M., 1977, Control mechanism of lymphocyte traffic. A study of the action of two sulphated polysaccharides on the distribution of ^{51}Cr and [^{3}H]adenosine-labeled mouse lymph node cells, *Cell. Immunol.* **31**:62.

Freitas, A. A., Rocha, B., Chiao, J. W., and de Sousa, M., 1978, Divergent actions of monomeric, dimeric and tetrameric concanavalin A on lymphocyte traffic, *Cell. Immunol.* **35**:59.

Frost, H., Cahill, R. N. P., and Trnka, Z., 1975, The migration of recirculating autologous and allogeneic lymphocytes through single lymph nodes, *Eur. J. Immunol.* **5**:839.

Frost, P., 1974, Further evidence for the role of macrophages in the initiation of lymphocyte trapping, *Immunology* **27**:609.

Fuks, Z., Strober, S., and Kaplan, H. S., 1976, Interaction between serum factors and T lymphocytes in Hodgkin's disease, *New Engl. J. Med.* **295**:1273.

Gadzar, A. F., Beitzel, W., and Talal, N., 1971, The age related response of New Zealand mice to a murine sarcoma virus, *Clin. Exp. Immunol.* **8**:501.

Gelfland, M. D., and Steinberg, A. D., 1973, Mechanism of allograft rejection in New Zealand mice. I. Cell synergy and its age dependent loss, *J. Immunol.* **110**:1652.

Gershon, R. K., 1974, T cell control of antibody production, in: *Contemporary Topics in Immunobiology* (M. D. Cooper and N. L. Warner, eds.), Vol. 3, pp. 1–40, Plenum Press, New York.

357

ECOTAXIS,
ECOTAXOPATHY,
AND LYMPHOID
MALIGNANCY:
TERMS, FACTS AND
PREDICTIONS

Gesner, B. M., and Ginsburg, V., 1964, Effect of glycosidases on the fate of transfused lymphocytes, *Proc. Natl. Acad. Sci. U.S.A.* **52**:750.

Gillette, R. W., McKenzie, G. O., and Swanson, M. H., 1973, Effect of concanavalin A on the homing of labelled T lymphocytes, *J. Immunol.* **111**:1902.

Goldschneider, M. D., and McGregor, D. D., 1968, Migration of lymphocytes and thymocytes in the rat. II. Circulation of lymphocytes and thymocytes from blood to lymph, *Lab. Invest.* **18**:397.

Goos, M., Kaiserling, E., and Lennert, K., 1976, Mycosis fungoides: Model for T lymphocyte homing to the skin?, *Br. J. Dermatol.* **94**:221.

Goudie, R. B., MacFarlane, P. S., and Lindsay, M. K., 1974, Homing of lymphocytes to non-lymphoid tissues, *Lancet* **1**:292.

Gowans, J. L., 1966, Life-span, recirculation and transformation of lymphocytes, *Int. Rev. Exp. Pathol.* **5**:1.

Gowans, J. L., and Knight, E. J., 1964, The route of recirculation of lymphocytes in the rat, *Proc. R. Soc. London Ser. B.* **109**:257.

Greaves, M. F., Owen, J. J. T., and Raff, M. C., 1974, *T and B Lymphocytes: Origin, Properties and Roles in Immune Responses,* Excerpta Medica, Amsterdam.

Green, I., Jaffe, I., Shevach, E., *et al.,* 1975, *Determination of the Origin of Malignant Reticular Cells by the Use of Surface Markers,* International Academy of Pathology Monograph, p. 282, Williams and Wilkins, Baltimore.

Hall, J. G., and Morris, B., 1965, The immediate effect of antigens on the cell output of a lymph node, *Br. J. Exp. Pathol.* **46**:450.

Hansen, J. A., and Good, R. A., 1974, Malignant disease of the lymphoid system in immunological perspective, *Hum. Pathol.* **5**:568.

Hansen, M. M., 1973, Chronic lymphocytic leukemia: Clinical studies based on 189 cases followed for a long time, *Scand. J. Haematol. Suppl.* **18**:3; cited in Lutzner *et al.* (1975).

Herman, P. G., Yamamoto, I., and Mellins, H. Z., 1972, Blood microcirculation in the lymph node during the primary immune response, *J. Exp. Med.* **136**:697.

Hoefschmit, E. C. M., 1974, Mononuclear phagocytes, reticulum cells, and dendritic cells in lymphoid tissues, in: *Mononuclear Phagocytes in Immunity, Infection and Pathology* (R. van Furth, ed.), p. 129, Blackwell Scientific Publications, Oxford.

Hoefschmit, E. C. M., and Gerver, J. A. M., 1975, Epithelial cells and macrophages in the normal thymus, in: *The Biological Activity of Thymic Hormones* (D. W. van Bekkum, ed.), Kooyker Scientific Publications, Rotterdam.

Howard, J., 1972, The life span and recirculation of marrow derived small lymphocytes from rat thoracic duct, *J. Exp. Med.* **135**:185.

Hughes, R. C., and Mautner, V., 1973, Interaction of adeno-virus with host cell membranes, in: *Membrane Mediated Information,* Vol. 1 (P. W. Kent, ed.), p. 104, MTP Medical and Technical Publishing Co., Lancaster, England.

Hurley, J. V., 1963, An electron microscopic study of leucocytic emigration and vascular permeability in rat skin, *Aust. J. Exp. Biol. Med. Sci.* **41**:171.

Jandl, H. J., Jones, A. R., and Castle, R. B., 1957, The destruction of red cells by antibodies in man. I. Observations on the sequestration and lysis of red cells altered by immune mechanisms, *J. Clin. Invest.* **36**:1428.

Kaartinen, M., Kosunen, T. U., and Makela, O. 1973, Complement and immunoglobulin levels in the serum and thoracic duct lymph of the rat, *Eur. J. Immunol.* **3**:556.

Kaur, J., Spiers, A. S. D., Catovsky, D., and Dalton, D. A. G., 1974, Increase of T lymphocytes in the spleen in Hodgkin's disease, *Lancet* **2**:800.

Kimber, R. J., and Lander, H., 1964, The effect of heat on human red cell morphology, fragility and subsequent survival *in vivo, J. Lab. Clin. Med.* **64**:922.

Lance, E. M., and Frost, P., 1974, Role of lymphocyte dynamics in regulation of the immune response, in: *Progress in Immunology II* (L. Brent and J. Holborrow, eds.), p. 157, North-Holland, New York.

Levy, R., and Kaplan, H. S., 1974, Impaired lymphocyte function in untreated Hodgkin's disease, *N. Engl. J. Med.* **290**:181.

Longmire, R. L., McMillan, R., Yelenosky, R., Armstrong, S., Lang, E., and Craddock, C. G., 1973, *In vitro* splenic IgG synthesis in Hodgkin's disease, *New Engl. J. Med.* **289**:763.

Lutzner, M., Edelson, R., Schein, P., Green, I., Kirkpatrick, C., and Ahmed, A., 1975, Cutaneous T cell lymphomas: The Sézary syndrome, mycosis fungoides and related disorders (NH conference), *Ann. Intern. Med.* **83**:449.

MacKay, I. R., and Smalley, M., 1966, Results of thymectomy in systemic lupus erythematosus: Observations on clinical course and serological reactions, *Clin. Exp. Immunol.* **1**:129.

MacKie, R., Sless, F., Cochran, R., and de Sousa, M., 1976, Lymphocyte abnormalities in mycosis fungoides, *Br. J. Dermatol.* **94**:173.

Malpighi, M., 1686, *Marcelli Malpighi Opera Omnia,* London.

Marchesi, V. T., and Gowans, J. L., 1964, The migration of lymphocytes through the endothelium of venules in lymph nodes: An electron microscopy study, *Proc. R. Soc. London Ser. B* **159**:283.

Marsh, G. W., Lewis, S. M., and Szur, L., 1966, Use of ^{51}Cr labelled heat damaged red cells to study splenic function. 1. Evaluation of method, *Br. J. Haematol.* **12**:161.

Martin, W. J., 1969, Assay for the immunosuppressive capacity of antilymphocyte serum. I. Evidence for opsonization, *J. Immunol.* **103**:979.

Matchett, K. M., Huang, A. T., and Kremer, W. B., 1973, Impaired lymphocyte transformation in Hodgkin's disease: Evidence for depletion of circulating T lymphocytes, *J. Clin. Invest.* **52**:1908.

Mellors, R. C., 1966a, Autoimmune disease in NZB/B1 mice. II. Autoimmunity and malignant lymphoma, *Blood* **27**:435.

Mellors, R. C., 1966b, Autoimmune and immunoproliferative diseases of NZB/B1 mice and hybrids, *Int. Rev. Exp. Pathol.* **5**:217.

Mellors, R. C., Aioki, T., and Huebner, R. J., 1969, Further implications of murine leukemia-like virus in the disorders of NZB mice, *J. Exp. Med.* **129**:1045.

Mikata, A., and Niki, R., 1971, Permeability of post-capillary venules of the lymph nodes: An electron microscopy study, *Exp. Mol. Pathol.* **14**:289.

Mongini, P. K. A., and Rosenberg, L. T., 1976, Inhibition of lymphocyte trapping by a passenger virus in murine ascitic tumours: Characterisation of lactic dehydrogenise virus (LGV) as the inhibitory component and analysis of the mechanism of inhibition, *J. Exp. Med.* **143**:100.

Morell, A. G., Gregoriadis, G., Scheinberg, I. H., Hickman, J., and Ashwell, G., 1971, The role of sialic acid in determining the survival of glycoproteins in the circulation, *J. Biol. Chem.* **246**:1461.

Morris, P. J., Cooper, I. A., and Madigan, J. P., 1975, Splenectomy for hematological cytopenias in patients with malignant lymphomas, *Lancet* **2**:250.

Moroz, C., Giler, S., Kupfer, B., and Urca, I., 1977, Lymphocytes bearing surface ferritin in patients with Hodgkin's disease and breast cancer, *N. Engl. J. Med.* **296**:1172.

Morse, S. I., 1964, Studies on the lymphocytosis induced in mice by *Bordetella pertussis, J. Exp. Med.* **121**:49.

Morse, S. I., and Riester, S. K., 1967, Studies on the leukocytosis and lymphocytosis induced by *Bordetella pertussis.* II. The effect of pertussis vaccine on the thoracic duct lymph and lymphocytes in mice, *J. Exp. Med.* **125**:619.

Nash, D. R., and Heremans, J. F., 1972, Intestinal mucosa as a source of serum IgA in the rat, *Immunochemistry* **9**:461.

Order, S. E., Porter, M., and Hellman, S., 1971, Hodgkin's disease: Evidence for a tumour associated antigen, *N. Engl. J. Med.* **285**:471.

Palmer, D. W., Dauphinée, M. J., Murphy, E., and Talal, N., 1976, Hyperactive T cell function in young NZB mice. Increased proliferative response to allogenic cells, *Clin. Exp. Immunol.* **23**:578.

Parker, E. Jr., Jackson, H., Jr., Fitzburgh, G., and Spies, T. D., 1932, Studies of diseases of lymphoid and myeloid tissues. IV. Skin reactions to human and avian tuberculin, *J. Immunol.* **22**:277.

Parrott, D. M. V. and de Sousa, M. A. B., 1967, The persistence of donor-derived cells in thymus grafts, lymph nodes and spleens of recipient mice, *Immunology* **13**:193.

Parrott, D. M. V., and de Sousa, M. A. B., 1971, Thymus-dependent and thymus-independent populations: Origin, migratory patterns and life-span, *Clin. Exp. Immunol.* **8**:663.

Parrott, D. M. V., de Sousa, M. A. B., and East, J., 1966, Thymus dependent areas in the lymphoid organs of neonatally thymectomized mice, *J. Exp. Med.* **123**:191.

Paulus, H. E., Machleder, H., Bangert, R., Stratton, J. A., Goldberg, L., Whitehouse, M. W., Yu, D., and Pearson, C. M., 1973, A case report: Thoracic duct lymphocyte drainage in rheumatoid arthritis, *Clin. Immunol. Immunopathol.* **1**:173.

Payne, S. F., Jones, D. B., Haegert, D. G., Smith J. C., and Wright, D. H., 1976, T and B lymphocytes and Reed-Sternberg cells in Hodgkin's disease lymph nodes and spleen, *Clin Exp. Immunol.* **24**:280.

Pearson, L. D., Simpson-Morgan, M. W., and Morris, B., 1976, Lymphopoiesis and lymphocyte recirculation in the sheep fetus, *J. Exp. Med.* **143**:167.

359

ECOTAXIS,
ECOTAXOPATHY,
AND LYMPHOID
MALIGNANCY:
TERMS, FACTS AND
PREDICTIONS

Phillips, J. L., 1976, Specific binding of zinc transferrin to human lymphocytes, *Biochem. Biophys. Res. Commun.* **72**:634.

Playfair, J. H. L., 1968, Strain differences in the immune response of mice. I. The neonatal response to sheep red cells, *Immunology* **15**:35.

Schlesinger, M., and Israel, E., 1974, The effect of lectins on the migration of lymphocytes *in vivo*, *Cell. Immunol.* **14**:66.

Schoefl, G. I., and Miles, R. E., 1972, The migration of lymphocytes across the vascular endothelium in lymphoid tissue: A re-examination, *J. Exp. Med.* **136**:568.

Schreiber, A. D., and Frank, M. M., 1972, The role of antibody and complement in the immune clearance and destruction of erythrocytes. 1. *In vivo* effects of IgG and IgM complement fixing sites, *J. Clin. Invest.* **51**:575.

Sprent, J., 1974, Migration and life-span of circulating B lymphocytes of nude (*nu/nu*) mice, in: *Proceedings of the First International Workshop on Nude Mice* (J. Rygaard and C. O. Povlsen, eds.), pp. 11–22, Gustav Fisher Verlag, Stuttgart.

Spry, C. J., 1972, Inhibition of lymphocyte recirculation by stress and corticotropin, *Cell. Immunol.* **4**:86.

Staples, P. J., and Talal, N. J., 1969, Relative inability to induce tolerance in adult NZB and NZB/NZW F mice, *J. Exp. Med.* **129**:123.

Steiner, P. E., 1934, Etiology of Hodgkin's disease: Skin reactions to avian and human tuberculin proteins in the Hodgkin's disease, *Arch. Intern. Med.* **54**:11.

Tada, T., Okumura, K., and Taniguchi, M., 1973, Regulation of homocytotropic antibody formation in the rat. VIII An antigen-specific T cell factor that regulates anti-hapten homocytotropic antibody response, *J. Immunol.* **111**:952.

Talal, N., and Steinberg, A. D., 1974, The pathogenesis of auto-immunity in New Zealand Black mice, *Curr. Top. Microbiol. Immunol.* **64**:79.

Tan, R. S. H., Butterworth, C. M., McLaughlin, H., Malka, S., and Samman, P. D., 1974, Mycosis fungoides—a disease of antigen persistence, *Br. J. Dermatol.* **91**:607.

Taub, R. N., Rosett, W., Adler, A., and Morse, S. I., 1972, Distribution of labelled lymph node cells in mice during the lymphocytosis induced by *Bordetella pertussis*, *J. Exp. Med.* **136**:1581.

Trentin, J. J., McGarry, M. P., Jenkins, V. K., Gallagher, M. T., Speirs, R. S., and Wolf, N. S., 1971, Role of inductive microenvironments or haemopoietic (and lymphoid?) differentiaion, and role of thymic cells in the eosinophilic granulocyte response to antigen, *Adv. Exp. Med. Biol.* **12**:289.

Vaerman, J. P., Andre, C., Bazin, H., and Heremans, J. F., 1973, Mesenteric lymph as a major source of serum IgA in guinea pigs and rats, *Eur. J. Immunol.* **3**:500.

van Ewijk, U., Brons, N. H., and Rozing, J., 1975, Scanning electron microscopy of homing and recirculating lymphocyte populations, *Cell. Immunol.* **19**:245.

van Snick, J. L., and Massom, P. L., 1976, The binding of lactoferrin to mouse peritoneal cells, *J. Exp. Med.* **144**:1568.

Veerman, A. J. P., 1974, On the interdigitating cells in the thymus-dependent area of the rat spleen: A relation between the mononuclear phagocyte system and T lymphocytes, *Cell Tissue Res.* **148**:247.

Veldman, J. E., 1970, Histophysiology and electron microscopy of the immune response, Ph.D. thesis, University of Groningen.

Wolf, N. S., and Trentin, J. J., 1968, Haemopoietic colony studies. V. Effect of haemopoietic organ stroma on differentiation of pluripotent stem cells, *J. Exp. Med.* **127**:205.

Woodruff, J. J., 1974, Role of lymphocyte surface determinants in lymph node homing, *Cell Immunol.* **13**:378.

Woodruff, J. J., and Gesner, B. M., 1968, Lymphocytes: Circulation altered by trypsin, *Science* **161**:176.

Woodruff, J. J., and Gesner, B. M., 1969, The effect of neuraminidase on the fate of transfused lymphocytes, *J. Exp. Med.* **129**:551.

Woodruff, J. J., and Woodruff, J. F., 1974, Virus-induced alterations of lymphoid tissues. IV. The effect of Newcastle disease virus on the fate of radiolabelled thoracic duct lymphocytes, *Cell. Immunol.* **10**:78.

Zacharie, H., Ellegaard, J., Grunnet, E., Søgaard, H., and Thulin, H., 1975, T and B cells and IgE in mycosis fungoides, *Acta Derm.-Venereol.* **55**:466.

Zatz, M. M., and Lance, E. M., 1971, The distribution of ^{51}Cr labelled lymphocytes in antigen stimulated mice: Lymphocyte trapping, *J. Exp. Med.* **134**:224.

Zatz, M. M., Mellors, R. C., and Lance, E. M., 1971, Changes in lymphoid populations of ageing CBA and NZB mice, *Clin. Exp. Immunol.* **8**:491.

12

Immunoglobulins in the Normal State and in Neoplasms of B Cells

EDWARD C. FRANKLIN and JOEL BUXBAUM

1. Introduction

The major function of plasma cells, and to a lesser extent of lymphocytes, is to produce immunoglobulins (Ig's). Since these molecules play a major role in the defense of the body against a variety of infectious agents, it does not come as a surprise that there is no other group of molecules with such extreme heterogeneity. This heterogeneity can be viewed on several levels. First, in most vertebrate species, there are several major classes and subclasses of Ig's. In man, these are IgG, IgA, IgM, IgD, and IgE. The properties of the major classes and subclasses are listed in Table 1. In the case of IgG, we know of four well-recognized subclasses (IgG1, -2, -3, and -4). There are two subclasses of IgA (IgA1 and -2). Subclasses of IgM and IgD are as yet less well defined, but it would appear that for IgM there may be several, and in the case of IgD, there appear to be two. As yet, no subclasses have been recognized for IgE. These major classes and subclasses of Ig's appear to have evolved one from the other as manifested by the striking structural homologies among them (Natvig and Kunkel, 1973; Fudenberg *et al.*, 1972; Solomon and McLaughlin, 1973). The next level of heterogeneity is somewhat more subtle, in that it reflects genetic polymorphisms that have been recognized for several of the Ig classes and subclasses and presumably exist for all of them (Fudenberg *et al.*, 1972). Last is the very complex heterogeneity related to antibody specificity (Wu and Kabat, 1970; Capra and Kehoe, 1975; Pawlak *et al.*, 1973; Rudikoff *et al.*, 1973). It is now well recognized that all antibodies differ one from the other in their

EDWARD C. FRANKLIN • Irvington House Institute, Rheumatic Diseases Study Group, Department of Medicine, New York University Medical Center, New York, New York 10016.   **JOEL BUXBAUM** • Research Service, Department of Medicine, Manhattan Veterans Administration Hospital, New York, New York 10010.

EDWARD C.
FRANKLIN AND JOEL
BUXBAUM

TABLE 1. Classes and Subclasses of Immunoglobulins

Property	IgG	IgM	IgA	IgD	IgE
Concentration (mg/ml)	12	1	2	0.03	0.005
Molecular weight	160,000	900,000	170,000	180,000	200,000
Structure	$\gamma_2 L_2$	$(\mu_2 L_2)_5$	$(\alpha_2 L_2)_{1-5}$	$\delta_2 L_2$	$\epsilon_2 L_2$
Homogeneous component in neoplasms	G myeloma	Macroglobulin	A myeloma	D myeloma	E myeloma
Subclasses	$\gamma_{1,2,3,4}$	Several	$\alpha_{1,2}$	$\delta_{1,2}$	?
Special properties	Placental passage Immunological memory +++ Cytophilia Complement fixation	Primary response IgM$_s$ ($\mu_2 L_2$) on lymphocytic membrane Complement fixation	Secretory immune system (local protection)	Lymphocyte membrane	Reagins ?Defense against parasitic infections
J chain	–	+	+	–	–
Secretory component	–	–	+	–	–
Genetic factor	Gm	–	Am	–	–

363

IMMUNOGLOBULINS
IN THE NORMAL
STATE AND IN
NEOPLASMS OF B
CELLS

primary amino acid sequence. While the mechanisms by which this heterogeneity is generated are not yet understood, we have learned a great deal about the structural features of these molecules and are quite certain that this heterogeneity is directly related to the specificity of different antibodies.

On a cellular level, this heterogeneity is reflected by a high degree of specialization of the antibody-producing cells. As postulated in the clonal selection theory, a plasma cell and all its progeny generally produce only one kind of Ig, namely, a molecule consisting of one kind of heavy chain and one kind of light chain (see Section 2). The reason for the heterogeneity that is apparent in the serum is that there are many different clones of plasma cells, all producing Ig's.

Over the years, this enormous and unprecedented degree of heterogeneity has made structural studies of Ig's and elucidation of the factors that control their biosynthesis exceedingly difficult. Only with the recognition that tumors of plasma cells and lymphocytes reflect the proliferation of individual clones, each producing a homogeneous Ig, has it been possible to use these molecules as models of antibodies and to investigate certain aspects of Ig biosynthesis. In this chapter, we will discuss some of the principles that regulate the synthesis and assembly of Ig's in normal and neoplastic plasma cells and factors that regulate their concentration, including the rates of synthesis, secretion, and catabolism. We will also describe examples of mutants, especially those that occur naturally in man, in which the plasma cells no longer produce intact Ig's, but rather produce fragments or incomplete molecules. Last, we will discuss some of the biological properties of the antibodies produced by the neoplastic cells, which are of great biological and often also of profound clinical significance.

Many if not all myeloma proteins appear to have antibody activity against known or unknown antigens (Rudikoff et al., 1973; Seligmann and Brouet, 1973; Freedman et al., 1976). Occasionally, when they are directed against host antigens or if they possess certain unusual physical properties, which alter their solubility or cause them to interact with themselves or other substances, they can result in tissue injury. For example, polymerization, especially of macroglobulins, may give rise to the hyperviscosity syndrome or cause them to precipitate in the cold. Sometimes, in the case of cold agglutinins, IgM antibodies combine with the patients' erythrocytes and cause hemolytic episodes. Bence Jones proteins or their fragments can result in renal tubular damage or may be deposited in the form of amyloid fibrils. Some proteins can combine with the surface of platelets or vascular endothelium or with some of the proteins involved in the clotting cascade or cause hemorrhagic phenomena (Lackner, 1973). Last, it is apparent that the plasma cell tumors can, in ways that are not yet fully understood, exert an immunosuppressive effect, thus causing hypogammaglobulinemia and increased susceptibility to infection (Zolla, 1972), and that they can also liberate certain substances that act on osteoclasts, causing osteoporosis (Mundy et al., 1974).

2. Structure of Immunoglobulins

The basic structure of all classes and subclasses of Ig's is the same (see Figure 1). They are composed of two types of polypeptide chains: the larger one, known as the heavy (H) chain, and the smaller one, known as the light (L) chain. The basic subunit of every class and subclass of Ig consists of two identical H chains and two

EDWARD C.
FRANKLIN AND JOEL
BUXBAUM

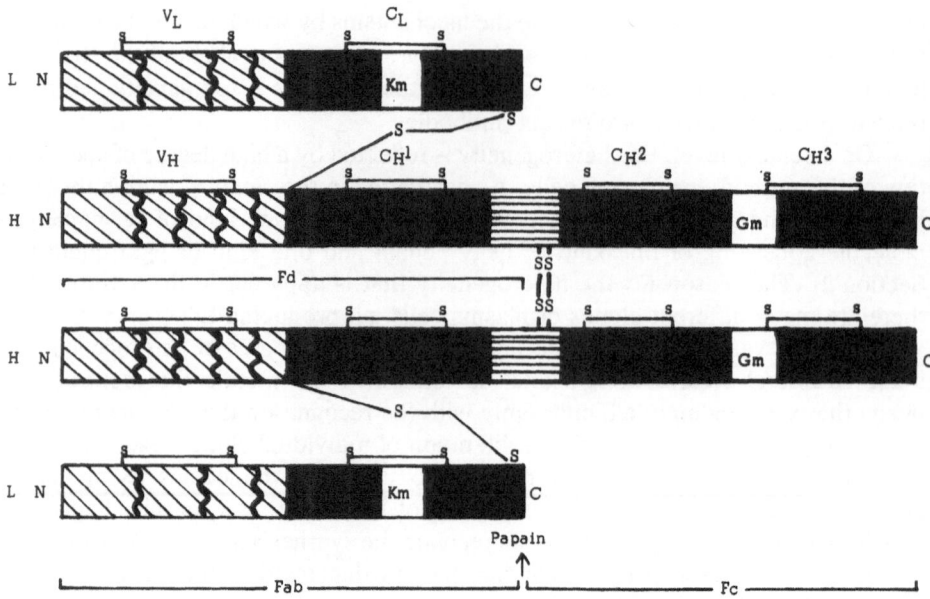

Figure 1. Schematic diagram of human IgG globulin. The solid black areas represent invariant (constant) regions, the diagonally striped areas represent regions of variability among different proteins, the horizontally striped areas represent hinges, and the vertical squiggly lines represent hypervariable regions. (C) Carboxy end; (N) amino end; (H) heavy chain; (L) light chain; (S———S) disulfide bond; (Gm,Km) genetic polymorphisms.

identical L chains. The L chains—of which there are two major types, one known as κ and one known as λ—are found in all classes and subclasses of Ig's. The H chains, on the other hand, differ one from the other in structure and are presumably responsible for the functional differences among the classes and subclasses of Ig's. They are known as γ, α, μ, δ, and ϵ (Pink *et al.*, 1971; Natvig and Kunkel, 1973; Frangione, 1975). Frequently in the case of IgA and always in the macroglobulins, the monomeric subunits are assembled in the form of polymers that contain, in addition, another type of polypeptide chain known as the joining (J) chain (Koshland, 1975). IgM exists as pentamers, while IgA subunits may form dimers, trimers, tetramers, and pentamers. Abundant structural, functional, and genetic information now exists to provide a very clear picture of the structural features of the various classes of Ig's. The L chains have molecular weights of about 25,000. When they exist unassembled in an Ig molecule, they are referred to as *Bence Jones proteins.* They are composed of approximately 215 amino acid residues, and because of certain structural and functional features, they can be divided into two major halves: (1) The *variable (V) region,* or domain, encompasses the amino terminal half and is related to antibody specificity (Hilschmann and Craig, 1965; Kohler *et al.*, 1970; Solomon, 1976). The variable regions of the different subclasses of κ and λ chains have been most strongly conserved during evolution and can be distinguished on the basis of their amino acid sequence and, in many instances, also on the basis of their antigenic properties (Solomon, 1976). The variability in amino acid sequence is most striking in several stretches known as the *hypervariable regions,* which are clearly involved in forming the antigen-binding site of a given molecule

(Wu and Kabat, 1970; Capra and Kehoe, 1975). (2) The *constant (C) region*, which differs in structure for κ and λ L chains, is the same for all molecules belonging to either the κ or the λ L chains, except for minor differences that have recently been described and that have raised the possibility of the existence of subclasses as well, and the subtle differences related to allotypes (Fudenberg *et al.*, 1972; Frangione, 1975; Fett and Deutsch, 1976). As is true also of the H chains, each domain contains within it a rather characteristic and rigidly conserved intrachain disulfide bridge encompassing approximately 60 amino acid residues that folds the molecule into a globular shape. The L chains are joined to the H chains by an interchain disulfide bridge involving the carboxy terminal cysteine residue (Edelman *et al.*, 1969; Gally, 1973).

365

IMMUNOGLOBULINS
IN THE NORMAL
STATE AND IN
NEOPLASMS OF B
CELLS

The H chains are somewhat more complex than the L chains in view of their larger size. Like that of the L chain, the amino terminal quarter of the H chain is known as the variable region or domain (Natvig and Kunkel, 1973; Rudikoff *et al.*, 1973; Frangione, 1975). As is the case for the L chains, there are several structurally and antigenically distinct H-chain V regions (Frangione, 1975; Gally, 1973). It is of interest that the same V regions are found associated with all known constant H-chain classes and subclasses, a finding that provided strong support for the concept of multigenic control of Ig polypeptide chains (Dreyer *et al.*, 1967). As is the case for the L chain, the V region contains a number of hypervariable regions that have been shown, on the basis of structural, antigenic, and, above all, X-ray diffraction studies, to be intimately involved in forming the antigen-binding site (Wu and Kabat, 1970; Capra and Kehoe, 1975; Davies *et al.*, 1975; Rudikoff *et al.*, 1973; Amzel *et al.*, 1974; Poljak *et al.*, 1973). The hypervariable regions of both H and L chains can be readily recognized by their antigenic properties, known as *idiotypes* or *idiotypic determinants* (Pawlak *et al.*, 1973; Rudikoff *et al.*, 1973). The constant regions have 3 or 4 domains, each consisting of approximately 110 amino acid residues (Frangione *et al.*, 1969a; Poljak *et al.*, 1973; Davies *et al.*, 1975), each with an intrachain disulfide bridge that folds them into a globular form. The function of each region is difficult to determine with absolute certainty at the moment; it seems likely, however, that the C regions play a significant role in delineating the unique structural and functional features characteristic of each class or subclass of Ig (Davis *et al.*, 1975; Cunningham *et al.*, 1969). For example, the C_H2 region appears to be responsible for complement fixation, C_H3 for cytophilic properties, and C_H2 for regulating the catabolic properties (Yasmeen *et al.*, 1976; Spiegelberg, 1974). Although they may have a common evolutionary origin, the H chains differ from the L chain in a number of ways. First, they are larger; second, in all classes and subclasses, with the exception of IgM, there exists in the middle of the H chain a region known as the *interdomain* or *hinge region* (Michaelsen *et al.*, 1977). Unlike the other regions, which show striking homologies one to the other among different subclasses and even among classes, the hinge is structurally unique in being rich in proline and cysteine residues that are involved in the interchain disulfide bridges joining the H chains to each other. On the basis of structural homologies, it seems possible that the hinge may have been subject to independent evolutionary forces (Wolfenstein-Todel *et al.*, 1976). Due to differences in the number and the location of these interchain disulfide bridges, it is possible to distinguish one subclass or class from the other by chemical means, a feature that is often of great value in distinguishing myeloma proteins when appropriate antisera are not readily available

EDWARD C.
FRANKLIN AND JOEL
BUXBAUM

(Frangione *et al.*, 1969b). The hinge is of great interest for a number of reasons. First, it appears to be unique in its structure and perhaps in its evolution. Second, it shows striking homologies in the various subclasses and classes that are not necessarily parallel to the homologies in the remainder of the H chain (Michaelsen *et al.*, 1977; Wolfenstein-Todel *et al.*, 1976). Third, it is a region in which a number of duplications seem to have occurred in several classes and subclasses. This is particularly striking in the case of the α and even more so in the case of the $\gamma3$ H chain, in which the hinge encompasses approximately 65 residues and appears to be the site of a series of quadruplications involving three cysteine residues. Last, the hinge is often the site at which deletions begin or end in some of the Ig variants to be described in Section 3 (Franklin and Frangione, 1975).

A great deal of recent information suggests that the genetics of Ig's is exceedingly complicated (Natvig and Kunkel, 1973; Fudenberg *et al.*, 1972; Frangione, 1975). The various H chains appear to be controlled by a series of closely linked loci. The L chains are controlled by separate genes that are unlinked to the H-chain genes and are located on a different chromosome. In the case of the κ L chains, the various subclasses of γ chains, and one of the subclasses of IgA (IgA2), genetic polymorphisms are now recognized, and it seems possible that additional polymorphisms exist for the other classes and subclasses as well (Natvig and Turner, 1971). The genetics of the Ig's, however, is even more complicated than could have been anticipated. There is a dogma in molecular biology that states that one gene controls the synthesis of one polypeptide chain. In the case of both the H and the L polypeptide chains, there is now abundant evidence that the situation is more complex. On the basis of genetic as well as structural studies, there is little doubt that at least two genes control the synthesis of the L polypeptide chains, and in the case of the H chains the possibility of even greater complexity has been raised. One set of genes is clearly involved in regulating the synthesis of the V regions common to the H chains, and another set controls the synthesis of the V region of each kind of L chain. The synthesis of the C region of each class of L polypeptide chain, and, in the case of the H chains, perhaps even each domain, is under the control of yet additional genes. The situation is even further complicated by suggestive evidence supporting the idea that perhaps the hypervariable regions and also the hinge may be controlled separately and inserted into the Ig polypeptide by as yet unknown mechanisms (Frangione, 1975; Wolfenstein-Todel *et al.*, 1976). While the mechanisms by which the V- and the C-region genes are joined are not understood, it seems more likely that this occurs at the level of the DNA or the RNA, rather than at the level of the polypeptide chain, since some studies clearly suggest that the polypeptide chain is synthesized as a single unit starting at the amino terminus (Fleischman, 1971). To date, most of the information bearing on these points has been generated from studies of homogeneous monoclonal proteins and plasma-cell tumors. The mechanism by which the diversity necessary for antibody function is generated is not clearly understood, and there is a great deal of controversy among those who favor a germ line basis and those who advocate somatic mutation mechanisms (Farnsworth *et al.*, 1976; Cohn, 1971; Edelman and Gall, 1969).

Although the basic structure of the classes and subclasses of Ig's is grossly similar, there are sufficient structural differences to allow us to distinguish one from the other. These differences, together with the functional differences among the

367

IMMUNOGLOBULINS
IN THE NORMAL
STATE AND IN
NEOPLASMS OF B
CELLS

various classes and subclasses of Ig's, suggest that this heterogeneity may have evolved to serve certain specialized functions. Unique functional properties have now been clearly defined for each class, and also for certain of the subclasses of IgG and IgA. These differences will not be discussed in detail, but will only be alluded to in passing (Natvig and Kunkel, 1973; Frangione, 1975; Spiegelberg, 1974). The IgG fraction is the major class of Ig involved in immunological memory. It is the major Ig that traverses the placenta from the maternal to the fetal circulation and consequently provides immunity to the newborn. The IgA fraction is of great interest, since it is the major Ig synthesized in various organs of secretion and thus serves as a first line of defense against a variety of infections. IgA antibodies that are part of the "secretory immune system" are predominantly synthesized locally in these sites and appear to have evolved a special mechanism that involves the joining of the Ig to another protein known as the *secretory component* that is synthesized in the epithelial cells (Tomasi, 1971) (see Section 6). Secretory component may play a role in protecting the IgA against degradation or in attracting IgA-bearing lymphoid cells to these tissues (Brown *et al.*, 1970; Poger and Lamm, 1974). Because of its greater resistance to proteolytic digestion, the IgA2 subclass seems to be particularly well adapted to fulfill these functions. IgM seems to be the major Ig produced during the primary immune response, and thus serves as the major antibody immediately after stimulation (Uhr *et al.*, 1962; Nossal *et al.*, 1964). In addition, the IgM monomer together with IgD seem to be the major Ig's on the surface of lymphocytes, presumably involved in antigen triggering of lymphoid cells (Rowe *et al.*, 1973; Fu *et al.*, 1974; Vitetta and Uhr, 1975). Last, the IgE fraction, which until now has been considered to be primarily a nuisance since it includes reaginic antibodies that are harmful to persons with a variety of allergies, may also play a protective role in certain infections, especially those of a parasitic nature, perhaps by increasing vascular permeability to allow other antibodies to interact with the parasites, and by specifically sensitizing macrophages necessary to kill them (Vitetta and Uhr, 1975; Bennich and Dorrington, 1972; Franklin, 1976). Thus, there can be little doubt that during the course of evolution, each of the Ig's has emerged and survived to provide special functions at specific sites in the body.

If we consider some of the subclasses of IgG, it becomes obvious that they differ in their ability to fix complement and to interact with cell surfaces, in their catabolism, and in several other properties that are very important in assuring the proper function and distribution of the antibody molecule (Spiegelberg, 1974). Since most of these secondary functions are of necessity located in the constant half of the molecule, it is this part of the molecule that is of great importance in assuring the proper location and function of various kinds of Ig's.

Antibodies have now been recognized in every class and subclass of Ig. For reasons again not yet understood, some antibodies are predominantly associated with one or another of the classes and subclasses of Ig's. Because of the existence of many thousands of antibodies differing in specificity, each class and subclass is heterogeneous and composed of a large number of different antibody molecules. Since myeloma proteins synthesized by a single clone of plasma cells or lymphocytes are much more homogeneous, they have served as very useful models for studying the Ig's and have provided us with the bulk of the structural information that is now available concerning these molecules. Each myeloma protein, many of which have now been shown to have antibody activity, can be classified as belonging to a class and subclass of Ig, and in general their frequency parallels that of a normal Ig. With this as background, it is now possible to consider factors that regulate the synthesis and assembly of Ig's and some of the unusual properties of Ig's produced in plasma-cell and lymphoid neoplasms.

3. Immunoglobulin Variants

Since structural studies of many myeloma proteins and macroglobulins during the last 15 years have clearly indicated their similarity to or perhaps even identity with normal Ig's, rigorous attempts were initiated in many laboratories in an effort to detect antibody activity in the monoclonal proteins. As a consequence, antibody activity has been identified in an ever-increasing number of homogeneous proteins, especially in the myeloma proteins of mice, a result that comes as somewhat of a surprise if one considers that there are many thousands of potential antigens with which antibodies can react (Rudikoff *et al.*, 1973; Seligmann and Brouet, 1973; Freedman *et al.*, 1976). Table 2 lists the most commonly encountered antigens that appear to react specifically with human myeloma proteins (Seligmann and Brouet, 1973; Freedman *et al.*, 1976). These include, in addition to certain bacterial antigens, many haptens such as DNP, phosphorylcholine, and others; as well as an unusually high frequency of autologous antigens such as the I antigen; and serum proteins such as Ig's, lipoproteins, and a variety of others. Analyses of the interaction of myeloma proteins with some of these antigens has indicated striking similarities to classic antigen–antibody reactions observed with induced antibodies (Eisen *et al.*, 1967). They often have the same binding constants as induced antibodies, the Fab fragment always binds the antigen, and many antibodies having similar specificities have common idiotypic and group-specific determinants (Capra and Kehoe, 1975; Pawlak *et al.*, 1973; Rudikoff *et al.*, 1973). On the basis of these features of human and murine myeloma proteins as well as homogeneous antibodies to streptococci and pneumococci induced by prolonged antigenic stimulation in mice and rabbits (Krause, 1970; Jaton *et al.*, 1973), it would appear that many, if not all, myeloma proteins might ultimately be shown to have antibody activity if it were possible to find the appropriate antigens for testing.

While the majority of proteins produced by plasma-cell tumors appear to be identical to normal Ig's, there has been increasing evidence in recent years that structurally abnormal Ig's or polypeptide chains can also be observed. Such *immunoglobulin variants,* as they have been called recently, were first noted in patients with γ-heavy-chain disease in man and, shortly after, in a few murine plasmacyto-

TABLE 2. Substances That React with Human Homogeneous Immunoglobulins[a]

I antigen	IgG	α2 Macroglobulin
Other red cell antigens	Antigen–antibody complexes	DNP derivatives
Streptolysin O	Fibrin	Cardiolipids
Staphylolysin	Transferrin	Heparin
Bacterial antigens (Klebsiella, Brucella)	Albumin	Phosphorylcholine
Rubella	Factor VIII	Riboflavin

[a]Adapted from Seligmann and Brouet, 1973.

mas as well. In the past 12 years, a variety of Ig variants have been described in man (Franklin and Frangione, 1975; Franklin et al., 1964), and it has become apparent that such molecules occur with an unexpectedly high frequency in murine plasmacytomas carried in long-term tissue culture (Milstein et al., 1974; Scharff, 1973–1974).

Studies of such molecules have been pursued with the hope that they may provide clear insights into the genetic control of Ig's. The most striking and also the most commonly observed Ig variants in man are the heavy-chain-disease (HCD) proteins. Three types of heavy-chain diseases have now been observed. These are γ-heavy-chain disease, the first of these disorders to be described (Franklin et al., 1964); α-heavy-chain disease, the most commonly encountered one (Seligmann et al., 1969); and μ-heavy-chain disease, which in most instances accompanies chronic lymphocytic leukemia (Franklin, 1975b). The clinical features associated with these diseases are described in Chapters 14 and 21, and we will limit ourselves to a description of the proteins produced. Though δ- and ε-heavy-chain diseases have not yet been reported and are likely to be rare, one should nevertheless search for them, especially in regions in which the population may be predisposed, as might be the case for ε-heavy-chain disease in ares of the world with a high incidence of parasitic infections that increase the number of IgE-producing cells.

The discovery of these mutant molecules is in part dependent on a certain amount of clinical intuition, but primarily the result of systematic immunoelectrophoretic workup of pathological sera with a battery of specific antisera. This workup must on occasion be supplemented with additional physicochemical or biochemical analyses such as molecular-weight determinations of the native and reduced protein to be certain of the results (Cohn, 1971). While all the H-chain variants currently recognized could be detected by these techniques, the possibility is far from remote that additional, more subtle, abnormalities are even more frequent, but that they will require more precise biochemical techniques for their recognition.

As was the case with Bence Jones proteins, the synthetic origin of which was recognized in 1955 (Osserman et al., 1957; Putnam and Hardy, 1955), there is now abundant evidence that HCD proteins are, in all but a few instances, biosynthetic products (Buxbaum, 1973). This conclusion is based on the normal turnover of Ig's observed in patients with γ-heavy-chain disease (Franklin et al., 1964), biosynthetic studies in short-term tissue culture in γ-, α-, and μ-heavy-chain diseases (Buxbaum, 1973), and the structural features of the HCD molecules (Franklin and Frangione, 1975).

Figure 2 lists the major types of HCD variants that have now been recognized.

3.1. γHCD Proteins

Structural studies have been most complete for γHCD proteins, and have demonstrated them to be a heterogeneous group of molecules, most commonly with a variety of internal deletions (Franklin and Frangione, 1975). In general, the sedimentation coefficient lies between 3.5 and 4 S, and the molecular weight ranges from 45,000 to 80,000 for the dimer. Electrophoretically, they usually migrate as a broad band in the fast β region, and the molecules tend to be rich in carbohydrate, a feature that may account for their apparent heterogeneity. Among the proteins

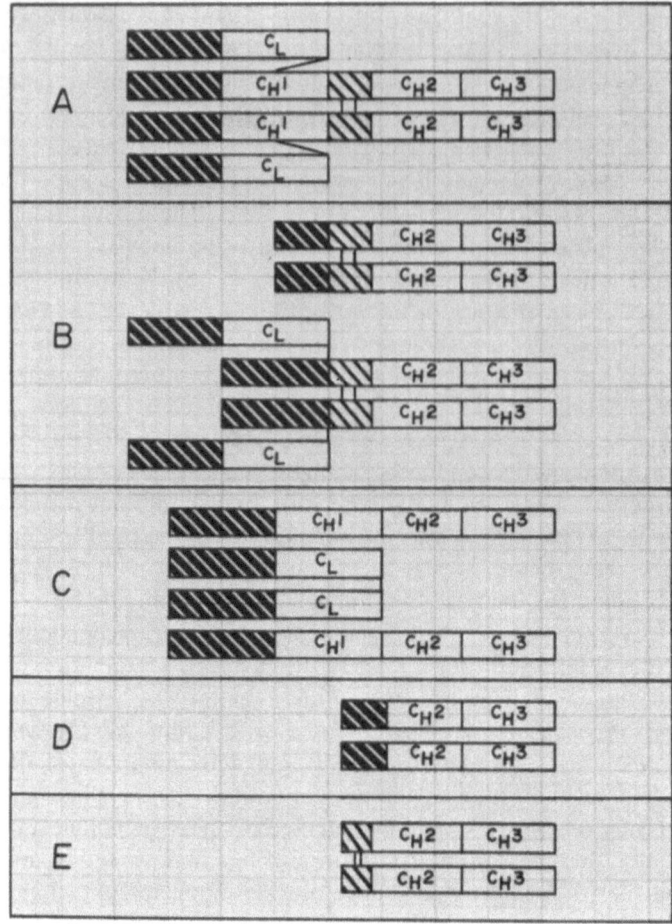

Figure 2. Schematic models of normal IgG (H_2L_2). (A), The most common type of γ and αHCD protein and an unusual murine myeloma with an internal deletion of C_H1 up to the hinge (B), myeloma protein with a deletion of the hinge only (C), γHCD protein with an internal deletion of part of V_H, C_H1, and the hinge (D), and γHCD proteins beginning in the hinge, where proteolysis cannot be excluded (E). The white-hatched black rectangles represent the V region; the black-hatched white rectangles, the hinge; and the open rectangles, the C region (C_H1, C_H2, C_H3, C_L). The lines between the H chains denote the H–H bridge; the line joining the H and L chains is the H–L bridge.

studied, there is an unexpectedly high incidence of $\gamma3$ proteins, though all four subclasses of γ chains are represented. None of the γHCD proteins has been shown to possess antibody activity.

To date, there has been only one example of a HCD molecule that appears to encompass the entire H chain (Lyons *et al.*, 1975; Franklin and Frangione, unpublished). As shown in Figure 2B, four proteins, Zuc ($\gamma3$), Cra ($\gamma1$), and Gif ($\gamma2$) and Yok ($\gamma1$) (Nabeshima *et al.*, 1976), resemble each other in having an internal deletion with resumption of the normal sequence with glutamic acid at residue 216. One of these, Zuc (Frangione and Milstein, 1969), is a $\gamma3$ protein that starts with the first 18 normal amino terminal residues, after which there is a deletion that includes

371

IMMUNOGLOBULINS
IN THE NORMAL
STATE AND IN
NEOPLASMS OF B
CELLS

the rest of the V_H and all the C_H1 regions, and a major part of the extended hinge normally present in $\gamma3$ H chains (Michaelsen *et al.*, 1977). The protein becomes identical to the invariant sequence of $\gamma3$ from a glutamic acid residue corresponding to 216 at the middle of the H chain. Cra (Franklin and Frangione, 1971) is a $\gamma1$ protein that lacks almost the entire Fd fragment. The amino terminal is heterogeneous, and after 10 or 11 residues that do not resemble any of the known H-chain V-region subclasses, there is a deletion of a size similar to that in Zuc. As was the case with Zuc, normal synthesis resumes at the glutamic acid residue at position 216 ($\gamma1$ numbering) (Edelman *et al.*, 1969). Gif is a $\gamma2$ protein that has a blocked NH_2-terminal and contains much of the Fd V region. It has a smaller deletion of about 100 residues corresponding to the Fd C region, and as in the other two, the normal sequence again starts at a glutamic acid residue that is homologous to residue 216 at the beginning of the hinge (Cooper *et al.*, 1972). Yok is a $\gamma1$ molecule that appears to have a similar type of deletion (Nabeshima *et al.*, 1976), and a recently reported $\gamma3$ molecule (CHI) with an intact hinge may also behave similarly (Frangione, 1976).

Four other proteins have an internal deletion that includes part of the V region, the C_H1 region, and, in addition, the hinge (Figure 2D). As a result, these molecules dissociate into monomers in the absence of reducing agents, a fact that readily suggests this type of a structural defect. One protein in this group (Hal), a $\gamma4$ HCD protein, has been studied carefully (Frangione *et al.*, 1973). Normal sequence resumes at a methionine residue at position 252. Three other proteins with internal deletions, probably including the hinge, have not been as carefully studied. Hi probably lacks the C_H1 region and the hinge (Terry and Ein, 1972). The other two (Smith *et al.*, 1973; Calvanico *et al.*, 1972) have not been studied sufficiently to map the deletion precisely. Perhaps methionine, at 252, may turn out to be another favored site at which normal sequence resumes.

The results with Cra and unpublished studies of three other HCD proteins with blocked *N*-termini as well as protein Hal have detected amino terminal sequences not previously reported for any human Ig's, a finding that raises several intriguing possibilities such as the existence of unexpressed subclasses, mutations, or the fusion of the Ig gene with a foreign DNA, perhaps introduced by an infectious agent.

Apparently almost as common are γHCD proteins that begin at the hinge, a site that is very susceptible to proteolysis by a variety of enzymes. While it is quite possible that they are the result of proteolytic digestion of a larger precursor molecule, the possibility that they too are synthetic products has not been excluded. Two examples of this type have been published, and we have personally observed three additional ones (Franklin and Frangione, 1975) (Figure 2E). In these proteins, the larger precursor was never found, nor was it possible to discover an increase in proteolytic activity in the serum. However, recent studies of one such patient (Omm) who has an intact $\gamma3\lambda$ myeloma protein as well as a 40,000-dalton fragment suggest that it may be a synthetic product due to a mutation, since it is synthesized by a clone of cells in long-term culture (Adlersberg *et al.*, 1975, 1978; Buxbaum and Franklin, unpublished).

While it seems likely that these functionless deleted proteins are abnormal, and the results of structural mutations, the significance of the γHCD protein in terms of a normal counterpart remains uncertain, since a recent and as yet unconfirmed paper (Lam and Stevenson, 1973) reported the isolation from a large pool of normal serum of a small amount of a 35,000-molecular-weight H chain with a normal amino terminal sequence PCA Val-Gln and presumably an internal deletion. If this finding should prove to be correct, it would raise the distinct possibility that these molecules are present normally in trace amounts, a possibility that would infinitely complicate the factors involved in the regulation of H- and L-chain synthesis.

A very significant observation that is difficult to explain in view of the fact that the H and L chains are under separate genetic control is the failure of L-chain synthesis in all the HCD patients with γ- and α-heavy-chain disease. It seems possible that the abnormal H chain interferes in some way with the normal regulatory mechanisms for L-chain synthesis (Franklin and Frangione, 1975).

There are two unusual crystalline myeloma proteins of the $\gamma 1$ type that resemble the HCD proteins in that they have a small deletion involving only the hinge (Fett *et al.*, 1973; Lopes and Steiner, 1973). These proteins, both belonging to the $\gamma 1$ subclass, appear to have a molecular weight of 145,000 daltons in nondissociating solvents, but yield an L-chain dimer and two free H chains with a mean molecular weight of 50,000 daltons when subjected to acid treatment or 8 M urea. In both these proteins, McG and Dow, the deletion has been clearly mapped and shown to involve residues 216–230 (Figure 2C). Not all crystalline proteins have such a deletion, since two crystalline molecules studied in our laboratory, one belonging to the IgG1 subclass, the other to the IgG2 fraction, had an intact hinge (Franklin and Frangione, 1975).

3.2. αHCD Proteins

All αHCD proteins studied to date belong to the $\alpha 1$ subclass and resemble the γHCD proteins in being smaller than the intact α chain, in being rich in carbohydrate, and in lacking a major part of the amino terminal half (Seligmann *et al.*, 1969). Only two molecules have been studied in detail, and like the γHCD proteins, they have been shown to have an internal deletion of the V_H and C_H1 regions, with return to normal at the valine residue at the beginning of the hinge, which may well correspond to the glutamic acid at 216 in the γHCD molecules (Wolfenstein-Todel *et al.*, 1974, 1975) (Figure 2B). These molecules are discussed in greater detail in Chapter 14.

3.3. μHCD Proteins

Less is known about the structure and nature of μHCD proteins, since they have proved more difficult to isolate. Most of these molecules appear to exist in the serum as pentamers similar to the $(Fc\mu)_5$ fragments with a sedimentation rate of 11.5 S and a molecular weight of 180,000–300,000, a feature that explains the general failure to find these molecules in the urine (Franklin and Frangione, 1975; Franklin, 1975b). The mechanisms for polymer formation remain to be explained, since J chain was not found in every case, possibly due to proteolytic digestion (Koshland, personal communication).

Patients with μHCD differ from those with the other types of HCD in that large amounts of unassembled L chains were synthesized in more than half (Franklin, 1975b). Since in the one instance studied by immunofluorescence, the L chains were found in the same cell as the H chains (Zucker-Franklin and Franklin, 1971), it

373

IMMUNOGLOBULINS
IN THE NORMAL
STATE AND IN
NEOPLASMS OF B
CELLS

was suggested that the part of the C_H1 region that contains the H–L bridge is missing, so that the L chains could not be linked to the H chains. Recent chemical studies have demonstrated that this is not the case, however, since the initial μHCD protein Gli has a deletion of the first 130 residues and begins with residue 131. It contains the cysteine residue at position 140, which, instead of being linked to an L chain, appears to be involved in an extra inter-H-chain disulfide bridge (Franklin *et al.*, 1976). Since the serum contained polymers of μ chains, monomers of L chains bound to cysteine, and disulfide-bridged dimers of L chains, this represents an instance of failure of assembly of an incomplete H chain and intact L chain for reasons that remain to be determined (Frangione *et al.*, 1976). One additional μHCD protein (Bur), which differed from the others in being smaller (mol. wt. 35,000 daltons), has been studied. This molecule started at residue 338 of the normal μ chain except for the presence of alanine instead of valine and lacked the region normally involved in the H–L bridge (Lebreton *et al.*, 1975).

3.4. Other Variants

In addition to the defects seen in HCD proteins, there are other rare examples of abnormal H and L polypeptide chains. Among these are several instances of IgG and IgA half-molecules, only one of which has been studied in some detail and shown to have a partial deletion of the C_H3 region (Spiegelberg *et al.*, 1975), an IgA myeloma lacking the C_H3 region (Despont *et al.*, 1974), and one instance of an F(ab')$_2$ fragment of IgM that lacked the Fc region (DeCoteau *et al.*, 1973). Since the precise nature of most of these deletions has not been delineated, and because they have been noted only in isolated instances, these molecules will not be described in detail.

Structural alterations of L chains occur more rarely, perhaps because there is less DNA involved in coding for the L polypeptide chain or because L-chain mutants may be more lethal. A number of examples have been noted, however, in which there are small deletions in either the C or the V region of the L polypeptide chain (Amzel *et al.*, 1974). Two striking examples of myeloma proteins having internal deletions of the major part of the V region have been noted. In both instances, the H chain has also been abnormal, most probably due to postsynthetic degradation (Smithies *et al.*, 1971; Isobe and Osserman, 1974).

It seems likely that future careful surveys of proteins from patients with plasma-cell tumors will identify additional examples of structurally altered molecules.

4. Symptoms Related to Proteins with Unusual Physical or Chemical Properties

It is important to emphasize that the symptoms in patients with plasma-cell neoplasms are generally due to the presence of a malignant tumor and are only rarely the result of the abnormal Ig. There are, however, a number of instances in which the protein itself can be damaging to the patient, as is the case in the hyperviscosity syndrome, cryoglobulinemia, cold agglutinins, Bence Jones protein, nephropathy, amyloidosis, and protein–protein interactions, resulting in bleeding and clotting disorders. These disorders will now be described.

EDWARD C.
FRANKLIN AND JOEL
BUXBAUM

4.1. Hyperviscosity Syndrome*

Hyperviscosity due to the increased concentration of serum Ig's is seen most often in the case of macroglobulinemia and occasionally in IgA myelomas in which larger polymers exist, and is associated only rarely with IgG molecules. The causes for the hyperviscosity can be several, the most common being the presence in the serum of large amounts of asymmetrical molecules. Symptoms usually make their appearance once the serum viscosity is greater than 5 times normal. Most often, the initial manifestations involve the CNS, with headaches, confusion, dizziness, blindness, and in some instances sudden deafness. The diagnosis can be readily suspected by funduscopic examination, which reveals markedly dilated vessels, hemorrhages, exudates, and rouleaux formation. More rarely, the major manifestations involve the circulatory system, with congestive heart failure, pleural effusions, or peripheral vascular insufficiency. The serum viscosity relative to normal serum or saline can be readily determined with a simple viscosimeter. The hyperviscosity syndrome is a medical emergency requiring vigorous plasmapheresis to reduce the viscosity, since death, usually due to a cerebral accident, can result quickly. Once the serum viscosity has been brought under control by vigorous plasmapheresis, the patient is usually placed on a maintenance program at intervals determined by the regular monitoring of the serum viscosity. At the same time, it is advisable to initiate proper chemotherapy to control the underlying disease.

4.2. Cryoglobulins†

Cryoglobulins were originally described about 30 years ago in patients with multiple myeloma. Since that time, molecules that precipitate in the cold have been observed in a variety of diseases. Several recent studies indicate that only a quarter of the cryoglobulins occur in patients with myeloma and macroglobulinemia; the majority appear to exist in various kinds of neoplasms of lymphoid cells, certain connective tissue diseases, certain autoimmune conditions, and an idiopathic form known as the mixed cryoglobulin syndrome. In the case of myeloma and macroglobulinemia, the cryoglobulins are usually monoclonal in nature and present in very large amounts. Nevertheless, despite their high concentration, they frequently do not give rise to symptoms. When symptoms occur, they usually include peripheral vascular insufficiency, cold intolerance, Raynaud's phenomena, gangrene, and other cutaneous manifestations including skin ulcerations. It is quite remarkable that large amounts of cryoglobulins can be present in these patients without giving rise to symptoms and that symptoms are frequently not related to the external temperature. In contrast, the predominant type of cryoglobulin now recognized is of the mixed type, composed of two Ig's—most often IgM and IgG, but occasionally also IgM and IgA, or IgA and IgG—and in rare instances of three immunoglobulins. All these mixed cryoglobulins behave as rheumatoid factors in that one of the components, most frequently the IgM fraction, appears to be an antibody to Ig's. These mixed cryoglobulins frequently are polyclonal, although in about half of them the IgM component may be monoclonal. Unlike the cryoglobulins seen in patients with myeloma and macroglobulinemia, they are usually present in very small

*For general references on the hyperviscosity syndrome, see Fahey (1963) and Bloch and Maki (1973).
†For general references on cryoglobulins, see Grey and Kohler (1973), Meltzer et al. (1966a,b), and Brouet et al. (1974).

amounts (<250 mg/dl). Though often slow in precipitating in whole serum, once isolated, they precipitate almost instantaneously. The mixed cryoglobulins commonly give rise to a characteristic symptom complex that is readily diagnosed (Meltzer et al., 1966; Brouet et al., 1974). Most patients with mixed cryoglobulins suffer from purpura and a long history of arthralgias. In many instances, the patients have hepatomegaly and splenomegaly, and evidence of hepatic dysfunction, a history of Sjögren's syndrome, thyroiditis, thrombocytopenia, and other manifestations of autoimmune diseases. Of utmost importance clinically is the very high incidence of renal disease, often of a very rapidly progressive nature. There is little doubt that the lesions are analogous to those of antigen–antibody complex vasculitis, since the vessels and the lesions contain the Ig's present in the cryoglobulin in association with complement, and since in certain instances specific antibodies and antigens have been recovered in the complex.

375

IMMUNOGLOBULINS
IN THE NORMAL
STATE AND IN
NEOPLASMS OF B
CELLS

Laboratory workup of such patients easily identifies the cryoglobulins that usually give a positive rheumatoid factor test, and in many instances, low levels of serum complement are found. Since the onset of renal disease is difficult to predict, it is important to watch these patients carefully. Over the years, we have found that in the prerenal stage, aspirin and mild antiinflammatory agents are sufficient to control the symptoms. Once renal disease begins, it is frequently necessary to start these patients on steroids and immunosuppressive agents. Despite this therapy, they frequently go on to develop a rapidly progressive form of renal disease or die of vasculitis involving other vessels such as the coronaries.

In studying these proteins, it is important to determine whether the IgM is monoclonal or polyclonal, since a monoclonal protein is more suggestive of underlying neoplasm. The mixed cryoglobulins are examples of antibodies directed against a host-constituent, since in all instances they seem to be Ig's directed against the patient's own IgGs. In many instances, the production of these proteins is initiated by an infection, most commonly with Hepatitis B virus (Levo et al., 1977). Closely related to cryoglobulins, but symptomatically less significant, are occasional examples of pyroglobulins. Because of their tendency to precipitate on heating, these molecules are detected accidentally during a routine laboratory procedure and are of little, if any, clinical significance.

4.3. Cold Agglutinins*

Not infrequently in patients with macroglobulinemia, IgM antibodies directed against the I antigen of the red cell appear. These antibodies have unusual properties in that they cause hemolysis only at low temperatures. Frequently, this leads to a severe degree of hemolytic anemia, which requires steroids, immunosuppressives, and, in some instances, splenectomy for control.

4.4. Bence Jones Proteins†

The effect of Bence Jones proteins in the serum and urine is variable. In some instances, these proteins can circulate for long periods of time without causing any damage. Other proteins that are indistinguishable chemically, physically, or immu-

---

*For a general reference on cold agglutinins, see Schubothe (1967).
†For general references on Bence Jones proteins, see Solomon (1976) and Williams et al. (1966).

nologically cause tubular damage, presumably during the reabsorption of these low-molecular-weight molecules that are filtered by the glomeruli. The renal symptoms that accompany Bence Jones protein nephropathy are generally proteinuria, which, when it is severe, results in the nephrotic syndrome. Therapy includes chemotherapy for the underlying myelomatous process and, in addition, management of the renal problem by standard procedures that cannot be detailed here due to space limitations. Not infrequently, this type of renal lesion is also associated with renal tubular acidosis, and instances of Fanconi syndrome have been reported.

4.5. Amyloidosis

A great deal of work has been undertaken in recent years to study the nature of amyloid. As a result of our ability to isolate the amyloid fibrils in a state of purity, it is now possible to divide them into several major categories (Franklin and Zucker-Franklin, 1972). One of these, most often seen in patients with primary amyloidosis and the type of amyloidosis associated with myeloma, consists largely of L chains or L-chain fragments. This conclusion is based largely on the work of Glenner and Terry (1973), who demonstrated that the amino acid sequence of the L chains was identical to that of the amyloid subunits, that amyloid fibrils could be produced by the proteolytic digestion of L chains, and that there is a cross-reactivity between antisera to amyloid subunits and the L polypeptide chains. Since the molecular weight of the amyloid subunit ranges between 8,000 and 25,000, it would appear that amyloid fibrils consist of partial or entire L polypeptide chains. For reasons that remain to be determined, λ polypeptide chains are more commonly involved in the genesis of amyloid than κ polypeptide chains, even though the κ chains occur with a much higher frequency. Another common kind of amyloid, which will not be discussed here, is that found in patients with secondary amyloidosis. It consists primarily of a protein known as the AA protein and contains little, if any, L polypeptide chains (Franklin, 1975a). Recent studies strongly suggest that amyloid may turn out to be a generic term that describes a large number of proteins that can assume the characteristic fibrillar appearance of amyloid (Sletten *et al.*, 1976).

4.6. Interactions of Myeloma Proteins with Other Serum Proteins and Cells

The interactions of myeloma proteins with other serum proteins and cells, such as platelets, or vascular endothelium, frequently give rise to bleeding and clotting disorders in these patients. Since these proteins can interact with virtually every clotting factor, the manifestations and the precise nature of these clotting disorders are highly variable. In addition, a few examples have been noted in which calcium is bound by myeloma proteins (Lackner, 1973).

Lest the reader be left with the impression that the complications secondary to the abnormal proteins are common, it is important to emphasize at this point that the examples cited in this section are relatively rare, and that in most instances, the proteins do not cause significant clinical problems. Immunodeficiency is not discussed here, since it is not the result of the abnormal protein and since it is covered in detail elsewhere in this volume.

5. Regulation of Immunoglobulin Levels

The serum concentration of Ig's is determined by the balance between synthesis and catabolism. The synthetic rate is a function of the number of cells producing

377

IMMUNOGLOBULINS
IN THE NORMAL
STATE AND IN
NEOPLASMS OF B
CELLS

a given Ig at a given time and of the amount of Ig produced per cell. Under normal circumstances, these quantities remain constant, accounting for the relatively small variations among normal persons. While each mature plasma cell probably produces about the same amount of IgA or IgG, Ig production is not constant throughout the cell cycle. A number of studies carried out with cell lines established from human peripheral blood lymphocytes or murine myeloma cells have demonstrated that Ig is usually synthesized and secreted in the late G_1 and early S phases of the cell cycle (Buell and Fahey, 1969; Garatun-Tjeldsto *et al.*, 1976; Cowan and Milstein, 1972). In one human IgM-producing line (1788), there was an additional burst of synthesis in early G2 (Watanabe *et al.*, 1973). It was not determined whether this burst was directly related to the class of Ig produced or was a property of the particular cell line. It is assumed at present that normal antibody-producing cells *in vivo* behave similarly.

IgM is produced by both lymphocytes and plasma cells. The quantity synthesized and secreted is dependent on the stage of maturation of the cell, however, and increases as the cell responds to stimuli that initiate differentiation. As B cells respond to antigen or mitogens (e.g., lipopolysaccharide in the mouse or pokeweed mitogen in man), the amount of IgM produced, its distribution within the cell, and the proportion that is secreted from the cell change markedly (Melchers *et al.*, 1975). Hence, IgM production varies not only with cell cycle but also with developmental stages in the IgM-producing cell population. Initially, after stimulation, the bulk of newly synthesized monomeric IgM is incorporated into the membrane; later, most of the new molecules are secreted as pentameric IgM. At present it is not clear whether surface IgM and secreted IgM arise from the same intracellular pool of polypeptides.

Numerous factors control the number of cells that synthesize any class of Ig. The regulation of both the amount and the type of antibody produced is complex. Most important is the environment of the host, which determines its antigenic exposure. Germ-free animals have much lower serum Ig levels than genetically identical members of the species that are conventionally reared (Sell, 1964). Hence, the intensity and variety of an individual animal's immunological experience, both past and present, influence the level of total Ig synthesis. Of almost equal importance is the quality of the experience. Most antigens engender a primary immune response that consists of IgM antibodies. Subsequently, the response shifts so that the major Ig species produced throughout the immune response is IgG (Uhr and Finkelstein, 1967). At any moment, therefore, the number of cells synthesizing IgG and IgM depends on the proportion of cells engaged in an early primary, late primary, or secondary response. Some antigens, however, seem to stimulate a predominantly IgM response, no matter what the duration or intensity of exposure (Howard *et al.*, 1973). Since many of these are the so-called "thymus-independent antigens" (see Chapter 11 and below), the number of cells producing IgM and the IgM level will depend in part on the host's exposure to thymus-independent antigens.

The cells that synthesize IgA are found predominantly in lymphoid tissue associated with secretory surfaces, particularly the gut-associated lymphoid tissue; consequently, antigens presented to these surfaces generally result in an IgA response. Although the bulk of the IgA antibody produced is secreted into luminal spaces, some of it finds its way, presumably via an enterosystemic circulatory pathway, into the serum, and contributes to the total serum IgA level (Tomasi, 1969).

EDWARD C.
FRANKLIN AND JOEL
BUXBAUM

Recent studies have indicated that Ig-producing B cells and their precursors reflect the influence of a variety of factors other than the antigens to which they are sensitive and their route of administration. Different populations of thymus-derived cells (T cells) appear to exert both positive and negative effects on the humoral immune response. Hence, both helper and suppressor populations of T cells influence the total serum Ig concentration by acting on the cells responding to individual antigens. Some of these regulatory activities may be carried out by humoral factors, while others may be mediated by cell-to-cell contact. The degree of antigen specificity of these regulatory factors also varies; in general, positive "helper" activity seems quite specific, while suppressor activity may be more general. The reader is referred to Chapter 11 for a comprehensive discussion of these regulatory influences.

Evidence has accumulated that the serum IgM level may be partially under control of the X chromosome. In groups of patients in whom serum Ig levels have been measured, females have statistically higher IgM levels than males. Subsequent studies in persons with three X chromosomes indicate that these persons have still higher IgM levels (Grundbacher, 1972). It is not certain whether this phenomenon represents control at the synthetic or the degradative level.

The catabolism of human serum Ig has been extensively studied, and a number of features of the process seem well established. In both normal and myelomatous humans, the rate of catabolism of IgG is directly related to its serum concentration (Fahey and Robinson, 1963). In most studies, serum IgG had a half-life of about 20 days, but in some, the $t_{1/2}$ was somewhat shorter (Spiegelberg et al., 1968). When the catabolic rates of the different IgG subclasses were examined, IgG3 was clearly the most rapidly degraded in vivo, with a $t_{1/2}$ of 8 days, compared to a mean of 11.5–12 days for the other three classes and 12.3 days for unfractionated IgG. IgG3 is also the most labile of the IgG proteins in vitro. The rate of catabolism is related to the properties of the Fc fragment of the H chains, in particular the Cγ2 region. The survival of enzymatically formed Fc fragments and Fc-related proteins isolated from the serum and urine of patients with γHCD is similar to that of the intact molecules (Spiegelberg, 1970).

Hypogammaglobulinemia is usually a result of decreased Ig synthesis. As a result, the rate of IgG catabolism is markedly reduced except in certain exceptional cases in which hypercatabolism is totally or partially responsible for the reduction in serum IgG levels (i.e., myotonic muscular dystrophy, Wiskott–Aldrich syndrome, or GI losses) (Strober et al., 1970). Under certain circumstances, antibodies directed against the IgG will increase its fractional catabolic rate. The serum levels are unaffected if the increased turnover is accompanied by an increased synthetic rate that overcomes the increased degradation.

Serum IgA has a much shorter $t_{1/2}$ than IgG. Two analyses have indicated that the $t_{1/2}$ is 5–6 days, with approximately 25% of the intravascular pool catabolized daily (Strober et al., 1968). The rate seems to be independent of the serum concentration, and is increased only by the presence of anti-IgA antibodies (Barth et al., 1964). The latter are frequently found in patients who have been transfused or have received frequent injections of γ-globulin (i.e. patients who are already hypogammaglobulinemic). The increased turnover in these patients is presumably related to immune clearance of IgA–anti-IgA complexes.

IgM proteins are confined primarily to the intravascular space (75–95%); they equilibrate most quickly in the experimental situation and are the easiest to mea-

379

IMMUNOGLOBULINS
IN THE NORMAL
STATE AND IN
NEOPLASMS OF B
CELLS

sure. In most studies, the $t_{1/2}$ is 4–6 days, with some 10–20% of the IgM being catabolized daily. As with IgA, the catabolic rate is independent of the total serum IgM concentration. It has been suggested that the rate of IgM catabolism may be increased in patients with active rheumatoid arthritis whose sera contain elevated levels of IgM and rheumatoid factor. These data are difficult to interpret, since patients with an increased turnover did not necessarily have high titers of rheumatoid factor as measured by latex fixation. No attempt was made to determine the presence of immune complexes in these patients (Rossing *et al.*, 1973).

An additional study in patients with rheumatoid disease suggested that IgG catabolism was increased independently of the serum IgG level. Inadequate data were obtained to offer any insight into the mechanism of accelerated catabolism. One can easily envision immune complex formation followed by rapid immune elimination in these patients, but there is insufficient experimental support for such a hypothesis (Watkins and Swannell, 1973).

IgD and IgE are present in extremely low concentrations in the serum. As the concentration increases, the fractional catabolic rate tends to go down (Rogentine *et al.*, 1961; Ogawa *et al.*, 1971). This type of behavior suggests that the mechanism reponsible for catabolism of these proteins (like that for IgM) can be saturated. Several investigators have attempted to explore the mechanism responsible for the apparently well-controlled rate of degradation of Ig's. To date, the precise site responsible is not well defined, though it appears to be close to the intravascular space. The hypothetical mechanisms so far proposed are not consistent with all the experimental data. The most widely accepted model is the one proposed by Brambell, in which a saturable system of receptors exists to protect circulating Ig's and which assumes that only unbound Ig molecules are accessible to degradation (Brambell *et al.*, 1964).

Free L chains are synthesized to slight excess in normal persons, in greater excess in some patients with systemic lupus erythematosus, and in enormous excess in 20–50% of patients with multiple myeloma (Epstein and Tan, 1966; Stone and Frenkel, 1975). The major site of L-chain catabolism is the normal kidney. In patients with renal damage, this site is lost to a variable extent, and more free L chains are seen in the serum and in the urine. In experimental animals, the $t_{1/2}$ of injected L chains can be markedly prolonged by nephrectomy, yet remains close to normal in animals after acute ureteral ligation (Wochner *et al.*, 1967). There are few equivalent data concerning the site of catabolism of intact Ig's.

6. Sites of Synthesis of Immunoglobulins and Factors Involved in Regulation of Synthesis

Immunofluorescent studies have demonstrated that most cells that secrete large amounts of Ig's synthesize only one H chain and one L chain at any time, and that the synthesis of H and L chains is approximately balanced (Bernier and Cebra, 1964). Several analyses of cultured human lymphoblastoid lines have shown synthesis and secretion of small amounts of Ig's of multiple classes (Takahashi *et al.*, 1969; Finegold *et al.*, 1967; Fahey and Lawrence, 1963). It is uncertain whether this has an *in vivo* analogue or whether it is an anomaly of the regulation of gene expression seen in cultured cells.

The quantitative distribution of spleen and lymph node cells that synthesize the different classes of Ig is similar to that seen in normal serum (Fahey and Lawrence,

1963; Bernier and Cebra, 1965; Van Furth *et al.*, 1966). In lymph nodes, the majority of Ig-producing cells are IgG producers, with IgM producers in the minority. IgA-producing plasma cells are found in the subepithelial regions of the gut, the GU tract, the sublabial salivary glands, mammary tissue, and the respiratory tree (Crabbe and Heremans, 1966; Anderson *et al.*, 1972; Lawton and Mage, 1970; Tomasi *et al.*, 1969). This distribution seems to be established early in ontogeny or in the neonatal period by the migration of cells that are programmed to synthesize IgA (Fichtelius, 1969). It is not certain what feature of the IgA-synthesizing cell is responsible for its ability to either recognize or be recognized by the nonlymphoid cells occupying its potential homing site.

Proper location is critical for cells that synthesize IgA, since IgA is the major Ig found in bodily secretions (Tomasi, 1971; Poger and Lamm, 1974). As the secretory Ig, the $\alpha_2 L_2$ molecule is found as a dimer linked to both the J chain, which may play a role in polymer formation, and secretory component (SC), a molecule synthesized by the nonlymphoid epithelial cells (Koshland, 1975; Lawton and Mage, 1970; Tomasi *et al.*, 1969). The linkage between SC and the $\alpha_2 L_2$ molecule takes place either within or at the surface of the SC-synthesizing epithelial cell. The kinetics and details of assembly have not been worked out, nor is the precise function of SC fully understood. Some authors feel that SC protects the functional portion of IgA from intraluminal proteolysis (Tomasi *et al.*, 1969).

IgD has been found in a small number of spleen cells, half of which also stain for λ L chains (Pernis *et al.*, 1966). Cells that stain for IgE have been demonstrated in bronchial mucosa, but not unexpectedly, the number of cells involved in the synthesis of the two minor Ig classes is small (Tada and Ishizaka, 1970). The origin of the small excess of L chains excreted in the urine by normal humans remains unclear. Biosynthetic studies performed with marrow cells obtained from persons with polyclonal hyperglobulinemia have not revealed excess L-chain synthesis (Buxbaum, unpublished). Metabolic balance studies have indicated that in some humans, 8–18 mg/kg body weight of excess L chains may be synthesized per day (Waterhouse *et al.*, 1973). It may be that the biosynthetic studies of the marrow reflect a sampling error that for some reason selected for cells with balanced synthesis. It could also indicate that an insufficient number of samples were studied. In the hyperimmune mouse and rabbit, spleen cells synthesize a small excess of L chains. It is not known whether this excess is due to the presence of some cells that synthesize only L chains or whether there is unbalanced synthesis in all the cells.

7. Molecular Events in the Synthesis and Assembly of Immunoglobulins

Biochemical analyses of cells undergoing an immune response have indicated that RNA and protein synthesis increase prior to DNA synthesis in response to antigen. Consistent with these observations are studies of mouse spleen cells responding to sheep erythrocytes, which can sometimes form IgM hemolytic plaques without undergoing division (Sulitzneanu *et al.*, 1973). Because of the qualitative and temporal heterogeneity of the normal response, there have been few precise molecular studies, and most available information has been derived from analyses of plasma-cell tumors.

There is now abundant evidence that H and L chains are synthesized on

381

IMMUNOGLOBULINS
IN THE NORMAL
STATE AND IN
NEOPLASMS OF B
CELLS

separate membrane-bound polyribosomes (Shapiro *et al.*, 1966; Askonas and Williamson, 1966). Some studies have shown some Ig synthesis on free polysomes, but this synthesis has always represented a minor portion of the total cellular Ig synthesis (Vassalli, 1967). There are few data concerning mRNA synthesis, processing, or transport in the normal immune response. Data available from studies with mouse myeloma cells indicate that L-chain mRNA is longer than is necessary to code for a protein the size of L chain (Swan *et al.*, 1972; Brownlee *et al.*, 1973). It has a segment of polyadenylic acid, 150–200 residues long, at the 3′ end of the molecule, a feature common to most mammalian mRNAs. In the mouse tumors that have been studied, the 5′ end of the mRNA molecule had a terminal methylated guanine residue and several other methylated bases in the region that does not code for the protein structure (Cory and Adams, 1975; Milstein and Brownlee, 1972). This also appears to be common to most mammalian mRNAs. When L-chain mRNA is translated in cell-free systems derived from either ascites cells, reticulocytes, or wheat germ, a peptide is synthesized that carries all the antigenic determinants of L chains but is longer by approximately 20 amino acid residues (Milstein and Brownlee, 1972). It appears that many mammalian proteins that are synthesized for secretion have the additional residues present at the amino terminus (Devillers-Thiery *et al.*, 1975). Since these longer pro-L chains are not detectable in the intact cell or in cell-free systems that contain microsomal membranes, it has been suggested that the membranes contain an enzyme that removes the additional residues when the chains are nascent on the polyribosomes, and that the propeptide may be involved in the membrane attachment and secretion steps. It has been further hypothesized that the additional residues are necessary to bind the molecule to the membrane and should be found in all proteins made for export. Some of these precursor peptides have been sequenced and found to be highly hydrophobic. The propeptides for different proteins, however, appear to vary in sequence (Devillers-Thiery *et al.*, 1975; Campbell and Blobel, 1976).

The mechanisms responsible for the coordination of H- and L-chain synthesis have not yet been elucidated. Early studies suggested that L chains were necessary to release H chains from the polyribosomes, since the hyperimmune rabbit lymph node always synthesized a small excess of L chains and L-chain-synthesizing polysomes contained only L chains, while both H and L chains in noncovalent linkage could be isolated from the polysomes that synthesized the H chains (Shapiro *et al.*, 1966; Askonas and Williamson, 1966). Subsequent experiments revealed that free H chains could be isolated from cytoplasmic lysates in certain murine and human plasma-cell tumors, thus proving that covalent linkage with L chains was not necessary for ribosomal release of H chains (Weitzman *et al.*, 1976).

Postribosomal events have been studied in the hyperimmune rabbit lymph node and the immune murine spleen. In the rabbit, the major assembly pathway appeared to be via H_2 and H_2L intermediates (Baumal and Scharff, 1973). In the murine spleen, all the possible assembly intermediates were noted, i.e., HL, H_2, and H_2L, suggesting that a variety of pathways were utilized. Polypeptide-chain assembly has been studied most thoroughly in the mouse myeloma system and to a lesser extent in human tumors. Tumor cells producing all the subclasses of IgG, IgA, and IgM have been incubated with radioactive amino acids and their intra- and extracellular Ig's isolated by immunological precipitation and analyzed to determine the nature and sequence of polypeptide-chain assembly. It has been found that there are three basic pathways of assembly of the H_2L_2 molecule: (1) $H + L \rightarrow HL$, $HL + HL \rightarrow H_2L_2$; (2) $H + L \rightarrow HL + H \rightarrow H_2L + L \rightarrow H_2L_2$; and (3) $H + H \rightarrow H_2 + L \rightarrow H_2L + L \rightarrow H_2L_2$. The major pathway appears to correlate with the Ig subclass. Since each IgG subclass has a characteristic number and location of inter-H-chain disulfide bonds, these bonds may play a role in determining the assembly pathway (DePreval *et al.*, 1970; Frangione *et al.*, 1969a). Recent experiments performed with isolated monoclonal Ig's that had been reduced and allowed to reoxidize *in vitro* demonstrated that the nature of the *in vitro* assembly strongly resembles that seen *in vivo*, and that the cell probably supplies a favorable chemical milieu for the reaction to take place (Petersen and Dorrington, 1974; Sears *et al.*, 1975).

Intracellular polymers larger than H_2L_2, e.g., those seen in IgM-producing cells, are seldom seen in the mouse, but are frequently seen in cells obtained from humans with macroglobulinemia (Buxbaum *et al.*, 1971b). The additional polymerization takes place with the incorporation of J chain and may also utilize a disulfide-interchange enzyme. These two substances have been shown to be necessary in some systems for complete quantitative *in vitro* assembly of murine IgA and IgM (Della-Corte and Parkhouse, 1973; Parkhouse and Della-Corte, 1973). Additional data obtained in the rabbit suggest that the production of the enzyme may be associated with the IgM response to antigen in this species (Delamette *et al.*, 1975).

Antibody H chains are glycosylated (Abel *et al.*, 1968). Although some myeloma patients excrete L chains that are glycosylated, the L-chain constituents of antibody molecules generally do not carry sugar moieties. The initial, or core, sugars are added to the H chain via a dolichol intermediate while it is still on the polyribosome (Waechter and Lennarz, 1976). The later sugars are added while assembly is taking place in the cisternae of the rough endoplasmic reticulum, and the final sugars are attached at the time of secretion in the Golgi zone (Melchers and Knopf, 1967; Zagury *et al.*, 1970). Lymphoid cells contain a number of glycosyl transferases to carry out this function (Schenkein and Uhr, 1970). At present, it does not appear that glycosylation is necessary for either the assembly or the secretion of IgG or IgM proteins, although some studies suggests that it may be necessary for transport from the endoplasmic reticulum to the Golgi apparatus (Weitzman and Scharff, 1976; Melchers, 1973).

The studies described above indicate what takes place in normal Ig-synthesizing cells, although many of the more detailed analyses were carried out with cells synthesizing monoclonal Ig's. Malignant disorders of Ig-producing cells demonstrate some aspects of Ig synthesis that either do not occur in normal cells or occur at such low frequencies that they are only rarely detectable with even a great deal of effort.

Cells from at least 75% of patients with IgG myelomas synthesize L chains in excess of the number of H chains synthesized (Zolla *et al.*, 1970). The incidence may be as high as 90–95% in IgA-producing myeloma cells (Buxbaum *et al.*, 1974). Approximately 20–25% of all patients with the clinical diagnosis of multiple myeloma synthesize only L chains (Stone and Frenkel, 1975). These chains are usually found intracellularly as monomers and dimers with monomers dominant. They are secreted with a 20-min lag. The dimer is the dominant form extracellularly, and only rarely are polymers larger than dimers found in the serum (Grey and Kohler, 1968). One study has indicated that in one such patient, an intracellular tetramer was formed (Buxbaum, unpublished). In the mouse, intracellular degradation of excess L chains was shown to occur in several tumors (Weitzman *et al.,* 1976).

383

IMMUNOGLOBULINS
IN THE NORMAL
STATE AND IN
NEOPLASMS OF B
CELLS

Analyses of amyloid proteins (see Section 4.5) found in myeloma or in primary amyloidosis have established that the major component of the deposits is identical to either L-chain fragments or whole L chain present in the patients' serum or urine (Glenner and Terry, 1973). Biosynthetic studies using cells obtained from several patients with this type of amyloid have failed to show a common synthetic pathway. One patient polymerized his L chains to a tetrameric state intracellularly, but this was not true in all cases (Buxbaum, unpublished).

More unusual than excess L-chain production is the production of H-chain fragments in patients with the several recognized types of HCDs. Studies of cells derived from patients with each type of HCD have indicated that the abnormal proteins are synthetic, not degradative, products (Buxbaum, 1973; Buxbaum and Preud'homme, 1972; Buxbaum *et al.,* 1971a). They are synthesized and secreted much like intact Ig's. Their degree of polymerization appears to reflect the primary structure of the intact Fc portion of the protein. L-chain synthesis has not been observed in any of the γ- or αHCD patients, but has been seen in most patients with μHCD. The cells of one of these patients have been extensively studied and have revealed little, if any, μ–L interaction intracellularly, although amino acid sequence analysis of the isolated fragment revealed the presence of cysteine 140, which usually participates in the formation of the H–L disulfide (see Section 3.3). This observation suggests that cysteine 140 may require additional residues to stabilize it for H–L interaction (Franklin *et al.,* 1976; Frangione *et al.,* 1976).

A small number of patients with multiple myeloma seem to secrete no H or L chains. A variety of mechanisms seem to be responsible. In some cases, there is clearly an abnormality of the rough endoplasmic reticulum necessary for Ig synthesis (Gach *et al.,* 1971). Some appear to be normal by electron microscopy, but exhibit peculiar patterns of immunofluorescence when analyzed by both the direct and indirect techniques, suggesting a variation in the antigenicity of the intracytoplasmic Ig (Preud'homme *et al.,* 1976). Others clearly seem to accumulate Ig in the cytoplasm, sometimes in a crystalline form (Cawley *et al.,* 1976).

To date, biosynthetic studies with cells obtained from these patients have not defined the precise defects. The cells incorporate radioactive amino acids into Ig's more slowly than do myeloma cells that make intact proteins. Most seem to synthesize excess L chains. Some also contain molecules that have H-chain antigenic determinants. The small amounts of Ig's synthesized have thus far precluded accurate antigenic or structural analyses. They may represent structurally defective H chains or H chains that are not properly glycosylated. It is not yet clear how these chains relate to normal Ig synthesis and secretion.

8. Conclusion

In conclusion, this cursory review of normal and pathological Ig's and the mechanisms involved in the regulation of their biosynthesis leaves little room for doubt that similar processes occur in both, and that study of one will contribute to an understanding of the other. In this area, more than most others, there is an intimate interrelationship between our understanding of normal and disease processes. Advances in each case are immediately applicable to the other.

EDWARD C.
FRANKLIN AND JOEL
BUXBAUM

Dr. Franklin's research is supported by USPHS grants AM 01431 and 02594, by the Irvington House Research Program, and by The Michael and Helen Schaffer Fund.

Dr. Buxbaum's research is supported by N.C.I. grant CA 12512 and by research funds from the Veterans Administration.

References

Abel, C. A., Spiegelberg, H. L., and Grey, H. M., 1968, The carbohydrate content of fragments and polypeptide chains of human γG myeloma proteins of different heavy chain subclasses, *Biochemistry* **7**:1271–1278.

Adlersberg, J. A., Franklin, E. C., and Frangione, B., 1975, Repetitive hinge region sequences in human IgG3: Isolation of an 11,000 dalton fragment, *Proc. Natl. Acad. Sci. U.S.A.* **72**:723–727.

Adlersberg, J. A., Franklin, E. C., Frangione, B., Zucker Franklin, D., and Grann, V., 1978, An unusual case of plasma cell neoplasm with an IgG_3 λ myeloma and a $γ_3$ heavy chain disease protein, *Blood* (in press).

Amzel, L. M. Poljak, R. J., Saul, F., Varga, J. M., and Richards, F. F., 1974, The three-dimensional structure of a combining region–ligand complex of immunoglobulin NEW at 3.5 Å resolution, *Proc. Natl. Acad. Sci. U.SA,* **71**:1427–1430.

Anderson, L. G., Cummings, N. A., Asofsky, R., Hylton, M. B., Tarplen, T. M., Tomasi, T. B., Jr., Wolf, R. O., Schall, G. L., and Talal, N., 1972, Salivary gland immunoglobulin and rheumatoid factor synthesis in Sjögren's syndrome: Natural history and response to treatment, *Am. J. Med.* **53**:456–463.

Askonas, B. A., and Williamson, A., 1966, Biosynthesis of immunoglobulins on polyribosomes and assembly of the IgG molecule, *Proc. R. Soc. London Ser. B* **166**:232–243.

Baumal, R., and Scharff, M. D., 1973, Synthesis, assembly and secretion of mouse immunoglobulin, *Transplant. Rev.* **14**:163–183.

Barth, W. F., Wochner, R. D., Waldmann, T. A., and Fahey, J. L., 1964, Metabolism of human gamma macroglobulins, *J. Clin. Invest.* **43**:1036.

Bennich, H., and Dorrington, K., 1972, Structure and conformation of immunoglobulin E (IgE), in: *Biological Role of the Immunoglobulin E System* (K. Ishizaka and D. H. Dayton, J., eds.), pp. 19–78, National Institute of Child Health and Human Development, Bethesda, Maryland.

Bernier, G. M., and Cebra, J. J., 1964, Polypeptide chains of human gamma globulin: Cellular localization by fluorescent antibody, *Science* **144**:1590.

Bernier, G. M., and Cebra, J. J., 1965, Frequency distribution of α, γ, κ and λ polypeptide chains in human lymphoid tissue, *J. Immunol.* **95**:246–253.

Bloch, K. J., and Maki, D. G., 1973, Hyperviscosity syndrome associated with immunoglobulin abnormalities, *Semin. Hematol.* **10**:113–124.

Brouet, J. C., Clauvel, J. P., Danon, F., Klein, M., and Seligmann, M., 1974, Biologic and clinical significance of cryoglobulins: A report of 86 cases, *Am. J. Med.* **57**:775–788.

Brown, W. R., Newcomb, R. W., and Ishizaka, K., 1970, Proteolytic degradation of exocrine and serum immunoglobulins, *J. Clin. Invest.* **49**:1374–1380.

Brownlee, G. G., Cartwright, E. M., Cowan, N. R., Jarvis, J. M., and Milstein, C., 1973, Purification and sequence of messenger RNA for immunoglobulin light chains, *Nature (London) New Biol.* **244**:235–240.

Brambell, F. W. R., Hemmings, W. A., and Morris, I. G., 1964, A theoretical model of gamma globulin catabolism, *Nature* **203**:1352.

Buell, D. N., and Fahey, J. L., 1969, Limited periods of gene expression in immunoglobulin synthesizing cells, *Science* **164**:1524.

Buxbaum, J. N., 1973, The biosynthesis, assembly and secretion of immunoglobulins, *Semin. Hematol.* **10**:33–52.

Buxbaum, J., and Preud'homme, J.-L., 1972, Alpha and gamma heavy chain diseases in man: Intracellular origin of the aberrant polypeptides, *J. Immunol.* **109**:1131–1137.

385

IMMUNOGLOBULINS
IN THE NORMAL
STATE AND IN
NEOPLASMS OF B
CELLS

Buxbaum, J., Franklin, E. C., and Scharff, M. D., 1971a, Immunoglobulin M heavy chain disease: Intracellular origin of the μ chain fragment, *Science* **169**:770–773.

Buxbaum, J., Zolla, S., Scharff, M. D., and Franklin, E. C., 1971b, Synthesis and assembly of human immunoglobulins by malignant human plasmacytes and lymphocytes. II. Heterogeneity of assembly in cells producing IgM proteins, *J. Exp. Med.* **133**:1118–1130.

Buxbaum, J., Zolla, S., Scharff, M. D., and Franklin, E. C., 1974, The synthesis and assembly of human immunoglobulins by malignant human plasmacytes. III. Heterogeneity in IgA polymer assembly, *Eur. J. Immunol.* **4**:367–369.

Calvanico, B. R., Plaut, A., and Tomas, T. B., 1972, Studies on a new gamma heavy chain disease protein, *Fed. Proc. Fed. Am. Soc. Exp. Biol.* **31**:3124 (abstract).

Campbell, P. N., and Blobel, G., 1976, The role of organelles in the chemical modification of the primary translation products of secretory proteins, *FEBS Lett.* **72**:215–226.

Capra, J. D., and Kehoe, J. M., 1975, Hypervariable regions, idiotypes and the antibody-combining site, *Adv. Immunol.* **20**:1–40

Cawley, J. C., Smith, J., Goldstone, A. H., Emmines, J., Hamblin, J. and Hough, L., 1976, IgA and IgM cytoplasmic inclusions in a series of cases of chronic lymphocytic leukemia, *Clin. Exp. Immunol.* **23**:78–82.

Cohn, M., 1971, The take-home lesson—1971, *Ann. N. Y. Acad. Sci.* **190**:529–584.

Cooper, S., Franklin, E. C., and Frangione, B., 1972, Molecular defect in a $\gamma 2$ heavy chain, *Science* **176**:187–189.

Cory, S., and Adams, J. M., 1975, The modified 5' terminal sequences in messenger RNA of mouse myeloma cells, *J. Mol. Biol.* **99**:519–547.

Cowan, N. J., and Milstein, C., 1972, Automatic monitoring of biochemical parameters in tissue culture. Studies on synchronously growing mouse myeloma cells, *Biochem. J.* **128**:445.

Crabbe, P. A., and Heremans, J. F., 1966, The distribution of immunoglobulin containing cells along the human gastrointestinal tract, *Gastroenterology* **51**:305–316.

Cunningham, B. A., Pflumm, M. N., Rutishauser, U., and Edelman, G. M., 1969, Subgroups of amino acid sequences in the variable regions of immunoglobulin heavy chains, *Proc. Natl. Acad. Sci. U.S.A.* **64**:997–1003.

Davies, D. R., Padlan, E. A., and Segal, D. M., 1975, Immunoglobulin structure at high resolution, in: *Contemporary Topics in Molecular Immunology*, Vol. 4 (F. P. Inman and W. J. Mandy, eds.), pp. 127–155, Plenum Press, New York.

DeCoteau, W. E., Calvanico, N. J., and Tomasi, T. B., 1973, Malignant lymphoma with a monoclonal F(ab) mu fragment, *Clin. Immunol. Immunopathol.* **1**:190–202.

Delamette, F., Marty, M. L., and Panijel, J., 1975, *In vitro* IgM polymerization, *Cell. Immunol.* **19**:262–275.

Della-Corte, E., and Parkhouse, R. M. E., 1973, Biosynthesis of IgA and IgM requirement for J-chain and a disulfide exchange enzyme for polymerization, *Biochem. J.* **136**:597–606.

DePreval, C., Pink, J. R. L., and Milstein, C., 1970, Interchain bridges of mouse IgG2a and IgG2b, *Nature (London)* **228**:930–932.

Despont, J.-P. J., Abel, C. A., Grey, H. M., and Penn, G. M., 1974, Structural studies on a human IgA1 myeloma protein with a carboxy-terminal deletion, *J. Immunol.* **112**:1517–1525.

Devillers-Thiery, A., Kindt, T., Scheele, G., and Blobel, G., 1975, Homology in amino terminal sequence of precursors to pancreatic secretory proteins, *Proc. Natl. Acad. Sci. U.S.A.* **72**:5016–5020.

Dreyer, W. S., Gray, W. R., and Hood, L., 1967, The genetic, molecular and cellular basis of antibody formation: Some facts and a unifying hypothesis, *Cold Spring Harbor Symp. Quant. Biol.* **32**:353–367.

Edelman, G. M., and Gall, W. E., 1969, The antibody problem, *Annu. Rev. Biochem.* **38**:415–466.

Edelman, G. M., Cunningham, W. E., Gall, P. D., Gottlieb, H., Rutishauser, H., and Waxdal, M. J., 1969, The covalent structure of an entire γG immunoglobulin molecule, *Proc. Natl. Acad. Sci. U.S.A.* **63**:78–85.

Eisen, H. N., Little, J. R., Osterland, K., and Simms, E. S., 1967, A myeloma protein with antibody activity, *Cold Spring Harbor Symp. Quant. Biol.* **32**:75–81.

Epstein, W. F., and Tan, M., 1966, Increase of L chain proteins in the sera of patients with sytemic lupus erythematosus and the synovial fluid of patients with peripheral rheumatoid arthritis, *Arthritis and Rheum.* **9**:713.

Fahey, J. L., 1963, Serum protein disorders causing clinical symptoms in malignant neoplastic disease, *J. Chron. Dis.* **16**:703–713.

Fahey, J. L., and Lawrence, M. E., 1963, Quantitative determination of 6.6 S γ immunoglobulin, β_2A-globulins, and γl macroglobulins in human serum, *J. Immunol.* **91**:597–603.

Fahey, J. L., and Robinson, A. C., 1963, Factors controlling serum γ-globulin concentration, *J. Exp. Med.* **118**:845.

Farnsworth, V., Goodfliesh, R., Rodkey, S., and Hood, L., 1976, Immunoglobulin allotypes of rabbit kappa chains: Polymorphism of a control mechanism regulating closely linked duplicated genes?, *Proc. Natl. Acad. Sci. U.S.A.* **73**:1293–1296.

Fett, J. W., and Deutsch, H. F., 1976, The variability of human λ-chain constant regions and some relationships to V-region sequences, *Immunochemistry* **13**:149–155.

Fett, J. W., Deutsch, H. F., and Smithies, O., 1973, Hinge-region deletion localized in the IgG-globulin Mcg, *Immunochemistry* **10**:115–118.

Fichtelius, K., 1969, Homing of lymphocytes to the gut epithelium, in: *Cellular Recognition* (R. T. Smith and R. A. Good, eds.), pp. 71–78, Appleton-Century-Crofts, New York.

Finegold, I., Fahey, J. L., and Granger, H., 1967, Synthesis of immunoglobulins by human cell lines in tissue culture, *J. Immunol.* **99**:839–848.

Fleischman, J. B., 1971, A partial amino acid sequence in the heavy chain of a rabbit antibody to Group C streptococcal carbohydrate, *Biochemistry* **10**:2753–2761.

Frangione, B., 1975, Structure of human immunoglobulins and their variants, in: *Immunodeficiency and Immunogenetics* (B. Benacerraf, ed.), pp. 2–53, Medical & Technical Publishing Co., Lancaster, England.

Frangione, B., 1976, A new immunoglobulin variant: γ3 Heavy chain disease protein CHI, *Proc. Natl. Acad. Sci. U.S.A.* **73**:1552–1555.

Frangione, B., and Milstein, C., 1969, Partial deletion in the heavy chain disease protein ZUC, *Nature (London)* **224**:597–599.

Frangione, B., Franklin, E. C., and Prelli, F., 1976, μ Heavy chain disease—a defect in immunoglobulin assembly: Structural studies of the κ chain, *Scand. J. Immunol.* **5**:623–627.

Frangione, B., Milstein, C., and Pink, J. R. L., 1969a, Structural studies of immunoglobulin G, *Nature (London)* **221**:145–148.

Frangione, B., Milstein, C., and Franklin, E. C., 1969b, Chemical typing of immunoglobulins, *Nature (London)* **221**:149–151.

Frangione, B., Lee, L., Haber, E., and Bloch, K., 1973, Protein HAL: Partial deletion of a γ-immunoglobulin gene(s) and apparent re-initiation at an internal AUG codon, *Proc. Natl. Acad. Aci. U.S.A.* **70**:1073–1077.

Franklin, E. C., 1975a, Amyloidosis, *Bull. Rheum. Dis.* **26**:832.

Franklin, E. C., 1975b, μ-Chain disease, *Arch. Intern. Med.* **135**:71–72.

Franklin, E. C. 1975c, Electrophoresis and immunoelectrophoresis in the diagnosis of dysproteinemias, in: *Laboratory Diagnosis of Immunologic Disorders* (G. N. Vyas, D. P. Stites, and G. Brecher, eds.), p. 3, Grune & Stratton, New York.

Franklin, E. C., 1976, Some impacts of clinical investigation on immunology: Surface IgD, IgE and heavy chain variants, *N. Engl. J. Med.* **294**:531–537.

Franklin, E. C., and Frangione, B., 1971, The molecular defect in a protein (CRA) found in γl heavy chain disease, and its genetic implications, *Proc. Natl. Acad. Sci. U.S.A.* **68**:187–191.

Franklin, E. C., and Frangione, B., 1975, Structural variants of human and murine immunoglobulins, in: *Contemporary Topics in Molecular Immunology,* Vol. 4 (F. P. Inman and W. J. Mandy, eds.), pp. 89–126, Plenum Press, New York.

Franklin, E. C., and Zucker-Franklin, D., 1972, Current concepts of amyloid, *Adv. Immunol.* **15**:249.

Franklin, E. C., Lowenstein, J., Bigelow, B., and Meltzer, M., 1964, Heavy chain (7 S γ-globulin) disease: A new clinical entity, *Am. J. Med.* **37**:332–350.

Franklin, E. C., Frangione, B., and Prelli, F., 1976, The defect in μ-heavy chain disease protein GLI, *J. Immunol.* **116**:1194–1195.

Freedman, M., Merrett, R., and Pruzanski, M., 1976, Human monoclonal immunoglobulins with antibody-like activity, *Immunochemistry* **13**:193–202.

Fu, S. M., Winchester, R. J., and Kunkel, H. G., 1974, Occurrence of surface IgM, IgD and free light chains on human lymphocytes, *J. Exp. Med.* **139**:1451–1456.

Fudenberg, H. H., Pink, J. R. L., Stites, D. P., and Wang, A.-C., 1972, *Basic Immunogenetics,* p. 214, Oxford University Press, New York.

387

IMMUNOGLOBULINS
IN THE NORMAL
STATE AND IN
NEOPLASMS OF B
CELLS

Gach, J., Simar, L., and Salmon, J., 1971, Multiple myeloma without μ-type proteinemia: Report of a case with immunologic and ultrastructural studies, *Am. J. Med.* **50**:835–844.

Gally, J. A., 1973, Structure of immunoglobulins, in: *The Antigens* (M. Sela, ed.), pp. 162–298, Academic Press, New York.

Garatun-Tjeldsto, O., Pryme, I. F., Weltman, J. K., and Dowben, R. M., 1976, Synthesis and secretion of light chain immunoglobulin in two successive cycles of synchronized plasma cells, *J. Cell Biol.* **68**:232.

Glenner, G. G., and Terry, W. D., 1973, Amyloidosis: Its nature and pathogenesis, *Semin. Hematol.* **10**:65.

Grey, H. M., and Kohler, P., 1968, A case of tetramer Bence-Jones proteinemia, *Clin. Exp. Immunol.* **3**:277–285.

Grey, H. M., and Kohler, P. F., 1973, Cryoimmunoglobulins, *Semin. Hematol.* **10**:87–112.

Grundbacher, F. J., 1972, Human X-chromosome carries quantitative genes for immunoglobulin M, *Science* **176**:311.

Hilschmann, N., and Craig, L. C., 1965, Amino acid sequence studies with Bence-Jones proteins, *Proc. Natl. Acad. Sci. U.S.A.* **53**:1403–1409.

Howard, J. G., Miranda, J. J., Zola, H., and Christie, S. H., 1973, Characteristics of B-cell tolerance induced with T-independent polysaccharides, in: *Microenvironmental Aspects of Immunity* (B. D. Jankovic and K. Iskavic, eds.), p. 369, Plenum Press, New York.

Isobe, T., and Osserman, E. F., 1974, Plasma cell dyscrasia associated with the production of incomplete (? deleted) IgG molecules, gamma heavy chains, and free lambda chains containing carbohydrate: Description of the first case, *Blood* **43**:505–526.

Jaton, J.-C., Braun, D. G., Strosberg, A. D., Haber, E., and Morris, J. E., 1973, Restricted rabbit antibodies: Amino acid sequences of rabbit H chains of allotype $\alpha 1$, $\alpha 2$, and $\alpha 3$ in the region 80 to 94, *J. Immunol.* **111**:1838–1843.

Kohler, H., Shimuzu, A., Paul, C., Moore, V., and Putnam, F. W., 1970, Three variable-gene pools common to IgM, IgG and IgA immunoglobulins, *Nature (London)* **227**:1318–1320.

Koshland, M. E., 1975, Structure and function of the J chain, *Adv. Immunol.* **20**:41–69.

Krause, R. M., 1970, The search for antibodies with molecular uniformity, *Adv. Immunol.* **12**:1.

Lackner, H., 1973, Hemostatic abnormalities associated with dysproteinemias, *Semin. Hematol.* **10**:125–133.

Lam, C. W. K., and Stevenson, G. T., 1973, Detection in normal plasma of immunoglobulin resembling the protein of γ-chain disease, *Nature (London)* **246**:419–421.

Lawton, A. R., and Mage, R. G., 1970, The synthesis of secretory IgA in the rabbit. I. Production of alpha, light and T-chains by *in vitro* cultures of mammary tissues, *J. Immunol.* **104**:388–396.

Lebreton, J., Ropartz, C., Rousseaux, J., Rouseel, P., Dautrevaux, M., and Biserte, G., 1975, Immuno-chemical and biochemical studies of a human Fcμ-like fragment (μ-chain disease), *Eur. J. Immunol.* **5**:179.

Levo, Y., Gorevic, P., Kassab, H., Zucker-Franklin, D., and Franklin, E. C., 1977, Association between Hepatitis B virus and essential mixed cryoglobulinemia, *N. Engl. J. Med.* **296**:1501.

Lopes, A. D., and Steiner, L. A., 1973, A structural defect in a crystallizable myeloma protein, *Fed. Proc. Fed. Am. Soc. Exp. Biol.* **32**:1003 (abstract).

Lyons, R. M., Chaplin, H., Tillack, T. W., and Majerus, P. W., 1975, Gamma heavy chain disease: Rapid, sustained response to cyclophosphamide and prednisone, *Blood* **46**:1–9.

Melchers, F., 1973, Biosynthesis, intracellular transport, and secretion of immunoglobulins: Effect of 2 de-oxy glucose in tumor cells producing and secreting IgG, *Biochemistry* **12**:1471–1476.

Melchers, F., and Knopf, P. M., 1967, Biosynthesis of the carbohydrate portion of immunoglobulin chains: Possible relation to secretion, *Cold Spring Harbor Symp. Quant. Biol.* **32**:255–262.

Melchers, F., Cone, R. E., Von Boehmer, H., and Sprent, J., 1975, Immunoglobulin turnover in B lymphocyte subpopulations, *Eur. J. Immunol.* **5**:382.

Meltzer, M., and Franklin, E. C., 1966, Cryoglobulinemia—a study of 29 patients. I. IgG and IgM cryoglobulins and factors affecting cryoprecipitability, *Am. J. Med.* **40**:828.

Meltzer, M., Franklin, E. C., Elias, K., McCluskey, R. T., and Cooper, N., 1966, Cryoglobulinemia—a clinical and laboratory study. II. Cryoglobulins with rheumatoid factor activity, *Am. J. Med.* **40**:837.

Michaelsen, T. E., Frangione, B., and Franklin, E. C., 1977, Primary structure of the "hinge" region of human IgG3: Probable quadruplication of a 15 amino acid residue basic unit, *J. Biol. Chem.* **252**:883–889.

Milstein, C., and Brownlee, G. G., 1972, A possible precursor of immunoglobulin light chains, *Nature (London) New Biol.* **239**:117–120.

Milstein, C., Adetugbok, K., Cowan, N. J., and Secher, D. S., 1974, Clonal variants of myeloma cells, *Prog. Immunol. II* **1**:157–168.

Mundy, G. R., Raisz, L. G., Cooper, R. A., Schechter, G. P., and Salmon, S. E., 1974, Evidence for the secretion of an osteoclast stimulating factor in myeloma, *New Engl. J. Med.* **291**:1041–1046.

Nabeshima, Y., Ikenaka, T., and Arima, T., 1976, N- and C-terminal amino acid sequences of a γ-heavy chain disease protein YOK, *Immunochemistry* **13**:245–249.

Natvig, J. B., and Kunkel, H. G., 1973, Human immunoglobulins: Classes, subclasses, genetic variants, and idiotypes, *Adv. Immunol.* **16**:1–59.

Natvig, J. B., and Turner, M. W., 1971, Localization of Gm markers to different molecular regions of the Fc fragment, *Clin. Exp. Immunol.* **8**:685–700.

Nossal, G. J. V., Szenbeg, A., Ada, G. L., and Austin, C. M., 1964, Single cell studies on 19 S antibody production, *J. Exp. Med.* **119**:485–502.

Ogawa, M., McIntyre, O. R., Ishizaka, K., Ishizaka, T., Terry, W. D., and Waldmann, T. A., 1971, Biologic properties of E myeloma proteins, *Amer. J. Med.* **51**:193.

Osserman, E. F., Graff, A., Marshall, M., Lawlor, D., and Graff, S., 1957, Incorporation of N^{15}-L-aspartic acid into the abnormal serum and urine proteins of multiple myeloma (studies of the interrelationships of these proteins), *J. Clin. Invest.* **36**:352–360.

Parkhouse, R. M. E., and Della-Corte, E., 1973, Biosynthesis of IgA and IgM: Control of polymerization by J chain, *Biochem. J.* **136**:607–609.

Pawlak, L., Hart, D. A., and Nisonoff, A., 1973, Requirements for prolonged suppression of an idiotypic specificity in adult mice, *J. Exp. Med.* **137**:1442–1458.

Pernis, B., Chiappino, G., and Rowe, D. S., 1966, Cells producing IgD immunoglobulins in human spleen, *Nature (London)* **211**:424–425.

Petersen, J. G. L., and Dorrington, K. J., 1974, An *in vitro* system for studying the kinetics of interchain disulfide bond formation in immunoglobulin G, *J. Biol. Chem.* **249**:5633–5641.

Pink, J. R. L., Wang, A.-C., and Fudenberg, H. H., 1971, Antibody variability, *Annu. Rev. Med.* **22**:145.

Poger, M. E., and Lamm, M. E., 1974, Localization of free and bound secretory component in human intestinal epithelial cells: A model for the assembly of secretory IgA, *J. Exp. Med.* **139**:629–642.

Poljak, R. J., Amzel, L. M., Avey, H. P., Chen, B. L., Phizackerley, R. P., and Saul, F., 1973, Three-dimensional structure of the Fab' fragment of human immunoglobulin at 2.8 Å resolution, *Proc. Natl. Acad. Sci. U.S.A.* **70**:3305–3310.

Preud'homme, J.-L., Hurez, D., Danon, F., Brouet, J. C., and Seligmann, M., 1976, Intracytoplasmic and surface bound immunoglobulins in "non-secretory" and Bence-Jones myeloma, *Clin. Exp. Immunol.* **25**:428–436.

Putnam, F. W., and Hardy, S., 1955, Proteins in multiple myeloma. III. Origin of Bence-Jones protein, *J. Biol. Chem.* **212**:361–369.

Rogentine, G. N., Jr., Rowe, D. S., Bradley, J., Waldmann, T. A., and Fahey, J. L., 1961, Metabolism of human immunoglobulin D, *J. Clin. Invest.* **45**:1467.

Rossing, N., Mouridsen, H. T., Baerentsen, O., and Jensen, K. B., 1973, Immunoglobulin (IgG and IgM) metabolism in patients with rheumatoid arthritis, *Scand. J. Lab. Inv.* **32**:15.

Rowe, D. S., Hug, K., Forni, L., and Pernis, B., 1973, Immunoglobulin D as a lymphocyte receptor, *J. Exp. Med.* **138**:965–972.

Rudikoff, S., Mushinski, E. B., Potter, M., Glaudemans, C. P. J., and Jolley, M. T., 1973, Six BALB/c IgA myeloma proteins that bind β-(1–6)-D-galactan: Partial amino acid sequences and idiotypes, *J. Exp. Med.* **138**:1095–1106.

Scharff, M. D., 1973–1974, The synthesis, assembly and secretion of immunoglobulins: A biochemical and genetic approach, *Harvey Lect.* **69**:125–142.

Schenkein, I., and Uhr, J. W., 1970, Glycosyl transferases of mouse IgG, *J. Immunol.* **105**:271–273.

Schubothe, H., 1967, The paraproteinaemia-like features of cold and warm autoantibody anaemias, in: *Gamma Globulins* (J. Killander, ed.), *Nobel Symposium 3*, pp. 555–572, Interscience, New York.

Sears, D., Mohler, J., and Beychock, S., 1975, A kinetic study *in vitro* of the reoxidation of interchain disulfide bonds in a human IgG1κ: Correlation between sulfhydryl disappearance and intermediates in covalent assembly of H_2L_2, *Proc. Natl. Acad. Sci. U.S.A.* **72**:353–357.

Seligmann, M., and Brouet, J. C., 1973, Antibody activity of human myeloma globulins, *Semin. Hematol.* **10**:163–177.

389

IMMUNOGLOBULINS
IN THE NORMAL
STATE AND IN
NEOPLASMS OF B
CELLS

Seligmann, M., Mihaesco, E., Hurez, D., Mihaesco, C., Preud'homme, J.-L., and Rambaud, J.-C., 1969, Immunochemical studies in four cases of alpha chain disease, *J. Clin. Invest.* **48**:2374–2389.

Sell, S., 1964, Gamma globulin metabolism in germ-free guinea pigs, *J. Immunol.* **92**:559.

Shapiro, A. L., Scharff, M. D., Maizel, J. V., and Uhr, J., 1966, Polyribosomal synthesis and assembly of the H and L chains of gamma globulin, *Proc. Natl. Acad. Sci. U.S.A.* **56**:216–221.

Sletten, K., Westermark, P., and Natvig, J., 1976, Characterization of amyloid fibril proteins from medullary carcinoma of the thyroid, *J. Exp. Med.* **143**:993.

Smith, L. L., Barton, B. P., Garver, F. A., Lutcher, C. L., and Fauget, G. B., 1973, Physiological and immunological characterization of a new IgG1 (γ1) heavy chain disease protein, *Fed. Proc. Fed. Am. Soc. Exp. Biol.* **32**:840 (abstract).

Smithies, O., Gibson, D., Fanning, E. M., Goodfliesch, R. M., Gilman, J. G., and Ballantyne, D. L., 1971, Quantitative procedures for use with the Edman–Begg sequenator: Partial sequences of two unusual immunoglobulin light chains, Rzf and Sac, *Biochemistry* **10**:4912–4921.

Solomon, A., 1976, Bence-Jones proteins and light chains of immunoglobulins, *N. Engl. J. Med.* **294**:17–23, 91–98.

Solomon, A., and McLaughlin, C. L., 1973, Immunoglobulin structure determined from products of plasma cell neoplasms, *Semin. Hematol.* **10**:3–17.

Spiegelberg, H. L., 1970, The submolecular site related to the rate of catabolism of IgG globulins, in: *Plasma Protein Metabolism* (M. A. Rothschild and T, Waldmann, eds.), p. 307, Academic Press, New York.

Spiegelberg, H. L., 1974, Biological activities of immunoglobulins of different classes and subclasses, *Adv. Immunol.* **19**:259.

Spiegelberg, H. L., Fishkin, B. G., and Grey, H. M., 1968, Catabolism of human γG immunoglobulins of different heavy chain subclasses, *J. Clin. Invest.* **47**:2323.

Spiegelberg, H. L., Heath, V., and Lang, J. E., 1975, Human myeloma IgG half-molecules. I. Structural and antigenic analyses, *Biochemistry* **14**:2157.

Stone, M. J., and Frenkel, E. P., 1975, The clinical spectrum of light chain myeloma: A study of 35 patients with special reference to the occurrence of amyloidosis, *Am. J. Med.* **58**:601–619.

Strober, W., Wochner, R. D., Barlow, M. H., McFarlane, D. E., and Waldmann, T. A., 1968, Immunoglobulin metabolism in ataxia telangiectasia, *J. Clin. Invest.* **47**:1905.

Strober, W., Blaese, R. M., and Waldmann, T. A., 1970, Abnormalities of immunoglobulin metabolism, in: *Plasma Protein Metabolism* (M. A. Rothschild and T. Waldmann, eds.), p. 287, Academic Press, New York.

Sulitzneanu, D., Marbrook, J., and Haskill, J. S., 1973, Direct conversion of precursors of PFC's into active PFC's *in vitro* without prior cell division, *Immunology* **24**:707–710.

Swan, D., Aviv, H., and Leder, P., 1972, Purification and properties of biologically active messenger RNA for a myeloma light chain, *Proc. Natl. Acad. Sci. U.S.A.* **69**:1967–1971.

Tada, T., and Ishizaka, K., 1970, Distribution of gamma E forming cells in lymphoid tissue of human and monkey, *J. Immunol.* **104**:377–387.

Takahashi, M., Yagl, Y., Moore, G. E., and Pressman, D., 1969, Pattern of immunoglobulin production in individual cells of human hematopoietic origin in established cultures, *J. Immunol.* **102**:1274–1283.

Terry, W., and Ein, D., 1972, Structural studies of γ heavy chain disease proteins, *Ann. N. Y. Acad. Sci.* **190**:467–471.

Tomasi, T. B., Jr., 1969, The concept of local immunity and the secretory system, in: *The Secretory Immunologic System* (D. H. Dayton, Jr., P. A. Small, Jr., R. M. Chanock, H. E. Kaufman, and T. B. Tomasi, Jr., eds.), U.S. Dept. Of Health, Education and Welfare.

Tomasi, T. B., Jr., 1971, The gamma A globulins: First line of defense, in: *Immunobiology* (R. A. Good, and D. W. Fisher, eds.), pp. 76–83, Sinauer, Stamford, Connecticut.

Tomasi, T. B., Bull, D., Tourville, D., Montes, M., and Yurchak, A., 1969, Distribution and synthesis of human secretory components, in: *The Secretory Immunologic System* (D. H. Dayton, Jr., P. A. Small, Jr., R. M. Chanock, Jr., H. E. Kaufman, and T. B. Tomasi, Jr., eds.), pp. 41–48, U.S. Department of Health, Education and Welfare, Washington, D.C.

Uhr, J. W., and Finkelstein, M. S., 1967, The regulation of antibody synthesis, *Prog. Allergy* **10**:37.

Uhr, J. W., Finkelstein, M. S., and Baumann, J. B., 1962, Antibody formation. III. The primary and secondary antibody response to bacteriophage φX 174 in guinea pigs, *Proc. Natl. Acad. Sci. U.S.A.* **115**:655–670.

Van Furth, R., Schuit, H. R. E., and Hijmans, W., 1966, The formation of immunoglobulins by human tissues *in vitro*. III. Spleen, lymph nodes, bone marrow and thymus, *Immunology* **11**:19–28.

Vassalli, P., 1967, Studies on cell free synthesis of rat immunoglobulins. I. A cell free system for protein synthesis prepared from lymph node microsomal vesicles, *Proc. Natl. Acad. Sci. U.S.A.* **58**:2117–2124.

Vitetta, E. S., and Uhr, J. W., 1975, Immunoglobulin-receptors revisited: A model for the differentiation of bone marrow-derived lymphocytes is described, *Science* **189**:964–969.

Waechter, C. J., and Lennarz, W. J., 1976, The role of the polyprenol-linked sugars in glycoprotein synthesis, *Annu. Rev. Biochem.* **45**:95.

Watanable, S., Yagi, Y., and Pressman, D., 1973, Immunoglobulin production in synchronized cultures of human hematopoietic cell lines, *J. Immunol.* **111**:797.

Waterhouse, C., Abraham, G., and Vaughan, J., 1973, The relationship between L-chain synthesis and γ-globulin production, *J. Clin. Invest.* **52**:1067–1077.

Watkins, J., and Swannell, A. J., 1973, Catabolism of human serum IgG in health, rheumatoid arthritis and active tuberculosis. Possible influence of IgG structure, *Ann. Rheum. Dis.* **32**:247.

Weitzman, S., and Scharff, M. D., 1976, Mouse myeloma mutants blocked in the assembly, glycosylation and secretion of immunoglobulin, *J. Mol. Biol.* **102**:237–252.

Weitzman, S., Marguilies, D., and Scharff, M. D., 1976, Mutations in mouse myeloma cells: Implications for human multiple myeloma and the production of immunoglobulins, *Ann. Intern. Med.* **85**:110–116.

Williams, R. C., Jr., Brunning, R. D., and Wollheim, F. A., 1966, Light-chain disease: An abortive variant of multiple myeloma, *Ann. Intern. Med.* **65**:471–486.

Wochner, R. D., Strober, W., and Waldmann, T. A., 1967, The role of the kidney in the catabolism of Bence-Jones proteins and immunoglobulin fragments, *J. Exp. Med.* **126**:207.

Wolfenstein-Todel, C., Mihaesco, E., and Frangione, B., 1974, "Alpha chain disease" protein DEF: Internal deletion of a human immunoglobulin α1 heavy chain, *Proc. Natl. Acad. Sci. U.S.A.* **71**:974–978.

Wolfenstein-Todel, C., Mihaesco, E., and Frangione, B., 1975, Variant of a human immunoglobulin: "Alpha chain disease" protein AIT, *Biochem. Biophys. Res. Commun.* **65**:47–53.

Wolfenstein-Todel, C., Franklin, E. C., and Frangione, B., 1976, Structural and evolutionary relationships of the hinge region of the major immunoglobulin classes and subclasses, *Ricerca* **6**:136–142.

Wu, T. T., and Kabat, E. A., 1970, An analysis of the sequences of the variable regions of Bence-Jones proteins and myeloma light chains and their implications for antibody complementarity, *J. Exp. Med.* **132**:211–250.

Yasmeen, D., Ellerson, J. R., Dorrington, K. J., and Painter, R. H., 1976, The structure and function of immunoglobulin domains. IV. The distribution of some effector functions among the Cγ2 and Cγ3 homology regions of human immunoglobulin G, *J. Immunol.* **116**:518–526.

Zagury, D., Uhr, J. W., Jamieson, J. D., and Palade, G. E., 1970, Immunoglobulin synthesis and secretion. II. Radioautographic studies of sites of addition of carbohydrate moieties and intracellular transport, *J. Cell Biol.* **46**:52–63.

Zolla, S., Buxbaum, J., Franklin, E. C., and Scharff, M. D., 1970, Synthesis and assembly of immunoglobulins by malignant plasmacytes. I. Myelomas producing γ chains and light chains, *J. Exp. Med.* **132**:148–162.

Zolla, S., Tanapatlhaiyapong, P., and Sullivan, B., 1976, Immunodeficiency induced by plasma cell tumors, in: *Neoplasm Immunity: Mechanisms* (R. G. Crispen, ed.), p. 15, Proceedings 4th Annual Chicago Symposium., Publ. Institute of Tuberculosis.

Zucker-Franklin, D., and Franklin, E. C., 1971, Ultrastructural and immunofluorescence studies of the cells associated with μ-chain disease, *Blood* **37**:257–271.

13

Burkitt's Lymphoma and Infectious Mononucleosis

DENNIS H. WRIGHT

We carry with us the wonders we seek without us:
there is all Africa and her prodigies in us.
Sir Thomas Browne
1605–1682

1. Introduction*

Two apparently disparate diseases form the subject of this chapter: infectious mononucleosis, an acute and usually self-limiting disease of adolescence and young adult life, and Burkitt's lymphoma, a rapidly progressive malignant lymphoma of children and occasionally of young adults that shows remarkable epidemiological features. The link between these two entities is the Epstein–Barr virus, which is now known to be the causative agent of infectious mononucleosis and is suspected of having a major etiological role in Burkitt's lymphoma. Following a presentation of the evidence linking the Epstein–Barr virus with infectious mononucleosis and Burkitt's lymphoma, one of the objectives of this chapter will be to explore the ways in which a single agent, if indeed the Epstein–Barr virus is a single agent, can evoke such different responses in different hosts.

---

*Abbreviations used in this chapter: (ADLC) antibody-dependent lymphocyte cytotoxicity; (BL) Burkitt's lymphoma; (CMI) cell-mediated immunity; (D) diffuse component of EA; (DNCB) dinitrochlorobenzene; (EA) early antigen; (EBNA) EBV-determined nuclear antigen; (EBV) Epstein–Barr virus; (IM) infectious mononucleosis; (MA) membrane antigen; (NPC) nasopharyngeal carcinoma; (PHA) phytohemagglutinin; (R) restricted component of EA; (SRBC) sheep erythrocytes; (VCA) viral capsid antigen.

DENNIS H. WRIGHT • University of Southampton Medical School, Southampton SO9 4XY, England.

2. Burkitt's Lymphoma

DENNIS H. WRIGHT

2.1. Historical Background

Documentary evidence of Burkitt's lymphoma in Uganda, in the form of the meticulous case notes of the missionary doctor Sir Albert Cook, go back to the turn of this century. His detailed clinical descriptions and drawings leave little doubt that he was seeing the same tumor syndrome that we now know as Burkitt's lymphoma (BL). Distorted West African wooden face masks have been adduced as proof of greater antiquity for the tumor (Pulvertaft, 1964). This evidence, however, is open to other interpretations. Even if the grotesque faces are meant to represent tumors and not merely to horrify, there are several other tumors of the jaws that are prevalent in tropical Africa, and perhaps the more slowly growing neoplasms of adults would be more likely to be depicted in the native art than the transient disfigurement of a dying child. Nevertheless, although BL has been shown to exhibit periodic fluctuations (Morrow *et al.*, 1976a), there is no reason it should not have been present in Africa for centuries.

Burkitt (1959) wrote his first paper on the tumor syndrome that bears his name in 1959. This article noted the clinicopathological identity of the patients with and without jaw involvement, whereas these two forms had previously been regarded as separate entities, and sketched the beginnings of the epidemiological studies that he pursued so vigourously over the next decade. By 1963, the clinical, pathological, and epidemiological features of the tumor, then usually referred to as the African childhood lymphoma, were more fully documented. At an international symposium in Paris that year, it was agreed that the eponymous title *Burkitt's tumor* (later changed to *Burkitt's lymphoma*) should be applied to this neoplasm, partly because the titles African lymphoma or African childhood lymphoma were not satisfactory in view of the known occurrence of the tumor in Papua and in occasional adults, but also as a tribute to Denis Burkitt, who, under seemingly impossible conditions, had done so much to delineate the clinical and epidemiological features of this neoplasm and was pioneering treatment with chemotherapy as an alternative to the often mutilating and usually futile surgical maneuvers that were the only available treatment until that time.

2.2. Pathology

Burkitt's lymphoma is composed of undifferentiated lymphoid cells with a characteristic cytology (Wright, 1963, 1970b) and with histological features that enable it to be differentiated from other malignant lymphomas in good-quality preparations (Berard *et al.*, 1969). The clinical and anatomical features of the tumor may be closely mimicked by those of other neoplasms (Ziegler *et al.*, 1971), or they may be similar to those seen with other lymphomas, e.g., retroperitoneal masses, which precludes definition of the tumor on these criteria alone. In general, the histopathological definition of the tumor has proved to be the most reliable means of identifying and categorizing BL and has usually correlated well with the characteristic anatomical features (Wright, 1966). Problems arise with a small proportion of cases that are histologically typical but have atypical clinical and anatomical features and, conversely, with those that show characteristic clinical and anatomical features but exhibit histological or cytological atypia (Magrath *et al.*, 1974). This problem is not, of course, unique to BL among neoplasms nor yet is it of sufficient magnitude to preclude the use of microscopic criteria for the identification of the tumor in epidemiological, etiological, and therapeutic studies.

One must nevertheless recognize that morphological identity does not necessarily imply etiological identity. It has been shown that many non-African and occasional African cases of BL identified by histological and cytological criteria lack EBV DNA (Klein, G., 1975). It would be premature to conclude that BL should be defined on the basis of the presence of EBV DNA in the tumor cells, particularly since EBV DNA has now been demonstrated in a case of immunoblastic lymphadenopathy (Bornkamm *et al.*, 1976). In a study of 20 American cases of BL, Ziegler *et al.* (1976) noted that 5 of their patients had serological profiles similar to those seen in African patients, and that these patients had a favorable prognosis compared with the others in the group. EBV-associated BL may be inversely proportional to endemicity (see Section 4.1.7).

The anatomical distribution of BL is in most patients strikingly different from that seen in other malignant lymphomas, and it was the more bizarre features that first drew attention to the tumor and formed the basis of the early epidemiological studies. The gross pathology has been well reviewed (Wright, 1964, 1970a, 1971). The salient features are:

1. Involvement of one or more quadrants of the jaw. This is an age-related phenomenon, being maximal at the age of 3 years and falling progressively thereafter (Burkitt and Wright, 1966), the overall incidence of jaw involvement in Ugandan patients being approximately 50%. The earliest radiological lesion appears around the apices of erupted or developing teeth (Cockshott, 1970). Jaw involvement is considerably in excess of lesions in other bones.
2. Of every 5 females with BL in Uganda, 4 had ovarian tumors, which were invariably bilateral. As for males, 4–10% have testicular tumors, which are bilateral in approximately one third of cases.
3. Involvement of abdominal viscera is common, almost all cases having renal tumors.
4. Endocrine glands are commonly infiltrated by tumor.
5. Massive bilateral involvement of the breasts is a dramatic manifestation of BL in young women during pregnancy and lactation (Shepherd and Wright, 1967).
6. Retroperitoneal masses may present as abdominal swellings or may cause paraplegia by interfering with the blood supply to the spinal cord.
7. Involvement of the brain, meninges, and cranial nerves may be apparent at presentation or may be the cause of relapse following chemotherapy.
8. The tumor rarely involves the thymus or peripheral lymph nodes. The spleen was involved in approximately one third of cases coming to postmortem in Uganda, but the tumor burden was often trivial compared with that seen in other organs in the same patient.

The widespread distribution of tumor seen in untreated cases of BL is undoubtedly due in part to blood-borne metastases. Small intravascular collections of tumor cells can often be seen in association with larger nodules in the liver and kidneys. It is difficult, however, to envisage metastatic spread giving rise to tumors in all four quadrants of the jaw in the absence of widespread skeletal involvement. It was for this reason that many of the early workers considered BL to be multicentric in origin. If one accepts that BL is monoclonal (Fialkow *et al.*, 1970, 1973), how can one account for the bizarre distribution of the tumor? Apart from CNS involvement, the sites of predilection are not immunologically privileged, though in a negative sense the lack of involvement of lymph nodes and spleen may be due to the hostile immunological environment at these sites. Two possible mechanisms to account for the localization of tumor deposits could be the provision of a favorable environment in terms of possible growth-promoting factors or ecotaxis. It is tempting to explain the massive bilateral breast tumors seen in pregnant and lactating women with BL on the basis of ecotaxis, since there is a migration of lymphocytes into the breast in late pregnancy. Could the jaw and ovarian tumors be similarly explained? Is there a migration of lymphocytes into the jaw at the stage of maximum tooth development? These localizations could equally well be accounted for if the developing tooth or pregnancy breast provided local factors that enhanced tumor growth.

2.3. Cytoidentity

By morphological criteria alone, BL cells are categorized as lymphoblasts. The cytoplasm is rich in polyribosomes, but contains scanty, rough endoplasmic reticulum. Gross anatomical features such as the infrequency of thymic involvement (Wright, 1964) or the histopathological observation of early infiltration of follicular areas of lymph nodes (Braylan *et al.*, 1975) suggested a B-cell origin for the tumor.

The presence of surface membrane IgM on a high proportion of BL cells and the presence of C3 and Fc receptors on tumor cells and EBV-transformed lymphocytes indicates that they are of B-cell lineage (Pattengale *et al.*, 1974; Binder *et al.*, 1975; Flandrin *et al.*, 1975; Epstein, A. L., *et al.*, 1976). Moreover, it has been shown that EBV receptors are a reliable marker of B cells (Greaves *et al.*, 1975). These receptors appear to be closely associated with the C3 receptor in that they show overlapping and cocapping and similar kinetic patterns (Yefenof *et al.*, 1976).

2.4. Monoclonal Origin

Most malignant lymphomas that bear immunoglobulins on the cell surface have been shown to be monotypic for heavy- and light-chain class, and are assumed to be monoclonal in origin. Approximately 60% of African cases of BL have surface IgM (Fialkow *et al.*, 1973). Unfortunately, one of the light-chain antisera used in this study was unsatisfactory, making it uncertain whether the surface immunoglobulin was monotypic. Most cell lines established from BL tissue have been shown to be monotypic with regard to surface immunoglobulins, a feature that distinguishes them from lymphoblastoid cell lines grown from the peripheral blood or lymph nodes of EBV-positive persons. The latter are polyclonal with respect to their surface immunoglobulin, show greater morphological variation, and have cytogenic differences from BL cell lines (Klein, E., *et al.*, 1972; Nilsson and Ponten, 1975).

Fialkow *et al.* (1973) studied isoenzymes of glucose 6-phosphate dehydrogenase 6-GPD in females heterozygous for the A and B form of this enzyme as a marker of monoclonality in BL. Of 34 tumors from 19 heterozygotes, 33 had a single phenotype. When multiple tumors from individual patients were studied, these were in general concordant for surface immunoglobulin and 6-GPD phenotype. Similarly, 36 early recurrent tumors were concordant; of 9 late recurrences, however, 3 were discordant, suggesting reinduction of a second malignant clone (Fialkow *et al.*, 1972, 1973). It should be noted, however, that the isoenzyme technique cannot detect minor cell populations of the order of 5–10% so that the recurrence could be due to outgrowth of a previously undetected minor clone (Fialkow, 1972). This degree of inexactitude casts a small degree of doubt on the now widely accepted dogma that BL is monoclonal.

There is still need for a study to establish whether within an individual patient all tumors are monotypic for the markers studied. The number of multiple tumors so far studied has been small, and the distribution of the lesions has been such that in many instances one could be metastatic from the other. It would be of particular interest to study multiple jaw tumors from the same patient.

2.5. Cytogenetics

A characteristic chromosomal abnormality that appears to involve a translocation from a number 8 to a number 14 chromosome has been demonstrated in direct biopsy cells and cultured cells from BL tumors (Manalov and Manalova, 1972; Jarvis *et al.*, 1974; Zech *et al.*, 1976). This abnormality has been found in 30 of 33 BL tumors studied and in two cell lines of non-BL origin. It was not present in peripheral blood lymphocytes of patients with BL and does not appear to be EBV-associated, since it was present in EBV-negative cell lines and could not be produced by infection of cell lines in which it was absent. Other less specific abnormalities such as trisomy have been found in biopsy and cultured BL cells (Zech *et al.*, 1976).

3. Infectious Mononucleosis—Pathology

Since lymph node biopsy is regarded as a complication of infectious mononucleosis (IM), not as a deliberate diagnostic procedure, it is not surprising that the experience of any one pathologist with such material is usually very limited. There have been, however, a number of excellent reviews of the histopathology of IM based on referred surgical and autopsy material (Downey and Stasney, 1936; Gall and Stout, 1940; Harrison, 1966; Lukes and Cox, 1958; Carter and Penman, 1969; Carter, 1972; Gowing, 1975).

''First the most striking morphological feature of this disease is the wild hyperplasia of lymphoreticular elements'' (Carter and Penman, 1969). The salient features of this hyperplasia consist of a variable follicular hyperplasia, giving way as the disease progresses to gradual replacement of the germinal follicles by amorphous and eosinophilic material. A more constant feature is an intense proliferation of blast cells in the T-dependent paracortex, these cells exhibiting marked cytoplasmic pyroninophilia. There is a concomitant proliferation of blast cells in the medullary cords, these cells in general being smaller than those in the paracortex, but exhibiting greater pleomorphism. Among these blast cells, occasional Reed–Sternberg-like cells may be seen (Lukes *et al.*, 1969), though Dorfman and Warnke (1974) believe there are subtle morphological differences between these cells and classic Reed–Sternberg cells. Carter and Penman (1969) remarked on the paucity of plasma cells in the medullary cords even in the late stages of IM, and suggested that the IgM response in this disease results from the synthetic activity of lymphoid cells. Other authors, however, state that the number of plasma cells varies, but may be abundant (Downey and Stasney, 1936; Tindle *et al.,* 1972; Gowing, 1975).

The tendency of the spleen to rupture in IM has made this organ available for histopathological study almost as frequently as lymph nodes. The lymphoid follicles are not hyperplastic, and reaction centers are inconspicuous (Gowing, 1975). There is a marked proliferation of lymphoid cells in the splenic cords, sometimes leading to obliteration of the sinusoids. Similar cells infiltrate the walls of blood vessels and may be seen in the subendothelial lymphatics of veins. Small areas of necrosis and of subcapsular and intrasplenic hemorrhage are frequently seen.

Tonsils show changes similar to those seen in lymph nodes, with proliferation of blast cells including bizarre multinucleate forms in the interfollicular areas (Carter and Penman, 1969; Tindle *et al.,* 1972). This proliferation may mimic malignant lymphoma.

In autopsied cases, widespread involvement of many tissues and organs may be found, with focal infiltrations of mononuclear cells. Such infiltrates in the liver may be associated with hepatitis and in the heart with clinical evidence of myocarditis. The CNS may be directly infected, giving an acute encephalomyelitis, or patients may develop a postinfective demyelinating encephalomyelitis (Guillain–Barré syndrome).

4. Epstein–Barr Virus

Epstein–Barr virus (EBV) was originally identified in lymphoblasts cultured from a Ugandan patient with BL (Epstein, M. A., *et al.,* 1964). It is now generally accepted to be the cause of IM (for reviews, see Klein, G., 1973; Miller, 1974; Henle, W., and Henle, 1972; Henle, W., *et al.,* 1974). One of the most impressive features of EBV is the ability to immortalize lymphoid cells so that they grow indefinitely in tissue culture (Miller, 1974). Different strains of EBV vary in their ability to immortalize lymphocytes, though no consistent difference has been detected between EBV isolated from IM, BL, or nasopharyngeal carcinoma (NPC) patients. Cell lines vary in their response to EBV, some being permissive and allowing viral replication, others responding not at all or producing only the early antigens of the viral replication cycle (for a review, see Klein, G., 1973).

4.1. Fingerprints of Epstein–Barr Virus

4.1.1. Virus Particles

EBV particles can be regularly visualized by electron microscopy in a small proportion of cells of producer BL or lymphoblastoid cell lines. The virus-containing cells exhibit a variety of degenerative changes (Epstein, M. A., *et al.,* 1965; Rabson *et al.,* 1966; Pope *et al.,* 1968), indicating that, as with other herpes virus infections, productively infected cells die. The number of virus-producing cells can be increased by manipulation of the cultures in various ways (Klein, G., 1973).

4.1.2. Epstein–Barr Viral Capsid Antigen

397

BURKITT'S
LYMPHOMA AND
INFECTIOUS
MONONUCLEOSIS

Viral capsid antigens (VCA) were recognized in virus-synthesizing cell lines by G. Henle and Henle (1966). Acetone-fixed cells from producer lines are used as the substrate, and sera are tested by the indirect immunofluorescence technique. Individually fluorescing cells contain virus particles when isolated and examined by electron microscopy, whereas nonfluorescing cells do not (Zur Hausen *et al.*, 1967). Sera that were positive by the immunofluorescence test coated isolated viral nucleocapsids and caused them to agglutinate, whereas fluorescence-negative sera did not (Henle, G., and Henle, 1966; Mayyasi *et al.*, 1967). Antibodies to VCA have been most widely used to study the epidemiology of EBV.

4.1.3. EBV-Determined Membrane Antigens

G. Klein *et al.* (1967) demonstrated a membrane antigen (MA) on viable cells from BL biopsies using the indirect immunofluorescence test with sera from BL patients and others. Bone marrow cells used as a control did not exhibit this antigen. MA can also be demonstrated on a proportion of virus-producer cultured cells derived from both BL and lymphoblastoid cell lines (Klein, G., *et al.*, 1967, 1968).

4.1.4. EBV-Induced Early Antigens

Exposure of nonproducer lines to EBV results in an abortive infection in which early antigens (EA) may be demonstrated by immunofluorescence, but virus particles and VCA are not produced (Henle, W., *et al.*, 1970). Similarly, exposure of producer lines to iododeoxyuridine or 5-bromodeoxyuridine leads to the production of EA only (Gerber, 1972; Hampar *et al.*, 1972).

Two patterns of immunofluorescence have been detected for EA. In one, there is diffuse (D) staining of the nucleus and cytoplasm, whereas the other shows restricted (R) cytoplasmic aggregates (Henle, G., *et al.*, 1971a). Both antigens are formed in the same cell, the D component appearing slightly in advance of the R component.

4.1.5. Soluble Complement-Fixing Antigen

EBV-genome-carrying cells contain a soluble complement-fixing antigen (Gerber and Deal, 1970; Pope *et al.*, 1969; Reedman *et al.*, 1972; Vonka *et al.*, 1970). It is probable that EBNA and the S antigen represent the same specificity (Klein, G., and Vonka, 1974).

4.1.6. EBV-Determined Nuclear Antigen

The EBV-determined nuclear antigen (EBNA) is demonstrated by exposing appropriately fixed cells to sera containing antibody in the presence of human complement and staining with fluorescein-conjugated antibody to β_1C-globulin (Reedman and Klein, 1973). The presence of EBNA is strictly correlated with the presence of the EBV genome. EBNA appears to be a virally determined or a virally changed chromosomal protein (Brown *et al.,* 1974; Reedman and Klein, 1973).

4.1.7. Epstein–Barr Virus

Various techniques of nucleic acid hybridization have been used to detect EBV DNA in tumor cells. Zur Hausen *et al.* (1970) introduced the technique of DNA–DNA hybridization on membrane filters. Radiolabeled viral complementary RNA made *in vitro* can be used as a sensitive probe capable of detecting approximately 2 EBV genomes per cell (Nonoyama and Pagano, 1971). The reassociation of radiolabeled DNA with cellular DNA in a liquid medium is the most sensitive method and can detect 0.2 EBV genome per cell (Nonoyama and Pagano, 1973). Initial studies suggested that EBV DNA was present in all African cases of BL and in all cultured B-cell lines, and that it was absent from all cases of BL occurring outside the endemic areas. All these assumptions have now been shown to be incorrect. EBV DNA was detected in approximately 80 cases of African BL by hybridization techniques (Zur Hausen, 1976). On average, each cell contains approximately 38 EBV genome equivalents (Klein, G., 1974). Two apparently typical cases of African Burkitt's lymphoma with serum antibodies to EBV VCA, but in which the tumor cells contained neither EBNA nor EBV DNA, were reported (Klein, G., quoted by Zur Hausen, 1976). The first of these cases gave rise to an EBV-negative lymphoblastoid cell line (BJA-B), the first such cell line established from an African case of BL (Menezes *et al.,* 1975). This cell line could be superinfected with EBV to produce EBNA-positive cells or EBNA- and EA-positive cells, depending on the strain of EBV used. Three such cell lines with B-cell characteristics derived from human lymphomas but lacking EBV genome have now been reported (Klein, G., *et al.,* 1974).

The majority of American BL have been negative when tested for EBV DNA; however, two cases containing multiple viral genome equivalents per cell were recently reported (Gravell *et al.,* 1976; Andersson *et al.,* 1976). Andersson and colleagues also reported a borderline case with approximately 2 genome equivalents per cell. In a further report that includes the cases reported by Andersson and colleagues, studies on 20 American patients with BL are recorded. Of these 20 cases, 15 had low or absent antibody titers to EBV VCA, and 5 had titers greater than 1:80, though only one or possibly two of the latter had EBV DNA in their tumor cells. A further patient in this series developed IM during treatment for BL and seroconverted. Despite this, the tumor remained EBV-negative (Ziegler *et al.,* 1976).

In a study of a large number of lymphomas in Germany, one patient with a histologically typical BL was found to have 15 EBV genome equivalents per cell (Bornkamm *et al.,* 1976; Zur Hausen, 1976). More than 50 B-cell lymphomas and more than 40 biopsies from patients with Hodgkin's disease contained no detectable amounts of EBV DNA when tested by nucleic acid hybridization. A surprising finding was the presence of 2–3 genome equivalents of EBV DNA in a biopsy from a patient with immunoblastic lymphadenopathy. The significance of this finding is uncertain, nor is it known which cells contain the EBV DNA. The amount of EBV DNA in these cells is probably higher than that indicated, since in the biopsy they would be diluted with stromal and inflammatory cells.

The observation that the majority of African cases of BL are EBV-genome-positive and that the majority of American and European cases are EBV-genome-negative led Ziegler *et al.* (1976) to suggest, as mentioned in Section 2.2, that EBV-associated BL is inversely proportional to endemicity. Zur Hausen (1975) proposed that the term Burkitt's lymphoma be abandoned in favor of the term *EBV-associated lymphoma,* and stated that there can be little doubt that the expression of virus-specific antigens within nuclei and membranes of EBV-carrying cells renders them profoundly different from virus-free cells of similar origin. While it is true that there are major differences between BL in endemic and nonendemic areas, when the diagnosis is based on histological criteria alone (Arseneau *et al.,* 1975; Banks *et al.,* 1975), there are also similarities and features that differentiate these patients from those with other types of malignant lymphomas (Wright, 1966). Furthermore, although Ziegler *et al.* (1976) showed that in American patients with BL high antibody titers to EBV VCA carried a favorable prognosis, comparable to that of the African patients, in the majority of their cases this was not associated with the expression of virus-specific antigens within nuclei and membranes of the tumor cells.

4.2. Immune Response to Epstein–Barr Virus

4.2.1. Anti-VCA IgM

Specific IgM antibodies to EBV can be determined using a sandwich technique with fluorescein-labeled anti-human IgM as the first layer (Banatvala *et al.,* 1972; Schmitz and Scherer, 1972). This test becomes positive in the acute phase of IM, but is rarely detectable 6 months later (Edwards and McSwiggan, 1975), in contrast to the IgG antibody response to VCA, which persists indefinitely. EBV-specific IgM is therefore a useful test in identifying recent infection with EBV.

4.2.2. Anti-VCA IgG*

The peak titer of this antibody is reached during the acute phase of IM. It declines slightly thereafter, and then in most communities remains at a relatively constant level indefinitely. G. Klein (1974) argued that this level of persisting antibody is determined by the number of virus-harboring cells converted during the early stages of the illness prior to the development of neutralizing antibodies, and that subsequent recruitment of virus-carrying cells is prevented by antibody. The steady antibody levels would imply that converted cells are maintained as a relatively constant proportion of the lymphoid cell population. If this reasoning is correct, the very high levels of antibodies to EBV VCA seen in young children in Uganda (de Thé *et al.,* 1975) would be associated with a large population of converted cells, a factor that might increase the chances of subsequent neoplastic development. This is also the one population group studied in which antibody titers are not maintained and in a certain proportion of children fall to unmeasurable levels. This may be related to the young age at which the children are infected, or possibly to other environmental factors such as malaria.

*See W. Henle *et al.* (1968) for a discussion.

4.2.3. EBV-Specific IgA Antibodies

Patients with NPC have been shown to have raised IgA antibodies to EBV VCA and EA (D). The incidence and titers of these antibodies were much higher than those seen with BL or other head and neck carcinomas. Titers fell in NPC patients following successful therapy. Some patients with IM showed a transient EBV-specific IgA response at low titers (Henle, G., and Henle, 1976).

4.2.4. Antibodies to Early Antigens

The majority of IM patients show a transitory antibody response to EBV-induced EA that is usually to the D component and rarely to the R component (Henle, W., *et al.,* 1974). Persistent high levels of antibodies to EA following IM are associated with severe and protracted disease (Horowitz *et al.,* 1975).

Antibodies to EA are not usually found in the normal population, though occasional patients with high levels to anti-VCA antibodies may exhibit antibodies to D or R or both. Antibodies to EA appear to be associated with continuing lymphoproliferation, and probably reflect the death of nonproducer abortively infected cells with release of intracellular antigens. A remarkable difference is observed in the antibody response to EA seen in NPC and BL. It is directed mainly against the D component in the former and against the R component in the latter (Henle, G., *et al.,* 1971a). The titers of antibodies to EA in both BL and NPC showed an increase with the stage of the disease (Henle, W., *et al.,* 1973). BL patients with low or declining titers of anti-R become long-term survivors, whereas persistence or development of high titers of antibodies to EA usually presages multiple and often fatal relapses (Henle, G., *et al.,* 1971b; Henle, W., *et al.,* 1973). A similar relationship between EA antibodies and lymphoproliferation was found with Herpesvirus saimiri infection in monkeys (Klein, G., *et al.,* 1973).

4.2.5. Neutralizing Antibodies

Several tests have been devised to detect EBV-neutralizing antibodies. These tests have been based on prevention of abortive infection of cells from nonproducer lines measured by inhibition of EA synthesis (Pearson *et al.,* 1970), cytopathic effects (Durr *et al.,* 1970), or inhibition of colony formation by the test cells (Rocchi and Hewetson, 1973), or prevention of transformation of cord-blood lymphocytes (Miller *et al.,* 1972). It is probable that neutralizing antibodies are closely related to antibodies to MA (Pearson *et al.,* 1970; Silvestre *et al.,* 1971), the viral envelope being composed of cell membrane altered by the virus. Since the MA is composed of several components, however, and probably antibodies to only one component are necessary to neutralize the virus, discordant results for these two antibody systems are occasionally obtained. De Schryver *et al.* (1976) found that splitting of immune complexes in serum from patients with BL or NPC increased the titer of anti-MA antibodies, but did not alter the level of neutralizing antibodies, supporting the hypothesis that these two antibody systems are directed, at least in part, to different antigens.

4.2.6. Antibodies to Membrane Antigens

Antibodies to MAs appear in the acute phase of IM slightly later than anti-VCA antibodies and, like the latter, persist indefinitely (Klein, G., et al., 1968). To avoid confusion with isoantibodies, it is usual to perform a blocking test in which the test serum is assayed for its ability to block a known MA-positive serum (Mutua) (Gunven and Klein, 1971). Since, however, the MA consists of a complex of at least three antigens, and since in any one serum antibodies may be present to only one or two of these, such sera will give a false negative result in the blocking test (since one antigen will be kept unblocked to react with the Mutua serum) and result in apparent discordance between the anti-VCA and anti-MA antibodies (Svedmyr et al., 1970).

The titers of anti-MA antibodies, like the titers of anti-VCA antibodies, are substantially higher in most patients with BL than in African controls (Gunven et al., 1970). Irradiation of BL and NPC leads to a rise in antibodies to MA and VCA (Einhorn, 1972; Einhorn et al., 1972). Antibody titers to MAs also show a disease-related pattern in BL.

4.3. Soluble Complement-Fixation Antigens(s) and EBV-Associated Nuclear Antigens

It appears that EBNA is the major, but not the sole, component in s-antigen preparations (Henle, W., and Henle, 1975). Antibodies to both antigens appear during late convalescence from IM and persist thereafter (Vonka et al., 1972). This persistence of antibody may be due to the release of antigens from latent nonproducer cells or to the periodic activation of virus production (Klein, G., 1973). Anti-EBNA titers vary widely in patients with BL; very low titers may be seen not only in moribund patients, but also in long-term survivors (Henle, W., and Henle, 1975). The antigen may be released into the circulation and stimulate antibody production as the result of active cell-mediated immunity (CMI), but also as the result of nonspecific tumor necrosis related to metabolic or vascular factors.

4.4. Cell-Mediated Reactivity Against EBV-Infected Cells: Cytotoxic T Cells

Unfractionated peripheral blood lymphocytes from patients with IM are cytotoxic, as measured by ^{51}Cr-release assay, to a range of lymphoid cell lines whether or not these lines carry the EBV genome. Similarly, peripheral blood lymphocytes stimulated in vitro with autologous EBV-genome-positive lymphoblastoid cells show indiscriminate cytotoxicity. If, however, the lymphocytes bearing complement receptors are first removed from the peripheral blood lymphocytes of patients in the acute phase of IM, the residual (T) lymphocytes show specific cytotoxicity against EBV-genome-carrying cell lines (Svedmyr and Jondal, 1975). The residual lymphocytic population from normal cell donors have no such effect. T lymphocytes isolated from a large biopsy of BL showed a similar cytotoxicity against EBV-genome-carrying lymphoblastoid cell lines, and also against the autochthonous tumor biopsy cells in vitro (Jondal et al., 1975). Previous cytotoxicity studies using unfractionated peripheral blood lymphocytes from patients with IM and BL had been negative (Hewetson *et al.*, 1972a) or equivocal (Rosenberg *et al.*, 1974), though cells from draining lymph nodes from two BL patients proved to be highly cytotoxic (Hewetson *et al.*, 1972a).

4.5. Antibody-Dependent Lymphocyte Cytotoxicity

Two recent reports (Jondal, 1976; Pearson and Orr, 1976) showed that antibodies present in the sera of EBV-positive but not EBV-negative persons were capable of inducing lymphocyte-mediated lysis of cells bearing EBV-induced MA, but not of uninfected Raji, or of Daudi cell lines that did not bear MA. These antibodies were absent from the sera of patients in the acute phase of IM. Antibody titers to EBV-induced MA were considerably higher by this assay than by the usual fluorescence test for MA. Preliminary studies showed no significant relationship between this antibody-dependent lymphocyte cytoxicity (ADLC) and BL, NPC, or other tumors. High titers were noted in every category including normal controls. It would be of considerable interest to know the relationship of ADLC to disease status and tumor burden in patients with BL.

5. Immune Responses in Infectious Mononucleosis and Burkitt's Lymphoma

5.1. Immune Response in Infectious Mononucleosis and Termination of the Disease

In a review of IM, Carter (1972) suggested that the outstanding question had changed from "What starts the disease?" to "What stops it?" Dameshek (1969) noted that "infectious mononucleosis is disturbingly similar to acute leukemia and shows several features of a generalised uncontrolled and self perpetuating proliferation of one of the white cell series; but why in contrast to acute leukemia is the abnormal process always reversible?" Lymph nodes from patients with IM show an often alarming proliferation of immature lymphoid cells that may closely mimic immunoblastic sarcoma or other lymphoid malignancies (Carter, 1972; Gowing, 1975), and in fatal cases there are often widespread lymphoid infiltrates in many tissues and organs (Carter, 1972). Lymphoblastoid cell lines can be readily established from the peripheral blood lymphocytes of patients with IM (Diehl *et al.*, 1968; Junge *et al.*, 1971), and can often be cloned directly in soft plasma clot substrates without preadaptation to tissue culture (Hewetson, quoted by Klein, G., 1973). Such lymphoblastoid cell lines can be transplanted to neonatal or immunosuppressed experimental animals with relative ease (Adams *et al.*, 1967, 1970; Southam *et al.*, 1969). Were it not that the patients almost invariably recover, these observations would probably be interpreted as indicating a malignant lymphoid proliferation.

Lymphocyte marker studies have shown that the majority of atypical cells seen in the peripheral blood of patients with IM are T cells, since they form spontaneous rosettes with sheep erythrocytes (SRBC) (Sheldon *et al.*, 1973; Papamichail *et al.*, 1974). The number of "atypical" lymphocytes usually outnumbers the T- or the B-cell population identified by marker techniques, however, indicating that both contribute to the pool of "atypical" cells (Giuliano *et al.*, 1974; Mangi *et al.*, 1974).

The ratio of T to B cells in the peripheral blood varies during the course of the disease. B cells are elevated during the first week and fall to normal at 3–4 weeks. T cells peak at 10–14 days and return to normal levels at 5–6 weeks (Mangi *et al.*, 1974). This sequence is in keeping with the concept that the T blasts are reacting to altered B blasts, as well as with the pattern of involvement seen in the lymph nodes in IM, in which the most marked lymphoblastoid proliferation takes place in the T-dependent paracortical areas (Carter, 1972; Gowing, 1975).

Some of the blastoid cells seen in the sinuses and medullary cords of the lymph nodes are presumably B cells that have been transformed by EBV. G. Klein *et al.* (1976) were able to demonstrate EBNA-positive blast cells in the peripheral blood of 5 patients in the acute phase of IM. Both the EBNA-positive cells and EBV-specific T cells disappeared from the blood after the acute phase. Much of the morphologically alarming lymphoid proliferation seen in IM is in fact host-T-cell response to EBV-infected B lymphoid cells and is self-limiting insofar as it terminates when all or most of the stimulating cells are eliminated. Many of the clinical manifestations of IM are probably related to this violent host response to EBV-infected lymphoid cells. The trivial or inapparent nature of EBV infections in young children is presumably due to the fact that they do not mount such a vigorous reaction, possibly due to relative immunological immaturity, though this is speculative. To some extent, the common exanthemata of infancy show a similar behavior, being much more debilitating when they occur in adolescents and young adults.

In answer to Carter's question "What stops IM?" a number of mechanisms have been identified that are probably contributory. Antibodies to VCA, MA, and neutralizing antibodies presumably stop the horizontal spread of the EBV and prevent infection of more B lymphocytes. Nonspecific enhanced destruction of lymphoid cell lines by peripheral blood lymphocytes has been demonstrated in the acute phase of IM (Hutt *et al.*, 1975; Royston *et al.*, 1975). This reactivity may be due at least in part to nonspecific activation of the peripheral blood leukocytes. Of greater significance is the demonstration of T cells specifically cytotoxic for EBV-genome-positive lymphoblastoid cells in the peripheral blood of patients with acute IM (Svedmyr and Jondal, 1975). These cells are cytotoxic for producer and non-producer cell lines, and therefore are presumably recognizing surface antigens other than MA. It is likely that these cells play an important role in the elimination of EBV-positive cells in patients with IM. Although they disappear from the peripheral blood during convalescence, it is probable that memory T cells, capable of reactivation under appropriate stimulus, persist. It is not known whether or to what extent similar EBV-specific cytotoxic T cells develop in children infected with EBV at a young age.

Antibodies directed against MA are capable of inducing ADLC (Pearson and Orr, 1976; Jondal, 1976). Such antibodies are not seen in the acute phase of IM, but develop during convalescence and are present in all sera from EBV-positive persons. ADLC would provide a mechanism for the elimination of EBV producer cells expressing MA, and would thus suppress recurrent infections. It would not, however, enable the host to eliminate EBV-genome-positive nonproducer cells.

With such a formidable array of humoral and cellular immune mechanisms directed against EBV and EBV-infected cells, it is not surprising that IM is a self-limiting disease. It may appear more surprising that EBV-genome-carrying cells are able to survive in the patient as demonstrated by the persistence of antibodies to

VCA at a constant level, the ability to grow EBV-positive lymphoblastoid lines from the peripheral blood of almost all EBV-positive donors provided sufficient quantities of blood are available (Diehl *et al.*, 1968; Gerber and Monroe, 1968; Moore *et al.*, 1967), and the oral excretion of EBV by normal subjects (Gerber *et al.*, 1973). Presumably, most EBV-genome-positive cells in these patients are nonproductive and are therefore unaffected by antibody or ADLC, though presumably a few cells are in the productive cycle maintaining the antigenic stimulus for anti-VCA production. Cytotoxic T lymphocytes may be unable to eliminate all EBV-genome-carrying cells either because the latter are being continually produced at a rate that exceeds the rate of destruction or because some cells do not have the antigens on their surface that are recognized by the cytotoxic T lymphocytes. The possibility that EBV replicates at some other site (e.g., nasopharyngeal mucosa) and continuously reinfects lymphoid cells merits further investigation.

The familial occurrence of fatal IM in males has been reported by a number of authors (Bar *et al.*, 1974; Purtilo, 1976). In some of these families, siblings or male cousins have also developed malignant lymphomas. The fatal IM is accompanied by a heterophile antibody response, but despite normal levels of immunoglobulins, the patients do not produce EBV-specific antibodies. Purtilo proposes that these may be one phenotypic manifestation of an X-linked recessive lymphoproliferative syndrome that includes agammaglobulinaemia following IM, and various malignant lymphomas including American BL. He suggests that the pathogenesis of this syndrome may be a defect in B cells resulting in unrestricted proliferation without the formation of antibodies to EBV. His alternative hypothesis of defective suppressor-T-cell activity is unlikely to be the entire explanation, in view of lack of production of antibodies to EBV by these patients. These families are clearly of the greatest interest in relation to both the immunological control of EBV infection and the etiology of malignant lymphomas.

5.2. General Immunological Reactivity of Patients with Infectious Mononucleosis

A bewildering range of antibodies develop during the course of an attack of IM, including antibodies to a wide variety of animal red cells, best exemplified by the heterophile reaction to SRBC that forms the basis of the Paul Bunnell diagnostic test (Fince, 1969), other animal antigens, and bacterial and viral antigens (Davidsohn and Lee, 1969). The transient appearance of antibodies to human antigens includes positive tests for rheumatoid factor (Dresner and Trombly, 1959; Holborow *et al.*, 1963; Carter, 1966; Kaplan, 1968), antinuclear factors (Johnson and Holborow, 1963; Wollheim and Williams, 1966; Carter, 1966; Kaplan and Tan, 1968), and antibodies to smooth muscle (Holborow *et al.*, 1973), platelets (Smith *et al.*, 1963), erythrocytes (Sawitsky *et al.*, 1950), lymphocytes, and thymocytes (Thomas, 1972).

Cutaneous anergy to a number of allergens has been demonstrated in the acute phase of IM, returning to normal with recovery (Haider *et al.*, 1973; Mangi *et al.*, 1974). A depressed response of blood lymphocytes to phytohemagglutinin (PHA), pokeweed mitogen, and candida, and in the mixed lymphocyte reaction, has also been shown (Mangi *et al.*, 1974; Papamichail *et al.*, 1974). Cooper *et al.* (1967) similarly showed a poor mitotic response of blood lymphocytes from IM patients compared with normal blood lymphocytes when stimulated by PHA, and Cooper (1969) concluded that the bulk of the atypical monocytes in the blood of patients with IM are either in G_1 or out of cycle. Papamichail *et al.* (1974) noted that the peripheral blood lymphocytes from patients with IM were able to bind fluorescein-conjugated PHA, and they concluded that the likely explanation of refractoriness to this mitogen is that the majority of cells have already been stimulated *in vivo* and thus rendered unresponsive to further stimulation. This conclusion is in keeping with the high spontaneous DNA and RNA synthesis by peripheral blood leukocytes in the first 2 weeks of IM (Rubin, 1966; Mangi *et al.*, 1974).

Recently, immune complexes were demonstrated in a patient in the acute phase of IM with an urticarial skin rash (Wands *et al.*, 1976). These complexes contained IgG, IgM, and IgA, as well as several complement components. They showed antibody activity to EBV and VCA, and on electron microscopy, particles resembling EBV were seen in the complexes. Immune complex formation is presumably an unusual and transient feature of IM, but might account for some of the less common features of the illness such as arthralgia and skin rashes.

The transient anergy seen in IM might be due to antibody coating of lymphocytes (Thomas, 1972), but is more likely to be due to antigenic competition and the precommitment of T lymphocytes both in the peripheral blood and in local lymph nodes. A similar depression of cutaneous reactivity is seen in other viral infections (Finkel and Dent, 1973; Kupers *et al.*, 1970).

5.3. General Immunological Reactivity of Patients with Burkitt's Lymphoma

Patients with BL show no increased susceptibility to intercurrent infection as is seen in other lymphomas associated with defects in the immune system. Ziegler *et al.* (1970), studying patients in Uganda, found that the delayed hypersensitivity response to dinitrochlorobenzene (DNCB) and the *in vitro* response of blood lymphocytes to PHA was the same in all stages of Burkitt's lymphoma as in control subjects. Stjernsward *et al.* (1970), however, found impaired reactivity to DNCB and deficient response of blood lymphocytes to PHA in untreated Kenyan cases of BL with a large tumor burden. Patients in remission had a normal response in both these tests.

Children with untreated BL have an impaired antibody response to a polysaccharide antigen isolated from *Escherichia coli* in comparison with age-matched controls and patients in remission (Ziegler *et al.*, 1970). This impaired humoral response correlates with lowered levels of serum IgM found in patients with untreated BL (Ziegler *et al.*, 1970; Ngu *et al.*, 1966). This lowering of serum IgM appears to be related to the presence of active tumor, rather than to an underlying defect of the BL patient. It may reflect a disturbance of homeostatic mechanisms caused by the presence of IgM-bearing tumor cells.

The role of malaria in any immunological disturbances in patients with BL must be considered, although the control children in the study by Ziegler and colleagues probably had the same exposure to this parasite as the BL patients. Children with acute malaria were found to have a diminished antibody response to the O antigen of *Salmonella typhi* and to tetanus toxoid. Their antibody response to the H antigen of *S. typhi* and their cutaneous cellular immune responses were normal (Greenwood *et al.*, 1972). These findings suggest minor immunological disturbances in acute malaria, but antibody responses and cutaneous reactivity are relatively crude measures of humoral and cellular immunity, and subtle changes could remain undetected.

5.4. Immune Response to Burkitt's Lymphoma

Clinical observations of spontaneous regressions (Burkitt and Kyalwazi, 1967; Ngu *et al.*, 1970), regression of tumor following apparent nonspecific therapy (David and Burkitt, 1968), or manifestly inadequate therapy (Burkitt *et al.*, 1965) suggested that patients with BL may exhibit host antitumor activity. Similarly, the excellent response to chemotherapy and the long-term remission seen in a high proportion of patients with BL could be related to host immunological reactivity to the tumor cells (Klein, G., 1975). BL has been shown to have an extremely fast growth rate, with a potential doubling time on the order of 48 hr (Cooper *et al.*, 1966; Iversen *et al.*, 1974). It may well be that only by proliferating at this rate is the tumor able to establish itself in a hostile immunological environment. The widespread dissemination of many untreated tumors, in contrast to the localization of recurrent tumors in single sites, often the CNS, could also be interpreted as evidence of host antitumor reactivity. At autopsy, patients with recurrent tumor frequently show infiltrations of lymphocytes and plasma cells in sites of previous tumor deposits (Wright, 1971).

Transient diminution of tumor size was reported in patients with BL given an injection of plasma from patients in remission (Burkitt, 1967; Ngu, 1967). In a double-blind trial, Fass *et al.* (1970a) were unable, however, to demonstrate any effect of convalescent serum, and they suggested that the results obtained by Burkitt and Ngu were fortuitous. Early studies of cutaneous delayed hypersensitivity reactions to membrane extracts of autologous BL cells showed that positivity in untreated cases was associated with a small tumor burden and in posttreatment cases it correlated with long-term remission, whereas patients with a negative reaction showed early relapse (Fass *et al.*, 1970b). Further studies of this phenomenon have not been reported.

Antibodies to various EBV-associated antigens, other than MA, probably have no direct anti-tumor-cell activity. High levels of anti-VCA antibodies seen in patients with BL do not appear to be related to tumor burden. They probably result from the continuous release of virus from productively infected cells. These are possibly tumor cells that are rapidly eliminated, since virus particles are never visualized in direct biopsy cells and VCA is rarely detected in such preparations. However, since MA occurs only in productively infected cell lines, and since it is present on biopsy cells from BL, it may well be that some of these cells are productive *in vivo*. Alternative explanations are that EBV is replicating at some other site (cf. replication of Marek's disease virus in feather follicles of chickens) or that the presence of tumor results in an abnormally marked humoral response to a small load of virus (Miller, 1974).

Antibodies to EA presumably play no part in tumor-cell destruction since this is an internal cell antigen. Nevertheless, as discussed previously, levels of anti-EA antibodies are correlated with tumor load and do have prognostic significance. Similarly, anti-MA antibodies have predictive significance; long-term survivors following chemotherapy show persistent high levels of anti-MA, whereas patients with recurrent tumors often show a fall in titer some time prior to the time that the tumor becomes clinically apparent (Gunven *et al.*, 1974). Such recurrent tumors may become coated with IgG, which on elution shows anti-MA activity (Hewetson *et al.*, 1972b) and virus-neutralizing properties (Klein, G., 1975). The fall in antibodies to MA that occurs before recurrent tumor is clinically apparent does not appear to be due to absorption of antibody by tumor cells, since in a case reported by G. Klein *et al.* (1969), in which anti-MA antibodies fell 6 months before recurrence, after a remission lasting 4½ years, the tumor cells were uncoated with IgG at a time when the anti-MA antibodies were still low. Following recurrence, the anti-MA antibodies rose. The sequence suggests that the fall in titer may be the cause rather than the result of tumor recurrence. These observations could be due, however, to the shedding of antibody–MA complexes from the tumor cells, since such complexes have been demonstrated in the serum of patients prior to clinical relapse. It would be of interest to measure the ADLC activity of the serum from these patients. If the serum retains this property, or, more particularly, if antibody eluted from tumor cells has this property, any defect of host antitumor activity must reside with patients' lymphocytes, a hypothesis that could be tested by using them as effector cells in ADLC reactions. It is possible that in such patients they are inhibited by blocking factors (Hellström and Hellström, 1970).

Cytotoxic T cells similar to those identified by Svedmyr and Jondal (1975) in the blood of patients with acute IM may have an important role in any host antitumor activity exhibited by patients with BL. Jondal *et al.* (1975) isolated T cells from a biopsy of BL and demonstrated cytotoxicity of these cells against EBV-carrying cell lines as well as the autologous biopsy tumor cells. This cytotoxicity was dose-dependent; significant killing was obtained with apparent lymphocyte tumor cell ratios of 15:1, though since the T-lymphocyte preparation was diluted with 50% unlabeled tumor cells, this ratio must have been much lower. The original tumor biopsy contained approximately 1% T lymphocytes; Gross *et al.* (1975), however, showed from 3.7 to 38% T lymphocytes in BL biopsies. Since they counted their rosette preparations in a chamber, they did not record the morphology of these cells. Histological and electron-microscopic preparations of BL biopsies certainly do not reveal large numbers of small lymphocytes; however, T lymphoblasts could easily be confused with BL tumor cells. Further studies are needed on the presence of cytotoxic T cells in BL tissue and their relationship to therapeutic response and survival. Although the ratio of these cells to tumor cells may be too low to be effective in the original tumor, it is possible that much higher effective ratios are obtained following chemotherapy with a substantial tumor-cell kill.

6. Association of Epstein–Barr Virus with Other Lymphoproliferative Disorders

Elevated antibody titers to EBV VCA have been reported in a number of lymphoproliferative disorders, though in none of these disorders is the association so constant or the mean titers so high as those seen in BL. Raised antibody levels to EBV-associated antigens are frequently encountered in patients with Hodgkin's disease, particularly in those with the lymphocyte-depleted subtypes (Johansson *et al.*, 1970; Levine *et al.*, 1971). Raised anti-VCA and anti-MA titers were encountered in approximately 40% of patients with chronic lymphocytic leukemia (Johansson *et al.*, 1971). Variable and conflicting reports of antibody levels to EBV in a number of nonneoplastic disorders have been published (for a review, see Klein, G., 1973).

The association of raised antibody levels to EBV with the lymphocyte-depleted subtypes of Hodgkin's disease suggests that this may be due to suppression of CMI or some other derangement of the immune system, rather than to the virus being carried as a passenger in the lymphoid cells of the tumor. There are two conflicting reports on the association of elevated EBV titers with depressed CMI in lymphoma patients. Levine *et al.* (1975) reported data that strongly indicated that the elevated EBV titers in lymphoma patients are not related to a specific or nonspecific depression of CMI, whereas Johansson *et al* (1975) concluded that a relationship exists between the immune defect and the high anti-VCA titers. Perhaps the most persuasive evidence relating raised anti-VCA titers to defective CMI is provided by the patient with a T-cell deficit reported by Businco *et al.* (1975) with raised EBV antibody levels that fell to normal following thymus grafting. A similar unpublished case is noted by these authors. Prolonged excretion of EBV was reported in renal transplant patients treated with immunosuppressive drugs (Strauch *et al.*, 1974).

The major difference in the association between EBV and BL and its association with other lymphoproliferative diseases is that in BL, the tumor cells are almost invariably EBV-genome-positive and exhibit various EBV-determined antigens, whereas with the exception of one case of immunoblastic lymphadenopathy, all other lymphomas have been found to be EBV-genome-negative (Zur Hausen, 1976). This latter study included tissue from more than 40 patients with Hodgkin's disease, though it should be borne in mind that in Hodgkin's tissue, the tumor cells are usually considerably outnumbered by reactive cells that would tend to dilute any EBV DNA present and might make it undetectable by the techniques used.

7. Epstein–Barr-Virus-Associated Lymphoma in Nonhuman Primates

Old World monkeys with the exception of gibbons cannot be infected by EBV, and the lymphocytes from these animals are resistant to infection *in vitro* (Frank *et al.*, 1976). In contrast, New World monkeys are susceptible to infection, and their lymphocytes can be immortalized by EBV *in vitro* (Miller, 1974). EBV-infected marmoset lymphoid cells in culture are particularly productive, releasing 1000-fold more virus than the human cells that contained the parent viral strain (Miller and Lipman, 1973).

When marmosets are infected with EBV, a variety of responses are obtained. There is a group of animals with lymphoma development, another group develops hyperplastic abdominal lymph nodes and antibodies to EBV, a third group seroconverts with inapparent infection, and a few animals show no antibody response (G. Miller, quoted by Klein, E., *et al.*, 1976). The group with hyperplastic lymph nodes has some resemblance to human IM, in that, whereas the peripheral lymph nodes and spleen are involved in humans, only the abdominal lymph nodes enlarge in marmosets (Shope, 1975). This reaction can be abrogated by human serum containing antibodies to EBV. A further difference between the response to EBV in marmosets and humans is that whereas EBV can be detected in cultured lymphocytes from man for many years and perhaps indefinitely following an attack of IM, in marmosets this is possible only during the acute stage of the disease.

Malignant lymphomas are produced regularly in a proportion of marmosets infected with EBV (Shope *et al.*, 1973; Miller, 1974; Werner *et al.*, 1975), though tumor induction varies with the species of marmoset and the strain of EBV used (Deinhardt *et al.*, 1975). The tumors differ from BL in that, as judged by the production of different classes of immunoglobulin, they appear to be polyclonal (Deinhardt *et al.*, 1975). M. A. Epstein *et al.* (1973a,b) observed a lymphoproliferative disease in one of three owl monkeys infected with an extract of EBV. Leibold *et al.* (1976) observed undifferentiated EBNA-positive malignant lymphomas in three squirrel monkeys injected with EBV-infected autologous lymphoid cells; these animals had also been splenectomized and infected with malaria. Tumors were not seen previously in squirrel monkeys injected with EBV-transformed autologous leukocytes (Shope and Miller, 1973), or in newborn and juvenile rhesus monkeys or gibbons inoculated with EBV (Miller, 1974). The antibody levels to EBV VCA and EA in tumor-bearing marmosets was fourfold higher than in nontumor-bearing animals, a parallel with BL, in which high levels of these antibodies are found (Miller, 1974).

8. Epidemiological Studies

8.1. Epidemiology of Epstein–Barr Virus Infection

Seroepidemiological surveys have established that EBV infection occurs throughout the world, even in remote areas such as the North Pole (Tischendorf *et al.*, 1970) and among isolated South American tribes (Black *et al.*, 1970; de Thé *et al.*, 1975; Evans, 1974; Niederman and Evans, 1973). The pattern of acquisition of antibodies with age varies, however, in different communities. Tropical climates and populations of low socioeconomic standard are associated with exposure to the virus early in life, while in temperate climates and in populations of high socioeconomic standard, the prevalence of antibodies may be less than 50% by young adult life (Evans and Niederman, 1972). Heterophile-positive IM occurs in the seronegative teenage and young adult members of the latter groups (Niederman *et al.*, 1968, 1970; Sawyer *et al.*, 1971).

There appears to be a low efficiency of transmission of the virus in family groups and among college students (Wahren *et al.*, 1970; Joncas and Mitnyan, 1970; Sawyer *et al.*, 1971) that contrasts with the high efficiency of spread found in a nursery (Pereira *et al.*, 1969) and an orphanage (Tischendorf *et al.*, 1970). These observations are consistent with the hypothesis that spread is effected mainly through saliva, which is readily transferred among young children in institutions, whereas among older groups this transference is effected mainly by the more passionate forms of kissing. It has been shown that the saliva of patients with IM contains EBV during the clinical illness and for a long time thereafter (Gerber *et al.*, 1973). A higher proportion (52%) of immunosuppressed patients previously exposed to the virus shed EBV in their throat washings than serologically positive controls (18%) (Strauch *et al.*, 1974). EBV is also found in the saliva of patients with BL and in a large proportion of healthy individuals in areas in which BL is prevalent (Gerber, quoted by de Thé, 1976a).

De Thé (1976a) compared the age specific prevalence of antibodies to EBV VCA in Uganda Africans, Singapore Chinese, Singapore Indians, and Caucasians from Nancy, France. He showed remarkable differences between these groups up to the age of 5 years. At age 2–3 years, almost all the Uganda children were VCA-positive, whereas in Singapore, only 20% of the Chinese and 37% of the Indians showed VCA antibodies. At 10 years, there was no great difference between the Uganda and Singapore groups, though the Caucasian group was only 60% positive at this time. Similar patterns were seen when antibodies to the complement-fixing soluble antigen of EBV were studied (de Thé *et al.*, 1975).

All Ugandan children in the 3- to 5-year-old groups are EBV-VCA-antibody-positive; in the 5- to 9- and 10- to 14-year-old groups, however, 1% and 5%, respectively, were found to be negative (de Thé *et al.*, 1975). The incidence of undetectable antibodies was greater among boys than among girls. This phenomenon had previously been noted by Kafuko *et al.* (1972) on a different group of children from the West Nile District of Uganda, making it unlikely that this is a cohort phenomenon. It appears likely, therefore, that some individuals, particularly boys, having had antibodies to VCA become antibody-negative. It should be noted, however, that this negativity is relative to the sensitivity of the test indicating a titer of less than 1:10, rather than an absolute loss of antibodies.

The geometric mean titers (GMT) of antibodies to VCA also differed among the four ethnic groups studied by de Thé. The Uganda children had an unexpectedly high level of antibodies in the first and second year of life, with a GMT of 423, similar to that seen in patients with Burkitt's lymphoma. Thereafter, the GMT fell to 60 in the 10- to 14-year-old age groups, a level below that seen in other ethnic groups at this age. de Thé speculates whether the very early infection with EBV seen in Ugandan children at a time of immunological immaturity results in heavy and prolonged viral replication, and that this might be significant in the etiology of Burkitt's lymphoma. It is not known why Ugandan children have such an early exposure to EBV. Transmission of saliva among children, which might account for the high prevalence of infection in toddlers in nurseries, would be unlikely in these very young children living in small family units. Transmission of infected lymphoid cells by biting insects is a possibility that might explain some of the epidemiological features of BL if EBV is an etiological agent. In this respect, a seroepidemiological study of EBV in highland areas of Uganda would be of particular interest. A further possible mode of spread of EBV to these very young children is the transmission of EBV-infected lymphoid cells in breast milk. Colostrum is known to contain large numbers of lymphoid cells (Beer and Billingham, 1975), and EBV-carrying lymphoblastoid cell lines have been established from human milk (W. Feller, cited by de Thé, 1976a). It would be of interest to know whether young African mothers secrete more EBV-carrying cells in their breast milk than mothers of other ethnic groups.

8.2. Epidemiology of Burkitt's Lymphoma

The observation by Burkitt (1962a,b) that the distribution of Burkitt's lymphoma in tropical Africa appears to be dependent on temperature and humidity led to the hypothesis that the tumor may be caused by an infectious agent. Early studies concentrated on arboviruses as likely candidates for this role until the discovery of EBV and the accumulation of evidence linking this virus with the tumor. The known worldwide distribution of EBV does not explain, however, the restricted distribution of "endemic" Burkitt's lymphoma to certain wet tropics. This led to the development of an alternative hypothesis suggesting that holoendemic falciparum malaria acts as a cocarcinogen either by causing immunosuppression or by stimulating intense lymphoproliferation (Burkitt, 1969; O'Conor, 1970). Any hypothesis must take into account the following observations:

1. Burkitt's lymphoma is the most common childhood malignancy in tropical Africa and Papua, and in both these locales, its distribution appears to be dependent on temperature and humidity (Wright, 1967). The incidence of the tumor in tropical Africa is in the region of 40 cases per million per year up to the age of 15 years; i.e. approximately 1 in 2000 children born will get Burkitt's lymphoma by the age of 16 (Pike and Morrow, 1972). The tumor, defined by histological and clinical features, occurs sporadically elsewhere in the world, but at a much lower incidence.

2. Burkitt's lymphoma is rare under the age of 3 years and has a peak incidence at approximately 7 years. Thereafter, the incidence falls rapidly, and the tumor is uncommon after the age of 15. The cumulative age incidence curve suggests that if Burkitt's lymphoma is due to an infectious agent, the indigenous population has met that agent and possibly acquired immunity to it by the early teens (Haddow, 1964).

3. Late teenage and adult cases of Burkitt's lymphoma are rare in tropical Africa, and tend to occur in immigrants from highland areas where the tumor is uncommon (Burkitt and Wright, 1966; Morrow et al., 1976a).

4. The age of onset of Burkitt's lymphoma appears to be inversely related to the frequency of the tumor in any population group (Morrow et al., 1976a).

5. The tumor has exhibited time–space clustering in the West Nile District (Pike et al., 1967; Williams et al., 1969) and Bwamba Country, Uganda (Morrow et al., 1971), though this was sought but not found in Mengo District, Uganda (Morrow et al., 1976a), and North Mara District, Tanzania (Brubaker et al., 1973). It has also been stated that the clustering effect declined in the West Nile District in 1968–1971 (Smith, quoted by Morrow et al., 1976a).

6. Epidemic drift of the tumor was observed in the West Nile District between 1961 and 1965 (Pike et al., 1967).

7. Burkitt's lymphoma shows seasonal variation in the West Nile District (Williams et al., 1974) and in Mengo District (Morrow et al., 1976a).

8. Three sibling pairs of BL were recorded with onsets of tumor within months of each other despite, in one instance, wide disparity in age (Pike and Morrow, 1972).

9. The incidence of BL showed a substantial decline in Mengo District, Uganda, over the decade 1959–1968 (Morrow et al., 1976a).

10. The male/female sex incidence is approximately 2 : 1, though under the age of 5 years, the incidence in females is greater than in males (Morrow et al., 1976a).

It is difficult to relate the forgoing observations on the epidemiology of Burkitt's lymphoma to the known epidemiology of EBV infection. The pattern of acquisition of antibodies to EBV may be of significance in the etiology of Burkitt's lymphoma, as proposed by de Thé (1976a), though it is unlikely to explain the geographical restriction of the tumor. It would be of interest to know the pattern of acquisition of antibodies to EBV in highland areas of East Africa in comparison with those found in the West Nile District of Uganda. Early exposure to EBV with an initial marked antibody response followed by a fall, possibly below detectable levels, may "prime" patients for the subsequent development of Burkitt's lymphoma, but would not explain time–space clustering, epidemic drift, seasonal variation, adult immigrant cases, and the age discordance of sibling pairs. These events suggest an environmental factor of limited duration, followed by a latent period of months rather than years for development of the tumor.

The known distribution of holoendemic malaria would explain the geographical restriction of Burkitt's lymphoma in tropical Africa and Papua (Dalldorf et al., 1964; Burkitt, 1969). The distribution of Burkitt's lymphoma in West Nile may also be related to holoendemic malaria (Kafuko et al., 1969), and the fall in incidence of Burkitt's lymphoma in Mengo District may be attributed to the increased use of antimalarial drugs (Morrow et al., 1976b). The observation that sickle cell trait, which gives some protection against malaria, also appears to protect against BL (Pike et al., 1970) lends weight to the hypothesis that malaria is a cofactor in the etiology of this tumor. A recent study reported from Nigeria, however, showed no relationship between sickle cell trait and protection against BL (Nkrumah and Perkins, 1976).

Unprotected African children living in areas of malarial holoendemicity show a maximum incidence of parasitaemia at 1 or 2 years of age. Parasitemia subsequently falls as the level of serum antibodies rises (McGregor, 1964). Since it appears on the available evidence that virtually all African children living in areas in which Burkitt's lymphoma is common are infected with EBV (de Thé, 1976a) and malaria (McGregor, 1964) before the age of 2–3, a further factor must presumably be implicated to account for the relatively low incidence of the tumor (40 per million per year). Adult cases and sibling pairs suggest that the time relationship of the two infections to each other is not critical. If Burkitt's lymphoma has a latent period of months, as suggested by some of the epidemiological features, why is the peak incidence at age 7 or 8 years?

It is difficult to explain time–space clustering, epidemic drift, and sibling pairs on the basis of EBV and malaria alone unless one invokes sudden recrudescence of malaria or reinfection with EBV as being significant factors. These inconsistences should encourage us to keep an open mind to the possibility of a third factor in the etiology of Burkitt's lymphoma or the possibility that EBV or malaria or both are not etiological factors.

Addendum. Since the completion of this chapter, the following information from the prospective study of EBV in relation to BL in the West Nile District of Uganda has come to hand. Of the 42,000 children bled in the main collection, 12 have subsequently developed BL after periods of 7–31 months. Sera from 10 of these cases have been analyzed. Of these, 6 showed significantly raised anti-VCA titres compared with neighborhood controls, 2 showed average values, and 2 were below average. Tumor tissue from one of the latter pair and one of the average pair contained no detectable EBV DNA when tested by hybridization techniques, though in one case this may have been due to inadequate material being available.

These preliminary results suggest that:

1. Antibodies directed against EBV 7–31 months prior to onset do not protect against BL development.
2. On the contrary, high VCA titers seem to be a factor that favors development of BL.
3. The rise in EA antibody titers observed in 7 of 10 cases at the time of BL development probably reflects a reactivation of a heavy and chronic EBV infection (de Thé, 1976b).

9. Discussion

It is now possible to propose a credible model for the pathogenesis of IM. Epidemiological studies suggest that the virus is shed in saliva, either in lymphocytes or in nasopharyngeal epithelial cells, and in adolescents and young adults spreads from person to person mainly as the result of kissing. Seronegative persons become infected, the virus colonizing the nasopharyngeal lymphoid tissue either directly or via the epithelial cells. Replication of the virus proceeds and spreads to B lymphocytes throughout the body until host responses limit its spread and eliminate the bulk of the infected cells. Anti-VCA and neutralizing antibodies develop early in the disease and prevent further horizontal spread of the virus. Antibodies to internal cell antigens such as EA and EBNA develop when cells containing these antigens die and release them; they may therefore reflect the intensity and extent of the infection, but play no part in limiting it. Antibodies to MA will mediate the destruction of productively infected cells through the mechanism of ADLC, leaving T cells specifically cytotoxic for EBV-genome-positive cells to eliminate those cells that carry nonproductive infection. It is this intense host immunological response, approximately 40 days after infection, that is presumably responsible for the various manifestations of the disease. The infection is not totally eliminated, however, as evidence by the prolonged excretion of EBV in saliva and the indefinite persistence of EBV-genome-positive cells in the peripheral blood and lymphoid tissue. These cells must presumably escape surveillance by cytotoxic T memory cells, or be continuously produced in areas that are inaccessible to such cells, possibly nasopharyngeal or oropharyngeal epithelium.

Much less is known of the clinically silent EBV infections that occur in childhood. Since these children are never identified, the kinetics of virus replication and of the host response remain a mystery. The lack of clinical symptoms is not due to tolerance, since all the host immunological responses except cytotoxic T cells have been identified in people infected in childhood, and the failure to detect the latter is probably due entirely to the fact that these cells are found only in the acute stage of infection. G. Klein (1975) pointed out that EBV is a highly successful virus in that it colonizes most of the human race and by maintaining a low profile sustains a productive infection in all or most of its hosts. IM may be a relatively new disease that has emerged as increased sophistication of certain societies has resulted in a large proportion of the population escaping the childhood mode of transmission to which the virus had adapted. That mode of transmission is still ill-understood.

Is there any difference in the residual immunity to EBV in those people who have clinically silent childhood infections and those who have had IM? A comparative study of these two groups would be of interest. One group of children that appears to show a difference in immune response from all other groups studied is that from West Nile. No other population has shown such an early and intense response to the virus as measured by the anti-VCA titers. Also, whereas in all other groups studied the anti-VCA titers are maintained at a constant level for the remainder of the person's life, in the West Nile children, there is a marked fall in titers, which in some reach undetectable levels. Since this has been observed independently by two different groups, it is presumably not a cohort effect, though a longitudinal study of a single group is needed to establish this point. This observation is the only response to EBV that appears to differentiate a population in an area of BL endemicity from other areas of the world. Do similar patterns of antibody response occur in other parts of Africa, in particular in those areas such as Southwest Uganda where the tumor is rare? Such questions are easier to ask than to answer in view of the enormous problems involved in mounting serological surveys of infant populations. Nevertheless, the question is of fundamental importance.

How is EBV transmitted to such very young infants in West Nile? Two possibilities are immediately apparent. One is that EBV-infected lymphocytes are transmitted to the infant via breast milk. In comparison with Europeans and North Americans, rural Africans are more likely to breast-feed their infants, and this feeding is likely to be maintained for a longer period of time. Prolonged breast-feeding until after the time that maternal antibodies disappear from the infant's blood may allow transmission of the virus by this route. Is there such a marked difference, however, between the feeding habits of mothers in West Nile and in the Indian and Chinese communities of Singapore? The second possibility is that the virus is transmitted by biting insects. Mosquitos interrupted in their feeding on one patient can transmit malaria by purely mechanical means, without replication of the parasite. Similarly, mosquitos have been shown to transmit a transplantable reticulum-cell sarcoma to newborn hamsters (Banfield et al., 1965). Is there a species of mosquito found only in the wet tropics that is particularly able to effect the transmission of EBV-infected lymphocytes?

Is the response to EBV different in those children infected in early infancy from those infected later in childhood? Two factors appear to differentiate these children. First, they develop very high titers of antibodies to EBV VCA. This probably indicates an intense infection of many cells throughout the body, a situation that might prime a large population for subsequent neoplastic development. Second, antibody levels to VCA fall during childhood, in some instances to undetectable levels. Does this reflect immunological immaturity or the elimination of most of the productively infected cells? Does the intense humoral response compensate for deficient cell-mediated responses? It is those T-cell responses that eliminate the nonproductively infected cells that may give rise to neoplasms, since productively infected cells die.

The evidence implicating EBV in the etiology of BL is now substantial, but not conclusive. High titers of antibodies to VCA and other EBV-determined antigens are found in almost all African patients with BL and in a proportion of non-African cases. Similarly, EBV DNA is found in almost all African cases of BL, which suggests that even if the virus has no etiological role, the tumor almost invariably arises in an EBV-genome-positive clone of cells. The suggestion that EBV is merely a passenger taking advantage of the expansion of a neoplastic B-cell clone appears unlikely. The virus is absent from all non-BL lymphomas studied to date. EBV-genome-negative cell lines were established from lymphomas in patients with antibodies to VCA, and it was possible to infect these cell lines with EBV *in vitro* (Klein, G., 1975).

A number of properties of EBV support the concept that it has oncogenic potential, in particular its ability to immortalize lymphocytes from EBV-negative donors. Such lymphocytes will replicate indefinitely in culture and can be transplanted to suitably conditioned experimental animals. The production of lymphomas in nonhuman primates by EBV is strong supportive evidence in favor of an oncogenic role in humans. This should be tempered, however, by the observation that tumors in marmosets are polyclonal. Are these tumors more akin to uncontrolled IM, rather than BL?

The significance of the characteristic cytogenetic abnormality found in almost all BL biopsies and cell lines has yet to be determined. It has been found in other lymphomas, and is thus lymphoma-associated rather than BL-associated. It is not found in EBV-positive lymphoblastoid cell lines nor in lymphoma-derived cell lines superinfected with EBV. Does it indicate genetic susceptibility to chromosome breakages or the intervention of another virus capable of causing such breakages? It is possible that EBV causes chromosome breakages in a small proportion of cells, and that expansion of this clone results in BL. The postulated role of malaria in the etiology of BL is that it either causes the expansion of a susceptible pool of B-cells before EBV infection or acts as a promoting factor after EBV infection, stimulating expansion and finally neoplastic transformation of a primed clone of cells. Alternatively, by immune depression or reticuloendothelial blockade, it might allow the growth of a neoplastic clone of cells that would otherwise be eliminated by immune surveillance.

In the search for a plausible hypothesis for the etiology of BL, the various potential combinations of EBV and malaria with or without other factors are legion. The final proof that EBV is oncogenic appears to be always just out of reach. Ethical considerations preclude direct human experimentation, and the results of animal experiments are not necessarily applicable to man. The case for EBV being implicated in the etiology of BL would be greatly strengthened if the seroepidemiology of the virus could be correlated with the epidemiology of the tumor. In this respect, the findings of de Thé and his colleagues in West Nile are encouraging. Vaccination programs, if successful, would also help to incriminate the virus; however, apart from logistic difficulties, such programs are probably not ethically justified given our present state of knowledge (Morrow *et al.,* 1976b).

References

Adams, R. A., Foley, G. E., and Uzman, B. G., 1967, Leukemia: Serial transplantation of human leukemic lymphoblasts in the newborn Syrian hamster, *Cancer Res.* **27**:772–782.

Adams, R. A., Foley, G. E., and Farber, S., 1970, Serial transplantation of Burkitt's tumors (EB3) cells in newborn Syrian hamsters and its facilitation by antilymphocyte serum, *Cancer Res.* **30**:338–345.

Andersson, M., Klein, G., Ziegler, J. L., and Henle, W., 1976, Association of Epstein–Barr viral genomes with American Burkitt lymphoma, *Nature (London)* **260**:357–359.

Arseneau, J. C., Canellos, G. P., Banks, P. M., Berard, C. W., Gralnick, H. R., and DeVita, V. T., 1975, American Burkitt's lymphoma: A clinicopathological study of 30 cases. I. Clinical factors relating to prolonged survival, *Am. J. Med.* **58**:314–321.

Banatvala, J. E., Best, J. M., and Weller, D. K., 1972, Epstein–Barr virus-specific IgM in infectious mononucleosis, Burkitt lymphoma and nasopharyngeal carcinoma, *Lancet* **1**:1205–1208.

Banfield, W. G., Woke, P. A., MacKay, C. M., and Cooper, H. L., 1965, Mosquito transmission of a reticulum cell sarcoma of hamsters, *Science* **148**:1239–1240.

Banks, P. M., Arseneau, J. C., Gralnick, H. R., Canellos, G. P., DeVita, V. T., and Berard, C. W., 1975, American Burkitt's lymphoma: A clinicopathologic study of 30 cases. II. Pathologic correlations. *Am. J. Med.* **58**:322–329.

Bar, R. S., Delor, C. J., Clausen, K. P., Hurtubise, P., Henle, W., and Hewetson, J. F., Fatal infectious mononucleosis in a family, *N. Engl. J. Med.* **290**:363–367.

Beer, A. E., and Billingham, R. S., 1975, Immunologic benefits and hazards of milk in maternal–perinatal relationship, *Ann. Intern. Med.* **83**:865–871.

Berard, C., O'Conor, G. T., Thomas, L. B., and Torloni, H., 1969, Histopathological definition of Burkitt's tumour, *Bull. W.H.O.* **40**:601–607.

Binder, R. A., Jencks, J. A., Chum, B., and Rath, C. E., 1975, "B" cell origin of malignant cells in a case of American Burkitt's lymphoma, *Cancer* **36**:161–168.

Black, F. L., Woodall, J. P., Evans, A. S., Lebhaver, H., and Henle, G., 1970, Prevalence of antibody against viruses in the Tiriyo, an isolated Amazon tribe, *Am. J. Epidemiol.* **91**:430–438.

Bornkamm, G. W., Stein, H., Lennert, K. , Ruggeberg, F., Bartels, H., and Zur Hausen, H., 1976, Attempts to demonstrate virus-specific sequences in human tumors. IV. EB viral DNA in European Burkitt lymphoma and immunoblastic lymphadenopathy with excessive plasmacytosis. *Int. J. Cancer* **17**:177–181.

Braylan, R. C., Jaffe, E. S., and Berard, C. W., 1975, Malignant lymphomas: Current classification and new observations, in: *Hematologic and Lymphoid Pathology Decennial 1966–1975* (S. C. Sommers, ed.), pp. 333–390, Appleton-Century-Crofts, New York.

Brown, T. D. K., Ernberg, I., Lannon, E. W., and Klein, G., 1974, Detection of Epstein–Barr virus (EBV)-associated nuclear antigen in human lymphoblastoid cell lines using an ^{125}I-IgG binding assay, *Int. J. Cancer* **13**:785–792.

Brubaker, G., Geser, A., and Pike, M. C., 1973, Burkitt's lymphoma in the North Mara District of Tanzania 1964–70: Failure to find evidence of time–space clustering in a high risk isolated rural area, *Br. J. Cancer* **28**:469–472.

Burkitt, D., 1959, Sarcoma involving jaws in African children, *Br. J. Surg.* **46**:218–233.

Burkitt, D., 1962a, A children's cancer dependent on climatic factors, *Nature (London)* **194**:232–234.

Burkitt, D., 1962b, Determining the climatic limitations of a children's cancer common in Africa, *Br. Med. J.* **2**:1019–1023.

Burkitt, D. P., 1967, Clinical evidence suggesting the development of an immunological response against African lymphoma, in: *Treatment of Burkitt's Tumour* (J. H. Burchenal and D. P. Burkitt, eds.), UICC Monogr. Ser. **8**:197–203, Springer-Verlag, Berlin.

Burkitt, D. P., 1969, Etiology of Burkitt's lymphoma—An alternative to a vectored virus, *J. Natl. Cancer. Inst.* **42**:19–28.

Burkitt, D. P., and Kyalwazi, S. K., 1967, Spontaneous remission of African lymphoma, *Br. J. Cancer* **21**:14–16.

Burkitt, D. P., and Wright, D., 1966, Geographical and tribal distribution of the African lymphoma in Uganda, *Br. Med. J.* **1**:569–573.

Burkitt, D. P., Hutt, M. S. R., and Wright, D. H., 1965, The African lymphoma: Preliminary observations on response to therapy, *Cancer* **18**:399–410.

Businco, L., Rezza, E., Giunchi, G., and Ainti, F., 1975, Thymus transplantation: Reconstitution of cellular immunity of a four-year-old patient with T-cell deficiency, *Clin. Exp. Immunol.* **21**:32–38.

Carter, R. L., 1966, Antibody formation in infectious mononucleosis. II. Other 19 S antibodies and false-positive serology, *Br. J. Haematol.* **12**:268.

Carter, R. L., 1972, The pathology of infectious mononucleosis—A review, in: *Oncogenesis and Herpes Viruses* (P. M. Biggs, G. de Thé, and L. N. Payne, eds.), pp. 230–238, International Agency for Research on Cancer, Lyon, France.

Carter, R. L., and Penman, H. G., 1969, Histopathology of infectious mononucleosis in: *Infectious Mononucleosis* (R. L. Carter and H. G. Penman, eds.), Blackwell, Oxford.

Cockshott, W. P., 1970, Radiological features, in: *Burkitt's Lymphoma* (D. P. Burkitt and D. H. Wright, eds.), pp. 23–33, E & S Livingstone, Edinburgh.

Cooper, E. H., 1969, Experimental studies of the atypical mononuclear cells in infectious mononucleosis in: *Infectious Mononucleosis* (R. L. Carter and H. G. Penman, eds.), pp. 121–145, Blackwell, Oxford.

Cooper, E. H., Frank, G. L., and Wright, D. H., 1966, Cell proliferation in Burkitt tumours, *Eur. J. Cancer* **2**:377–384.

Cooper, E. H., Hale, A. J., and Milton, J. D., 1967, The proliferation of infectious mononucleosis lymphocytes *in vitro, Acta Haematol.* **38**:19.

Dalldorf, G., Linsell, C. A., Barnhart, F. E., and Martyn, R., 1964, An epidemiological approach to the lymphomas of African children and Burkitt's sarcoma of the jaws, *Perspect. Biol. Med.* **7**:435–449.

Dameshek, W., 1969, Speculations on the nature of infectious mononucleosis, in: *Infectious Mononucleosis* (R. L. Carter and H. G. Penman, eds.), pp. 225–240, Blackwell, Oxford.

David, J., and Burkitt, D. P., 1968, Burkitt's lymphoma: Remissions following seemingly non-specific therapy, *Br. Med. J.* **4**:288–291.

Davidsohn, I., and Lee, C. L., 1969, The clinical serology of infectious mononucleosis, in: *Infectious Mononucleosis* (R. L. Carter and H. G., Penman, eds.), pp. 177–200, Blackwell, Oxford.

Deinhardt, F., Falk, L., Wolfe, L. G., Paeiga, J., and Johnson, D., 1975, Response of marmosets to experimental infection with Epstein–Barr virus, in: *Oncogenesis and Herpes Viruses,* Vol. 2 (G. de Thé, M. A. Epstein, and H. Zur Hausen, eds.), pp. 161–168, International Agency for Research on Cancer, Lyon, France.

De Schryver, A., Rosen, A., Gunven, P., and Klein, G., 1976, Comparison between two antibody populations in the EBV system: Anti MA versus neutralizing antibody activity, *Int. J. Cancer* **17**:8–13.

De Thé, G., 1976a, Epstein–Barr virus behaviour in different populations and implications for control of Epstein–Barr virus associated tumors, *Cancer Res.* **36**:692–695.

De Thé, G., 1976b, Seventh Annual Report, International Agency for Cancer Research, Lyon, France.

De Thé, G., Day, H. E., Geser, A., Ho, J. H. C., Lavoué, M. F., Simons, M., Sohier, J., Tukei, P., Vonka, V., and Zavadova, H., 1975, Sero-epidemiology of the Epstein–Barr virus: Preliminary analysis of an international study, in: *Oncogenesis and Herpesviruses II* (G. de Thé, M. A. Epstein, and H. Zur Hausen, eds.), IARC Scientific Publication No. 11, Vol. 2, pp. 3–16, International Agency for Research on Cancer, Lyon, France.

Diehl, V., Henle, G., Henle, W., and Kohn, G., 1968, Demonstration of a herpes group virus in cultures of peripheral leukocytes from patients with infectious mononucleosis, *J. Virol.* **2**:663–669.

Dorfman, R. F., and Warnke, R., 1974, Lymphadenopathy simulating the malignant lymphomas, *Hum. Pathol.* **5**:519–550.

Downey, H., and Stasney, J., 1936, The pathology of the lymph nodes in infectious mononucleosis, *Folia Haematol.* **54**:417–423.

Dresner, E., and Trombly, P., 1959, The latex fixation reaction in nonrheumatic diseases, *N. Engl. J. Med.* **261**:981.

Durr, F. E., Monroe, J. H., Schmitter, R., Traul, K. A., and Hirshaut, Y., 1970, Studies on the infectivity and cytopathology of Epstein–Barr virus in human lymphoblastoid cells, *Int. J. Cancer* **6**:436–449.

Edwards, J. M. B., and McSwiggan, D. A., 1975, Studies on the significance of Epstein–Barr virus-specific IgM in human sera, in: *Oncogenesis and Herpesviruses II* (G. de Thé, M. A. Epstein, and H. Zur Hausen, eds.), pp. 59–62, IARC Scientific Publication, Lyon, France.

Einhorn, N., 1972, Effect of local radiotherapy on the level of EBV-associated membrane-reactive antibodies in the sera of patients with certain malignant tumors, *Cancer* **29**:714–723.

Einhorn, N., Henle, G., Henle, W., Klein, G., and Clifford, P., 1972, Effects of local radiotherapy on the antibody levels against EBV-induced early and capsid antigens (EA and VCA) in patients with certain malignant tumours, *Int. J. Cancer* **9**:182–192.

Epstein, A. L., Henle, W., Henle, G., Hewetson, J. F., and Kaplan, H. S., 1976, Surface marker characteristics and Epstein–Barr virus studies of two established North American Burkitt's lymphoma cell lines, *Proc. Natl. Acac. Sci. U.S.A.* **73**:228–232.

Epstein, M. A., Achong, B. G., and Barr, Y. M., 1964, Virus particles in cultured lymphoblasts from Burkitt's lymphoma, *Lancet* **1**:702–703.

Epstein, M. A., Henle, G., Achong, B. G., and Barr, Y. M., 1965, Morphological and biological studies on a virus in cultured lymphoblasts from Burkitt's lymphoma, *J. Exp. Med.* **121**:761–770.

Epstein, M. A., Hunt, R. D., and Rabin, H., 1973a, Pilot experiments with EB-virus in owl monkeys (*Aotus trivirgatus*). I. Reticuloproliferative disease in an inoculated animal, *Int. J. Cancer* **12**:309–318.

Epstein, M. A., Rabin, H., Ball, G., Rickinson, A. B., Jarvis, J., and Melendez, L. V., 1973b, Pilot experiments with EB-virus in owl monkeys (*Aotus trivirgatus*). II. EB-virus in a cell line from an animal with reticuloproliferative disease, *Int. J. Cancer* **12**:319–332.

Evans, A. S., 1974, New discoveries in infectious mononucleosis, *Mod. Med.* **1**:18–24.

Evans, A. S., and Niederman, J. C., 1972, Epidemiology of infectious mononucleosis: A review, in: *Oncogenesis and Herpesviruses* (P. M. Biggs, G. de Thé, and L. N. Payne, eds.), pp. 351–356, IARC Publication No. 2, Lyon, France.

Fass, L., Herberman, R. B., Ziegler, J., and Morrow, R. H., 1970a, Evaluation of the effect of remission plasma on untreated patients with Burkitt's lymphoma, *J. Natl. Cancer Inst.* **44**:145–149.

Fass, L., Herberman, R. B., and Ziegler, J., 1970b, Delayed cutaneous hypersensitivity reactions to autologous extracts of Burkitt lymphoma cells, *N. Engl. J. Med.* **282**:776–780.

Fialkow, P. J., 1972, Use of genetic markers to study cellular origin and development of tumors in human females, *Adv. Cancer Res.* **15**:191–226.

Fialkow, P. J., Klein, G., Gartler, S. M., and Clifford, P., 1970, Clonal origin for individual Burkitt tumours, *Lancet* **1**:384–386.

Fialkow, P. J., Klein, G., and Clifford, P., 1972, Second malignant clone underlying a Burkitt tumour exacerbation, *Lancet* **2**:629–631.

Fialkow, P. J., Klein, E., Klein, G., Clifford, P., and Singh, S., 1973, Immunoglobulin and glucose-6-phosphate dehydrogenase as markers of cellular origin in Burkitt lymphoma, *J. Exp. Med.* **138**:89–102.

Finch, S. C., 1969, Laboratory findings in infectious mononucleosis, in: *Infectious Mononucleosis* (R. L. Carter and H. G. Penman, eds.), pp. 47–62, Blackwell, Oxford.

Findel, A., and Dent, P. B., 1973, Abnormalities in lymphocyte proliferation in classical and atypical measles infection, *Cell. Immunol.* **6**:41–48.

Flandrin, G., Brovet, J. C., Daniel, M. T., and Preud'homme, J. L., 1975, Acute leukaemia with Burkitt's tumour cells: A study of six cases with special reference to lymphocyte surface markers, *Blood* **45**:183–188.

Frank, A., Andiman, W. A., and Miller, G., 1976, Epstein–Barr virus and nonhuman primates: Natural and experimental infection, *Adv. Cancer Res.* **23**:171–201.

Gall, E. A., and Stout, H. A., 1940, The histological lesion in lymph nodes in infectious mononucleosis, *Am. J. Pathol.* **16**:433–443.

Gerber, P., 1972, Activation of Epstein–Barr virus by 5-bromodeoxy-uridine in "virus-free" human cells, *Proc. Natl. Acad. Sci. U.S.A.* **69**:83–85.

Gerber, P., and Deal, D. R., 1970, Epstein–Barr virus-induced viral and soluble complement-fixing antigens in Burkitt lymphoma cell cultures, *Proc. Soc. Exp. Biol. Med.* **134**:748–751.

Gerber, P., and Monroe, J. H., 1968, Studies on leukocytes growing in continuous culture derived from normal human donors, *J. Natl. Cancer Inst.* **40**:855–866.

Gerber, P., Nonoyama, M., Lucas, S., Perlin, E., and Goldstein, L. I., 1973, Oral excretion of Epstein–Barr virus by healthy subjects and patients with infectious mononucleosis, *Lancet* **2**:988–989.

Giuliano, V. J., Jasin, H. E., and Ziff, M., 1974, The nature of the atypical lymphocyte in infectious mononucleosis, *Clin. Immunol. Immunopathol.* **3**:90–98.

Gowing, N. F. C., 1975, Infectious mononucleosis: Histopathological aspects, in: *Hematologic and Lymphoid Pathology Decennial 1966–1975* (S. C. Sommers, ed.), pp. 261–280, Appleton-Century-Crofts, New York.

Gravell, M., Levine, P. H., McIntyre, R. F., Laud, V. J., and Pagane, J. S., 1976, Epstein–Barr virus in an American patient with Burkitt's lymphoma: Detection of viral genome in tumor tissue and establishment of a tumor-derived cell line (NAB), *J. Natl. Cancer Inst.* **56**:701–704.

Greaves, M. F., Brown, G., and Rickinson, A. B., 1975, Epstein–Barr virus binding sites on lymphocyte subpopulations and the origin of lymphoblasts in cultured lymphoid cell lines and in the blood of patients with infectious mononucleosis, *Clin. Immunol. Immunopathol.* **3**:514–524.

Greenwood, B. M., Bradley-Moore, A. M., Palit, A., and Bryceson, A. D. M., 1972, Immunosuppression in children with malaria, *Lancet* **1**:169–172.

Gross, R. C., Steel, C. M., Levin, A. G., Singh, S., and Brubaker, G., 1975, *In vitro* immunological studies on East African cancer patients. III. Spontaneous rosette formation by cells from Burkitt lymphoma biopsies, *Int. J. Cancer* **15**:139–143.

Gunven, P., and Klein, G., 1971, Blocking of direct membrane immunofluorescence in titration of membrane-reactive antibodies associated with EBV, *J. Natl. Cancer Inst.* **47**:539–548.

Gunven, P. G., Klein, G., Henle, G., Henle, W., and Clifford, P., 1970, Antibodies to EBV-associated membrane and viral capside antigens in Burkitt lymphoma patients, *Nature (London)* **228**:1053.

Gunven, P., Klein, G., Clifford, P., and Singh, S., 1974, Epstein–Barr virus-associated membrane reactive antibodies during long term survival after Burkitt's lymphoma, *Proc. Natl. Acad. Sci. U.S.A.* **71**:1422–1426.

Haddow, A. J., 1964, Age incidence in Burkitt's lymphoma syndrome, *E. Afr. Med. J.* **41**:1–6.

Haider, S., Coutinho, M. de L., Edmond, R. T. D., and Sutton, R. N. P., 1973, Tuberculin anergy and infectious mononucleosis, *Lancet* **2**:74.

Hampar, B., Derge, J. G., Martos, L. M., and Walker, J. L., 1972, Synthesis of Epstein–Barr Virus after activation of the viral genome in a "virus-negative" human lymphoblastoid cell (Raji) made resistant to 5-bromodeoxyuridine, *Proc. Nat. Acad. Sci.* **69**:78–82.

Harrison, C. V., 1966, Lymph nodes in infectious mononucleosis, in: *Recent Advances in Pathology* (C. V. Harrison, ed.), p. 210, J. & A. Churchill, London.

Hellström, I., and Hellström, K. F., 1970, Colony inhibition studies on blocking and non-blocking serum effects on cellular immunity to Moloney sarcomas, *Int. J. Cancer* **5**:195–201.

Henle, G., and Henle, W., 1966, Immunofluorescence in cells derived from Burkitt's lymphoma, *J. Bacteriol.* **91**:1248–1256.

Henle, G., and Henle, W., 1976, Epstein–Barr virus specific IgA serum antibodies as an outstanding feature of nasopharyngeal carcinoma, *Int. J. Cancer* **17**:1–7.

Henle, G., Henle, W., and Diehl, V., 1968, Relation of Burkitt's tumor associated herpes-type virus to infectious mononucleosis, *Proc. Natl. Acad. Sci. U.S.A.* **59**:94–101.

Henle, G., Henle, W., and Klein, G., 1971a, Demonstration of two distinct components in the early antigen complex of Epstein–Barr virus infected cells, *Int. J. Cancer* **8**:272–278.

Henle, G., Henle, W., Klein, G., Gunven, P., and Clifford, P., 1971b, Antibodies to early Epstein–Barr virus induced antigens in Burkitt's lymphoma, *J. Natl. Cancer Inst.* **46**:861–871.

Henle, W., and Henle, G., 1972, Epstein–Barr virus: The cause of infectious mononucleosis—a review, in: *Oncogenesis and Herpesviruses* (G. de Thé, P. M. Biggs, and L. N. Payne, eds.), pp. 296–274, IARC Scientific Publications, Lyon, France.

Henle, W., and Henle, G., 1975, Host responses to herpesviruses: A review, in: *Oncogenesis and Herpesviruses II* (G. de Thé, M. A. Epstein and H. Zur Hausen, eds.), pp. 215–224, IARC Scientific Publications, Lyon, France.

Henle, W., Henle, G., Zajac, B. A., Pearson, G., Wanbke, R., and Scriba, M., 1970, Differential reactivity of human serums with early antigens induced by Epstein–Barr virus, *Science* **169**:188–190.

Henle, W., Henle, G., Gunven, P., Klein, G., Clifford, P., and Singh, S., 1973, Patterns of antibodies to Epstein–Barr virus-induced early antigens in Burkitt's lymphoma: Comparison of dying patients with long-term survivors, *J. Natl. Cancer Inst.* **50**:1163–1173.

Henle, W., Henle, G. E., and Horwitz, C. A., 1974, Epstein–Barr virus specific diagnostic tests in infectious mononucleosis, *Hum. Pathol.* **5**:551–565.

Hewetson, J. F., Golub, S. H., Klein, G., and Singh, S., 1972a, Cellular reactions against Burkitt lymphoma cells. I. Colony inhibition with effector cells from patients with Burkitt's lymphoma, *Int. J. Cancer* **10**:142–149.

Hewetson, J. F., Gothoskar, B., and Klein, G., 1972b, Radioiodine labelled antibody test for the detection of membrane antigens associated with Epstein–Barr virus, *J. Natl. Cancer Inst.* **48**:87–94.

Holborow, E. J., Asherson, G. L., Johnson, G. D., Barnes, R. D. S., and Carmichael, D. J., 1963, Antinuclear factor and other antibodies in blood and liver diseases, *Br. Med. J.* **1**:656.

Holborow, E. J., Hemsted, E. H., and Mead, S. V., 1973, Smooth muscle antibodies in infectious mononucleosis, *Br. Med. J.* **3**:323.

Horowitz, C. A., Henle, W., Henle, G., and Schmitz, H., 1975, Clinical evaluation of patients with infectious mononucleosis and development of antibodies to the R component of the Epstein–Barr virus-induced early antigen complex, *Am. J. Med.* **58**:330–338.

Hutt, L. M., Huang, Y. T., and Dascomb, H. E., 1975, Enhanced destruction of lymphoid cell lines by peripheral blood leukocytes taken from patients with acute infectious mononucleosis, *J. Immunol.* **115**:243–248.

Iversen, O. H., Iversen, U., Ziegler, J. L., and Bluming, A. Z., 1974, Cell kinetics in Burkitt's lymphoma, *Eur. J. Cancer* **10**:155–163.

Jarvis, J. E., Ball, G., Rickinson, A. B., and Epstein, M. A., 1974, Cytogenetic studies in human lymphoblastoid cell lines from Burkitt's lymphomas and other sources, *Int. J. Cancer* **14**:716–721.

Johansson, B., Klein, G., Henle, W., and Henle, G., 1970, Epstein–Barr virus (EBV)-associated antibody patterns in malignant lymphomas and leukemia. I. Hodgkin's disease, *Int. J. Cancer* **6**:450–462.

Johansson, B., Klein, G., Henle, W., and Henle, G., 1971, Epstein–Barr virus (EBV)-associated antibody patterns in malignant lymphoma and leukemia. II. Chronic lymphocytic leukemia and lymphocytic lymphoma, *Int. J. Cancer* **8**:475–486.

Johansson, B., Klllander, D., Holm, G., Mellstedt, H., Henle, G., Henle, W., Klein, G., and Soderberg, G., 1975, Epstein–Barr virus (EBV) associated antibody patterns in relation to the deficiency of cell-mediated immunity in patients with Hodgkin's disease, in: *Oncogenesis and Herpesviruses II* (G. de Thé, M. A. Epstein, and H. Zur Hausen, eds.), pp. 237–247, International Agency for Research on Cancer, Lyon, France.

Johnson, G. D., and Holborow, E. J., 1963, Immunofluorescent test for infectious mononucleosis, *Nature (London)* **198**:1316.

Joncas, J., and Mitnyan, C., 1970, Serological response of the EBV antibodies in pediatric cases of infectious mononucleosis and their contacts, *Can. Med. Assoc. J.* **102**:1260–1263.

Jondal, M., 1976, Antibody-dependent cellular cytotoxicity (ADCC) against Epstein–Barr virus-determined membrane antigens. I. Reactivity in sera from normal persons and from patients with acute infectious mononucleosis, *Clin. Exp. Immunol.* **25**:1–5.

Jondal, M., Svedmyr, E., and Klein, E., 1975, Killer T cells in a Burkitt's lymphoma biopsy, *Nature (London)* **255**:405–407.

Junge, U., Hoekstra, J., and Deinhardt, S., 1971, Stimulation of peripheral lymphocytes by allogenic and autochthonous mononucleosis cell lines, *J. Immunol.* **106**:1306–1315.

Kafuko, G. W., Baingana, N., and Knight, E. M., 1969, Association of Burkitt's tumour and holoendemic malaria in West Nile District, Uganda—Malaria as a possible aetiologic factor, *E. Afr. Med. J.* **46**:414–436.

Kafuko, G. W., Henderson, B. E., and Kirya, B. G., 1972, Epstein–Barr virus antibody levels in children from the West Nile District of Uganda, *Lancet* **1**:706–709.

Kaplan, M. E., 1968, Cryoglobulinaemia in infectious mononucleosis: Quantitation and characterization of the cryoproteins, *J. Lab. Clin. Med.* **71**:754.

Kaplan, M. E., and Tan, E. M., 1968, Antinuclear antibodies in infectious mononucleosis, *Lancet* **1**:561.

Klein, E., van Furth, R., and Johnasson, B., 1972, Immunoglobulin synthesis as cellular marker of malignant lymphoid cells, in: *Oncogenesis and Herpesviruses* (P. M. Biggs, G. de Thé, and L. N. Payne, eds.), pp. 253–257, IARC Scientific Publications, Lyon, France,

Klein, E., Klein, G., and Levine, P. H., 1976, Immunological control of human lymphoma: Discussion, *Cancer Res.* **36**:724–727.

Klein, G., 1973, The Epstein–Barr virus, in: *The Herpesviruses* (A. S. Kaplan, ed.), pp. 521–555, Academic Press, New York.

Klein, G., 1974, Studies on the Epstein–Barr virus genome and the EBV-determined nuclear antigen in human malignant disease, in: *Tumor Viruses: Cold Spring Harbor Symp. Quant. Biol.* **39**:783–796.

Klein, G., 1975, The Epstein–Barr virus and neoplasia, *N. Engl. J. Med.* **293**:1353–1357.

Klein, G., and Vonka, V., 1974, Relationship between the Epstein–Barr (EBV)-determined complement fixing antigen and the nuclear antigen (EBNA) detected by anticomplement fluorescence, *J. Natl. Cancer Inst.* **53**:1645–1646.

Klein, G., Clifford, P., Klein, E., Smith, R. T., Minowada, J., Kourilsky, F. M., and Burchenal, J. H., 1967, Membrane immunofluorescence reaction of Burkitt lymphoma cells from biopsy specimens and tissue cultures, *J. Natl. Cancer Inst.* **39**:1027–1044.

Klein, G., Pearson, G., Nadkarni, J. S., Nadkarni, J. J., Klein, E., Henle, G., Henle, W., and Clifford, P., 1968, Relation between Epstein–Barr viral and cell membrane immunofluorescence of Burkitt tumor cells. I. Dependence of cell membrane immunofluorescence on presence of EB virus, *J. Exp. Med.* **128**:1011–1020.

Klein, G., Clifford, P., Henle, G., Henle, W., Geering, G., and Old, L. J., 1969, EBV-associated serological patterns in a Burkitt lymphoma patient during regression and recurrence, *Int. J. Cancer* **4**:416–421.

Klein, G., Pearson, G., Rabson, A., Ablashi, D. V., Falk, L., Wolfe, L., Deinhardt, F., and Rabin, H., 1973, Antibody reactions to Herpesvirus saimiri (HVS)-induced early and late antigens (EA and LA) in HVS-infected squirrel, marmoset and owl monkeys, *Int. J. Cancer* **12**:270–289.

Klein, G., Lindahl, T., Jondal, M., Leibold, W., Menezes, J., Nilsson, K., and Sundstrom, C., 1974, Continuous lymphoid cell lines with characteristics of B-cells (bone-marrow-derived) lacking the

Epstein–Barr virus genome and derived from three human lymphomas, *Proc. Natl. Acad. Sci. U.S.A.* **71**:3283–3286.

Klein, G., Svedmyr, E., Jondal, M., and Persson, P. O., 1976, EBV-determined nuclear antigens (EBNA)-positive cells in the peripheral blood of infectious mononucleosis patients, *Int. J. Cancer* **17**:21–26.

Kupers, T. A., Petrich, J. M., Holloway, A. W., and St. Geme, J. W., 1970, Depression of tuberculin delayed hypersensitivity by live attenuated mumps virus, *J. Pediatr.* **76**:716–721.

Leibold, W., Huldt, G., Flanagan, T. D., Andersson, M., Dalens, M., Wright, D. H., Voller, A., and Klein, G., 1976, Tumorigenicity of Epstein–Barr virus (EBV)-transformed lymphoid line cells in autologous squirrel monkeys, *Int. J. Cancer* **17**:533–541.

Levine, P. H., Ablashi, D. V., Berard, C. W., Carbone, P. P., Waggoner, D. E., and Malan, L., 1971, Elevated antibody titres to Epstein–Barr virus in Hodgkin's disease, *Cancer* **27**:416–421.

Levine, P. H., Connelly, R. R., Herberman, R. G., McCoy, J. L., and Fabrizio, P. L., 1975, Humoral and cellular immunity to EBV and lymphoid cell line antigens in human lymphoma, in: *Oncogenesis and Herpesviruses II* (G. de Thé, M. A. Epstein, and H. Zur Hausen, eds.), pp. 225–235, International Agency for Research on Cancer, Lyon, France.

Lukes, R. J., and Cox, F. H., 1958, Clinical and morphologic findings in 30 fatal cases of infectious mononucleosis, *Am. J. Pathol.* **34**:586–590.

Lukes, R. J., Tindle, B. H., and Parker, J. W., 1969, Reed–Sternberg-like cells in infectious mononucleosis, *Lancet* **2**:1003.

Magrath, I. T., Ziegler, J. L., and Templeton, A. C. 1974, A comparison of clinical and histopathologic features of childhood malignant lymphoma in Uganda, *Cancer* **33**:285–294.

Manalov, G., and Manalova, Y., 1972, Marker band in one chromosome 14 from Burkitt lymphomas, *Nature (London)* **237**:33–34.

Mangi, R. J., Niederman, J. C., and Kelleher, J. E., Jr., 1974, Depression of cell mediated immunity during acute infectious mononucleosis, *N. Engl. J. Med.* **291**:1149–1153.

Mayyasi, S. A., Schidlovsky, G., Bulfone, L. M., and Buscheck, F. T., 1967, The coating reaction of the herpes-type virus isolated from malignant tissues with an antibody present in sera, *Cancer Res.* **27**:2020–2024.

McGregor, I. A., 1964, Acquisition of immunity to *Plasmodium falciparum* infections in Africa, *Trans. R. Soc. Trop. Med. Hyg.* **58**:80–92.

Menezes, J., Leibold, W., Klein, G., and Clements, G., 1975, Establishment and characterization of an Epstein–Barr virus (EBV)-negative lymphoblastoid B cell line (BJA-B) from an exceptional EBV-genome-negative African Burkitt's lymphoma, *Biomedicine* **22**:276–284.

Miller, G., 1974, The oncogenicity of Epstein–Barr virus, *J. Infect. Dis.* **130**:187–205.

Miller, G., and Lipman, M., 1973, Release of infectious Epstein–Barr virus by transformed marmoset leukocytes, *Proc. Natl. Acad. Sci. U.S.A.* **70**:190–194.

Miller, G., Niederman, J. C., and Stitt, D. A., 1972, Infectious mononucleosis: Appearance of neutralizing antibody to Epstein–Barr virus measured by inhibition of formation of lymphoblastoid cell lines, *J. Infect. Dis.* **125**:403–406.

Moore, G. E., Gerner, R. E., and Franklin, H. A., 1967, Culture of normal human leukocytes, *J. Am. Med. Assoc.* **199**:519–524.

Morrow, R. H., Pike, M. C., Smith, P. G., Ziegler, J. L., and Kisuule, A., 1971, Burkitt's lymphoma: A time–space cluster of cases in Bwamba country of Uganda, *Br. Med. J.* **2**:491–492.

Morrow, R. H., Kisuule, A., Pike, M. C., and Smith, P. G., 1976a, Burkitt's lymphoma in the Mengo Districts of Uganda: Epidemiologic features and their relationship to malaria, *J. Natl. Cancer Inst.* **56**:479–483.

Morrow, R. H., Gutensohn, N., and Smith, P. G., 1976b, Epstein–Barr virus: Malaria interaction models for Burkitt's lymphoma—implications for preventive trials, *Cancer Res.* **36**:667–669.

Ngu, V., 1967, Host defences to Burkitt's tumour, *Br. Med. J.* **1**:345–347.

Ngu, V., McFarlane, H., Osunkoya, B. O., and Udeozo, I. O. K., 1966, Immunoglobulins in Burkitt's lymphoma, *Lancet* **2**:414–416.

Ngu, V. A., Burkitt, D. P., and Osunkoya, B. O., 1970, Clinical and related evidence of host defence mechanisms, in: *Burkitt's Lymphoma* (D. P. Burkitt and D. H. Wright, eds.), pp. 158–163, E & S Livingstone, Edinburgh.

Niederman, J. C., and Evans, A. S., 1973, Infectious mononucleosis, in: *Serological Epidemiology* (J. R. Paul and C. White, eds.), pp. 119–132, Academic Press, New York.

Niederman, J. C., McCollum, R. W., Henle, G., and Henle, W., 1968, Infectious mononucleosis: Clinical manifestation in relation to EB virus antibodies, *J. Amer. Med. Assoc.* **203**:205–229.

Niederman, J. C., Evans, A. S., Subrahmanyan, M. S., and McCollum, R. W., 1970, Prevalence, incidence and persistence of EB virus antibody in young adults, *N. Engl. J. Med.* **282**:361–365.

Nilsson, K., and Ponten, J., 1975, Classification and biological nature of established human hematopoietic cell lines, *Int. J. Cancer* **15**:321–341.

Nkrumah, F. K., and Perkins, I. V., 1976, Sickle cell trait, hemoglobin C trait, and Burkitt's lymphoma, *Am. J. Trop. Med. Hyg.* **25**:633–636.

Nonoyama, M., and Pagano, J. S., 1971, Detection of Epstein–Barr viral genome in nonproductive cells, *Nature (London) New Biol.* **233**:103–106.

Nonoyama, M., and Pagano, J. S., 1973, Homology between Epstein–Barr virus DNA and viral DNA from Burkitt's lymphoma and nasopharyngeal carcinoma determined by DNA–DNA reassociation kinetics, *Nature (London)* **242**:44–47.

O'Conor, G. T., 1970, Persistent immunologic stimulation as a factor in oncogenesis with special reference to Burkitt's tumor, *Am. J. Med.* **48**:279–285.

Papamichail, M., Sheldon, P. J., and Holborow, E. J., 1974, T- and B-cell subpopulations in infectious mononucleosis, *Clin. Exp. Immunol.* **18**:1–11.

Pattengale, P. K., Smith, R. W., and Gerber, P., 1974, B-cell characteristics of human peripheral and cord blood lymphocytes transformed by Epstein–Barr virus, *J. Natl. Cancer Inst.* **52**:1081–1086.

Pearson, G. R., and Orr, T. W., 1976, Antibody-dependent lymphocyte cytotoxicity against cells expressing Epstein–Barr virus antigens, *J. Natl. Cancer Inst.* **56**:485–488.

Pearson, G., Dewey, F., Klein, G., Henle, G., and Henle, W., 1970, Relation between neutralization of Epstein–Barr virus and antibodies to cell-membrane antigens induced by the virus, *J. Natl. Cancer Inst.* **45**:989–995.

Pereira, M. S., Blake, J. M., and Macrae, A. D., 1969, EB virus antibody at different ages, *Br. Med. J.* **4**:526–527.

Pike, M. C., and Morrow, R. H., 1972, Some epidemiological problems with "EBV + malaria gives BL"—A review, in: *Oncogenesis and Herpesviruses* (P. M. Biggs, G. de Thé, and L. N. Payne, eds.), pp. 349–350, IARC, Lyon, France.

Pike, M., Williams, E. H., and Wright, B., 1967, Burkitt's tumour in the West Nile District of Uganda, 1961–65, *Br. Med. J.* **2**:395–399.

Pike, M., Morrow, R. H., Kisuule, A., and Mafigiri, J., 1970, Burkitt's lymphoma and sickle cell trait, *Br. J. Prev. Soc. Med.* **24**:39–41.

Pope, J. H., Achong, B. G., and Epstein, M. A., 1968, Cultivation and fine structure of virus-bearing lymphoblasts from a second New Guinea Burkitt lymphoma: Establishment of sublines with unusual cultural properties, *Int. J. Cancer* **3**:171–182.

Pope, J. H., Norne, M. K., and Wetters, E. J., 1969, Significance of a complement-fixing antigen associated with herpes-like virus and detected in the Raji cell line, *Nature (London)* **222**:186–187.

Pulvertaft, R. J. V., 1964, A study of malignant tumours in Nigeria by short term tissue culture, *J. Clin. Pathol.* **18**:261–283.

Purtilo, D. T., 1976, Pathogenesis and phenotypes of an X-linked recessive lymphoproliferative syndrome, *Lancet* **2**:882–885.

Rabson, A. S., O'Conor, G. T., Baron, S., Whang, J. J., and Legallais, F. Y., 1966, Morphologic, cytogenetic and virologic studies *in vitro* of a malignant lymphoma from an African child, *Int. J. Cancer* **1**:89–106.

Reedman, B. M., and Klein, G., 1973, Cellular localisation of an Epstein–Barr virus (EBV-associated complement-fixing antigen) in producer and nonproducer lymphoblastoid cell lines, *Int. J. Cancer* **11**:499–520.

Reedman, B. M., Pope, J. H., and Moss, D. J., 1972, Identity of the soluble EBV-associated antigens of human lymphoid cell lines, *Int. J. Cancer* **9**:172–181.

Rocchi, G., and Hewetson, J. F., 1973, A practical and quantitative microtest for determination of neutralizing antibodies against Epstein–Barr virus, *J. Gen. Virol.* **18**:385–391.

Rosenberg, E. B., McCoy, J. L., Green, S. S., Donnelly, F. C., Siwarski, D. F., Levine, P. H., and Heberman, R. B., 1974, Destruction of human lymphoid tissue-culture cell lines by human peripheral lymphocytes in ^{51}Cr-release cytotoxicity assays, *J. Natl. Cancer Inst.* **52**:345–352.

Royston, I., Sullivan, J. L., Periman, P. O., and Perlin, E., 1975, Cell-mediated immunity to Epstein–

Barr-virus-transformed lymphoblastoid cells in acute infectious mononucleosis, *N. Engl. J. Med.* **293**:1159–1163.

Rubin, A. D., 1966, Lymphocyte RNA synthesis in infectious mononucleosis: The response to phyto-hemagglutinin *in vitro*, *Blood* **28**:602.

Sawitsky, A., Papps, J. P., and Weiner, L. M., 1950, The demonstration of antibody in acute hemolytic anemia complicating infectious mononucleosis, *Am. J. Med.* **8**:260.

Sawyer, R. N., Evans, A. S., Niederman, J. C., and McCollum, R. W., 1971, Prospective studies of a group of Yale University freshmen. I. Occurrence of infectious mononucleosis, *J. Infect. Dis.* **123**:263–270.

Schmitz, H., and Scherer, M., 1972, IgM antibodies to Epstein–Barr virus in infectious mononucleosis, *Arch. Gesamte Virusforsch.* **37**:332–339.

Sheldon, P. J., Papamichail, M., Hemsted, E. H., and Holborow, E. J., 1973, Thymic origin of atypical lymphoid cells in infectious mononucleosis, *Lancet* **1**:1153–1155.

Shepherd, J. J., and Wright, D. H., 1967, Burkitt's tumour presented as bilateral swelling of the breast in women of child-bearing age, *Br. J. Surg.* **54**:776–780.

Shope, T. C., 1975, Prevention of Epstein–Barr virus (EBV)-induced infection in cotton-topped marmosets by human serum containing EBV neutralizing activity, in: *Oncogenesis and Herpesviruses II* (G. de Thé, M. A. Epstein, and H. Zur Hausen, eds.), pp. 153–159, International Agency for Research on Cancer, Lyon, France.

Shope, T., and Miller, G., 1973, Epstein–Barr virus: Heterophile responses in squirrel monkeys inoculated with virus-transformed autologous leukocytes, *J. Exp. Med.* **137**:140–147.

Shope, T., Deichario, D., and Miller, G., 1973, Malignant lymphoma in cotton-topped marmosets following inoculation of Epstein–Barr virus, *Proc. Natl. Acad. Sci. U.S.A.* **10**:2487–2491.

Silvestre, D., Kourilsky, F. M., Klein, G., Yata, Y., Neupont-Sautes, C., and Levy, J. P., 1971, Relationship between the EBV-associated membrane antigen on Burkitt lymphoma cells and the viral envelope, demonstrated by immunoferritin labelling, *Int. J. Cancer* **8**:222–233.

Smith, D. S., Abell, J. D., and Cast, I. P., 1963, Autoimmune haemolytic anaemia and thrombocytopenia complicating infectious mononucleosis, *Br. Med. J.* **2**:1210.

Southam, C. M., Burchenal, J. H., and Clarkson, B., 1969, Heterotransplantation of human cell lines from Burkitt's tumors and acute leukemia into newborn rats, *Cancer* **23**:281–299.

Stjernsward, J., Clifford, P., and Svedmyr, E., 1970, General and tumour-distinctive cellular immunological reactivity, in: *Burkitt's Lymphoma* (D. P. Burkitt and D. H. Wright, eds.), pp. 164–171, E & S Livingstone, Edinburgh.

Strauch, B., Andrews, L. L., Siegel, N., and Miller, G., 1974, Oropharyngeal excretion of Epstein–Barr virus by renal transplant recipients and other patients treated with immunosuppressive drugs, *Lancet* **1**:234–237.

Svedmyr, E., and Jondal, M., 1975, Cytotoxic effector cells specific for B cell lines transformed by Epstein–Barr virus are present in patients with infectious mononucleosis, *Proc. Natl. Acad. Sci. U.S.A.* **72**:1622–1626.

Svedmyr, A., Demissie, A., Klein, G., and Clifford, P., 1970, Antibody patterns in different human sera against intracellular and membrane–antigen complexes associated with Epstein–Barr virus, *J. Natl. Cancer Inst.* **44**:595–610.

Thomas, D. B., 1972, Antibodies to membrane antigen(s) common to thymocytes and a subpopulation of lymphocytes in infectious mononucleosis sera, *Lancet* **1**:399.

Tindle, B. H., Parker, J. W., and Lukes, R. J., 1972, "Reed–Sternberg-cells" in infectious mononucleosis, *Am. J. Clin. Pathol.* **58**:607.

Tischendorf, P., Shramek, G. J., Balagtas, R. C., Deinhardt, F., Knospe, W. H., Noble, G. R., and Maynard, J. E., 1970, Development and persistence of immunity to Epstein–Barr virus in man, *J. Infect. Dis.* **122**:401–409.

Vonka, V., Benyesh-Melnick, M., Lewis, R. T., and Wimberly, I., 1970, Some properties of the soluble (s) antigen of cultured lymphoblastoid cell lines, *Arch. Gesamte Virusforsch.* **31**:113–124.

Vonka, V., Vlčková, I., Závadová, H. Kouba, K., Lazovská, J., and Duben, J., 1972, Antibodies to EB virus capsid antigen and to soluble antigen of lymphoblastoid cells in infectious mononucleosis patients, *Int. J. Cancer* **9**:529–535.

Wahren, B., Lantorp, K., Sterner, G., and Espmark, A., 1970, Antibodies in family contacts of patients with infectious mononucleosis, *Proc. Soc. Exp. Biol. Med.* **133**:934–939.

Wands, J. R., Perrotto, J. L., and Isselbacher, K. J., 1976, Circulating immune complexes and complement sequence activation in infectious mononucleosis, *Am. J. Med.* **60**:269–272.

Werner, J., Woolf, H., Apodaca, J., and Zur Hausen, H., 1975, Lymphoproliferative disease in a cotton-topped marmoset after inocluation with infectious mononucleosis-derived Epstein–Barr virus, *Int. J. Cancer* **15**:1000–1008.

Williams, E. H., Spit, P., and Pike, M. C., 1969, Further evidence of space–time clustering of Burkitt's lymphoma patients in the West Nile District of Uganda, *Br. J. Cancer* **23**:235–246.

Williams. E. H., Day, N. E., and Geser, A. G., 1974, Seasonal variation in onset of Burkitt's lymphoma in the West Nile District of Uganda, *Lancet* **2**:19–22.

Wollheim, F. A., and Williams, R. C., 1966, Studies on the macroglobulins of human serum. I. Polyclonal immunoglobulin class M (IgM) increase in infectious mononucleosis, *N. Engl. J. Med.* **274**:61.

Wright, D. H., 1963, Cytology and histochemistry of the Burkitt lymphoma, *Br. J. Cancer* **17**:50–55.

Wright, D. H., 1964, Burkitt's tumour: A post-mortem study of 50 cases, *Br. J. Surg.* **51**:245–251.

Wright, D. H., 1966, Burkitt's tumour in England: A comparison with childhood lymphosarcoma, *Int. J. Cancer* **1**:503–514.

Wright, D. H., 1967, The epidemiology of Burkitt's tumor, *Cancer Res.* **27**:2424–2438.

Wright, D. H., 1970a, Gross distribution and haematology, in: *Burkitt's Lymphoma* (D. P. Burkitt and D. H. Wright, eds.), pp. 64–81, E & S Livingstone, Edinburgh.

Wright, D. H., 1970b, Microscopic features, histochemistry, histogenesis and diagnosis, in: *Burkitt's Lymphoma* (D. P. Burkitt and D. H. Wright, eds.), pp. 82–102, E & S Livingston, Edinburgh.

Wright, D. H., 1971, Burkitt's lymphoma: A review of the pathology, immunology and possible etiologic factors, in: *Pathology Annual* (S. C. Sommers, ed.), pp. 337–363, Appleton-Century-Crofts, New York.

Yefenof, E., Klein, G., Jondal, M., and Oldstone, M. B. A., 1976, Surface markers on human B- and T-lymphocytes. IX. Two-color immunofluorescence studies on the association between EBV receptors and complement receptors on the surface of lymphoid cell lines, *Int. J. Cancer* **17**:693–700.

Zech, L., Haglund, U., Nilsson, K., and Klein, G., 1976, Characteristic chromosomal abnormalities in biopsies and lymphoid-cell lines from patients with Burkitt and non-Burkitt lymphomas, *Int. J. Cancer* **17**:47–56.

Ziegler, J. L., Cohen, M. H., Morrow, R. H., Kyalwazi, S. K., and Carbone, P. P., 1970, Immunologic studies in Burkitt's lymphoma, *Cancer* **25**:734–739.

Ziegler, J. L., Wright, D. H., and Kyalwazi, S. K., 1971, Differential diagnosis of Burkitt's lymphoma of the face and jaws, *Cancer* **27**:503–514.

Ziegler, J. L., Andersson, M., Klein, G., and Henle, W., 1976, Detection of Epstein–Barr virus DNA in American Burkitt's lymphoma, *Int. J. Cancer* **17**:701–706.

Zur Hausen, H., 1975, Oncogenic herpes viruses, *Biochim. Biophys. Acta* **417**:25–53.

Zur Hausen, H., 1976, Biochemical approaches to detection of Epstein–Barr virus in human tumors, *Cancer Res.* **36**:678–680.

Zur Hausen, H., Henle, W., Hummeler, K., Diehl, V., and Henle, G., 1967, Comparative study of cultured Burkitt tumor cells by immunofluorescence, autoradiography and electron microscopy, *J. Virol.* **1**:830–837.

Zur Hausen, H., Schulte-Holthausen, H., Klein, G., Henle, W., Henle, G., Clifford, P., and Santesson, L., 1970, EBV DNA in biopsies of Burkitt's tumours and anaplastic carcinomas of the nasopharynx, *Nature (London)* **228**:1056–1058.

14

α-Chain Disease: A Possible Model for the Pathogenesis of Human Lymphomas

MAXIME SELIGMANN and JEAN-CLAUDE RAMBAUD

1. Introduction

α-Chain disease (α-CD) is a proliferative disorder of B lymphoid cells involving primarily the IgA secretory system, in which plasma cells produce a presumably homogeneous population of immunoglobulin (Ig) molecules consisting of incomplete α chains devoid of light (L) chains. Since the first description of this new Ig abnormality (Seligmann *et al.*, 1968) in a young Syrian patient affected with malabsorption and diffuse plasmacytic infiltration of the small intestine (Rambaud *et al.*, 1968), more than 150 cases have been recognized to our knowledge. Thus, α-CD appears to be by far the most frequent of the heavy (H)-chain diseases.

In three patients, α-CD was apparently confined to the respiratory tract. All the other patients were affected with the digestive form of α-CD, which is localized mainly in the small intestine and the mesenteric lymph nodes.

α-CD appears to proceed in two stages. The early stage is characterized by a possibly nonmalignant diffuse and extensive plasma-cell infiltration, whereas the latter stage is characterized by overt malignancy and supervening immunoblastic lymphoma. The elucidation of this sequence of events and of the natural history of the disease may offer a revealing insight into the development of lymphomas in man. Moreover, the sociogeographic distribution of the digestive form of α-CD shows a clear predilection for underprivileged populations living in areas with a high

MAXIME SELIGMANN • Laboratory of Immunochemistry and Immunopathology (INSERM U 108), Research Institute on Blood Diseases, Hôpital Saint-Louis, Paris 10, France. JEAN-CLAUDE RAMBAUD • Department of Gastroenterology and Research Unit on Physiopathology of Digestion (INSERM U 54), Hôpital Saint-Lazare, Paris 10, France.

degree of infestation by intestinal pathogens. This finding, as well as the evidence for complete remissions achieved in early stage by oral antibiotic therapy (see Section 4), imply that environmental factors (which do not exclude the possible role of predisposing genetic factors) play a presumably crucial role in the pathogenesis of this disorder. α-CD may thus constitute a model providing unique opportunities for research into the pathogenesis of human lymphomas.

2. Immunoglobulin Abnormalities

2.1. Laboratory Diagnosis

The diagnosis of α-CD relies entirely on laboratory studies including immunochemical analysis of the serum proteins, and, as previously emphasized (Seligmann et al., 1969, 1971), it may offer some difficulties in a routine laboratory. The diagnosis can easily be missed on the serum protein electrophoregram; the pathological protein was not noticeable in this test in half the 90 cases studied in our laboratory. When detected by electrophoresis, the pathological α-CD protein shows an abnormal broad band usually in the $\alpha 2$ and β regions (Figure 1). The characteris-

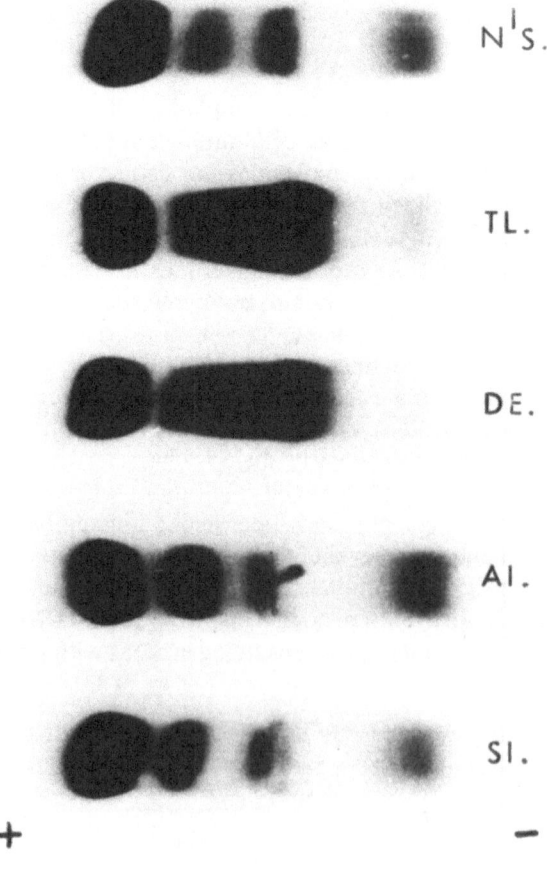

Figure 1. Agar gel electrophoretic pattern of the serum of four patients with α-CD, compared with normal serum (N'S.). In patients TL and DE, an abnormal very broad band is observed. In patient Al, there is only an increase in $\alpha 2$ globulins. In patient SI, the pathological protein is not noticeable. Reproduced from Seligmann et al. (1969) with the permission of the *Journal of Clinical Investigation*.

tic narrow band, which is suggestive of a monoclonal Ig abnormality, is always lacking. In most of the cases in which the pathological protein was not noticeable, serum electrophoresis showed only a decrease in serum albumin and a moderate to severe hypogammaglobulinemia (Figure 1).

427

α-CHAIN DISEASE: A
POSSIBLE MODEL
FOR THE
PATHOGENESIS OF
HUMAN
LYMPHOMAS

The diagnosis is usually suspected or established by the immunoelectrophoretic analysis of the serum of these patients (Figure 2). In many cases, the protein abnormality escaped detection by routine immunoelectrophoresis using polyvalent antiserum to normal human serum; analysis with monospecific antisera to IgA is essential. The abnormal component usually gives an abnormal precipitin line either extending from the α1 globulins to the slow β2 region or showing a faster electrophoretic mobility than normal IgA. In a few patients, however, the α-CD protein had a slow electrophoretic mobility. The anomalous component does not, of course, precipitate with antisera to L chains. It should be emphasized, however, that this lack of precipitation with anti-κ and anti-λ antisera is not a sufficient criterion for the diagnosis of α-CD, since a number of IgA myeloma proteins, even though they contained L chains (mainly λ chains), failed to precipitate with such antisera.

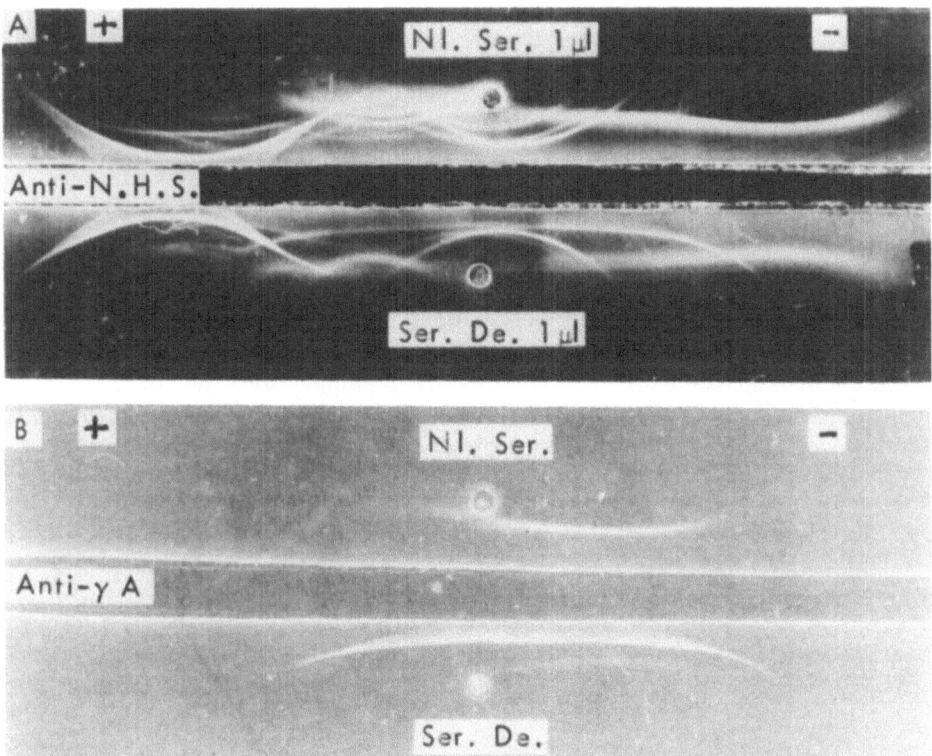

Figure 2. Immunoelectrophoretic analysis of the serum of a patient with α-CD (De) compared with normal serum (Nl. Ser.) developed with a polyvalent antiserum to whole normal human serum (anti-N.H.S.) (A) and an antiserum to α chains (anti-γ A) (B). Note the abnormal broad precipitin line. The line given by this abnormal component was not revealed by antisera to κ or λ L chains. Reproduced from Seligmann *et al.* (1971) with the permission of the *Annals of the New York Academy of Sciences*.

Selected antisera to IgA, which contain antibodies related to the conformational specificity of the Fab region, which precipitate only with α and L chains combined, were found to be very useful for the diagnosis of α-CD by immunoelectrophoresis (Figure 3) or the Ouchterlony technique (Figure 4) (Seligmann et al., 1969). The immunoselection technique of Radl combined with immunoelectrophoresis (Doe et al., 1972) is a little more sensitive and is also of great help when potent and carefully selected antisera to light chains are available. In all doubtful cases, the pathological protein should be purified, reduced, and alkylated, and the lack of L chains should be demonstrated directly by starch or polyacrylamide gel electrophoresis or by gel filtration after dissociating the molecule.

The serum levels of normal IgA, IgG, and IgM molecules are usually depressed. These decreases are not due solely to a protein-losing enteropathy, as shown by the disproportionate depression of serum Ig levels relative to the serum albumin concentration. Deficiencies of humoral immunity, as well as of cellular immunity, have been demonstrated in a few patients (Rambaud et al., 1970; Manousos et al., 1974). To our knowledge, no functional tests of the secretory immune system have been performed in these patients.

The diagnosis of α-CD is made more difficult by the very low concentration of pathological protein in the urine. In most patients, however, it could be detected in concentrated urine and had the same electrophoretic and immunochemical characteristics as that in the serum. Bence Jones proteinuria was never found. The pathological protein was also found in significant amounts in jejunal fluid in the digestive form of α-CD, as expected from the involvement of the intestine, whereas the secretory IgA in the parotid saliva of these patients was normal (Seligmann et al., 1969).

In patients with a clinicopathological pattern analogous to that of α-CD but without detectable α-CD protein in the serum, the search for the abnormal Ig should be systematically performed in the secretions, i.e., in the intestinal fluid in the digestive form of the disease. In those patients without detectable α-CD protein, in neither the serum nor the secretions, the production of α-CD protein by the proliferating cells should be searched for by immunofluorescence or biosynthetic studies (Seligmann et al., 1969; Buxbaum and Preud'homme, 1972), since nonsecretory forms of α-CD may exist analogous to nonsecretory human and murine

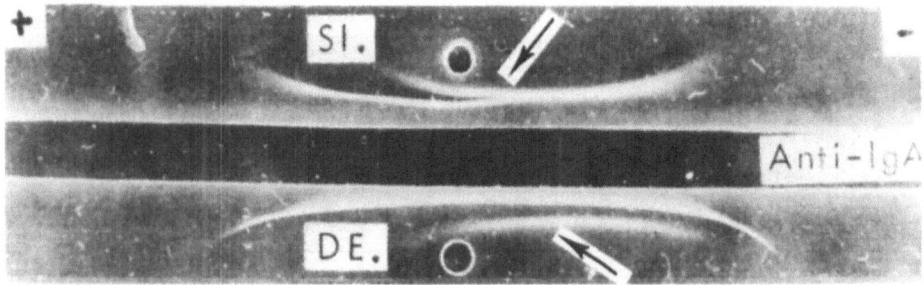

Figure 3. Immunoelectrophoretic analysis of two α-CD sera using a specific antiserum to IgA that contains, after absorption with L chains, precipitating antibodies reacting with the L–H chain combination. The precipitin line corresponding to normal IgA is shown by the arrows. This line spurs over the α-CD protein line of serum Sl, whereas it is inside the α-CD protein line in serum DE. Reproduced from Seligmann et al. (1971) with the permission of the Annals of the New York Academy of Sciences.

429

α-CHAIN DISEASE: A
POSSIBLE MODEL
FOR THE
PATHOGENESIS OF
HUMAN
LYMPHOMAS

Figure 4. Ouchterlony test for identification of α-CD protein. The selected antiserum to IgA in the center well is that used in Figure 3. It shows that the serum under study (X) contains an α-CD protein, since the precipitin line is deficient when compared with normal IgA (N¹S.) and with IgA1 myeloma proteins of both L-chain types (δA1 L., γA1 K.), while it is in identity with the reference α-CD protein (TL). Reproduced from Seligmann *et al.* (1969) by permission of the *Journal of Clinical Investigation.*

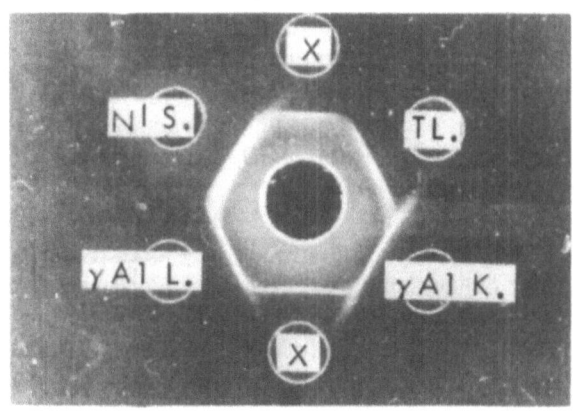

myeloma. Immediate degradation of the incomplete α chains may occur in these forms.

Interesting exceptions to the usual Ig findings in α-CD have been reported. A small homogeneous IgG component was found in addition to α-CD protein in serum in two cases (Seligmann, 1975a). The sera from two patients with the clinicopathological pattern of the digestive form of α-CD were found to contain an entire IgA myeloma globulin; Bence Jones protein was also present in the urine of one of these two cases (Chantar *et al.*, 1974; Tangun *et al.*, 1975). In another young girl presenting with the typical clinicopathological features of intestinal α-CD, a γ-CD protein was demonstrated in the serum and in the intestinal biopsy (Seligmann, 1975b).

2.2. Structural and Cellular Studies

α-CD is defined as the production of a population of molecules consisting of incomplete heavy α chains and devoid of L chains.

The striking and unexpected electrophoretic heterogeneity of these presumably monoclonal α-CD proteins may be related to their high carbohydrate content (Seligmann *et al.*, 1971) and to their high tendency to polymerize. Indeed, on ultracentrifugation, α-CD proteins appear to consist of dimers with a 3–4 S sedimentation constant and, in most instances, of larger polymers of various sizes (Seligmann *et al.*, 1969). Joining (J) chain was found in all α-CD proteins so far studied (Seligmann, 1975a). The electric charge heterogeneity of α-CD proteins is certainly due in part to the fact that the *N*-terminal sequences of several such proteins are heterogeneous, as shown by Seligmann *et al.* (1971). Even for some proteins with a single *N*-terminal amino acid residue, marked heterogeneity became apparent after two steps in degradation. Attempts to obtain the *N*-terminal sequence on an automated sequencer were unsuccessful. The *N*-terminal residues were different from those found in any of the subgroups of the variable (V) regions of normal H chains. This heterogeneity is probably the consequence of a limited intracellular proteolysis occurring after the synthesis of an incomplete α H chain. That the *N*-terminal residues found in the seven proteins studied were valine or isoleucine or both suggests that the degradation stops at this level for some reason, which could be enzyme specificity, steric hindrance, or the presence of a carbohydrate moiety. An analogous limited intracellular postsynthetic proteolysis of the

NH_2-terminus of an incomplete protein was described for a non-sense mutant of alkaline phosphatase produced by *Escherichia coli* (Natori and Garen, 1970). Alternatively, postsynthetic cleavage may occur extracellularly. In one case of γ-CD, the nascent abnormal chain in the cytoplasm and in the culture fluid during biosynthetic studies had a molecular weight of 36,000, in contrast to the molecular weight of the serum γ-CD protein, which was 28,000 daltons (Buxbaum and Preud'homme, 1972).

The molecular weight of the monomeric polypeptide subunit of several serum α-CD proteins was found to vary between 29,000 and 34,000 (Dorrington *et al.*, 1970; Seligmann *et al.*, 1971). The length of these chains was thus greater than half but smaller than three quarters of normal $\alpha 1$ H chains. Antigenic analysis (Seligmann *et al.*, 1969) and chemical studies (Seligmann *et al.*, 1971) indicated that the entire Fc fragment was present in α-CD proteins, that their *C*-terminus was identical with that of normal $\alpha 1$ chains, and that the H–L peptide was missing. The hinge region was shown by chemical methods to be present in all eight proteins so far studied. All attempts to raise individually specific antibodies to α-CD proteins have failed, indicating the paucity of antigenic determinants in the V region of the chain. In view of these results and of the molecular-weight data, the missing portion of the chain is located in the Fd segment and involves both the V_H and C1 regions.

The demonstration of a large internal deletion in a γ-HCD protein (Frangione and Milstein, 1969) led us to postulate that in α-CD we were dealing with a similar primary deletion followed and obscured by a secondary proteolysis of limited degree (Seligmann *et al.*, 1971). This hypothesis has been supported to some extent by biosynthetic and structural studies. Cellular biosynthetic studies in a case of α-CD excluded the possibility of the synthesis of a *normal α* chain with subsequent degradation to a smaller fragment after its release from the ribosomes (Buxbaum and Preud'homme, 1972). The amino acid sequence of the hinge region of the protein of this patient (DEF), compared with that of another α-CD protein (AIT) and with that of a normal $\alpha 1$ chain, is shown in Figure 5 (Wolfenstein-Todel *et al.*, 1974, 1975). Normal synthesis resumes in both α-CD proteins at a valine residue in the hinge region just preceding a segment that contains a partially duplicated fragment and the inter-H-chain disulfide bonds. Starting with this valine residue and with the exception of a substitution of threonine for serine at residue 12 of protein DEF, the sequence is completely identical to that of a normal $\alpha 1$ chain. It is of interest that this valine residue at position 9 of the tryptic hinge peptide could represent the counterpart of glutamine at position 216 of γ chains, the site at which normal synthesis resumes in several γ-CD proteins with internal deletions (Frangione and Franklin, 1973; Franklin and Frangione, 1975). Figure 5 indicates that the first eight residues of the peptide of protein DEF differ from the sequence that normally precedes the valine in $\alpha 1$ chains. These short segments were thought to correspond to the V region. If this assumption proves to be correct, the primary defect in these α-CD proteins would be an internal deletion encompassing most of the V_H and $C_H 1$ regions, which are under independent genetic control. It is not excluded, however, that the segment preceding the valine that marks the beginning of the normal sequence is not a portion of the normal V region, but rather corresponds to an unusual repair of broken DNA or to a noncleaved polypeptide (?precursor, ?viral genome). It therefore appears essential to obtain N-terminal sequences of several α-CD proteins despite the heterogeneity that precluded success in previous attempts.

431

α-CHAIN DISEASE: A
POSSIBLE MODEL
FOR THE
PATHOGENESIS OF
HUMAN
LYMPHOMAS

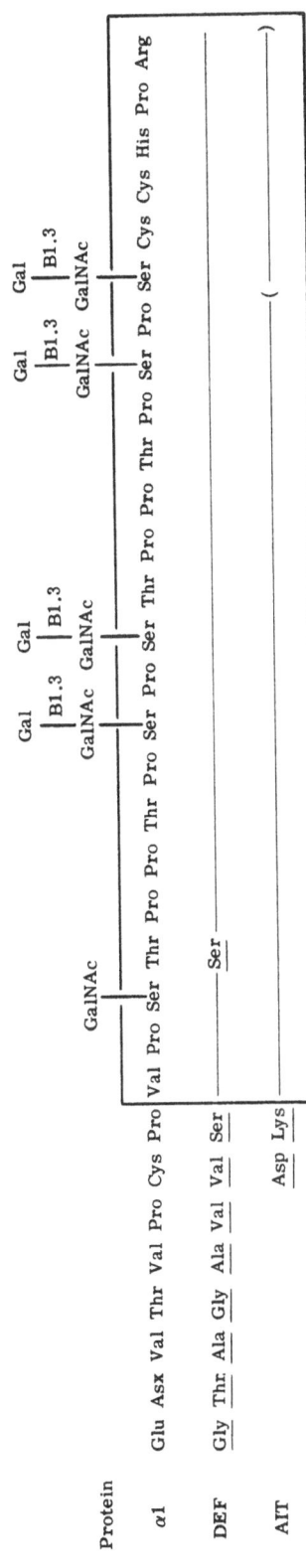

Figure 5. Comparison of the hinge region of a myeloma α1 chain and of α-CD proteins DEF and AIT. Identical residues are in the rectangle. Nonhomologous residues are underlined. A horizontal line in the rectangle indicates a sequence identical to that shown in the top peptide. Reproduced from Wolfenstein-Todel *et al.* (1975).

MAXIME SELIGMANN
AND JEAN-CLAUDE
RAMBAUD

All 70 α-CD proteins that have been typed to date in our laboratory belong to the $\alpha 1$ subclass. The absence of a single case of $\alpha 2$-HCD in this series is probably not accidental, since 10% of the normal serum IgA and 30% of the normal secretory IgA molecules belong to the $\alpha 2$ subclass (Grey *et al.*, 1968). The meaning of this finding is unknown. The possibility exists that α-CD proteins belonging to the $\alpha 2$ subclass could be very rapidly degraded at the intracellular or extracellular level. That all the molecules of α-CD protein in a given patient belong to only one IgA subclass and the finding of a single amino acid substitution in position 12 of protein DEF (Figure 5), as well as the results of structural studies of several γ-CD proteins strongly suggest that α-CD proteins are monoclonal. This assumption cannot be confirmed, however, because an essential criterion for monoclonality, i.e., structural homogeneity of the V region, could not be demonstrated. It should also be noted that in a young Norwegian patient affected with a digestive disease bearing some similarities to α-CD, polyclonal IgA molecules with κ and λ L chains and with both $\alpha 1$ and $\alpha 2$ H chains were produced (Brandtzaeg and Baklien, 1974).

Cultures of jejunal biopsy specimens from α-CD patients in medium containing ^{14}C-labeled amino acids have established that the α-CD protein is synthesized *in vitro* by the proliferating cells (Seligmann *et al.*, 1968). Radioimmunoelectrophoretic analysis of protein synthesized *in vitro* by cells teased from mesenteric nodes also demonstrated the production of labeled α-CD proteins (Seligmann *et al.*, 1969). Immunofluorescent studies of intestinal mucosa and mesenteric nodes revealed variable and sometimes weak staining in the cytoplasm of cells composing the cellular infiltrate (Seligmann *et al.*, 1969). Membrane-bound α chains were not found on the surface of α-CD-protein-synthesizing cells in the patients initially studied (Preud'homme and Seligmann, 1972), but were detected in several subsequent patients (Preud'homme *et al.*, unpublished).

Immunofluorescent studies failed to detect any L-chain production in the cells that secrete α-CD proteins (Seligmann *et al.*, 1969). No free labeled L chains were found in radioimmunoelectrophoretic analysis of proteins synthesized *in vitro* by intestinal or mesenteric node proliferating cells (Seligmann *et al.*, 1969). This failure of L chain synthesis was confirmed by biosynthetic studies of nascent Ig subunits in such patients (Buxbaum and Preud'homme, 1972). Since L and H chains are under the control of unlinked genes, this peculiar situation raises a puzzling problem for the cellular geneticist. The possibility remains that the L chain is transcribed but not translated. Studies looking for the presence or absence of its messenger are warranted, since Cowan *et al.* (1974) detected an inactive L-chain mRNA in the cells of a nonsecreting variant of a mouse myeloma that contained an abnormally short H chain and failed to synthesize L chain.*

3. Clinicopathological Features

3.1. Digestive Form of α-Chain Disease

The clinical features of intestinal α-CD are markedly uniform (Table 1). The disease usually presents with a severe malabsorption syndrome. Its onset may be

---

*In one patient whose cells were recently studied in our laboratory, monotypic light chains were synthesized but not secreted, as shown by immunofluorescence and biosynthesis experiments (Preud'homme *et al.*, unpublished).

433

α-CHAIN DISEASE: A
POSSIBLE MODEL
FOR THE
PATHOGENESIS OF
HUMAN
LYMPHOMAS

TABLE 1. Main Clinical Findings in 34 Cases of α-Chain Disease[a]

Finding	Incidence
Chronic diarrhea	100%
With overt steatorrhea	47%
Watery appearance	24%
Type not precise	29%
Abdominal pains	93%
Diffuse	38%
Epigastric	16%
Periumbilical	6%
Right-sided	6%
Site unknown	34%
Weight loss	97%
Finger-clubbing	47%
Vomiting	41%
Tetany	38%
Edemas	24%
Abdominal mass(es)	24%
Fever	21%
Ascites	12%

[a]The cases presented in this table include cases referenced in the text, cases reported by Irunberry et al. (1970), Zlotnick and Levy (1971), Bernadou et al. (1972), Guardia et al. (1972), Henry et al. (1974), Metrass et al. (1974), Pittman et al. (1975), and Shahid et al. (1975), and personal unpublished cases.

insidious or abrupt. In most cases, the first and main symptom of the disease is chronic diarrhea. Steatorrhea is usually obvious, and the stools often appear watery and are sometimes very copious. Patients complain of abdominal pains of variable intensity and localization, and vomiting is frequent. Several patients first experienced localized, acute pains with vomiting; some patients have been operated on with the diagnosis of appendicitis or acute pancreatitis. The time from appearance of the first symptom to diagnosis has ranged from 1 month to 6 years. In some cases (Bognel et al., 1972; Bonomo et al., 1972), the usual clinical pattern of α-CD was preceded by a protracted prodromic period with symptoms simulating the irritable colon syndrome. The spontaneous course of α-CD may be continuous, but often proceeds as exacerbations separated by more or less complete improvements.

The abdomen is usually distended and tender, and some ascitic fluid may be present. Hypertrophied mesenteric lymph nodes may be palpated as abdominal masses. Signs of chronic small bowel obstruction with or without palpable abdominal mass(es), or surgical emergencies, such as intestinal intussuception or perforation, or epiploic infarction, or both, may reveal the presence of the disease (Bonomo et al., 1972; unpublished data). These "tumoral" symptoms are more often observed, however, in the later stages of α-CD. Nasopharyngeal, gastric, and rectal localizations of the lymphoid proliferation have occasionally been described. It should be emphasized that hepatosplenomegaly is usually not observed and that peripheral lymphadenopathy is a very rare sign at presentation.

Finger-clubbing appears more frequently than with any other intestinal disease. Fever is uncommon. Asthenia and loss of weight, often rapid and severe, are consistently observed. Severe protein malnutrition may be evidenced by edemas, alopecia, and amenorrhea.

MAXIME SELIGMANN
AND JEAN-CLAUDE
RAMBAUD

The main biological abnormalities are summarized in Table 2. Low serum albumin levels and creatorrhea are nearly constant features, and a search for protein-losing enteropathy is usually positive. Dehydration and electrolyte imbalance may need emergency intravenous fluid replacement. The severity of diarrhea has led on occasion to hypokalemic nephropathy with polyuria. Tetany is frequently observed and may be the major presenting symptom. Hypocalcemia, which is often severe, is secondary to magnesium, rather than to vitamin D, deficiency (Dent *et al.*, 1968; Rambaud *et al.*, 1978). Hemorrhagic syndromes and overt osteomalacia are absent. The frequent high levels of serum alkaline phosphatase are usually accounted for by the increase in intestinal isoenzyme (Doe *et al.*, 1972). Anemia of variable type, with low serum levels of any or all of iron, folate, and B_{12}, remains mild or moderate. Total serum lipids and cholesterol are low, even in the frequent eventuality of mild steatorrhea. Xylose, glucose, folic acid, and vitamin B_{12} absorption tests (even with exogenous intrinsic factor) are indicative of malabsorption in

TABLE 2. Main Laboratory and Radiological Findings Related to Intestinal Involvement in 34 Cases of α-Chain Disease[a]

Finding	Incidence[b]
Laboratory data	
Hemoglobin	
10–13 g/dl	54% (28)
<10 g/dl	14% (28)
Serum potassium <3.5 mEq/liter	55% (20)
Serum albumin	
2.5–3.5 g/liter	46% (28)
<2.5 g/liter	46% (28)
Serum cholesterol <0.15 g/dl	89% (19)
Serum calcium <9.0 mg/dl	71% (28)
Raised serum alkaline phosphatase	81% (21)
Intestinal studies	
Fecal fats (24-hr output)	
<6 g	5% (22)
6–15 g	45% (22)
>15 g	50% (22)
Abnormal D-xylose test	83% (18)
Abnormal oral glucose tolerance test	93% (13)
Abnormal Schilling test	56% (9)
Protein-losing enteropathy	71% (7)
Intestinal bacteriology and parasitiology	
Jejunal fluid bacteria overgrowth	80% (5)
Stool and/or jejunal fluid parasites	
Giardia lamblia	24% (34)
Ascaris	3% (34)
Hookworm	3% (34)
Trichuris trichiura	3% (34)
Coccidia	3% (34)
Schistosoma mansoni	3% (34)
Small-intestinal X rays	
Hypertrophic folds	
("pseudopolypoid" pattern)	86% (28)
Strictures and/or defects	43% (28)

[a]The cases are those presented in Table 1.
[b]The figures in parentheses are the numbers of cases for which data were available.

most instances. Bone marrow aspirates and biopsies are usually normal, with the exception that occasional α-CD-producing plasma cells are detectable by immunofluorescence studies in a few patients (Seligmann *et al.*, 1969).

Small-intestinal X rays, with a thin and nonflocculable barium preparation, show very hypertrophic and pseudopolypoid folds in duodenal and jejunal mucosa, sometimes associated with stricture or filling defects, suggesting extrinsic compression by hypertrophic peripancreatic or mesenteric lymph nodes or both (Figure 6). Mediastinal adenopathy is usually not observed. Abdominal lymphangiography

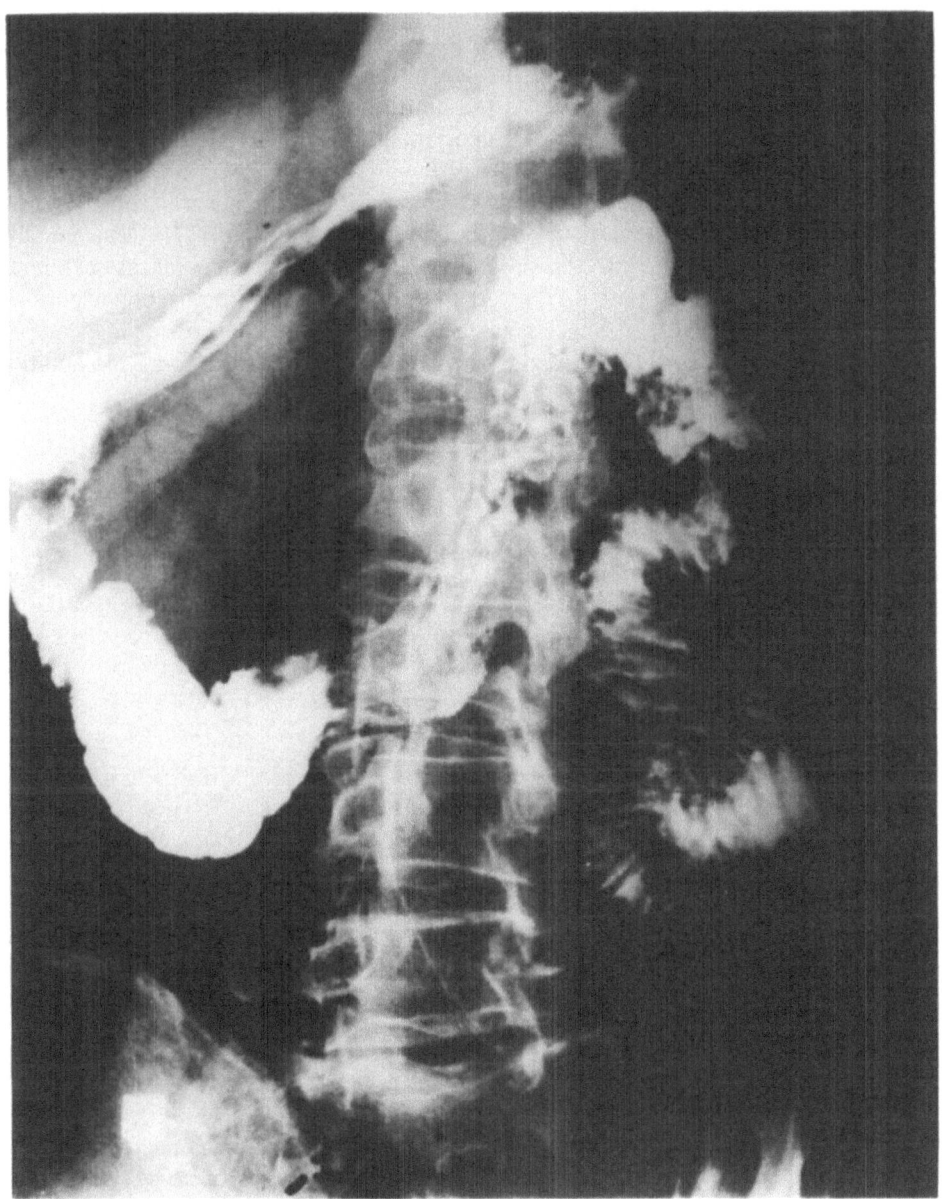

Figure 6. Barium meal in a patient with α-CD. Note the enlarging of the duodenal loop, the narrowing of D2, and the hypertrophy of duodenal and proximal jejunal folds.

MAXIME SELIGMANN
AND JEAN-CLAUDE
RAMBAUD

may reveal an involvement of the retroperitoneal lymph nodes. Radiological features of osteomalacia are absent, and skeletal surveys show no evidence of osteolytic lesions.

Limited bacteriological studies of stools have not revealed the consistent presence of any particular pathogens. In several patients, overgrowth of aerobes and anaerobes has been demonstrated in jejunal fluid, often associated with bile salt deconjugation and high indicanuria. Evidence of parasitic infestation is common but not constant. A variety of parasites have been found, giardiasis being the most frequent (Table 2).

The intestinal lesions of α-CD usually predominate in the duodenum and jejunum, in contrast to the other, more common lymphomas of the digestive tract, which have a predilection for the stomach, terminal ileum, and colorectal areas. The entire length of the small intestine is most often involved. Its serosal surface, apart from possible lymphatic dilatation, often appears normal without nodular formation. Its wall is mildly thickened at palpation. Intestinal ulcerations are rare. The mesenteric nodes are often greatly enlarged.

Multiple biopsies taken during laparotomy or with a peroral capsule show massive infiltration of the lamina propria by round cells (Figure 7). Occasionally, these infiltrates penetrate into the submucosa. Most cells in this infiltrate belong to the plasma-cell series (Figure 8A), as confirmed by electron microscopy (Scotto *et al.*, 1970; Doe *et al.*, 1972). These plasma cells do not usually show cellular atypia. In some instances, small lymphocytes and transitional forms are found, in addition

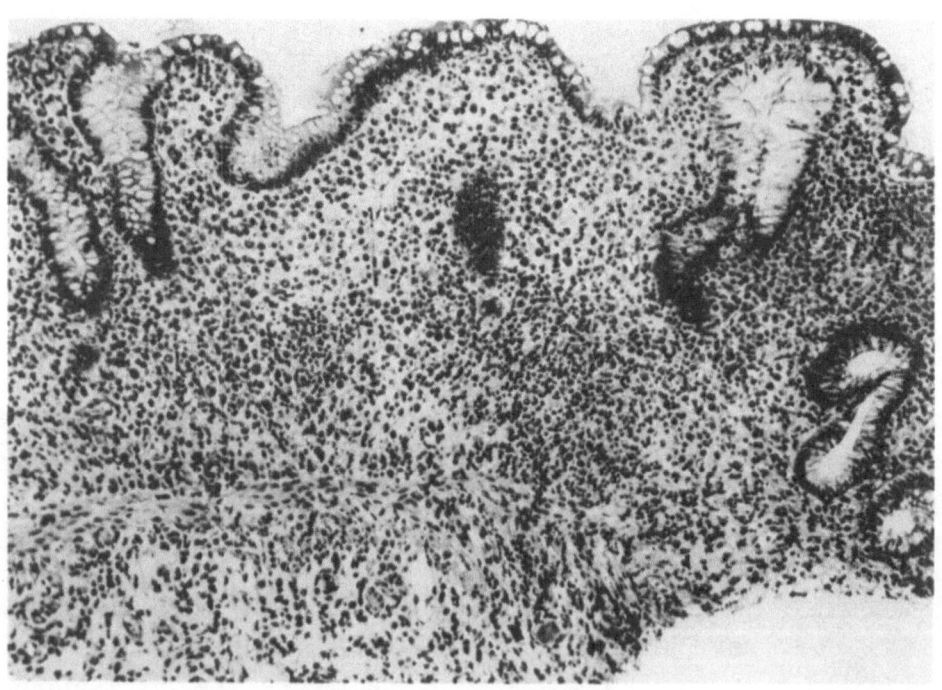

Figure 7. Jejunal peroral biopsy. Note the subtotal villous atrophy, the increased number of goblet cells, and the sparsity and the destruction of the crypts by the massive lamina propria infiltrate, which extends slightly to the submucosa. Hematoxylin–eosin. × 125. Reproduced from Rambaud *et al.* (1972) with permission of the *Annales de Gastroenterologie et d'Hepatologie.*

437

α-CHAIN DISEASE: A
POSSIBLE MODEL
FOR THE
PATHOGENESIS OF
HUMAN
LYMPHOMAS

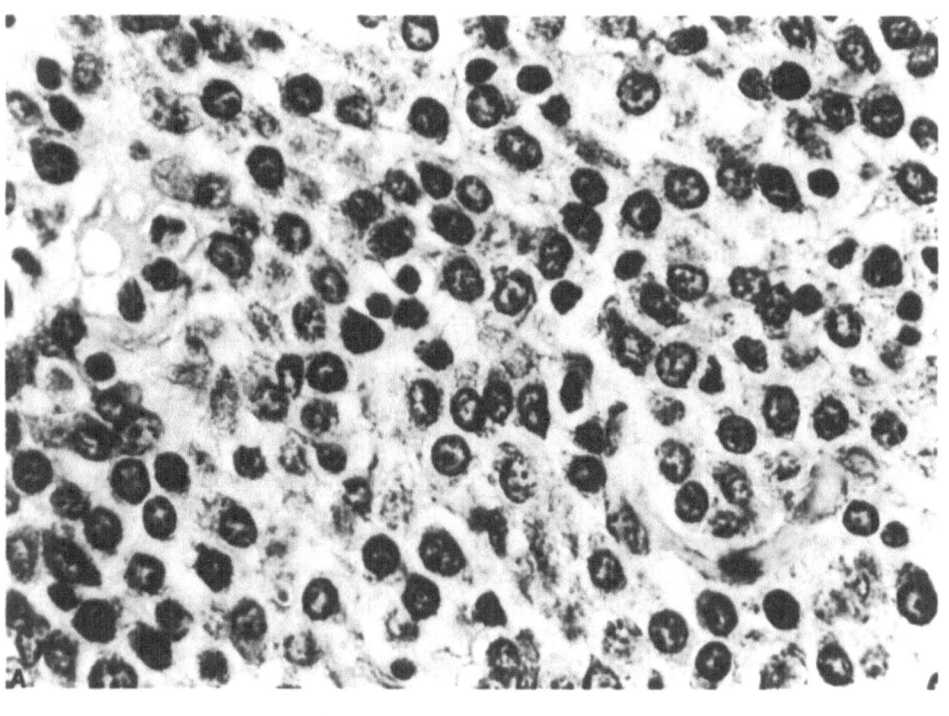

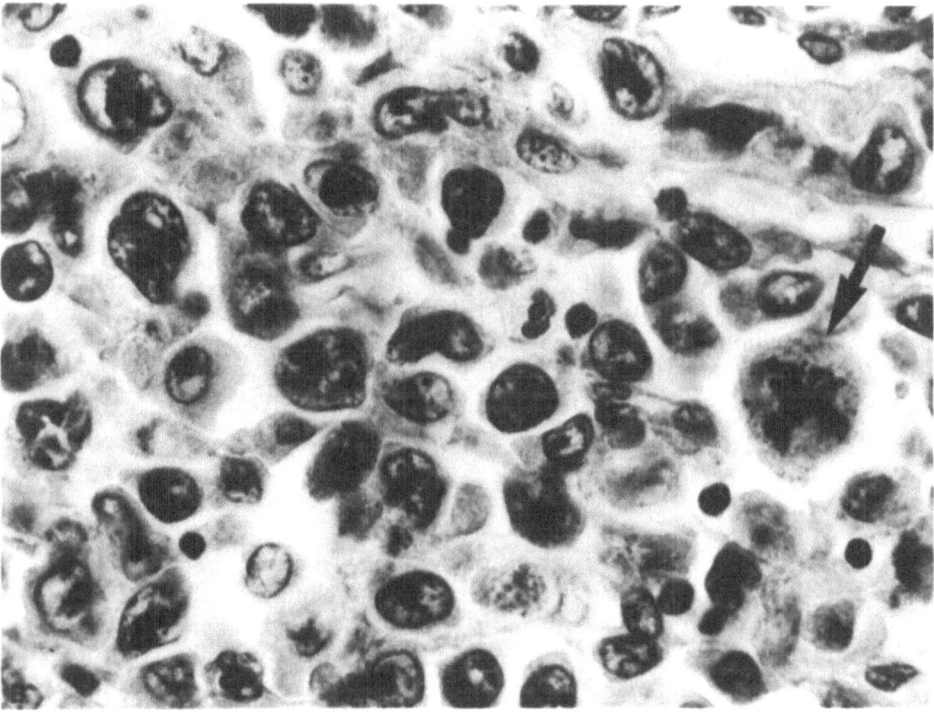

Figure 8. Details of the lamina propria infiltrate. Hematoxylin–eosin. × 1200. (A) At the time of diagnosis, most cells are plasma cells, sometimes mature, often young but not dystrophic. (B) At a later stage of the disease (immunoblastic lymphoma), all cells appear dystrophic, and some are large, with a polysegmented nucleus containing multiple nucleoli and with occasional mitoses (arrow). Reproduced from Rambaud *et al.* (1972) with permission of the *Annales de Gastroenterologie et d'Hepatologie*.

to the plasma cells. The plasma-cell infiltration is usually massive, causing wide separation and sparsity of the crypts and obliteration of the villous architecture without significant impairment of the integrity of the surface epithelium (see Figure 7). The villous atrophy may be incomplete and focal areas may remain, in which the villous architecture is preserved with heavy infiltration of the villous stroma by plasma cells or lymphocytes or both.

In some instances, the infiltrate extends to deep submucosa and even muscularis propria. In these areas, plasma cells are often atypical, and large pyroninophilic immunoblastlike cells are scattered within the plasmacytic infiltrate, either isolated or gathered in small islets or even large nodules (Galian *et al.*, 1977).

Mesenteric lymph nodes very often show the same cellular infiltrate as small-intestinal lamina propria, leading often to an obliteration of the normal architecture, especially when immunoblastic cells are present.

In some cases (Bognel *et al.*, 1972; Bonomo *et al.*, 1972), a first biopsy of jejunal or mesenteric lymph nodes or both merely showed a nonspecific hyperplastic lymphoid infiltration. In subsequent biopsies, the typical plasma-cell infiltration became apparent. In the absence of appropriate immunological studies, one cannot assume that these initial findings were truly related to an early stage of α-CD.

In some patients, who frequently presented with the "tumoral" symptoms mentioned above, pathological evidence of a truly malignant lymphoma is found in the gut (Figure 8 B) or the mesenteric nodes or both. In the small intestine, the lymphoma cells may form single (Novis *et al.*, 1973) or multiple (Rappaport *et al.*, 1972; Bonomo *et al.*, 1972; Montoro-Marin *et al.*, 1974; Manousos *et al.*, 1974; Teulières, 1975) circumscribed tumors. In some of these cases, the characteristic plasma-cell infiltration of α-CD might not be recognized if intestinal biopsies are not performed at a site distant from the tumoral formation(s). In other cases, the malignant lymphoma cells are intermingled with the plasma-cell proliferation and invade the deeper layers of the gut wall (Bognel *et al.*, 1972; Bonomo *et al.*, 1972; Chadli *et al.*, 1973; Galian *et al.*, 1977). Histologically, the malignant lymphoma is composed of large neoplastic cells. These tumors have been called reticulum-cell sarcomas or histiocytic lymphomas, according to the older classifications. The features of these cells strongly suggest, however, that we are dealing with the so-called "immunoblastic" lymphoma. Cells resembling Reed–Sternberg cells may be part of the infiltrate of the tumor, but they usually have a pyroninophilic cytoplasm.

Extensive histological studies have failed to reveal evidence of amyloid deposition.

3.2. Respiratory form of α-Chain Disease

Three of the reported patients with α-CD were considered to be probably affected with the respiratory form of the disease. Unfortunately, the pathological changes were poorly documented in these cases. The first patient described (Stoop *et al.*, 1971) was an 8-year-old Dutch girl who showed diffuse infiltrative pulmonary changes with enlarged mediastinal lymph nodes, dyspnea, and impaired diffusion associated with a marked eosinophilia and a typical α-CD protein in the serum. There was no obvious involvement of the small intestine. She developed a pharyngeal tumor with the histological characteristics of a paragranuloma, and there were no indications of synthesis of the α-CD protein by this tumor.

The second case (Faux *et al.*, 1973) was described in Boston in a 3-year-old boy with recurrent respiratory infections and hypogammaglobulinemia. The authors stated that he had no significant pulmonary changes, but X rays were not described and biopsies were not performed. The α-CD protein in serum was shown to be associated with J chain. This young patient is doing well under γ-globulin therapy, and the α-CD protein has gradually disappeared (F. Rosen, 1976, personal communication).

The third case (Florin-Christensen *et al.*, 1974) is that of a 76-year-old man presenting with dyspnea, mottling on chest X ray, and a low CO transfer factor. The mediastinal nodes were enlarged at postmortem. Histological reports were available only for the lung and kidney, and there was no evidence of malignancy. The serum IgA component did not precipitate with antisera to L chains, either before or after reduction, and reacted with rat mitochondria in immunofluorescence studies.

The IgA abnormality described by Moroz *et al.* (1971) in an Israeli adult female and her relatives appears to be different from α-CD. We believe that further cases of the respiratory form of α-CD with well-documented plasmacytic infiltration in the bronchi and mediastinal nodes, as well as cases involving the salivary glands and other sites of secretory IgA synthesis, will be described in the future.

4. Natural History

The natural history of α-CD is probably of utmost importance, but has not yet been fully elucidated.

The digestive form of the disease appears to proceed in two stages. The early "premalignant" stage is characterized by diffuse and extensive plasma-cell infiltration. In the absence of therapy, there is progressive deterioration, usually culminating in frank malignancy with immunoblastic tumors. Death is usually due either to cachexia and infection or to complications of the localized tumors.

Patients with well-documented initial status and adequate long-term follow-up are still scarce. In two patients who were regularly followed until death, however, it was possible to observe the progressive passage from mature plasmacytic proliferation to overt malignant lymphomas (Bognel *et al.*, 1972; Galian *et al.*, 1977). In the gut, foci of large malignant cells first appeared in the deep mucosa and in the submucosa, and all transitional forms between these cells and the plasma cells were observed. At any stage during the development of the lymphoma, mesenteric lymph nodes showed a noticeably higher degree of malignancy than the intestinal wall.

α-CD clearly involves the small-intestine-associated lymphoid system. The extensive plasma-cell infiltration almost always remains confined to the enteromesenteric area. Involvement of the large intestine, or of the stomach and the liver and/or spleen, is very rare. Plasma-cell infiltration of mediastinal or peripheral lymph nodes, or of the bone marrow, has been exceptionally noted. Even at the second stage of the disease, dissemination of the immunoblastic tumors outside the abdomen is a rare and late event.

Several lines of evidence strongly suggest that if we assume that the plasmacytic proliferation of α-CD is monoclonal in nature, the large cells of the immunoblastic lymphoma that arise in the late course of the disease are derived from the same B-cell clone as the initial plasma-cell proliferation. Both types of proliferations can be found intermingled in tissues of the lymph nodes and the gut (Bognel *et al.*,

1972). Rough endoplasmic reticulum may be found by electron microscopy in the apparently poorly differentiated malignant cells (Doe, 1975). All transitional forms between the large undifferentiated malignant cells and the mature plasma cells may be found in some patients. Intracytoplasmic α-CD protein may be undetectable by immunofluorescence in the most malignant and undifferentiated cells (Bognel *et al.*, 1972; Teulières, 1975). It must also be emphasized that the α-CD protein may disappear from serum and tumor tissues as the lymphoma develops (Teulières, 1975). However, α-CD protein has been identified in one patient in the perinuclear cisternae of the large lymphomatous cells found in the bone marrow (Reyes, personal communication). Furthermore, the study of membrane-bound Ig's has provided conclusive evidence that the sarcomatous cells of morphologically similar lymphomas arising in two other immunoproliferative disorders, i.e., chronic lymphocytic leukemia (CLL) and Waldenström's macroglobulinaemia (WM), originate from the same clone as the previous lymphoid proliferation (Brouet *et al.*, 1975). Alpha chains were recently found on the surface of the large lymphomatous cells in one patient with α-CD (Brouet *et al.*, 1977), and very recent studies of Ig biosynthesis provide evidence that these lymphomatous cells do indeed derive from the same clone as the plasma-cell proliferation (Ramot *et al.*, 1977; unpublished results from our laboratory).

Whether the plasmacytic phase of α-CD is truly benign is open to question. The hypothesis of a benign process seems unlikely in those patients with high and rising serum levels of the pathological protein (if its monoclonal nature is confirmed). This hypothesis is also unlikely when the plasma-cell proliferation invades deeply into the submucosa and possibly the muscularis propria, or completely disorganizes the architecture of the mesenteric lymph nodes and shows atypical forms with an admixture of large "immunoblastic" cells. This pleomorphic invasive proliferation probably represents the early stage of the malignant lymphoma. In most cases, however, the plasma cells of the infiltrate appear to be mature and well differentiated with scarce mitoses. This does not necessarily militate against malignancy, since in other malignant lymphoproliferative disorders, such as CLL and WM, the proliferating cells are normal in appearance. Karyotypic studies of plasma cells taken from the intestinal infiltrate during the "benign" phase may help to resolve this question. The truly benign nature of α-CD at its initial stage is a real possibility, since apparently complete remission of the disease was achieved in several patients treated only with oral antibiotics (Roge *et al.*, 1970; Monges *et al.*, 1975; Rambaud *et al.*, 1978; Ramot, personal communication). Disappearance of the α-CD protein from the serum and intestinal fluid was noted in these patients, together with a normal histological appearance and negative immunofluorescent studies. It should be emphasized that in one patient (Roge *et al.*, 1970), complete remission does persist 5 years after withdrawal of therapy. It is also noteworthy that in the three published cases, the initial serum level of α-CD protein was relatively low.

5. Treatment

Since relatively few data are available to date, we can give only our present and provisional opinion on the main therapeutic guidelines in the digestive form of the disease.

441

α-CHAIN DISEASE: A
POSSIBLE MODEL
FOR THE
PATHOGENESIS OF
HUMAN
LYMPHOMAS

All patients in whom α-CD has been diagnosed and in whom signs of overt malignancy were not found on peroral biopsies should be submitted to laparotomy, if there is no major contraindication, in order to perform multiple large transmural biopsies of the small intestine and of several mesenteric lymph nodes and liver.

Patients without any evidence of a sarcomatous process should first be treated with oral antibiotics alone. The same could perhaps apply to patients with suspected but not documented malignancy (i.e., patients with submucosal infiltration, complete obliteration of nodal architecture, or scattered immunoblastlike cells). Unless the antibiotic choice could be directed by repeated quantitative bacteriological studies of jejunal fluid and antibiograms, tetracycline should be given at a dosage of 2 g/day. Since a dramatic improvement in clinical and biological symptoms of malabsorption may occur with such a treatment without any significant changes in intestinal lesions (Teulières, 1975; Galian *et al.*, 1977) or without disappearance of the α-CD protein (Rambaud *et al.*, 1978; Seligmann and Danon, unpublished), evaluations of response to therapy should be based mainly on intestinal biopsies (with immunofluorescence studies whenever possible) and on repeated search for α-CD protein in blood and, if negative, in jejunal fluid. If no marked improvement is observed after 3 months of antibiotic therapy or if complete remission is not achieved after 9–12 months, cyclophosphamide should be administered at a dose of 200 mg/m² i.m. or i.v. weekly. In those patients in whom the disease remains stable or progressive or in whom a recurrence occurs, multiple intestinal biopsies should be performed, and a second laparatomy may be advisable.

In patients with overt malignant lymphoma diagnosed at onset or later in the course of the disease and localized to the enteromesenteric area, total abdominal irradiation should be performed after a short course of tetracycline, prednisone, and possibly chemotherapy. A maximum dosage of 3500 rads over the entire abdominal cavity seems to be required. Liver and kidneys should be protected as usual, and the weekly dosage should not exceed 750 rads. After a 1-month rest, irradiation should be followed by polychemotherapy for residual disease. Polychemotherapy should be given first to patients with malignant lymphomas involving the liver or extraabdominal nodes or viscera. A subsequent abdominal irradiation may be indicated in these patients for focal residual tumor. The most advisable polychemotherapy seems to be a combination of cyclophosphamide, adriamycin, vincristine, and prednisone (CHOP protocol) administered in cycles at monthly intervals for at least 6 months.

At all stages of the disease, supportive therapy is essential and should include fluid and electrolyte replacement given intravenously, blood or serum albumin infusions, vitamins and iron, and an appropriate diet.

6. Epidemiology and Relationship to So-Called "Mediterranean Lymphoma"

The age distribution of α-CD is in sharp contrast to that of multiple myeloma and of intestinal lymphoma occurring in Western Europe, since the great majority of patients affected with α-CD are between 10 and 30 years old (Seligmann, 1975a). The sex distribution shows a moderate prevalence of males, with a 3:2 ratio (Seligmann, 1975a).

MAXIME SELIGMANN
AND JEAN-CLAUDE
RAMBAUD

The geographic origins of 100 patients affected with α-CD (diagnosed or confirmed in our laboratory in the vast majority of cases) are listed in Table 3. Although early reports of α-CD concerned mainly patients living in the Mediterranean region, there now appears to be a wide spectrum of racial or ethnic origin, and cases have now been described in many parts of the world. Four cases were recently recognized in Central Africa. It should be emphasized that the three patients from the Netherlands, Great Britain, and the United States were those with a presumably respiratory form of the disease and without detectable intestinal involvement. The digestive form of the disease appears to be extremely rare in Western "developed" countries. The case reported in a Finnish boy (Savilahti and Brandtzaeg, 1973) was atypical, since the disease involved mainly the colon and terminal ileum, whereas the plasma-cell population of the jejunal mucosa appeared to be normal. Most patients originated from and had been living in areas with a high degree of infestation by intestinal microorganisms and were exposed to conditions of poor hygiene in low socioeconomic circumstances.

There appears to be no strong predilection for cases to cluster in families. No clear Ig abnormalities were found in a limited number of sera from close relatives of patients (Seligmann *et al.*, 1971; Ramot and Hulu, 1975; Lewin *et al.*, 1976).

The so-called "Mediterranean lymphoma," i.e., primary diffuse intestinal lymphoma associated with malabsorption, was first reported in Israel (Ramot *et al.*, 1965; Eidelman *et al.*, 1966). This syndrome, which affects underprivileged young adults, has since been described in Iran (Nasr *et al.*, 1970), Iraq (Al-Bahrani and Bakir, 1971), and South Africa (Novis *et al.*, 1973). In Israel, these lymphomas are found relatively frequently among Arabs and first- and second-generation Jewish immigrants from Middle Eastern and North African countries, but almost never affect Israeli Jews of Ashkenazi origin. A variety of histological types have been described, and there was much confusion in the literature about the pathology of these lymphomas. In fact, it is likely that most cases could be described under the heading "immunoblastic" lymphoma. Initial reports of these so-called "Mediterra-

TABLE 3. Geographic Origins of 100 Patients with α-Chain Disease

Africa		South and Central America	
Tunisia	20	Colombia	1
Algeria	18	North Argentina	1
South Africa	2	Mexico	1
Morocco	1	Europe	
Middle East		Spain	9
Iran	10	South Italy	5
Israel	8	Turkey	6
Lebanon	2	Yugoslavia	2
Syria	1	Greece	2
Libya	1	Portugal	1
Iraq	1	Finland	1
Far East		Netherlands	1[a]
Pakistan	2	Great Britain	1[a]
Cambodia	1	North America	
India	1	United States	1[a]

[a]Respiratory form.

443

α-CHAIN DISEASE: A
POSSIBLE MODEL
FOR THE
PATHOGENESIS OF
HUMAN
LYMPHOMAS

nean'' lymphomas did not include Ig studies. Recent evidence suggests that they often begin as an apparently benign infiltration of the small intestine by plasma cells. As mentioned above, α-CD patients have been observed over several years to progress from an apparently benign plasmacytic stage to a malignant intestinal lymphoma identical to the so-called "Mediterranean lymphoma." A retrospective pathological study from a group of 20 patients suffering from "Mediterranean lymphoma" revealed that in 16 cases, a diffuse plasma-cell infiltrate was present in association with the malignant lymphoma (Rappaport *et al.*, 1972). The remaining four patients showed a purely plasmacytic proliferation in the small intestine, without histological evidence for malignancy.

The true incidence of α-CD among the so-called "Mediterranean lymphomas" is still open to discussion. Our hypothesis (Seligmann and Rambaud, 1969) that many of these lymphomas are in fact α-CD (provided their definition is restricted to cases showing a diffuse plasma-cell proliferation with or without superimposed sarcoma) has been confirmed by the study of serum Ig's in numerous such patients. α-CD protein was found in the serum in several cases classified histologically as reticulum-cell sarcoma (Ramot and Hulu, 1975). We and others have been unable, however, to detect the α-CD protein in the sera of some such patients. Such a failure may reflect the insensitivity of techniques used or the advanced undifferentiated stage of the malignancy. Careful prospective studies should include a systematic search for the abnormal protein in jejunal fluid and, in negative cases, at the intracellular level, as discussed in Section 2.1. Current findings suggest that the majority of cases of diffuse "Mediterranean lymphoma" represent the late malignant phase of α-CD.

7. Pathogenesis

The very peculiar geographic distribution of α-CD patients and the clear predilection of α-CD for underprivileged populations suggest that environmental factors providing a local and protracted antigenic stimulation may play an important role in the pathogenesis of this disease (Seligmann *et al.*, 1971). The occurrence of complete and lasting remissions after administration of antibiotics only (see Section 4) should also be recalled. One common factor among susceptible populations of various ethnic origins is their exposure to an environment of poor hygiene in areas with a high degree of infestation by intestinal pathogens. Studies conducted in some affected populations (e.g., in Shiraz) have shown that chronic GI infection and diarrhea are common, and serial intestinal biopsies in healthy people have shown an increased lymphocytic and plasma-cell infiltration within the lamina propria of the small bowel. Since orally ingested microorganisms are known to be a powerful proliferative stimulus to the secretory IgA system, the early phase of α-CD could represent an aberrant humoral immune response following sustained topical antigenic stimulation of the intestinal mucosa. The specific or nonspecific nature of the postulated stimulating microorganisms is open to question. Limited bacteriological, parasitic, and virological studies have not revealed evidence of a specific agent associated with α-CD. The postulated antigenic stimulation, however, may have occurred many years before α-CD became clinically manifest. The clinical onset of the disease has occurred in some patients more than 10 years after withdrawal from the environmental factors. Microorganisms involved in the pathogenesis of α-CD

MAXIME SELIGMANN
AND JEAN-CLAUDE
RAMBAUD

may be present only during childhood and absent in identifiable form years later at the time of diagnosis. Unfortunately, the absence of Fab in α-CD protein precludes its use for identifying putative antigenic stimuli.

These environmental factors could trigger the clonal proliferation directly. Alternatively, they may be only predisposing factors causing a nonspecific stimulation of immunocytes that could then potentiate the oncogenic effect of a virus interfering with genes controlling IgA synthesis (Rambaud and Matuchansky, 1973). In either case, it is remarkable that the plasma-cell proliferation resulting from the postulated antigenic stimulation appears to lead to H-chain diseases rather than to myeloma. This fact suggests the following hypotheses (WHO Meeting Report 1976). An abnormal B-cell clone synthesizing the α-CD protein could be produced in the gut through a series of recombinant events during embryogenesis. Another possibility is that a somatic mutation event gives rise to a cell that produces the α-CD protein permitting it to enter into the gut-associated lymphoid system and to home into lamina propria. In either case, the abnormal clone would overgrow in abnormal microenvironmental situations and could, for instance, be susceptible to the proliferation stimulus of bacterial lipopolysaccharide in the intestinal lumen. In addition, the abnormal clone could have a selective advantage for proliferation because of the lack of antibody activity of its Ig product, possibly resulting in the suppression of a feedback mechanism.

The postulated environmental antigenic stimulus might be associated with an underlying immunodeficiency. This could be a defect rendering the host more susceptible to infection with oncogenic organisms or a basic defect of the feedback mechanisms controlling the cellular proliferative response to stimulation. Immunodeficiency could be due to malnutrition, especially in early infancy, as suggested by Dutz *et al.,* (1971), or to genetic factors.

In fact, the role of environmental factors does not exclude the possibility of predisposing genetic factors. Although limited family studies have failed to reveal consistent Ig abnormalities, a search for genetic markers may help to identify predisposed subjects. Raised serum levels of the intestinal isoenzyme of alkaline phosphatase were reported in patients with α-CD and Mediterranean lymphoma and in their healthy relatives (Ramot and Streifler, 1966, Doe *et al.,* 1972; Lewin *et al.,* 1976). The histocompatibility antigens of the patients and their relatives should be determined.

8. Conclusion

In conclusion, α-CD raises a number of interesting problems related to the structure of the abnormal Ig and to cellular genetics, to the compartmentalization of the plasmacytic proliferation to the small-intestine IgA system, and to the probable role of intestinal microorganisms in its pathogenesis. In addition, α-CD may constitute a model of a lymphoma characterized by a continuous sequence of events ranging from a possibly benign hyperplastic process reversible by the administration of antibiotics to an overt neoplastic proliferation.

References

Al-Bahrani, Z. R., and Bakir, F., 1971, Primary intestinal lymphoma—Challenging problem in abdominal pain, *Ann. R. Coll. Surg. Engl.* **49**:103–113.

445

α-CHAIN DISEASE: A
POSSIBLE MODEL
FOR THE
PATHOGENESIS OF
HUMAN
LYMPHOMAS

Bernadou, A., Segond, P., Bilski-Pasquier, G., Mihaesco, E., Preud'homme, J. L., and Bousser, J., 1972, La maladie des chaines alpha: A propos d'une observation, *Nouv. Rev. Fr. Hematol.* **12**:333.

Bognel, J. C., Rambaud, J. C., Modigliani, R., Matuchansky, C., Bognel, C., Bernier, J. J., Scotto, J., Hautefeuille, P., Mihaesco, E., Hurez, D., Preud'homme, J. L., and Seligmann, M., 1972, Etude clinique, anatomo-pathologique et immunochimique d'un nouveau cas de maladie des chaines alpha suivi pendant cinq ans, *Rev. Eur. Etud. Clin. Biol.* **17**:362–374.

Bonomo, L., Dammacco, F., Marano, R., and Bonomo, G. M., 1972, Abdominal lymphoma and alpha chain disease, *Am. J. Med.* **52**:73.

Brandtzaeg, P., and Baklien, K., 1974, Bowel diseases involving local immunoglobulin systems, *Acta Pathol. Microbiol. Scand. Sect. A* **248**:43–60.

Brouet, J. C., Labaume, S., and Seligmann, M., 1975, Evaluation of T and B lymphocyte membrane markers in human non-Hodgkin malignant lymphomas, *Br. J. Cancer* **31** (*Suppl. 2*):121–127.

Brouet, J. C., Mason, D. Y., Danon, F., Preud'homme, J. L., Seligmann, M., Reyes, F., Navab, F., Galian, A., René, E., and Rambaud, J. C., 1977, Alpha chain disease: Evidence for a common clonal origin of intestinal immunoblastic lymphoma and plasmacytic proliferation, *Lancet* **1**:861.

Buxbaum, J. N., and Preud'homme, J. L., 1972, Alpha and gamma heavy chain diseases in man: Intracellular origin of the aberrant polypeptides, *J. Immunol.* **109**:1131–1137.

Chadli, A., Hafsia, M., Maamouri, M. T., Haddad, N., and Ayed, K., 1973, Lymphome mediterranéen avec maladie des chaines alpha: Etude anatomo-patho-logique à propos du premier cas tunisien, *Arch. Anat. Pathol.* **21**:199–210.

Chantar, C., Escartin, P., Plaza, A. G., Corugedo, A. F., Arenas, J. I., Sanz, E., Anaya, A., Bootello, A., and Segovia, J. M., 1974, Diffuse plasma cell infiltration of the small intestine with malabsorption associated to IgA monoclonal gammapathy, *Cancer* **34**:1620–1630.

Cowan, N. J., Secher, D. S., and Milstein, C., 1974, Intracellular immunoglobulin chain synthesis in non-secreting variants of a mouse myeloma: Detection of inactive light-chain messenger RNA, *J. Mol. Biol.* **90**:691–701.

Dent, C. E., Norris, T. St. M., Smith, R., Sutton, R. A. L., and Temperley, J. M., 1968, Steatorrhoea with striking increase of plasma alkaline-phosphatase of intestinal origin, *Lancet* **1**:1333–1336.

Doe, W. F., 1975, Alpha chain disease: Clinicopathological features and relationship to so-called Mediterranean lymphoma, *Br. J. Cancer* **31** (*Suppl. 2*):350–355.

Doe, W. F., Henry, K., Hobbs, J. R., Avery Jones, E., Dent, C. E., and Booth, C. C., 1972, Five cases of alpha-chain disease, *Gut* **13**:947–957.

Dorrington, K. J., Mihaesco, E., and Seligmann, M., 1970, The molecular size of three α-chain disease proteins, *Biochim. Biophys. Acta* **221**:647–649.

Dutz, W., Asvadi, S., Sadri, S., and Kohout, E., 1971, Intestinal lymphoma and sprue: A systematic approach, *Gut* **12**:804–810.

Eidelman, S., Parkins, A., and Rubin, C., 1966, Abdominal lymphoma presenting as malabsorption: A clinicopathologic study of 9 cases in Israel and a review of the literature, *Medicine (Baltimore)* **45**:111–137.

Faux, J. A., Crain, J. D., Rosen, F. S., and Merler, E., 1973, An alpha heavy chain abnormality in a child with hypogammaglobulinemia, *Clin. Immunol. Immunopathol.* **1**:282–290.

Florin-Christensen, A., Doniach, D., and Newcomb, P. B., 1974, Alpha chain disease with pulmonary manifestations, *Br. Med. J.* **2**:413–415.

Frangione, B., and Franklin, E. C., 1973, Heavy chain diseases: Clinical features and molecular significance of the disordered immunoglobulin structure, *Semin. Hematol.* **10**:53–64.

Frangione, B., and Milstein, C., 1969, Partial deletion in the heavy chain disease protein ZUC, *Nature (London)* **224**:597–599.

Franklin, E. C., and Frangione, B., 1975, Structural variants of human and murine immunoglobulins, *Contemp. Top. Mol. Immunol.* **4**:89–126.

Galian, A., Lecestre, M. J., Scotto, J., Bognel, C., Matuchansky, C., and Rambaud, J. C., 1977, Pathological study of alpha-chain disease, with special emphasis on evolution, *Cancer* **39**:2081–2101.

Grey, H. M., Abel, C. A., Yount, W. J., and Kunkel, H. G., 1968, A subclass of human γA-globulins (γA2) which lacks the disulfide bonds linking heavy and light chains, *J. Exp. Med.* **128**:1223.

Guardia, J., Moragas, A., Pedreira, J. D., Ferragut, A., Gomez-Perez, J., Martinez-Vasquez, J. M., and Llorens, V., 1972, Enfermedad de las cadenas pesadas alfa (enfermedad de Seligmann), *Rev. Clin. Esp.* **127**:923–926.

Henry, K., Bird, R. G., and Doe, W. F., 1974, Intestinal coccidiosis in a patient with alpha-chain disease, *Br. Med. J.* **1**:542–543.

Irunberry, J., Benallegue, A., Illoul, G., Timsit, G., Abbadi, M., Benabdallah, S., Boucekkine, T., Ould-Aoudia, J. P., and Colonna, P., 1970, Trois cas de maladie des chaines alpha observés en Algérie, *Nouv. Rev. Fr. Hematol.* **10**:609–616.

Lewin, K. J., Kahn, L. B., and Novis, B. H., 1976, Primary intestinal lymphoma of "Western" and "Mediterranean" type, alpha chain disease and massive plasma cell infiltration: A comparative study of 34 cases, *Cancer* **38**:2511–2528.

Manousos, O. N., Economidou, J. C., Georgiadou, D. E., Pratsika-Ougourloglou, K. G., Hadziyannis, S. J., Merikas, G. E., Henry, K., and Doe, W. F., 1974, Alpha-chain disease with clinical, immunological and histological recovery, *Br. Med. J.* **2**:409–412.

Metrass, M. J., Virella, G., Baptista-Cunha, M. A., and Alfonso, G., 1974, Linfoma intestinal productor de cadenas alfa, *Sangre* **19**:418–434.

Monges, H., Aubert, L., Chamlian, A., Remacle, J. P., Mathieu, B., Cougard, A., and Arroyo, H., 1975, Maladie des chaines alpha à forme intestinale: Présentation d'un cas traité par antibiotherapie avec rémission clinique, histologique et immunologique, *Arch. Fr. Mal. Appar. Dig.* **64**:223–231.

Montoro-Marin, F., Bermejo, M. R., Monzonis Torres, M. C., and Perez Pena, F., 1974, Aspectos evolutivos y necropsicos de un caso de linfoma mediterraneo con enfermedad de cadenas alfa, *Med. Clin.* **62**:158–161.

Moroz, C., Amir, J., and De Vries, A., 1971, A hereditary immunoglobulin A abnormality—absence of light–heavy-chain assembly: Study of immunoglobulin synthesis in tonsillar cells, *J. Clin. Invest.* **50**:2726–2733.

Nasr, K., Haghighi, P., Bakhshandeh, K., and Haghshenas, M., 1970, Primary lymphoma of the upper small intestine, *Gut* **11**:673–678.

Natori, S., and Garen, A., 1970, Molecular heterogeneity in the amino-terminal region of alkaline-phosphatase, *J. Mol. Biol.* **49**:577–588.

Novis, B. H., Kahn, L. B., and Bank, S., 1973, Alpha-chain disease in Subsaharan Africa, *Am. J. Dig. Dis.* **18**:679–688.

Pittman, F. E., Tripathy, K., Isobe, T., Bolanos, O. M., Osserman, E. F., Pittman, J. C., and Lotero, H. R., 1975, IgA heavy chain disease: A case detected in the Western hemisphere, *Am. J. Med.* **58**:424–430.

Preud'homme, J. L., and Seligmann, M., 1972, Surface-bound immunoglobulins as a cell marker in human lymphoproliferative diseases, *Blood* **40**:777–794.

Rambaud, J. C., and Matuchansky, C., 1973, Alpha-chain disease: Pathogenesis and relation to Mediterranean lymphoma, *Lancet* **1**:1430–1432.

Rambaud, J. C., Bognel, C., Prost, A., Bernier, J. J., Le Quintrec, Y., Lambling, A., Danon, F., Hurez, D., and Seligmann, M., 1968, Clinico-pathological study of a patient with "Mediterranean" type of abdominal lymphoma and a new type of IgA abnormality ("alpha chain disease"), *Digestion* **1**:321–336.

Rambaud, J. C., Matuchansky, C., Bognel, J. C., Bognel, C., Bernier, J. J., Scotto, J., Perol, C., Ferrier, J. P., Mihaesco, E., Hurez, D., and Seligmann, M., 1970, Nouveau cas de maladie des chaînes alpha chez un Eurasien. *Ann. Méd. Interne* **121**:135–148.

Rambaud, J. C., Matuchansky, C., Bognel, C., Galian, A., Le Quintrec, Y., and Bernier, J. J., 1972, La maladie des chaines alpha: Rapport avec le "lymphome méditerranéen": Diagnostic et orientations thérapeutiques actuelles, *Ann. Gastro-enterol. Hepatol.* **8**:481–494.

Rambaud, J. C., Piel, J. L., Galian, A., Leclerc, J. P., Danon, F., Girard-Pipeau, F., Modigliani, R., and Illoul, G., 1978, Rémission complète clinique, histologique et immunologique d'un cas de maladie des chaines alpha traité par antibiothérapie orale, *Gastro-enterol. Clin. Biol.* **2**:49–61.

Ramot, B., and Hulu, N., 1975, Primary intestinal lymphoma and its relation to alpha heavy chain disease, *Br. J. Cancer* **31**(Suppl. 2):343–349.

Ramot, B., and Streifler, C., 1966, Raised serum-alkaline phosphatase, *Lancet* **2**:587.

Ramot, B., Shanin, N., and Bubis, J. J., 1965, Malabsorption syndrome in lymphoma of small intestine, *Isr. J. Med. Sci.* **1**:221–226.

Ramot, B., Levanon, M., Hahn, Y., Lahat, N., and Moroz, C., 1977, The mutual clonal origin of the lymphoplasmocytic and lymphoma cell in alpha-heavy chain disease, *Clin. Exp. Immunol.* **27**:440–445.

Rappaport, H., Ramot, B., Hulu, N., and Park, J. K., 1972, The pathology of so-called Mediterranean abdominal lymphoma with malabsorption, *Cancer (Philadelphia)* **29**:1502–1511.

447

α-CHAIN DISEASE: A
POSSIBLE MODEL
FOR THE
PATHOGENESIS OF
HUMAN
LYMPHOMAS

Roge, J., Druet, P., and Marche, C., 1970, Lymphome méditerranéen avec maladie des chaines alpha: Triple rémission clinique, anatomique et immunologique, *Pathol. Biol.* **18**:851–858.

Savilahti, E., and Brandtzaeg, P., 1973, An atypical case of alpha-chain disease, *Scand. J. Immunol.* **2**:322 (abstract).

Scotto, J., Stralin, H., and Caroli, J., 1970, Ultrastructural study of two cases of α-chain disease, *Gut* **11**:782–788.

Seligmann, M., 1975a, Immunochemical, clinical and pathological features of α-chain disease, *Arch. Intern. Med.* **135**:78–82.

Seligmann, M., 1975b, Alpha chain disease, *J. Clin. Pathol.* **28**(*Suppl. Assoc. Clin. Pathol.*):6:72–76.

Seligmann, M., and Rambaud, J. C., 1969, IgA abnormalities in abdominal lymphoma (α-chain disease), *Isr. J. Med. Sci.* **5**:151–157.

Seligmann, M., Danon, F., Hurez, D., Mihaesco, E., and Preud'homme, J. L., 1968, Alpha-chain disease: A new immunoglobulin abnormality, *Science* **162**:1396–1397.

Seligmann, M., Mihaesco, E., Hurez, D., Mihaesco, C., Preud'homme, J. L., and Rambaud, J. C., 1969, Immunochemical studies in four cases of alpha chain disease, *J. Clin. Invest.* **48**:2374–2389.

Seligmann, M., Mihaesco, E., and Frangione, B., 1971, Studies on alpha chain disease, *Ann. N. Y. Acad. Sci.* **190**:487–500.

Shahid, M. J., Alami, S. Y., Nassar, V. H., Balikian, J. B., and Salem, A. A., 1975, Primary intestinal lymphoma with paraproteinemia, *Cancer* **35**:848–858.

Stoop, J. W., Ballieux, R. E., Hijmans, W., and Zegers, B. J. M., 1971, Alpha chain disease with involvement of the respiratory tract in a Dutch child, *Clin. Exp. Immunol.* **9**:625–635.

Tangun, Y., Saracbasi, Z., Inceman, S., Danon, F., and Seligmann, M., 1975, IgA myeloma globulin and Bence-Jones proteinuria in a diffuse plasmacytoma of small intestine, *Ann. Intern. Med.* **83**:673.

Teulières, J. P., 1975, La maladie des chaines lourdes alpha, M. D. thesis, Claude Bernard University, Lyon, France.

WHO Meeting Report, 1976, Alpha-chain disease and related small intestinal lymphoma, *Arch. Fr. Mal. Appar. Dig.* **65**:591–607.

Wolfenstein-Todel, C., Mihaesco, E., and Frangione, B., 1974, "Alpha chain disease" protein Def: Internal deletion of a human immunoglobulin A₁ heavy chain, *Proc. Natl. Acad. Sci. U.S.A.* **71**:974–978.

Wolfenstein-Todel, C., Mihaesco, E., and Frangione, B., 1975, Variant of a human immunoglobulin: α-Chain disease protein AIT, *Biochem. Biophys. Res. Commun.* **65**:47–53.

Zlotnick, A., and Levy, M., 1971, α-Heavy chain disease: A variant of Mediterranean lymphoma, *Arch. Intern. Med.* **128**:432–436.

15

Lymphoreticular Disorders of the Gastrointestinal Tract: Roentgenographic Features

RICHARD H. MARSHAK, ARTHUR E. LINDNER, and DANIEL MAKLANSKY

1. Introduction

The lymphoreticular disorders of the gastrointestinal tract are of particular concern in the small bowel, and we will therefore begin this chapter with a discussion of the technique of radiological examination of the small bowel and some comments on the appearance of the normal small intestine. This will lead us to a description of the appearance of the small bowel in immunoglobulin-deficiency syndromes and in small-intestinal lymphocytic lymphoma. We conclude with considerations of lymphocytic lymphoma involving the stomach and the colon.

2. Roentgen Examination of the Small Bowel—Technique

For many years, the small bowel was neglected in the roentgen examination of the GI tract. Barium moved with inconvenient slowness through this lengthy structure, and there appeared to be very few important diseases that affected the small intestine. In recent years, however, techniques have been developed to improve the speed and quality of the examination, and it has become apparent that accurate diagnosis of many GI and systemic diseases can be established by radiographic study of the small bowel.

RICHARD H. MARSHAK and DANIEL MAKLANSKY • The Mount Sinai School of Medicine, New York, New York 10029.   ARTHUR E. LINDNER • New York University School of Medicine, New York, New York 10016.

Patients are examined after an overnight fast. Whenever possible, all medications are discontinued the day before the examination. Anticholinergics and ganglionic-blocking agents tend to cause dilatation and to mimic the sprue pattern, and narcotics affect both motility and the appearance of the small-bowel folds.

A preliminary film of the abdomen prior to the administration of barium is often helpful. In adults without disease, the small bowel may contain scattered amounts of gas, but visualization of an entire segment or a loop is an abnormal finding, and large amounts indicate ileus or an obstruction. Gas in the lumen can serve as a contrast medium on a plain film of the abdomen and very effectively demonstrate an area of pathology within the small bowel. The total absence of air from the small intestine is abnormal.

The small bowel is examined following administration of a mixture that is half barium sulfate, by volume, with an adequate suspending agent, and half water.

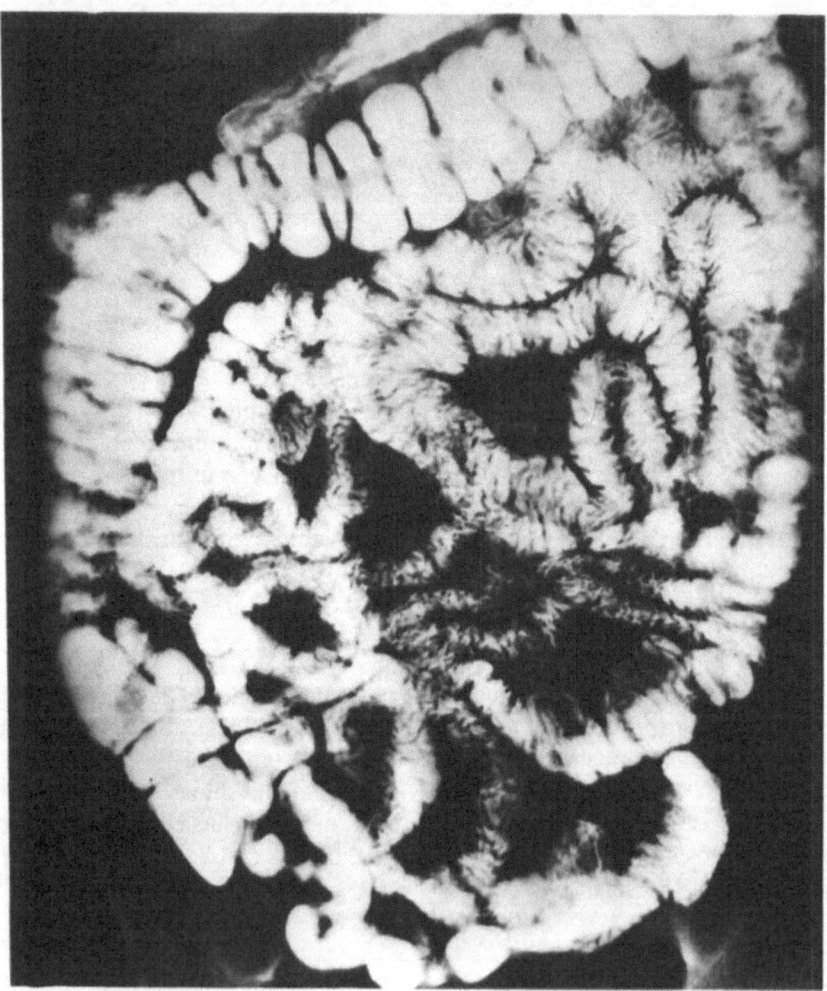

Figure 1. Normal small intestine. Note that the column of barium is continuous and that the loops have an undulating, serpentine appearance.

451

LYMPHORETICULAR
DISORDERS OF THE
GASTROINTESTINAL
TRACT:
ROENTGENO-
GRAPHIC FEATURES

Commercial preparations today are usually manufactured with such an agent incorporated in the mixture. At least 16 oz. of the mixture is used, and often 20 oz. or more is required. Use of smaller amounts of barium may cause incomplete filling of loops and simulate an abnormality. This large volume of barium is especially valuable in the interpretation of diffuse lesions of the small bowel. Many intestinal loops may be visualized simultaneously and in continuity, so that the relationship of one segment to another can be evaluated.

3. The Normal Small Bowel

In almost all patients, the jejunum is located in the left upper quadrant and the ileum in the right lower quadrant. Occasionally, as in congenital malrotations and in paraduodenal hernias, the relationships may be altered. The valvulae conniventes are well developed in the jejunum and therefore appear as prominent folds that persist even in the presence of distal obstructions. The caliber of the jejunum (2–3 cm) is slightly greater than that of the ileum (1.5–2.5 cm).The small intestine has an undulating, coiled appearance. The loops of bowel touch one another, and there is no persistent separation of the loops (Figure 1). The barium column in the normal small bowel is continuous, but identification of an occasional area of segmentation or of some fragmentation does not indicate disease. Such minor findings may be related to the physical characteristics of the barium or to the presence of slightly more fluid in the lumen than is usually seen.

4. The Small Bowel in Immunoglobulin-Deficiency Syndromes

Soon after Bruton's first description of congenital agammaglobulinemia (Bruton, 1952), it became apparent that common variable hypogammaglobulinemia is a much more frequent disorder, and that it is commonly associated with GI disturbances. In fact, diarrhea and steatorrhea were features of the first reported case of this type of hypogammaglobulinemia (Sanford *et al.*, 1954). Within a few years, the association of hypogammaglobulinemia with sprue (Cohen *et al.*, 1962), and with pernicious anemia and atrophic gastritis (Lewis *et al.*, 1957; Twomey *et al.*, 1969), was recognized. A unique group of hypogammaglobulinemic patients was then identified (Hermans *et al.*, 1966), characterized by nodular lymphoid hyperplasia of the small bowel, diarrhea, and an unusual susceptibility to infection with *Giardia lamblia*. Infection with this parasite has since been detected with undue frequency in other immunodeficiency syndromes (Ament and Rubin, 1972).

The enteropathic immunoglobulin (Ig) deficiencies are predominantly of acquired adult-onset type, since the congenital forms are uncommonly associated with GI symptoms (Ament *et al.*, 1973). The disease may be either primary (idiopathic) or secondary to some other process involving the bowel, such as the exudative enteropathies and various lymphoreticular malignancies.

4.1. Clinical Classification of Immunoglobulin-Deficiency Syndromes

For the purposes of this discussion, it is useful to classify the various Ig disorders associated with GI manifestations into the following principal groups:

I. Primary immunoglobulin disorders with GI manifestations
   A. Variable immunoglobulin deficiency
      1. Hypogammaglobulinemic sprue (Cohen *et al.*, 1962; Eidelman *et al.*, 1968). Uniform depression of all Ig levels, with malabsorption and villous atrophy, but with absence of plasma cells in the lamina propria and no response to excluding gluten from the diet.
      2. Hypogammaglobulinemia with pernicious anemia (Twomey *et al.*, 1969) and atrophic gastritis, but with absence of antibodies to parietal cells and intrinsic factor, frequent lack of response of the B_{12} malabsorption to exogenous intrinsic factor, and lack of the expected elevation of the

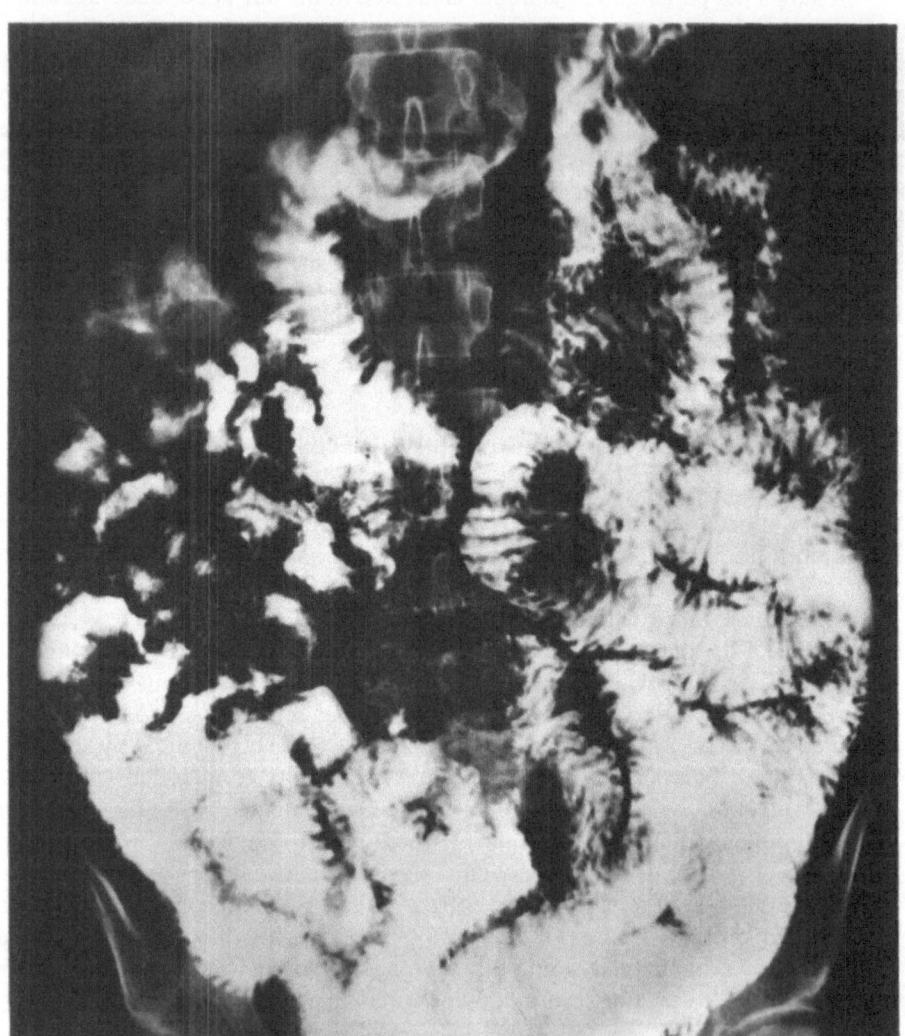

Figure 2. Hypogammaglobulinemic sprue. The roentgen alterations are indistinguishable from celiac sprue. They include dilatation, especially of the jejunum, associated with fragmentation, segmentation, and increased secretions. Hypogammaglobulinemic sprue is rare, and a diagnosis cannot be made by roentgen examination alone.

453

LYMPHORETICULAR
DISORDERS OF THE
GASTROINTESTINAL
TRACT:
ROENTGENO-
GRAPHIC FEATURES

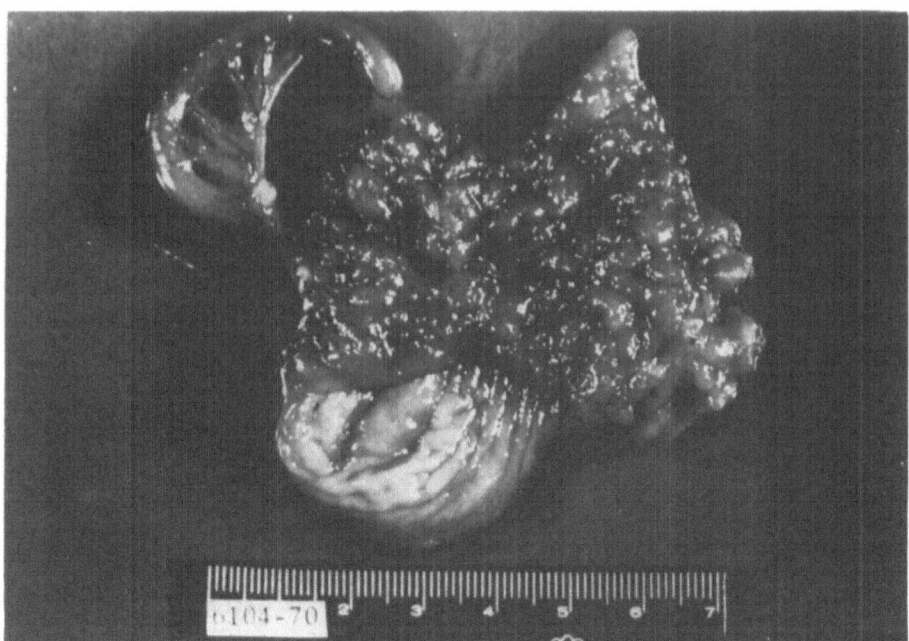

Figure 3. Specimen of distal ileum demonstrating nodular lymphoid hyperplasia. Histological sections revealed marked lymphoid hyperplasia. The appendix is visualized and is normal.

fasting serum gastrin level (Hughes *et al.*, 1972). There is villous atrophy and lack of plasma cells in the small bowel.

3. Nodular lymphoid hyperplasia of the small bowel (Hermans *et al.*, 1966). The Ig defect is incomplete and affects especially IgA and IgM in most cases. There is malabsorption and a high incidence of intestinal infection with *Giardia lamblia, Strongyloides, Candida,* bacteria, and possibly viruses. Respiratory infections are frequent. The villi appear normal on small-bowel biopsy, but there are few or no plasma cells found; lymphoid aggregates are seen.

B. Selective IgA deficiency

1. IgA-deficient sprue (Mawhinney and Tomkin, 1971). Isolated IgA deficiency with gluten enteropathy, villous atrophy, and presence of ample plasma cells in the lamina propria, although these cells are abnormal in that they contain IgM and no IgA. There is no unusual susceptibility to infection.

2. Isolated IgA deficiency with nodular lymphoid hyperplasia also occurs (Gryboski *et al.*, 1968), although it is more commonly associated with variable Ig deficiency.

It must be noted that in some instances, a single patient will show a combination of features, such as nodular lymphoid hyperplasia and giardiasis together with spruelike villus atrophy, rendering his disease difficult to classify according to the scheme outlined above. There is an increased incidence of gastric (Hermans and Huizenga, 1972) and colonic (Hodgson *et al.*, 1967) carcinoma, as well as lym-

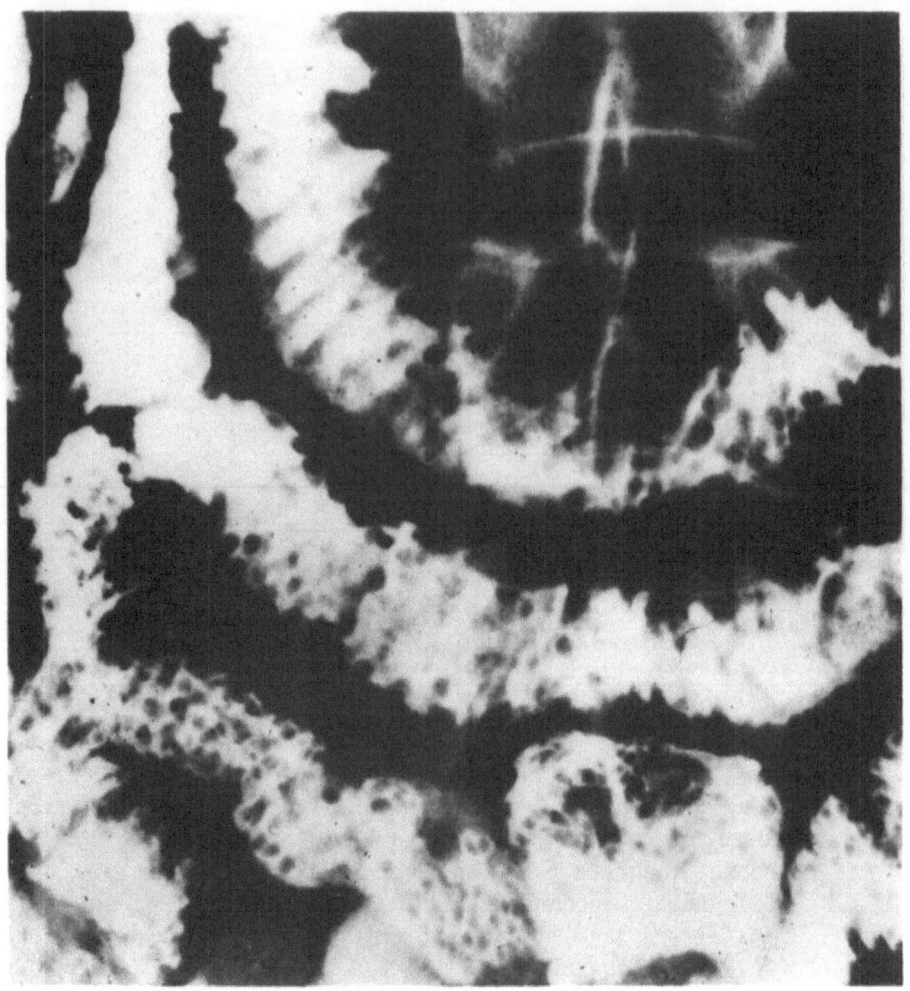

Figure 4. Common variable immunoglobulin deficiency (magnified view). Symmetrical small nodules are identified. This is an excellent example of the typical nodules of nodular lymphoid hyperplasia.

phoma of the bowel, in all these enteropathic types of Ig deficiency, especially in children (Shackelford and McAlister, 1975).

One or more of the following factors may contribute to the etiology of the malabsorption that is so frequent in primary hypogammaglobulinemia: intramural intestinal infection, intraluminal bacterial overgrowth, *Giardia lamblia,* gastric achlorhydria, pancreatic insufficiency, and gluten sensitivity. The intestinal mucosal alterations may be secondary to infection by bacteria or parasites, and often improve after their eradication (Ament and Rubin, 1972).

II. Secondary immunoglobulin disorders with GI manifestations
    A. Decreased Ig synthesis or increased synthesis of abnormal Ig fragments, or both. These disorders are exemplified by Waldenström's macroglobulinemia, α-chain disease, and other plasma cell dyscrasias. They have also been found in well-differentiated lymphocytic lymphoma and chronic lymphocytic leukemia.

455

LYMPHORETICULAR
DISORDERS OF THE
GASTROINTESTINAL
TRACT:
ROENTGENO-
GRAPHIC FEATURES

α-Chain disease (''Mediterranean lymphoma'') is a condition characterized by a diffuse plasma-cell proliferation affecting the IgA secretory system
(Bonomo *et al.*, 1972; Rambaud and Matuchansky, 1973; Seligmann, 1975).
The cells synthesize an abnormal Ig fragment that is part of the heavy chain
of IgA (α chain). In nearly all cases, the plasma-cell infiltrate involves the
entire length of the small intestine and mesenteric lymph nodes, although a
respiratory form of the disease has also been reported. The clinical picture is
usually that of a severe malabsorption syndrome affecting males or females,
generally in their second or third decades. The serum contains free α chain
with reduced levels of IgG, IgM, and albumin. The pathological counterpart
is an abdominal lymphoma, originally termed ''Mediterranean lymphoma''
because of the peculiar ethnographic distribution of most of the earlier
reported cases. Whether α-chain disease starts as a benign hyperplastic
process or is malignant from its onset has not been determined.

B. Increased Ig breakdown and loss secondary to exudative gastroenteropa-
thies, including intestinal lymphangiectasia (Shimkin *et al.*, 1970). The effect
is similar to the losses that occur with the nephrotic syndrome and exfolia-

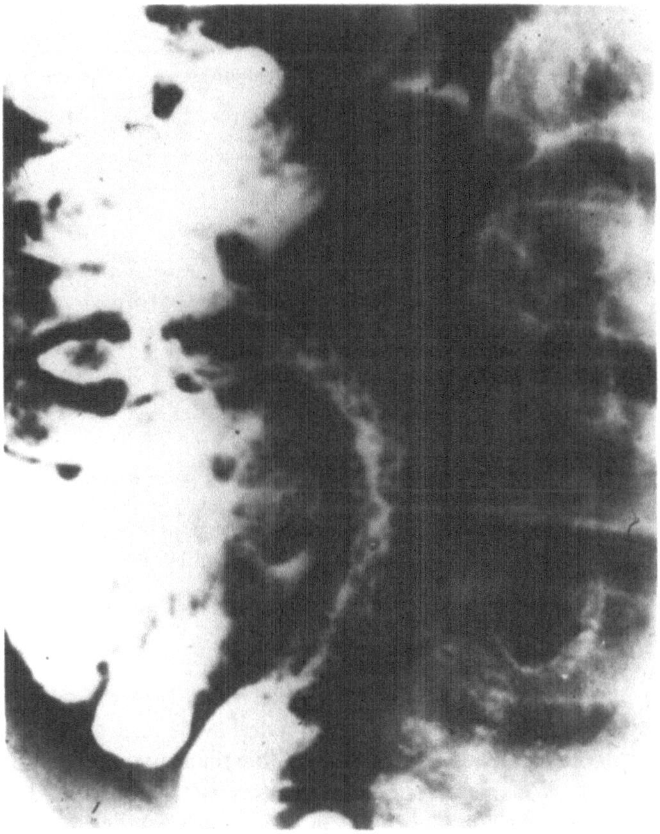

Figure 5. Terminal ileum with nodular lymphoid hyperplasia. This patient had no immunoglobulin
deficiencies. The alterations were confined to the terminal ileum and consisted of small nodular filling
defects. When nodular lymphoid hyperplasia is restricted to the terminal ileum in young people, it is
rarely of significance.

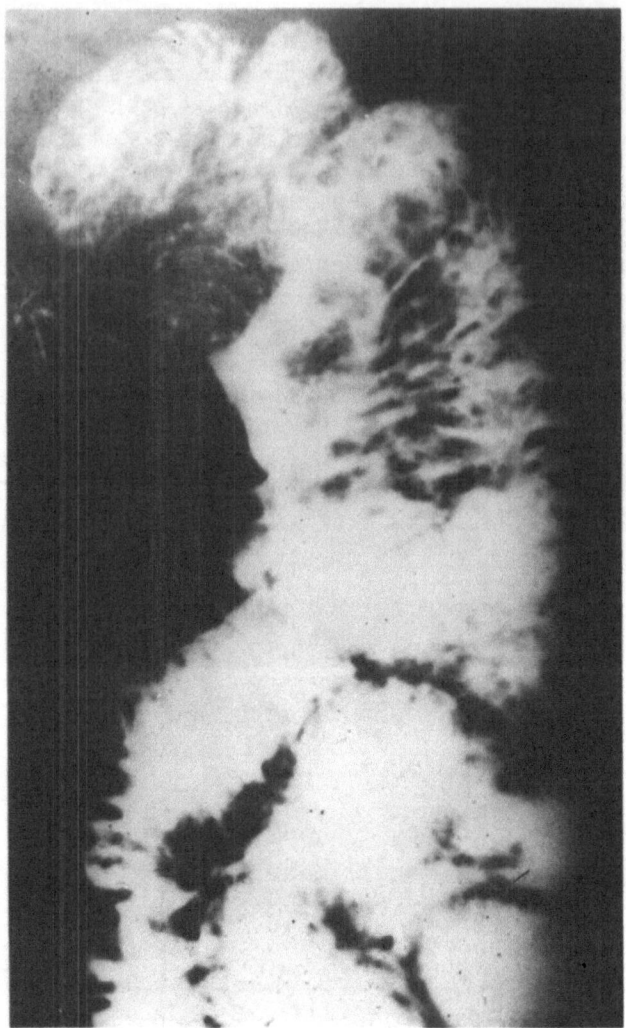

Figure 6. Lymphocytic lymphoma. There is a segment in the midjejunum measuring 3 inches in length in which the mucosa is ulcerated, with a nodular configuration along the contours. There is no obstruction. Some of the tiny defects previously described are seen in adjacent loops of bowel. At surgery, almost the entire small bowel was involved with lymphosarcoma. Courtesy of Dr. Roger Blahut.

tive dermatitides. The major fall here is in IgG (presumably because of its relatively small molecular size) associated with loss of albumin, together with lymphopenia when secondary to intestinal lymphangiectasia.

C. Amyloidosis. Nonspecific Ig abnormalities such as elevated or depressed serum levels of IgA, IgG, and IgM are frequently encountered in all types of amyloidosis (Glenner *et al.*, 1972). M components are found in the serum or urine of most patients with amyloidosis associated with lymphoproliferative disorders.

457

LYMPHORETICULAR
DISORDERS OF THE
GASTROINTESTINAL
TRACT:
ROENTGENO-
GRAPHIC FEATURES

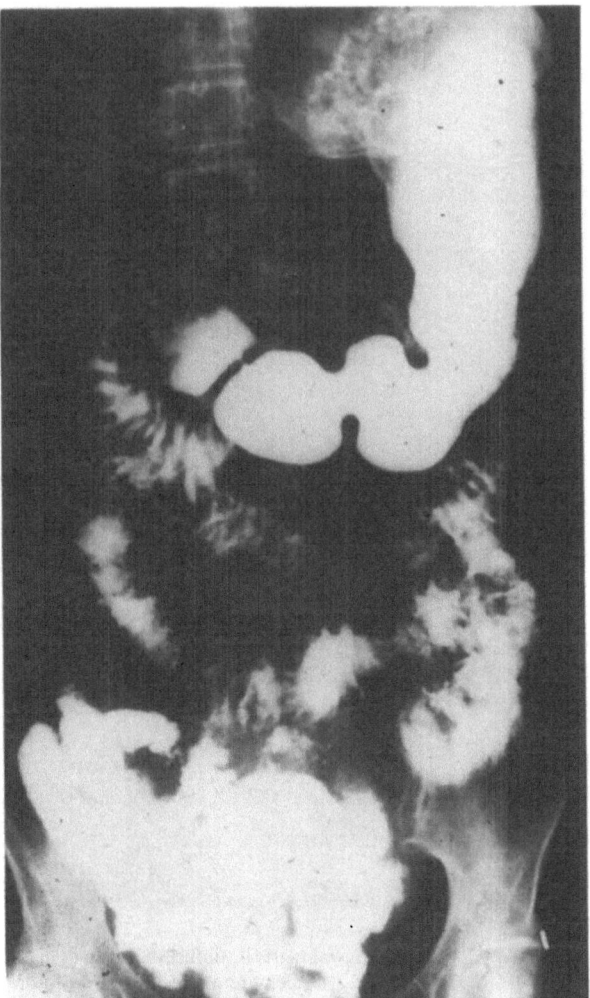

Figure 7. Giardiasis. There is spasm and irritability of the jejunum, associated with narrowing of the lumen and increased secretions. The valvulae conniventes are thickened. The findings are secondary to inflammatory edema. The ileum is within normal limits.

4.2. Roentgen Features

With this clinical classification in mind, we have organized the roentgeno-graphic manifestations of the enteropathic immunoglobulin-deficiency syndromes into the following groups:

1. *Sprue (malabsorption) pattern,* as seen in hypogammaglobulinemic sprue and in IgA-deficient sprue
2. *Multiple nodular defects*
3. *Inflammatory changes* secondary to giardiasis

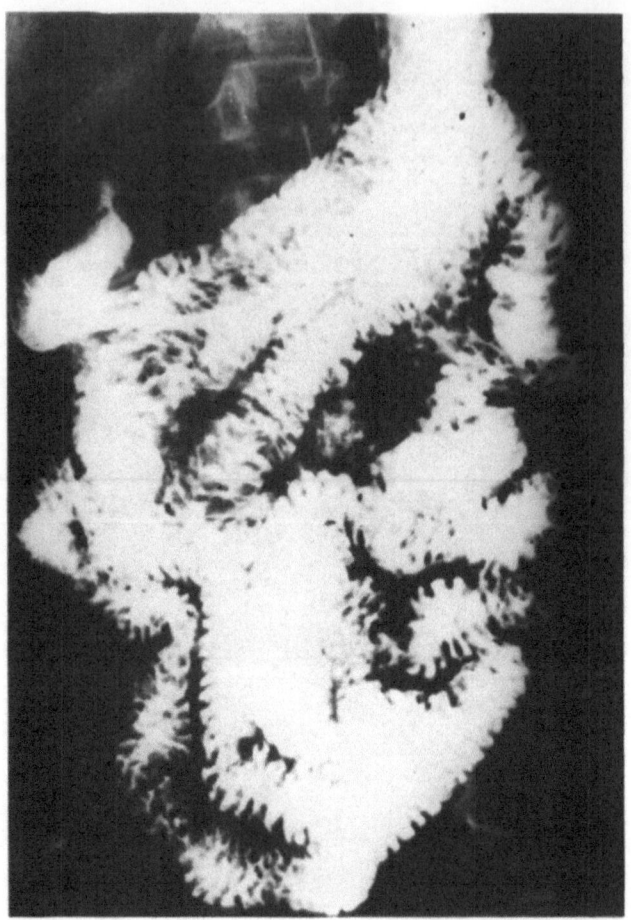

Figure 8. Amyloidosis. There is a striking, symmetrical, diffuse, sharply demarcated thickening of the valvulae conniventes. Dilatation is minimal. Segmentation and fragmentation are absent. There is no evidence of an inflammatory process.

4. *Thickening of the small-intestinal folds,* as in amyloidosis, lymphoma, macroglobulinemia, α-chain disease, and intestinal lymphangiectasia

The roentgen alterations are not necessarily confined to just one of these findings, and a patient may exhibit more than one of these features either simultaneously or on successive examinations.

4.2.1. Sprue (Malabsorption) Pattern

The roentgen findings in hypogammaglobulinemic sprue and in IgA-deficient sprue are indistinguishable from those seen in celiac sprue, with dilatation of the small bowel, segmentation, fragmentation, and scattering of the barium column, and hypersecretion causing dilution of barium distally (Figure 2). Transient nonobstructive intussusceptions may be observed.

459

LYMPHORETICULAR
DISORDERS OF THE
GASTROINTESTINAL
TRACT:
ROENTGENO-
GRAPHIC FEATURES

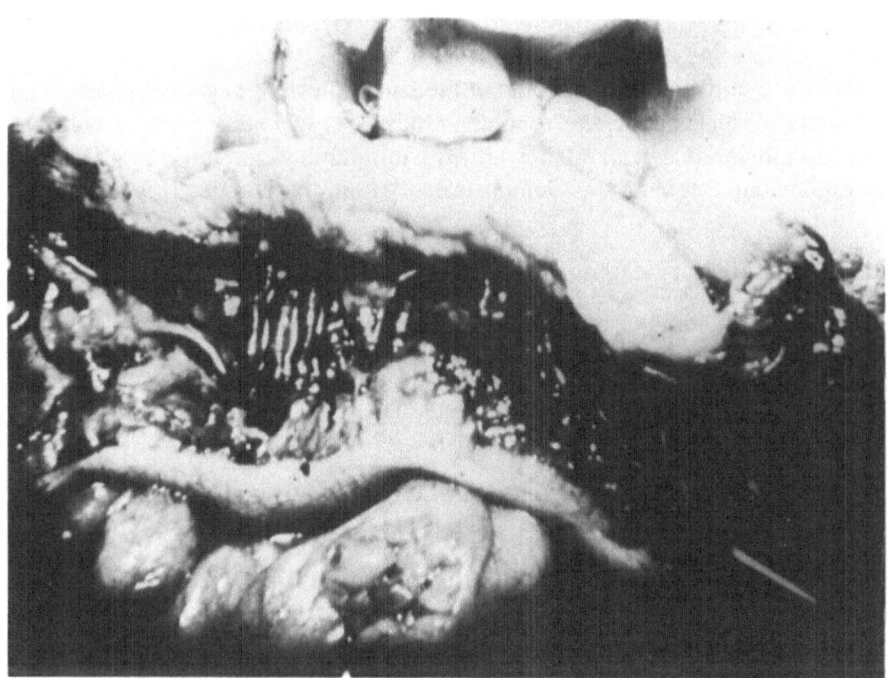

Figure 9. Amyloidosis. Gross specimen reveals marked thickening of the wall. This thickening is responsible for the roentgen findings described in Figure 10.

Rarely, a sprue pattern is seen in diffuse intestinal lymphocytic lymphoma. In such patients, the distinctive roentgen features of lymphocytic lymphoma are also present, such as nodularity, ulceration and irregular thickening of the folds.

4.2.2. Multiple Nodular Defects

Multiple nodular defects (nodular lymphoid hyperplasia) are most commonly seen in variable Ig deficiency with *Giardia* in the stool and in isolated IgA deficiency.

Nodular lymphoid hyperplasia associated with hypogammaglobulinemia affects predominantly the small intestine (Figure 3). Less frequently, the colon and rectum are involved. The characteristic roentgen feature is a uniform distribution throughout the involved segment of intestine of innumerable tiny, smooth, nodular filling defects measuring 1–3 mm in diameter (Hodgson *et al.*, 1967) (Figure 4). The nodules are round and regular in outline, and are not associated with other mucosal alterations. The small bowel is not dilated, and the valvulae conniventes are not thickened or blunted. Microscopic examination of a peroral small-bowel biopsy specimen reveals the characteristic enlarged lymphoid follicles within the lamina propria, causing effacement of the villus pattern of the overlying mucosa and imparting a nodular or polypoid appearance.

Although it is true that nodular lymphoid hyperplasia is usually associated with Ig abnormalities, it can be seen in the absence of such serum alterations. In children and young adults, the terminal ileum alone may demonstrate multiple small symmetrical nodules as a normal finding (Figure 5).

Diffuse lymphocytic lymphoma of the small intestine may also result in multiple nodules visualized on the roentgen study. These nodules are usually larger, irregular, and variable in size. They are both intraluminal and intramural in location. Ulcerations can frequently be demonstrated within the nodules (Figure 6).

4.2.3. Inflammatory Changes Secondary to Giardiasis

The roentgen findings in *Giardia lamblia* infection are inflammatory in character and are usually limited to the duodenum and jejunum (Marshak *et al.*, 1968). There is spasm and irritability, and slight narrowing of the lumen with thickening and distortion of the folds. Increased intestinal secretions frequently cause blurring

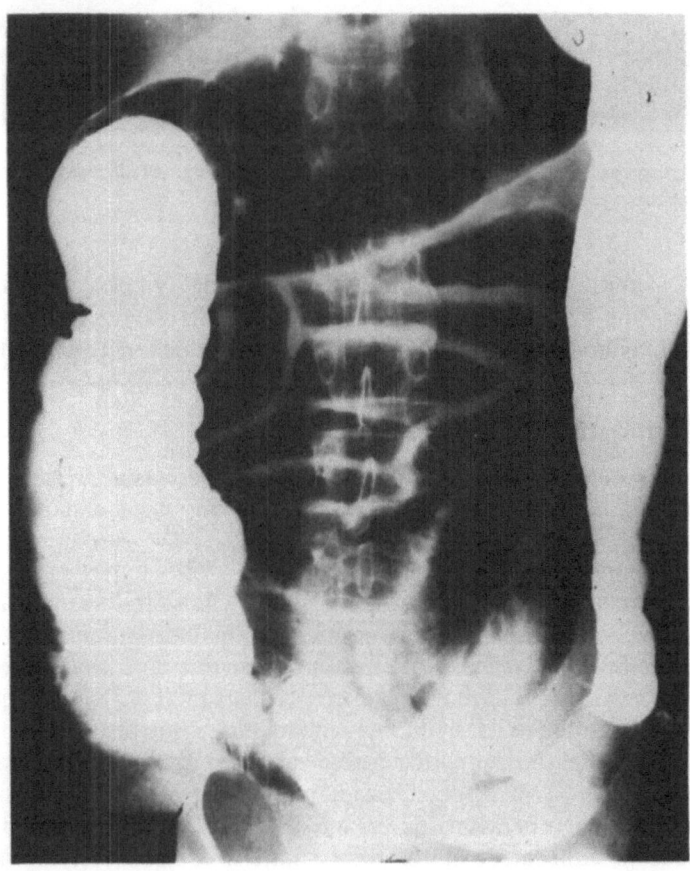

Figure 10. Amyloidosis. There is a complete absence of the haustral markings throughout the colon, and the configuration resembles that of ulcerative colitis. The air-filled loops of small bowel are separated by the presence of fluid in the abdomen.

461

LYMPHORETICULAR
DISORDERS OF THE
GASTROINTESTINAL
TRACT:
ROENTGENO-
GRAPHIC FEATURES

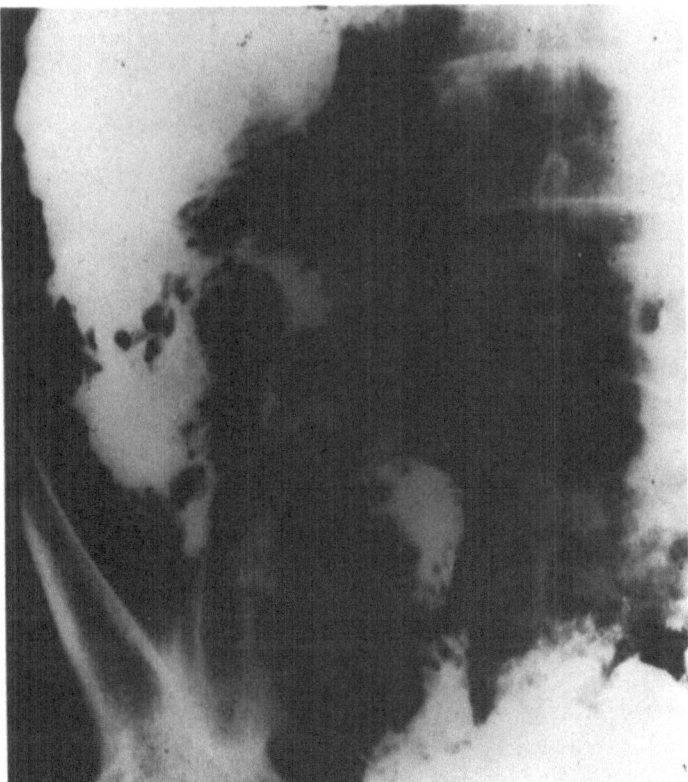

Figure 11. Lymphocytic lymphoma. Multiple tumor nodules of varying size are present in the terminal ileum, cecum, and ascending colon. The terminal ileum is slightly dilated. The nodules are obviously larger and less symmetrical than those of nodular lymphoid hyperplasia.

of the folds and sometimes fragmentation and slight segmentation of the barium column. Transit through the jejunum may be rapid. The ileum usually appears normal (Figure 7).

When giardiasis complicates a hypogammaglobulinemic enteropathy, the roentgen changes described above may be associated with the multiple tiny filling defects of nodular lymphoid hyperplasia or, less commonly, with the sprue (malabsorption) pattern. Eradication of the parasite results in return of the fold pattern to normal, as well as improvement of the villus structure in hypogammaglobulinemic sprue, regression of diarrhea, steatorrhea, and malabsorption, and of lactose intolerance and abnormal intestinal protein loss. The number and size of the nodular follicles are not affected, however, by treatment of the *Giardia* infection.

It is important to note that the presence of *Giardia lamblia* in the stool does not necessarily mean that the small-bowel roentgen study will be abnormal. Indeed, small-bowel changes are not seen in most patients with giardiasis.

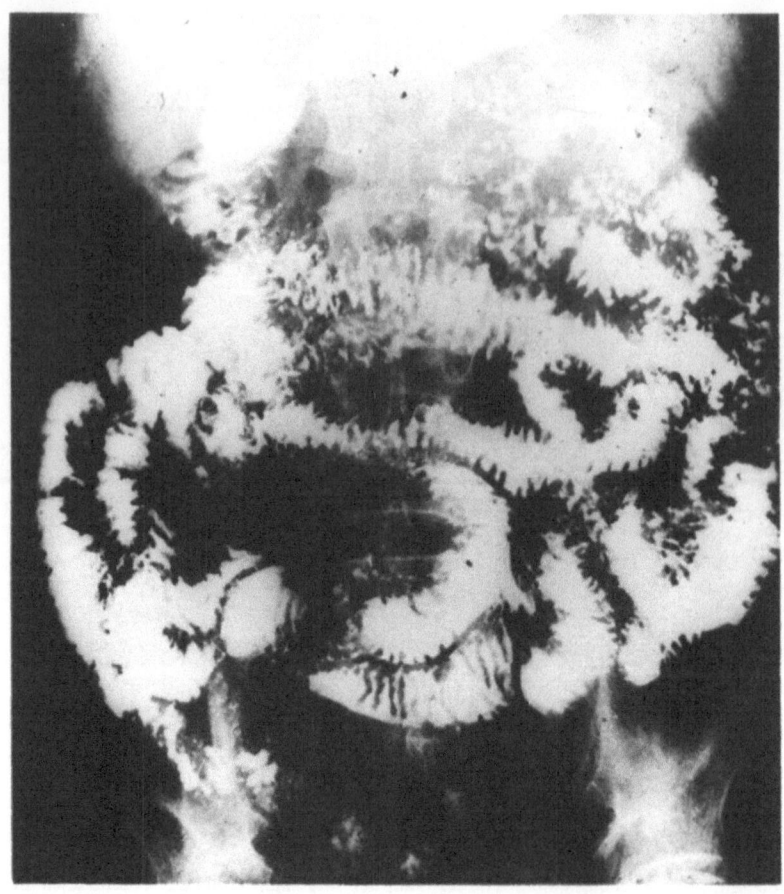

Figure 12. α-Chain disease. This entity was previously described as Mediterranean lymphoma. Not enough cases have yet been studied to delineate a definitive roentgen pattern. In this case, there is thickening of the folds, associated in some areas with minimal narrowing of the lumen. No other abnormalities are noted. In some cases, flat nodules along the contour of the bowel have been described.

4.2.4. Thickening of the Small-Intestinal Folds

Thickening of the small-bowel folds is not characteristic of the primary enteropathic immunodeficiencies, as classified in Section 3.1, except for superimposed *Giardia lamblia* infection. It is, however, a feature of the secondary Ig disorders.

a. Amyloidosis. By infiltration of the bowel wall, amyloidosis produces conspicuous thickening of the folds, and this process tends to be uniform throughout the entire small bowel on roentgen study. Enlargement of the folds in the ileum gives an appearance resembling the normal feathery pattern of the jejunum, a configuration that has been termed *jejunization of the ileum.* There is no significant dilatation or increased secretions, and nodules are not present (Figure 8).

When amyloidosis involves the colon, it produces roentgen alterations that are similar to those of chronic ulcerative colitis, with absent haustral markings but no significant shortening (Figures 9 and 10). Ascites is often present and can be

463

LYMPHORETICULAR
DISORDERS OF THE
GASTROINTESTINAL
TRACT:
ROENTGENO-
GRAPHIC FEATURES

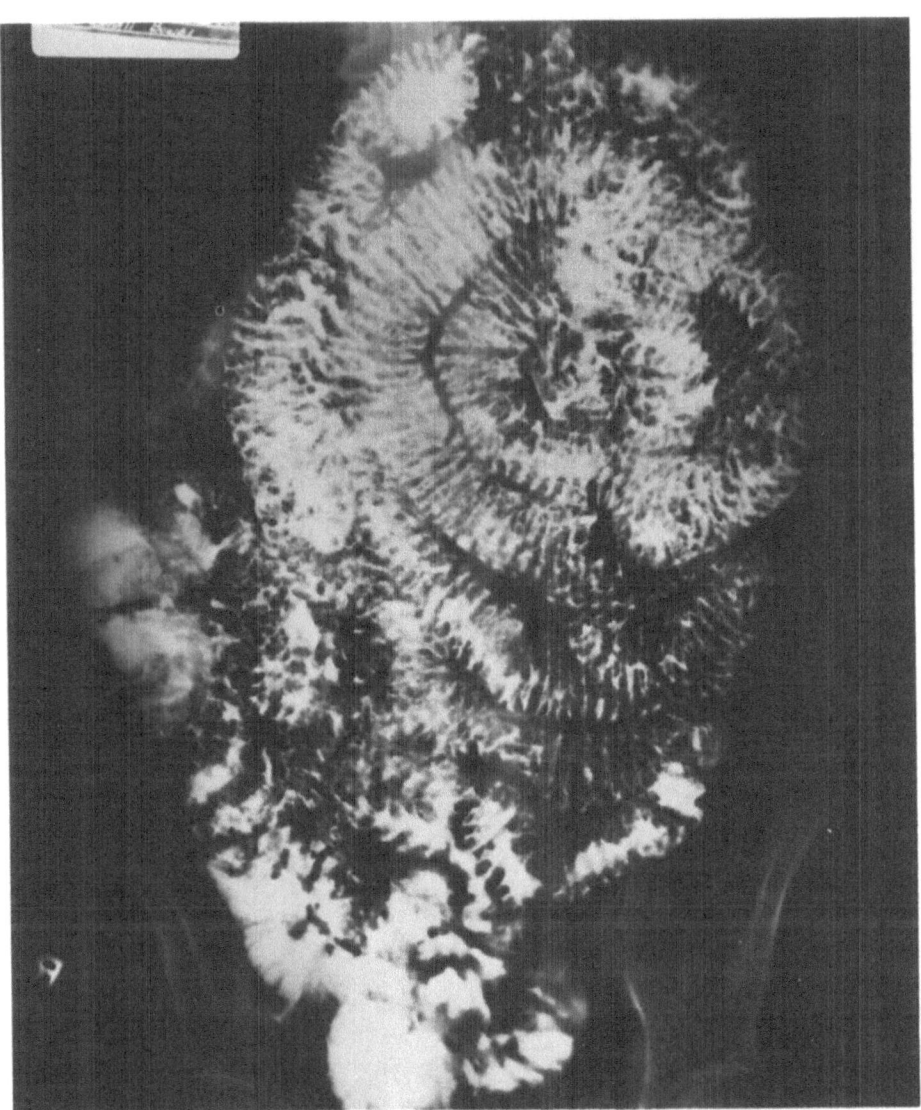

Figure 13. Waldenström's macroglobulinemia. There is diffuse thickening of the valvulae conniventes associated with a granular mucosal surface. In some areas, it appears almost nodular.

RICHARD H.
MARSHAK *ET AL.*

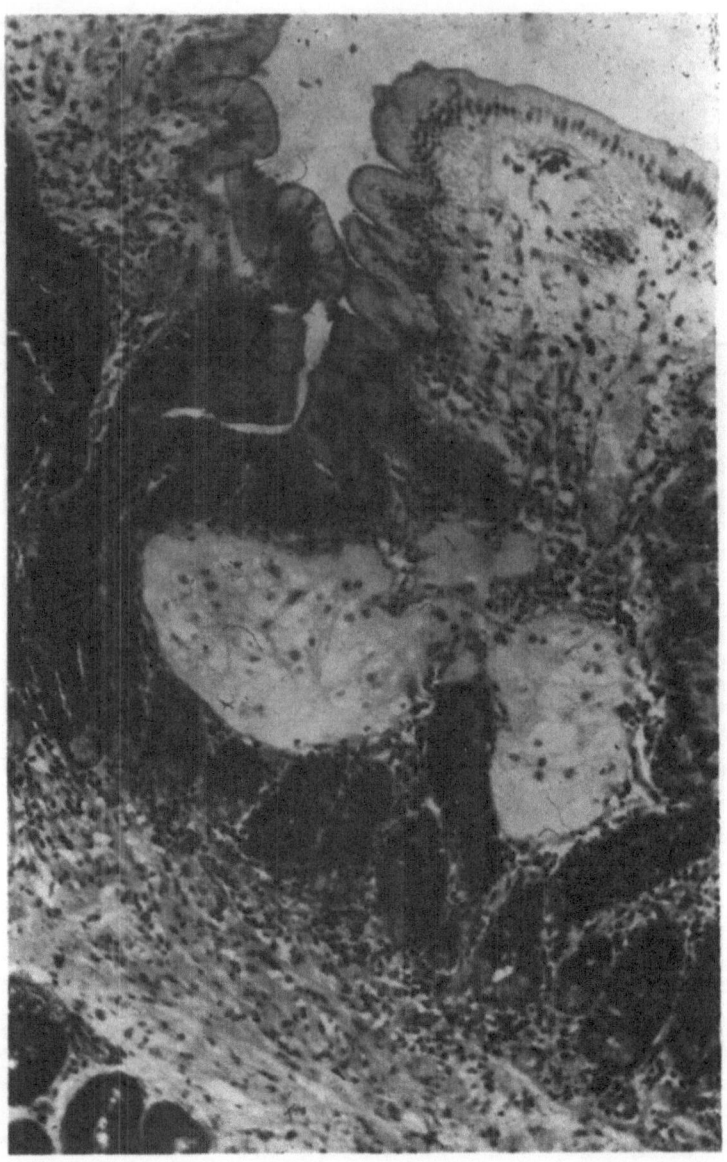

Figure 14. Intestinal lymphangiectasia. Histological sections demonstrate marked dilatation of the lymphatics as well as edema of the mucosa.

465

LYMPHORETICULAR
DISORDERS OF THE
GASTROINTESTINAL
TRACT:
ROENTGENO-
GRAPHIC FEATURES

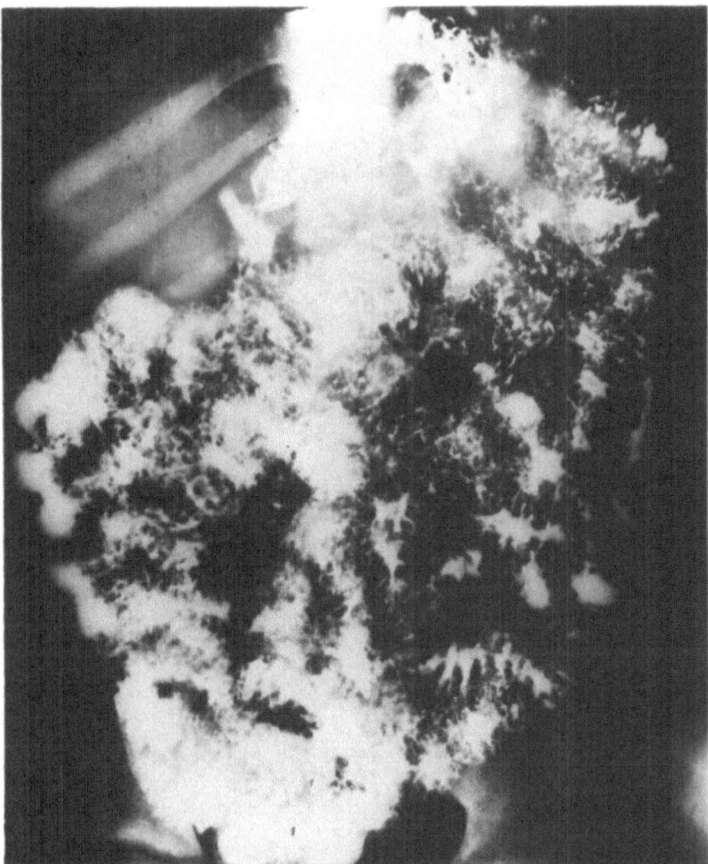

Figure 15. Intestinal lymphangiectasia. The entire small bowel is involved. There is minimal segmentation and fragmentation, associated with diffuse thickening of the valvulae conniventes and moderate secretions. There is no dilatation. The serum albumin in this patient was 1 g/dl. The alterations described are probably due to intestinal edema secondary to hypoalbuminemia.

recognized by separation of the loops of small bowel. In the stomach, amyloid infiltration produces a polypoid tumor or features similar to those of scirrhous carcinoma.

b. Lymphocytic Lymphoma. Lymphocytic lymphoma may also appear as a smooth, diffuse thickening of the intestinal folds throughout the small bowel, without hypersecretion. The thickened folds are more commonly irregularly nodular, and coarse marginal scalloping of the bowel contour may be seen (Figure 11).

c. α-Chain Disease. The roentgenographic features of this disease are variable. The small-intestinal folds may be irregularly thickened (Figure 12). Multiple nodular defects may be demonstrated having the same characteristics as other lymphomas and involving the entire length of the small bowel.

There have been described a group of patients with marked plasma-cell and

RICHARD H.
MARSHAK *ET AL.*

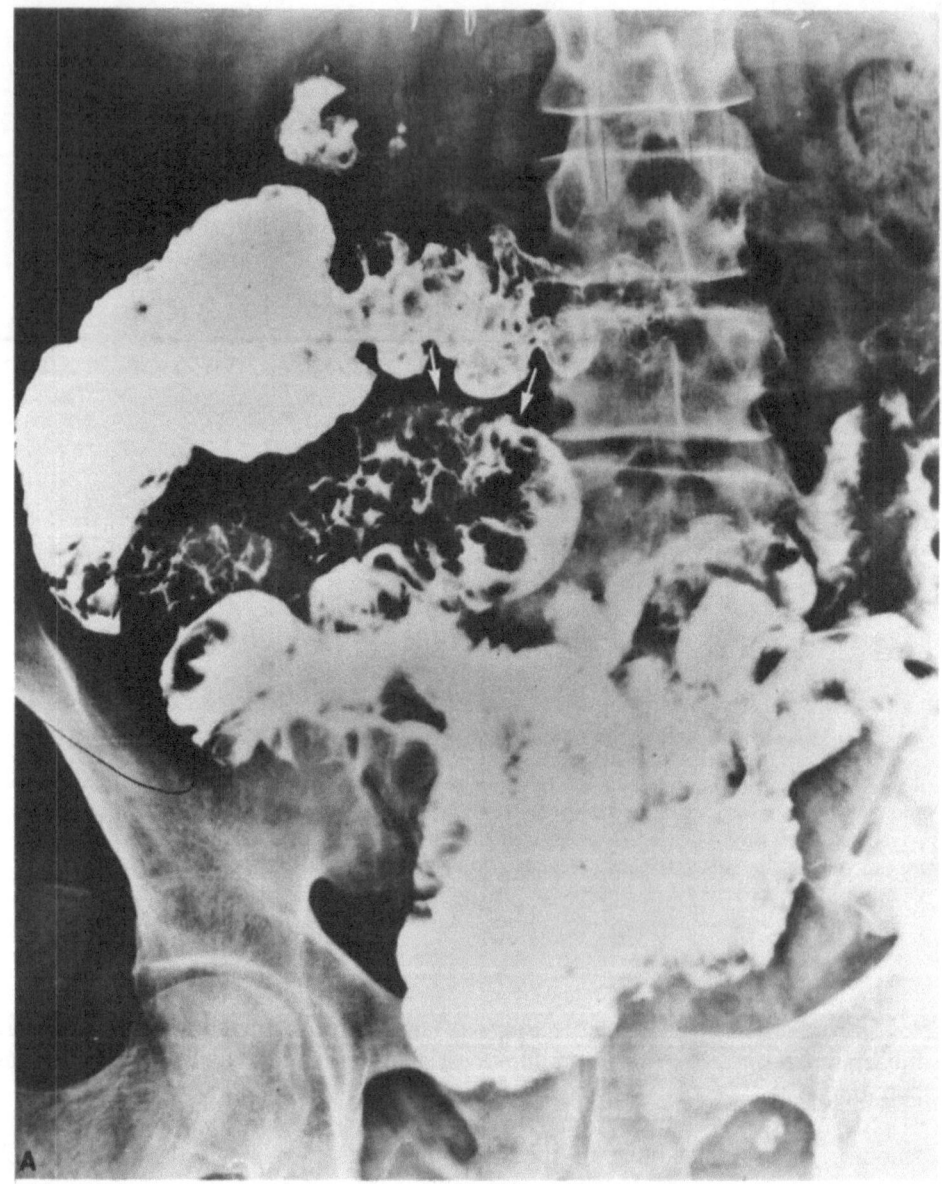

Figure 16A. Lymphocytic lymphoma. The mucosal pattern is replaced by numerous polypoid intramural and intraluminal defects that alter the caliber of the bowel lumen. There is no evidence of obstruction.

467

LYMPHORETICULAR
DISORDERS OF THE
GASTROINTESTINAL
TRACT:
ROENTGENO-
GRAPHIC FEATURES

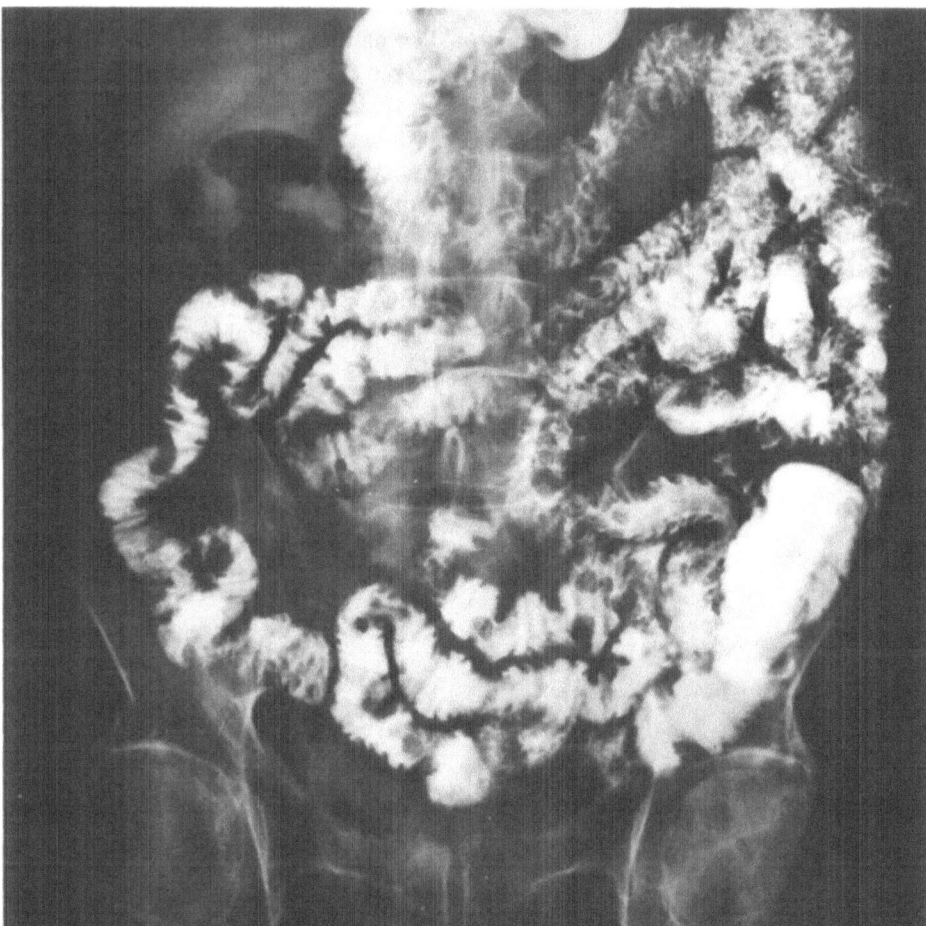

Figure 16B. Lymphocytic lymphoma (nodular form). Numerous small polypoid intramural and intraluminal defects are distributed throughout the small bowel.

lymphocyte infiltration of the small bowel, but without progression to lymphoma during a period of follow-up. Such patients have a variety of serum Ig defects ranging from deficiency to excessive levels. This group probably represents a heterogeneous collection of abnormalities that await classification. They have in common, however, the roentgen alterations of thickening of the folds and at times submucosal or intraluminal nodules (Ruoff *et al.*, 1971). Patients with these findings frequently present clinically with diarrhea and malabsorption.

d. **Waldenström's Macroglobulinemia.** Uniform thickening of the folds of the small bowel is also found in some cases of Waldenström's macroglobulinemia. The wall of the intestine is thickened, as evidenced by separation of the loops on small bowel series, and the lumen may be moderately dilated (Khilnani *et al.*, 1969). The mucosal surface itself may have a fine granular appearance (Figure 13).

e. Intestinal Lymphangiectasia. This is an exudative, protein-losing enteropathy with gross dilatation of the lymphatics of the lamina propria of the small bowel reflecting a generalized disorder of the development of lymphatic channels. Hypogammaglobulinemia, mainly affecting IgG, is associated with a fall in serum albumin and, to a lesser degree, other proteins, as well as with the loss of lymphocytes into the bowel lumen. Enlargement of folds on roentgen examination usually affects both the jejunum and the ileum. The pattern of fold enlargement is uniform, orderly, and symmetrical in a given loop. A stacked-coin appearance is common, and the folds may have a regular biconvex appearance (Figures 14 and 15). Excessive intestinal secretions result in dilution of the barium column, at times in association with segmentation and fragmentation. Dilatation is minimal or absent.

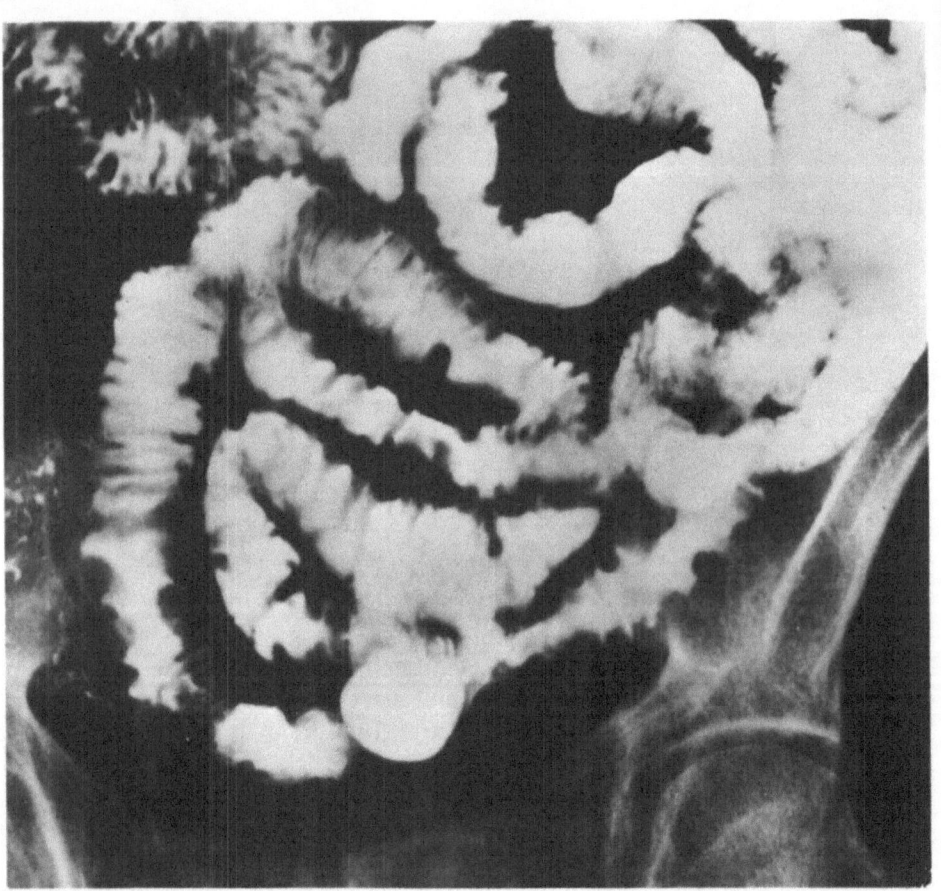

Figure 17. Lymphocytic lymphoma. There is thickening and blunting of the folds with some encroachment on the bowel lumen, but no obstruction. In some areas, small bowel nodules can be identified along the contour of the bowel lumen. The nonstenotic phase of regional enteritis is simulated.

469

LYMPHORETICULAR
DISORDERS OF THE
GASTROINTESTINAL
TRACT:
ROENTGENO-
GRAPHIC FEATURES

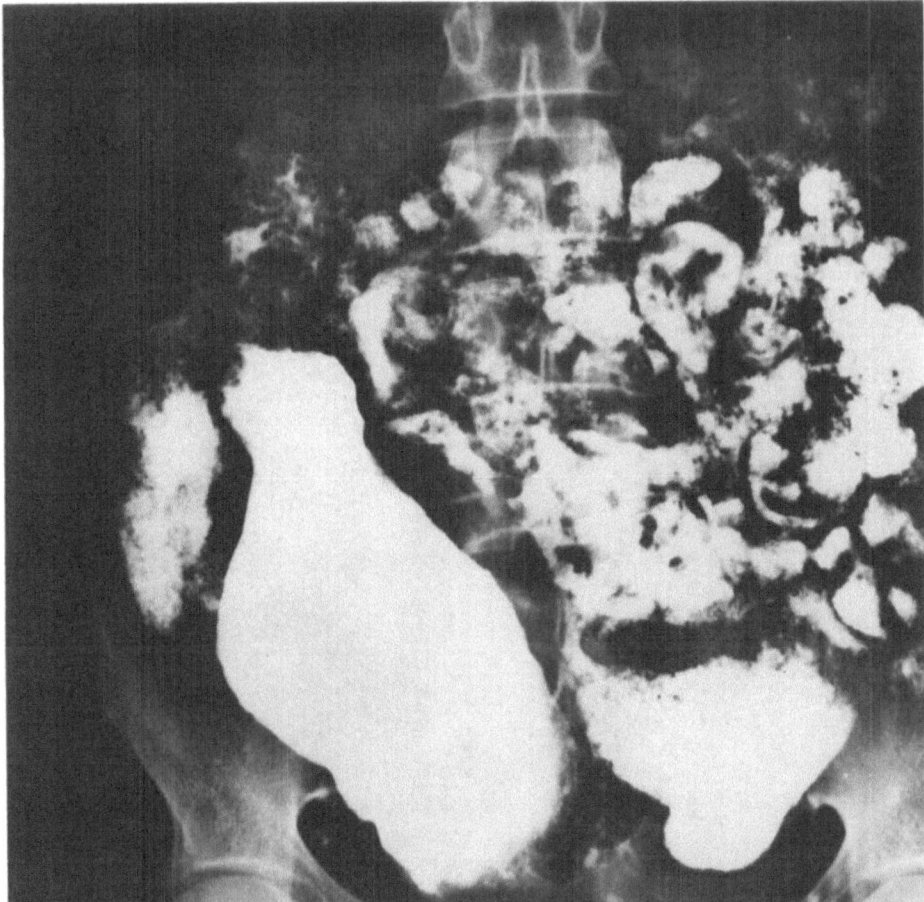

Figure 18. Lymphocytic lymphoma. Marked aneurysmal dilatation of the ileum. The increased thickness of the bowel wall is indicated by the increased distance between the involved bowel and the adjacent loops.

The thickening of the folds noted radiologically in intestinal lymphangiectasia in part represents mucosal and submucosal edema secondary to hypoproteinemia.

5. Lymphocytic Lymphoma of the Small Bowel

We have classified the roentgenological changes in lymphosarcoma of the small bowel (Marshak and Lindner, 1976) as follows:

1. Multiple nodular defects
2. Infiltrating form
3. Polypoid form
4. Endoexoenteric form with excavation and fistula formation
5. Predominantly invasion of the mesentery with (A) large extraluminal masses or (B) production of the sprue pattern

RICHARD H.
MARSHAK *ET AL.*

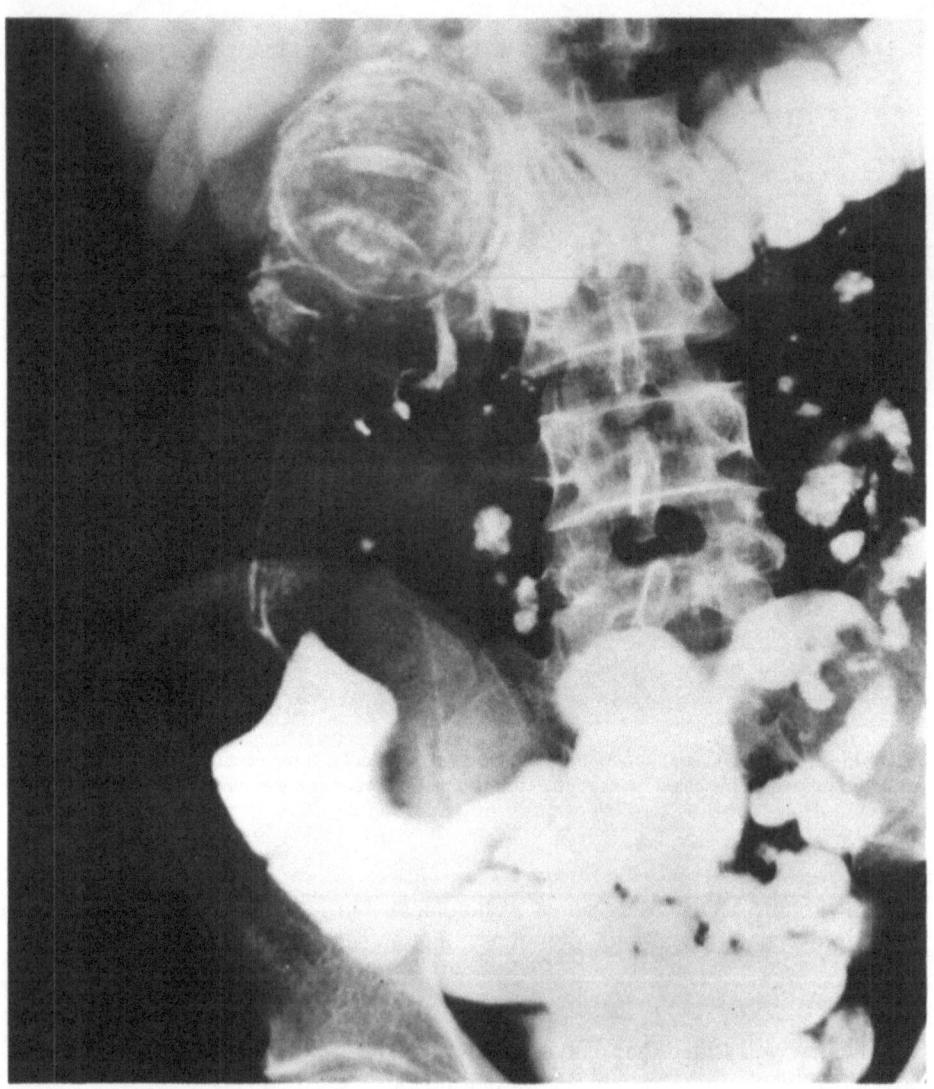

Figure 19. Lymphocytic lymphoma. Polypoid lymphosarcoma of the terminal ileum, resulting in an ileocecal intussusception with minimal obstruction. The lesion is obscured by the intussusception.

5.1. Multiple Nodular Defects

471

LYMPHORETICULAR
DISORDERS OF THE
GASTROINTESTINAL
TRACT:
ROENTGENO-
GRAPHIC FEATURES

These defects appear as multiple intraluminal nodules or intramural defects of varying size that alter the mucosal pattern and produce an irregular, coarse scalloping of the bowel contour (Figures 16A, 16B). Ulceration may be seen within the nodules because of central necrosis. The bowel lumen is of normal or even increased caliber. These changes are more often found in the ileum and involve segments varying from one to several feet in length. The altered segments retain their pliability and are not fixed in position. This type may occur as sole manifestation of lymphosarcoma, or it may be associated with other intestinal changes. Not infrequently when the terminal ileum is involved, nodules extend into the cecum and ascending colon. In some cases, the nodules are tiny and difficult to identify.

5.2. Infiltrating Form

The bowel wall becomes diffusely infiltrated and thickened. The degree of thickening varies from area to area, producing irregular segments of narrowing and relative dilatation. The degree of narrowing is never as marked as that observed in carcinoma or inflammatory disease. The mucosal folds may become flattened and effaced, or they may be thickened and thrown up into irregular, nodular projections, producing coarse, irregular scalloping of the bowel contour with intraluminal filling defects of different size (Figure 17). The mural thickening causes separation and straightening of the intestinal loops, which stand out clearly from the closely approximated normal small intestine. The barium column sometimes has a mottled appearance because of the increased secretions within the lumen of the affected segment. The infiltration may be limited to short segments, either single or multiple, which appear as short areas of eccentric narrowing of the bowel lumen with effacement or thickening of the mucosal folds and evidence of tumor formation. Lymphocytic lymphoma is primarily a medullary tumor and produces no desmoplastic reaction. Thus, marked rigidity of the involved segment is uncommon, and there is usually insufficient stenosis to produce proximal dilatation of the small intestine. Stricture formation sufficient to cause intestinal obstruction has been noted, however, in association with ulceration and secondary infection. Occasionally, a discrete ulceration within a mass can evoke mechanical intestinal obstruction by producing spasm or by completely encircling the lumen of the bowel.

Another form of segmental infiltration of the bowel wall in lymphocytic lymphoma is characterized by marked localized dilatation. This has been referred to as aneurysmal dilatation (Figure 18). The increased thickness of the bowel wall is demonstrated by increased separation from adjacent loops. Barium tends to pool within the widened lumen, and no mucosal pattern can be seen. The contours of the dilated segment may be smooth or coarsely irregular, or show scalloping and nodularity due to intramural tumor formation. The adjacent mucosa may appear intact or thickened and nodular. In an occasional form of lymphocytic lymphoma diffuse thickening of the folds throughout the small bowel is seen with little evidence of nodularity or intraluminal defects.

5.3. Polypoid Form

When a tumor has grown to a size sufficient to produce a discrete intraluminal mass and is without intramural extension, it may be drawn forward by peristalsis to

RICHARD H.
MARSHAK *ET AL.*

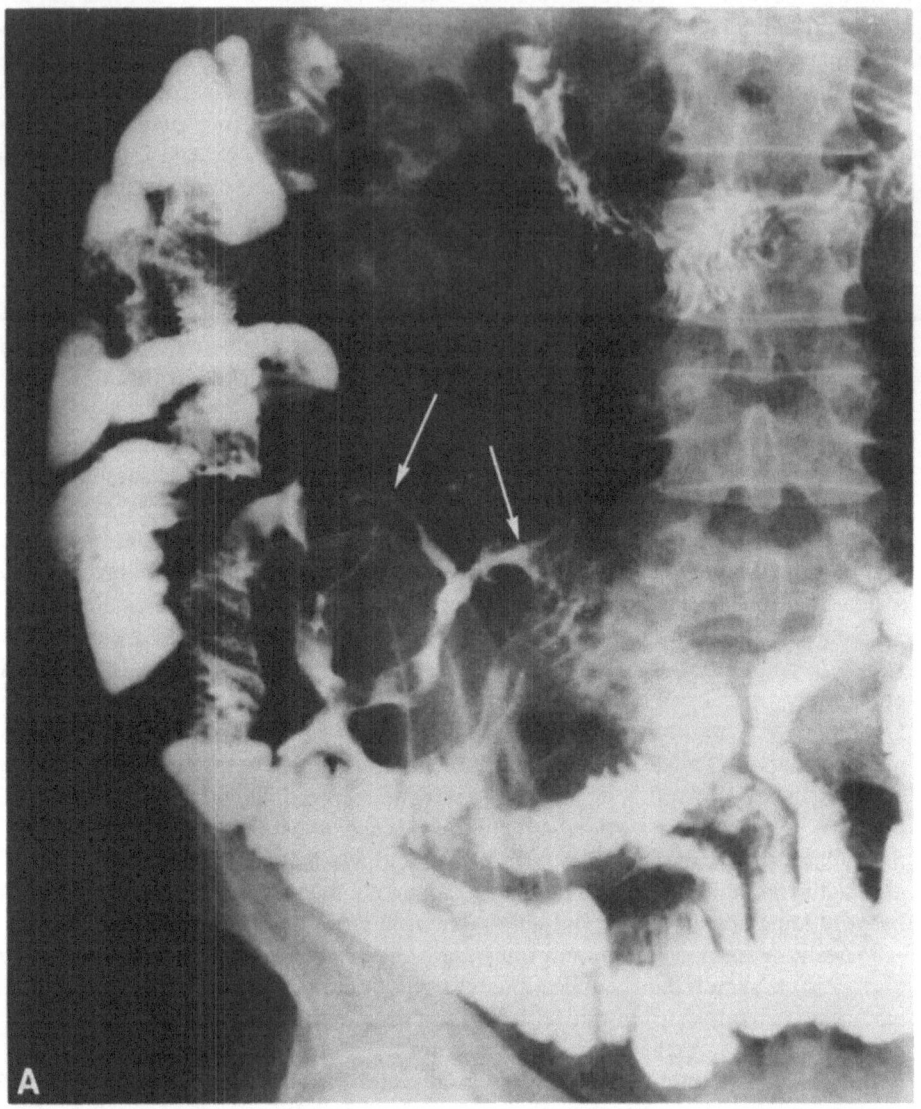

Figure 20A. Lymphocytic lymphoma. Endoexoenteric lymphosarcoma of the distal ileum. The normal bowel lumen is replaced by many intercommunicating, tortuous tracts throughout the tumor. The arrows indicate the nodular mucosal pattern proximal to the mass. The lumen of the segment is not narrowed.

473

LYMPHORETICULAR
DISORDERS OF THE
GASTROINTESTINAL
TRACT:
ROENTGENO-
GRAPHIC FEATURES

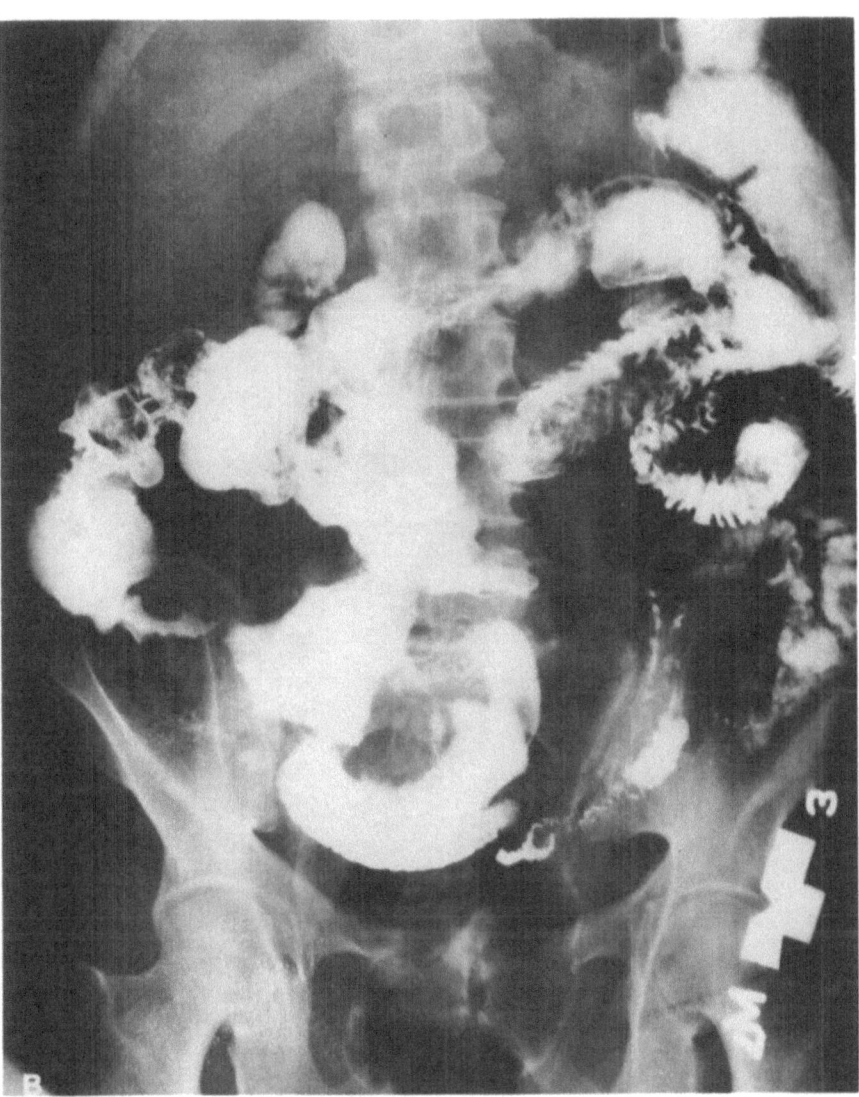

Figure 20B. Lymphocytic lymphoma (same case as in Figure 20A, 3 months later). There is a large, irregular, triangular excavated area within the lumen containing an amorphous collection of barium. The mucosal pattern and the adjacent small-intestinal loops are considerably thickened.

RICHARD H.
MARSHAK *ET AL.*

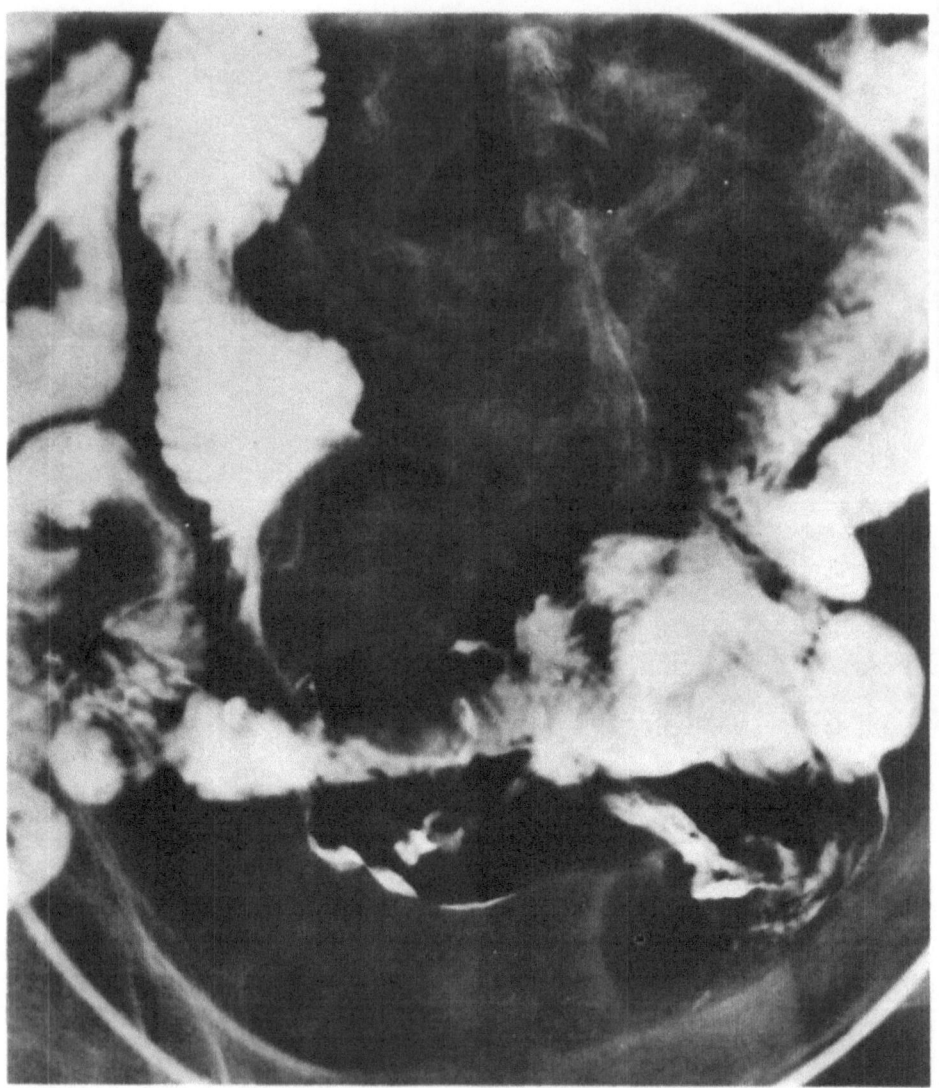

Figure 21. Lymphocytic lymphoma. There is a single, smooth, submucosal defect in the distal jejunum.

475

LYMPHORETICULAR
DISORDERS OF THE
GASTROINTESTINAL
TRACT:
ROENTGENO-
GRAPHIC FEATURES

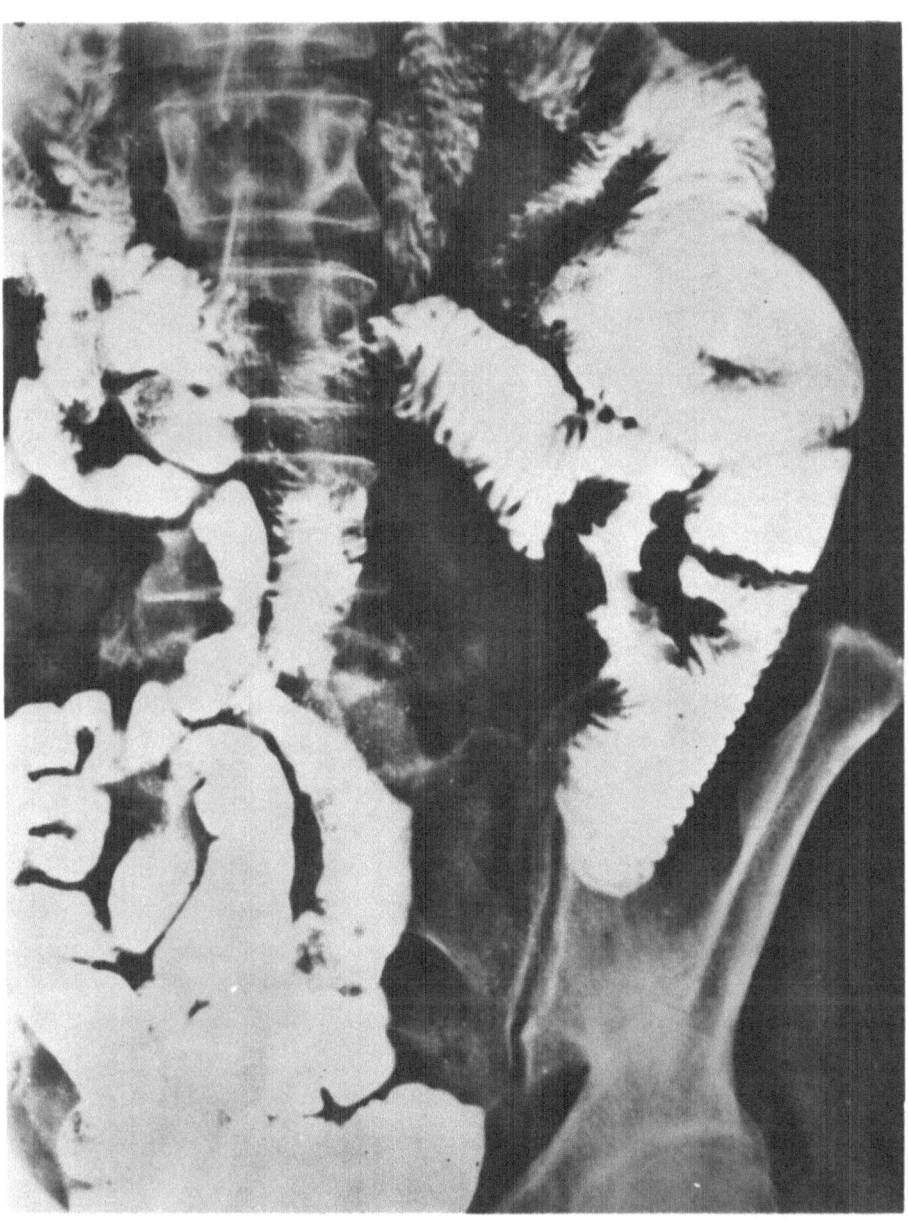

Figure 22. Hodgkin's disease. There is a segment of midjejunum that is narrowed and rigid for a distance of approximately 5 cm. The contours are scalloped with multiple nodular masses intruding on the lumen of the bowel. The proximal bowel is slightly dilated.

RICHARD H.
MARSHAK *ET AL.*

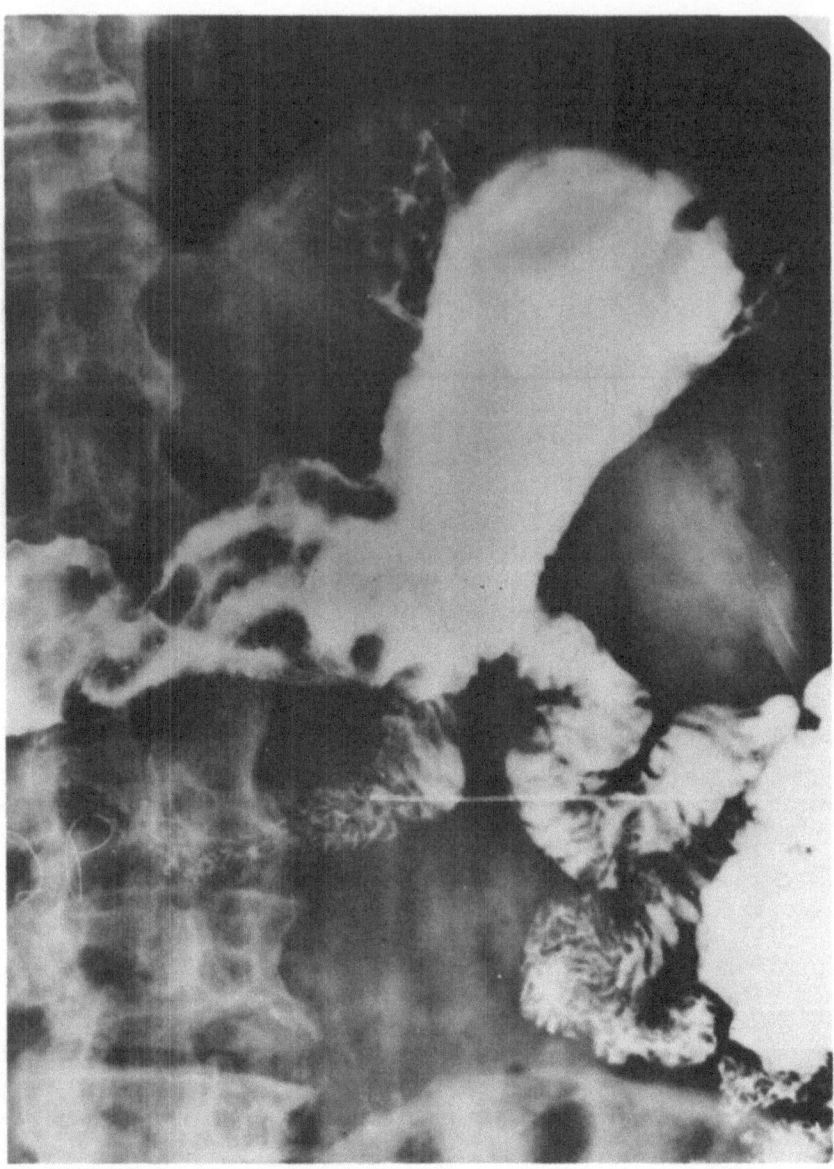

Figure 23. Lymphocytic lymphoma of the stomach. The folds in the distal half of the stomach are irregularly thickened, rigid, and nodular. The duodenal bulb is similarly involved. There is some loss of pliability. No definite ulceration is identified. The proximal two thirds of the stomach is normal.

477

LYMPHORETICULAR
DISORDERS OF THE
GASTROINTESTINAL
TRACT:
ROENTGENO-
GRAPHIC FEATURES

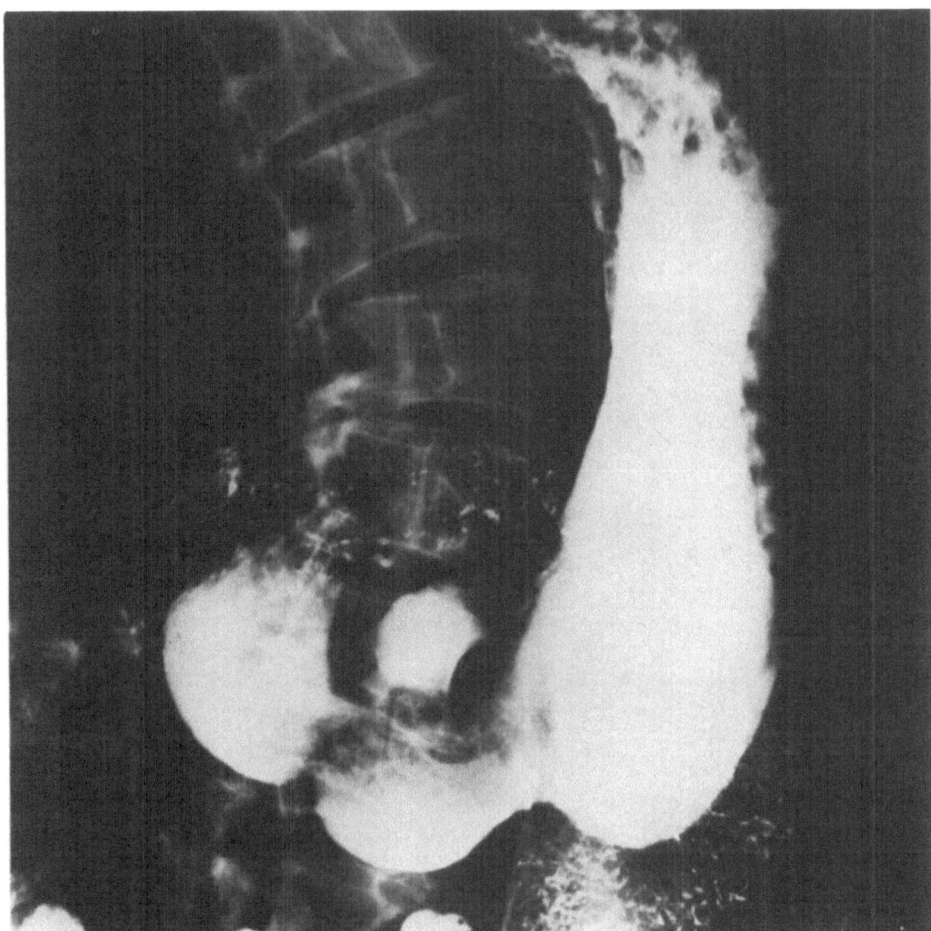

Figure 24. Lymphocytic lymphoma of the stomach. There is a large ulcer extending from the lesser curvature aspect of the reentrant angle of the stomach. Irregular masses project into the base of the ulcer crater. The surrounding folds are not enlarged. Differentiation from an ulcerating carcinoma is difficult.

form a pseudopedicle. It may become the lead point of an intussusception (Figure 19). Unless there are other clues to the nature of the underlying lesion, the cause of the intussusception cannot be determined from the roentgenogram. At times, the polypoid tumor is large, bulky, and presents predominantly as an intraluminal lesion without intussusception.

5.4. Endoexoenteric Form with Excavation

In this instance, a large, irregular ulceration with multiple fistulas communicating with the adjacent bowel is seen. The roentgen findings are bizarre. Characteristically, there is an extensive, irregular, amorphous patch of barium that does not conform to the intestinal lumen and communicates with the surrounding bowel.

RICHARD H.
MARSHAK *ET AL.*

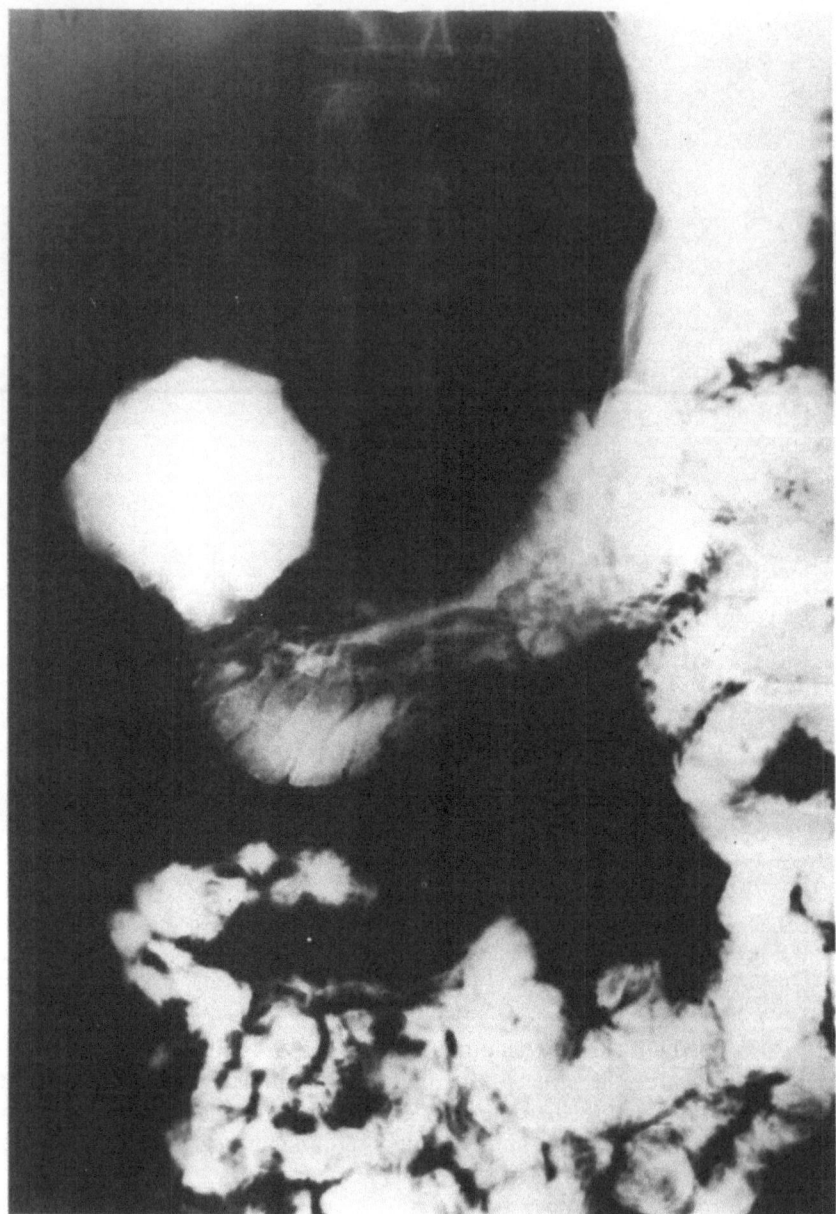

Figure 25. Lymphocytic lymphoma extending into the duodenal bulb. The duodenal bulb is replaced by a large, amorphous, irregular crater. Numerous nodular indentations, due to tumor, are identified.

479

LYMPHORETICULAR
DISORDERS OF THE
GASTROINTESTINAL
TRACT:
ROENTGENO-
GRAPHIC FEATURES

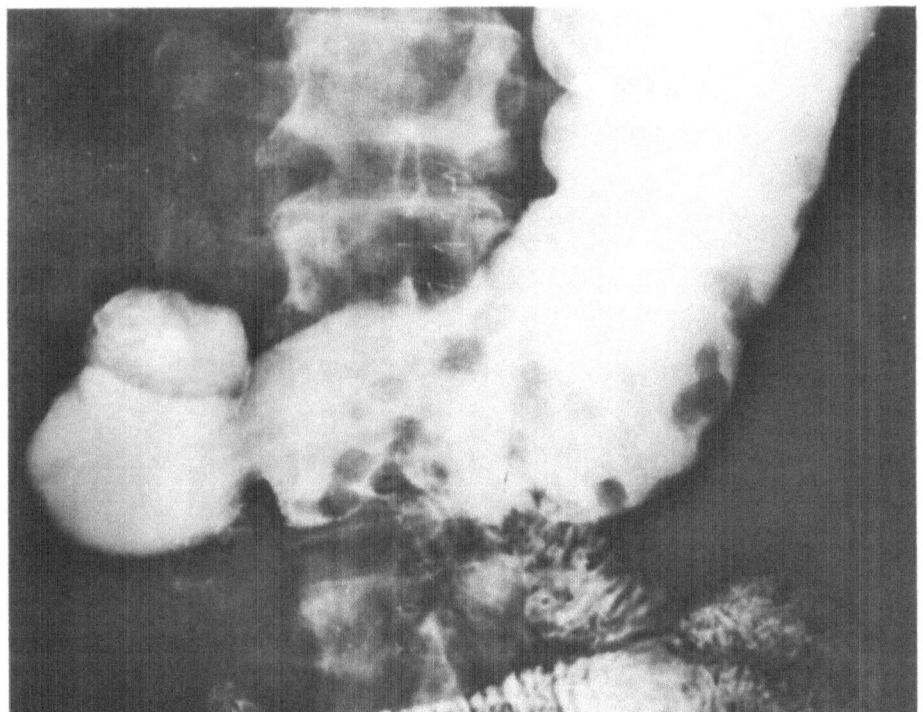

Figure 26. Lymphocytic lymphoma of the stomach. There are multiple irregular polypoid defects involving the distal half of the stomach. No discrete ulceration is identified. There is no narrowing. Differentiation from multiple benign polyposis of the stomach may be difficult.

Adjacent loops are displaced by the large mass. Fistulas are frequent (Figures 20A and B). Before massive excavation occurs, the tumor and the involved portion of small intestine may be criss-crossed by many intercommunicating channels connecting the tumor with the lumen of the small intestine. These channels appear as amorphous barium streaks of different caliber. In the early cases, the presence of altered intestinal loops and fistulas may suggest regional enteritis. Subsequent events produce massive excavation of the involved area and indicate the presence of a necrotic neoplasm.

In lymphocytic lymphoma, many features may be combined and seen simultaneously. The lesion is usually multiple, and sometimes the nodular, the infiltrating, and the endoexoenteric forms are seen at one time.

5.5. Predominantly Invasion of the Mesentery

Large extraluminal masses are identified. The greater portion of the tumor grows centrifugally and produces tumors that can attain huge proportions and even extend into the retroperitoneum. These manifest themselves roentgenologically by displacement of the abdominal organs, pressure defects on the adjacent viscera, and

RICHARD H.
MARSHAK *ET AL.*

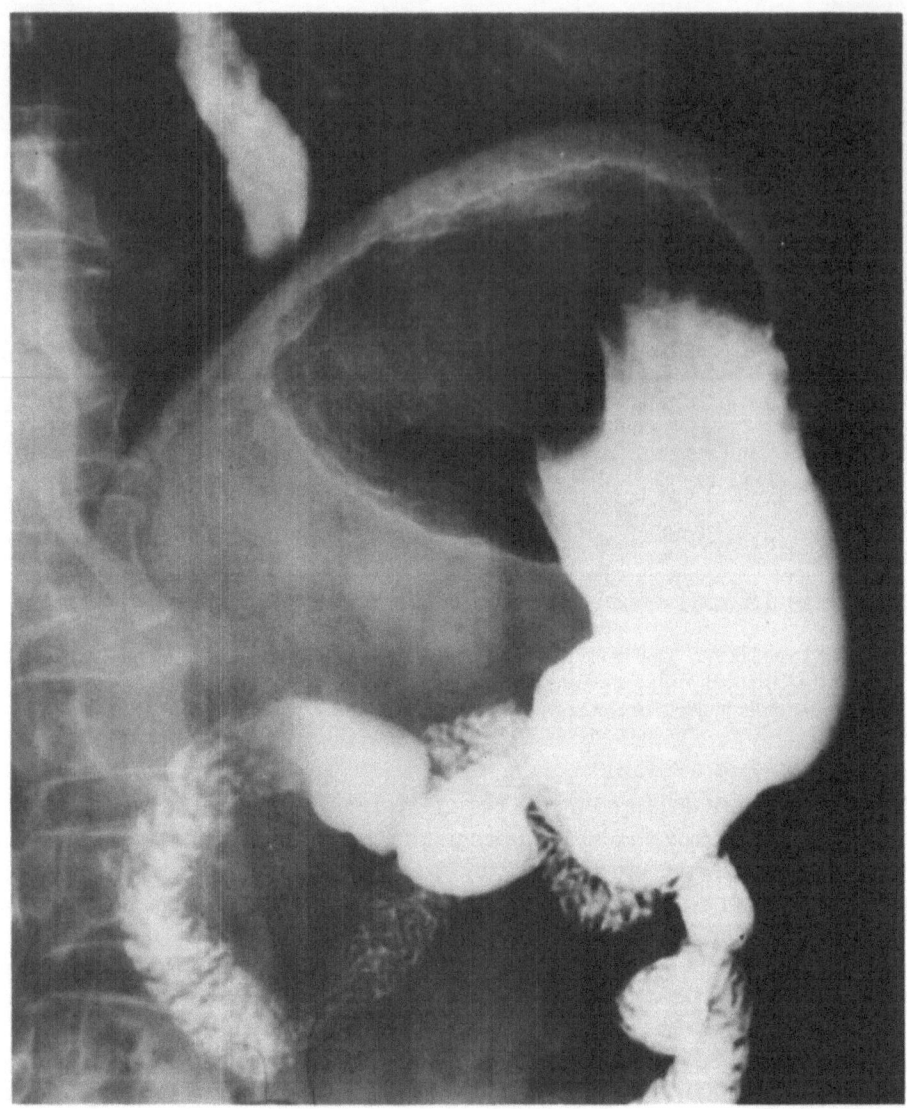

Figure 27. Lymphocytic lymphoma of the stomach. There is a large polypoid lesion involving the fundus of the stomach. This type of lesion may also be seen frequently in myosarcoma. Against a diagnosis of carcinoma is the absence of splitting of the barium stream even though the huge mass extends to the esophagogastric junction. No ulceration is seen.

481

LYMPHORETICULAR
DISORDERS OF THE
GASTROINTESTINAL
TRACT:
ROENTGENO-
GRAPHIC FEATURES

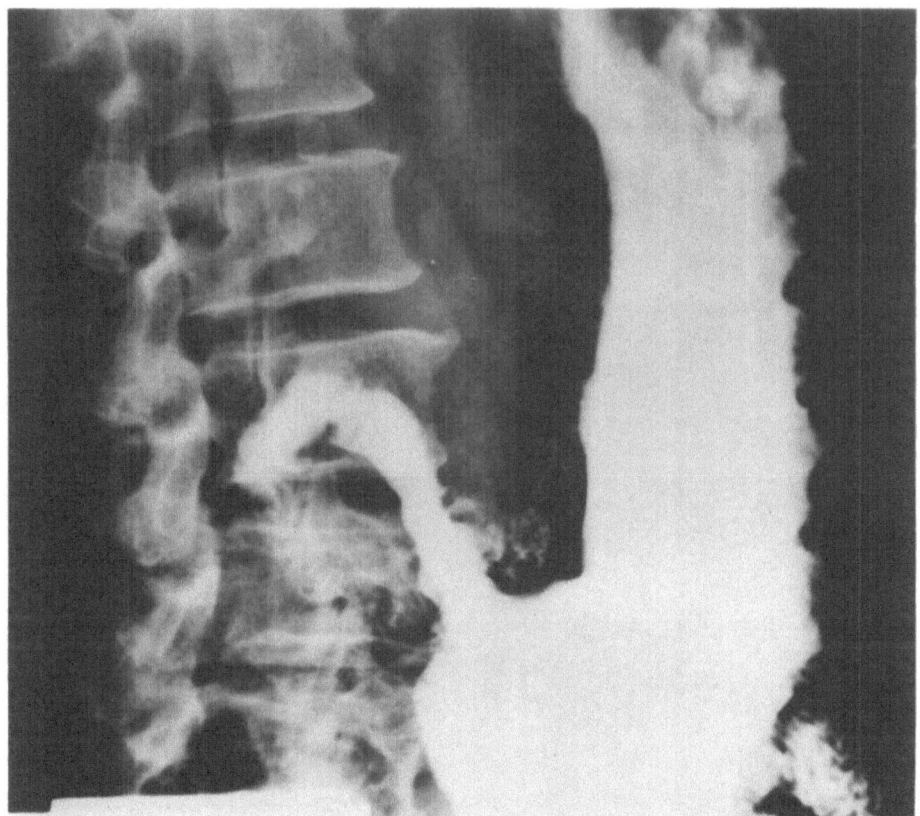

Figure 28. Hodgkin's disease of the stomach. There is narrowing of the distal third of the stomach by a large irregular mass. The findings are those usually associated with a carcinoma of the stomach, but the diagnosis in this case was Hodgkin's disease. Hodgkin's disease, Crohn's disease of the stomach, and atypical forms of gastritis may narrow the antral portion of the stomach, producing a similar configuration. Hodgkin's disease can also produce a form of linitis plastica, sometimes with multiple ulcerations.

invasion of the intestinal wall (Figure 21). Unlike metastatic carcinoma, the loops of intestine are not fixed, angulated, or obstructed. Also in contrast to metastatic carcinoma, the folds are not stretched, deformed or separated.

In another form of the invasion of the mesentery, the sprue pattern is produced.

5.6. Hodgkin's Disease

Hodgkin's disease produces the same kinds of lesions of the small intestine as lymphocytic lymphoma, but excavation, fistulas, and aneurysmal dilatation are not as frequent. Unlike lymphocytic lymphoma, Hodgkin's disease can cause marked fibrosis of the bowel wall with constriction of the lumen. Roentgenographically (Figure 22), there is eccentric narrowing of the bowel lumen, which tapers in a

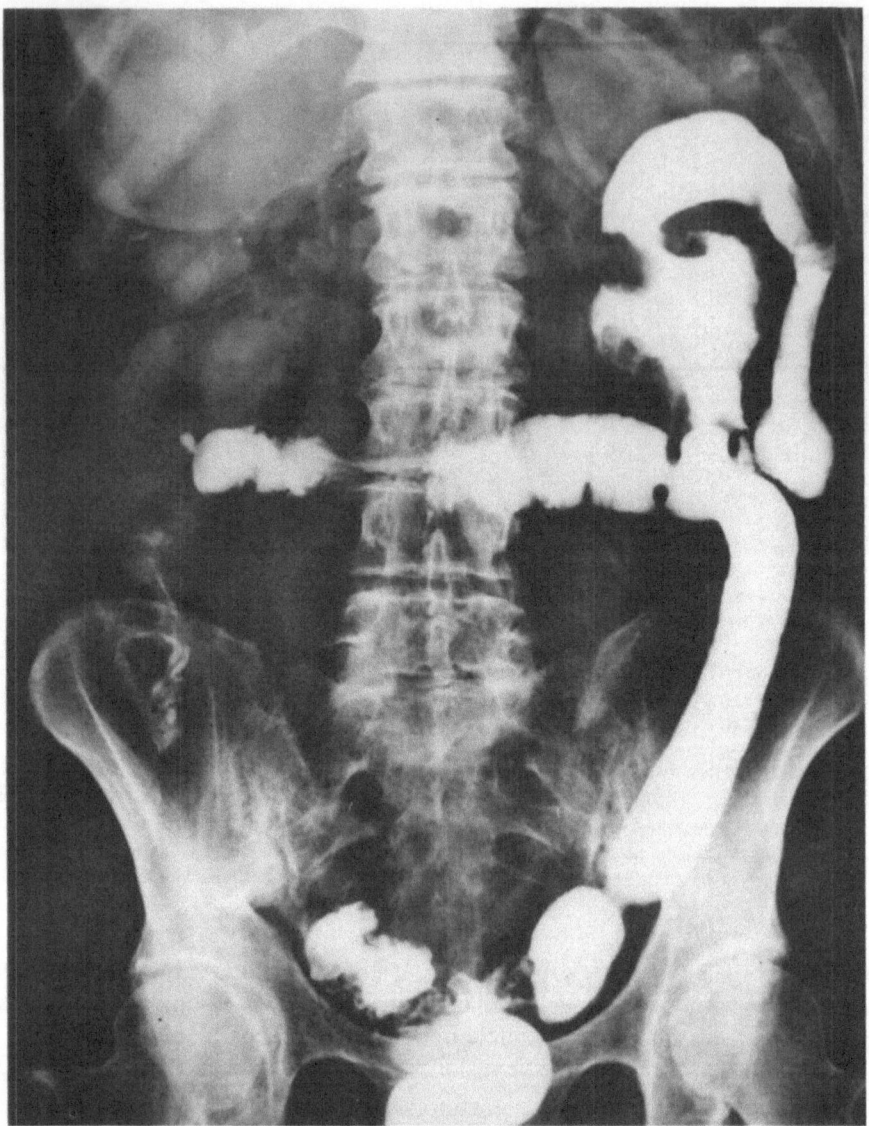

Figure 29. Lymphocytic lymphoma of the colon. A discrete mass is present in the region of the splenic flexure. This measures approximately 3½ inches in length with moderate narrowing at each end. The central portion of the mass is more dilated than the actual lumen of the bowel. The contours are irregular and scalloped, secondary to pressure from tumor. It is difficult to state whether the dilatation is due to a large ulceration or to aneurysmal dilatation of the bowel wall.

483

LYMPHORETICULAR
DISORDERS OF THE
GASTROINTESTINAL
TRACT:
ROENTGENO-
GRAPHIC FEATURES

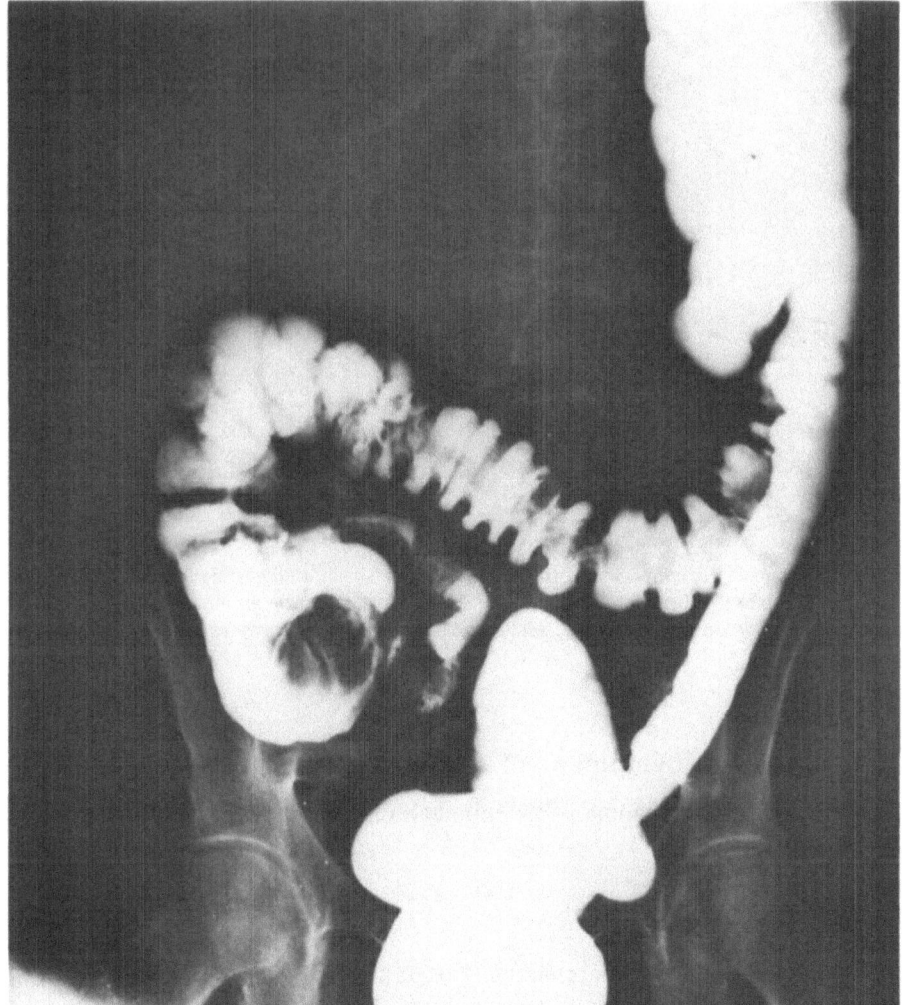

Figure 30. Lymphocytic lymphoma of the colon. There is a slightly lobulated polypoid tumor mass measuring 3 cm in diameter in the cecum. A single diagnosis is impossible in this case. A polypoid carcinoma is the most likely diagnosis, but lymphocytic lymphoma should always be considered when a tumor mass is present in this region.

fusiform manner. There are no overhanging edges at the margin of the lesion, which is frequently longer than that seen in carcinoma. The contour of the bowel lumen is irregular due to nodularity of the bowel wall. The frequent narrowing associated with Hodgkin's disease mandates a differential diagnosis from other constricting lesions such as inflammation, infarction, and carcinoma. Occasionally, Hodgkin's disease may present a ribbonlike appearance with some degree of rigidity, narrowing, and evidence of extrinsic pressure. The folds adjacent to this segment are often thickened and blunted.

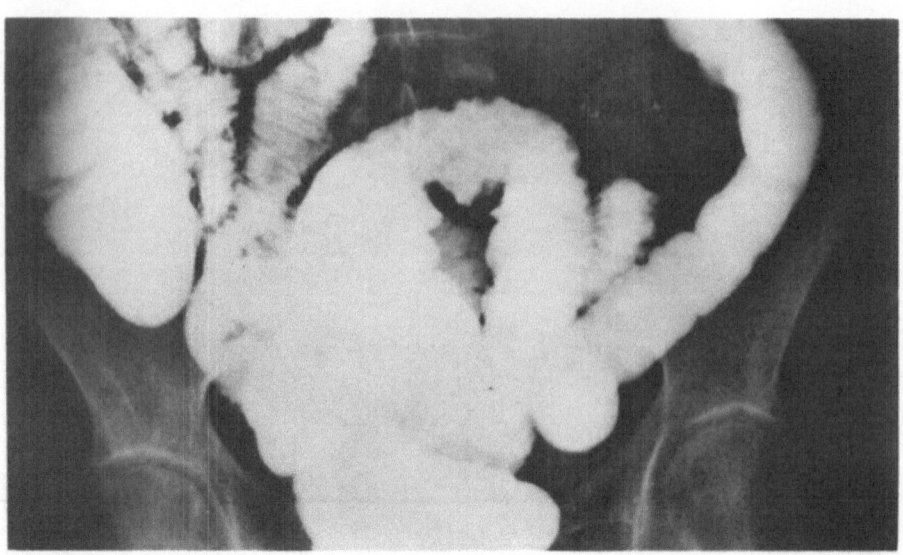

Figure 31. Lymphocytic lymphoma of the colon. Multiple small, scalloped defects are seen along the contour of the bowel. There is no evidence of spasm, irritability, or an inflammatory process. The diagnosis was made on sigmoidoscopy. Multiple, small moundlike structures without ulceration were identified.

6. Lymphocytic Lymphoma of the Stomach

Lymphocytic lymphoma of the stomach may be classified into the subgroups discussed below.

6.1. Infiltrating Form

This is one of the more characteristic types of lymphocytic lymphoma. The process may be segmental, diffuse (involving the entire stomach), and sometimes extending into the duodenal bulb. The folds are rigid; at times, however, they retain some pliability, and frequently they have a nodular or polypoid configuration. These nodules may become confluent, producing an appearance suggesting multiple polyps (Figure 23). Small ulcerations due to superficial erosions are not infrequent. The differential diagnosis of the infiltrating form of lymphocytic lymphoma includes benign segmental hyperrugosity, benign diffuse hyperrugosity, and Menetrier's disease. In benign segmental hyperrugosity of the stomach, the large folds characteristically involve the greater curvature aspect of the stomach from the fundus to the antrum, sparing the latter region. The digital markings on the greater curvature have a symmetrical and regular configuration. The diffuse form of hyperrugosity (so-called "hypertrophic gastritis") may be associated with a duodenal ulcer. It usually involves the entire stomach. Menetrier's disease may be associated with protein-losing enteropathy. It typically involves the greater curvature aspect of the stomach, sparing the antrum. It may also involve the lesser curvature of the

485

LYMPHORETICULAR
DISORDERS OF THE
GASTROINTESTINAL
TRACT:
ROENTGENO-
GRAPHIC FEATURES

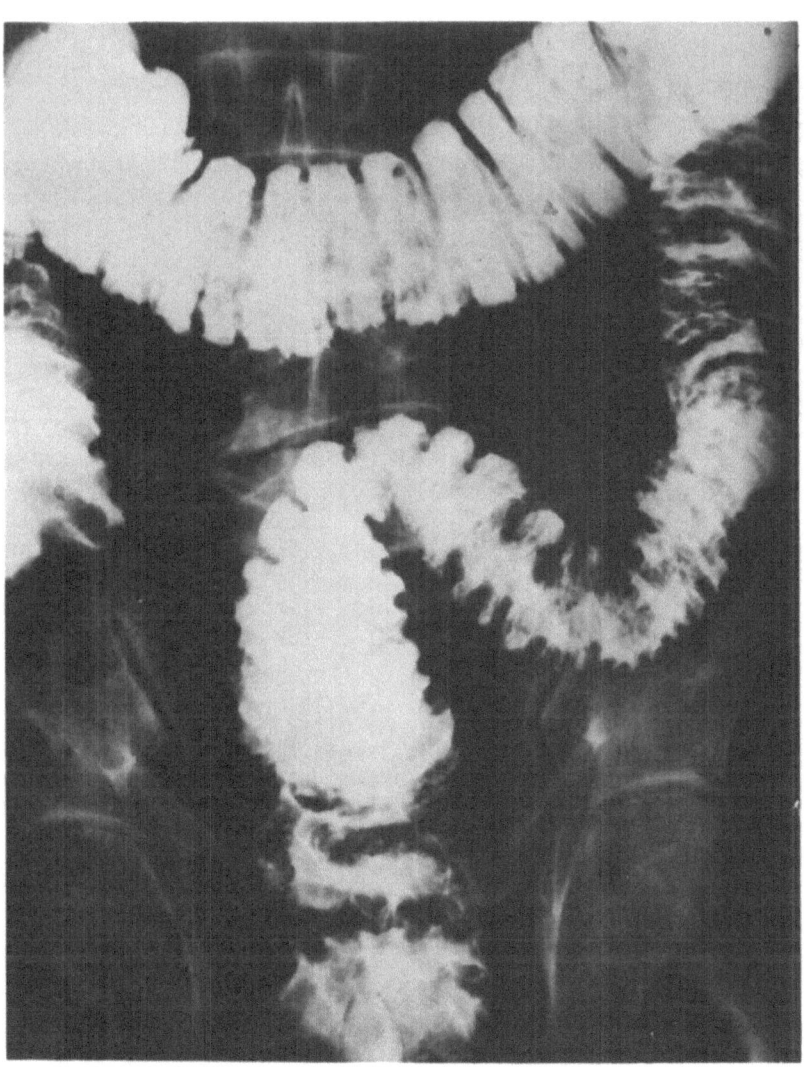

Figure 32. Lymphocytic lymphoma of the colon. Multiple large, irregular folds are seen in the rectum and sigmoid, associated with intraluminal defects. There is no evidence of spasm, irritability, or shortening of the colon. The bowel appears to be more distensible than is usually noted, probably secondary to the tumor masses. The entire colon is involved.

RICHARD H.
MARSHAK *ET AL.*

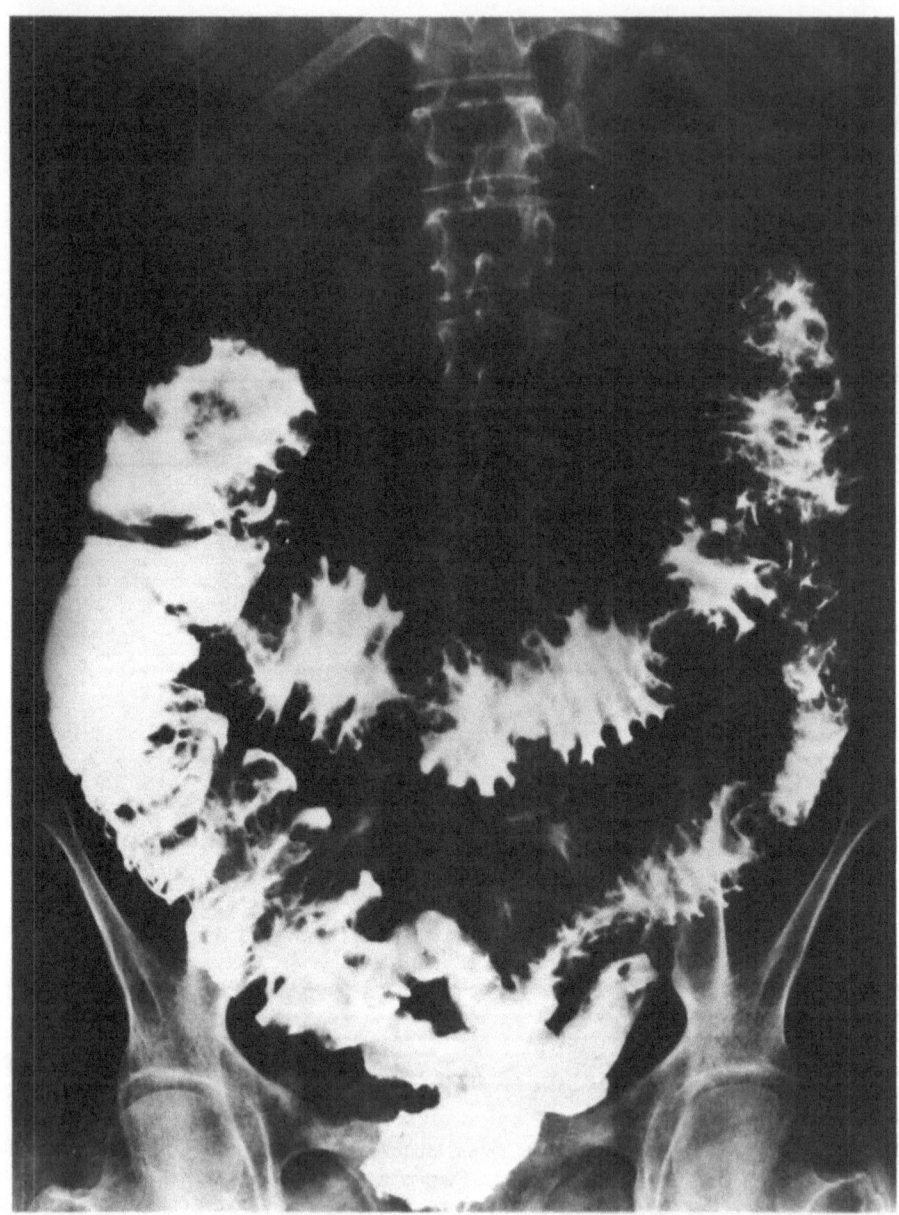

Figure 33. Lymphocytic lymphoma of the colon. Evacuation film of Figure 32. The bowel still retains a considerable amount of barium. Multiple fingerlike projections are seen extending from the contour of the bowel associated with small defects. Numerous small polypoid lesions are also present.

stomach, usually to a lesser degree. In these cases, the antrum may be involved. At times, the folds in Menetrier's disease are so large that differential diagnosis from lymphocytic lymphoma requires biopsy. It is important in those cases with large folds to administer considerable amounts of barium to demonstrate distensibility of the stomach, a procedure that the endoscopist utilizes when he injects air to determine whether the folds are rigid or pliable.

487

LYMPHORETICULAR
DISORDERS OF THE
GASTROINTESTINAL
TRACT:
ROENTGENO-
GRAPHIC FEATURES

6.2. Ulcerating Type

Single or multiple ulcers of the stomach occur in lymphocytic lymphoma. These ulcers may be seen in conjunction with the infiltrative and polypoid forms of the disease. The ulcers vary considerably in size. When they are small or medium, they frequently have a saucerlike configuration surrounded by a tumor mass and are indistinguishable from carcinoma (Figure 24). Only the multiplicity of the lesions suggests lymphocytic lymphoma. Sometimes the ulcers project from the contour of the stomach and simulate an indeterminate ulcer. In a few cases, the surrounding thickened folds suggest the presence of lymphocytic lymphoma. When an ulcer becomes huge, irregular, and aneurysmal (exceeding the diameter of the adjacent gastric lumen), the lesion is highly characteristic of lymphosarcoma (Figure 25). The ulcer frequently extends beyond the contours of the stomach, and tumor masses projecting into the ulcer can be identified. Such ulcerations may be markedly irregular because multiple nodules indent and surround the ulcerating tumor. Perforation occurs frequently. The large ulcers are frequently seen in association with an extraluminal mass. The combination of mass and excavations within the tumor produce a bizarre configuration resembling extraluminal extravasation of barium.

6.3. Polypoid Form

The polyps vary in size. When small or medium, they are frequently multiple, and they mimic multiple polyposis of the stomach (Figure 26). Usually they are irregular and ulcerated. The folds between the polyps may be thickened. When a single large polypoid mass is identified, the differential diagnosis from polypoid carcinoma, giant benign polyp, and myoma or myosarcoma can be impossible (Figure 27). This lesion may be combined with the infiltrative form, so the association of thickened folds and multiple polypoid defects is not unusual.

6.4. Simulating Carcinoma

There is a large ulceration with a surrounding mass (see Figure 24). The findings usually suggest carcinoma, and only on cut pathological sections can a diagnosis of lymphocytic lymphoma be made.

6.5. Endoexogastric Variety

In this form, either the endogastric or the exogastric portion, or both, may be huge. Ulcerations are frequent and can be large and irregular. Some of the largest tumors involving the stomach belong to this category.

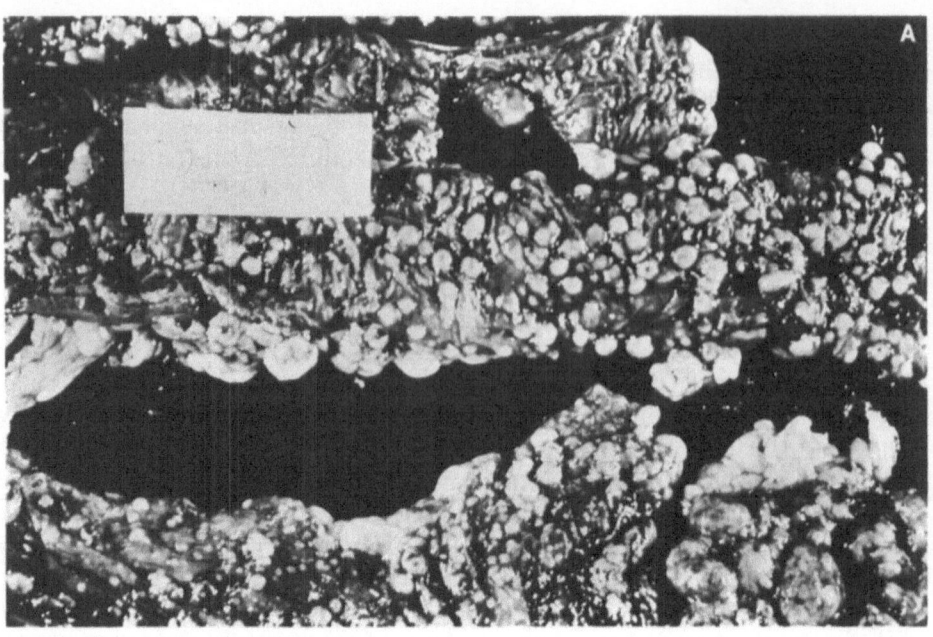

Figure 34A. Lymphocytic lymphoma of the colon. A remarkable case of diffuse lymphosarcoma mimicking familial polyposis. There are numerous polyps distributed throughout the colon. A large polypoid tumor mass is identified in the cecal region. This type of tumor mass is more commonly seen in lymphosarcoma than in familial polyposis.

6.6. Hodgkin's Disease

Hodgkin's disease of the stomach is uncommon in comparison with the incidence of lymphocytic lymphoma, and it is rarely primary. Because the lesion is often characterized by a desmoplastic reaction, it may mimic scirrhous carcinoma (Figure 28). In another form, multiple ulcers occur in association with a narrowed stomach. In a third form, the typical features of lymphocytic lymphoma of the stomach are present, and differential diagnosis is impossible.

7. Lymphocytic Lymphoma of the Colon

Lymphocytic lymphoma of the colon occurs in two principal forms: (1) a discrete, or localized type, which presents as a single mass; and (2) an extensive, diffuse, infiltrating tumor that extends over long segments of the bowel (Wychulis *et al.*, 1966).

The localized variety of lymphocytic lymphoma may present as an area of narrowing with little or no obstruction, with the roentgen changes of carcinoma of the colon, and the pathological diagnosis often comes as a surprise. In another form of localized lymphocytic lymphoma, aneurysmal dilatation of a short segment of colon occurs (Figure 29). In a third type of localized lymphocytic lymphoma, there is a single polypoid mass indistinguishable from polypoid carcinoma. This type is most frequently seen in the cecal area (Figure 30). In considering all these localized forms, it should be noted that at times, lymphocytic lymphoma extends through the bowel, producing a mass with both an intraluminal and an extramural component.

489

**LYMPHORETICULAR
DISORDERS OF THE
GASTROINTESTINAL
TRACT:
ROENTGENO-
GRAPHIC FEATURES**

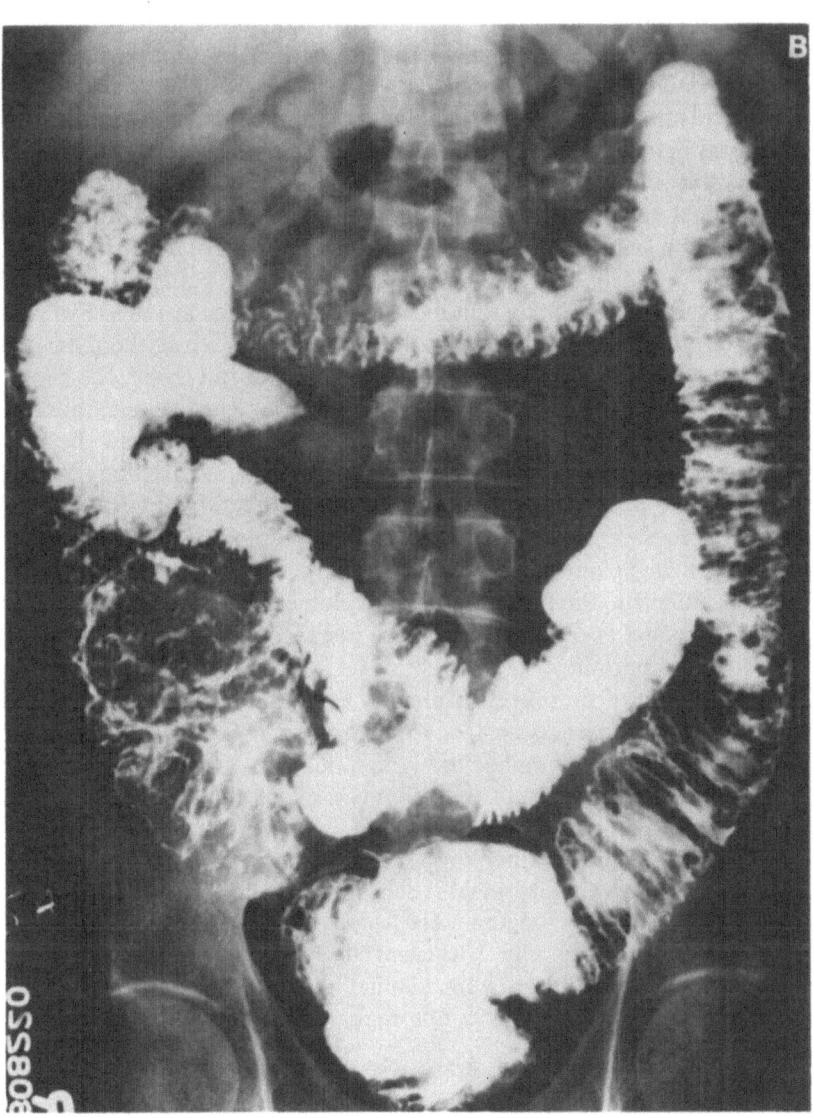

Figure 34B. Lymphocytic lymphoma of the colon (same case as Figure 34A). The specimen bears a remarkable resemblance to familial polyposis. On a superficial examination, differential diagnosis is impossible. The presence of the large mass in the cecum suggests lymphosarcoma. The polyps in this case are also of interest because they all proved to be pedunculated.

In the diffuse type of lymphocytic lymphoma, the entire colon or long segments are involved (Wolf and Marshak, 1960; Hazzi *et al.*, 1973). Frequently, the process is associated with concomitant disease of the terminal ileum. In its earliest form, small discrete nodules are seen along the contour of the bowel presenting as scalloped, irregular filling defects (Figure 31). These defects may be found throughout the colon or confined to a short segment. When the bowel is fully distended with barium, the nodules may be partially effaced, but usually some evidence of these small contour defects can be identified.

In more advanced disease, barium enema examination shows a transformation of the mucosal pattern into an extremely irregular, nodular appearance with many coarse folds and fingerlike projections into the bowel lumen (Figure 32). These findings are most apparent on evacuation films (Figure 33). The tumor masses and the lack of desmoplastic reaction cause the colon to be more distensible than would be anticipated. For similar reasons, the bowel fails to collapse after emptying. Despite the presence of so many tumors and the large irregular folds (Figures 33 and 34A,B), there is little irritability or spasm of the bowel during the introduction of barium. The haustral pattern tends to be maintained at this stage, the bowel is not shortened, and there are no intraluminal secretions or mucosal ulcerations. When the bowel is completely filled, the intraluminal projections may be obscured, although numerous closely spaced polypoid indentations persist along the contours. Pedicles can rarely be identified in the polypoid tumors of lymphocytic lymphoma.

As the process continues and submucosal tumor becomes extensive, the haustral pattern disappears and is replaced by large irregular folds resembling giant rugae in the stomach. Such thick folds are not easily effaced, but they can be obscured if the colon is distended. In these instances, the evacuation film is once more extremely important.

Intussusception, if present, is ordinarily easily reduced, although a mass may persist in the region of the ileocecal valve and prevent filling of the terminal ileum.

In the final stages of lymphocytic lymphoma, the folds may become so large and bulky that complete filling of the colon is difficult and areas of bowel obstruction secondary to tumor may be encountered.

Lymphocytic lymphoma involving small bowel, mesentery, or regional lymph nodes may produce large, bulky masses causing extrinsic compression on the colon.

Hodgkin's Disease. Hodgkin's disease involving the colon is so rare that we have seen only three cases. One was associated with ulcerative colitis. The other two demonstrated marked narrowing, simulating metastatic carcinoma rather than lymphocytic lymphoma. We have not seen a patient with primary Hodgkin's disease of the colon.

References

Ament, M. E., and Rubin, C. E., 1972, Relation of giardiasis to abnormal intestinal structure and function in gastrointestinal immunodeficiency syndromes, *Gastroenterology* **62**:216–226.

Ament, M. E., Ochs, H. D., and Davis, S. D., 1973, Structure and function of the gastrointestinal tract in primary immunodeficiency syndromes: A study of 39 patients, *Medicine (Baltimore)* **52**:227–248.

Bonomo, L., Dammacco, F., Marano, R., and Bonomo, G. M., 1972, Abdominal lymphoma and alpha chain disease, *Am. J. Med.* **52**:73–86.

Bruton, O. C., 1952, Agammaglobulinemia, *Pediatrics* **9**:722–728.

Cohen, N., Paley, D., and Janowitz, H. D., 1962, Acquired hypogammaglobulinemia and sprue: Report of a case and review of the literature, *J. Mt. Sinai Hosp.* **28**:421–427.

491

LYMPHORETICULAR
DISORDERS OF THE
GASTROINTESTINAL
TRACT:
ROENTGENO-
GRAPHIC FEATURES

Eidelman, S., Davis, S. D., and Rubin, C. E., 1968, Immunologic studies in "hypogammaglobulinemic sprue," *Clin. Res.* **16**:117.

Glenner, G. G., Ein, D., and Terry, W. D., 1972, The immunoglobulin origin of amyloid, *Am. J. Med.* **52**:141–147.

Gryboski, J. D., Self, T. W., Clemett, A., and Herskovic, T., 1968, Selective immunoglobulin. A deficiency and intestinal nodular lymphoid hyperplasia: correction of diarrhea with antibiotics and plasma, *Pediatrics* **42**:833–837.

Hazzi, C. G., Lindner, A. E., and Marshak, R. H., 1973, Diffuse lymphosarcoma of the intestine, *Am. J. Gastroenterol.* **60**:74–80.

Hermans, P. E., and Huizenga, K. A., 1972, Association of gastric carcinoma with idiopathic late-onset immunoglobulin deficiency, *Ann. Intern. Med.* **76**:605–609.

Hermans, P. E., and Huizenga, K. A., Hoffman, H. N., Brown, A. L., and Markowitz, H., 1966, Dysgammaglobulinemia associated with nodular lymphoid hyperplasia of the small intestine, *Am. J. Med.* **40**:78–89.

Hodgson, J. R., Hoffman, H. N., II, and Huizenga, K. A., 1967, Roentgenologic features of lymphoid hyperplasia of the small intestine associated with dysgammaglobulinemia, *Radiology* **88**:883–888.

Hughes, W. S., Brooks, P. F., and Conn, H. O., 1972, Serum gastrin levels in primary hypogammaglobulinemia and pernicious anemia: Studies in adults, *Ann. Intern. Med.* **77**:746–750.

Khilnani, M. T., Keller, R. J., and Cuttner, J., 1969, Macroglobulinemia and steatorrhea: Roentgen and pathologic findings in the intestinal tract, *Radiol. Clin. North Am.* **7**:43–55.

Lewis, E. C., II, and Brown, H. E., Jr., 1957, Agammaglobulinemia associated with pernicious anemia and diabetes mellitus, *Arch. Intern. Med.* **100**:296–299.

Marshak, R. H., and Lindner, A. E., 1976, *Radiology of the Small Intestine,* 2nd edition, pp. 409–450, Saunders, Philadelphia.

Marshak, R. H., Ruoff, M., and Lindner, A. E., 1968, Roentgen manifestations of giardiasis, *Am. J. Roentgenol.* **104**:557–560.

Mawhinney, H., and Tomkin, G. H., 1971, Gluten enteropathy associated with selective Ig-A deficiency, *Lancet* **2**:121–124.

Rambaud, J. D., and Matuchansky, C., 1973, Alpha-chain disease: Pathogenesis and relation to Mediterranean lymphoma, *Lancet* **1**:1430–1432.

Ruoff, M., Lindner, A. E., and Marshak, R. H., 1971, Malabsorption syndrome with plasma cell infiltration of the small bowel, *Am. J. Gastroenterol.* **55**:602–608.

Sanford, J. P., Favour, C. B., and Tribeman, M. S., 1954, Absence of serum gamma globulins in an adult, *N. Engl. J. Med.* **250**:1027–1029.

Seligmann, M., 1975, Immunological, clinical and pathological features of alpha-chain disease, *Arch. Intern. Med.* **135**:78–82.

Shackelford, G. D., and McAlister, W. H., 1975, Primary immunodeficiency diseases and malignancy, *Am. J. Roentgenol Radium Ther. Nucl. Med.* **123**:144–153.

Shimkin, P. M., Waldmann, T. A., and Krugman, R. L., 1970, Intestinal lymphangiectasia, *Am. J. Roentgenol.* **110**:827–841.

Twomey, J. J., Jordan, P. H., Jarrold, T., Trubowitz, S., Ritz, N. D., Conn, H. O., 1969, The syndrome of immunoglobulin deficiency and pernicious anemia, *Am. J. Med.* **47**:340–350.

Wolf, B. S., and Marshak, R. H., 1960, Roentgen features of diffuse lymphosarcoma of the colon, *Radiology* **76**:733–740.

Wychulis, A. R., Beahrs, O. H., and Woolner, L. B., 1966, Malignant lymphoma of the colon, *Arch. Surg.* **93**:215–225.

16

Proliferative Disorders of the T-Cell Series

BIJAN SAFAI

1. Introduction

Advances in immunobiology have provided important insight into the cellular structure of the immune system. In-depth studies of cell function and correlation of these functions with membrane properties have helped define lymphocyte physiology. It has been shown that in inbred mice impairment or arrest of differentiation may result in various forms of lymphoid malignancies.

The traditional classification of lymphoproliferative disorders, based as it is on morphological criteria, does not provide an accurate or reproducible system. It does not offer prognostic value or correlate with modern concepts of immunology. In contrast, the application of immunological methodology has facilitated classification and assessment of prognosis.

The term *T-cell neoplasia* is an oversimplification. With improved knowledge of the lymphocyte subpopulations and the molecular bases for their normal function, various disorders of lymphocyte subpopulations will be understood better. The newly acquired knowledge should provide important clues regarding etiology and new therapeutic measures.

The subject of this chapter is the proliferative disorders of the T-cell series. Emphasis will be focused on the well-recognized cutaneous T-cell lymphomas.

2. Cutaneous T-Cell Lymphomas

2.1. Mycosis Fungoides

2.1.1. History and Definition

Mycosis fungoides (MF) is an uncommon chronic disease of the lymphoreticular system. It is normally confined to the skin for a long period of time, and may

---

BIJAN SAFAI • Memorial Sloan-Kettering Cancer Center, New York, New York 10021.

then progress to involve the lymph nodes and internal organs with a fatal outcome. Most investigators consider it neoplastic, although a few still believe that it is reactive (granulomatous) process.

Alibert (1806) described the first case and later renamed it *mycosis*, depicting its mushroomlike tumors. The histological picture of MF was described by Ranvier (1872), while Bazin (1862) described its three clinical stages. Bazin named the disease *mycosis fungoides* and recognized its malignant nature. Vidal and Brocq (1885) described a second form of MF, *mycosis fungoides d'emblée*, of which tumorous lesions are the only clinical manifestations. Some consider the *d'emblée* form to be a variant of lymphocytic or histiocytic lymphoma (Vidal and Brocq, 1895; Bluefarb, 1959; Epstein *et al.*, 1972; Fuks *et al.*, 1973). Hallopeau and Besnier (1892) described a third form of MF in which erythroderma is the main clinical finding. It is believed that erythrodermatous MF is a clinical manifestation of a number of diseases, including some lymphoproliferative disorders (see Section 2.2.4) (Epstein *et al.*, 1972; Hallopeau and Besnier, 1892; Klein *et al.*, 1973).

2.1.2. Clinical Manifestations

Classic MF is manifested by the sequential development of (1) scaly, eczematous, erythematous patches; (2) infiltrated lichenified plaques; and (3) tumors and ulcers. These clinical manifestations have been classified in three stages: premycotic, infiltrative, and tumorous. These stages are morphologically variable. The interval between the development of different stages could be weeks or years; different stages may overlap.

The initial clinical and histological pictures of MF are nonspecific and may simulate eczema, psoriasis, parapsoriasis en plaques (see Section 2.1.2a), or poikiloderma (see Section 2.1.2b). The premycotic eruption may be preceded by a severe, persistent pruritus that normally continues through the first two stages of the disease. A polymorphic-type eruption with a multiplicity of clinical manifestations, characteristic of the premycotic stage, gradually subsides to be replaced by infiltrated plaques characteristic of stage II MF. During stage II disease, the cutaneous lesions rapidly change. New infiltrations appear, while the old ones heal, leaving only some hyperpigmentation and, rarely, atrophy or scars. Generalized lymphadenopathy may occur with stage II disease. As the disease progresses, the tumoral lesions of stage III disease gradually develop in the infiltrated plaques or in previously normal skin. These tumors increase in both size and number and give a fungating appearance; some of these tumors spontaneously regress. Mucous membranes are rarely involved. The general health of the patient declines during the tumor stage. Extracutaneous involvement progresses with fever, weight loss, night sweats, diarrhea, cachexia, and ultimately death.

Disappearance of the tumors following concurrent diseases such as erysipelas and pneumonia has been reported. Temporary improvement of the cutaneous lesions has occurred during an attack of influenza. These concurrent diseases may activate host resistance against the underlying MF. Pruritus persists until the rapidly progressive stage or until intrinsic host defenses against the abnormal cells in the skin are severely impaired.

a. Parapsoriasis en Plaques. Brocq (1902) first used the term *parapsoriasis* to classify a large group of cutaneous disorders, among which was the so-called "*parapsoriasis en plaques*." Some are of the opinion that most if not all cases of parapsoriasis en plaques develop into MF (Keil, 1942; Lapiere, 1949), while others believe that parapsoriasis en plaques remains as such without resulting in MF (Montgomery and Burkhart, 1942; Ormsby and Montgomery, 1954) or other lymphomatous diseases. The reason for this uncertainty is largely that parapsoriasis en plaques is usually diagnosed by clinical criteria (Osmundsen, 1968). The histological changes are not diagnostic, nor are there any laboratory studies that would support this diagnosis. The premycotic stage of MF is so variable that it may mimic many dermatoses. The matter is even further complicated because the term parapsoriasis en plaques has been used to designate various clinical pictures. In addition, the term parapsoriasis en plaques is used interchangeably with the term poikiloderma atrophicans vascularis and is considered to include two unrelated conditions, one benign and the other potentially malignant (Samman, 1972). Others, however, consider the two as separate entities (Osmundsen, 1968; Samman, 1964; Fleischmajer *et al.*, 1965).

Irrespective of the confusing nomenclature, it is clear that at least a small proportion of patients with parapsoriasis en plaques progress to develop MF; the majority continue to have only parapsoriasis en plaques. Considering the great similarities between the premycotic stage of MF and parapsoriasis en plaques, it is an attractive hypothesis to consider parapsoriasis en plaques an early stage of MF in persons who possess the potential to combat the development of abnormal neoplastic processes of MF. The outcome of this battle may decide whether a given person develops MF or remains with parapsoriasis en plaques.

b. Poikiloderma Atrophicans Vascularis. Jacobi (1908) gave the name *poikiloderma atrophicans vascularis* (PAV) to a condition that was later considered by Dowling and Freudenthal (1938) to be a form of dermatomyositis. Clinically, PAV consists of large reddish-brown skin markings composed of spotty hyper- and hypopigmentation, fine telangiectasia, fine scaling, wrinkling, and atrophy (Bluefarb, 1959; Mehregan and Pinkus, 1976; Braverman, 1970). The histological picture of PAV is diagnostic and consists of varying degrees of epidermal and dermal changes. The dermal infiltrate is mainly lymphocytic, but atypical cells as well as occasional epidermal invasion by mononuclear cells may be seen. The histological picture rarely suggests the presence of MF. Poikilodermatous changes have been described in association with lupus erythematosus, dermatomyositis, chronic radiodermatitis, and various lymphomas, as well as MF. PAV should therefore be related to the underlying diseases that cause this cutaneous picture.

Some authors use PAV interchangeably with parapsoriasis en plaques and believe that while lesions may clear permanently with or without treatment, a small potential exists for malignant transformation (Samman, 1972). Poikilodermatous changes, however, are encountered so repeatedly in MF that the prognosis must be guarded whenever prereticulotic poikiloderma is observed (Samman, 1972). It is now generally accepted that PAV is only a descriptive term for a particular clinical manifestation, not a separate entity (Mehregan and Pinkus, 1976; Block *et al.*, 1963a).

2.1.3. Histopathology

The histological picture of MF is similar to its clinical appearance in that it is quite variable and changes considerably from one stage to another. Various histological presentations can be seen by simultaneous samplings of different lesions or by repeated biopsies of the same lesion as it progresses over a period of time. Confusion regarding the pathology of MF has resulted mainly from the variable histopathology during the different stages of the disease and the lack of easily identifiable cells in all phases.

In the earliest stage, the histological picture is usually nonspecific and consists of a perivascular infiltrate. As the disease progresses, there appears a bandlike polymorphous, cellular infiltrate that involves mainly the upper dermis, but later extends to involve its entire thickness. The infiltrate consists of pleomorphic atypical cells admixed with polymorphous inflammatory elements such as normal-appearing lymphocytes, plasma cells, histiocytes, and eosinophils (Van Scott and Haynes, 1971; Allen, 1967; Lever and Schaumburg-Lever, 1975). A lymphomatous process is suspected only when one sees cells that seem to vary from the norm with enlarged nuclei or increased stainability (Van Scott and Haynes, 1971). Thereafter, the number of atypical cells increases considerably to occupy the entire dermis and progresses to dominate the epidermis; this would correspond to the clinical tumor stage of MF. Similar infiltration may be observed in internal organs as well as skin appendages. The characteristic MF cells are described as mononuclear cells with hyperchromatic, folded, and indented nuclei (Mehregan and Pinkus, 1976; Allen, 1967; Lever and Schaumburg-Lever, 1975) (Figure 1). The MF cells, having sparse basophilic cytoplasm, are larger and more deeply stainable than histiocytes (Lever and Schaumburg-Lever, 1975). These cells may be demonstrated in pre-MF only with difficulty.

The inflammatory infiltrate has been considered by some to represent an immunological reaction of the host to the proliferating atypical cells. The proportion of atypical cells increases relative to the inflammatory cells as the disease progresses. Tumor cells predominate the entire field in advanced MF (Rappaport and Thomas, 1974).

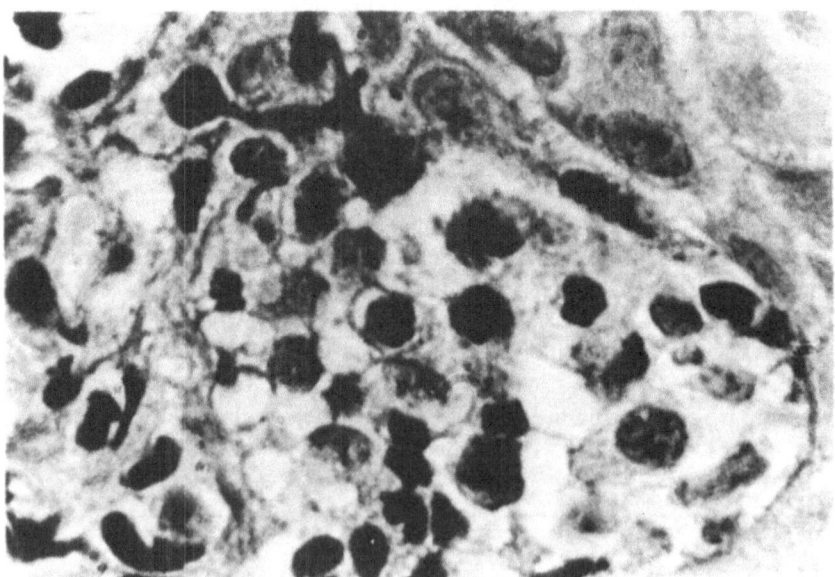

Figure 1. High-power view of involved skin showing typical abnormal MF cells with large, hyperchromatic, infolded, indented nuclei and sparse basophilic cytoplasm. Hematoxylin and eosin. Magnification ×800.

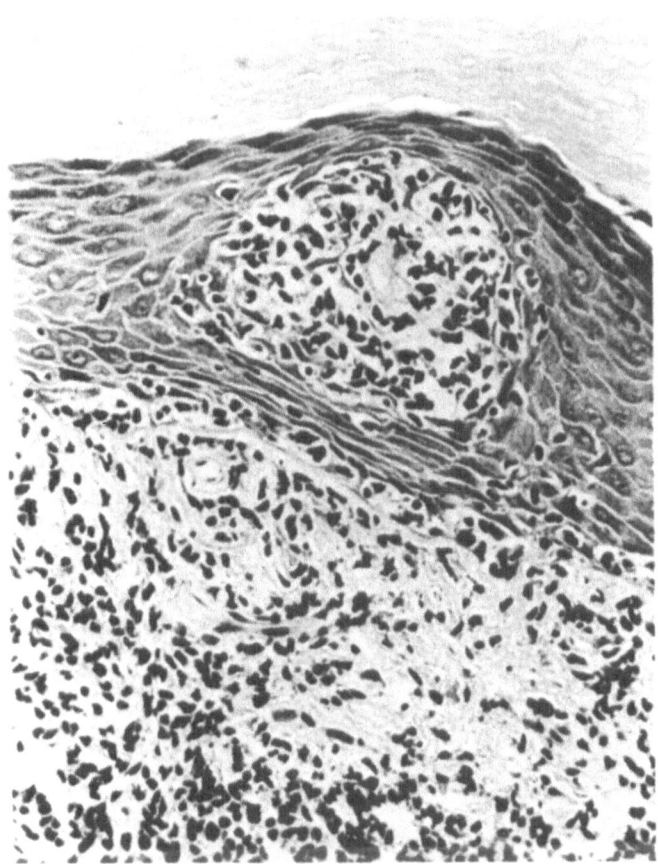

Figure 2. Focal intraepidermal collection of lymphoreticular cells (Pautrier's microabscess). Hematoxylin and eosin. Magnification × 200.

The focal intraepidermal collection of lymphoreticular cells (Pautrier's microabscesses) (Figure 2) is considered highly characteristic if not pathognomonic for MF. The absence of Pautrier's abscesses, however, does not exclude the diagnosis. The number of these cells increases with the progression of the disease and the infiltration extends into upper epidermal levels (Lever and Schaumburg-Lever, 1975; Van Scott and Haynes, 1971; Rappaport and Thomas, 1974). Infiltration of atypical cells into the epidermis singly, in cluster, or in diffuse form reflects the affinity of the atypical MF cells for epithelial structures (epitheliotrophy) and is considered diagnostic for MF (Rappaport and Thomas, 1974; Sandbank, 1971). Aside from MF, Pautrier's microabscesses have been reported only once with histiocytic lymphoma of the skin (Kim *et al.*, 1963).

2.1.4. Ultrastructural Studies

The ultrastructural features of MF cells described first by Lutzner and Jordan (1968) have been repeatedly confirmed (Sandbank, 1971; Lutzner *et al.*, 1971; Brownlee and Murad, 1970) and are now well accepted by others (Labaze *et al.*, 1972; Variakojis *et al.*, 1974; Rosas-Uribe *et al.*, 1974; Orbaneja *et al.*, 1972). These investigators studied the ultrastructure of MF cells in the skin, lymph nodes, peripheral blood, and other organs, and concluded that these atypical convoluted cells are highly characteristic of MF and also of Sézary syndrome (SS). More recently, two different cell types (small and large variants) were observed in both MF and SS infiltrates (Lutzner *et al.*, 1973).

The ultrastructure of MF cells consists of large, infolded, convoluted, serpentine, and cerebriform nuclei (Figure 3), scant cytoplasm with few organelles, clustered mitochondria, dense homogeneous chromatin, and prominent nucleoli. The nuclear envelope shows multiple infoldings that produce fingerlike projections of the nucleoplasm.

Although some believe MF cells to be of the histiocytic series (Fisher *et al.*, 1972), most observers believe that they are of lymphoid-cell origin. Ultrastructural studies of lymphocytes from patients with infectious mononucleosis (Schumacher *et al.*, 1969) and phytohemagglutinin (PHA)-stimulated normal lymphocytes and chronic lymphocytic leukemia (CLL) lymphocytes (Biberfeld, 1971) have reported that such lymphocytes show similar ultrastructural changes. It has been shown that MF cells may be readily found in cutaneous lesions of MF patients, and that they might be abnormal lymphoid cells (Flaxman *et al.*, 1971; Brownlee and Murad, 1970; Orbaneja *et al.*, 1972). The lymphocytic nature of MF cells is further proved by the study of surface markers that indicate that circulating SS cells, as well as neoplastic cells obtained from cutaneous lesions of MF, have characteristics of thymus-derived lymphocytes (Rabinowitz *et al.*, 1976; Lutzner *et al.*, 1975; Broome *et al.*, 1973; Brouet *et al.*, 1973a; Edelson *et al.*, 1974a). It has been suggested that MF and SS cells possibly represent transformed lymphocytes (Labaze *et al.*, 1972).

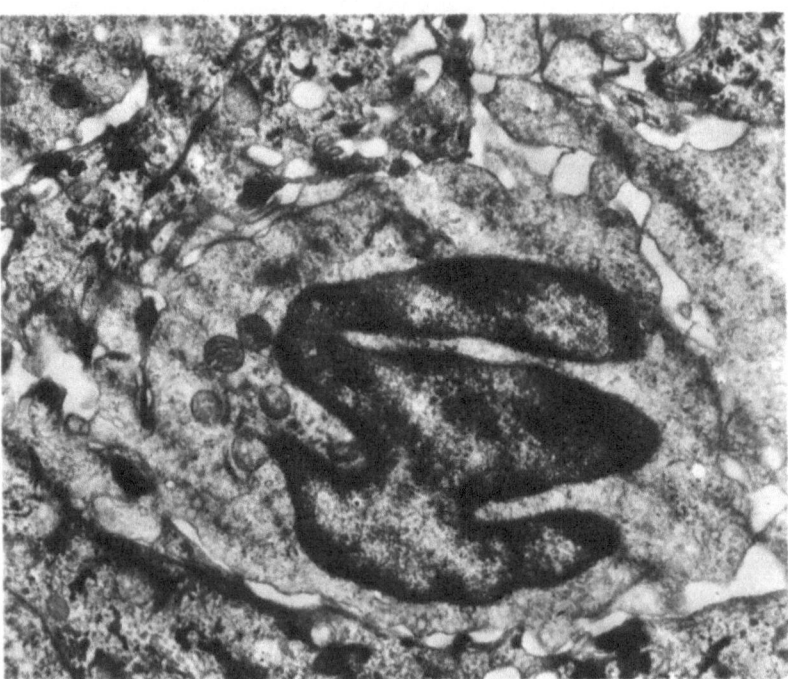

Figure 3. Electron micrograph of involved skin showing typical MF cell with large infolded, convoluted, and serpentine nucleus. Magnification × 4000.

Phagolysosome characteristics of histiocytes have not been observed in MF cells (Lutzner *et al.*, 1971). Moreover, the fine structure of MF cells differs from that of histiocytosis X (Gionotti and Caputo, 1969), leukemic histiocytic lymphoma (Schnitzer and Kass, 1973), acute monocytic leukemia (Freeman and Journey, 1971), hairy cell leukemia (Ghadially and Skinnider, 1972), CLL, and lymphocytic lymphoma (Schrek, 1972).

The observation of these cells has not been limited to MF and SS. Occasional atypical cells identical to MF cells have been seen in electron-microscopic studies not only of parapsoriasis, but also of various other skin disorders (Lutzner *et al.*, 1971; Flaxman *et al.*, 1971).

An intensive ultrastructural study of the skin, peripheral blood, lymph nodes, and spleen from patients with clinical and histological diagnoses of MF demonstrated the presence of more than occasional atypical MF cells, singly or in clusters (Rosas-Uribe *et al.*, 1974). When MF cells are found with diseases other than MF, they are rarely observed more frequently than as single cells. Poorly differentiated lymphocytic lymphoma with nodular patterns is reported to be the only extracutaneous neoplasm in which clusters of these atypical cells are frequently seen in lymph nodes (Rosas-Uribe *et al.*, 1974). This disease is not likely to be confused with MF either clinically or histologically. The ability to adhere to and penetrate viable cells (emperipolesis) both *in vivo* and *in vitro* (Ioachin, 1965; Shelton and Dalton, 1959) is one of the characteristic features of lymphoid cells that has been observed in MF (Rosas-Uribe *et al.*, 1974). It is concluded that atypical MF cells are most likely of lymphocytic origin and that the presence of more than occasional cells with convoluted nuclei in clusters or sheets viewed electron-microscopically is characteristic and highly suggestive of MF and SS (Rosas-Uribe *et al.*, 1974). Nevertheless, there is no definitive marker cell, and the diagnosis of MF is still based on cumulative rather than single features (Rappaport and Thomas, 1974; Escovitz *et al.*, 1974).

2.1.5. Cytogenetic Studies

Spiers and Baikie (1970) were the first to report on a cytogenetic study of lymph nodes in MF. A more extensive cytogenetic study of skin, lymph nodes, spleen, blood, and bone marrow was reported by Erkman-Balis and Rappaport (1974). They were able to show an abnormal karyotype with a modal chromosome number ranging from 44 to 50. These abnormalities were consistent in each case and remained unchanged over periods of up to 18 months. The abnormal findings differed, however, among the cases studied. Karyotypic deviations were related neither to the PHA stimulation nor to therapy, since they were present in both treated and untreated patients. These investigators demonstrated that cytogenetic studies of involved tissues have diagnostic value in that when the histological examinations were negative or doubtful, the cytogenetic studies of lymph nodes and bone marrow showed the presence of abnormal cells. The presence of abnormal karyotype in separated cells from skin lesions, lymph nodes, and bone marrow of patients with MF supports the existence of a neoplastic disorder that may extend to extracutaneous tissues. The chromosome abnormalities were numerical or morphological, or both, showing mostly diploid ranges (Erkman-Balis and Rappaport, 1974), and are therefore comparable to the diploid ranges seen with other lymphomas (Erkman-Balis and Conen, 1972; Millard, 1968; Spiers and Baikie, 1970).

Most cases of SS studied from a cytogenetic view have exhibited near-tetraploid ranges (Brouet *et al.*, 1973a; Lutzner *et al.*, 1973). In dermatopathic lymphadenitis, approximately 26% of the mitotic cells showed abnormal karyotypes. In contrast, at least 50% of mitotic cells in lymph nodes histologically diagnosed as MF showed abnormal karyotypes. Erkman-Balis and Rappaport (1974) concluded that the chromosome alteration apparently arose in one of these lesions, with subsequent regional and systemic dissemination of the abnormal cells. Once an abnormal cell line is established, subsequent changes, if any, are very small (Erkman-Balis and Rappaport, 1974). It is thought that mitotic cells in dermal infiltrates are indicative of *in situ* proliferation of MF cells, and are not the result of infiltration by outside cells (Brownlee and Murad, 1970).

A recent report on HLA in MF indicates a high frequency of HLA-B8 (46.6%) as well as a high frequency of antigens of the "W19" complex, in particular AW31 and AW32 (Dick *et al.*, 1976). Our ongoing HLA studies of patients with MF do not as yet show any statistically significant association.

2.1.6. Extracutaneous Involvement

While some authors believe that extracutaneous dissemination of MF is rare (Allen, 1967), others are of the opinion that it is frequent and involves not only lymph nodes but also other viscera (Block *et al.*, 1963b; Cawley *et al.*, 1951; Cyr *et al.*, 1966; Epstein *et al.*, 1972; Long and Mihm, 1974).

The incidence of extracutaneous disease ranges from 14% (Allen, 1954) to 100% (Long and Mihm, 1974), with an overall incidence of 73% (Long and Mihm, 1974; Levi and Wiernik, 1975). In three major reviews, the rate of extracutaneous involvement was placed at 23% (Fuks *et al.*, 1973), 35% (Epstein *et al.*, 1972), and 71% (Rappaport and Thomas, 1974). The main reason for this frequency variance is the lack of definitive diagnostic criteria for extracutaneous involvement. However, increased awareness of extracutaneous dissemination and better methodology for its recognition have resulted in a much higher incidence of reported cases of MF with internal involvement.

Extracutaneous dissemination of MF is associated with a poor prognosis; these patients follow a rapid downhill course, with a mean survival of 11–12 months from the time of diagnosis (Epstein *et al.*, 1972; Rappaport and Thomas, 1974; Fuks *et al.*, 1974). Systemic dissemination was considered to represent transformation from MF to a malignant lymphoma of histiocytic or poorly differentiated lymphocytic type or to Hodgkin's disease (Cawley *et al.*, 1951; Cyr *et al.*, 1966; Larsen, 1968; Rauschkolb, 1961). Moreover, there have been controversial reports on the clinicohistopathological features of extracutaneous dissemination of MF (McDonald, 1969; Orbaneja *et al.*, 1972; Rappaport *et al.*, 1968; Levi and Wiernik, 1975). With the application of newer criteria and the use of electron microscopy and cytogenetical analysis, however, many investigators have been able to demonstrate that the involved lymph nodes and viscera of MF patients have a characteristic if not specific cellular composition closely resembling that of the cutaneous lesions (Rappaport and Thomas, 1974; Erkman-Balis and Rappaport, 1974; Long and Mihm, 1974). The presence of MF cells is essential for the differentiation of extracutaneous MF from other lymphomas, and has been found in the majority of patients with MF at autopsy (Rappaport and Thomas, 1974). An impressive morphological similarity has been shown to exist between atypical cells of MF in both skin and extracutaneous lesions (Brownlee and Murad, 1970; Flaxman *et al.*, 1971; Lutzner *et al.*, 1971; Sandbank, 1971; Rappaport and Thomas, 1974). The neoplastic cellular proliferations in both cutaneous and extracutaneous tissues are distinct and differ from those of other lymphoid or histiocytic neoplasms (Lever and Schaumburg-Lever, 1975; Rappaport and Thomas, 1974). On the basis of the observations reported above, the extracutaneous dissemination of MF is recognized at present as a distinct clinicopathological phase in the natural history of the disease (Rappaport and Thomas, 1974).

A major problem in the diagnosis of extracutaneous dissemination of MF is the controversial histological picture seen by light microscopy in the enlarged lymph nodes—the so-called "dermatopathic lymphadenitis"—which is not considered diagnostic for MF. However, recent ultrastructural studies of lymph nodes showing histological features of dermatopathic lymphadenitis have helped somewhat to clarify the confusion. MF cells are shown ultrastructurally in the dermatopathic lymphadenopathy of patients with MF (Lutzner *et al.*, 1971), but not in that of other dermatoses (Jimbow *et al.*, 1969). Further investigations have demonstrated that the ultrastructural findings of clusters or sheets of atypical cells of MF are indicative of actual lymph node involvement by MF (Rosas-Uribe *et al.*, 1974). The only exception to this is the poorly differentiated lymphocytic lymphoma with nodular (follicular) patterns in which atypical cells similar to and occasionally indistinguishable from MF cells are seen (Rosas-Uribe *et al.*, 1974). Abnormal karyotypes identical to those found in skin biopsy specimens were observed in lymph nodes histologically diagnosed as dermatopathic lymphadenitis (Erkman-Balis and Rappaport, 1974).

One may underdiagnose extracutaneous dissemination of MF if only light microscopy is used. Significant visceral involvement seen postmortem was often undetected before death (Epstein *et al.*, 1972). Electron-microscopic and cytogenetic studies of suspected tissues give promising results not only in better detection of extracutaneous dissemination, but also in earlier diagnosis, improved prognosis, and more effective therapy.

Many investigators now realize that the presence of enlarged lymph nodes, whether or not MF is demonstrable in its sections, is highly suggestive of extracutaneous dissemination (Rappaport and Thomas, 1974). Lymphadenopathy also indicates that the barrier to the spread of MF from the skin has broken down (Rappaport and Thomas, 1974; Variakojis *et al.*, 1974). It is now apparent that the systemic dissemination of MF can be as extensive as that of any other lymphoma (Epstein *et al.*, 1972; Block *et al.*, 1963b; Rappaport and Thomas, 1974; Cyr *et al.*, 1966). There is a definite correlation between the severity of cutaneous disease and the occurrence of visceral MF (Epstein *et al.*, 1972). The most common site of extracutaneous dissemination is believed to be the lymph nodes (Levi and Wiernik, 1975). The distribution of extracutaneous MF differs from that of other lymphomas: Lung involvement is reported to be greater than spleen, liver, or bone marrow involvement. In contrast to Hodgkin's disease, pulmonary MF is usually not associated with prominent mediastinal masses (Rappaport and Thomas, 1974). Consistent absence of radiological evidence of MF in bone has been reported (Thomas, L. B., *et al.*, 1964); gross lesions in bone marrow are reported to be rare in MF in contrast to CLL. Microscopic bone marrow involvement with MF, however, is relatively frequent (Rappaport and Thomas, 1974).

It is important to determine extracutaneous MF and its extent for more accurate staging, which influences the choice of therapy. Although histological examination of palpable lymph nodes has not been very helpful, revealing only nonspecific or dermatopathic changes in 42–66% of cases (Block *et al.*, 1963b; Clendenning *et al.*, 1964; Epstein *et al.*, 1972; Fuks *et al.*, 1973), ultrastructural (Lutzner *et al.*, 1971) and cytogenetic (Spiers and Baikie, 1970; Erkman-Balis and Rappaport, 1974) studies of the palpable lymph nodes seem to be promising procedures in accurately detecting extracutaneous dissemination of MF during earlier stages of the disease.

Lymphangiographic studies have revealed abnormal changes in the size and internal structure of paraaortic and iliac nodes in over one third of MF patients (Fuks *et al.*, 1974). Lymphography may detect clinically unsuspected nodal involvement in a significant number of patients (Escovitz *et al.*, 1974). There is no lymphographic pattern pathogonomonic of MF that would distinguish it from the other lymphomas (Escovitz *et al.*, 1974). So far, lymphangiography has had a limited role in the staging of MF.

Surgical staging, a well-established procedure in Hodgkin's disease, has rarely been applied in MF. Involvement of the spleen, lymph nodes, and liver was shown in one report (Variakojis *et al.*, 1974). It was demonstrated that the results of clinical and radiological diagnostic procedures correlated well with laparotomy findings in patients with MF (Griem *et al.*, 1975).

2.1.7. Staging Classification

A variety of staging classifications have been suggested for MF, based on cutaneous and extracutaneous involvement (Escovitz *et al.*, 1974; Fuks *et al.*, 1974; Griem *et al.*, 1975). There is still no satisfactory classification, however, due to the lack of proper diagnostic procedures with early disease when clinical and histological findings are nonspecific. In addition, there are difficulties in the determination of extracutaneous involvement.

Recent progress in the diagnosis and treatment of other lymphomas has prompted many investigators to use the same procedures for MF. Lymphangiography, various radioisotope studies, bone marrow aspirations and biopsies, as well as liver and lymph node biopsies, are gradually being introduced in the evaluation of patients with MF (Escovitz *et al.*, 1974; Fuks. *et al.*, 1974; Griem *et al.*, 1975). The use of these procedures is likely to become more frequent.

Electron-microscopic (Brownlee and Murad, 1970; Rosas-Uribe *et al.*, 1974; Orbaneja *et al.*, 1972) and cytogenetic (Erkman-Balis and Rappaport, 1974) studies of the skin, spleen, lymph nodes, bone marrow, and peripheral blood have shown excellent results, and are being tried in the evaluation and staging of MF. Immunological evaluation of the patient's status with studies of surface markers has been very fruitful (Mackie *et al.*, 1976), and is being used more frequently. Laparoscopy and laparotomy have been used with considerable success in other lymphomas, and are now being introduced for MF (Variakojis *et al.*, 1974).

Once such extensive investigations have been carried out, an accurate clinicopathological staging classification will be available that would supply both prognostic and therapeutic indices for MF.

2.1.8. Natural History, Course, and Prognosis

It is widely accepted that MF is a form of lymphoma with clinicopathological features distinct from those of other lymphoid neoplasms (Bluefarb, 1959; Levi and

Wiernik, 1975; Rappaport and Thomas, 1974). Most, if not all, agree that MF has its primary origin in the skin, and eventually progresses to involve internal organs (Block *et al.*, 1963b; Cawley *et al.*, 1951; Cyr *et al.*, 1966; Bazin, 1862; Rappaport and Thomas, 1974). It occurs more commonly in males than in females, with a ratio ranging from 1.3:1 to 2:1 (Epstein *et al.*, 1972; Fuks *et al.*, 1973); it is less common in blacks than in Caucasians (Epstein *et al.*, 1972). The skin lesions appear most often in the fifth decade of life. Most patients present with the classic form of MF (Alibert, 1806) and go through all three clinical stages of the disease. There is a definite correlation between the more severe clinical picture and more extensive visceral involvement (Epstein *et al.*, 1972).

Mycosis fungoides is an uncommon illness. It has been estimated that 1000–2000 cases are now affected in the United States (Escovitz *et al.*, 1974), with fewer than 200 resultant deaths recorded per year (Burbank, 1971). These figures reflect underdiagnosis of MF in earlier years. The age of the patient at diagnosis and the presence of skin tumors, ulceration, peripheral lymphadenopathy, and overt visceral dissemination all have prognostic significance (Block *et al.*, 1963b; Cyr *et al.*, 1966; Epstein *et al.*, 1972; Fuks *et al.*, 1973; Levi and Wiernik, 1975). The duration of the disease, particularly in its early stages, is extremely variable (Variakojis *et al.*, 1974). The median duration of the nonspecific cutaneous manifestation before a definite diagnosis is made has been reported to be 4–10 years, ranging from a few months to 50 years (Bluefarb, 1959). Once the histological diagnosis is confirmed, however, the median survival is less than 5 years (Block *et al.*, 1963b; Cyr *et al.*, 1966; Epstein *et al.*, 1972; Fuks *et al.*, 1973; Levi and Wiernik, 1975). The presence of skin tumors, ulcers, and enlarged lymph nodes indicates that the median survival appears to be less than 2.5 years (Epstein *et al.*, 1972; Fuks *et al.*, 1973).

Lymphadenopathy in patients with MF is associated with poor prognosis due to the high incidence of visceral dissemination (Long and Mihm, 1974; Fuks *et al.*, 1973; Epstein *et al.*, 1972). The survival of these patients is approximately 1.5–2 years (Block *et al.*, 1963b; Epstein *et al.*, 1972; Escovitz *et al.*, 1974). Often, enlarged lymph nodes in patients with MF show benign hyperplasia or dermatopathic lymphadenitis (Bluefarb, 1959). Even in this group, there is a higher risk as compared with the patients without lymph node enlargement (Escovitz *et al.*, 1974). The mean survival in ME patients with the diagnosis of dermatopathic lymphadenitis is 34 months (Block *et al.*, 1963b; Epstein *et al.*, 1972). Once extracutaneous disease develops, mean survival is less than 1 year (Block *et al.*, 1963b; Cyr *et al.*, 1966; Epstein *et al.*, 1972; Fuks *et al.*, 1973). A 67% survival is reported in patients suffering from MF without evidence of lymphadenopathy, as compared with 43% for those with enlarged lymph nodes during 5–10 years of follow-up after therapy (Fuks *et al.*, 1974).

Bone marrow is not usually involved in MF (Block *et al.*, 1963b; Cyr *et al.*, 1966). Lymphopenia develops, however, in up to 67% of patients (Cyr *et al.*, 1966). Lymphocytopenia suggests a poor prognosis (Fuks *et al.*, 1973). In this respect, MF resembles Hodgkin's disease.

Although symptomatic improvement is achieved with various therapeutic programs, none has prolonged survival (Epstein *et al.*, 1972; Klein *et al.*, 1973). Extracutaneous involvement represents a major cause of death. These patients usually die within 1 year despite treatment (Epstein *et al.*, 1972; Fuks *et al.*, 1973).

Recent reports suggest that aggressive treatment with either topical nitrogen mustard (Van Scott and Kalmanson, 1973) (see Section 2.3.2) or electron-beam irradiation (Fuks *et al.*, 1973) results in long-term disease-free remissions. However, this is valid only for patients with disease confined to the skin. Improved prognosis with advanced MF depends in part on early identification of premalignant as well as extracutaneous involvement (Fuks *et al.,* 1974; Griem *et al.,* 1975). Most investigators have come to realize that therapeutic programs must be based on the extent of the disease.

2.1.9. Immunological Studies

Host resistance may play a major role in determining the progression of MF. In citing determinants, specific immune responses and factors such as lymphocyto-penia that lead to the overcoming by the disease of intrinsic host resistance are important considerations concerning MF. The origin, nature, and antigenic specific-ity of the MF cell are important subjects for future investigation.

Delayed hypersensitivity responses are reported to be unchanged in the major-ity of patients with MF until the terminal stages of the disease (Blaylock *et al.,* 1966; Clendenning and Van Scott, 1965; Mackie *et al.,* 1976). Low numbers of circulating T and B cells are observed in MF patients (Mackie *et al.,* 1976). Low T-cell and high-null cell values as well as impaired cell-mediated immunity (as measured by *in vivo* skin testing with common antigens) are reported in patients with advanced MF (Nordqvist and Kinney, 1976). Likewise, lymphoproliferative responses to mito-gens and antigens in culture are also impaired only in advanced disease. Serum IgA levels are reported to be elevated in some cases (Blaylock *et al.,* 1966). Our unpublished observations confirm other reports (Tan, R. S. H., *et al.,* 1974; Mackie *et al.,* 1976) of elevated serum levels of IgE in some MF cases. The significance of increased serum IgA and IgE in MF patients is not clear. It may be due to faulty interaction of T and B cells, or perhaps to the effect of neoplastic MF T cells on the function of immunoglobulin-secreting cells.

A recent report (Umbert *et al.,* 1976), as well as our own observations, demonstrate a high level of leukocyte migration-inhibiton factors (LMIF) in the serum of some patients with MF. The presence of these factors has also been reported in patients with SS (Yoshida *et al.,* 1975; Umbert *et al.,* 1976). We postulate that these mediators are released from the patient's normal T lymphocytes in response to stimulation by neoplastic MF-cell antigens. In addition, our prelimi-nary studies suggest the presence of high levels of serum thymic factors in the serum of patients with MF.

2.2. Sézary Syndrome

2.2.1. History

Sézary syndrome (SS) was first described by a French dermatologist bearing that name (Sézary and Bouvrain, 1938). The clinical and pathological features of this syndrome were further delineated by Sézary and Bolgart (1942). They sug-gested that the *cellules monstreuses* present in the blood were reticular in nature and released from the skin into the blood circulation and proposed the name *paramycosis hemotrope.*

2.2.2. Clinical Manifestations and Course

Sézary syndrome is characterized by generalized exfoliative erythroderma, intensive pruritus, and the presence of atypical cells in peripheral blood as well as in the cellular infiltrate of the skin. Cutaneous lesions include infiltrated plaques, nodules, tumors, and ulcers, as well as edema, lichenification, purpura, and hypo- and hyperpigmentation. Hyperkeratosis of the palms and soles, dystrophic nails, and diffuse alopecia may be seen. Edema and infiltration of the periorbital tissues produce a characteristic leonine or masklike face. Conjunctivitis, blepharitis, and ectropion can occur. Peripheral lymphadenopathy is seen. The enlarged lymph nodes are firm, nontender, and freely moveable. Hepatomegaly is present in some cases, and is usually not related to the course of the disease. The spleen is rarely enlarged (Winkelmann and Linman, 1973). Cases of SS have been reported from all continents; however, this syndrome has not been seen in children.

The onset of the disease is usually insidious (Fleischmajer and Eisenberg, 1964); the clinical manifestations may follow a nonspecific dermatitis or an infiltrative erythema (Winkelmann and Linman, 1973). Involvement of the skin is transient in the early stages, and spontaneous remissions and exacerbation are common (Taswell and Winkelmann, 1961).

In the late stages of the disease, anorexia, loss of weight, and rapid rise in both peripheral blood leukocytes and abnormal cell counts are followed by rapid physical deterioration (Fleischmajer and Eisenberg, 1964). The disease is usually fatal (Fleischmajer and Eisenberg, 1964). The duration of the disease is varied, having been reported to be from 6 months to 16 years (Fleischmajer and Eisenberg, 1964; Brouet et al., 1973a). The average life expectancy is about 5 years (Taswell and Winkelmann, 1961). Men usually die within 5 years of onset, women within 8 to 10 years.

Leukocytosis is a prominent hematological feature that may be absent in the early stages of the disease. While the number of polymorphonuclear leukocytes may be decreased, the lymphocyte count is increased, and peripheral blood smears reveal the presence of abnormal cells with large nuclei and scant cytoplasm (Fleischmajer and Eisenberg, 1964). Absolute lymphocytosis has been reported (Winkelmann and Linman, 1973). Atypical lymphocytes accounting for 10% of peripheral blood cells are compatible with the diagnosis of SS (Winkelmann, 1974).

Although it has been widely accepted that the bone marrow is usually spared with SS (Edelson et al., 1974a), bone marrow involvement does occur (Rosas-Uribe et al., 1974; Bureau et al., 1959). In SS, fewer than 50% of the nucleated cells in bone marrow are lymphocytes. Hematopoietic cell lines are well preserved. This supports the possibility that Sézary cells are of extramedullary origin (Edelson et al., 1974a).

2.2.3. Histopathology

The histological findings in SS consist of a polymorphic infiltrate in the upper dermis, primarily with Sézary cells (S cells), but also with lymphoid cells, histiocytes, eosinophils, neutrophils, and plasma cells. The picture is identical to that of MF. The S cell is indistinguishable from the MF cell as seen in the cutaneous infiltrates. The epidermis is frequently thickened; hyperkeratosis and parakeratosis are observed. Exocytosis of normal and atypical lymphocytes into the epidermis is seen, and Pautrier's microabscesses containing abnormal lymphocytes as seen in MF are often present (Fleischmajer and Eisenberg, 1964; Edelson et al., 1974a; Lever and Schaumburg-Lever, 1975). At times, the cells are hyperchromatic and mitotic figures are rare (Winkelmann and Linman, 1973).

The enlarged peripheral lymph nodes may only show nonspecific inflammatory changes, giving a picture of dermatopathic lymphadenitis (Fleischmajer and Eisenberg, 1964). In other instances, however, the normal architecture is completely replaced by atypical cells (Tedeschi and Lansinger, 1965; Edelson *et al.*, 1974a). It may be difficult to distinguish reactive from noeplastic changes in involved lymphoid tissues (Fleischmajer and Eisenberg, 1964). There is no histological evidence of thymic tissue involvement (Edelson *et al.*, 1974b).

2.2.4. Sézary Syndrome: Its True Nature and Relationship to Mycosis Fungoides

There has been a great deal of controversy in the literature as to whether SS is a clinical and pathological entity distinct from MF and whether it represents a true malignancy. The malignant nature of SS was originally described by Sézary himself, and was based on the fact that all his reported cases died of their illness within a 4-year period. Some investigators considered SS as a separate entity (Wilson, H. T. H., and Fielding, 1953). Others (Winkelman, 1974; Tedeschi and Lansinger, 1965) regarded this disorder as a hyperplastic nonneoplastic process of the reticuloendothelial system that may be seen in association with various lymphoreticular malignancies such as Hodgkin's disease, histiocytic lymphoma, CLL, and MF, and may precede their onset; they considered the visceral involvement as a malignant transformation, and believed that patients with SS may develop malignant lymphomas (Paradinas and Harrison, 1974; Winkelmann, 1974).

Sézary syndrome was also considered by some investigators to be a separate lymphoreticular disorder with a distinctive pattern (Winkelmann and Linman, 1973; Taswell and Winkelmann, 1961). Present evidence indicates, however, that SS is a variant of cutaneous T-cell lymphomas. In contrast to the views discussed above, the majority regard SS as a leukemic variant of MF, a well-recognized form of lymphoma (Block *et al.*, 1963b; Epstein *et al.*, 1972; Clendenning *et al.*, 1964; Lutzner *et al.*, 1975). It is suggested that SS is the erythrodermic type of MF (Lutzner *et al.*, 1975; Bureau *et al.*, 1959; Schein *et al.*, 1976) (see Section 2.1.1). There are many case reports in the literature describing the presence of circulating S cells in patients with typical MF (Block *et al.*, 1963b; Miura and Shima, 1954; Clendenning *et al.*, 1964). Clinical and histological studies of patients with SS disclosed no essential differences between this syndrome and MF (Clendenning *et al.*, 1964; Allen, 1954; Saito *et al.*, 1964; Braverman, 1970; Fleischmajer and Eisenberg, 1964). Circulating abnormal mononuclear cells have been found in as many as 20% of patients with typical MF (Clendenning *et al.*, 1964; Lutzner *et al.*, 1971). These circulating atypical cells were indistinguishable from S cells (Block *et al.*, 1963b; Cyr *et al.*, 1966; Clendenning *et al.*, 1964; Lutzner and Jordan, 1968; Orbaneja *et al.*, 1972; Labaze *et al.*, 1972). Sézary cells in skin infiltrates are indistinguishable from MF cells and show a hyperchromatic irregularly shaped nucleus (Lutzner and Jordan, 1968; Lutzner *et al.*, 1971). Pautrier microabscesses are often present in the involved skin of patients with SS just as in MF and contain S cells (Edelson *et al.*, 1974a; Fleischmajer and Eisenberg, 1964). It is widely reported that patients with SS die as a result of either an intercurrent disease, particularly infection, or the development of MF in viscerae (Winkelmann and Linman, 1973; Tedeschi and Lansinger, 1965; Paradinas and Harrison, 1974; Fleischmajer and Eisenberg, 1964). Sézary syndrome has been reported to occur in patients who have previously had classic MF (Van Scott and Haynes, 1971). The ultrastructural studies of S cells and MF cells have demonstrated identical features (Lutzner *et al.*, 1971; Brownlee and Murad, 1970; Rosas-Uribe *et al.*, 1974; Orbaneja *et al.*, 1972; Flaxman *et al.*, 1971). The early appearance of atypical cells in peripheral blood is the main difference between SS and MF. Recent analyses of the cell-surface determinants and functional studies have demonstrated that the abnormal cells in both SS and MF possess T-cell properties. On the basis of the aforementioned data, SS and MF appear to represent different clinical expressions of the same disease process, with progressive involvement of skin and internal organs. They are both caused by the proliferation of neoplastic T lymphocytes, one with a leukemic phase and the other without it.

2.2.5. The Sézary Cell

a. Lymphoid Nature. Main *et al.* (1959) were the first to consider the Sézary cell (S cell) as an abnormal lymphocyte. Morphological, cytochemical, ultrastructural, and immunological data have confirmed that S cells are most likely abnormal lymphocytes of thymus-derived origin and refuted the possibility that these cells represent reticulohistiocytes or monocytes (Lutzner *et al.*, 1971; Brouet *et al.*, 1973a; Zucker-Franklin *et al.*, 1974; Crossen *et al.*, 1971).

S cells and normal lymphocytes are often indistinguishable by light microscopy. In electron microscopy the S cell is distinguished from the normal lymphocyte by the largely convoluted nucleus, the cytoplasmic fibrils, large amounts of glycogen, and variability in size (Zucker-Franklin *et al.*, 1974). Heterogeneity in nuclear shape and size has been observed within the same patient and from patient to patient (Lutzner *et al.*, 1973). Further evidence supporting the nature and function of the S cell will be reviewed in other sections.

b. Ultrastructural Studies. Lutzner and Jordan (1968) were the first to report on the ultrastructure of these cells. They demonstrated that in cut sections, the nucleus of the S cell is highly serpentine, while three-dimensionally it is cerebriform and convoluted and appears to have a circular outline with highly convoluted sheets or folds (Figure 4). The chromatin is irregularly condensed at the periphery of the nuclear membrane and in dense aggregates throughout the nucleus. These findings were further amplified by other investigators (Lutzner *et al.*, 1973; Zucker-Franklin *et al.*, 1974). It was shown that the hyperchromatic folded nuclei are surrounded by a small rim of cytoplasm that contains a network of cytoplasmic fibrils (Zucker-Franklin *et al.*, 1974). More recently, the presence of S cells was demonstrated in patients with MF and parapsoriasis en plaques (Lutzner *et al.*, 1971).

Using light and electron microscopy, cytophotometry, and cytogenetic studies, Lutzner *et al.* (1973) were the first to describe a small-cell variant of the S cell. These smaller cells are 7–9 μm in diameter and feature indented nuclei hyperdiploidy or pseudiploidy in chromosome counts, diploidy of DNA values, and marker chromosomes (Brouet *et al.*, 1973a; Zucker-Franklin *et al.*, 1974). It was also demonstrated that aside from ultrastructural and cytogenetic similarities, the small-cell type shares membrane properties similar to those of T lymphocytes with the classic large-cell type (Brouet *et al.*, 1973a).

A recent ultrastructural study of patients with lymphomatoid papulosis revealed the presence of cells with serpentine nuclei in the tissues studied (Schneiderman *et al.*, 1975). Ultrastructural studies of skin specimens taken from patients

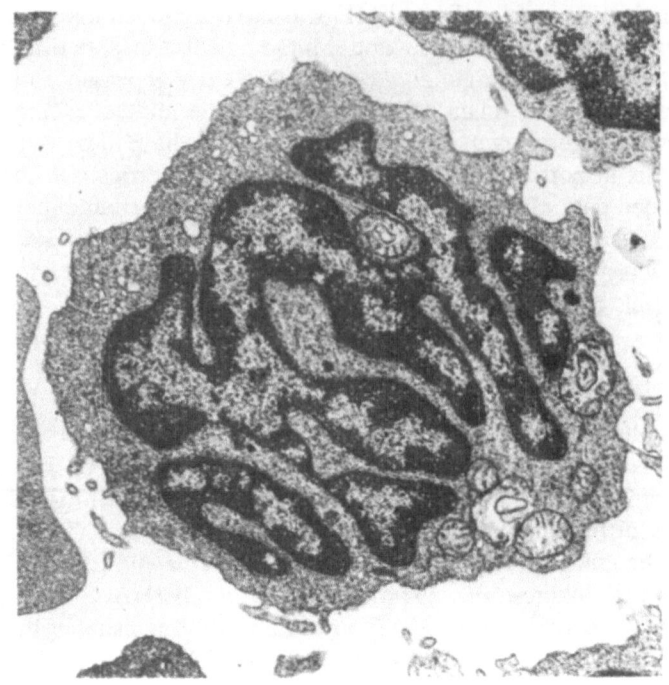

Figure 4. Electron micrograph of peripheral blood of a patient with Sézary syndrome showing typical S cell with large, highly convoluted cerebriform, infolded, and serpentine nucleus with sparse cytoplasm. Magnification × 4000.

with lichen planus, histiocytic lymphoma, and some other skin disorders revealed the presence of cells with serpentine nuclei (Lutzner *et al.*, 1971; Flaxman *et al.*, 1971). Detection of cells with convoluted serpentine nuclei in tissues therefore cannot be used as a definitive diagnostic criterion for SS or MF (Lutzner *et al.*, 1971). It has been demonstrated, however, that the cells with convoluted nuclei are diagnostic for MF if they are seen in sheets and clusters (Rosas-Uribe *et al.*, 1974; Rappaport and Thomas, 1974; Variakojis *et al.*, 1974; Orbaneja *et al.*, 1972; Brownlee and Murad, 1970). It is also pointed out that the detection of cells with serpentine nuclei in involved viscera is a valuable clue for the diagnosis of extracutaneous involvement in SS and MF.

Freeze–etch electron microscopy, which allows examination of the shape and distribution of both cytoplasmic and nuclear-membrane configuration without the artifacts of fixation, was used to study the S cell. The cerebriform and spherical nature of the cell was confirmed, and the nucleus appears fuller than appreciated by regular electron microscopy (Tan, H. K., *et al.*, 1974). These findings generally support the conclusions of previous investigators (Lutzner and Jordan, 1968; Lutzner *et al.*, 1973) about the nuclear topology of S cells and MF cells.

Quantitative determination of the nuclear shape has been achieved using the nuclear contour index (the ratio of the nuclear circumference to the square root of the nuclear cross-sectional area) developed by Schrek (1972). It has been shown that S cells have indices higher than those of normal lymphocytes, while CLL lymphocytes have the smallest indices (Litovitz and Lutzner, 1974).

c. Cytogenetic Studies.   Crossen *et al.* (1971) first demonstrated that S-cells contained chromosomal abnormalities both in number and in structure. They showed two abnormal cell lines—one with a chromosome number of 76 with a distinctive marker and the other with a chromosome number of 98–100 with another characteristic marker. Further cytogenetic studies demonstrated that major changes in the karyotype of S cells consist of heteroploidy, hyperdiploidy, pseudodiploidy, and a consistent presence of chromosomal markers (Crossen *et al.*, 1971; Brouet *et al.*, 1973a; Lutzner *et al.*, 1973; Prunieras, 1974; Dewald *et al.*, 1974). The large-cell variants were hyperploid or pseudodiploid (Brouet *et al.*, 1973a; Lutzner *et al.*, 1973). Some patients with SS were reported to have minute chromosomal fragments (Lutzner *et al.*, 1973). In one case, hypodiploidy, rather than hyperdiploidy and marker chromosomes, was observed (Dewald *et al.*, 1974). In another series, the chromosome number ranged widely in each patient, and there was no consistent clone of abnormal cells (Lutzner *et al.*, 1973). In patients with SS, chromosome markers are frequently seen independent of chromosome numbers or chromosomal breakage and seem to represent stable aberrations (Lutzner *et al.*, 1973). These markers seem to indicate some similarities among various patients with SS (Prunieras, 1974). Some are of the opinion that marker chromosomes may be related to the pathogenesis of SS (Dewald *et al.*, 1974). Similar chromosomal markers, however, are seen in other neoplastic cells. Karyotypic abnormalities present in blood leukocytes are not demonstrable in studies on bone marrow from the same patients (Lutzner *et al.*, 1973). Cytophotometric measurements of S cells appear to correlate closely with cytogenetic findings, and indicate that the abnormal cells exist in peripheral blood before cultivation (Lutzner *et al.*, 1973; Crossen *et al.*, 1971).

The resemblance between chromosomal aberrations of long-term cultures of lymphoblastoid cell lines and chromosomal changes of S cells has been noted and taken as possible support for the hypothesis that S cells represent abnormal lymphocytes that escape from immune surveillance (Prunieras, 1974). These studies suggest that S cells are malignant and have some similarities to MF cells (Lutzner *et al.*, 1973).

d. Cytochemical Studies.   Strong β-glucoronidase activity was shown in a large proportion of normal lymphocytes (Yam and Mitus, 1968). The cytochemical evaluation of the S cells revealed β-glucoronidase activity much higher than in normal lymphocytes. S cells also stain positively for periodic acid–Schiff stain (PAS) and negatively for peroxidase and monocyte-specific esterase (Yam *et al.*, 1971; Brouet *et al.*, 1973a; Flandrin and Daniel, 1974).

e. Cell-Surface Properties and Functional Studies.   Normal lymphocytes are stimulated to synthesize DNA and RNA and to undergo mitosis when cultured with PHA (Ling, 1968). Peripheral blood leukocytes from patients with SS, containing S cells, responded normally to PHA (Crossen *et al.*, 1971; Broome *et al.*, 1973; Lutzner *et al.*, 1973; Zucker-Franklin *et al.*, 1974). Other reports indicated, however, that lymphoproliferative hyporesponsiveness in culture with mitogens and antigens may occur in SS (Labaze *et al.*, 1972; Lutzner *et al.*, 1975). These *in vitro* responses correlated well with the skin reactivity to the same antigens (Lutzner *et al.*, 1975; Nordqvist and Kinney, 1976). Leukocytes from patients with SS may also be good or poor stimulators or responders in the mixed leukocyte culture reaction (Lutzner *et al.*, 1975; Gorski *et al.*, 1977). It should be remembered, however, that T cells (and perhaps S cells) lack membrane antigens that stimulate this reaction.

The loss of PHA responsiveness while the property of spontaneous rosette formation is still present (Brouet et al., 1973a; Labaze et al., 1972) suggests that there may be a dissociated loss of S-cell function without loss of membrane markers (Kalden et al., 1974). In addition, PHA responsiveness of S cells was lost after chemotherapy (Zucker-Franklin et al., 1974).

Transformation of normal lymphocytes is inhibited by adrenocorticosteroids (Elves et al., 1964). In SS, the inhibition of hyperdiploid lines by prednisone was much more profound than that of diploid lines (Crossen et al., 1971). Recently, a case of small-cell variant of SS was reported with spontaneously dividing diploid lymphocytes in unstimulated 24-hr cultures but depressed responsiveness to PHA and concanavalin A, while responses to pokeweed mitogen and allogeneic lymphocytes were in the normal range (Vance et al., 1975).

It has been demonstrated that S cells are neither phagocytic nor adhesive (Brouet et al., 1973a; Zucker-Franklin et al., 1974). These observations are entirely consistent with their lymphocytic origin. Both PAS-positive diastase-soluble and diastase-resistant granules have been reported in S cells (Labaze et al., 1972; Clendenning et al., 1964). These granules, however, do not seem to be a characteristic feature of S cells.

Studies of the membrane properties of the S cells revealed that these cells are devoid of membrane-bound immunoglobulins. These cells also lacked membrane receptors for Fc or complement. Like normal T cells, however, they did form spontaneous rosettes with sheep erythrocytes (SRBC) (Brouet et al., 1973a; Preud'homme and Seligmann, 1972; Broome et al., 1973; Froland et al., 1971; Lutzner et al., 1973).

The comparison of percentages of abnormal cells and rosette-forming cells leads to the conclusion that the majority of S cells, but not all, form spontaneous rosettes with SRBC (Brouet et al., 1973a; Zucker-Franklin et al., 1974). Most blood mononuclear cells (65–90%) showed spontaneous rosette formation in patients with both large and small variants of SS (Brouet et al., 1973a). In SS, however, low T-cell and high null-cell values were also reported (Nordqvist and Kinney, 1976). In all patients studied, the proportion of B lymphocytes was strikingly low, with normal distribution of light- and heavy-chain classes (Brouet et al., 1973a; Zucker-Franklin et al., 1974).

Electron-microscopic studies clearly demonstrated the presence of the S cell in most though not all erythrocyte rosettes and its absence in erythrocyte–antibody–complement rosettes (Zucker-Franklin et al., 1974). These studies also indicated that S cells are not B lymphocytes and favored their belonging to the thymus-derived lymphocyte series (Brouet et al., 1973a; Lutzner et al., 1973; Zucker-Franklin et al., 1974; Broome et al., 1973; Brouet et al., 1973b). The percentage of S cells decreased with chemotherapy, while the number of B cells remained low (Zucker-Franklin et al., 1974).

Cells with the appearance of S cells extracted from skin infiltrates, lymph nodes, and lung tissues in patients with SS were identified as T cells (Lutzner et al., 1975; Rabinowitz et al., 1976). In addition, the cellular infiltrates of some other skin disorders were shown to carry membrane properties of the T cells (Lutzner et al., 1975).

Further characterization of S cells as thymus-derived lymphocytes has been achieved by the use of a specific rabbit anti-human T-cell antiserum, cytotoxic for T lymphocytes. These experiments indicated that S cells are antigenically similar to T cells (Brouet *et al.*, 1973a), and may represent altered or transformed T lymphocytes (Labaze *et al.*, 1972). Rabbit anti-human B-cell antiserum adsorbed with human thymocytes was shown to be cytotoxic only for fewer than 10% of lymphocytes from patients with SS (Lutzner *et al.*, 1975). S cells therefore lack B-cell-specific antigens. S cells, whether of the large- or small-cell variants, manifest similar characteristics (Brouet *et al.*, 1973a).

There have been reported cases of SS that have demonstrated a decrease in or absence of *in vitro* and *in vivo* responsiveness to various mitogens and antigens (Lutzner *et al.*, 1973; Edelson *et al.*, 1974a; Nordqvist and Kinney, 1976). Attempts have been made to determine whether the defective response of these patients is due to the presence of inhibitory factors or is secondary to an intrinsic defect of the S cell itself (Lutzner *et al.*, 1975). There has been no evidence of any factors in the sera of these patients that could inhibit the mitogenic response of the S cells or normal lymphocytes. The supernatant fluid of the cultured S cells in the presence of various mitogens also lacked evidence of inhibitory factors (Lutzner *et al.*, 1975). It was concluded that the lack of mitogenic responses in these patients is not due to the release of inhibitory factors. It was also demonstrated that radioactively labeled mitogens bind to S cells as well as to normal lymphocytes. The lack of response to nonspecific mitogens is therefore not due to defective binding processes. These investigators further demonstrated that in contrast to the results with CLL lymphocytes (Abel *et al.*, 1970), prolonged incubation of unresponsive S cells with mitogens does not produce a significant response (Lutzner *et al.*, 1975). These investigators were also able to show that although normal lymphocytes were stimulated by rabbit anti-human thymocyte globulin, purified anti-T-cell antibody, or rabbit anti-S-cell antiserum, the S cells could not be made to transform by the use of these antisera (Lutzner *et al.*, 1975).

Blastogenic factor is produced from normal human lymphocytes stimulated by antigens, and is capable of transforming normal nonsensitive lymphocytes into blast cells. It was demonstrated that in contrast to normal lymphocytes, S cells failed to transform in the presence of blastogenic factor (Lutzner *et al.*, 1975).

Although macrophage inhibitory factor (MIF)-like activity was observed in the sera of patients with SS (Yoshida *et al.*, 1975; Lutzner *et al.*, 1975; Umbert *et al.*, 1976), cells from patients with SS failed to produce MIF in response to various stimuli (Lutzner *et al.*, 1975). Antibody-coated target cells were not killed by S cells (Lutzner *et al.*, 1975).

Unlike the case with normal mononuclear cells, leukocyte chemotactic activity was not detected in the supernatant of S-cell cultures (Gallin and Kirkpatrick, 1974); this lack may compromise the ability of the patient to mobilize normal leukocytes to infected and necrotic regions (Epstein *et al.*, 1972; Lutzner *et al.*, 1975). Elevated levels of IgE and IgA were reported in both SS and MF (Lutzner *et al.*, 1975; Epstein *et al.*, 1972; MacKie *et al.*, 1976; Blaylock *et al.*, 1966; Tan, R. S. H., *et al.*, 1974).

The capacity of S cells to act as helper T cells was demonstrated in cocultures of these cells with normal lymphocytes (Broder *et al.*, 1976; Waldmann *et al.*, 1976). These studies showed that at least some cases of SS represent proliferation of T lymphocytes that can act as helper T cells in the production of immunoglobulins. We have observed suppressor activity in one patient, helper in another, and no activity in the remaining cases of MF and SS to be expressed, using both a coculture technique and a specific surface marker for detection of helper and suppressor T cells (Gupta *et al.*, 1978).

2.2.6. Pathogenesis and Future Prospects

In the early stages of the disease, neoplastic elements in the skin are rare, and an inflammatory reaction, composed of immunocompetent cells, dominates the histological picture (Rappaport and Thomas, 1974); this inflammatory reaction may be attempting to contain the neoplastic process. This early nonspecific histological picture corresponds with the early stage of the clinical presentation, i.e., nonspecific skin eruptions, severe pruritus, and sometimes erythroderma. Ultrastructural studies of involved skin at this stage have shown the presence of abnormal cells with folded serpentine nuclei that are not evident by light microscopy. This process usually remains stationary for many years. Eventually, the balance is tilted in favor of neoplastic expansion.

Thus, large numbers of neoplastic cells come to dominate the histological picture, while inflammatory cells become scant, producing a characteristic pleomorphic dermal infiltrate, easily diagnosed by light microscopy. This corresponds to the clinical plaque stage of the disease. It has been postulated that immunological barriers in the skin control the spread of the disease, and that once these barriers are lost, the malignant cells proliferate in an unlimited fashion (Rappaport and Thomas, 1974). Thereafter, the extracutaneous phase of the disease begins and follows a similar progressive course, and the patient usually expires from sepsis.

A series of reactions between the neoplastic cells and immunocompetent cells in skin and peripheral blood may initiate the release of cytotoxic substances and certain other mediators (e.g., MIF) (Yoshida *et al.*, 1975; Umbert *et al.*, 1976). Moreover, it is probably the reflection of these cellular interactions and their products in the blood and skin that produces persistent pruritus, erythroderma, exfoliation, and other evidence of the disease.

It has been suggested that the spillover from the skin is the reason for circulating abnormal cells observed in SS and in 20% of MF cases. One may speculate, however, that the presence of an abnormal membrane marker on the surface of these cells may be the reason for the circulation of the neoplastic S cells in the peripheral blood (see Chapter 11). It is postulated that mutational clones of lymphocytes are constantly produced but are kept under control by immunocompetent cells (Burnet, 1973). On the basis of this hypothesis, the questions have been raised whether SS is a manifestation of the effect of aging on the immune surveillance (Prunieras, 1974) and whether the S cells are abnormal T cells. Their proliferation may contribute to the depletion of normal populations of immunocytes that control mutational clones. It seems very unlikely that aging is an important factor; however, the enhancement of immune surveillance by neoplastic S cells may cause inadequacies of immunocompetent cells.

It is agreed by most observers that clinical manifestations of MF and SS invariably start in the skin, and that they either are or have the potential to become malignant neoplastic diseases; a proportion of the patients eventually develop visceral involvement (Rappaport and Thomas, 1974). The question has been raised whether the transformation of normal T lymphocytes to S cells is initiated by a certain antigenic stimulus in skin (Ding *et al.*, 1975).

It is generally recognized that the interaction among cells is basically conducted through the plasma membrane, and that various cells, through their surface membrane, relate to their environment and to each other. Boyse and Old (1977) recently described their findings in regard to immunogenetics of T-cell differentiation in mice. They found that during the course of the development of an organism, cells pass from one compartment of differentiation into the next developing new displays of molecules in the form of newly expressed surface antigens. They demonstrated that cell-surface components, which are recognized as specific surface antigens, are determined and regulated by selective gene action. Adult bone marrow cells migrate to the thymus, where a new phenotype is induced. The induction of a set of genes reconstitutes the cell surface, and the new displays of molecules are then expressed as new surface antigens. This process is followed by mitosis leading to activation of a second set of genes, and so on. These induced cells must follow regulated morphogenetic movements that are based on the cell-surface discrimination before they can manifest their destined function. These investigators also showed that leukemia viruses can be incorporated into the cytoplasmic membrane of thymocytes independent of virus production, and be inherited as a Mendelian character. The expression of this leukemia virus, along with the thymocyte surface phenotype, are governed by the thymus.

In the light of these experimental works, one may speculate that lymphoid cells, passing through various steps of differentiation and under the control of the thymus, may develop certain abnormal surface antigens. These cells may give rise to a fairly well differentiated neoplastic cell line, capable of exhibiting certain neoplastic features such as abnormal chromosomes, defective function, and altered surface characteristics. This could perhaps explain the pathogenic mechanisms involved in the development of MF and S cells.

Studies on the distribution and kinetics of lymphocytes (ecotaxis) have helped the understanding of lymphocyte circulation and tumor-cell homing patterns (see Chapter 11). Ecotaxis is defined as the capacity of lymphoid cell populations to migrate and arrange themselves in a clearly defined microenvironment. Alteration of the cell surface may result in maldistribution (ecotaxopathy) of the involved lymphocytes. The neoplastic cell lines of SS and MF, influenced by their abnormal surface properties and under the discipline of ecotaxis, may exhibit altered distribution patterns and special affinity for the skin. This epitheliotropism, which is one of the characteristic histological features of SS and MF, is accounted for by the presence of abnormal cells in the epidermis either singly (exocytosis) or in cluster (Pautrier's microabscesses). This affinity for the skin may result in the removal of abnormal cells from other lymphoid organs and their sequestration in the skin. Thus, the relative sparing of bone marrow and other lymphoid organs may be readily explained.

It is likely that a peculiar relationship exists among prethymocytes, thymus-derived cells, and epithelial cells. The presence of cornifying squamous epithelium identical to the skin in the thymus (Hassal's corpuscles) (Mandel, 1968) speaks in favor of this relationship. Moreover, it has been demonstrated that thymopoietin produced by thymic epithelium governs the differentiation and maturation of the thymus-derived lymphocytes (Goldstein, 1975) Perhaps abnormal lymphocytes produced in the normal sites of hemopoiesis pass through the thymus and are then attracted to the skin, where they continue their differentiation under the influence of as yet unknown epidermal factors. Moreover, the presence of high concentrations of serum-thymic factors in sera of MF patients observed in our preliminary studies speaks in favor of this hypothesis. The reported success of total-body electron-beam therapy in MF patients may be the result of correction of abnormal skin environment (Goos *et al.*, 1976) or removal of faulty interaction between the infiltrating cells and the skin. Much work must be done before the etiology and pathogenesis of cutaneous T-cell lymphomas are clearly understood.

2.3. Therapeutic Approaches to Cutaneous T-Cell Lymphomas

Treatment of cutaneous T-cell lymphomas has varied considerably. The cutaneous lymphomas have been considered by the majority to be diseases that may extend over decades and may remain stationary for long periods of time, whether treated or not. Thus, with a few exceptions (Fuks *et al.*, 1973; Van Scott and Kalmanson, 1973; Levi and Wiernik, 1975), the therapeutic approach has been generally conservative and predominantly palliative. Owing to the satisfactory control of the skin manifestations, extracutaneous extension of the disease is encountered more and it presents a major therapeutic problem (Fuks *et al.*, 1973).

2.3.1. Topical Agents

Topical applications of a variety of agents have produced some improvement in the early stages of the disease. Application of various corticosteroid preparations has resulted in significant responses lasting up to 6 months (Farber *et al.*, 1968). Topical applications of nitrosourea compounds in cases resistant to nitrogen mustard (HN_2) have been effective (Zackheim, 1972). Methotrexate and 5-fluorouracil have been used topically with poor results (Luikart, 1969).

2.3.2. Nitrogen Mustard

The successful treatment of cutaneous lesions of MF with topical application of nitrogen mustard (HN_2, mechlorethamine) was first described in 1956 (Sipos and Jakso, 1956), and has been confirmed by a number of investigators. These authors reported that in a number of patients with cutaneous MF, topical applications of HN_2 were very effective over long periods and without serious complications (Arundell and Chan, 1968; Van Scott and Kalmanson, 1973; Waldorf *et al.*, 1967, 1968). Complete responses (free of detectable disease) were achieved in over 50% (30–73%) of patients with plaque-stage disease and in 30% of patients with erythroderma (Arundell and Chan, 1968; Van Scott and Kalmanson, 1973; Waldorf *et al.*, 1967, 1968). Resolution of tumorous lesions following whole-body application of HN_2 was also observed (Van Scott and Kalmanson, 1973). With continuous maintenance HN_2 therapy, a substantial number of patients have been reported to be free of detectable disease for over 2 years; relapses have occurred whenever maintenance thereapy was too infrequent. The use of sustained applications of HN_2 for a minimum period of 3 years is therefore recommended to maintain a disease-free state (Van Scott and Kalmanson, 1973). The initial response and survival after treatment with HN_2 has been correlated with the stage of disease at the time of therapy and with the percentage of S cells in the peripheral blood in erythrodermic disease. The response to topical HN_2 in patients with a high percentage of circulating S cells is less favorable than that of erythrodermic patients without circulating S cells. The likelihood of complete remission is greater if treatment is started with early disease, rather than in the tumor stage (Vonderheid *et al.*, 1977).

Intralesional injections of HN$_2$ may also cause regression of skin tumors (Van Scott and Kalmanson, 1973). Frequent low doses of intravenous HN$_2$ were reported to be effective in the late stages of MF and to produce a 78% clinical remission rate and a 35% disease-free status (Van Scott et al., 1975).

HN$_2$ has been used effectively for up to 12 months in the treatment of patients who relapsed following total-skin electron-beam therapy. Moreover, following therapy with HN$_2$, these patients may return and benefit from additional electron-beam irradiation (Levi and Wiernik, 1975).

There is no evidence that topical HN$_2$ causes systemic toxicity. Other internal malignancies were observed, however, in a group of patients treated for long periods with topical HN$_2$ (Vonderheid et al., 1977). Delayed hypersensitivity reactions develop in about 34% of patients treated topically with HN$_2$ (Levi and Wiernik, 1975). This reaction is seen only in patients with intact immune responsiveness. Weekly intravenous injections of small doses of HN$_2$ prior to its topical use proved helpful by inducing immunological tolerance to HN$_2$ (Van Scott and Kalmanson, 1973). This tolerance is transient, however, and develops in only a small proportion of the patients (Vonderheid et al., 1977). Patients who repeatedly relapse eventually develop HN$_2$ resistance and require other forms of therapy (Vonderheid et al., 1977).

2.3.3. Immunotherapy

Immunotherapeutic modalities are being used increasingly in the treatment of various neoplasms. In MF, topical applications of dinitrochlorobenzene (DNCB) or S,2-aminoethylisothiuronium (AET) induced delayed hypersensitivity reactions on plaque lesions and resulted in short-lived partial or complete remission (Ratner et al., 1968; Klein et al., 1973; Van Scott and Kalmanson, 1973; Stewart, 1969; Stjernsward and Levin, 1971). This mode of immunotherapy has been extensively used in the management of skin cancers (Klein et al., 1973, 1975). Inflammation produced by application of primary irritant substances such as sodium lauryl sulfate did not result in lesion regression. Thus, it is concluded that the mechanism of action of DNCB and AET is most likely due to induction of delayed hypersensitivity (Ratner et al., 1968). In the same manner, spontaneous delayed hypersensitivity to topical HN$_2$ in some MF cases may benefit patients with the disease (Van Scott and Kalmanson, 1973). Increases in the proportion of lymphocytes and decreases in the number of atypical MF cells were observed in skin sections following induction of delayed hypersensitivity reaction on MF lesions (Waldorf et al., 1968).

Spontaneous regression of MF has also been reported (Cawley et al., 1951). Complete resolution of all MF lesions produced in this fashion usually lasted for only a few months (Van Scott and Kalmanson, 1973). The erythrodermic type of MF is not responsive to immunotherapy (Vonderheid et al., 1977). It therefore appears that the rate and duration of remission are related to the severity and stage of the disease at the time of allergic reaction (Vonderheid et al., 1977).

2.3.4. Radiation Therapy

Lymphoid cells are generally radiosensitive. Various forms of radiation have been applied extensively in the treatment of cutaneous lymphomas since 1902 (Scholtz, 1902). Small-field, low-kilovoltage (100–140 kV, 50% depth dose at approximately 10 mm) irradiation is of great value, and is still applied to severely infiltrated plaques and tumors (Szur, 1964; Trump *et al.*, 1953). Its use is limited, however, not only because it can cover only small fields, but also because of possible side effects such as radiodermatitis and myelosuppression (Levi and Wiernik, 1975). Very-low-voltage X ray (10–15 kV) and systemic administration of radioactive isotopes such as ^{24}Na, ^{32}P, and ^{76}As are of little value (Szur, 1964).

Due to generalized cutaneous involvement in MF and SS, total-skin irradiation is a more logical approach. Low-voltage X ray from beryllium window units (teleroentgen radiation) (Goldschmidt, 1962) or linear accelerators (Fuks and Bagshaw, 1971) have been used for whole-body irradiation. The beta rays from strontium 90 penetrate only to a depth of 4 mm and are therefore not very effective (Trump *et al.*, 1953). Trump *et al.* (1953) reported the first use of high-energy electrons in the treatment of superficial malignant lesions. Since then, many investigators have repeatedly confirmed the effectiveness of electron-beam therapy in the management of cutaneous lymphomas (Fuks *et al.*, 1973; Van Scott and Kalmanson, 1973; D'Angio *et al.*, 1975; Szur, 1975). Electrons are basically homogeneous in energy and direction and give uniform radiation, the penetration of which is controllable and sharply limited, being approximately 10 mm for each two million volts of energy (Trump *et al.*, 1953). Total-skin electron irradiation is relatively simple and does not affect the hematopoietic system (D'Angio *et al.*, 1975; Szur, 1975). Recent modifications of technique have reduced the concomitant delivery of X ray to only 1–2% of the full electron dose (Szur, 1975).

The rate of complete remission is dose-dependent and inversely related to the extent of the disease (Fuks *et al.*, 1973; D'Angio *et al.*, 1975). Higher doses of irradiation (more than 2000 rads in a single course) were therefore used in recently reported series and resulted in long-term control of cutaneous manifestations (Levi and Wiernik, 1975; Fuks *et al.*, 1973; D'Angio *et al.*, 1975). In one series, 58% of MF cases showed complete remission following total-skin electron-beam therapy; some patients achieved disease-free survival for 3–14 years after a single course of therapy (Fuks *et al.*, 1973). Following total-skin electron-beam therapy, extracutaneous involvement was observed in none of the patients with eczematous and limited plaques, in 15% with the lichenified form, in 20% with generalized plaques, in 35% in the erythematous group, and in 60% with cutaneous tumors (Fuks *et al.*, 1973). Perhaps cure may be achieved with aggressive use of electron irradiation in early stages of MF (Fuks *et al.*, 1973).

Apart from being possibly curative in early stages of the disease, aggressive use of electron irradiation is reported to produce prompt relief of symptoms and disappearance of all types of MF lesions, thus providing a potent palliative measure for incurable cases (Fuks *et al.*, 1973; D'Angio *et al.*, 1975). Repeated courses of total-skin electron irradiation are also beneficial. As the number of courses increased, however, significant side effects appeared, including skin atrophy, telangiectasia, xerosis, transient erythema, onycholysis, hair loss, and temporary hyperpigmentation (Szur, 1975; Van Scott and Kalmanson, 1973; Fuks *et al.*, 1973; D'Angio *et al.*, 1975). Following improvements in the apparatus and modification of the technique of administration, only mild, transient lymphopenia and thrombocytopenia were seen (Szur, 1975), and pancytopenia, reported in earlier series, is not encountered today.

2.3.5. Chemotherapy

The effectiveness of various chemotherapeutic agents for the treatment of cutaneous lymphoma is the subject of several reviews (Levi and Wiernik, 1975;

Epstein *et al.*, 1972). Although topical HN$_2$ and total-skin electron therapy have provided a suitable control of skin manifestations, this form of therapy does not prevent the development of extracutaneous extension of the disease (Levi and Wiernik, 1975; Fuks *et al.*, 1973; Epstein *et al.*, 1972).

A variety of chemotherapeutic agents have been used to treat advanced cutaneous and extracutaneous diseases unresponsive to other modes of therapy (Levi and Wiernik, 1975). Various single chemotherapeutic agents have proved ineffective (Fuks *et al.*, 1973; Epstein *et al.*, 1972). The initial favorable response to corticosteroids is usually followed by the rapid development of disease resistance (Epstein *et al.*, 1972; Wright *et al.*, 1964).

Among the various alkylating agents used, cyclophosphamide is the most effective, producing response rates of 62–100% (Epstein *et al.*, 1972; Van Scott *et al.*, 1962). Chlorambucil has been reported to be effective if used in combination with prednisone (Winkelmann and Linman, 1973) or as adjuvant therapy with total-skin electron irradiation.

The most effective agents among the antimetabolites have been reported to be methotrexate (Wright *et al.*, 1964) and 6-azaribine (McDonald and Calabresi, 1971). Of the cytotoxic antibiotics, bleomycin has been reported promising for the treatment of MF (Co-operative Group for Leukemia and Reticulocytosis, 1972; Spigel and Coltman, 1973), especially since it is concentrated in high levels in both the skin and the lungs. The response to bleomycin, however, has usually lasted less than 3 months (Levi and Wiernik, 1975). Combination chemotherapy has been infrequently used; the results do not seem to be much different from those with other modes of therapy.

In general, the wide variety of chemotherapeutic agents thus far used for the treatment of cutaneous lymphoma have been effective only temporarily (rarely longer than 6 months). Even with maintenance therapy, a continued response is only occasionally achieved for longer than 1 year (Levi and Wiernik, 1975; Epstein *et al.*, 1972). There is no evidence that any of these therapeutic modalities has increased the survival rate; the survival for each mode of therapy did not vary from the corrected survival of all patients (Epstein *et al.*, 1972).

It is apparent that if an improved prognosis is to be gained, aggressive treatment must be pursued in the early stages of the disease (Levi and Wiernik, 1975). In addition, extracutaneous extension should be diagnosed as early as possible and followed by the aggressive use of multiple therapeutic modalities. Moreover, combination of topical HN$_2$ or total-skin electron irradiation with multiple-drug chemotherapy, total nodal irradiation, and various immunotherapeutic approaches may provide a better prognosis and control of the disease.

2.3.6. Leukapheresis

Recently, Edelson *et al.* (1974c) formulated a new concept that there is an equilibrium in SS between the circulating abnormal cells and those in skin infiltrates. Following the removal of the circulating cells, a relative migration of the cells from the tissue back into the blood would occur. Thus, repeated leukapheresis would deplete abnormal cells from the skin. Continuous-flow centrifugation has been used, in which leukocytes are selectively removed from the blood and the other constituents are returned to the patient. This procedure has been said to be effective in decreasing the size of affected lymph nodes and enlarged spleens in some patients with a leukemic phase (L. Reich, Memorial Sloan-Kettering Institute, personal communication). Repeated leukapheresis has been reported to be effective as a maintenance therapy in two cases of SS (Edelson *et al.*, 1974c; Tan, R. S. H., *et al.*, 1975). We observed no favorable results, however, in 5 MF and 1 SS patients thus treated (Safai *et al.*, 1978).

2.4. Lymphomatoid Papulosis

Lymphomatoid papulosis is a cutaneous disorder characterized by recurrent, self-healing skin eruptions, a malignant-appearing histological picture, and the absence of systemic involvement. Although there had been some reports in the literature describing this condition, it was not until 1968 that Macaulay (1968) first termed this disorder *lymphomatoid papulosis*.

The disease resembles Mucha–Habermann disease clinically and seems to pursue a benign but protracted clinical course with recurrent exacerbations and remissions, while the patient's general health remains unaffected. It may last from a few weeks to several years (Macaulay, 1968; Valentino and Helwig, 1973; Black and Wilson-Jones, 1972; Marks *et al.*, 1972). The age at onset has ranged from 8 to 60 years, but the disease usually occurs in the first half of life. Males are affected more often than females (Valentino and Helwig, 1973).

The diagnosis of lymphomatoid papulosis is based on both clinical and histological findings. The predominant skin lesions are papules and occasional nodules, which eventually heal with some scarring and hyperpigmentation. The eruption is usually asymptomatic, but mild pruritus may be present.

The general histological picture is one of dermal polymorphous infiltrate and occasionally epidermal invasion by large pleomorphic hyperchromatic bizarre cells. The cytoplasm of these cells is basophilic and relatively scant, while the nuclei are hyperchromatic, round or irregular, and lobulated or kidney-shaped (Valentino and Helwig, 1973); they contain more DNA than normal nuclei (Verallo and Fand, 1969). The cells are usually mononuclear and vary in size from 25 to 40 μm, which is much larger than MF cells; some are multinucleated and closely resemble Reed–Sternberg cells. Mitotic figures are often present (Macaulay, 1968). Various numbers of small lymphocytes and monocytes are mixed with these abnormal cells, giving a polymorphic pattern (Macaulay, 1968; Valentino and Helwig, 1973; Black and Wilson-Jones, 1972). The dermal infiltrate is usually perivascular in distribution, and dermal edema and extravasated red blood cells are present (Macaulay, 1968; Black and Wilson-Jones, 1972). Epidermotropism of these bizarre cells is an outstanding histological feature (Macaulay, 1968). The large atypical cells are consistently prominent in the infiltrate and give an overall impression of malignant lymphoma (Macaulay, 1968; Black and Wilson-Jones, 1972). The infiltrate in lymphomatoid papulosis is often more pleomorphic and less diffuse than that seen in MF (Valentino and Helwig, 1973).

Electron-microscopic study of lymphomatoid papulosis showed paramyxoviruslike particles (Sandbank and Feurman, 1972). This report awaits confirmation. The atypical cells of lymphomatoid papulosis have been proved to possess ultrastructural characteristics similar to those of S cells (Schneiderman *et al.*, 1975; Flaxman *et al.*, 1971). A recent report presented evidence that most of these cells carry surface characteristics of thymus-derived lymphocytes (Lutzner *et al.*, 1975; Schneiderman *et al.*, 1975). It was suggested that lymphomatoid papulosis also be grouped as a cutaneous T-cell lymphoma (Lutzner *et al.*, 1975; Schneiderman *et al.*, 1975).

Until recently, lymphomatoid papulosis has not been associated with systemic lymphoreticular disorders. In two such cases, however, disseminated lymphomas, with eventually fatal outcomes, have now been observed, (Kawada *et al.*, 1969; Muller and Schulze, 1971).

3. Other Proliferative Disorders of the T-Cell Series—Disorders with Both T- and B-Cell Markers

Various other T-cell abnormalities are covered extensively in other chapters. It is of particular importance to discuss briefly in this section only the peculiar lymphoproliferative syndromes characterized by cells that possess both T- and B-cell markers.

Normally, a small percentage of human peripheral blood lymphocytes is demonstrated to carry both sets of markers (Marchalonis *et al.*, 1973; Bentwich *et al.*, 1973; Shevach *et al.*, 1974; Chiao and Good, 1976; Mendes *et al.*, 1974). While forming spontaneous rosettes with SRBC, this subset of lymphocytes may carry one or few of the B-cell markers. The term *D lymphocyte* has been used for these doubly marked lymphoid cells (Chiao and Good, 1976). The presence of D lymphocytes in patients who lack antibody-producing B cells on a genetic basis indicates the possibility that D cells are independent of the plasma-cell line and the B-cell population (Chiao *et al.*, 1975).

The surface immunoglobulins detected on freshly drawn cells may represent an antibody directed toward the cell-surface determinants (Brouet and Prieur, 1974). Such situations have been encountered in patients with systemic lupus erythematosus (Wernet and Kunkel, 1973), in CLL (Preud'homme and Seligmann, 1972), in infectious mononucleosis (Thomas, D. B., 1972), and also in NZB mice (Shirai *et al.*, 1973). In addition, in a series of more than 100 CLL cases, two patients were found to exhibit both T- and B-cell characteristics. On analysis of these two patients, however, one case proved to be B-CLL in which surface immunoglobulins had anti-SRBC antibody activity leading to immune rosette formation, and the other case was shown to be T-CLL with leukemic cells incapable of *in vitro* synthesis of membrane-bound immunoglobulins (Brouet and Prieur, 1974). One must therefore be careful in interpreting such data, and multiple use of several markers is of utmost importance to properly classify lymphoproliferative diseases as T- or B-cell disorders.

In a few murine malignant lymphomas, the neoplastic cells were reported to exhibit characteristics of both T and B lymphocytes (Harris *et al.*, 1973; Grey *et al.*, 1972; Greenberg and Zatz, 1975). In humans, there are only a few case reports describing the simultaneous presence of both T- and B-cell markers on the surface of the malignant lymphoid cells (Brouet *et al.*, 1975; Hsu, 1976; Shevach *et al.*, 1974; Sandilands *et al.*, 1974; Siegal *et al.*, 1976).

In a case of lymphosarcoma cell leukemia, while the majority of the leukemic cells exhibited T-cell receptors, a progressive increase in the number of blast cells carrying both sets of markers was reported (Hsu *et al.*, 1975). Similar increase in surface immunoglobulins on leukemic T cells in mice was also observed (Greenberg and Zatz, 1975). Chiao *et al.* (1975) reported a reduced proportion of peripheral D lymphocytes in some patients with lymphocytic leukemia. The presence of a small population of doubly marked lymphocytes was recently described in the peripheral blood of all four patients with X-linked infantile agammaglobulinemia (Chiao *et al.*, 1975).

Leukemic proliferation of cells with dual markers, normally found in peripheral blood, is thought to result in this type of presentation (Siegal *et al.*, 1976; Sandilands *et al.*, 1974; Shevach *et al.*, 1974). Contrary to this view, it is postulated that the activation of B-cell genes during the process of malignant differentiation of the neoplastic T cells gives rise to cells with both sets of surface markers (Hsu *et al.*, 1975; Nowell *et al.*, 1976). It is also speculated that cells with dual markers arise from precursor cells that have the potential of expressing both sets of receptors or from the unmasking of cryptic receptor sites during malignant transformation (Magrath, 1974). The neoplastic lymphocytes from a case with leukemic lymphosarcoma were shown to bind both SRBC and complement-coated erythrocytes, while they lacked other cell-surface receptors. These cells carried a particular chromosomal abnormality that is considered a clue to the chromosomal origin of some lymphocyte surface markers in man (Siegal *et al.*, 1976).

4. Hypereosinophilic States

There is growing evidence that a relationship exists between eosinophils and thymus-derived lymphocytes, and that the actual mechanism of eosinophilia may be largely mediated by immunological processes (Gupta, 1977). This new knowledge is based on experimental work by Basten and Beeson (1970), which is discussed later in this section.

Eosinophilia is described in conjunction with numerous clinical syndromes (Panush *et al.*, 1971; Benvenisti and Ultman, 1969; Chusid *et al.*, 1975; Hardy and Anderson, 1968). It is noted most frequently in allergic conditions and parasitic infestations (Chusid *et al.*, 1975; Jacob *et al.*, 1964; Snyder, 1961). Occasionally, eosinophilia occurs with autoimmune diseases (Panush *et al.*, 1971; Wilson, K. S., and Alexander, 1945), blood dyscrasia (Theologides, 1972), and malignancies (Bengtsson, 1968; Benevenisti and Ultman, 1969; Liao *et al.*, 1972), or as a leukemoid reaction (Rickles and Miller, 1972). Benign familial eosinophilia has been reported (Naiman *et al.*, 1964).

A clinicohistopathological entity was first described by Kimura (Kimura *et al.*, 1948; Kawada and Takahashi, 1966) as characterized by eosinophilia and subcutaneous nodules. The histological findings include capillary proliferation, eosinophilic infiltration, and lymphoreticular hyperplasia leading to lymphoid follicle formation. This report from Japan was supported by reports of a similar disorder from Europe (Wells and Whimster, 1968) and the United States (Mehregan and Shapiro, 1971).

Persistent and marked eosinophilia occurs with diffuse eosinophilic infiltration of various organs (heart, lungs, CNS); this is associated with hematological abnormalities and with significant morbidity and mortality. The etiology of these syndromes is not known. They have been referred to as eosinophilic leukemia (Block *et al.*, 1963a), Loeffler's fibroblastic endocarditis (Brink and Weber, 1963), and disseminated eosinophilic collagen disease (Odeberg, 1965). However, the existence of each of these as a distinct clinical entity is debatable (Bently *et al.*, 1961; Benvenisti and Ultman, 1969; Rickles and Miller, 1972; Chusid *et al.*, 1975). Moreover, due to considerable overlap of the clinical and laboratory findings, it was suggested that they be referred to collectively as the *hypereosinophilic syndrome*

(Hardy and Anderson, 1968). In addition, many authors believe that there is a continuum of hypereosinophilic states, with eosinophilic leukemia being at one pole (Hardy and Anderson, 1968; Roberts *et al.*, 1970; Chusid *et al.*, 1975). Loeffler's endocarditis, Loeffler's syndrome, disseminated eosinophilic collagen disease, and polyarteritis nodosa are among the nonmalignant disorders included in the hypereosinophilic syndrome that may clinically simulate eosinophilic leukemia (Engfeldt and Zetterstrom, 1956; Snyder,1961; Benvenisti and Ultman, 1969).

The majority of patients with these syndromes do not appear to have eosinophilic leukemia. However, malignant proliferation may occur in the eosinophil as in any other cell line (Chusid *et al.*, 1975).

While its existence as a separate entity is still debated (Benvenisti and Ultman, 1969; Bently *et al.*, 1961; Chen and Smith, 1960), eosinophilic leukemia is classified on the basis of cell type as blastic-, immature-, and mature-cell variants (Benvenisti and Ultman, 1969). The risk of developing acute blastic leukemia is much increased when immature cells are present (Benvenisti and Ultman, 1969). Determinations of leukemic markers (serum B_{12} and folate, leukocyte alkaline phosphatase levels, basophilia, and chromosome analysis) have proved to be of predictive value in terms of symptomatology and response to therapy (Chusid *et al.*, 1975). The clinical spectrum of eosinophilic leukemia varies considerably and may manifest features of the myeloproliferative as well as the hyperallergic disorders (Yam *et al.*, 1972; Benvenisti and Ultman, 1969).

The hypereosinophilic syndrome is primarily a disease of middle age, with a male predominance (Chusid *et al.*, 1975). Aside from one series (Chusid *et al.*, 1975), the average survival in most reviews is estimated to be less than 1 year (Bently *et al.*, 1961; Benvenisti and Ultman, 1969; Rickles and Miller, 1972), indicating that eosinophilic leukemia is a rapidly fatal disease. The clinical findings include persistent eosinophilia associated with organ damage, hepatosplenomegaly, lymphadenopathy, anemia, weight loss, anorexia, fatigue, and a generally poor response to therapy (Chusid *et al.*, 1975). Corticosteroid therapy is reported to have eosinopenic effects (Rebhun, 1974; Benvenisti and Ultman, 1969). Treatment of eosinophilic leukemia has been disappointing.

Cytogenetic studies demonstrated aneuploidy in cultured cells; 2 of 5 cases had a C-group deletion (Chusid *et al.*, 1975). Four cases were reported with the Philadelphia chromosome (Gruenwald *et al.*, 1965; Kauer and Engle, 1964; Chusid *et al.*, 1975). Eosinophils can be recognized only after promyelocytes acquire specific granules. A mutation may take place at this stage of differentiation affecting only the eosinophils. This may explain why the Philadelphia chromosome is seen only rarely in these cases (Zucker-Franklin, 1971). These findings may suggest that some cases of hypereosinophilic syndrome represent a chronic myeloproliferative disorder that resembles classic chronic granulocytic leukemia.

Whether eosinophils are present as a response to tissue damage or whether their presence itself produces tissue damage is not clear (Chusid *et al.*, 1975; Benvenisti and Ultman, 1969). Eosinophilic leukemoid reactions secondary to drugs and parasites, and prolonged eosinophilia, as well as all subgroups of hypereosinophilic syndrome regardless of their etiology, may result in cardiac injury (Chusid *et al.*, 1975; Yam *et al.*, 1972). Endocardial lesions are reported in at least 20% of cases with eosinophilic leukemia (Benvenisti and Ultman, 1969). It therefore appears that endocardial lesions are the result of eosinophilia and their presence does not exclude a diagnosis of eosinophilic leukemia (Yam *et al.*, 1972). It is not clear whether eosinophilic granules contain substances that produce cardiac damage (Zucker-Franklin, 1971, 1974). Eosinophils are rich in histamine, hydrolases, and coagulation factors (Graham *et al.*, 1955; Barnhart and Riddle, 1963). Destruction of eosinophils *in situ* may cause local release of these enzymes, which may then produce the endocardial inflammation and injury (Yam *et al.*, 1972). Thus, the excess of eosinophils may be directly responsible for the various findings in these disorders (Benvenisti and Ultman, 1969).

The process of fibrinolysis at the site of inflammation and facilitation of wound-healing are among the activities of eosinophils (Riddle and Barnhart, 1965). Eosinophils were shown to demonstrate antiheparin and lipid cofactor activity in the Venum-plasma clotting tests (Archer, R. K., 1963), which are not specific for them (Benvenisti and Ultman, 1969). Eosinophils also show cyanide-resistant peroxidase activity (Yam *et al.*, 1971), but do not contain alkaline phosphatase or chloracetate esterase (Kaplow, 1968). Aside from their hydrolytic enzymes, the eosinophilic granules contain substances that neutralize histamine, bradykinin, and serotonin, suggesting that in some situations, these cells may actually have a healing effect on the inflammatory response (Zucker-Franklin, 1971, 1974).

Recent studies demonstrated that 45–70% of eosinophils bind two types of complement receptors: (1) immune-adherence-type receptors, which are specific for C4 or C3b; and (2) C3d-type receptors, which are specific for C3d (Gupta *et al.*, 1976). Eosinophils differ from fully matured neutrophils in having C3d receptors and relatively weak immune-adherence (C4 or C3b) receptors, while the neutrophils lack C3d receptors and have strong immune-adherence receptors. Receptors for IgGFC (by the aggregated IgG method) are present on only 17% of eosinophils. Eosinophils are believed to lack surface immunoglobulins (Gupta *et al.*, 1976; Ishizaka *et al.*, 1970). Hubscher (1975), however, reported the presence of IgE on the surface of 25–30% of eosinophils. Eosinophils do not bind to mouse or sheep erythrocytes.

Experimental evidence suggests that eosinophils accumulate at sites of antigen injection and antibody production (Speirs, 1958); they phagocitize antigen–antibody complexes and play a major role in processing immune complexes (Litt, 1963, 1964a,b; Sabesin, 1967; Zucker-Franklin, 1971, 1974). For these reasons, some investigators have suggested that hypereosinophilic reactions are due to a profound antigenic stimulus of unknown variety (Hardy and Anderson, 1968; Rickles and Miller, 1972). Phagocytosis of erythrocyte–antibody complexes is reported to be increased in patients with transient eosinophilia (Tai and Spry, 1976).

A number of factors are described as chemotactic for eosinophils; among them are complement components and antigen–antibody complexes (Litt, 1964a; Kay, 1970; Archer, G. T., and Hirsch, 1963). In the absence of serum, immune complexes are not chemotactic for eosinophils (Ward, 1969). Aggregated IgG and IgM are also reported to be chemotactic for eosinophils (Laster and Gleich, 1970). It has been demonstrated that stimulated or sensitized lymphocytes release biologically active substances that interact with immune complexes and generate eosinophilic chemotactic factors that are antigen-specific (Basten and Beeson, 1970; Basten *et al.*, 1970; Cohen and Ward, 1971; Torisu *et al.*, 1973). The presence of eosinophilic chemotactic factors of anaphylaxis (Kay *et al.*, 1971) and similar factors in certain tumors (Wasserman *et al.*, 1974) has also been described (Chusid *et al.*, 1975). A metabolic derangement of normal plasma inhibitors or activators for eosinophilic chemotactic factors may therefore produce an outpouring of eosinophils from bone marrow (Chusid *et al.,* 1975). Relatively little is known about the kinetics of eosinophils. For example, it is only suggested that corticosteroids can cause eosinopenia by redistribution of these cells (Anderson, 1969).

Although the pathogenesis of eosinophilia in various clinical syndromes as well as its role in immunological events are unclear (Panush *et al.,* 1971), experimental work suggests that immunological mechanisms may be involved in the pathogenesis of eosinophilia (Speirs, 1958; Litt, 1963, 1964b; Sebesin, 1967; Basten *et al.,* 1970; Basten and Beeson, 1970; Cohen and Ward, 1971).

Basten and Beeson (1970) showed that *Trichinella spiralis* larvae are capable of evoking eosinophilia in rats and mice, and that these animals produce much greater eosinophilia on rechallenge. Thoracic duct lymphocytes from sensitized donors can transfer the stimulus for induction of eosinophilia to normal syngeneic recipients. Adult rats treated with antilymphocyte serum and rats thymectomized at birth do not develop eosinophilia after introduction of the parasites. Reconstitution with syngeneic bone marrow and thoracic duct lymphocytes from normal and sensitized donors in irradiated rats resulted in the animals' ability to respond to the parasitic stimulus. The factors inducing eosinophilia may be transferred to unstimulated animals by sensitized lymphocytes enclosed in millipore chambers, which suggests that active humoral agent(s) may be released from sensitized lymphocytes (Basten and Beeson, 1970; Basten *et al.,* 1970).

The production of eosinophils in the bone marrow can be divided into inductive and proliferative phases. The inductive phase is reported to last 24 hr after injection of *T. spiralis;* it is suppressed by antilymphocyte serum, but is not affected by cytotoxic drugs. In the proliferative phase, the increase in eosinophils is 16 to 64 fold; this phase is not affected by antilymphocyte serum, but is sensitive to cytotoxic drugs (Basten and Beeson, 1970).

On the basis of the aforementioned observations, it appears that T lymphocytes play an essential role in the development of eosinophilia. This hypothesis is further supported by the presence of eosinophilia reported in patients with agammaglobulinemia (Huntley and Cotas, 1965). Eosinophilia was also observed in patients with thymic dysplasia (Duic *et al.,* 1970) and patients with bronchial asthma with low T lymphocytes (absolute counts) (Gupta *et al.,* 1975). It is therefore possible that the T cells exercise a helper or a suppressor effect on the eosinophils (Gupta, 1977).

In addition to the studies cited above that suggest the relationship of thymus-derived lymphocytes and eosinophilia, occasional clinical and histological observations have also attested to the link between eosinophils and lymphoid cells. Eosinophils are observed in fetal thymus, especially in the 14-week-old human embryo (Schaffer, 1891) and in the interlobular septa of the thymus medulla (Bhathal and Campbell, 1965). Eosinophils are routinely found in human thoracic duct (Zucker-Franklin, 1963). Infiltration of eosinophils in the thymus-dependent area of the lymph nodes in a patient with hypereosinophilic syndrome has been reported (Rebhun, 1974).

5. Conclusion and Outlook

The T-cell types of lymphoid malignancies have received somewhat less attention than those of the B-cell class. In a short time, however, the rapidly developing knowledge of macromolecular engineering has yielded new insight into the nature of this group of neoplasms.

Analysis of the basic structural details and molecular definition of lymphoid-cell differentiation and interaction have already generated an exciting interplay between the clinic and fundamental science in this branch of medicine. Application of this information in the maintenance and possibly in the repair of the lymphoid-cell machinery will have a major influence in reducing or eliminating many of the diseases of mankind. Clearly, we are at the initial stage of this scientific journey, and much has to be learned before the complete picture of lymphoid malignancies is revealed.

References

Abel, C. W., Camp, C. W., and Johnson, L. D., 1970, Effects of phytohemagglutinin and isoproterenol on DNA synthesis in lymphocytes from normal donors and patients with chronic lymphocytic leukemia, *Cancer Res.* **30**:717–723.

Alibert, J. L. M., 1806, *Déscription des Maladies de la Peau Observées à L'Hôpital St. Louis*, pp. 157–158, Barrois, Paris.

Allen, A. C., 1954, *Mycosis Fungoides in the Skin*, p. 1010, C. V. Mosby, St. Louis.

Allen, A. C., 1967, *The Skin—A Clinicopathologic Treatise*, 2nd Ed., Grune & Stratton, New York.

Anderson, V., 1969, Autoradiographic studies of eosinophil kinetics: Effect of cortisol, *Cell Tissue Kinet.* **2**:139.

Archer, G. T., and Hirsch, J. G., 1963, Motion picture studies on degranulation of horse eosinophils during phagocytosis, *J. Exp. Med.* **118**:287–293.

Archer, R. K., 1963, *The Eosinophil Leukocytes*, p. 150, Blackwell Scientific Publications, Oxford.

Arundell, F. D., and Chan, W. M., 1968, Mycosis fungoides: Topical use of nitrogen mustard in recurrent cases, *Calif. Med.* **109**:461–468.

Barnhart, M. I., and Riddle, J. M., 1963, A role for eosinophils in fibrinolysis, in: *Proceedings of the 9th Congress of the European Society of Haematology*, p. 1330, S. Karger, Lisbon, Basel, and New York.

Basten, A., and Beeson, P. B., 1970, Mechanism of eosinophilia. II. Role of the lymphocyte, *J. Exp. Med.* **131**:1288–1305.

Basten, A., Boyer, M. H., and Beeson, P. B., 1970, Mechanism of eosinophilia. I. Factors affecting the eosinophil response of rats to *Trichinella spiralis*, *J. Exp. Med.* **131**:1271–1287.

Bazin, P. A. E., 1862, *Leçons Thériques et Cliniques sur les Affections Cutanées Artificielles*, p. 372, A. Delahaye, Paris.

Bengtsson, E., 1968, Eosinophilic leukemia, an immunopathological reaction?, *Acta. Pediatr. Scand.* **57**:245–249.

Bently, H. P., Reardon, A. E., and Knoedler, J. P., 1961, Eosinophilic leukemia, *Am. J. Med.* **30**:310–322.

Bentwich, Z., Douglas, S. D., Siegal, F. P., and Kunkel, H. G., 1973, Human lymphocyte–sheep erythrocyte rosette formation: Some characteristics of the interaction, *Clin. Immunol. Immunopathol.* **1**:511–522.

Benvenisti, D. S., and Ultman, J. E., 1969, Eosinophilic leukemia: Report of five cases and review of literature, *Ann. Intern. Med.* **71**:731–745.

Bhathal, P. S., and Campbell, P., 1965, Eosinophil leukocytes in the child's thymus, *Aust. Ann. Med.* **14**:210–213.

Biberfeld, P., 1971, Morphogenesis in blood lymphocytes stimulated with phytohemagglutinin (PHA)—A light and electron microscope study, *Acta Pathol. Microbiol. Scand. (Suppl. A)* **223**:1–70.

Black, M. M., and Wilson-Jones, E., 1972, "Lymphatoid" pityriasis lichenoides: A variant with histological features simulating a lymphoma, *Br. J. Dermatol.* **86**:329–347.

Blaylock, W. K., Clendenning, W. E., Carbone, P. P., and Van Scott, E. J., 1966, Normal immunologic reactivity in patients with the lymphoma mycosis fungoides, *Cancer* **19**:233–236.

Block, J. B., Carbone, P. P., Oppenheim, J. J., and Frei, E., 1963a, The effect of treatment in patients with chronic myelogenous leukemia: Biochemical studies, *Ann. Intern. Med.* **59**:629–636.

Block, J. B., Edgcomb, J., Eisen, A., and Van Scott, E. J., 1963b, Mycosis fungoides: Natural history and aspects of its relationship to other malignant lymphomas, *Am. J. Med.* **34**:228–235.

Bluefarb, S. M., 1959, *Cutaneous Manifestations of the Malignant Lymphomas,* pp. 5–219, Charles C. Thomas, Springfield, Illinois.

Boyse, E. A., and Old, L. J., 1977, The immunogenetics of differentiation in the mouse, Harvey lecture, 1976.

Braverman, I. M., 1970, Mycosis fungoides, in: *Skin Signs of Systemic Disease,* pp. 76–92, W. B. Saunders, Philadelphia.

Brink, A. J., and Weber, H. W., 1963, Fibroblastic parietal endocarditis with eosinophilia, *Am. J. Med.* **34**:52–70.

Brocq, L., 1902, Les parapsoriasis, *Ann. Dermatol. Syphiligr.* **3**:433.

Broder, S., Edelson, R. L., Lutzner, M. A., Neson, D. L., MacDermott, R. P., Durm, M. E., Goldman, C. K., Meade, B. D., and Waldmann, T. A., 1976, The Sézary syndrome: A malignant proliferation of helper T cells, *J. Clin. Invest.* **58**:1297–1306.

Broome, J. D., Zucker-Franklin, D., Weiner, M. S., Bianco, C., and Nussenzweig, V., 1973, Leukemic cells with membrane properties of thymus derived (T) lymphocytes in case of Sézary syndrome: Morphologic and immunologic studies, *Clin. Immunol. Immunopathol.* **1**:319–329.

Brouet, J. C., and Prieur, A.-M., 1974, Membrane markers on chronic lymphocytic leukemia cells: A B-cell leukemia with rosettes due to anti-sheep erythrocyte antibody activity of the membrane bound IgM and a T-cell leukemia with surface Ig, *Clin. Immunol. Immunopathol.* **2**:481–487.

Brouet, J. C., Flandrin, G., and Seligmann, M., 1973a, Indications of the thymus-derived nature of the proliferating cells in six patients with Sézary syndrome, *N. Engl. J. Med.* **289**:341–344.

Brouet, J. C., Flandrin, G., and Seligmann, M., 1973b, Démonstration d'une prolifération de cellules lymphocytaires thymodependantes dans le syndrome de Sézary, *C. R. Acad. Sci. (Paris)* **276**:247–249.

Brouet, J. C., LaBaume, S., and Seligmann, M., 1975, Evaluation of T and B lymphocyte membrane markers in human non-Hodgkin's malignant lymphomata, *Br. J. Cancer* **31**(*Suppl. 2*):121–127.

Brownlee, T. R., and Murad, T. M., 1970, Ultrastructure of mycosis fungoides, *Cancer* **26**:686–698.

Burbank, F., 1971, Patterns in cancer mortality in the United States, 1950–1967, NCI Monograph No. 33, pp. 496–504.

Bureau, Y., Barrière, H., and Guenel, J., 1959, La réticulose erythrodermique avec réticulémic de Sézary, *Presse Med.* **67**:2276–2278.

Burnet, M., 1973, Aging and immunological surveillance, *Triangle* **12**:159–162.

Cawley, E. P., Curtis, A. C., and Leach, J. E. K., 1951, Is mycosis fungoides a reticuloendothelial neoplastic entity?, *Arch. Dermatol. Syphilol.* **64**:255–272.

Chen, H. P., and Smith, H. S., 1960, Eosinophilia leukemia, *Ann. Intern. Med.* **52**:1343–1352.

Chiao, J. W., and Good, R. A., 1976, Studies of the presence of membrane receptors for complement, IgG and the sheep erythrocyte rosetting capacity on the same human lymphocytes, *Eur. J. Immunol.* **6**:157–162.

Chiao, J. W., Pantic, V. S., and Good, R. A., 1975, Human lymphocytes bearing both receptors for complement components and SRBC, *Clin. Immunol. Immunopathol.* **4**:545–555.

Chusid, M. J., Dale, D. C., West, B. C., and Wolff, S. M., 1975, The hypereosinophilic syndrome: Analysis of fourteen cases with review of the literature, *Medicine* **54**:1027.

Clendenning, W. E., and Van Scott, E. J., 1965, Skin autografts and homografts in patients with the lymphoma mycosis fungoides, *Cancer Res.* **25**:1844–1853.

Clendenning, W. E., Brecher, G., and Van Scott, E. J., 1964, Mycosis fungoides: Relationship to malignant cutaneous reticulosis and the Sézary syndrome, *Arch. Dermatol.* **89**:785–792.

Cohen, S., and Ward, P. A., 1971, *In vitro* and *in vivo* activity of a lymphocyte and immune complex-dependent chemotactic factor for eosinophils, *J. Exp. Med.* **133**:133–146.

Cooperative Group for Leukemia and Reticulocytosis, 1972, Bleomycin in the reticuloses (trial of the European Organization for Research on the Treatment of Cancer), *Br. Med. J.* **1**:285–286.

Crossen, P. E., Mellor, J. E. L., Finley, A. G., Ravich, R. B., Vincent, P. C., and Gunz, F. W., 1971, The Sézary syndrome: Cytogenetic studies and identification of the Sézary cell as an abnormal lymphocyte, *Am. J. Med.* **50**:24–34.

Cyr, D. P., Geokas, M. C., and Worsley, G. H., 1966, Mycosis fungoides: Hematologic findings and terminal course, *Arch. Dermatol.* **94**:558–573.

D'Angio, G. J., Nisce, L. Z., and Kim, J. H., 1975, Weekly total skin electron beam therapy for mycosis fungoides and other cutaneous lymphomata: Further experience, *Br. J. Cancer* **31**(*Suppl. 2*):379–385.

Dewald, G., Spurbeck, J. L., and Vitek, H. A., 1974, Chromosomes in patient with Sézary syndrome, *Mayo Clin. Proc.* **49**:553–557.

Dick, H. M., Mackie, R., and de Sousa, M., 1976, HLA and mycosis fungoides, in: *International Symposium on HLA and Diseases, 1st, Paris, 1976. HLA and Disease: Predisposition to Disease and Clinical Implications; Abstracts.* (J. Dausset and A. Svejgaard, eds.), p. 99, Inserm, Paris.

Ding, J. C., Adams, P. B., Patison, M., and Cooper, I. A., 1975, Thymic origin of abnormal lymphoid cells in Sézary syndrome, *Cancer* **35**:1325–1332.

Dowling, G. B., and Freudenthal, W., 1938, Dermatomyositis and poikiloderma atrophicans vascularis: A clinical and histological comparison, *Br. J. Dermatol.* **50**:519–539.

Duic, A., Crozier, D. N., Lynch, M. J., and McClure, P. D., 1970, Swiss agammaglobulinemia with hypoglycemia, osseous changes and eosinophilia, *Can. Med. Assoc. J.* **103**:64–68.

Edelson, R. L., Kirkpatrick, C. H., Shevach, E. M., Schein, P. S., Smith, R. W., Green, I., and Lutzner, M. A., 1974a, Preferential cutaneous infiltration by neoplastic thymus-derived lymphocytes—Morphological and functional studies, *Ann. Intern. Med.* **80**:685–692.

Edelson, R. H., Lutzner, M. A., Kirkpatrick, C. H., Shevach, E. M., and Green, I., 1974b, Morphologic and functional properties of the atypical T lymphocytes of the Sézary syndrome, *Mayo Clin. Proc.* **49**:558–566.

Edelson, R., Facktor, M., Andrews, A., Lutzner, M., and Schein, P., 1974c, Successful management of the Sézary syndrome, *N. Engl. J. Med.* **291**:293–294.

Elves, M. W., Gough, J., and Israéls, M. C. G., 1964, The place of the lymphocyte in the reticulo-endothelial system: A study of the *in vitro* effect of prednisone on lymphocytes, *Acta Haematol. (Basel)* **32**:100–107.

Engfeldt, B., and Zetterstrom, R., 1956, Disseminated eosinophilic collagen disease, *Acta. Med. Scand.* **153**:337–353.

Epstein, E. H., Levin, D. L., Croft, J. D., and Lutzner, M. A., 1972, Mycosis fungoides: Survival, prognostic features, response to therapy and autopsy findings, *Medicine* **15**:61–72.

Erkman-Balis, B., and Conen, P. E., 1972, Consistent chromosome abnormalities in each of three cases of childhood lymphosarcoma, *Eur. J. Cancer* **8**:683–688.

Erkman-Balis, B., and Rappaport, H., 1974, Cytogenetic studies in mycosis fungoides, *Cancer* **34**:626–633.

Escovitz, E. S., Soulen, R. L., Van Scott, E. J., Kalmanson, J. D., and Barry, W. E., 1974, Mycosis fungoides: A lymphographic assessment, *Diagn. Radio.* **112**:23–27.

Farber, E. M., Zackheim, H. S., McClintock, R. P., and Cox, A. J., Jr., 1968, Treatment of mycosis fungoides with various strengths of fluocinolone acetonide cream, *Arch. Dermatol.* **97**:165–172.

Fisher, E. R., Horvath, B. L., and Wechsler, H. L., 1972, Ultrastructural features of mycosis fungoides, *Am. J. Clin. Pathol.* **58**:99–110.

Flandrin, G., and Daniel, M. T., 1974, β-Glucuronidase activity in Sézary cells, *Scand. J. Haematol.* **12**:23–31.

Flaxman, A., Zelazny, G., and Van Scott, E. J., 1971, Nonspecificity of characteristic cells in mycosis fungoides, *Arch. Dermatol.* **104**:141–147.

Fleischmajer, R., and Eisenberg, S., 1964, Sézary's reticulosis: Its relationship with neoplasias of the lymphoreticular system, *Arch. Dermatol.* **89**:69–79.

Fleischmajer, R., Pascher, F., and Sims, C. F., 1965, Parapsoriasis en plaques and mycosis fungoides, *Dermatologica* **131**:149–160.

Freeman, A. I., and Journey, L. J., 1971, Ultrastructural studies on monocytic leukemia, *Br. J. Haematol.* **20**:225–231.

Froland, S., Natvig, J. G., and Berdal, P., 1971, Surface-bound immunoglobulin as a marker of B lymphocytes in man, *Nature (London) New Biol.* **234**:251–252.

Fuks, Z., and Bagshaw, M. A., 1971, Total skin electron treatment of mycosis fungoides, *Radiology* **100**:145–150.

Fuks, Z., Bagshaw, M. A., and Farber, E. M., 1973, Prognostic signs and the management of mycosis fungoides, *Cancer* **32**:1385–1395.

Fuks, Z., Castellino, R. A., Carmel, J. A., Farber, E. M., and Bagshaw, M. A., 1974, Lymphography in mycosis fungoides, *Cancer* **34**:106–112.

Gallin, J. I., and Kirkpatrick, C. H., 1974, Chemotactic activity in dialyzable transfer factor, *Proc. Natl. Acad. Sci. U.S.A.* **71**:498–502.

Ghadially, F. N., and Skinnider, I. F., 1972, Ultrastructure of hairy cell leukemia, *Cancer* **29**:444–452.

Gianotti, F., and Caputo, R., 1969, Skin ultrastructure in Hand–Schuler–Christian disease: Report on abnormal Langerhans cells, *Arch. Dermatol.* **100**:342–349.

Goldschmidt, H., 1962, Teleroentgen irradiation in dermatologic therapy—Low voltage (soft) X-rays, in: *Proceedings of the XIIth International Congress of Dermatology* (D. M. Pillsbury and C. S. Livingood, eds.), Vol. I, pp. 643–646, Excerpta Medica, New York.

Goldstein, G., 1975, Isolation of thymopoietin (thymin), *Ann. N. Y. Acad. Sci.* **249**:177–183.

Goos, M., Kaiserling, E., and Lennert, K., 1976, Mycosis fungoides: Model for T-lymphocyte homing to the skin?, *Br. J. Dermatol.* **94**:221–222.

Gorski, A. J., Dupont, B., Hensen, J. H., Safai, B., Pahwa, S., and Good, R. A., 1977, Human immunodeficiency disease: Impairment of cellular interactions leading to mediator production in mixed lymphocyte culture production, *J. Immunol.* **118**:858–862.

Graham, H. T., Lowry, O. H., Wheelwright, F., Lenz, M. A., and Parish, H. H., Jr., 1955, Distribution of histamine among leukocytes and platelets, *Blood* **10**:467–481.

Greenberg, R. S., and Zatz, M. M., 1975, Spontaneous AKR lymphoma with T and B cell characteristics, *Nature (London)* **257**:314–316.

Grey, H. M., Colon, S., Campbell, P., and Rabellino, E., 1972, Immunoglobulins on the surface of lymphocytes. V. Quantitative studies on the question of whether immunoglobulins are associated with T cells in the mouse, *J. Immunol.* **109**:776–783.

Griem, M. L., Moran, E. M., Ferguson, D. J., Mettler, F. A., and Griem, S. F., 1975, Staging procedures in mycosis fungoides, *Br. J. Cancer* **31**(*Suppl. 2*):362–367.

Gruenwald, H., Kiossoglou, K. A., Mitus, W. J., and Dameshek, W., 1965, Philadelphia chromosomes in eosinophilic leukemia, *Am. J. Med.* **39**:1003–1010.

Gupta, S., 1977, Eosinophil, discovery, structure, function, and disorders, *Pol. Arch. Med. WEWN* **57**:435–445.

Gupta, S., Frenkel, R., Rosenstein, M., and Grieco, M. H., 1975, Lymphocyte subpopulations, serum IgE and total eosinophil counts in bronchial asthma, *Clin. Exp. Immunol.* **22**:438–445.

Gupta, S., Ross, G. D., Good, R. A., and Siegal, F. P., 1976, Surface markers of human eosinophils, *Blood* **48**:755–763.

Gupta, S., Safai, B., Good, R. A., 1978, Subpopulations of human T lymphocytes IV, quantitation and distribution in mycosis fungoides and Sézary syndrome, *Cell. Immunol.* (in press).

Hallopeau, H., and Besnier, F., 1892, On the erythrodermia of mycosis fungoides, *J. Cutaneous Genitourin. Dis.* **10**:453.

Hardy, W. R., and Anderson, R. E., 1968, The hypereosinophilic syndromes, *Ann. Intern. Med.* **68**:1220–1228.

Harris, A. W., Bankhurst, A. D., Mason, S., and Warner, N. I., 1973, Differentiated functions expressed by cultured mouse lymphoma cells. II. θ antigen, surface immunoglobulin and a receptor for antibody on cells of a thymoma cell line, *J. Immunol.* **110**:431–438.

Hsu, C. C. S., 1976, T and B lymphocytes in chronic lymphocytic leukemia, *N. Engl. J. Med.* **295**:505.

Hsu, C. C. S., Marti, G. E., Schrek, R., and Williams, R. C., Jr., 1975, Lymphocytes bearing B and T cell markers in patient with lymphosarcoma cell leukemia, *Clin. Immunol. Immunopathol.* **3**:385–395.

Hubscher, T., 1975, Role of the eosinophil in the allergic reactions. I. EDI- and eosinophil-derived inhibitor of histamine release, *J. Immunol.* **114**(4):1379–1388.

Huntley, C. C., and Cotas, M. C., 1965, Eosinophilia and agammaglobulinemia, *Pediatrics* **36**:425–428.

Ioachin, H. L., 1965, Emperipolesis of lymphoid cells in mixed cultures, *Lab. Invest.* **14**:1784–1795.

Ishizaka, T., Tomioka, H., and Ishizaka, T., 1970, Mechanisms of passive sensitization. I. Presence of IgE and IgG molecules on human leukocytes, *J. Immunol.* **105**:1459–1467.

Jacob, H. S., Sidd, J. J., Greenberg, B. H., and Lingley, J. F., 1964, Extreme eosinophilia with iodide hypersensitivity, *N. Engl. J. Med.* **271**:1138–1140.

Jacobi, E., 1908, Poikiloderma atriphicans vascularis, in: *Ikonographia Dermatologica* (A. Niesser and E. Jacobi, eds.), Vol. 3, p. 95, Urban and Schwarzenberg, Berlin.

Jimbow, K., Sato, S., and Kukita, A., 1969, Cells containing Langerhans granules in human lymph nodes of dermatopathic lymphadenopathy, *J. Invest. Dermatol.* **53**:295–299.

Kalden, J. R., Peter, H. H., Odriozola, J., Richter, W., and Richter, R., 1974, Sézary syndrome, *Lancet* **1**:688.

Kaplow, L. W., 1968, Leukocyte alkaline phosphatase cytochemistry: Application and methods, *Ann. N. Y. Acad. Sci.* **155**:911–947.

Kauer, G. L., and Engle, R. L., 1964, Eosinophilic leukemia with Ph_1-positive cells, *Lancet* **2**:1340.

Kawada, A., and Takahashi, A. T., 1966, Eosinophilic lymphfolliculosis of the skin (Kimura's disease), *J. Dermatol. Ser. B* **76**:61–72.

Kawada, A., Anekoji, K., Miyamoto, M., Nakai, T., and Mori, S., 1969, Unusual manifestation of malignant reticulosis of the skin: Cutaneous lesion simulating parapsoriasis gutta, *Dermatologica* **138**:369–378.

Kay, A. B., 1970, Studies on eosinophil leukocyte migration. II. Factors specifically chemotactic for eosinophils and neutrophils regenerated from guinea pig serum by antigen–antibody complexes, *Clin. Exp. Immunol.* **7**:723–737.

Kay, A. B., Stechschulte, D. J., and Austen, K. F., 1971, An eosinophilic leukocyte chemotactic factor of anaphylaxis, *J. Exp. Med.* **133**:602–619.

Keil, H., 1942, Relation of parapsoriasis to mycosis fungoides, *Arch. Dermatol. Syphilol.* **46**:950–951.

Kim, R., Winkelmann, R. K., and Dockerty, M., 1963, Reticulum cell sarcoma of the skin, *Cancer* **16**:646–655.

Kimura, T., Yoshimura, S., and Ishikawa, E., 1948, Unusual granulation combined with hyperplastic changes of lymphatic, *Trans. Soc. Pathol. Jpn.* **37**:179–180.

Klein, E., Burgess, G. H., and Helm, F., 1973, Neoplasms of the skin, in: *Cancer Medicine*, 1st ed. (J. F. Holland and E. Frei III, eds.), pp. 1789–1822, Lea & Febiger, Philadelphia.

Klein, E., Holtermann, O. A., Helm, F., Rosner, D., Milgrom, H., Adler, S., Stoll, H. L., Jr., Case, R. W., Prior, L., and Murphy, G. P., 1975, Immunologic approaches to the management of primary and secondary tumors involving the skin and soft tissue (review of a ten-year program), *Transplant. Proc.* **7**:297–315.

Labaze, J. J., Moscovic, E. A., Pham. T. D., and Azar, H. A., 1972, Histological and ultrastructural findings in a case of the Sézary syndrome, *J. Clin. Pathol.* **25**:312–319.

Lapiere, S., 1949, Evolution et pronostic du parapsoriasis en plaques, *Arch. Dermatol. Syphilol.* **9**:609–622.

Larsen, T. E., 1968, Mycosis fungoides—A restrospective investigation of 34 fatal cases, *Tidsskr. Nor. Laegeforen.* **88**:2248–2251.

Laster, C. E., and Gleich, G. J., 1970, Chemotaxis of eosinophils by aggregated immunoglobulins *Clin. Res.* **28**:427 (abstract).

Lever, W. F., and Schaumburg-Lever, G., 1975, *Histopathology of the Skin*, 5th Ed., pp. 697–703, J. B. Lippincott, Philadelphia.

Levi, J. A., and Wiernik, P. H., 1975, Management of mycosis fungoides—Current status and future prospects, *Medicine* **54**:73–88.

Liao, K. T., Rosai, J., and Dameshek, K., 1972, Malignant histiocytosis with cutaneous involvement and eosinophilia, *Am. J. Clin. Pathol.* **57**:438–448.

Ling, N. R., 1968, *Lymphocyte Stimulation*, p. 224, North-Holland Publishing Co., Amsterdam.

Litovitz, T. L., and Lutzner, M. A., 1974, Quantitative measurements of blood lymphocytes from patients with chronic lymphocyte leukemia and the Sézary syndrome, *J. Natl. Cancer Inst.* **53**:75–77.

Litt, M., 1963, Studies in experimental eosinophilia. V. Eosinophils in lymph nodes of guinea pigs following primary antigenic stimulation, *Am. J. Pathol.* **42**:529–547.

Litt, M., 1964a, Eosinophil and antigen–antibody reactions, *Ann. N. Y. Acad. Sci.* **116**:964–985.

Litt, M., 1964b, Studies in experimental eosinophilia. VI. Uptake of immune complexes by eosinophils, *J. Cell Biol.* **23**:355–361.

Long, J. C., and Mihm, M. C., 1974, Mycosis fungoides with extracutaneous dissemination: A distinct clinicopathological entity, *Cancer* **34**:1745–1755.

Luikart, R., II, 1969, Mycosis fungoides, *Arch. Dermatol.* **99**:376–378.

Lutzner, M. A., and Jordan, H. W., 1968, The ultrastructure of an abnormal cell in Sézary's syndrome, *Blood* **31**:719–726.

Lutzner, M. A., Hobbs, J. W., and Horvath, P., 1971, Ultrastructure of abnormal cells in Sézary's syndrome, mycosis fungoides, and parapsoriasis en plaque, *Arch. Dermatol.* **103**:375–386.

Lutzner, M. A., Emerit, I., Durepaire, R., Flandrin, G., Grupper, C. H., and Prunieras, M., 1973, Cytogenetic, cytophotometric and ultrastructural study of large cerebriform cells of the Sézary syndrome and description of a "small cell variant," *J. Natl. Cancer Inst.* **50**:1145–1162.

Lutzner, M., Edelson, R., Schein, P., Green I., Kirkpatrick, C., and Ahmed, A., 1975, Cutaneous T-cell lymphomas: The Sézary syndrome, mycosis fungoides and related disorders, *Ann. Intern. Med.* **83**:534–552.

Macaulay, W. L., 1968, Lymphomatoid papulosis, *Arch. Dermatol.* **97**:23–30.

Mackie, R., Sless, F. R., Cochran, R., and de Sousa, M., 1976, Lymphocyte abnormalities in mycosis fungoides, *Br. J. Dermatol.* **94**:173–178.

Magrath, I. T., 1974, Burkitt's lymphoma: A B or T cell tumor?, *Eur. J. Cancer* **10**:83–88.

Main, R. A., Goodall, H. B., and Swanson, W. C., 1959, Sézary's syndrome, *Br. J. Dermatol.* **71**:335–343.

Mandel, T., 1968, The development and structure of Hassall's corpuscles in the guinea pig: A light and electron microscopic study, *Z. Zellforsch. Mikrosk. Anat.* **89**:180–192.

Marchalonis, J. J., Atwell, J. L., and Cone, R. E., 1973, Isolation of surface immunoglobulin from lymphocytes from human and murine thymus, *Nature (London) New Biol.* **235**:240–242.

Marks, R., Black, M., and Wilson-Jones, E., 1972, Pityriasis lichenoides: A reappraisal, *Br. J. Dermatol.* **86**:215–225.

McDonald, C. J., 1969, Mycosis fungoides—A malignant cutaneous lymphoma, *Conn. Med.* **33**:37–41.

McDonald, C. J., and Calabresi, P., 1971, Azaribine for mycosis fungoides, *Arch. Dermatol.* **103**:158–167.

Mehregan, A. H., and Pinkus, H., 1976, *A Guide to Dermatohistopathology,* 2nd Ed. pp. 630–636, Appleton-Century-Crofts, New York.

Mehregan, A. H., and Shapiro, L., 1971, Angiolymphoid hyperplasia with eosinophilia, *Arch. Dermatol.* **103**:50–57.

Mendes, N. F., Miki, S. S. and Peixinko, Z. F., 1974, Combined detection of human T and B lymphocytes by rosette formation with sheep erythrocytes and zymosan C_3 complexes, *J. Immunol.* **113**:531–536.

Millard, R. E., 1968, Chromosome abnormalities in the malignant lymphomas, *Eur. J. Cancer* **4**:97–105.

Miura, M., and Shima, T., 1954, Malignant reticulosis of the skin. I. Two cases of mycosis fungoides, *Jpn. J. Dermatol.* **64**:419.

Montgomery, H., and Burkhart, R. J., 1942, Parapsoriasis: Its relation to mycosis fungoides and tuberculosis, *Arch. Dermatol. Syphilol.* **46**:673–690.

Muller, S. A., and Schulze, J. W. J. A., 1971, Mucha–Habermann disease mistaken for reticulum cell sarcoma, *Arch. Dermatol.* **103**:423–427.

Niaman, J. L., Oski, F. H., and Diamond, L. K., 1964, Hereditary eosinophilia: Report of a family and review of the literature, *Am. J. Hum. Genet.* **16**:195–203.

Nordqvist, B. C., and Kinney, J. P., 1976, T and B cells and cell-mediated immunity in mycosis fungoides, *Cancer* **37**:714–718.

Nowell, P., Daniele, R., Rowlands, D., Jr., and Winger, L., 1976, T and B lymphocytes in chronic lymphocytic leukemia, *N. Engl. J. Med.* **295**:504.

Odeberg, B., 1965, Eosinophilic leukemia, disseminated eosinophilic collagen disease—a distinct entity, *Acta Med. Scand.* **177**:129–144.

Orbaneja, J. G., Yus, E. S., Diaz-Flores, L., and Huarte, P. S., 1972, Cytology of the mycosis fungoides and the Sézary syndrome: Correlation between light and electron microscopy, *Br. J. Dermatol.* **87**:96–105.

Ormsby, O. S., and Montgomery, H., 1954, *Diseases of the Skin,* p. 328, Lea & Febiger, Philadephia.

Osmundsen, P. E., 1968, Parapsoriasis en plaques, *Acta Dermatol. Venerol.* **48**:345–354.

Panush, R. S., Franco, A. E., and Schur, P. H., 1971, Rheumatoid arthritis associated with eosinophilia, *Ann. Intern. Med.* **75**:199–205.

Paradinas, F. J., and Harrison, K. M., 1974, Visceral lesions in an unusual case of Sézary's syndrome, *Cancer* **33**:1068–1074.

Preud'homme, J. L., and Seligmann, M., 1972, Surface-bound immunoglobulins as a cell marker in human lymphoproliferation disease, *Blood* **40**:777–794.

Prunieras, M., 1974, DNA content and cytogenetics of the Sézary cells, *Mayo Clin. Proc.* **49**:548–552.

Rabinowitz, B., Naguchi, S., and Roenick, H. H., 1976, Tumor cell characterization in mycosis fungoides, *Cancer* **37**:1747–1753.

Ranvier, L. A., 1872, Rapport sur la candidature de M. Deboves au titre de membre adjoint—mycosis fongoide, *Soc. Anat. Paris, Bull. Ser. 3* **7**:477.

Rappaport, H., and Thomas, L. B., 1974, Mycosis fungoides: The pathology of extracutaneous involvement, *Cancer* **34**:1198–1229.

Rappaport, H., Edgcomb, J., and Thomas, L., 1968, Mycosis fungoides—A reevaluation of its position in the scheme of lymphoreticular neoplasms, *Am. J. Clin. Pathol.* **50**:625.

Ratner, A. C., Waldorf, D. S., and Van Scott, E. J., 1968, Alterations of lesions of mycosis fungoides lymphoma by direct imposition of delayed hypersensitivity reactions, *Cancer* **21**:83–88.

Rauschkolb, R. R., 1961, Mycosis fungoides—Discussion and clinical experience of the Cleveland Metropolitan Hospital, *Arch. Dermatol.* **83**:217–223.

Rebhun, J., 1974, Systemic eosinophilic infiltrative disease, *Ann. Allergy* **32**:86–93.

Rickles, F. R., and Miller, D. R., 1972, Eosinophilic leukemoid reactions, *J. Pediatr.* **80**:418–428.

Riddle, J. M., and Barnhart, M. I., 1965, The eosinophil as a source for profibrinolysin in acute inflammation, *Blood* **25**:776–794.

Roberts, W. C., Buja, L. M., and Ferrans, V. J., 1970, Loeffler's fibroplastic parietal endocarditis, eosinophilic leukemia, and Davie's endomyocardial fibrosis: The same disease at different stages, *Pathol. Microbiol.* **35**:90–95.

Rosas-Uribe, A., Variakojis, D., Molnar, Z., and Rappaport, H., 1974, Mycosis fungoides: An ultrastructural study, *Cancer* **34**:634–645.

Sabesin, S. S., 1967, A function of the eosinophil: Phagocytosis of antigen–antibody complexes, *Proc. Soc. Exp. Biol. Med.* **112**:667.

Safai, B., Reich, L., and Good, R. A., 1978, Failure of lymphapheresis in the treatment of Sézary syndrome and mycosis fungoides, *Clin. Res.* (in press).

Saito, T., Kojima, M., Sugawara, K., Kakinuma, Y., and Iijima, S., 1964, An autopsy case of Sézary's reticulosis, *Eukushima J. Med. Sci.* **11**:1–23.

Samman, P. D., 1964, Survey of reticuloses and premycotic eruptions, *Br. J. Dermatol.* **76**:1–9.

Samman, P. D., 1972, The natural history of parapsoriasis en plaques (chronic superficial dermatitis) and prereticulotic poikiloderma, *Br. J. Dermatol.* **87**:405–411.

Sandbank, M., 1971, Mycosis fungoides: Ultrastructural study with demonstration of atypical cells and nuclear bodies, *Arch. Dermatol.* **103**:206–213.

Sandbank, M., and Feurman, E. J., 1972, Lymphomatoid papulosis: An electron microscopic study of the acute and healing stages with demonstration of paramyxo-virus-like particles, *Acta Dermatol.* **52**:337–345.

Sandilands, G. P., Gray, K., Cooney, A., Browning, J. D., Grant, R. M., Anderson, J. R., Dagg, J. H., and Lucie, N., 1974, Lymphocytes with T and B cell properties in a lymphoproliferative disorder, *Lancet* **1**:903–904.

Schaffer, S., 1891, Über das Vorkommen eosinophiler Zellen der menschlichen Thymus, *Zentralbl. Med. Wiss.* **29**:401.

Schein, P. S., Macdonald, J. S., and Edelson, R., 1976, Cutaneous T-cell lymphoma, *Cancer* **38**:1859–1861.

Schneiderman, P., Edelson, R., Lutzner, M., and Green, I., 1975, Lymphomatoid papulosis: Immunologic and ultrastructural studies, *Clin. Res.* **23**:455 (abstract).

Schnitzer, B., and Kass, I., 1973, Leukemic phase of reticulum cell sarcoma (histiocytic lymphoma)—A clinicopathological and ultrastructural study, *Cancer* **31**:547–559.

Scholtz, W., 1902, Über den Einfluss der Roentgenstrahlen auf die Haut in gesunden und kranken Zustände, *Arch. Dermatol. Syph. (Berlin)* **59**:421–446.

Schrek, R., 1972, Ultrastructure of blood lymphocytes from chronic lymphocytic leukemia and lymphosarcoma cell leukemia, *J. Natl. Cancer Inst.* **48**:51–64.

Schumacher, H. R., McFeely, A. E., and Maugel, T. K., 1969, The mononucleosis cell, *Blood* **33**:833–842.

Sézary, A., and Bolgert M., 1942, Réticulose érythrodermique avec réticulémie, *Bull. Soc. Fr. Dermatol. Syphiligr.* **49**:355–356.

Sézary, A., and Bouvrain, Y., 1938, Erythrodermie avec presence de cellules monstreuses dans terme et dans sang circulant, *Bull. Soc. Fr. Dermatol. Syphiligr.* **45**:254–260.

Shelton, E., and Dalton, A. J., 1959, Electron microscopy of emperipolesis, *J. Biophys. Biochem. Cytol.* **6**:513–514.

Shevach, E., Edelson, R., Frank M., Lutzner, M., and Green I., 1974, Human Leukemia cells with both B and T cell surface receptors, *Proc. Natl. Acad. Sci. U.S.A.* **71**:863–866.

Shirai, T., Yoshiki, T., and Mellors, R. C., 1973, Effects of natural thymocytotoxic autotantibody of NZB mice and of specifically prepared antilymphocyte serum of the tissue distribution of ^{51}Cr-labeled lymphocytes, *J. Immunol.* **110**:517–523.

Siegal, F. P., Voss, R., Al-Mondhiry, H., Polliack, A., Hansen, J. A., Siegal, M., and Good, R. A., 1976, Association of a chromosomal abnormality with lymphocytes having both T and B markers in a patient with lymphoproliferative disease, *Am. J. Med.* **60**:157–166.

Sipos, K., and Jakso, G., 1956, A mustárnitrogén helyi alkalmazása néhány börbetegségben, *Borgyogy. Venerol. Sz.* **32**:198–203.

Snyder, C. H., 1961, Visceral larva migrans, 10 years experience, *Pediatrics* **28**:85–91.

Speirs, R. S., 1958, Advances in the knowledge of the eosinophil in relation to antibody formation, *Ann. N. Y. Acad. Sci.* **73**:283–306.

Spiers, A. S. D., and Baikie, A. G., 1970, A special role of the group 17, 18, chromosomes in reticuloendothelial neoplasia, *Br. J. Cancer* **24**:779–791.

Spigel, S. C., and Coltman, C. A., Jr., 1973, Therapy of mycosis fungoides with bleomycin, *Cancer* **32**:762–770.

Stewart, T. H. M., 1969, The regression of an inflammatory skin lesion by the induction of a delayed hypersensitivity reaction: A case report, *Cancer* **24**:117–121.

Stjernswärd, J., and Levin, A., 1971, Delayed hypersensitivity: Induced regression of human neoplasms, *Cancer* **28**:628–640.

Szur, L., 1964, Radiotherapy of the skin reticuloses, *Br. J. Dermatol.* **76**:10–20.

Szur, L., 1975, The treatment of mycosis fungoides and related conditions with particular emphasis on electron therapy, *Br. J. Cancer* **31**(*Suppl. 2*):368–378.

Tai, P. C., and Spry, C. J. F., 1976, Studies on blood eosinophils. I. Patients with a transient eosinophilia, *Clin. Exp. Immunol.* **24**:415–422.

Tan, H. K., Harrison, M., and Gralnik, H., 1974, Nuclear topography in the abnormal cell of Sézary syndrome: Observation by freeze–electron microscopy, *J. Natl. Cancer Inst.* **52**:1367–1371.

Tan, R. S. H., Butterworth, C. M., McLaughlin H., Malka, S., and Samman, P. D., 1974, Mycosis fungoides—A disease of antigen persistence, *Br. J. Dermatol.* **91**:607–616.

Tan, R. S. H., Oon, C. J., Barrett, A. J., and Hayes, J. P., 1975, Sézary syndrome: Treatment by leukophoresis, *Proc. R. Soc. Med.* **68**:648–649.

Taswell, H. F., and Winkelmann, R. K., 1961, Sézary syndrome—A malignant reticulemic erythroderma, *J. Am. Med. Assoc.* **177**:465–472.

Tedeschi, I. G., and Lansinger, D. T., 1965, Sézary syndrome: A malignant leukemic reticuloendotheliosis, *Arch. Dermatol.* **92**:257–262.

Theologides, A., 1972, Unfavorable signs in patients with chronic myelocytic leukemia, *Ann. Intern. Med.* **76**:95–99.

Thomas, D. B., 1972, Antibodies to membrane antigen(s) common to thymocytes and a subpopulation of lymphocytes in infectious mononucleosis sera, *Lancet* **1**:399–403.

Thomas, L. B., Frei, E., III, and Hilbish, T. F. 1964, Regional consideration of leukemia and lymphoma—The skeletal system, in: *Treatment of Cancer and Allied Diseases*, 2nd Ed. (G. Palk and I. Ariel, eds.), pp. 206–233, Hoeber Medical Division, Harper and Row, New York.

Torisu, M., Yoshida, T., Ward, P. A., and Cohen, S., 1973, Lymphocyte-derived eosinophil chemotactic factor. II. Studies on the mechanism of activation of the precursor substance by immune complex, *J. Immunol.* **111**:1450–1458.

Trump, J. G., Wright, K. A., Evans, W. W., Anson, J. H., Hare, H. F., Former, J. L., Jacque, G., and Horne, K. W., 1953, High energy electrons for the treatment of extensive superficial malignant lesions, *Am. J. Roentgenol. Radium Ther. Nucl. Med.* **69**:623–629.

Umbert, P., Belcher, R. W., and Winkelmann, R. K., 1976, Macrophage inhibitor factor (MIF) in cutaneous lymphoproliferative disease, *Br. J. Dermatol.* **95**:475–480.

Valentino, L. A., and Helwig, E. B., 1973, Lymphomatoid papulosis, *Arch. Pathol.* **96**:409–416.

Vance, C., Sabad, A., Kersey, J., Goltz, R., Gentry, W., and Cervenka, J., 1975, Lymphocyte abnormalities in the small cell variant of Sézary syndrome, *Clin. Res.* **23**:455 (abstract).

Van Scott, E. J., and Haynes, H. A., 1971, Cutaneous lymphomas, in: *Dermatology in General Medicine* (T. B. Fitzpatrick, K. A. Arndt, W. H. Clark, Jr., *et al.*, eds.), pp. 556–573, McGraw-Hill Book Co., New York.

Van Scott, E. J., and Kalmanson, J. D., 1973, Complete remissions of mycosis fungoides lymphoma induced by topical nitrogen mustard (HN₂), *Cancer* **32**:18–30.

Van Scott, E. J., Auerbach, R., and Clendenning, W. E., 1962, Treatment of mycosis fungoides with cyclophosphamide, *Arch. Dermatol.* **85**:107–109.

Van Scott, E. J., Grekin, D. A., Kalmanson, J. D., Vonderheid, E. C., and Barry, W. E., 1975, Frequent low doses of intravenous mechlorethamine for late-stage mycosis fungoides lymphoma, *Cancer* **36**:1613–1618.

Variakojis, D., Rosas-Uribe, A., and Rappaport, H., 1974, Mycosis fungoides—Pathologic findings in staging laparotomies, *Cancer* **33**:1589–1600.

Verallo, V. M., and Fand, S. B., 1969, DNA measurements in lymphomatoid papulosis: Evidence of this new entity, *J. Invest. Dermatol.* **53**:51–57.

Vidal, E., and Brocq, L., 1885, Étude sur le mycosis fongoide, *Fr. Med.* **2**:946, 957, 969.

Vonderheid, E. C., Van Scott, E. J., Johnson, W. C., Grekin, D. A., and Asbell, S. O., 1977, Topical chemotherapy and immunotherapy of mycosis fungoides, *Arch. Dermatol.* **113**:454–462.

Waldmann, T. A., Broder, S., Durm, M., Meade, B., Krakauer, B., Blackman, M., and Goldman, C., 1976, T cell suppression of pokeweed mitogen induced immunoglobulin production, in: *Mitogens in Immunobiology* (J. J. Oppenheim and D. L. Rosentreich, eds.), pp. 509–521, Academic Press, New York.

Waldorf, D. S., Haynes, H. A., and Van Scott, E. J., 1967, Cutaneous hypersensitivity and desensitization to mechlorethamine in patients with mycosis fungoides lymphoma, *Ann. Intern. Med.* **67**:282–290.

Waldorf, D. S., Ratner, H. C., and Van Scott, E. J., 1968, Cells in lesions of mucosis fungoides lymphoma following therapy: Changes in number and type, *Cancer* **21**:264–269.

Ward, P. A., 1969, Chemotaxis of human eosinophils, *J. Exp. Med.* **54**:121–128.

Wasserman, S. I., Goetzel, E. J., Ellman, L., and Austen, K. F., 1974, Tumor associated eosinophilotactic factor, *N. Engl. J. Med.* **290**:420–428.

Wells, G. C., and Whimster, I. W., 1968, Subcutaneous angiolymphoid hyperplasia with eosinophilia, *Br. J. Dermatol.* **89**:1–15.

Wernet, P., and Kunkel, H. G., 1973, Antibodies to a specific surface antigen of T cells in human sera inhibiting mixed leukocytic culture reaction, *J. Exp. Med.* **138**:1021–1026.

Wilson, H. T. H., and Fielding, J., 1953, Sézary's reticulosis with exfoliative dermatitis, *Br. Med. J.* **1**:1087–1089.

Wilson, K. S., and Alexander, H. L., 1945, The association of periarteritis nodosa, bronchial asthma and hypereosinophilia, *J. Lab. Clin. Med* **30**:361–363.

Winkelmann, R. K., 1974, Clinical studies of T cell erythroderma in the Sézary syndrome, *Mayo Clin. Proc.* **49**:519–525.

Winkelmann, R. K., and Linman, J. W., 1973, Erythroderma with atypical lymphocytes (Sézary syndrome), *Am. J. Med.* **55**:192–198.

Wright, J. C., Lyons, M. M., Walker, D. G., Golomb, F. M., Gumport, S. L., and Medrek, T. J., 1964, Observations on the use of cancer chemotherapeutic agents in patients with mycosis fungoides, *Cancer* **17**:1045–1062.

Yam, L. T., and Mitus, W. J., 1968, The lymphocyte β-glucoronidase activity in lymphoproliferative disorders, *Blood* **31**:480–489.

Yam, L. T., Li, C. Y., and Crosby, W. H., 1971, Cytochemical identification of monocytes and granulocytes, *Am. J. Clin. Pathol.* **55**:283–290.

Yam, L. T., Li, C. Y., Necheles, T. F., and Katayama, I., 1972, Pseudoeosinophilia, eosinophilic endocarditis and eosinophilic leukemia, *Am. J. Med.* **53**:193–202.

Yoshida, T., Edelson, R., Cohen, S., and Green, I., 1975, Migration inhibitory activity in serum and cell supernatants in patients with Sézary syndrome, *J. Immunol.* **114**:915–918.

Zackheim, H. S., 1972, Treatment of mycosis fungoides with topical nitrosourea compounds, *Arch. Dermatol.* **106**:177–182.

Zucker-Franklin, D., 1963, The ultrastructure of cells in human thoracic duct lymph, *J. Ultrastruct. Res.* **9**:325–339.

Zucker-Franklin, D., 1971, Eosinophilia of unknown etiology: A diagnostic dilemma, *Hosp. Pract.* **6**:119–127.

Zucker-Franklin, D., 1974, Eosinophil function and disorder, *Adv. Intern. Med.* **19**:1–25.

Zucker-Franklin, D., Melton, J. W., III, and Quagliatia, F., 1974, Ultrastructural, immunologic and functional studies on Sézary cells: A neoplastic variant of thymus-derived (T) lymphocytes, *Proc. Natl. Acad. Sci. U.S.A.* **71**:1877–1881.

17

Lymphoreticular Malignancies in Childhood

JOHN H. KERSEY and MARK E. NESBIT

1. Introduction

Malignancies of the lymphoid system of children are the most frequent form of childhood cancer (Warner, 1974). In the past, this group of diseases was very poorly understood and generally quite rapidly fatal. Recently, major advances have been made toward understanding the etiology, the pathogenesis, the prognostic features, and the immunological aspects of these lymphoid malignancies. An attempt to summarize recent advances in this field forms the basis of this chapter.

The lymphoid system of normal children is extremely active and complex. Lymphoid cells are normally found in nearly every organ of the body, but are especially active in the thymus, lymph nodes, bone marrow, and GI tract of children. Lymphocytes are of two major classes—those of the thymus-processed, or T-cell, system, and those processed in bone marrow, gut, liver, and other sites and known as the B-cell system (Warner, 1974; Kersey and Gajl-Peczalska, 1975). The major organs of the lymphoid system of the child include the thymus, tonsils, lymph nodes, and spleen; they tend to be large and active, probably in response to the large number of new antigens to which the child is exposed. With such intense proliferative activity in childhood, it is probably not surprising that lymphoid cells appear to be frequent targets for the malignant process.

2. Clinical Features of Lymphoreticular Malignancies

In recent years, a number of attempts have been made to distinguish physical and laboratory features that might be useful in understanding prognostic features around which therapy could be developed. From these studies, it has become apparent that these diseases can be divided into several groups that are useful, if not

JOHN H. KERSEY • Departments of Pediatrics, and Laboratory Medicine and Pathology, University of Minnesota, Minneapolis, Minnesota 55455. MARK E. NESBIT • Department of Pediatrics, University of Minnesota, Minneapolis, Minnesota 55455.

JOHN H. KERSEY AND
MARK E. NESBIT

for etiological understanding, at least for prognostication. Traditionally, the major distinction that has been made is between leukemia and lymphoma. By standard definition, a lymphoma is a malignancy that does not involve the marrow early in the course of the disease, whereas leukemia is a disease with significant early marrow involvement. While this traditional distinction is of some value and forms the basis for this discussion, it is only partially successful because (1) many patients present with evidence of extensive extranodal *and* bone marrow involvement (Sonley, 1972; Pinkel *et al.*, 1975); (2) lymphoma and acute leukemia are difficult if not impossible to distinguish on cytomorphological grounds (Sonley, 1972; Pinkel *et al.*, 1975); and (3) immunological analysis indicates that the cell of origin of a particular subset of the leukemias is identical to that of the "lymphomas" (see Section 5.2).

Despite these reservations, we considered it desirable to attempt to distinguish leukemia and lymphoma on *clinical* grounds, largely because a large body of literature has been collected with this perspective over the past 30 years.

3. Lymphoblastic Leukemia of Childhood: Prognostic Factors

3.1. Age

In 1942, Cooke (1942) reported that in 1500 cases of acute leukemia of all types, 40% were in the 3- to 5-year-old age group. Age appeared to be important in prognosis in that children under 2 or over 10 had a worse prognosis. Confirmatory observations by Pierce *et al.* (1969) indicated that acute lymphoid leukemia peaked in the 2–5 age group, and that the most favorable prognosis was in the 2–6 age group, especially when leukocyte counts were below 4000. This childhood peak in the incidence of leukemia is not found among black children (Ederer *et al.*, 1964).

3.2. Sex

Possible associations between sex of the child and leukemia type were examined in one study, and no significant differences were noted (Pierce *et al.*, 1969). Relationships between sex and survival were studied by Colebach (1975), who observed that females were more likely to be long-term survivors than were males; similar results were observed in some studies, but not in others, reviewed by Colebach. In studies by the Southwest Group, reviewed by George *et al.* (1973), no difference between females and males was observed, except in those patients younger than 1 year.

3.3. Maternal Factors

Much interest has centered around maternal factors associated with leukemia in an attempt to determine etiological factors that might be important. In 1972, Fedrick and Alberman (1972) reported a longitudinal study of almost 2000 infants born to mothers with a history of influenza; mothers with such a history had leukemic children more frequently than did mothers without influenza. More recently, a different study (Gibson and Graham, 1974) evaluated maternal factors that might be correlated with prognosis in acute leukemia. According to this study, short-term survivors are most likely to have been born to mothers who have a history of disease (viral and other), who are likely to have irradiation during pregnancy, who are likely to have borne the leukemic children as products of later pregnancies, and who had fewer complications during pregnancies with children who subsequently developed leukemia than with pregnancies with children who did not.

3.4. Morphological and Histochemical Features

Several attempts have been made to classify leukemia on the basis of morphological features. One study reported an inverse correlation between size of lymphoblasts and duration of remission (Pantazopoulos and Sinks, 1974). Mathé suggested that decreasing cell size (and presumed increased differentiation) resulted in improved prognosis (Mathé et al., 1971). Using the same criteria, another group was unable to correlate prognosis with cell size (Jacquillat et al., 1972). Nucleolar prominence was postulated by Lee and Glidewell (1973) to result in decreased survival. Lymphoblasts frequently stain positively with periodic acid–Schiff stain (PAS). Löffler et al. (1973) found that PAS-positive cells correlated with improved prognosis. On the other hand, a study by Humphrey et al. (1974) revealed no prognostic value in the PAS staining.

In summary, despite these attempts at classification using morphological and histochemical criteria, no standards have been developed that have been acceptable to the international medical community.

3.5. Cell Kinetics

It is possible that studies of the proliferative activity of leukemic cells would provide prognostic information. Early studies by Nesbit and Krivit (1968) suggested that rapid proliferation as predicted by labeling indices was associated with a more favorable chemotherapeutic result. More recent studies by Murphy and Mauer (1975) suggested that labeling indices are probably not prognostic in children with acute leukemia.

3.6. Extent of Involvement

The extent of organ involvement may influence prognosis in acute lymphoblastic leukemia (ALL). Studies by Hardisty and Till (1968) found that organomegaly in children with ALL is associated with shortened median survival time. More recently, Fitzpatrick et al. (1974) reported that nodal and organ involvement was associated with increased risk of CNS leukemia.

3.7. Familial Factors

In a death-certificate study of childhood cancers, Miller (1971) found seven pairs of presumably identical twins who had died of leukemia. In all instances, death occurred within a 7-month interval. Zuelzer and Cox (1969) reported that concordance for leukemia is almost 100% in identical twins who contract the disease before the age of 1.

Studies have also been performed on the risk of development of leukemia among other family members. Nora *et al.* (1968) reported that family members have about a fourfold increased risk for development of leukemia (16/3273 vs. 4/2909). Approximately the same fourfold risk was reported by Miller (1967). Miller reports the risk to leukemic siblings to be about 1/720.

4. Malignant Lymphoma of Childhood

4.1. General Aspects

Traditionally, childhood leukemias and lymphomas have been separated on the basis of the presence or absence of marrow involvement at diagnosis. In lymphoma cases without marrow involvement, the presumption is that the disease has origin in an extramedullary site. One group has concluded, however, that there is no meaningful distinction between leukemia and lymphoma on either clinical or morphological grounds, and that acute lymphoblastic leukemia is essentially a stage IV lymphoma (Pinkel *et al.*, 1975). On the other hand, there are data indicating that the combination of extramedullary disease with marrow involvement results in a worse prognosis than disease with marrow involvement alone (see Section 5.2).

4.2. Childhood vs. Adult Types

Clinical and pathological data indicate a clear difference between non-Hodgkin's lymphoma of childhood vs. that of adults. Whereas up to 75% of adults achieve 5-year survival, the average survival among children was found to be 6 months or less in two studies in the 1960's (Oettgen and Murphy, 1967; Burkitt, 1967). Histologically, differences between adult and childhood types are apparent; whereas the bulk of adult tumors are nodular, the vast majority of childhood lymphomas are diffuse (Murphy *et al.*, 1975). Immunological studies indicate that the cell of origin in adult lymphoma is generally the bone-marrow-derived (B) lymphocyte, whereas the cell of origin in childhood lymphoma is most often the thymus-derived (T) lymphocyte (Kersey *et al.*, 1974; Kaplan *et al.*, 1974). The results in adult lymphoma are discussed in more detail in Chapter 10 of this volume.

4.3. Prognostic Clinical and Histopathological Features

In a recent report, Pinkel *et al.* (1975) attempted to distinguish malignant lymphoma of childhood on the basis of histological type. The largest group was that in which the lymphoma was described as diffuse, "undifferentiated," non-Burkitt's, and "lymphoblastic"; this group comprised primarily boys under the age of 10. Median survival in this group was 1 year. The second largest group was that of diffuse, "poorly differentiated," and "histiocytic lymphoma"; this group comprised mainly boys older than 10. Median survival was only 6 months. Two patients had non-African Burkitt's-type lymphoma and died at 5 months and 10 months. In this study, a direct relationship was observed between stage of the disease and prognosis: according to the study, local irradiation was felt to be adequate for treatment of stage I disease; patients with stages II–IV should receive antileukemic therapy.

A recent report of 172 cases from France (Lemerle *et al.*, 1973) suggested that age, sex, and histological type of tumors were not important in prognosis. The initial stage was felt to have prognostic value. The overall 30-month survival rate was 27%. The survival rate was 58% for stage I patients, 24% for stage II patients, and 8% for stage IV patients.

5. Childhood Leukemias and Lymphomas

5.1. Immunological Classification: Background

As discussed above, attempts at classification of childhood lymphomas and lymphoid leukemias using morphological criteria have been less than satisfactory because of the subjective nature of the methodology employed. The development of new methodologies for evaluation of the surface-marker characteristics of lymphoid malignancies has permitted a new perspective in the classification of leukemias and lymphomas.

Various lymphoid subpopulations may be distinguished using surface-marker analyses. Thymus-derived (T) lymphocytes carry receptors for sheep erythrocytes (SRBC) and bear a surface antigen known as human T-lymphocyte antigen (HTLA) that is detectable using absorbed heterologous antithymocyte sera. The second major subpopulation, B lymphocytes, is formed in bone marrow, fetal liver, gut, and other sites; these cells carry surface immunoglobulin (SIg) (detectable by fluorescence), complement receptors, receptors for the Fc portion of the immunoglobulin molecule, and human B-lymphocyte antigen (HBLA), which is detectable using absorbed heterologous anti-B-cell sera. Recent studies from several laboratories indicate that these lymphoid subpopulations are not always mutually exclusive, and that a small population of double- (or triple-) marker cells exists (Dickler *et al.*, 1974; Gajl-Peczalska *et al.*, 1976). The significance of this double-marker population is not yet clear, although it is possible that they represent multipotential or stem cells.

5.2. Immunodiagnosis

Surface-marker analysis has permitted development of a new classification system for childhood lymphomas and leukemias. The methods employed for immunodiagnosis have been standardized in a number of laboratories using guidelines established by the WHO Committee for T- and B-Cell Analysis (WHO/IARC-Sponsored Workshop, 1974). This standardization has permitted a quantitative evaluation of the cellular origin of the childhood malignancies and, it is to be hoped, will result in a language that will be acceptable worldwide.

Childhood lymphoreticular malignancies can be divided into several major groups by immunodiagnostic methods. In our laboratory, we are currently dividing our subjects into three major groups on the basis of surface-marker analysis (Table 1). This classification provides, on one hand, an objective analysis of the leukemic cells and, on the other, information that correlates with prognosis.

Group I comprises patients with T-cell–E-rosette-positive leukemia–lymphoma. Patients in this group tend to have mediastinal masses (1), be males (2), and have high white counts. Tumor cells form SRBC rosettes and often complement

JOHN H. KERSEY AND
MARK E. NESBIT

TABLE 1. Childhood Lymphoid Malignancies: Minnesota Series (69 Patients)[a]

I. T-cell–E-rosette-positive group (10 patients)	II. B-cell, SIgM-positive group (7 patients)	III. "Null"-cell, rosette-negative-, SIgM-negative group (52 patients)
1. Mediastinal mass, probably thymus (7/10); possibly primary	1. Abdominal involvement—probably primaries (7/7)	1. Absence of mediastinal mass or involvement (51/52)
2. Predominance of males (7/10)	2. Predominance of males (6/7); characteristic age (8–16)	2. No age or sex predominance
3. Nodal masses (4/10) ?primary site; absence of bone marrow involvement at diagnosis in some cases (4/10)		3. Bone marrow involvement at diagnosis (52/52)
4. Tumor cells: a. Form SRBC rosettes (10/10) b. Form complement rosettes (2/4) c. Carry HTLA (5/5)	4. Tumor cells synthesize μ heavy-chain (5/5) or λ (3/5) or κ light-chain (2/5) Ig	
5. Morphology different from SIgM-positive (Burkitt's) subgroup, but similar to SRBC-rosette-negative subgroup	5. Characteristic morphology: "Burkitt cell," "stem cell"	5. Morphology distinguished from SIgM-positive (Burkitt's) subgroup, but not from SRBC-rosette-positive subgroup
6. "Sternberg sarcoma"; "poorly differentiated lymphocytic lymphoma"		6. Presence of HTLA-positive lymphoblasts (14/25) in some cases
7. Poor prognosis	7. Very poor prognosis	7. Survival dependent on white count at diagnosis: >100,000, poor <100,000, good

[a]The parenthetical numbers in the text refer to the correspondingly numbered features in this table.

rosettes (4). Morphologically, cells are different from those of the B-cell, IgM-positive group, but similar to those of the "null"-rosette-, SIgM-negative group (5). Prognosis is poor (7), and only 15% of patients are alive at 14 months (Coccia *et al.*, 1976). Other investigators have also confirmed the poor prognosis in this group (Sen and Borella, 1975; Tsukimoto *et al.*, 1976).

Group II is the B-cell, SIgM-positive group. In this group is a predominance of males and a characteristic age (2), abdominal involvement (1), and a characteristic morphology (5). Tumor cells synthesize μ heavy chains (4), and the prognosis is very poor (7); in our series, 100% of patients were dead at 6 months. The distinctive features of this group were also reported by Flandrin *et al.* (1975).

Group III is the "null"-cell, rosette-negative, SIgM-negative group. This group comprises the largest number of patients (52 in the Minnesota series). Almost all patients have bone marrow involvement (3); no age or sex predominance is observed (2). Tumor-cell morphology is distinguished from that of the SIgM-positive (Burkitt's group), but not from that of the rosette-positive group (5). In our series, lymphoblasts also carried HTLA in 14 of 25 cases (6). Survival in this group depends on white count at diagnosis (7). Patients with white counts above 100,000 had a very poor diagnosis. Of patients who had "null"-rosette-negative and SIgM-negative disease and had a white count below 100,000, more than 90% were alive at 30 months.

Table 2 presents a summary of the current state of the art in immunological classification of childhood lymphoid malignancies based on data from a number of laboratories, including ours. It is already apparent that Groups I–III can be further subdivided on the basis of immunological analysis. While a consensus has been reached on the prognostic importance of these three subgroups, it is not yet apparent whether further subdivision will be of prognostic value. The challenge to workers involved in attempts to provide clinical–immunopathological correlations is clear.

TABLE 2. Immunological Classification of Childhood Lymphoid Malignancies

	I. Rosette-positive subgroup	II. SIgM-positive subgroup	III. Rosette-negative, SIgM-negative subgroup
Immunology	Rosettes with: SRBC: almost always Complement: frequently	Surface IgM: Monoclonal K or λ	Carry HTLA heteroantigens in some instances Carry non-T (monocyte-B cell) alloantigens in some instances
Clinical	Males > females Adolescents frequently	Males > females, all ages	Males = females, 3–7
	Extramedullary mass: Mediastinal Lymph node	Abdominal mass	No mass
	If leukemia, high white count	Normal white count	Normal white count
	"Lymphoma"	"Lymphoma"	"Leukemia"
Histology–cytology	Distinguishable from SIgM-positive subgroup	Burkitt's lymphoma	Distinguishable from SIgM-positive subgroup
Prognosis	Poor	Very poor	Good

JOHN H. KERSEY AND
MARK E. NESBIT

5.3. Childhood Leukemias and Lymphomas Associated with Immunodeficiency Syndromes

Children with primary genetically determined immunodeficiency syndromes are known to be at increased risk for development of lymphoreticular malignancies, especially those that do not initially involve the bone marrow and would thus be termed lymphomas. The overall risk of development of malignancy in children with primary immunodeficiency syndromes is high; despite short life spans, 5–10% of children with various immunodeficiency syndromes develop malignancy (Kersey *et al.*, 1974). Included in this group are patients with severe combined immunodeficiency, X-linked (Bruton's) agammaglobulinemia, Wiskott–Aldrich syndrome, and ataxia–telangiectasia. The risk for development of malignancy in children with primary immunodeficiency is about 100 times that of the general population. In children with immunodeficiency syndromes, the majority of the increased risk is to the lymphoid system; the risk to nonlymphoid tissues is significantly lower. It is of interest that the organ that is itself deficient in function is also the target of the malignant process. The possible mechanisms for malignant adaptation under these circumstances are several and include the following: (1) basic cellular defects could result in both increased malignant transformation and decreased lymphoid function; (2) defective immune regulation could result in decreased "surveillance" against aberrant lymphoid cells; (3) defective immune surveillance of oncogenic viruses could result in enhanced spread of lymphotropic oncogenic viral agents. Attempts to culture oncogenic viruses from immunodeficient patients and attempts to understand the mechanism of growth control that is defective in the lymphoid system of these patients should yield data that can then be applied to the general population.

A major unanswered question is the extent to which immunological abnormalities may predispose to lymphoid malignancy in the vast majority of patients who do not have a history of increased infection, autoimmunity, or other putative risk factors. Data generated from experimental model systems indicate that certain histocompatibility-linked genes are associated with either high or low risk of malignancy. An example is the resistance Gross virus-1 (*RGV-1*) gene in the mouse. Similarly, susceptibility to leukemogenesis by the B/T virus is influenced by an *H-2*-associated gene. In both cases, non-responsiveness is associated with the H-2^k haplotype (reviewed by Schreffler and David, 1975). Several attempts have been made to demonstrate that specific *HLA* haplotypes are associated with enhanced susceptibility to leukemogenesis in humans. The initial observation of Walford *et al.* (1970) suggesting that *HLA A2-B12* is associated with acute leukemia of childhood was confirmed in one study, but not in several other studies.

6. Conclusions

Lymphoreticular malignancies continue to be the most frequent form of childhood cancer. Our immediate charge is to develop improved methods of diagnosis and prognostication. Evidence presented in this chapter indicates that immunodiagnostic classification will be a useful addition to the current list of factors known to influence prognosis. The use of immunodiagnostic and other methods for prognostication will undoubtedly result in stratification of treatment protocols.

The long-range challenge in childhood lymphoreticular malignancies is to understand the pathogenetic mechanisms involved. Why do certain malignancies involve T cells and others SIgM-bearing B cells? Why do cells that currently lack detectable surface markers (and might therefore be termed "less differentiated") have a better prognosis than those with easily detectable surface markers? Why does immunodeficiency result in more frequent malignancy? What is the role of viruses and external carcinogens in production of these malignancies? Will the suggestion from the mouse that T-cell malignancies are virally induced also hold true in humans? In the end, the answers to these and other questions will further our understanding to the point where we can begin to discuss prevention and perhaps immunoprophylaxis in these frequent childhood disorders.

ACKNOWLEDGMENT

This work was supported in part by grants from the USPHS (CA-16228, CA-08832, CA-15548, and CA-07306).

References

Burkitt, D., 1967, Long-term remissions following one and two-dose chemotherapy for African lymphoma, *Cancer* 20:756–759.

Coccia, P. F., Kersey, J. H., Gajl-Peczalska, K. J., Krivit, W., and Nesbit, M., 1976, Prognostic significance of surface marker analysis in childhood non-Hodgkin's lymphoproliferative malignancies, *Am. J. Hematology* 1:405–417.

Colebach, J. H., 1975, Five year survival in acute leukemia: Clinical, cytological and immunologic studies, *Wadley Med. Bull.* 5:12–28.

Cooke, J. V., 1942, Incidence of acute leukemia in children, *J. Am. Med. Assoc.* 119:547.

Dickler, H. B., Adkinson, N. F., and Terry, N. D., 1974, Evidence for individual human peripheral blood lymphocytes bearing both B and T cell markers, *Nature (London)* 247:213–214.

Ederer, F., Meyers, M. H., and Mantel, N., 1964, Statistical problem in space and time: Do leukemia cases come in clusters?, *Biometrics* 20:626–632.

Fedrick, J., and Alberman, E. D., 1972, Reported influenza in pregnancy and subsequent cancer in the child, *Br. Med. J.* 2:485–487.

Fitzpatrick, J., Lieberman, N., and Sinks, L., 1974, Staging of acute leukemia and the relationship to CNS involvement, *Cancer* 33:1376–1381.

Flandrin, G., Brouet, J. C., Daniel, M. T., and Preud'homme, J. L., 1975, Acute leukemia with Burkitt's tumor cells: A study of six cases with special reference to lymphocyte surface markers, *Blood* 45:183–188.

Gajl-Peczalska, K. J., Chartrand, S., Bloomfield, C. D., Corte, J., Coccia, P. F., Nesbit, M. E., and Kersey, J. H., 1976, Lymphocytes bearing multiple surface markers in 543 patients with neoplastic and nonneoplastic diseases *Clin. Immunol. Immunopathol.* 8:292–299.

George, S. L., Fernbach, D. J., Vietti, T. J., Sullivan, M. P., Lane, D. M., Haggard, M. E., Berry, D. H., Lonsdale, D., and Komp, D., 1973, Factors influencing survival in pediatric leukemia, *Cancer* 32:1542–1553.

Gibson, R. W., and Graham, S., 1974, Epidemiology of long term survival with acute leukemia, *N. Engl. J. Med.* 290:583–587.

Hardisty, R. M., and Till, M. M., 1968, Acute leukemia 1959–1964: Factors influencing prognosis, *Arch. Dis. Child.* 43:107–115.

Humphrey, G. B., Nesbit, M. E., and Brunning, R. D., 1974, Prognostic value of the periodic acid–Schiff reaction in acute lymphoblastic leukemia, *Am. J. Clin. Pathol.* 61:393–397.

Jacquillat, L., Flandrin, G., Weil, M., Auclerc, G., Gemon, M. F., Barron, M., and Bernard, J., 1972, Correlation between cytological varieties and prognosis in acute lymphocytic leukemia, *Proc. Am. Assoc. Cancer Res.* 14:2.

Kaplan, J., Mastrangelo, R., and Peterson, W. D., 1974, Childhood lymphoblastic lymphoma: A cancer of thymus-derived lymphocytes, *Cancer Res.* **34**:521–525.

Kersey, J., and Gajl-Peczalska, K. J., 1975, T and B lymphocytes in humans: A review, *Am. J. Pathol.* **81**:446–457.

Kersey, J. H., Nesbit, M. E., and Gajl-Peczalska, K. J., 1974, The lymphoid system: Abnormalities in immunodeficiency and malignancy, *J. Pediatr.* **84**:789–796.

Lee, S. L., and Glidewell, O., 1973, Cytology and survival in acute lymphatic leukemia of childhood, in: *Recent Results in Cancer Research* (G. Mathé, P. Pouillart, and L. Schwarzenberg, eds.), Vol. 43, pp. 28–34, Springer-Verlag, New York.

Lemerle, M., Gerrard-Marchant, R., Sarrazin, D., Sancho, H., Tchernia, G., Flamant, F., Lemerle, J., and Schweisguth, O., 1973, Lymphosarcoma and reticulum cell sarcoma in children: A retrospective study of 172 cases, *Cancer* **32**:1499–1507.

Löffler, H., 1973, Indications and limits of cytochemistry in acute leukemia, in: *Recent Results in Cancer Research* (G. Mathé, ed.), pp. 57–62, Springer-Verlag, New York.

Mathé, G., Pouillart, P., Sterescu, M., Amiel, J. L., Schwartzenberg, L., Schneider, M., Hayat, M., DeVassal, F., Jasmin, C., and Lafleur, M., 1971, Subdivision of classical varieties of acute leukemia: Correlation with prognosis and cure expectancy, *Eur. J. Clin. Biol. Res.* **16**:554–560.

Miller, R. W., 1967, Persons with exceptionally high risk of leukemia, *Cancer Res.* **27**:2420–2423.

Miller, R. W., 1971, Death from childhood leukemia and solid tumors among twins and other siblings in the U.S. 1960–1967, *J. Natl. Cancer Inst.* **46**:203–209.

Murphy, S. B., and Mauer, A. M., 1975, Staging of acute lymphoblastic leukemia, in: *Conflicts in Childhood Cancer* (L. Sinke, ed.), pp. 7–28, Alan Less, New York.

Murphy, S. B., Frizzera, G., and Evans, A. E., 1975, A study of childhood non-Hodgkin's lymphoma, *Cancer* **36**:2121–2131.

Nesbit, M. E., and Krivit, W., 1968, Sequential changes in proliferative activity of acute leukemia of childhood. Presented at the meeting of the 12th Int. Soc. Hematol., Sept. 1–6, 1968, New York.

Nora, A. H., Nora, J. J., and Fernbach, D. J., 1968, Hereditary predisposition to leukemia, in: *Proceedings of the International Congress of the Twelfth International Society of Hematology,* p. 23, New York.

Oettgen, H. F., and Murphy, M. L., 1967, Malignant lymphoma of childhood in the U.S. and Burkitt's tumor in Africa: Therapeutic results, in: *Treatment of Burkitt's Tumour* (J. H. Burchenal and D. P. Burkitt, eds.), pp. 105–108, Springer-Verlag, New York.

Pantazopoulos, N., and Sinks, L. F., 1974, Morphologic criteria for prognostication of acute leukemia, *Br. J. Haematol.* **27**:25–30.

Pierce, M. I., Borges, W. H., Heyn, R., Wolff, J. A., and Gilbert, E. S., 1969, Epidemiologic factors and survival experience in 1770 children with acute leukemia, *Cancer* **23**:1296–1304.

Pinkel, D., Johnson, W., and Aur, R. J. A., 1975, Non-Hodgkin's lymphoma in children, *Br. J. Cancer* **31**:298–323.

Schreffler, D. C., and David, C. S., 1975, *H-2* gene complex and *I* immune response region, *Arch. Immunol.* **20**:125–195.

Sen, L., and Borella, L., 1975, Clinical importance of lymphoblasts with T markers in childhood acute leukemia, *N. Engl. J. Med.* **292**:828–832.

Sonley, M., 1972, Lymphosarcoma in childhood, *Paediatrician* **1**:249–260.

Tsukimoto, I., Wong, K. Y., and Lampkin, B. C., 1976, Surface markers and prognostic factors in acute lymphoblastic leukemia, *N. Engl. J. Med.* **294**:245–248.

Walford, R. L., Finkelstein, S., Neerhout, R., Konrad, P., and Shanbrom, E., 1970, Acute childhood leukemia in relation to the *HL-A* human transplantation genes, *Nature (London)* **225**:461–462.

Warner, N. L., 1974, Membrane immunoglobulins and antigen receptors on B and T lymphocytes, *Adv. Immunol.* **19**:67–216.

WHO/IARC-Sponsored Workshop on Human B and T Cells, 1974, Identification, enumeration, and isolation of B and T lymphocytes from human peripheral blood, *Scand. J. Immunol.* **3**:521–532.

Zuelzer, W. W., and Cox, D. E., 1969, Genetic aspects of leukemia, *Semin. Hematol.* **6**:228–249.

18

Immunodeficiency States Associated with Acute Leukemias, Multiple Myeloma, and Waldenström's Macroglobulinemia

BENJAMIN KOZINER and ROBERT A. GOOD

1. Acute Leukemias

A relationship between oncogenesis and immunocompetence has been suggested by the growing recognition of altered immune responses in tumor-bearing animals and men. No evidence remains more supportive of this relationship than the frequent occurrence of various types of malignancy in cases of primary immunodeficiency. The development of acute leukemias—mostly of the lymphoid system—has been repeatedly observed under these circumstances (Gatti and Good, 1971).

Further adding to the possible role of immunological factors in acute leukemia, provocative findings have been reported in relatives of leukemic patients. Mothers of children with acute lymphoblastic leukemia (ALL) had significantly increased levels of serum IgA and IgG (Hann *et al.*, 1975) or IgM (Sutton, R. N. P., *et al.*, 1969; Snyder *et al.*, 1970). Santos *et al.* (1973) found evidence of humoral (cytotoxic antibody) or cellular [lymphocyte cytotoxicity and production of migration-inhibitory factor (MIF)] reactivity to leukemic cells in about a quarter of patients with acute leukemia. Lymphocyte reactivity against leukemic cells was also detected in HLA-identical siblings by way of lymphocyte cytotoxicity (Rosenberg, E. B., *et al.*, 1972) and the capacity to become stimulated in mixed leukocyte culture (MLC) (Santos *et al.*, 1973). The susceptibility of skin fibroblasts to undergo

BENJAMIN KOZINER and ROBERT A. GOOD • Memorial Sloan-Kettering Cancer Center, New York, New York 10021.

in vitro transformation by SV40 tumor virus was found to be greatly increased among the members of a family afflicted by 6 cases of acute myeloblastic leukemia (AML), suggesting the value of the test in the detection of persons at high risk for leukemia (Snyder *et al.*, 1970).

Juvenile myelomonocytic leukemia, an uncommon disorder affecting mostly infants and young children, has been associated with elevated levels of serum immunoglobulins (Ig's) of restricted heterogeneity. A high incidence of anti-nuclear and anti-human IgG antibodies was observed. Strikingly, when family members were studied, similar serological alterations were found to be particularly clustered in a few families (Cannat and Seligmann, 1973).

Presumptive "leukemia-associated antigens" were identified on blast cells of patients with acute leukemia (Harris, R., 1973). These changes in the antigenic phenotype of leukemic cell surfaces may relate to viral transformation or "oncofetal" differentiation, or may truly represent "tumor-specific" neoantigens (Alexander, 1972; Boyse and Old, 1976). Hypothetically, small accumulations of cells with neoplastic potential may periodically develop as a result of genetic mutation and, because of their altered surface antigenicity, undergo immunological attack and eventual regression. On failure of this mechanism of "immunological surveillance," malignant growth might be permitted to occur (Burnet, 1957, 1970; Thomas, 1959). The lack of suppressor activity, enabling neoplastic proliferation (Gershwin and Steinberg, 1973), the actual enhancement of tumor growth by an incipient immune reactivity (Prehn, 1972), or the "blocking" effect of new antigenic sites mediated by serum factors, which prevents self-responsiveness (Hellström *et al.*, 1969, 1971; Sjögren *et al.*, 1971), remain as possible legitimate mechanisms linking immunity to oncogenic development.

Adequate immunocompetence has been correlated with good prognosis in acute leukemia, presumably because it enhances the development of specific tumor immunity (Hersh *et al.*, 1971; Gutterman *et al.*, 1972, 1973a). On this basis, potentiation of immune reactivity was sought by the use of active immunotherapy during different phases of the leukemic processes (Mathé, 1971; Powles *et al.*, 1971).

Preceding antileukemic therapy, low neutrophil numbers (Silver *et al.*, 1957; Bodey *et al.*, 1966; Hughes and Smith, 1973) with concomitant impairment of neutrophil function (Rosner *et al.*, 1970; Goldman and Catovsky, 1972) are mostly responsible for the frequent occurrence of bacterial infection. In contrast, viral, fungal, and protozoal infections characteristically occur on treatment, and may be attributed to the depressed humoral and cellular immunity caused by intensive therapy (Hersh *et al.*, 1965a; Armstrong *et al.*, 1971; Levine *et al.*, 1972).

1.1. Effect of Antileukemic Therapy on the Immune Response

Immunosuppressive antimetabolite therapy may inhibit the development of delayed hypersensitivity, delay the occurrence of homograft rejection, and prevent the production of a local inflammatory response by interfering with its mononuclear cell phase (Hitchings and Elion, 1963; Gabrielsen and Good, 1967).

6-Mercaptopurine (6-MP) is a most potent inhibitor of the primary antibody response (Schwartz *et al.*, 1958, 1959; Sterzl, 1960). Short-term intensive chemotherapy with either methotrexate (MTX) or 6-MP suppressed the primary response

545

IMMUNO-
DEFICIENCY STATES
ASSOCIATED WITH
ACUTE LEUKEMIAS,
MULTIPLE
MYELOMA, AND
WALDENSTRÖM'S
MACRO-
GLOBULINEMIA

to tularemia, V_1, and pneumococcal antigens (Hersh *et al.*, 1965b). On cessation of therapy, there is a prompt recovery of immune responsiveness, with production of antibody within 24 hr (Hersh *et al.*, 1966).

The list of chemotherapeutic agents that affect the primary antibody response includes, in addition to MTX, vincristine, 6-thioguanine, and cyclophosphamide (Santos *et al.*, 1964). The secondary antibody response is also affected by 6-MP (LaPlante *et al.*, 1972; Rosenberg, S., and Calabresi, 1964). Inhibition of *in vitro* lymphocyte transformation that is initiated by phytohemagglutinin (PHA) or small-pox vaccine *in vitro* was also observed during chemotherapy with 6-MP and MTX with or without prednisolone (Hersh and Oppenheim, 1967). Delayed cutaneous hypersensitivity of patients treated with 6-MP remains generally intact (Hersh *et al.*, 1965b; Zweiman, 1973), although allograft rejection is depressed (Uphoff, 1961; Sutton, W. R. *et al.*, 1962). Maintenance chemotherapy with 6-MP and MTX caused depression of recall-antigen reactivity in children with ALL in remission, this depression being more pronounced with continuous, as opposed to intermittent, administration of the combination (Garay *et al.*, 1976).

6-MP causes marked inhibition of the mononuclear cell phase of the local inflammatory response without any major effect on the granulocyte phase (Page *et al.*, 1962a,b, 1964).

Vincristine and prednisone (either alone or in combination with other agents) also provoke a fall in the blastogenic response, which rises to normal or supranormal levels a few days after cessation of therapy, provided it has not been administered for longer than 1 week (Sacks *et al.*, 1975).

The mechanisms by which glucocorticosteroids interfere with the human immune response remain poorly defined, despite their overt immunosuppressive effects in clinical practice (Schwartz, 1968; Mannick and Egdahl, 1968). The administration of glucocorticosteroids causes immunosuppression mainly by interfering with the efferent limb of the cellular immune response. Monocytopenia of variable duration occurs either in relation to decreased cell production by precursor cells or, alternatively, to impaired release into circulation of bone marrow monocytes (Thompson and Van Furth, 1973). Furthermore, steroids interfere with the effect of MIF on monocyte function (Balow and Rosenthal, 1972). Steroid-induced lymphocytopenia is a result of lympholysis and suppression of lymphocyte production (Germuth, 1956). The administration of glucocorticosteroids also results in impairment of leukocyte mobilization (Peters *et al.*, 1972), intracytoplasmic killing of ingested organisms (Sbarra *et al.*, 1964), and neutrophil bactericidal activity (Jungi *et al.*, 1971). A short course of methylprednisolone also caused a significant decrease in the level of γ-globulin, and more particularly, of IgG. Both depressed production and increased catabolism of these proteins have been implicated (Butler and Rossen, 1973).

Cytarabine, a most useful agent in the treatment of acute myelocytic leukemias, interferes with both primary and secondary humoral responses, as well as with skin reactivity to dinitrochlorobenzene (DNCB). However, established delayed hypersensitivity to common antigens remains preserved (Mitchell *et al.*, 1969).

Chemotherapy may also transiently depress the MLC response, with eventual rebound of *in vitro* reactivity (Halterman and Leventhal, 1971; Leventhal *et al.*, 1972).

When craniospinal irradiation is added to a program of intensive chemotherapy for childhood ALL, further immunosuppression ensues. Lymphopenia at the expense of T cells, with decreased PHA responsiveness, develops. This decrease in the number and function of T cells appears to relate to an increase in the incidence of fatal infections during remission (Campbell, A. C. *et al.*, 1973).

1.2. Humoral Immunity

In general, the level of serum Ig's has been described as normal in untreated children with acute leukemia (Kiran and Gross, 1969; Ragab *et al.*, 1970; Gooch and Fernbach, 1971). Isolated increases of IgM (Foy *et al.*, 1975), and decreases in IgG (Chandra, 1972) or IgA (McKelvey and Carbone, 1965) with otherwise normal amounts of other Ig's, have been reported. Children with acute leukemia retain the capacity to produce Ig's in response to infection, in general, with IgG, IgM, and IgA fluctuating together in any given patient (Gooch and Fernbach, 1971).

After a 5-week course of vincristine and prednisone, all classes of Ig's were depressed in children with ALL. Those patients in long-term remission on maintenance chemotherapy had Ig levels that did not differ significantly from those of controls. Children who were relapsing and receiving reinduction therapy had significantly lower Ig levels than patients who remained in remission on maintenance treatment. No particular Ig pattern was observed in children who went from remission to relapse (Ragab *et al.*, 1970). Patients in remission from ALL and AML, who developed severe infections, had a more severe depression of Ig levels than those leukemic patients without infection (Graham-Pole *et al.*, 1975).

Untreated patients with acute leukemia have normal primary and secondary antibody responses (Larson and Tomlinson, 1953; Silver *et al.*, 1960; Heath *et al.*, 1964; Hersh *et al.*, 1966). The antibody response after immunization with type-specific pneumococcal capsular polysaccharides I and II was higher in untreated patients with acute leukemia than in a control group (Larson and Tomlinson, 1953). In 10 children with acute leukemia, the antibody response to typhoid–paratyphoid, influenza, and mumps vaccines and diphtheria and tetanus toxoids after immunization was significantly less than that of a group of normal controls. Although all patients except one responded to at least one of the antigens, significantly poorer responses could be demonstrated in leukemic patients only by comparing the overall antibody response to all antigens. No correlation could be made individually between the incidence of bacterial infection and the degree of antibody response (Silver *et al.*, 1960).

During induction therapy, antibody formation was found to be depressed, with 50% of the immunized patients failing to develop a measurable antibody response to poliovirus vaccine. Moreover, those patients who responded showed a higher antibody titer than control subjects (Dupuy *et al.*, 1971).

Primary antibody production to the hemagglutinin antigen of the Hong Kong influenza virus and the secondary response to the neuraminidase of the same virus were found to be depressed in children undergoing maintenance combination chemotherapy for ALL in remission. The primary humoral response, however, showed a greater degree of inhibition as compared with the secondary type. Of 20 children, 5 had low serum IgG levels and 3 of these 5 had no hemagglutination

547

IMMUNO-
DEFICIENCY STATES
ASSOCIATED WITH
ACUTE LEUKEMIAS,
MULTIPLE
MYELOMA, AND
WALDENSTRÖM'S
MACRO-
GLOBULINEMIA

inhibition antibody to the Hong Kong virus vaccine. Moreover, despite a normal response to PHA, low IgG titers and depressed antibody production were found after 2 years of continuous therapy (Borella and Webster, 1971).

Frommel *et al.* (1969) observed that long-term, intensive chemotherapy produced very marked reduction of levels of all major classes of Ig's in 3 children with lymphosarcoma. In 1 patient, cessation of immunosuppressive antimetabolite therapy at the time of pneumocystis carinii infection resulted in a tremendous increase of IgM to 1200 mg/dl. The findings argue that Ig determinations should be more widely used as an indicator of biological events occurring during treatment of leukemias.

A careful analysis of the kinetics of immunological recovery following discontinuation of long-term combination chemotherapy was provided by Borella *et al.* (1972). After cessation of chemotherapy in patients in continuous remission for $2\frac{1}{2}$–3 years, there was an increase in the number of peripheral blood and bone marrow lymphocytes, in IgG and IgM, and in the antibody titer to Hong Kong influenza virus without documented antigenic challenge. This pattern was frequent in the group of patients younger than 5 years, but not in older patients. On the basis of these observations, the investigators advise caution in the interpretation of early bone marrow lymphocytosis in these patients, since it may represent immunological recovery, rather than leukemic relapse. Moreover, a rise in antibody titer may be a manifestation of immunological rebound, rather than being secondary to extrinsic infectious stimulation.

The detection of cytotoxic antibody activity against ALL cells in the sera from 3 unimmunized normal subjects suggests the presence of specific antigenic determinants on the leukemic cell surface. Furthermore, this cytotoxic activity could be removed by absorption with leukemic cells, but not with remission leukocytes (Bias *et al.*, 1972).

Complement levels were reported to be normal in untreated patients with AML (Foy *et al.*, 1975).

1.3. Cellular Immunity

Normal cutaneous delayed hypersensitivity has been repeatedly described in untreated patients with acute leukemia (Miller, D. G., 1962; Good and Finstad, 1968; Dupuy *et al.*, 1971; Char *et al.*, 1973). Of patients with untreated leukemia, 96% reacted to at least one recall antigen of a battery of skin tests, but the number and size of the individual reactions tended to be diminished (Dupuy *et al.*, 1971).

In a group of untreated patients with AML, 7 of 25 were anergic to recall antigens, and 5 of these 7 failed to achieve a remission status, whereas 13 of 18 patients with normal delayed hypersensitivity to at least one skin antigen achieved a complete remission. The development of delayed hypersensitivity to keyhole limpet hemocyanin (KLH) was also a useful indicator of the likelihood of obtaining a complete remission. In general, those patients converting from immunoincompetence to immunocompetence during therapy achieved a remission, whereas those reverting to their previous immunoincompetence failed to do so (Hersh *et al.*, 1971).

Different conclusions were arrived at in a similar study of cell-mediated immunity, carried out in untreated patients with acute nonlymphocytic leukemias (Greene *et al.*, 1974). No correlation could be established between the capacity to respond to a battery of recall antigens or DNCB and various prognostic features (ability to achieve a complete remission, duration of remission, and survival).

Positive delayed cutaneous hypersensitivity elicited by autologous blast cell membranes from leukemia patients appeared to correlate with good prognosis, being seen more frequently during remission than in relapse. Furthermore, an increase in remission duration was observed in patients who had positive responses (Oren and Herberman, 1971; Char *et al.*, 1973; Herberman *et al.*, 1973).

1.4. Blastogenic Responses

The analysis of *in vitro* lymphocyte transformation is difficult to evaluate in acute leukemias due to the presence of circulating blast forms that may incorporate tritiated thymidine by themselves and increase the unstimulated background.

In a majority of untreated patients with acute leukemia, induction of morphological transformation of peripheral blood lymphocytes by PHA, as well as DNA synthesis, did not differ from the values observed in normal controls. RNA synthesis was decreased during the period preceding therapy, however, and increased on achievement of remission (Sutherland *et al.*, 1971). Patients with ALL and white cell counts lower than 20,000 responded normally to PHA, although those patients with white cell counts higher than 20,000 showed abnormal dose–response curves. A prognostic implication was suggested on the basis of these findings (Zusman *et al.*, 1975). The defective response to PHA *in vitro* may be related to the inhibitory effect of leukemic sera. This assumption is supported by the poor blastogenic response to PHA of normal allogeneic lymphocytes on incubation with sera from patients with AML (Walker *et al.*, 1973).

Of 25 patients with AML evaluated before and after intensive chemotherapy, two thirds showed normal *in vitro* blastogenic responses to PHA and streptolysin O. Those patients who underwent a significant tumor reduction had initially a normal *in vitro* lymphocyte response to PHA that remained unchanged after therapy. In contrast, a further drop in PHA responsiveness occurred in the group of patients who failed to achieve a therapeutic response (Hersh *et al.*, 1971). On cessation of chemotherapy, the decreased mitogenic responses undergo rapid recovery (Hersh *et al.*, 1974).

In general, a normal *in vitro* transformation of peripheral blood lymphocytes from children with ALL before therapy (Astaldi *et al.*, 1966) and in remission (Astaldi *et al.*, 1966; Kourilsky *et al.*, 1966) has been reported. Since a short remission was associated with a response of less than 40%, the prognostic significance of the test was stressed (Foy *et al.*, 1975).

Blastogenic responses to PHA and various antigens (KLH, *Candida albicans*, and influenza antigens) were also studied after termination of maintenance chemotherapy in patients who were in continuous remission for 2½–3 years. Although the *proportion* of responders by *in vitro* lymphocyte transformation increased following discontinuation of drugs, no significant differences in the *degrees* of PHA responsiveness were detected between values obtained during and after therapy. Conversely, the mean *in vitro* responses to KLH, *Candida*, or influenza antigen continued to increase for 13–36 weeks after termination of therapy. Both PHA and antigen-induced transformation showed different patterns in a comparative study of peripheral blood and bone marrow (Green and Borella, 1973).

549

IMMUNO-
DEFICIENCY STATES
ASSOCIATED WITH
ACUTE LEUKEMIAS,
MULTIPLE
MYELOMA, AND
WALDENSTRÖM'S
MACRO-
GLOBULINEMIA

The *in vitro* blastogenic response to pokeweed mitogen (PWM) was found to be similar to that of normal controls in children with ALL in remission who had not received intensive therapy. This response, however, was persistently impaired even several months after termination of intensive chemotherapy that had been accompanied by craniospinal radiation (Humphrey *et al.*, 1972).

Leukemic sera from newly diagnosed cases of childhood ALL with white cell counts greater than 50,000 caused significant inhibition of normal *in vitro* lymphocyte transformation to PWM. No inhibition was seen when sera from patients previously untreated, in remission, or in relapse with white cell counts below 50,000 were used. This effect was assumed to be related to the presence of an unidentified inhibitor (Humphrey *et al.*, 1975).

Remission peripheral blood lymphocytes have been repeatedly found to react with autologous blasts in the MLC reaction (Fridman and Kourilsky, 1969; Viza *et al.*, 1969; Powles *et al.*, 1971; Leventhal *et al.*, 1972). Greater blastogenic responses and MIF production were observed with myeloblasts than with lymphoblasts, on stimulation of autologous and allogeneic lymphocytes in MLC (Gutterman *et al.*, 1972; Cotropia *et al.*, 1976). Sheep erythrocyte (SRBC)-rosetting lymphoblasts failed to stimulate allogeneic donor lymphocytes in a similar system (Leventhal *et al.*, 1976; Tsukimoto *et al.*, 1976). Patients with acute leukemia also showed positive blastogenic responses to autologous soluble antigens obtained from leukemic cells and purified by extraction with KCl. A strong blastogenic response was in general correlated with good prognosis, presensitization apparently being required for this reaction to occur (Gutterman *et al.*, 1973b). Inhibition of the blastogenic response in patients with AML was found to be associated with bound IgG on the leukemic cells. Some patients, however, had facilitation of the blastogenic response in autologous but not in allogeneic serum (Gutterman *et al.*, 1973a).

The induction of blastogenesis in autologous peripheral blood lymphocytes also proved to be a good marker for residual leukemia in the bone marrow of patients presumed to be in complete remission. Of 17 patients whose cells failed to react, 15 remained in complete remission, while 5 of 8 patients whose peripheral blood lymphocytes were stimulated by the "remission" bone marrow subsequently relapsed (Gutterman *et al.*, 1974).

1.5. Neutrophil Function

Neutropenia and defective neutrophil functions can be implicated as the factors mostly responsible for the frequent occurrence of bacterial infections in patients with acute leukemia before chemotherapy is instituted.

Studies of the local exudative cellular response in patients with acute leukemia revealed a defective migration of leukocytes to inflammatory sites (Perillie and Finch, 1960, 1964; Holland *et al.*, 1971). A similar granulocytic response was observed in patients with both AML and ALL. The macrophage response, however, appeared to be more adequate in AML (Boggs, 1960).

The phagocytic ability of leukemic cells has been reported to be normal (Silver *et al.*, 1957; Sbarra *et al.*, 1965; Tornyos, 1967; Rosner *et al.*, 1970) or impaired (Groch *et al.*, 1965; Penny and Galton, 1966; Rosner *et al.*, 1970; Strauss *et al.*, 1970).

More recently, it has been shown that neutrophils from patients with active AML are capable of phagocytizing live yeast organisms, but are unable to carry on intracytoplasmic killing (Rosner *et al.*, 1970; Lehrer and Cline, 1971; Goldman and Th'ng, 1973; Cline, 1973). The abnormal neutrophil candidacidal function in AML may relate to decreased levels of activity of lysozyme or myeloperoxidase or both (Lehrer and Cline, 1971; Davis *et al.*, 1971; Catovsky *et al.*, 1972a), as well as to a deficiency or inhibitory factor of leukemic plasma (Goldman and Th'ng, 1973).

The phagocytic cells in ALL were found not only to be decreased in number, but also to be functionally unfit as indirectly determined by defective hexose monophosphate shunt activity (Skeel *et al.*, 1972; Pickering *et al.*, 1975) and other abnormalities in the metabolism of carbohydrates (Stjernholm *et al.*, 1970). Moreover, they appear to be excessively fragile (Nir *et al.*, 1970).

Bacteriolytic activity of leukemic sera against *Escherichia coli* was found to be lower than normal in ALL but normal in AML. Bactericidal activity, however, was higher in leukemic sera than in normal controls (Pruzanski *et al.*, 1973).

Variable values have been reported for nitroblue tetrazolium dye reduction test in unstimulated cells as well as after stimulation in acute leukemias (Miller, D. R., and Kaplan, 1970; Goldman and Catovsky, 1972; Tan *et al.*, 1973; Pickering *et al.*, 1975).

1.6. Surface Markers

In one fifth of the cases of childhood ALL, the presence of lymphoblasts with receptors for SRBC appears to correlate clinically with older age at presentation, mediastinal enlargement on X-rays, and a higher white cell count (Sen and Borella, 1975; Tsukimoto *et al.*, 1976). In most patients, though, lymphoblasts are "null" cells, since they lack conventional B- and T-cell markers. Further investigations of the nature of "null" cells in ALL have led to controversial interpretations regarding their being B (Fu *et al.*, 1975) or T (Kersey *et al.*, 1975) cells, although the presence of high levels of the enzyme terminal deoxynucleotidyltransferase, as also found in some cases of blastic chronic myeloid leukemia, argues in favor of their thymic-related lineage (McCaffrey *et al.*, 1975).

Jaffe *et al.* (1976) recently reported on the presence of receptors for complement on the cells of three cases with "childhood lymphoblastic lymphoma." In all these cases, receptors for both SRBC and complement were demonstrated simultaneously on the leukemic cells. The authors explained the heterogeneity of cellular types found as a reflection of altered differentiation of the neoplastic cells. Current surface-marker techniques have been unable to characterize the cells from cases of AML. In most of the reported cases, the leukemic cells did not have receptors of either monocytes, B, or T cells (Brown *et al.*, 1974; Samoilova *et al.*, 1975).

Decreased numbers of lymphocytes, and more particularly of T cells, have been repeatedly observed in leukemic patients in remission, and this decrease was related to long-standing chemotherapy (Sen and Borella, 1973; Garay *et al.*, 1976).

1.7. Summary: Acute Leukemias

In acute leukemias, the adaptive immune function remains generally intact, with adequate humoral and cellular defense mechanisms. The susceptibility to infection relates directly to the decreased number and defective function of neutrophils preceding therapy, and to the potent and universal immunosuppression that results from the administration of chemotherapy. Further progress in the treatment of these diseases will require either potentiation of immune reactivity against leukemic cells and intercurrent infection or the design of less immunosuppressive and more selective antileukemic therapy.

551

IMMUNO-
DEFICIENCY STATES
ASSOCIATED WITH
ACUTE LEUKEMIAS,
MULTIPLE
MYELOMA, AND
WALDENSTRÖM'S
MACRO-
GLOBULINEMIA

2. Multiple Myeloma

The study of myelomatous proteins has been most rewarding in facilitating the comprehensive understanding of the normal Ig system (Kunkel et al., 1951; Slater et al., 1955; Porter, 1973; Edelman, 1973).

Although multiple myeloma (MM) is characterized by the neoplastic proliferation of plasma cells, producing and releasing homogeneous Ig, sporadic cases of nonsecretory MM are known to occur (Hurez et al., 1970; Arend and Adamson, 1974). The homogeneity of these paraproteins argues in favor of these products being secreted by the progeny of a single neoplastic cell clone (Waldenström, 1962).

Despite the lack of antibody activity against 20 different antigens in 275 human samples of myelomatous proteins (Yoo and Franklin, 1971), a variety of antibody activities have been described to be present in Ig molecules of all classes. Antibody-combining specificities against streptolysin O and streptococcal hyaluronidase are of biological significance. Anti-IgG activity or rheumatoid factors, cold agglutinins, antibodies against coagulation factors (fibrin, factor VIII, fibrin monomers), serum proteins (transferrin, $\alpha_2 M$, albumin), lipoprotein, and certain haptenic groups such as dinitrophenol, phosphorocoline, 5'-acetourocil, and purine and pyrimidine nucleotides have all been described (Metzger, 1969; Eisen et al., 1970; Potter, 1971; Osterland and Espinoza, 1975). Despite these antibodylike activities, as would be expected the abnormal paraprotein remains functionally incapable of preventing the frequent occurrence of infections.

The impaired ability to produce adequate antibody levels and to mount an effective humoral response correlates with increased susceptibility to bacterial infection, mainly caused by extracellular pyogenic organisms (Zinneman and Hall, 1954; Good, 1957; Fahey et al., 1963). Pneumonia due to *Diplococcus pneumoniae* and *Staphylococcus aureus*, pyelonephritis caused by *Escherichia coli* and *Pseudomonas aureoginosa*, and episodes of septicemia frequently complicate and terminate the course of patients with MM (Zinneman and Hall, 1954; Glenchur et al., 1959; Salmon et al., 1967; Meyers et al., 1972).

IgG represents the most abundant serum Ig in the normal population, and paraproteins of the IgG class occur in over 50% of patients with MM (Ameis et al., 1976). The class of myelomatous paraprotein appears to correlate with certain patterns of bacterial susceptibility. Recurrent infections in patients with IgG myeloma are generally caused by single organisms of either gram-positive or gram-negative types, while multiple bacteria of both gram-positive and -negative types are implicated in cases of IgA myeloma (Allen and Peeler, 1972).

2.1. Humoral Immunity

Static determinations of the remaining polyclonal Ig's have shown low levels and defective antibody activity.

Of patients with MM, 80–90% had low titers of polyclonal Ig (Hobbs, 1968; Alexanian and Migliore, 1970; Cwynarski and Cohen, 1971). Mean levels were found to be decreased to 10–30% of normal (McKelvey and Fahey, 1965). On response to chemotherapy, normal levels of Ig may be observed (Alexanian and Migliore, 1970).

Although the capacity to mount a primary antibody response may be severely compromised, secondary responses to previously encountered antigens usually remain intact (Zinneman and Hall, 1954; Fahey *et al.*, 1963; Cone and Uhr, 1964).

On immunization with KLH, MM patients displayed a delayed induction time for IgM antibody formation, a rapid switch from IgM to IgG production, and a decline in the level of total antibody produced when compared with normal subjects. Patients with solitary plasmacytomas, however, generally had a normal immune response to KLH (Harris, J. E., *et al.*, 1971).

The primary response to bacteriophage ϕX174 was markedly reduced with absence of detectable antibody in a majority of patients, while a rise in antidiphtheria toxin measuring the secondary response occurred in almost all patients. Moreover, although comparison of responses between normal controls and MM patients showed significant differences when typhoid, diphtheria, and mumps antigens were tested, the response to influenza vaccine remained unimpaired (Cone and Uhr, 1964). Antibody production after challenge with the polysaccharides of *D. pneumoniae*, *Brucella*, and typhoid–paratyphoid vaccine occurred in inverse proportion to the total amount of abnormal serum Ig (Zinneman and Hall, 1954). Serum levels of staphylococcal α-antitoxin and antistreptolysin O were found to be low in a majority of patients with myelomatosis (Marks, 1953). Quantitative defects in agglutinin formation to *Salmonella typhosa*, *Paracolobactrum ballerup*, *E. coli*, SRBC, A and B human erythrocytes, and lysins for *S. typhosa*, *E. coli*, and sheep cells were originally reported. Complement activity was observed to be normal in all patients, but only one patient had normal antibodies (Lawson *et al.*, 1955).

The depressed levels of polyclonal (nonparaprotein) Ig's are mostly due to defective synthesis, though increased plasma volume and catabolic rate may be contributory factors (Solomon *et al.*, 1963).

To explain the defective B-cell function, it has been postulated that the neoplastic cells may produce "chalones" or specific mitotic inhibitors impeding the development of normal B-cell clones on antigenic stimulation (Salmon, 1973). Other mechanisms proposed to account for the impaired Ig production and humoral response in MM include the feedback inhibition of normal Ig production by the high levels of monoclonal paraprotein (Zolla, 1972), or simple crowding of the bone marrow by the malignant plasma cells displacing normal lymphocytes (Alexanian and Migliore, 1970).

Broder *et al.* (1975) found a marked depression in polyclonal Ig production *in vitro* by peripheral blood lymphocytes from patients with MM. Circulating mononuclear cells from 3 of 6 patients studied suppressed the Ig synthesis of normal lymphocytes in coculture. This suppressor activity was not mediated by isolated T cells, but removal of phagocytic cells (monocytes) from lymphocyte populations in 2 patients greatly enhanced polyclonal Ig production. It appears probable that suppressor cells normally regulate the degree of lymphoid hyperplasia and its released end products in response to various stimuli. On failure of the suppression mechanism, the disordered proliferation may eventually result in neoplastic growth (Gershwin and Steinberg, 1973).

553

IMMUNO-
DEFICIENCY STATES
ASSOCIATED WITH
ACUTE LEUKEMIAS,
MULTIPLE
MYELOMA, AND
WALDENSTRÖM'S
MACRO-
GLOBULINEMIA

2.2. Cellular Immunity

Delayed hypersensitivity to at least one of eight commonly encountered antigens was observed in all patients, but half failed to become sensitized to dinitrofluorobenzene (Cone and Uhr, 1964). Tuberculin sensitivity has been reported to be normal (Linton *et al.*, 1963; Glenchur *et al.*, 1959), decreased (Meyers *et al.*, 1972), and normal in patients with myeloma in good clinical condition, but impaired in poor-risk cases (Good *et al.*, 1962). Cutaneous reactivity to KLH, a newly encountered antigen, was also found to be impaired (Harris, J. E., *et al.*, 1971). Prolongation of skin-homograft survival could not be proved (Zinneman and Hall, 1954; Linton *et al.*, 1963). Low but detectable activity of serum MIF activity was found in 2 of 3 patients with MM. The production of serum MM activity in these patients could have been stimulated by virus infection, nonspecific mitogenic factors, or the proliferative response to the neoplastic cells, in addition to immunological activation (Cohen *et al.*, 1974).

2.3. Blastogenic Responses

Although *in vitro* lymphocyte response to PHA has been reported to be normal (Hersh *et al.*, 1970) or subnormal (Campbell, A. E. *et al.*, 1975), blastogenesis was significantly decreased using synchronized cell culture systems (Salmon and Fudenberg, 1969). Serial peripheral blood lymphocyte transformations showed that one third of the patients had reversed the original higher-PWM-than-PHA response, more likely due to the effect of chemotherapy (Campbell, A. E., *et al.*, 1975). *In vitro* lymphocyte responses to streptolysin O, vaccinia, and KLH were also decreased following immunization (Harris, J. E., *et al.*, 1969). Antibody-induced cytotoxicity of lymphocytes from untreated patients was normal or slightly elevated, while that of treated patients was markedly depressed. PHA-induced cytotoxicity and stimulation of lymphocytes by concanavalin A were normal, however, in all groups (Mellstedt and Holm, 1973).

Neoplastic plasma cells derived from subjects with plasma cell leukemia or plasmacytomas were unresponsive to PHA. These cells were also defective in their response and ability to stimulate allogeneic lymphocytes in a mixed lymphocyte–plasma-cell culture system (Beaulieu *et al.*, 1976).

The incubation of peripheral blood lymphocytes and bone marrow plasma cells from patients with MM with the individual idiotypic antisera was able to provoke proliferation with increased DNA synthesis not seen with isotypic antisera (Abdou and Abdou, 1972, 1975).

2.4. Neutrophil Function

When abnormal phagocytosis and neutrophil adhesiveness were found in patients with neoplastic paraproteins, the abnormality was observed to originate in the plasma, since it occurred in cross-mixing experiments of leukocytes with plasma containing M components, but failed to develop on testing with normal plasma (Penny and Galton, 1966). The abnormal paraprotein could also be partly responsible for the significantly elevated resting oxidative metabolism of leukocytes in MM (Selvaraj et al., 1967).

Wide variation in phagocytic activity measured by the blood clearance of injected ^{131}I-labeled aggregated human serum albumin was observed, this variation appearing to be unrelated to the extent of tissue involvement or previous therapy (Groch et al., 1965).

2.5. Complement Levels

Normal whole complement levels were originally reported (Lawson et al., 1955). The concentration of the complement protein C1q was found to be decreased in 45% of patients with IgG and IgA myeloma (Kohler and Müller-Eberhard, 1969). However, high levels of C2 have also been reported (Southam and Siegel, 1966).

2.6. Surface Markers

The analysis of B- and T-cell populations in MM has given conflicting results. Untreated patients have depressed counts of SRBC rosettes (T cells) (Jones and McFarlane, 1975). Although the proportion of peripheral blood lymphocytes bearing receptors for complement appears to be increased (Jones and McFarlane, 1975; Mellstedt et al., 1973), the percentage of B lymphocytes carrying surface Ig (SIg) has been repeatedly observed to be decreased (Lindström et al., 1973; Knapp et al., 1974; Abdou and Abdou, 1975).

Since patients with benign monoclonal gammopathies have normal percentages of SIg-bearing cells, these changes in membrane properties appear to be useful in the differentiation of cases of MM (Lindström et al., 1973). The use of antiidiotypic antisera raised against individual serum M-components rather than antiisotypic antisera enabled recognition of a greater proportion of monoclonal SIg-bearing cells that also stained autologous plasma cells (Mellstedt et al., 1974; Chen et al., 1975). After therapy, the number of Ig-bearing lymphocytes and bone marrow plasma cells idiotipically identified, as well as the serum gammopathy, decreased simultaneously (Mellstedt et al., 1974).

Recently, individual RNA-rich extracts (biochemically suggesting properties of messenger RNA) from the plasma of patients with MM appeared to be effective in the conversion of SIg, as indicated by the decrease in the proportion of cells with isotypic markers and the increase in cells with idiotypic ones. This effect was

555

IMMUNO-
DEFICIENCY STATES
ASSOCIATED WITH
ACUTE LEUKEMIAS,
MULTIPLE
MYELOMA, AND
WALDENSTRÖM'S
MACRO-
GLOBULINEMIA

described to be specific, since the RNA-rich preparation from one patient did not lead to the appearance of new SIg reactive to antiidiotypic antisera to another myeloma globulin (Chen *et al.*, 1975).

These changes in surface phenotype could eventually result in impaired antibody formation due to defective antigen recognition. Whether the immunological deficiency in MM is due to an abnormal clone of lymphocytes carrying the stigma of malignant transformation, or is caused by the acquired conversion of normal lymphocytes mediated by an RNA-containing factor released by the tumor, remains largely speculative at this writing.

3. Waldenström's Macroglobulinemia

After Waldenström's original description of the macroglobulinemia syndrome (Waldenström, 1944), the clinical association with increased susceptibility to bacterial infection was rapidly established (Imhof *et al.*, 1959; Glenchur *et al.*, 1958; Barandun *et al.*, 1958; Pachter and Havey, 1962; Fahey *et al.*, 1963). Although 20–30% of patients with Waldenström's macroglobulinemia (WM) suffer from severe and recurrent infections (Imhof *et al.*, 1957; Hobbs, 1968), the remainder show a lesser predisposition for infectious complications. Furthermore, despite similar serum protein abnormalities, patients with WM had less susceptibility to infection than patients with MM. In both entities, the incidence of infections was inversely correlated with the ability to mount an adequate antibody response (Fahey *et al.*, 1963).

3.1. Humoral Immunity

A genetic predisposition for the development of WM is suggested by the striking incidence of Ig abnormalities in families of patients affected by the disease. In a survey of 65 families of patients with WM, 7 were found to include 1 or 2 first-degree relatives with serum IgM-paraproteins, and some had clinical and hematological evidence of WM. Abnormal levels of polyclonal Ig's and antiglobulin factors were also frequently observed in first-degree relatives (Seligmann *et al.*, 1967).

The abnormal serum paraprotein is usually a pentamer of IgM, although a fraction of cases with monoclonal 7 S IgM also occur (Carter and Hobbs, 1971). The serum paraprotein may manifest clinically as cryoglobulin, cold agglutinin (Krajny and Pruzankski, 1976), anti-IgG rheumatoid factor activity (Bonomo *et al.*, 1970), true anti-antibody (Warner *et al.*, 1971), or false-positive VDRL reaction (Drusin *et al.*, 1974).

Approximately 60% of patients with WM had low levels of polyclonal Ig's (Hobbs, 1968; Salmon and Fudenberg, 1969). The titers of IgG and IgA were described as reduced to 65–80% of normal (McKelvey and Fahey, 1965; Krajny and Pruzanski, 1976). In general, the level of monoclonal IgM was found to be inversely related to the levels of remaining IgG and IgA (Cwynarski and Cohen, 1971).

Both primary and secondary antibody responses have been observed to be impaired in WM (Glenchur *et al.*, 1958; Barandun *et al.*, 1958; Pachter and Havey, 1962; Fahey *et al.*, 1963). The antibody responses to typhoid, diphtheria, and mumps immunizations were markedly decreased when compared with those of normal controls, and were similar to the abnormalities found in MM. The impairment in antibody response was detected even very early after diagnosis (Fahey *et al.*, 1963). The IgM-antibody response was more particularly affected than that of other Ig fractions, as demonstrated by the use of relatively weak antigens such as SRBC stroma, but not with stronger antigens, e.g., brucellin (Pitts and McDuffie, 1967).

3.2. Blastogenic Response

A subnormal *in vitro* blastogenic response to PHA in short-term culture was reported by Catovsky *et al.* (1972b) and further confirmed by Jenkins (1972) and Campbell, A. E., *et al.* (1975). *In vitro* stimulation with PHA of peripheral blood lymphocytes in 6 patients with WM showed a marked decrease in the incorporation of thymidine into DNA and uridine into RNA (Salmon and Fudenberg, 1969).

3.3. Complement Activity

Whole-serum complement and C2 levels were found to be diminished in less than one third and C1 and C3 levels in approximately 50% of patients with WM. Despite these abnormalities, no correlation could be established with the levels of serum Ig's, cryoglobulins, cold agglutinins, or antinuclear and antiglobulin antibodies (Glovsky and Fudenberg, 1970). Serum C1q titer was also found to be low in 2 of 4 patients with WM (Kohler and Müller-Eberhard, 1969).

3.4. Neutrophil Function

A normal inflammatory response was originally described when the skin-window cover-slip technique of Rebuck and Crowley (1955) was applied (Pachter and Havey, 1962). Neutrophil phagocytosis of yeast forms and adherence to glass were observed to be impaired in patients with WM. Although these defective functions were partly related to the concentration of plasma paraproteins, they were not corrected by incubation with normal plasma (Penny and Galton, 1966).

3.5. Surface Markers

In untreated patients with WM, a variable proportion of bone marrow and peripheral blood lymphoid cells display monoclonal SIgM of light-chain specificity similar to that of the secreted serum IgM (Marmont and Damasio, 1971; Preud'homme and Seligmann, 1972; Knapp *et al.*, 1974). A decrease in the percentage of Ig-bearing cells generally ensues on treatment (Preud'homme and Seligmann, 1972). The concomitant analysis of surface and intracytoplasmic Ig's in bone marrow plasma cells and pleomorphic lymphocytes reveals different stages of maturation of B cells in WM. The neoplastic cells may display Ig only on their surface, show both membrane and cytoplasmic Ig, or exclusively exhibit intracytoplasmic staining for Ig (Preud'homme and Seligmann, 1972; Knapp *et al.*, 1974). It is likely that WM represents a neoplastic proliferation of more differentiated B lymphocytes than the cells involved in chronic lymphocytic leukemia and other B-

557

IMMUNO-
DEFICIENCY STATES
ASSOCIATED WITH
ACUTE LEUKEMIAS,
MULTIPLE
MYELOMA, AND
WALDENSTRÖM'S
MACRO-
GLOBULINEMIA

cell lymphomas, since there is a more frequent further transition into a functional plasma cell stage.

3.6. Summary: Multiple Myeloma and Waldenström's Macroglobulinemia

The immunological deficiency observed in multiple myeloma and Waldenström's macroglobulinemia pertains selectively to the altered humoral antibody formation due to the production of monoclonal paraproteins. The primary antibody response is more affected than the secondary type, with decrease in the levels of the remaining polyclonal immunoglobulins. More rational and selective forms of therapy directed toward the paraprotein-producing cells and other cellular elements carrying the stigma of malignant transformation need to be defined. Recently, several new avenues might have been suggested by provocative immunological observations. Immunotherapy with specific antiidiotypic antisera, selective B-cell chemotherapy, and the hypothetical application of suppressive or permissive mediators of the immune response represent largely speculative therapeutic alternatives.

ACKNOWLEDGMENTS

The original studies reported herein have been supported by Public Service Research Grants CA-08748, CA-17404, and CA-19267 from the NCI; by the Zelda R. Weintraub Cancer Fund; and by the American Heart Association.

References

Abdou, N. I., and Abdou, N. L., 1972, Anti-immunoglobulins in multiple myeloma, *Clin. Exp. Immunol.* **11**:57.

Abdou, N. I., and Abdou, N. L., 1975, The monoclonal nature of lymphocytes in multiple myeloma: Effects of therapy, *Ann. Intern. Med.* **83**:42.

Alexander, P., 1972, Fetal "antigens" in cancer, *Nature (London)* **235**:137.

Alexanian, R., and Migliore, P. J., 1970, Normal immunoglobulins in multiple myeloma: Effect of melphalan chemotherapy, *J. Lab Clin. Med.* **75**:225.

Ameis, A., Ko, H. S., and Pruzanski, W., 1976, M components—A review of 1242 cases, *Can. Med. Assoc. J.* **22**:889.

Allen, J. C., and Peeler, R. N., 1972, A correlation between patterns of infection and immunoglobulin concentrations in multiple myeloma, *Ann. Intern. Med.* **76**:876.

Arend, W. P., and Adamson, J. W., 1974, Nonsecretory myeloma, *Cancer* **33**:721.

Armstrong, D., Young, L. S., Meyer, R. D., and Blevins, A. H., 1971, Infectious complications of neoplastic disease, *Med. Clin. North Am.* **55**:729.

Astaldi, G., Massimo, L., Airo, R., and Mori, P. G., 1966, Phytohemagglutinin and lymphocytes from acute lymphocytic leukemia, *Lancet* **1**:1265.

Balow, J. E., and Rosenthal, A. S., 1972, Mechanisms of steroid suppression of cellular immunity, *Clin. Res.* **20**:506.

Barandun, S., Huser, H. J., and Hässig, A., 1958, Klinische Erscheinungsformen des Antiköpermangel-syndroms, *Schweiz. Med. Wochenschr.* **88**:78.

Beaulieu, R., Pirofsky, B., and Davies, G. H., 1976, Immunologic studies of human plasma cells, *Am. J. Hematol.* **1**:325.

Bias, W. B., Santos, G. W., Burke, P. J., Mullins, G. M., and Humphrey, R. L., 1972, Cytotoxic antibody in normal human serums reactive with tumor cells from acute lymphocytic leukemia, *Science* **178**:304.

Bodey, G. P., Buckley, M., Sathe, Y. S., and Freireich, E. J., 1966, Quantitative relationships between circulating leukocytes and infections in acute leukemia, *Ann. Intern. Med.* **64**:328.

Boggs, D., 1960, The cellular composition of inflammatory exudates in human leukemias, *Blood* **15**:466.

Bonomo, L., Dammacco, F., Tursi, A., and Trizio, D., 1970, Waldenström's macroglobulinemia with anti-IgG activity: A series of five cases, *Clin. Exp. Immunol.* **6**:531.

Borella, L., and Webster, R. G., 1971, The immunosuppressive effects of long term combination chemotherapy in children with acute leukemia in remission, *Cancer Res.* **31**:420.

Borella, L., Green, A. A., and Webster, R. G., 1972, Immunologic rebound after cessation of long term chemotherapy in acute leukemia, *Blood* **40**:42.

Boyse, E. A., and Old, L. J., 1976, Some aspects of normal and abnormal cell surface genetics, *Annu. Rev. Genet.* **3**:269.

Broder, S., Humphrey, R., Durm, M., Blackman, M., Meade, B., Goldman, C., Strober, W., and Waldmann, T., 1975, Impaired synthesis of polyclonal (non-para-protein) immunoglobulins by circulating lymphocytes from patients with multiple myeloma: Role of suppressor cells, *N. Engl. J. Med.* **293**:887.

Brown, G., Greaves, M. F., Lister, T. A., Rapson, N., and Papamichael, M., 1974, Expression of human T and B lymphocyte cell surface markers on leukemic cells, *Lancet* **2**:753.

Burnet, F. M., 1957, Cancer: A biological approach, *Br. Med. J.* **1**:779.

Burnet, F. M., 1970, The concept of immunological surveillance, *Prog. Exp. Tumor Res.* **13**:1.

Butler, W. T., and Rossen, R. D., 1973, Effects of corticosteroids on immunity in man. I. Decreased serum IgG concentration caused by 3 or 5 days of high doses of methyl-prednisolone, *J. Clin. Invest.* **52**:2629.

Campbell, A. C., Hersey, P., MacLennan, I. C. M., Kay, H. E. M., Pike, M. C., and the Medical Research Council's Working Party on Leukemia in Childhood, 1973, Immunosuppressive consequences of radiotherapy and chemotherapy in patients with acute lymphoblastic leukemia, *Br. Med. J.* **2**:385.

Campbell, A. E., DeVine, J., Azam, L., Hamid, J., DeLamore, I. W., and McFarlane, H., 1975, Lymphocyte transformation in patients with paraproteinaemia, *Br. J. Haematol.* **29**:179.

Cannat, A., and Seligmann, M., 1973, Immunological abnormalities in juvenile myelomonocytic leukemia, *Br. Med. J.* **1**:71.

Carter, P. M., and Hobbs, J. R., 1971, Clinical significance of 7S IgM diseases, *Br. Med. J.* **2**:260.

Catovsky, D., Galton, D. A. G., and Robinson, J., 1972a, Myeloperoxidase-deficient neutrophils in acute myeloid leukemia, *Scand. J. Haematol.* **9**:142.

Catovsky, D., Tripp, E., and Hoffbrand, A. B., 1972b, Response to phytohaemagglutinin and pokeweed mitogen in chronic lymphocytic leukaemia, *Lancet* **1**:794.

Chandra, R. K., 1972, Serum immunoglobulin levels in children with acute lymphoblastic leukemia and their mothers and sibs, *Arch. Dis. Child.* **47**:618.

Char, D. H., Lepourhiet, A., Leventhal, B. G., and Herberman, R. B., 1973, Cutaneous delayed hypersensitivity responses to tumor associated and other antigens in acute leukemia, *Int. J. Cancer* **12**:409.

Chen, Y., Bhoopalam, N., Yakulis, V., and Heller, P., 1975, Changes in lymphocyte surface immunoglobulins in myeloma and the effect of an RNA-containing plasma factor, *Ann. Intern. Med.* **83**:625.

Cline, M. J., 1973, A new white cell test which measures individual phagocyte function in a mixed leukocyte population. I. A neutrophil defect in acute myelocytic leukemia, *J. Lab. Clin. Med.* **81**:311.

Cohen, S., Fisher, B., Yoshida, T., and Bettigole, R., 1974, Serum-migration inhibitory activity in patients with lymphoproliferative diseases, *N. Engl. J. Med.* **290**:882.

Cone, L., and Uhr, J. W., 1964, Immunological deficiency disorders associated with chronic lymphocytic leukemia and multiple myeloma, *J. Clin. Invest.* **43**:2241.

Cotropia, J. P., Gutterman, J. U., Hersh, E. M., Granatek, C. H., and Mavligit, G. M., 1976, Antigen expression and cell surface properties of human leukemic blasts, *Ann. N. Y. Acad. Sci.* **276**:146.

Cwynarski, M. T., and Cohen, S., 1971, Polyclonal immunoglobulin deficiency in myelomatosis and macroglobulinemia, *Clin. Exp. Immunol.* **8**:237.

Davis, A. T., Brunning, R. D., and Quie, P. G., 1971, Polymorphonuclear leukocyte myeloperoxidase deficiency in a patient with myelomonocytic leukemia, *N. Engl. J. Med.* **285**:789.

Drusin, L. M., Litwin, S. D., Armstrong, D., and Webster, B. P., 1974, Waldenström's macroglobulinemia in a patient with a chronic biologic false-positive serologic test for syphilis, *Am. J. Med.* **56**:429.

559

IMMUNO-
DEFICIENCY STATES
ASSOCIATED WITH
ACUTE LEUKEMIAS,
MULTIPLE
MYELOMA, AND
WALDENSTRÖM'S
MACRO-
GLOBULINEMIA

Dupuy, J. M., Kourilsky, F. M., Fradelizzi, D., Feingold, N., Jacquillat, C., Bernard, J., and Dausset, J., 1971, Depression of immunologic reactivity of patients with acute leukemia, *Cancer* **27**:323.

Edelman, G. M., 1973, Antibody structure and molecular immunology, *Science* **180**:830.

Eisen, H. N., Michaelides, M. C., Underdown, B. J., Schulenburg, E. P., and Simms, E. S., 1970, Myeloma proteins with antihapten antibody activity, *Fed. Proc. Fed. Am. Soc. Exp. Biol.* **29**:78.

Fahey, J. L., Scoggins, R., Utz, F. P., and Szwed, C. F., 1963, Infection, antibody response and gamma globulin components in multiple myeloma and macroglobulinemia, *Am. J. Med.* **35**:698.

Foy, A., Cauchi, M. N., and Whiteside, M. G., 1975, Non-specific immunological function in acute myeloblastic leukemia, *Pathology* **7**:117.

Fridman, W. H., and Kourilsky, F. M., 1969, Stimulation of lymphocytes by autologous leukemic cells in acute leukaemia, *Nature (London)* **224**:277.

Frommel, D., Good, R. A., and Hong, R., 1969, Immunoglobulin levels and protracted hematopoietic malignancy, *Helv. Paediatr. Acta (Suppl. XIX)* **24**:26.

Fu, S. M., Winchester, R. J., and Kunkel, H. G., 1975, The occurrence of the HL-B alloantigens on the cells of unclassified acute lymphoplastic leukemias, *J. Exp. Med.* **142**:1334.

Gabrielsen, A. E., and Good, R. A., 1967, Chemical suppression of adaptive immunity, *Adv. Immunol.* **6**:91.

Garay, G. E., Pavlovsky, S., Sasiain, M. C., Pizzolato, M. A., Binsztein, N., and Eppinger-Helft, M., 1976, Immunocompetence and prognosis in children with acute lymphoblastic leukemia: Combination of two different maintenance therapies, *Med. Pediatr. Oncol.* **2**:403.

Gatti, R. A., and Good, R. A., 1971, Occurrence of malignancy in immuno-deficiency diseases, *Cancer* **28**:89.

Germuth, F. G., Jr., 1956, Role of adrenocortical steroids in infection, immunity and hypersensitivity, *Pharmacol. Rev.* **8**:1.

Gershwin, M. E., and Steinberg, A. D., 1973, Loss of supressor function as a cause of lymphoid malignancy, *Lancet* **2**:1174.

Glenchur, H., Zinneman, H. H., and Briggs, D. R., 1958, Macroglobulinemia: Report of two cases, *Ann. Intern. Med.* **48**:1055.

Glenchur, H., Zinneman, H. H., and Hall, W. H., 1959, A review of fifty-one cases of multiple myeloma: Emphasis on pneumonia and other infections as complications, *Arch. Intern. Med.* **103**:173.

Glovsky, M., and Fudenberg, H. H., 1970, Reduced complement activity in sera of patients with Waldenström's macroglobulinemia, *J. Immunol.* **104**:1072.

Goldman, J. M., and Catovsky, D., 1972, The function of the phagocytic leucocytes in leukemia, *Br. J. Haematol.* **23**(Suppl.):223.

Goldman, J. M., and Th'ng, K. H., 1973, Phagocytic function of leucocytes from patients with acute myeloid and chronic granulocytic leukemia, *Br. J. Haematol.* **25**:299.

Gooch, W. M., and Fernbach, D. J., 1971, Immunoglobulins during the course of acute leukemia in children, *Cancer* **28**:984.

Good, R. A., 1957, Morphological basis of the immune response and hypersensitivity, in: *Host–Parasite Relationships in Living Cells* (H. Felton, ed.), p. 68, Charles C. Thomas, Springfield, Illinois.

Good, R. A., and Finstad, J., 1968, The development and involution of the lymphoid system and immunologic capacity, *Trans. Am. Clin. Climatol. Assoc.* **79**:69.

Good, R. A., Kelly, W. D., Rotstein, J., and Varco, R. L., 1962, Immunologic deficiency diseases, *Prog. Allergy* **6**:187.

Graham-Pole, J., Willoughby, M. L. N., Aitken, S., and Ferguson, A., 1975, Immune status of children with and without severe infection during remission of malignant disease, *Br. Med. J.* **2**:467.

Green, A. A., and Borella, L., 1973, Immunologic rebound after cessation of long term chemotherapy in acute leukemia. II. *In vitro* response to phytohemagglutinin and antigens by peripheral blood and bone marrow lymphocytes, *Blood* **42**:99.

Greene, W. H., Schimpff, S. C., and Wiernick, P. H., 1974, Cell-mediated immunity in acute nonlymphocytic leukemia: Relationship to host factors, therapy, and prognosis, *Blood* **43**:1.

Groch, G. S., Perillie, P. E., and Finch, S. C., 1965, Reticuloendothelial phagocytic function in patients with leukemia and multiple myeloma, *Blood* **26**:489.

Gutterman, J. U., Hersh, E. M., McCredie, K. B., Bodey, G. P., Sr., Rodriguez, V., and Freirich, R. J., 1972, Lymphocyte blastogenesis to human leukemia cells and their relationship to serum factors, immunocompetence and prognosis, *Cancer Res.* **32**:2524.

Gutterman, J. U., Hersh, E. M., Mavligit, G. M., Freirich, E. J., Rossen, R. D., Butler, W. T.,

McCredie, K. B., Bodey, G. P., and Rodriguez, V., 1973a, Cell mediated and humoral immune response to acute leukemia cells and soluble leukemia antigen—Relationship to immunocompetence and prognosis, *Natl. Cancer Inst. Monogr.* **37**:153.

Gutterman, J. U., Rossen, R. D., Butler, W. T., McCredie, K. B., Bodey, G. P., Freirich, E. J., and Hersh, E. M., 1973b, Immunoglobulin on tumor cells and tumor induced lymphocyte blastogenesis in human acute leukemia, *N. Engl. J. Med.* **288**:169.

Gutterman, J. U., Mavligit, G., Burgess, M. A., McCredie, K. B., Hunter, C., Freirich, E. J., and Hersh, E. M., 1974, Immunodiagnosis of acute leukemia—Detection of residual disease, *J. Natl. Cancer Inst.* **53**:389.

Halterman, R. H., and Leventhal, B. G., 1971, Enhanced immune response to leukemia, *Lancet* **2**:704.

Hann, H. W. L., London, W. T., Sutnick, A. I., Blumberg, B. S., Lustbader, E., Carim, H. M., Evans, A. E., Kay, H. E. M., and MacLennan, I. C. M., 1975, Studies of parents of children with acute leukemia, *J. Natl. Cancer Inst.* **54**:1299.

Harris, J. E., Alexanian, R., Hersh, E. M., and Migliore, P., 1969, Abnormal immune response to keyhole limpet hemocyanin with multiple myeloma, *Ann. Intern. Med.* **70**:1084.

Harris, J. E., Alexanian, R., Hersh, E. M., and Migliore, P., 1971, Immune function in multiple myeloma: Impaired responsiveness to keyhole limpet hemocyanin, *Can. Med. Assoc. J.* **104**:389.

Harris, R., 1973, Leukemia antigens and immunity in man, *Nature (London)* **241**:95.

Heath, R. B., Fairley, G. H., and Malpas, J. S., 1964, Production of antibodies against viruses in leukemia and related diseases, *Br. J. Haematol.* **10**:365.

Hellström, I., Hellström, K. E., and Evans, C. A., 1969, Serum-mediated protection of neoplastic cells from inhibition by lymphocytes immune to their tumor-specific antigens, *Proc. Natl. Acad. Sci. U.S.A.* **62**:362.

Hellström, I., Sjögren, H. O., Warner, G., and Hellström, K. E., 1971, Blocking of cell-mediated tumor immunity by sera from patients with growing neoplasma, *Int. J. Cancer* **7**:226.

Herberman, R. B., Hollinshead, A. C., Alford, T. C., McCoy, J. L., Halterman, R. H., and Leventhal, B. G., 1973, Delayed cutaneous hypersensitivity reactions to extracts of human tumors, *Natl. Cancer Inst. Monogr.* **37**:189.

Hersh, E. M., and Oppenheim, J. J., 1967, Inhibition of *in vitro* lymphocyte transformation during chemotherapy in man, *Cancer Res.* **27**:98.

Hersh, E. M., Bodey, G. P., Nies, B. A., and Freirich, E. J., 1965a, Causes of death in acute leukemia: A ten year study of 414 patients from 1954–1963, *J. Am. Med. Assoc.* **193**:105.

Hersh, E. M., Carbone, P. P., Wong, V. C., and Freirich, E. J., 1965b, Inhibition of the primary immune response in man by antimetabolites, *Cancer Res.* **25**:997.

Hersh, E. M., Carbone, P. P., and Frereich, E. J., 1966, Recovery of immune responsiveness after drug suppression in man, *J. Lab. Clin. Med.* **67**:566.

Hersh, E. M., Curtis, J. E., Harris, J. E., McBride, C., Alexanian, R., and Rossen, R., 1970, Host defense mechanisms in lymphoma and leukemia, in: *Leukemia–Lymphoma,* p. 149, Year Book Medical Publishers, Chicago.

Hersh, E. M., Whitecar, J. P., McCredie, K. B., Bodey, G. P., and Freirich, E. J., 1971, Chemotherapy, immunocompetence, immunosuppression and prognosis in acute leukemia, *N. Engl. J. Med.* **285**:1211.

Hersh, E. M., Gutterman, J. U., Mavligit, G. M., McCredie, K. B., Burgess, M. A., Matthews, A., and Freirich, E. J., 1974, Serial studies of immunocompetence of patients undergoing chemotherapy for acute leukemia, *J. Clin. Invest.* **54**:401.

Hitchings, G. H., and Elion, G. B., 1963, Chemical supression of the immune response, *Pharmacol. Rev.* **15**:365.

Hobbs, J. R., 1968, Secondary antibody deficiency, *Proc. R. Soc. Med.* **61**:883.

Holland, J. F., Senn, H., and Banerjee, T., 1971, Kinetic and comparative studies on localized leukocyte mobilization in acute leukemia, *Blood* **37**:499.

Hughes, W. T., and Smith, D. R., 1973, Infection during induction of remission in acute lymphocyte leukemia, *Cancer* **31**:1008.

Humphrey, G. B., Nesbit, M. E., Chary, K. K. N., and Krivit, W., 1972, Impaired lymphocyte transformation in leukemic patients after intensive therapy, *Cancer* **29**:402.

Humphrey, G. B., Peterson, L., Whalen, M., Parker, D. E., Lankford, J., Krivit, W., and Nesbit, M., 1975, Lymphocyte transformation in leukemic serum, *Cancer* **35**:1341.

561

IMMUNO-
DEFICIENCY STATES
ASSOCIATED WITH
ACUTE LEUKEMIAS,
MULTIPLE
MYELOMA, AND
WALDENSTRÖM'S
MACRO-
GLOBULINEMIA

Hurez, D., Preud'homme, J.-L., and Seligmann, M., 1970, Intracellular "monoclonal" immunoglobulins in non-secretory human myeloma, *J. Immunol.* **104**:263.

Imhof, J. W., Baars, H., and Verloop, M. D., 1959, Clinical and hematological aspects of macroglobuli-nemia Waldenström, *Acta Med. Scand.* **163**:349.

Jaffe, E. S., Braylan, R. C., Frank, M. M., Green, I., and Berard, C. W., 1976, Heterogeneity of immunologic markers and surface morphology in "childhood lymphoblastic lymphoma," *Blood* **48**:213.

Jenkins, E. C., 1972, Waldenström's macroglobulinemia and phytohaemagglutinin response, *Lancet* **2**:437.

Jones, S. V., and McFarlane, H., 1975, T and B cells in myelomatosis, *Br. J. Haematol.* **31**:545.

Jungi, W. F., Rhomberg, W. V., and Peters, W., 1971, Influence of corticosteroids on granulocyte function: Therapeutic implications, *Schweiz. Med. Wochenschr.* **101**:1790.

Kersey, J., Nesbit, M., Hallgreen, H., Sabad, A., Yunis, E., and Gajl-Peczalska, K., 1975, Evidence for origin of certain childhood acute lymphoblastic leukemias and lymphomas in thymus derived lymphocytes, *Cancer* **36**:1348.

Kiran, O., and Gross, S., 1969, The G-immunoglobulins in acute leukemia in children: Hematologic and immunologic relationships, *Blood* **33**:198.

Knapp, W., Schuit, R. E., Bolhuis, R. L. H., and Hijmans, W., 1974, Surface immunoglobulins in chronic lymphatic leukemia, macroglobulinemia and myelomatosis, *Clin. Exp. Immunol.* **16**:541.

Kohler, P. F., and Müller-Eberhard, H. J., 1969, Complement–immunoglobulin relation: Deficiency of C'1q associated with impaired immunoglobulin G synthesis, *Science* **163**:474.

Kourilsky, F. M., Lovric, L., and Levacher, A., 1966, Phytohemagglutinin and lympocytes from acute leukemia, *Lancet* **2**:856.

Krajny, M., and Pruzanski, W., 1976, Waldenström's macroglobulinemia: Review of 45 cases, *Can. Med. Assoc. J.* **114**:899.

Kunkel, H. G., Slater, R. J., and Good, R. A., 1951, Relation between certain myeloma proteins and normal gamma globulins, *Proc. Soc. Exp. Biol. Med.* **76**:190.

LaPlante, E. S., Condie, R. M., and Good, R. A., 1962, Prevention of the secondary immune response with 6-mercaptopurine, *J. Lab. Clin. Med.* **59**:542.

Larson, D. L., and Tomlinson, L. J., 1953, Quantitative antibody studies in man. III. Antibody response in leukemia and other malignant lymphomas, *J. Clin. Invest.* **32**:317.

Lawson, H. A., Stuart, C. A., Paull, A. M., Philips, A. M., and Philips, R. W., 1955, Observations on the antibody content of the blood in patients with multiple myeloma, *N. Engl. J. Med.* **252**:13.

Lehrer, R. I., and Cline, M. J., 1971, Leukocyte candidacidal activity and resistance to systemic candidiasis in patients with cancer, *Cancer* **27**:1211.

Leventhal, B. G., Halterman, R. H., Rosenberg, E. B., and Herberman, R. B., 1972, Immune reactivity of leukemia patients to autologous blast cells, *Cancer Res.* **32**:1820.

Leventhal, B. G., Leung, E., and Johnson, G. E., 1976, E-rosette forming lymphoblasts fail to stimulate allogeneic donors in mixed leukocyte culture (MLC), *Proc. Am. Soc. Clin. Oncol.* **17**:271.

Levine, A. S., Graw, R. S., and Young, R. C., 1972, Management of infections in patients with leukemia and lymphoma: Current concept and experimental approaches, *Semin. Hematol.* **9**:141.

Lindström, F. D., Hardy, W. R., Eberle, B. J., and Williams, R. C., 1973, Multiple myeloma and benign monoclonal gammopathy: Differentiation by immunofluorescence of lymphocytes, *Ann. Intern. Med.* **78**:837.

Linton, A. L., Dunnigan, M. G., and Thomson, J. A., 1963, Immune responses in myeloma, *Br. Med. J.* **2**:86.

Mannick, J. A., and Egdahl, R. H., 1968, Endocrinologic agents, in: *Human Transplantation* (F. T. Rapaport and J. Dausset, eds.), Vol. 29, p. 472, Grune & Stratton, New York.

Marks, J., 1953, Antibody formation in myelomatosis, *J. Clin. Pathol.* **6**:62.

Marmont, A. M., and Damasio, E. E., 1971, B-lymphocytes in macroglobulinaemia, *Lancet* **2**:1326.

Mathé, G., 1971, Active immunotherapy, *Adv. Cancer Res.* **14**:1.

McCaffrey, R., Smoler, D. F., Parkmann, R., and Baltimore, D., 1975, Terminal deoxynucleotidyl transferase activity in human leukemic cells and in normal human thymocytes, *N. Engl. J. Med.* **292**:775.

McKelvey, E. M., and Carbone, P. P., 1965, Serum immune globulin concentrations in acute leukemia during intensive chemotherapy, *Cancer* **18**:1292.

McKelvey, E. M., and Fahey, J. L., 1965, Immunoglobulin changes in disease: Quantitation on the basis of heavy polypeptide chains, IgG (gamma G), IgA (gamma A), and IgM (gamma M), and of light polypeptide chains type K (I) and type L (II), *J. Clin. Invest.* **44**:1178.

Mellstedt, H., and Holm, G., 1973, *In vitro* studies of lymphocytes from patients with plasma cell myeloma. I. Stimulation by mitogens and cytotoxic activities, *Clin. Exp. Immunol.* **15**:309.

Mellstedt, H., Jondal, M., and Holm, G., 1973, *In vitro* studies of lymphocytes from patients with plasma cell myeloma. II. Characterization by cell surface markers, *Clin. Exp. Immunol.* **15**:321.

Mellstedt, H., Hammarström, S., and Holm, G., 1974, Monoclonal lymphocyte population in human plasma cell myeloma, *Clin. Exp. Immunol.* **17**:371.

Metzger, H., 1969, Myeloma proteins and antibodies, *Am. J. Med.* **47**:837.

Meyers, B. R., Hirschman, S. Z., and Axelrod, J. A., 1972, Current patterns of infection in multiple myeloma, *Am. J. Med.* **52**:87.

Miller, D. G., 1962, Patterns of immunological deficiency in lymphomas and leukemias, *Ann. Intern. Med.* **57**:703.

Miller, D. R., and Kaplan, H. G., 1970, Decreased nitroblue tetrazolium dye reduction in the phagocytes of patients receiving prednisone, *Pediatrics* **45**:861.

Mitchell, M. S., Wade, M. E., DeConti, R. C., Bertino, J. R., and Calabresi, P., 1969, Immunosuppressive effects of cytosine arabinoside and methotrexate in man, *Ann. Int. Med.* **70**:535.

Nir, E., Efrati, P., and Danon, D., 1970, The osmotic fragility of human leucocytes in normal and in some pathological conditions, *Br. J. Haematol.* **18**:237.

Oren, M. E., and Herberman, R. B., 1971, Delayed cutaneous hypersensitivity reactions to membrane extracts of human tumor cells, *Clin. Exp. Immunol.* **9**:45.

Osterland, C. K., and Espinoza, L. R., 1975, Biological properties of myeloma proteins, *Arch. Intern. Med.* **135**:32.

Pachter, M. R., and Havey, Q. G., 1962, Antibody deficiency in macroglobulinemia, *Am. J. Clin. Pathol.* **37**:248.

Page, A. R., Condie, R. M., and Good, R. A., 1962a, Effect of 6-mercaptopurine on inflammation, *Am. J. Pathol.* **40**:519.

Page, A. R., Condie, R. M., and Good, R. A., 1962b, Clinical studies on the anti-inflammatory activity of 6-mercaptopurine, *Blood* **20**:118.

Page, A. R., Condie, R. M., and Good, R. A., 1964, Suppression of plasma cell hepatitis with 6-mercaptopurine, *Am. J. Med.* **36**:200.

Penny, R., and Galton, D. A. G., 1966, Studies on neutrophil function. II. Pathological aspects, *Br. J. Haematol.* **12**:633.

Perillie, P. E., and Finch, S. C., 1960, The local exudative cellular response in leukemia, *J. Clin. Invest.* **39**:1353.

Perillie, P. E., and Finch, S. C., 1964, Quantitative studies of the local exudative cellular reaction in acute leukemia, *J. Clin. Invest.* **43**:425.

Peters, W. P., Holland, J. F., Senn, H., Rhomberg, W., and Banerjee, T., 1972, Corticosteroid administration and localized leukocyte mobilization in man, *N. Engl. J. Med.* **286**:342.

Pickering, L. K., Anderson, D. C., Choi, S., and Feigin, R. D., 1975, Leukocyte function in children with malignancies, *Cancer* **35**:1365.

Pitts, N. C., and McDuffie, F. C., 1967, Defective synthesis of IgM antibodies in macroglobulinemia, *Blood* **30**:767.

Porter, R. R., 1973, Structural studies of immunoglobulins, *Science* **180**:713.

Potter, M., 1971, Myeloma proteins (M-components) with antibody-like activity, *N. Engl. J. Med.* **284**:831.

Powles, R. L., Balchin, L. A., Hamilton Fairley, G., and Alexander, P., 1971, Recognition of leukemia cells as foreign before and after autoimmunization, *Br. Med. J.* **1**:486.

Prehn, R., 1972, The immune reaction as a stimulator of tumor growth, *Science* **176**:170.

Preud'homme, J. L., and Seligmann, M., 1972, Immunoglobulins on the surface of lymphoid cells in Waldenström's macroglobulinemia, *J. Clin. Invest.* **51**:701.

Pruzanski, W., Leers, W.-D., and Wardlaw, A., 1973, Bactericidal and bacteriolytic activity of leukemic sera, *Cancer Res.* **33**:2048.

Ragab, A. H., Lindquist, J., Vietti, T. J., Choi, S. C., and Osterland, C. K., 1970, Immunoglobulin pattern in childhood leukemia, *Cancer* **26**:890.

563

IMMUNO-
DEFICIENCY STATES
ASSOCIATED WITH
ACUTE LEUKEMIAS,
MULTIPLE
MYELOMA, AND
WALDENSTRÖM'S
MACRO-
GLOBULINEMIA

Rebuck, J. W., and Crowley, J. H., 1955, A method of studying leukocyte function *in vivo, Ann. N. Y. Acad. Sci.* **59**:757.

Rosenberg, E. B., Herberman, R. B., Levine, P. H., Halterman, R. H., Meloy, J. L., and Wunderlich, J. R., 1972, Lymphocyte cytotoxicity reactions to leukemia associated antigens in identical twins, *Int. J. Cancer* **9**:648.

Rosenberg, S., and Calabresi, P., 1963, Enhanced suppression of the secondary immune response by combination of 6-mercaptopurine "Duazomycin A," *Nature (London)* **199**:1101.

Rosner, F., Valmont, I., Kozinn, P. J., and Caroline, L., 1970, Leukocyte function in patients with leukemia, *Cancer* **25**:835.

Sacks, K. L., Olweny, C., Mann, D. L., Simon, R., Johnson, G. E., Poplack, D. G., and Leventhal, B. G., 1975, A clinical trial of chemotherapy and RAJI immunotherapy in advanced acute lymphatic leukemia, *Cancer Res.* **35**:3715.

Salmon, S. E., 1973, Immunoglobulin synthesis and tumor kinetics of myeloma, *Semin. Hematol.* **10**:135.

Salmon, S. E., and Fudenberg, H. H., 1969, Abnormal nucleic acid metabolism of lymphocytes in plasma cell myeloma and macroglobulinemia, *Blood* **33**:300.

Salmon, S. E., Samal, B. A., Hayes, D. M., Hosley, H., Miller, S. P., and Schilling, A., 1967, Role of gamma globulin for immunoprophylaxis in multiple myeloma, *N. Engl. J. Med.* **277**:1336.

Samoilova, R. S., Bulicheva, T. I., and Skurkovich, S. V., 1975, Immunoglobulins on the surface of blast cells in human acute leukemia, *Blood* **46**:443.

Santos, G. W., Owens, A. H., and Sensenbrenner, L. L., 1964, Effects of selected cytotoxic agents on antibody production in man: A preliminary report, *Ann. N. Y. Acad. Sci.* **114**:404.

Santos, G. W., Mullins, G. M., Bias, W. B., Anderson, P. N., Graziano, K. D., Klein, D. L., and Burke, P. J., 1973, Immunologic studies in acute leukemia, *Natl. Cancer Inst. Monogr.* **37**:69.

Sbarra, A. J., Shirley, W., Selvaraj, R. J., Ouchi, E., and Rosenbaum, E., 1964, The role of the phagocyte in host–parasite interactions. I. The phagocytic capabilities of leukocytes from lympho-proliferative disorders, *Cancer Res.* **24**:1958.

Sbarra, A. J., Shirley, W., Selvaraj, R. J., McRipley, R. J., and Rosenbaum, E., 1965, The role of the phagocyte in host–parasite interactions. III. The phagocytic capabilities of leukocytes from myelo-proliferative and other neoplastic disorders, *Cancer Res.* **25**:1199.

Schwartz, R. S., 1968, Immunosuppressive drug therapy, in: *Human Transplantation* (F. T. Rapaport and J. Dausset, eds.) Vol. 28, p. 440, Grune & Stratton, New York.

Schwartz, R., Stack, J., and Damashek, W., 1958, Effect of 6-mercaptopurine on antibody production, *Proc. Soc. Exp. Biol. Med.* **99**:164.

Schwartz, R., Eisner, A., and Damashek, W., 1959, The effect of 6-mercaptopurine on primary and secondary immune responses, *J. Clin. Invest.* **38**:1394.

Seligmann, M., Danon, F., and Mihaesco, C., 1967, Immunoglobulin abnormalities in families of patients with Waldenström's macroglobulinemia, *Am. J. Med.* **43**:66.

Selvaraj, R. J., McRipley, R. J., and Sbarra, A. J., 1967, The metabolic activities of leukocytes from lymphoproliferative and myeloproliferative disorders during phagocytosis, *Cancer Res.* **27**:2287.

Sen, L., and Borella, L., 1973, Expression of cell surface markers on T- and B-lymphocytes after long-term chemotherapy of acute leukemia, *Cell. Immunol.* **9**:84.

Sen, L., and Borella, L., 1975, Clinical importance of lymphoblasts with T markers in childhood acute leukemia, *N. Engl. J. Med.* **292**:828.

Silver, R. T., Beal, G., Schneiderman, M., and McCullough, N., 1957, The role of the mature neutrophil in bacterial infections in acute leukemia, *Blood* **12**:814.

Silver, R. T., Utz, J. P., Fahey, J., and Frei, E., III, 1960, Antibody response in patients with acute leukemia, *J. Lab. Clin. Med.* **56**:634.

Sjögren, H. O., Hellström, I., Bansal, S. C., and Hellström, K. E., 1971, Suggestive evidence that the "blocking antibodies" of tumour-bearing individuals may be antigen–antibody complexes, *Proc. Nat. Acad. Sci. U.S.A.* **68**:1372.

Skeel, R. T., Yankee, R. A., and Henderson, E. S., 1971, Hexose monophosphate shunt activity of circulating phagocytes in acute lymphocytic leukemia, *J. Lab. Clin. Med.* **77**:975.

Slater, R. J., Ward, S. M., and Kunkel, H. G., 1955, Immunological relationships among the myeloma proteins, *J. Exp. Med.* **101**:85.

Snyder, A. L., Henderson, E. S., Li, F. P., and Todaro, G. J., 1970, Possible inherited leukemogenic factors in familial acute myelogenous leukemia, *Lancet* **1**:586.

Solomon, A., Waldmann, T. A., and Fahey, J. L., 1963, Metabolism of normal 6.6S γ-globulin in normal subjects and in patients with macroglobulinemia and multiple myeloma, *J. Lab. Clin. Med.* **62**:1.

Southam, C. M., and Siegel, A. H., 1966, Serum levels of second component of complement in cancer patients, *J. Immunol.* **97**:331.

Sterzl, J., 1960, Inhibition of the induction phase of antibody formation by 6-mercaptopurine examined by the transfer of isolated cells, *Nature (London)* **185**:256.

Stjernholm, R. L., Dimitrov, N. V., and Zito, S., 1970, Carbohydrate metabolism in leukocytes. XIII. Differentiation by metabolism of leukemic leukocytes into three groups, *J. Reticuloendothel. Soc.* **7**:539.

Strauss, R. R., Paul, B. B., Jacobs, A. A., Simmons, C., and Sbarra, A. J., 1970, The metabolic and phagocytic activities of leukocytes from children with acute leukemia, *Cancer Res.* **30**:480.

Sutherland, R. M., Inch, W. R., and McCredie, J. A., 1971, Phytohemagglutinin (PHA)-induced transformation of lymphocytes from patients with cancer, *Cancer* **27**:574.

Sutton, R. N. P., Bishun, N. P., and Soothill, J. F., 1969, Immunological and chromosomal studies in first-degree relatives of children with acute lymphoblastic leukemia, *Br. J. Haematol.* **17**:113.

Sutton, W. R., Griffith, H. B., and Preston, F. W., 1962, Effect of cancer chemotherapeutic agents on the survival of homografts of skin, *Surg. Forum* **12**:117.

Tan, C. V., Rosner, F., and Feldman, F., 1973, Nitroblue tetrazolium dye reduction in various hematologic disorders, *N. Y. State J. Med.* **73**:952.

Thomas, L., 1959, Discussion in: *Cellular and Humoral Aspects of the Hypersensitivity States* (H. S. Lawrence, ed.), p. 529, Hoeber-Harper, New York.

Thompson, J., and Van Furth, R., 1973, The effect of glucocorticosteroids on the proliferation and kinetics of promonocytes and monocytes of the bone marrow, *J. Exp. Med.* **137**:10.

Tornyos, K., 1967, Phagocyte activity of cells of the inflammatory exudate in human leukemia, *Cancer Res.* **27**:1756.

Tsukimoto, I., Wong, K. Y., and Lampkin, B. C., 1976, Surface markers and prognostic factors in acute lymphoblastic leukemia, *N. Engl. J. Med.* **294**:245.

Uphoff, D. E., 1961, Drug-induced immunological "tolerance" for homotransplantation, *Transplant. Bull.* **28**:12.

Viza, D. C., Bernard Degani, O., Bernard, C. L., and Harris, R., 1969, Leukaemia antigens, *Lancet* **2**:493.

Waldenström, J., 1944, Incipient myelomatosis or "essential" hypergammaglobulinemia with fibrinogenopenia—a new syndrome?, *Acta Med. Scand.* **117**:216.

Waldenström, J., 1962, Hypergammaglobulinemia as a clinical hematological problem: A study in the gammopathies, *Science* **148**:266.

Walker, J. S., Davis, D., Davies, P., Freeman, C. B., and Harris, R., 1973, Immunological studies in acute myeloid leukemia: PHA responsiveness and serum inhibitory factors, *Br. J. Cancer* **27**:203.

Warner, N. L., Mackenzie, M. R., and Fudenberg, H., 1971, Anti-antibody activity of a monoclonal macroglobulin, *Proc. Natl. Acad. Sci. U.S.A.* **68**:2846.

Yoo, T. J., and Franklin, E. C., 1971, Lack of antibody activity in human myeloma proteins, *J. Immunol.* **107**:365.

Zinneman, H. H., and Hall, W. H., 1954, Recurrent pneumonia in multiple myeloma and some observations on immunologic response, *Ann. Intern. Med.* **41**:1152.

Zolla, S., 1972, The effect of plasma cytomas on the immune response of mice, *J. Immunol.* **108**:1039.

Zusman, J., Nesbit, M., and Rundles, W., 1975, Abnormal lymphocyte function in acute lymphatic leukemia (ALL): Prognostic implications, *Proc. Am. Assoc. Cancer Res.* **16**:175.

Zweiman, B., 1973, Immunosuppression by thiopurines, *Transplant. Proc.* **5**:1197.

19

Immunodeficiencies Associated with Chronic Lymphocytic Leukemia and Non-Hodgkin's Lymphomas

SUDHIR GUPTA and ROBERT A. GOOD

1. Introduction

Chronic lymphocytic leukemia and non-Hodgkin's lymphomas represent a malignant proliferation of immunocytes. They are commonly associated with a variety of immune deficiency states. Some of these immune abnormalities are as characteristic as are hemodynamic disturbances in cardiac disorders. Since a classic immune response (comprised of afferent, central, and efferent limbs) involves humoral immunity, cellular immunity, phagocytic cell system, and amplifying systems (e.g., the complement system), an attempt is made to discuss the immune deficiencies associated with each of these disorders under these four broad categories.

2. Chronic Lymphocytic Leukemia

Patients with chronic lymphocytic leukemia (CLL) possess two distinct populations of lymphocytes (Hersh *et al.*, 1971). The first consists of normal T and B lymphocytes. The second population is that of leukemic cells, usually of B-cell type; however, a few cases of T-cell leukemia (Insel *et al.*, 1975; Yadoi *et al.*, 1974) and cases in which the leukemic cells have markers for both T- and B-cell type (Shevach *et al.*, 1974; Chiao *et al.*, 1975) have been reported. The leukemic cells most often carry surface immunoglobulin (Foulis *et al.*, 1973, Dickler *et al.*, 1973, Gupta *et al.*, 1976b), albeit in lower density than do normal B cells. They usually

SUDHIR GUPTA and ROBERT A. GOOD • Memorial Sloan-Kettering Cancer Center, New York, New York 10021.

SUDHIR GUPTA AND
ROBERT A. GOOD

form spontaneous rosettes with mouse erythrocytes (Stathopoulos and Elliott, 1974; Gupta and Grieco, 1975; Gupta *et al.*, 1976b), a marker for a subset of human B cells (Gupta *et al.*, 1975, 1976a). The leukemic B cells, however, are incapable of normal immune functions. It is the accumulation of such cells that in some way as yet unclear leads to the impaired adaptive immunity involving the normal lymphocyte population that results in the immunodeficiency often found in CLL.

2.1. Humoral Immunity

2.1.1. Serum Immunoglobulins

Deficiency in the amount of serum immunoglobulins (Ig) is fairly commonly observed in patients with CLL. Agammaglobulinemia and hypogammaglobulinemia are present in 35–50% of cases (Cone and Uhr, 1964; Harris and Bagai, 1972; Miller and Karnofsky, 1961; Hudson and Wilson, 1957; Prasad, 1958; Boggs and Fahey, 1960; Jim and Reinhard, 1956). The immunoelectrophoretic analysis of serum from these patients has demonstrated that serum IgM and IgA levels are more commonly reduced than are the levels of IgG (Leoncini *et al.*, 1968; Miller, 1962; Miller and Karnofsky, 1961; Cone and Uhr, 1964; Shaw *et al.*, 1960; Petermann *et al.*, 1948). The presence of hypogammaglobulinemia usually reflects a widely disseminated disease of long duration, relatively resistant to chemotherapy and associated with a poor prognosis. The hypogammaglobulinemia is not the result of chemotherapy, since many untreated patients develop hypogammaglobulinemia that varies in severity. Ultman *et al.* (1959) found that patients with CLL who do not have hypogammaglobulinemia survive twice as long as do patients with hypogammaglobulinemia. A low γ-globulin level has always been irreversible in this disease; Creyssel *et al.* (1958) referred to it as *signe permanent notices*. Hypogammaglobulinemia correlates with an increased frequency of bacterial infections (Shaw *et al.*, 1960; Miller and Karnofsky, 1961). Pisciotta *et al.* (1960) found that ^{131}I-labeled IgG γ-globulin had a normal half-life in a patient with CLL. In contradistinction to the situation with certain primary immunodeficiency diseases and myeloma, no one has yet reported that the hypogammaglobulinemia associated with CLL is secondary to increased "suppressor" activity of circulating leukocytes. It is therefore likely that hypogammaglobulinemia of CLL is due primarily to a failure of synthesis of γ-globulin by the B cells and plasma cells (Gamble and Cutting, 1966), rather than being secondary to increased catabolism of γ-globulin or alteration in the activity of regulatory T or adherent phagocytic cells. This relationship is likely a consequence of diminution in the numbers of normal B lymphocytes and consequent decrease in numbers of plasma cells, but its true basis is not clear.

2.1.2. Specific Antibody Formation

Many studies on the ability of patients with CLL to form specific circulating antibodies have been carried out. Usually, these patients are poor producers of specific antibodies. An absence of or marked decrease in isohemagglutinins is a common feature in CLL, but rather surprisingly Miller and Karnofsky (1961) found no correlation between low titers of isohemagglutinins and either the level of γ-

567

IMMUNO-
DEFICIENCIES
ASSOCIATED WITH
CHRONIC
LYMPHOCYTIC
LEUKEMIA AND
NON-HODGKIN'S
LYMPHOMAS

globulin or the history of susceptibility to infection. A poor response to immunization with typhoid–paratyphoid A and B vaccine (Miller and Karnofsky, 1961), as well as poor responses to pneumococcal antigens (Hickling and Sutliff, 1928), have been reported. In contrast, low antibody responses to typhoid–paratyphoid antigen appear to correlate well with the frequency of infections in patients with CLL. Antibody responses to mumps, influenza, streptokinase, and diphtheria antigens are also deficient (Howell, 1920; Larson and Tomlinson, 1953; Shaw *et al.*, 1960) and antibody responses to tularemia vaccine are markedly depressed (Saslaw *et al.*, 1961) in patients with CLL. Millian *et al.* (1965) and Heath *et al.* (1964) studied the complement-fixing viral antibody content of the serum of patients with a variety of lymphoproliferative disorders (including CLL). None of these patients had been given viral vaccine before the serum specimens were collected. The patients with CLL were, however, the most deficient in antibody content of any of the groups studied. Southam *et al.* (1951) found no heterophil antibody in patients with CLL; in contrast, such antibodies are commonly observed in patients with Hodgkin's disease and acute leukemia. Fiddes *et al.* (1972) reported that patients with CLL are poor antibody responders after both primary and secondary immunization. In the latter study, bacteriophage ϕX 174 was used as a primary antigenic stimulus and diphtheria toxoid as an antigen to reveal a secondary immune response in persons previously immunized with this antigen. The kinetics of immune response in CLL (using keyhole limpet hemocyanin as an antigen) seemed to be featured by a prolonged induction time for IgM antibody and by a delayed switchover from IgM and IgG production (Hersh *et al.*, 1970).

2.2. Cellular Immunity

2.2.1. *In Vitro* Lymphocyte Blastogenic Transformation

A decreased proportion of T lymphocytes has been recorded in the peripheral blood from patients with CLL; in patients with high leukocyte counts, however, the absolute number of T cells is usually normal (Oppenheim *et al.*, 1963). The reactivity to mitogens such as concanavalin A (Con A), phytohemagglutinin (PHA), and pokeweed mitogen (PWM), and to staphylococcal filtrate and purified protein derivative (PPD) has regularly been reduced when compared with the reactivity of normal lymphocytes to these stimuli (Blattner *et al.*, 1976; Catovsky *et al.*, 1972a; Froland and Staven, 1972; Libansky, 1969; Konig *et al.*, 1972; Norogrodsky *et al.*, 1972; Pegorara and Gavosto, 1973; Perera and Pegrum, 1974; Rubin *et al.*, 1976; Smith *et al.*, 1973; Utsinger, 1975; Winter *et al.*, 1964; Benezra *et al.*, 1971). Bouroncle *et al.* (1969) reported a long-term follow-up study of the transformation of lymphocytes to PHA in 25 patients with CLL. They observed lymphocyte transformation in culture for 11 consecutive days (in contrast to the conventional 3-day cultures) and demonstrated that the lymphocytes in patients with CLL differ functionally from normal lymphocytes in culture not only in that they are less responsive than normal to PHA stimulation, but also because the response that does occur is delayed. Maximum lymphocyte transformation was seen in cultures after 5–9 days, with an average time to maximal response being 7 days as compared with controls, for which the maximum was observed between 3 and 5 days. Such

SUDHIR GUPTA AND
ROBERT A. GOOD

abnormal response curves were seen in patients with both low and high leukocyte counts. Similar hyporesponsiveness and delayed response have also been reported by other investigators (Catovsky *et al.*, 1972a,b; Froland and Staven, 1972; Holm *et al.*, 1967; Konig *et al.*, 1972). That higher concentrations of PHA do not result in further increase in the lymphocytic transformation suggests that the abnormality is most likely due to a cellular defect; indeed, Bouroncle *et al.* (1969) found that the patients' serum did not exert an inhibitory effect.

Serum inhibitor(s) of blastogenesis have been reported, however, in occasional patients with CLL. Sugden (1974) demonstrated inhibition of PHA response by serum from a patient with CLL. Spengler and Stjernholm (1972) reported the presence in a patient with CLL of a transient heat-stable, complement-independent lymphotoxic serum factor that inhibited the blastogenesis of normal lymphocytes to stimulation with PHA. The appearance of this factor was synchronous with the cycling of leukocyte counts, the presence of the inhibitor being associated with inversion of a period of rising lymphocyte counts to a period of falling counts. Tavadia *et al.* (1974) demonstrated the presence of thermolabile factor in both the sera and the lymphocyte extracts from several patients with CLL. This factor inhibited the transformation of normal lymphocytes with PHA. Utsinger (1975) also reported the presence of a noncytotoxic blastogenic inhibitory factor in the sera of patients with CLL. This inhibitor is not a product of B cells, and inhibited the blastogenesis of normal lymphocytes with PHA and PWM. It therefore appears that in certain patients with CLL, abnormalities of blastogenic response to mitogen may be, in part, secondary to serum- or lymphocyte-derived inhibitors or both. The molecular definition of such factor(s) is yet to be accomplished, but could go far toward defining immunological perturbations in CLL.

Rubin (1971) studied RNA and DNA synthesis in PHA-stimulated lymphocytes from patients with CLL. The high-count CLL cells demonstrated delayed maximal increase in RNA synthesis after PHA stimulation. The addition of leukemic cells to cultures of normal lymphocytes did not retard the development of the normal response to PHA. Similar observations were reported by Havemann and Rubin (1968). Lymphocytes from patients with CLL who had low counts also showed a delayed response to PHA, but the abnormality observed was less marked than that of the high-count group. Impaired responses are commonly seen in patients who have high lymphocyte counts and at the same time have low levels of serum Ig's. There appears to be a defect in the mechanism involved in regulating the assembly of new ribosomes (Rubin, 1971). A failure to conserve 18 S RNA subunits may cause an aborted PHA-induced stimulation of 45 S RNA transcription, leading to an overall delay in RNA synthesis after 48 hr of PHA stimulation. Efficient conservation of 18 S RNA was observed, however, at 168 hr. The imbalance in ribosomal RNA metabolism was considered by Rubin (1971) to be responsible for the feeble and delayed DNA synthesis and proliferation of leukemic lymphocytes in response to PHA. That the increased RNA and DNA synthesis develop in a single wave after PHA stimulation in patients with CLL suggests that mainly one cohort or one population of cells is responding, and that very few circulating lymphocytes respond normally. Autoradiographic studies have demonstrated that the late-reacting lymphocytes in CLL belong to a discrete and abnormal population. The PHA-responsive leukemic lymphocytes yield a RNA isolation pattern different from that of PHA-responsive normal lymphocytes (Deutsch and Norden, 1971). It has been

569

IMMUNO-
DEFICIENCIES
ASSOCIATED WITH
CHRONIC
LYMPHOCYTIC
LEUKEMIA AND
NON-HODGKIN'S
LYMPHOMAS

suggested that the suboptimal and delayed responses observed may be due not only to the failure of leukemic lymphocytes to handle RNA synthesis in the normal way, but also to the presence of increased quantities of glycogen, which may interfere with the metabolic activities of these cells (Sagone *et al.*, 1972).

It has been shown that the peripheral blood lymphocytes from leukemic patients can become highly responsive to mitogen stimulation following splenic or total-body irradiation (Kagan and Johnson, 1967; Astaldi *et al.*, 1968). Leukemic bone marrow lymphocytes are also more reactive to mitogens than are peripheral blood cells. This characteristic could accord with the contention that the abnormal cells accumulate in the peripheral blood because they cannot leave the circulation (Hersh *et al.*, 1971; Stryckmans *et al.*, 1968). Bouroncle *et al.* (1969) observed that patients with CLL receiving Leukaran therapy reach a nearly complete hematological and clinical remission before the capacity for normal blastogenesis reappears. From all these studies, it must be inferred that patients with CLL have a mixed population of lymphocytes. These include neoplastic cells, which may be more sensitive to Leukaran therapy and which are poorly responsive to the plant lectins, and the normal, more responsive cells. As the former are progressively inhibited and then destroyed, the population of normal lymphocytes increases and finally predominates. Algom and Richter (1973), using a bovine serum albumin gradient, demonstrated in peripheral blood of patients with CLL the simultaneous existence of immunocompetent and immunoincompetent populations of lymphocytes. Two of the five fractions of isolated lymphocytes responded normally to PHA, PWM, and Con A, whereas the three other fractions of lymphocytes were essentially inert.

Since it has been suggested that hyporesponsiveness of lymphocytes from patients with CLL may be secondary to dilution of normal T cells by leukemic (B) cells, a number of studies have been done to examine the responses of purified fractions of T and B cells from patients with CLL to a variety of mitogens. Wybran *et al.* (1973) demonstrated normal blastogenesis to PHA and Con A of purified T cells from patients with CLL. Schultz *et al.* (1976) and Utsinger (1975), however, observed depressed and delayed responses of purified T and B lymphocytes to PHA and PWM. A decrease in the number of receptor sites for PHA and Con A has also been found to be a characteristic of leukemic lymphocytes (Norogrodsky *et al.*, 1972; Kornfeld, 1969). Thus, it is apparent that the hyporesponsiveness to phytomitogens observed in CLL cannot be attributed solely to a dilution effect, but rather that it represents a constellation of both cellular and extracellular factors.

Lymphocytes from patients with CLL are also hyporesponsive when stimulated *in vitro* with normal allogeneic leukocytes in mixed leukocyte culture (MLC); however, the capacity of leukemic lymphocytes as stimulators in this assay seemed to be intact (Ruhl *et al.*, 1976; Smith *et al.*, 1973; Pentycross, 1974). This abnormality does not seem to be secondary to a serum factor.

2.2.2. Cytotoxic Activity and Lymphokine Production

Holm *et al.* (1967) and Mellstedt and Pettersson (1974) demonstrated that the cytotoxic potential of lymphocytes from patients with CLL is impaired when compared with responses induced in lymphocytes from healthy persons. Perera and Pegrum (1974) found that PWM and Con A are equally ineffective in provoking leukemic lymphocytes to express cytotoxic activity. When leukemic lymphocytes were pretreated with bald nuclear material derived from leukemic lymphocytes treated with PHA, however, a marked cytotoxic effect on Chang liver cells was demonstrated. This response approached in magnitude that produced by normal lymphocytes. Mellstedt and Pettersson (1974) also observed impaired antibody-dependent cytotoxicity by lymphocytes from patients with CLL. This abnormality, however, may be due to a reduced number of or deficient function of the "third population" or so-called "K cells" (Gupta, unpublished).

Normal lymphocytes (predominantly T cells) stimulated with Con A or with allogeneic cells produce leucocyte migration-inhibition factor (LMIF) (Gorski *et al.*, 1975, 1976). When the LMIF production in MLC is studied, it is possible to evaluate the functions of cells for their capacity to stimulate (non-T cells) or respond (T cells) in the LMIF assay. Gorski *et al.* (1977) recently studied the Con-A- and MLC-induced LMIF production by CLL cells, as well as the capacity of lymphocytes of these patients to stimulate production of LMIF by normal cells in MLC. They observed that lymphocytes of 11 of 13 patients stimulated normal LMIF production by normal lymphoid cells. This finding is consonant with the view that production of certain lymphokines is an event independent of proliferation. Epstein and Cline (1974) reported impaired production of interferon by leukemic cells *in vitro* after stimulation with PHA and PWM.

2.2.3. Delayed Cutaneous Hypersensitivity and Allograft Rejection

Delayed hypersensitivity that has been established by known immunization and the ability to develop new delayed hypersensitivity reactions to a variety of antigens (e.g., tuberculin, histoplasmin, candida, mumps, streptokinase) appears to be quite intact in most patients with CLL (Cone and Uhr, 1964; Libansky, 1969; Miller and Karnofsky, 1961; Block *et al.*, 1969; Moayeri *et al.*, 1975). Some patients with CLL, however, cannot readily be sensitized to new antigens, e.g., 2,4-dinitro-1-fluorobenzene (Cone and Uhr, 1964). Delayed hypersensitivity may be transferred to negative reactors by intramuscular or intradermal injections of leukocytes obtained from donors with positive skin reactions. The capacity to reject skin allografts was reported by Miller *et al.* (1961) to be either normal or impaired. No clear correlation between acceptance of skin grafts and serum γ-globulin levels, specific antibody production, or capacity to develop or express delayed skin hypersensitivity was observed prior to treatment.

2.3. Biological Amplification System (Serum Complement)

Miller and Karnofsky (1961) reported normal levels of total hemolytic complement, its four components, and properdin in patients with CLL. No correlation was found with the level of γ-globulin or historical evidence of increased susceptibility to infection. Recently, however, Day *et al.* (1976) reported the presence of circulating immune complexes containing antilymphocyte antibody in a patient with CLL. This abnormality was associated with hypocomplementemia and with recurrent episodes of nonhereditary angioedema. Total hemolytic complement levels in this patient were very low. Immunochemical analysis of complement components showed C1q and C1s inhibitor to be very much decreased and C1r and C1s components to be undetectable. Hemolytic C1, C4, and C2 were less than 5% of

571

IMMUNO-
DEFICIENCIES
ASSOCIATED WITH
CHRONIC
LYMPHOCYTIC
LEUKEMIA AND
NON-HODGKIN'S
LYMPHOMAS

normal, and functional C1s inhibitor was lacking. High serum concentration of cold-reactive antilymphocyte antibody was also demonstrated, and this antibody was present in the cryoglobulin and in the 19 S fraction isolated from the cryoglobulin. Much more work with the newer methods for evaluating serum complement, complement components, circulating antigen–antibody complexes, and evidence of complement activation is needed in this disease. Initial studies indicate that antigen–antibody complement complexes may frequently be present in the serum.

2.4. Phagocytic Cell System

In CLL, the proportion of mature granulocytes in the peripheral blood is usually reduced; the absolute numbers of this class of phagocytic cells, however, are frequently normal. The cellular composition of inflammatory exudates studied at autopsy and studied clinically by the Rebuck skin window technique is also quite normal (Boggs, 1960). Biozzi et al. (1958) found normal phagocytic function of the reticuloendothelial system in patients with CLL from studies using measurement of clearance of denatured ^{131}I-labeled human albumin. In vitro phagocytic and bactericidal activity of leukocytes from patients with CLL, however, has been found to be impaired (Groch et al., 1965; Hirschberg, 1939; Sbarra et al., 1964). This abnormality may be corrected by replacing the serum of leukemic patients with normal serum in the culture system. This finding indicates that the defect observed is probably attributable to an opsonic defect, rather than a specific cellular defect.

2.5. Familial Chronic Lymphocytic Leukemia—Immunological Analysis

Recently, Blattner et al. (1976) studied immunological characteristics in 5 siblings, 4 of whom developed CLL. A familial tendency to CLL has been well documented (Fraumeni et al., 1969). Serum Ig's were usually normal, except that levels at the low range of normal were found for IgM in 3 of the siblings with leukemia. Other family members had normal Ig levels. In this study, all the siblings responded to at least one antigen in delayed cutaneous hypersensitivity testing. In vitro proliferative responses to PHA, Con A, PWM, SK-SD (streptokinase-streptodornase), Candida, tetanus, and allogeneic lymphocytes were abnormal in 4 leukemic siblings. The degree of abnormality paralleled the severity of the disease. Lymphocytes from 1 of these patients responded poorly to PHA and Con A, and those of 2 responded poorly to PWM, specific antigens, and allogeneic cells in MLC. Responses of the lymphocytes of the sibling who was free of leukemia were normal for all antigens studied. Mitogen-induced and antibody-dependent cytotoxicity were markedly impaired in all 4 leukemic siblings and normal in healthy siblings of this family.

2.6. Other Characteristics of Leukemic Cells

2.6.1. Lymphocyte Motility

Schrek (1963), using the slide-incubation method, demonstrated decreased mobility of CLL lymphocytes after 3 days in culture, but this assay did not detect mobility during the first 24 hr.

Recently, Jarvis *et al.* (1976) studied *in vitro* lymphocyte motility of lymphocytes from patients with CLL utilizing a modified Boyden chamber technique. They demonstrated that during short-term cultures, the lymphocytes from patients with CLL are significantly less mobile than are normal lymphocytes. Such motility appears to be a process involving active metabolism, since migration can be markedly inhibited by sodium azide and by decreasing the incubation temperature. Purified normal B cells are more mobile than are T cells and more mobile than combined B and T cells of normal persons. The mobility of CLL cells (B cells in origin) is markedly reduced compared with that of normal lymphocytes. This finding supports the concept that the mobility of CLL cells is intrinsically abnormal. Recently, Goldman *et al.* (1977) reported decreased numbers of mobile lymphocytes in CLL and found this abnormality to be correlated with the number of T lymphocytes.

2.6.2. Intracellular Nucleotides and Enzymes

The role of cyclic nucleotides in regulation of cell proliferation has been extensively investigated. Cyclic AMP (cAMP) inhibits the proliferation of a variety of cells, including human lymphocytes (Hadden *et al.*, 1970; Abell and Monahan, 1973). In earlier studies, the cAMP phosphodiesterase, an enzyme that degrades cAMP to 5'-AMP, of lymphocytes from patients with CLL was reported to be increased (Monahan *et al.*, 1975). This finding raised the possibility that the differences observed may reflect the presence of different proportions of distinct lymphocyte subpopulations. These observations, however, were based on a very small number of patients. Recently, Scher *et al.* (1976) found a slight, although statistically significant, decrease in mean cAMP phosphodiesterase activity in lymphocytes of untreated patients with CLL. The values for patients with treated CLL were intermediate. However, no correlation of cAMP phosphodiesterase levels with the percentages of B- and T- cells or with absolute lymphocyte counts could be ascertained. Their findings suggest that cAMP phosphodiesterase activity *per se* does not account for the low levels of cAMP in leukemic lymphocytes. The substrate saturation patterns are usually identical, providing evidence for similar kinetic behavior. Polgar *et al.* (1973) demonstrated that basal levels of adenylate cyclase are much lower in CLL than in normal lymphocytes; furthermore, the adenylate cyclase is less responsive to hormonal stimulation in leukemic lymphocytes than it is in normal lymphocytes. These findings probably account for low levels of cAMP in lymphocytes of patients with CLL without implicating changes in the concentration of phosphodiesterase.

Tung *et al.* (1976) studied adenosine deaminase (ADA) activity in lymphocytes from patients with CLL. They reported decreased specific activity of ADA in lymphocytes from untreated patients as compared with normals. This enzyme abnormality was not found when ADA concentrations in erythrocytes of patients with CLL and of normals were compared. Activity of diphosphopyridine nucleotide diaphorase is normal and sialyl transferase activity is elevated in lymphocytes of patients with CLL. The diminution of ADA activity is closely related to the increased lymphocyte count. The study of enzymatic activity of purified T and B cells demonstrated that the specific activity of ADA in B cells from CLL patients is significantly lower than that of their T cells and lower even than that of normal B cells. Indeed, the activity in T cells from CLL patients seemed to be significantly

greater than that in T cells from normal blood. This finding is particularly interesting
in light of a finding that high levels of ADA were present in the lymphocytes when
the CLL was of the T-cell variety.

573

IMMUNO-
DEFICIENCIES
ASSOCIATED WITH
CHRONIC
LYMPHOCYTIC
LEUKEMIA AND
NON-HODGKIN'S
LYMPHOMAS

2.6.3. Miscellaneous

Leukemic lymphocytes have cytoplasmic deoxycytidine deaminase, an
enzyme not found in normal lymphocytes (Scholar and Calabresi, 1973). Certain
other characteristics of leukemic cells seem worth mentioning. Leukemic cells from
patients with CLL are more sensitive to colchicine (Thomson and Robinson, 1967)
and α-asparaginase than are normal lymphocytes (Schrek et al., 1967). The CLL
cells also seem to be more resistant to radiation than are normal lymphocytes. They
also possess greater ability to absorb bacteria onto their cell membrane (Selvaraj et
al., 1967). CLL lymphocytes lack the normal capacity to circulate between vascular
and extravascular compartments (Stryckmans et al., 1968). Isoproterenol inhibits
in vitro responses of leukemic lymphocytes to PHA, but does not exert such an
effect on normal lymphocytes (Johnson and Abell, 1970). In comparison with
normal lymphocytes, leukemic lymphocytes consume less glucose and metabolize
less carbohydrate by way of the hexose monophosphate shunt pathway (Brody et
al., 1969) than do normal lymphocytes. Surprisingly, CLL lymphocytes have a
greater capacity to repair DNA damage produced by ultraviolet irradiation or X-
irradiation (Huang et al., 1972) than do normal lymphocytes. The leukemic cells
appear to contain a special DNA-binding protein of 24,000 daltons that appears to
be involved in DNA repair, and this protein is not found in normal lymphocytes
(Huang et al., 1975).

2.7. Associated Diseases

In addition to an increased susceptibility to infection, numerous other consequences of the disturbances of the immune system have been described in patients
suffering from CLL. Second, apparently primary, neoplasms occur more frequently
in patients who suffer from this neoplastic disorder than might be expected by
chance alone (Lawrence and Donald, 1959; Moertel and Hagedorn, 1957). The
increased incidence of tumors applies to tumors of the stomach, lung, and skin
(Lawrence and Donald, 1959). Coombs-positive autoimmune hemolytic anaemia
often occurs in patients with CLL who have greatly reduced Ig levels (Craig et al.,
1952). Allergic vasculitis, systemic lupus erythematosus, cryoglobulinemia, and
autoimmune thrombocytopenia—all of which are diseases or phenomena that
regulate, reflect, and involve circulating antigen–antibody complexes—may also
complicate CLL (Craig et al., 1952; Calabro, 1967; Ebbe et al., 1962). Finally, an
increased incidence of ampicillin hypersensitivity was reported in CLL (Cameron
and Richmond, 1971).

2.8. Summary

In summary, patients with chronic lymphocytic leukemia often develop irreversible hypogammaglobulinemia. This complication is of variable severity, but is
at outset progressive and commonly associated with advanced disease of prolonged
duration that is resistant to therapy and carries a poor prognosis. Hypogammaglob-

ulinemia is due to an inability to synthesize immunoglobulin normally, rather than to increased catabolism or to alterations in any regulatory ("suppressor" or "helper") cell activity. CLL lymphocytes respond slowly and less vigorously than do normal lymphocytes to mitogens, antigens, and allogeneic cells. Production of interferon and certain other lymphokines may be defective. Mitogen-induced cytotoxic potential is impaired. These impaired responses are due mainly to intrinsic defect of the lymphocytes of patients with this disease. In addition, inhibition of proliferative responses has been attributed to inhibitors present in serum or inhibitors derived from lymphocytes. Some immunodeficiencies described in CLL have been attributed simply to dilution of normally responding cells, with the less responsive CLL cells interfering especially with essential cooperative lymphocyte interactions.

Leukemic lymphocytes are strong stimulators in MLC. Delayed cutaneous hypersensitivity is usually intact. Complement components are usually present in normal amounts, and are probably functionally normal. The phagocytic cell system also seems to be quite normal in patients with CLL. Defects of phagocytosis and bactericidal activity that have been encountered in CLL are associated with hypogammaglobulinemia and appear to be secondary to deficiency of opsonins.

3. Non-Hodgkin's Lymphomas

Because of problems of precise staging and lack of generally acceptable histopathological classification, comprehensive and detailed studies of immunodeficiencies associated with non-Hodgkin's lymphomas are not available nearly so readily as they are for CLL and Hodgkin's disease. At the time of diagnosis, the malignant disease is usually already widespread and survival time is often short. As described in Chapters 9 and 10, nodular lymphomas and well-differentiated lymphocytic lymphomas are practically always composed of malignant B lymphocytes. In some cases, poorly differentiated lymphocytic lymphomas are made up of neoplastic T lymphocytes (Lukes and Collins, 1974; Peter *et al.*, 1974; Seligmann, 1974), but here too B-lymphocytic origin is predominant. A group of both nodular and diffuse non-Hodgkin's lymphomas derived from follicular center cells of B-cell origin (Leech *et al.*, 1975; Jaffe *et al.*, 1974) and "null-cell" lymphomas have been described (Brouet *et al.*, 1975). Lymphomas with both T- and non-T-cell characteristics have also been observed (Lukes and Collins, 1974). It is our opinion that these malignancies involve a T cell deviated to malignancy at a stage of its development when it also has certain surface markers that are shared by non-T cells.

3.1. Humoral Immunity

3.1.1. Serum Immunoglobulins

γ-Globulin values ranging from agammaglobulinemia to hypergammaglobulinemia have been observed in patients with lymphosarcoma (Arends *et al.*, 1954). Hypogammaglobulinemia is found in approximately 15% of patients with diseases diagnosed as lymphosarcoma and in 11% of those who have so-called "reticulum-cell sarcomas" (Miller, 1962). It is less frequent in lymphosarcomas than in CLL, but in patients with lymphosarcoma evolving into lymphatic leukemia—the leukolymphosarcoma (B-lymphocyte lymphoma) group—low γ-globulin levels are very common, and the degree of hypogammaglobulinemia is likely to be profound. In lymphomas, as in CLL, a monoclonal gammapathy may sometimes be present (Alexanian, 1974). In addition, cryoglobulinemia has been reported in a number of patients with lymphosarcoma (Miller, 1965).

575

IMMUNO-
DEFICIENCIES
ASSOCIATED WITH
CHRONIC
LYMPHOCYTIC
LEUKEMIA AND
NON-HODGKIN'S
LYMPHOMAS

3.1.2. Specific Antibodies

Primary and secondary antibody responses are usually depressed when studied in non-Hodgkin's solid-tissue lymphomas (Saslaw *et al.*, 1961; Larson and Tomlinson, 1953; Barr and Fairley, 1961). A poor response to immunization with typhoid–paratyphoid A and B vaccine and pneumococcal antigen has been observed in patients carrying the diagnosis of lymphosarcoma (Miller and Karnofsky, 1961; Hickling and Sutliff, 1928). Indeed, only 23.3% of patients with lymphosarcoma and reticulum-cell sarcoma, predominantly B-cell lymphomas, produced significant titers of antibody to tularemia vaccine (Saslaw *et al.*, 1961), in contrast to 94% of normal subjects. Millian *et al.* (1965) reported that antiviral antibody responses in lymphosarcoma and reticulum-cell sarcoma are poorer than those of normals or patients with Hodgkin's disease. These responses, however, were better than in patients with CLL, who are most deficient in viral antibody production. Heath *et al.* (1964) reported depressed antibody response to influenza vaccine. Southam *et al.* (1951) found heterophil antibody titers to be demonstrable in only 1 of 9 patients with lymphosarcoma, whereas demonstrable titers were regularly present in normals. Milgrom *et al.* (1973) demonstrated the presence of heterophile antigen in the splenic lymphocytes of patients with lymphosarcoma and reticulum sarcoma and suggested that the malignant transformation of human lymphocytes in certain patients with lymphoma may be accompanied by acquisition of heterophile antigens. Libansky (1969) reported normal antibody response to streptokinase in the group of patients with reticulum-cell sarcoma that he studied.

3.2. Cellular Immunity

3.2.1. *In Vitro* Lymphocyte Blastogenic Transformation

In cases of lymphosarcoma and reticulum-cell sarcoma, the PHA response of blood lymphocytes may be normal (Astaldi *et al.*, 1968; Twomey and Douglass, 1974) or depressed (Hersh and Irvin, 1969; Ruhl *et al.*, 1976; Noguchi *et al.*, 1976; Mendes *et al.*, 1974). Mavone and Stramignoni (1974) reported normal *in vitro* response of blood lymphocytes to PHA; however, impaired blastogenesis was observed with lymph node lymphocytes from patients with lymphosarcoma. Papac (1970) reported a wide range of PHA responsiveness (normal to markedly depressed) in patients with lymphosarcoma. Depressed PHA responses are most marked in older patients with disease of long duration and in patients with the small-cell type lymphosarcoma. In patients with reticulum-cell sarcoma the PHA response is quite markedly impaired. Depressed PHA responses do not correlate with total number of lymphocytes or T-cell proportions. Sagone *et al.* (1972), studying glucose metabolism, found significantly lower rates of glucose utilization and hexose monophosphate shunt activity in patients with lymphoma with poor

PHA response. In contrast, he observed normal glucose utilization in the group whose cells were responsive to PHA. This defect is similar to that found in lymphocytes from patients with CLL, and suggests that impaired glucose metabolism in CLL is characteristic of the functionally abnormal cells. Hansen *et al.* (1973) observed decreased *in vitro* responses of lymphocytes from patients with solid-tissue non-Hodgkin's lymphomas to PHA, PWM, *Candida albicans, Escherichia coli,* PPD, SK-SD, and *Staphylococcus aureus. In vitro* blastogenesis to normal allogeneic lymphocytes has been reported to be normal (Hansen *et al.,* 1973) or impaired (Ruhl *et al.,* 1976; Twomey and Douglass, 1974; Mendes *et al.,* 1974) in patients of this general group. The stimulator capacity of lymphoma lymphocytes in MLC, however, is usually intact (Ruhl *et al.,* 1976; Hansen *et al.,* 1973; Twomey and Douglass, 1974). The lymphocytes from patients with reticulum-cell sarcoma survive poorly in culture, and a lymphocytotoxic plasma factor may be implicated in this phenomenon.

3.2.2. Delayed Cutaneous Hypersensitivity and Allograft Rejection

Skin tests to a number of ubiquitous antigens are normal in the majority of patients with non-Hodgkin's lymphoma of short duration who have disease localized to one parenchymal organ or to regional lymph nodes. In patients with more widespread disease of long duration who are in poor general health, however, significantly higher frequency of anergy is observed. Lamb *et al.* (1962) found profound anergy in most patients with solid-tissue non-Hodgkin's lymphoma in poor critical condition. Approximately 75% of patients with localized or regional lymphosarcoma or reticulum-cell sarcoma have positive mumps skin test reactions (Sokal and Aungst, 1971). In contrast, only about 20% of those with disseminated disease have positive mumps skin test reactions. In this disease, as in Hodgkin's disease, a good correlation exists between positive skin test reactivity and survival. About 75% of patients with positive mumps skin test reactions were alive 3 years after skin testing, while the majority of those who had negative reactions had died before 3 years. Patients with lymphosarcoma whose reaction converted from negative to positive after vaccination with bacillus Calmette Guérin had a better prognosis than those remaining unresponsive. This correlation, however, did not hold well for reticulum-cell sarcoma. The rejection of skin allografts is usually delayed in patients with either reticulum-cell sarcoma or lymphosarcoma (Miller, 1962; Green and Corso, 1959).

3.3. Phagocytic Cell System

Reticuloendothelial phagocytic functions are normal in most patients with a variety of non-Hodgkin's solid-tissue lymphomas (Groch *et al.,* 1965). Biozzi *et al.* (1958) reported normal or accelerated phagocytic activity in patients with lymphoma and CLL, in contrast to reduced phagocytic indices in a few patients with acute leukemia. Delaloye and Cruchaud (1960) and Groch *et al.* (1965) also observed a reduced phagocytic index in patients with acute leukemia and normal or rapid phagocytosis in those with lymphoma and chronic leukemia. Selvaraj *et al.* (1967) studied metabolic activities of leukocytes from patients with lymphoma. With autologous serum, spontaneous respiration and glucose-1-^{14}C oxidation were both considerably greater than normal, although phagocytic stimulation of these metabolic activities was lower than that observed with normals. Normal serum raised the phagocytic stimulation of glucose-1-^{14}C oxidation to normal limits, causing both a decrease in resting metabolism and an increase in phagocytosis-induced burst of metabolism. Lactate production was similar to that of normals. The resting leukocytes from lymphosarcoma patients demonstrated higher respiratory and glucose-1-^{14}C oxidase activity than that seen in leukocytes of normals. Stimulation of respiration by killed *Staphylococcus albus* particles was slightly higher than with normal cells, but stimulation of the oxidation of glucose-1-^{14}C was considerably lower than normal. Substitution of normal serum for autologous serum had a small inhibitory effect on these metabolic parameters.

577

IMMUNO-
DEFICIENCIES
ASSOCIATED WITH
CHRONIC
LYMPHOCYTIC
LEUKEMIA AND
NON-HODGKIN'S
LYMPHOMAS

3.4. Familial Lymphoreticular Malignancies—An Immunological Analysis

Potolsky *et al.* (1971) studied 4 surviving sibs of a family in which 5 persons died of lymphoreticular neoplasms (3 with lymphoma and 2 with chronic leukemia). All 4 surviving sibs showed clear-cut abnormalities in one or more tests of cellular and humoral immunity. Each had a decreased level of IgG, and showed a significant depression in delayed cutaneous hypersensitivity against a battery of skin tests representing 23 fungal, viral, and bacterial antigens. Of the surviving 4 sibs, 2 had depressed lymphocyte responsiveness to PHA. Lymph node histopathology was abnormal in 2 sibs: one showed dilated lymphatics, small cortex, and absent germinal centers; the other had lymphocytic hyperplasia and a paucity of germinal centers. All 4 sibs had detectable antibody to two or three of five viruses (herpes, adenovirus, cytomegalovirus, measles, and psittacosis virus group) tested. There was no evidence of increased chromosomal breakage. One of these sibs subsequently went on to develop lymphosarcoma. The immunological abnormalities encountered in such a setting may reflect a premalignant state, could well be related to deficiency in dealing with the consequences of a virus infection or exposure to a chemical carcinogen.

3.5. Associated Diseases

The incidence of infectious complications in patients with lymphosarcoma and reticulum-cell sarcoma is higher than normal but only about half as great as that seen in CLL. Bacterial infection, particularly pneumonia, is common (Feld and Bodey, 1975). Cryptococcosis is associated with reticulum-cell sarcoma and lymphosarcoma with a frequency approaching that observed for Hodgkin's disease.

Lymphosarcoma may be associated with systemic lupus erythematosus, rheumatoid arthritis, dermatomyositis, and Sjögren's syndrome (Calabro, 1967). Lymphosarcoma and so-called reticulum-cell sarcomas occur in high incidence in patients with primary immunodeficiencies such as Wiskott–Aldrich syndrome, ataxia–telangiectasia, and common variable immunodeficiency (Gatti and Good, 1971; Kersey *et al.*, 1973, 1975; Spector *et al.*, 1978).

3.6. Summary

In summary, patients with non-Hodgkin's lymphomas often demonstrate impairment of both cellular and humoral immunity that is usually minimal in early stages of localized disease, but becomes more pronounced with progression of the

SUDHIR GUPTA AND
ROBERT A. GOOD

disease. Defects are usually more pronounced in patients with so-called reticulum cell sarcoma than in patients with lymphosarcoma. Depressed *in vitro* blastogenic response to mitogens is accompanied by abnormal glucose metabolism of lymphocytes. Reticuloendothelial phagocytic functions are generally intact. Familial studies demonstrate an apparent genetic relationship between immunological abnormalities and susceptibility to neoplasia of lymphoid tissue.

ACKNOWLEDGMENTS

This investigation was supported by Public Health Service Research Grants CA-1726, CA-08748, CA-17404, AI-11457, and AG-00451 from the National Institutes of Health, by the Zelda R. Weintraub Cancer Fund, by the Judith Harris Selig Memorial Fund, and by the Fund for the Advanced Study of Cancer.

References

Abell, C. W., and Monahan, T. M., 1973, The role of adenosine 3′,5′-cyclic monophosphate in the regulation of mammalian cell division, *J. Cell Biol.* **59**:549–558.

Alexanian, R., 1974, Monoclonal gammopathy in lymphoma, *Arch. Intern. Med.* **135**:62–66.

Algom, D., and Richter, M., 1973, Immunocompetent cells in man. I. The demonstration of the simultaneous existence of immunocompetent and immunoincompetent populations of lymphocytes in the circulation of patients with chronic lymphocytic leukemia and acquired hypogammaglobulinemia, *Lab. Invest.* **29**:587–594.

Arends, T., Coonrad, F. C., and Rundles, R. W., 1954, Serum proteins in Hodgkin's disease and malignant lymphoma, *Am. J. Med.* **16**:833–841.

Astaldi, G., Girando, L. C., and Marsani, F., 1968, Lymphocytes in reticulum cell sarcoma, *Lancet* **2**:410.

Barr, M., and Fairley, G. H., 1961, Circulating antibodies in reticuloses, *Lancet* **1**:1305–1310.

Benezra, D., Pitaro, R., Hochman, A., and Cividalli, G., 1971, *In vitro* activation of lymphocytes from patients with malignant diseases. II. Studies on the behaviour of stimulated lymphocytes from patients with leukemia, *Oncology* **25**:415–424.

Biozzi, G., Benecerraf, B., Halpern, B. N., Stiffel, C., and Hillemand, B., 1958, Exploration of the phagocytic function of the reticuloendothelial system with heat denatured human serum albumin labeled with ¹³¹I and application to the measurement of liver blood flow in normal man and in some pathologic conditions, *J. Lab. Clin. Med.* **51**:230–239.

Blattner, W. A., Strober, W., Muchmore, A. V., Blease, R. M., Broder, S., and Fraumeni, J. F., 1976, Familial chronic lymphocytic leukemia: Immunologic and cellular characterization, *Ann. Intern Med.* **84**:554–557.

Block, J. B., Haynes, H. A., Thompson, W. L., and Neiman, P. E., 1969, Delayed hypersensitivity in chronic lymphocytic leukemia, *J. Natl. Cancer Inst.* **42**:973–980.

Boggs, D., 1960, The cellular composition of inflammatory exudates in human leukemias, *Blood* **15**:466–475.

Boggs, D. R., and Fahey, J. L., 1960, Serum protein changes in malignant disease. II. The chronic leukemias, Hodgkin's disease and malignant melanoma, *J. Natl. Cancer Inst.* **25**:1381–1390.

Bouroncle, B. A., Clausen, K. P., and Aschenbrand, J. F., 1969, Studies of the delayed response to phytohemagglutinin (PHA) stimulated lymphocytes in 25 chronic lymphatic leukemia patients before and during therapy, *Blood* **34**:166–178.

Brody, J. I., Oski, F. A., and Singer, D. E., 1969, Impaired pentose phosphate shunt and decreased glycolytic activity in lymphocytes of chronic lymphocytic leukemia: Metabolic pathway, *Blood* **34**:421–429.

Brouet, J. C., Labaume, S., and Seligmann, M., 1975, Evaluation of T and B lymphocyte membrane markers in human non-Hodgkin's malignant lymphomata, *Br. J. Cancer* **31**(*Suppl. 2*):121–127.

Calabro, J. J., 1967, Cancer and arthritis, *Arthritis Rheum.* **10**:553–567.

Cameron, S. J., and Richmond, J., 1971, Ampicillin hypersensitivity in lymphatic leukemia, *Scot. Med. J.* **16**:425–427.

Catovsky, D., Holt, P. J. L., and Galton, D. A. G., 1972a, Lymphocyte transformation in immunoproliferative disorders, *Br. J. Cancer* **26**:154–163.

Catovsky, D., Tripp, E., and Hoffbrand, A. V., 1972b, Response to phytohemagglutinin and pokeweed mitogen in chronic lymphocytic leukemia, *Lancet* **1**:794–796.

Chiao, J. W., Pantic, V. S., and Good, R. A., 1975, Human lymphocytes bearing both receptors for complement components and SRBC, *Clin. Immunol. Immunopathol.* **4**:545–556.

Cone, L., and Uhr, J. W., 1964, Immunological deficiency disorders associated with chronic lymphocytic leukemia and multiple myeloma, *J. Clin. Invest.* **43**:2241–2248.

Craig, A. B., Waterhouse, C., and Young, L. E., 1952, Autoimmune hemolytic disease and cryoglobulinemia associated with chronic lymphatic leukemia, *Am. J. Med.* **13**:793–804.

Creysell, R., Morel, P., Pellet, M., Medard, J., Revol, L., and Croizat, P., 1958, Deficit en gammaglobulines et complications infectieuses des leucemies lymphoides chroniques, *Sang* **29**:383.

Day, N. K., Winfield, J. B., Gee, T., Winchester, R., Teshima, H., and Kunkel, H. G., 1976, Evidence for immune complexes involving antilymphocyte antibodies associated with hypocomplimentaemia in chronic lymphocytic leukemia (CLL), *Clin. Exp. Immunol.* **26**:189–195.

Delaloye, B., and Cruchaud, S., 1960, Measurement of the phagocytic activity of the RES in clinical practice by denatured human albumin labeled with ^{131}I: Consideration on the measurement of hepatic circulation in cirrhosis, *Schweiz. Med. Wochenschr.* **90**:1155–1160.

Deutsch, A., and Norden, A., 1971, Isolation and characterization of RNA from lymphocytes of chronic lymphocytic leukemia, *Scand. J. Haematol.* **8**:112–122.

Dickler, H. B., Siegal, F. P., Bentwich, Z. M., and Kunkel, H. G., 1973, Lymphocyte binding of aggregated IgG and surface Ig staining in chronic lymphocytic leukemia, *Clin. Exp. Immunol.* **14**:97–106.

Ebbe, S., Wittels, B., and Dameshek, W., 1962, Autoimmune thrombocytopenic purpura ("ITP" type) with chronic lymphocytic leukemia, *Blood* **19**:23–37.

Epstein, L. B., and Cline, M. J., 1974, Chronic lymphocytic leukemia: Studies on mitogen-stimulated lymphocyte interferon as a new technique for assessing T lymphocyte effector function, *Clin. Exp. Immunol.* **16**:553–563.

Feld, R., and Bodey, G. P., 1975, Significant infections in patients with malignant lymphoma treated with chemotherapy, *Proc. Am. Assoc. Cancer Res.* **16**:237.

Fiddes, P., Penney, R., and Wells, J. Z., 1972, Clinical correlations with immunoglobulin levels in chronic lymphatic leukemia, *Aust. N. Z. J. Med.* **4**:346–350.

Foulis, A. K., Cochran, A. J., and Anderson, J. R., 1973, Surface immunoglobulins of leukemic cells, *Clin. Exp. Immunol.* **14**:481–490.

Fraumeni, J. F., Jr., Vogel, C. L., and DeVita, T., 1969, Familial chronic lymphocytic leukemia, *Ann. Intern. Med.* **71**:279–284.

Froland, S. S., and Staven, P., 1972, Response to phytohemagglutinin and pokeweed mitogen in chronic lymphocytic leukemia, *Lancet* **1**:795–796.

Gamble, C. N., and Cutting, H. O., 1966, The production of gammaglobulin by lymphocytes in chronic lymphocytic leukemia: Immunocytotoxicity investigation of a case, *Blood* **27**:187–198.

Gatti, R. A., and Good, R. A., 1971, Occurrence of malignancy in immunodeficiency diseases, *Cancer* **28**:89–98.

Goldman, A. S., Schmalstieg, F. C., Harris, N. S., Rudloff, H. B., Goldblum, R. M., and Alperin, J. B., 1977, Lymphocyte motility in chronic lymphocytic leukemia and X-linked hypo-γ-globulinemia, *Clin. Res.* **25**:75A.

Gorski, A. J., Dupont, B., Hansen, J. A., and Good, R. A., 1975, Leukcoyte migration inhibitory factor (LMIF) induced by concanavalin A: A standardized microassay for production *in vitro, Proc. Natl. Acad. Sci. U.S.A.* **72**:3197–4000.

Gorski, A. J., Dupont, B., Hansen, J. A., and Good, R. A., 1976, Leukocyte migration inhibitory factor (LMIF) production in undirectional mixed lymphocyte cultures, *J. Immunol.* **117**:865–870.

Gorski, A. J., Dupont, B., Hansen, J. A., Safai, B., Pahwa, S., and Good, R. A., 1977, Human immunodeficiency disease: Impairment of cellular interactions leading to mediator production in mixed lymphocyte culture reaction, *J. Immunol.* **118**:858–862.

Green, I., and Corso, P. F., 1959, A study of skin homografting in patients with lymphomas, *Blood* **14**:235–245.

579

IMMUNO-
DEFICIENCIES
ASSOCIATED WITH
CHRONIC
LYMPHOCYTIC
LEUKEMIA AND
NON-HODGKIN'S
LYMPHOMAS

Groch, G. S., Perillie, P. E., and Finch, S. C., 1965, Reticuloendothelial phagocytic function in patients with leukemia, lymphoma and multiple myeloma, *Blood* **26**:489–499.

Gupta, S., and Grieco, M. H., 1975, Rosette formation with mouse erythrocytes. I. Probable marker for human B lymphocytes, *Int. Arch. Allergy Appl. Immunol.* **49**:734–742.

Gupta, S., Good, R. A., and Siegal, F. P., 1975, Spontaneous rosette-formation of mouse erythrocytes with human "B" lymphocytes, *Clin. Res.* **23**:411A.

Gupta, S., Good, R. A., and Siegal, F. P., 1976a, Rosette-formation with mouse erythrocytes. II. A marker for human B and non T lymphocytes, *Clin. Exp. Immunol.* **25**:319–328.

Gupta, S., Good, R. A., and Siegal, F. P., 1976b, Rosette-formation with mouse erythrocytes. III. Studies in primary immunodeficiency and lymphoproliferative disorders, *Clin. Exp. Immunol.* **26**:204–213.

Hadden, J. W., Hadden, E. M., and Middleton, E., Jr., 1970, Lymphocyte blast transformation. I. Demonstration of adrenergic receptors in human peripheral lymphocytes, *Cell. Immunol.* **1**:583–595.

Hansen, J. A., Bloomfield, C. D., Dupont, B., Gajlpeczalska, K., Kiszkiss, D., and Good, R. A., 1973, Lymphocyte subpopulations and immunodeficiency in lymphoproliferative malignancies, in: *Proceedings of the 8th Leukocyte Culture Conference* (K. Lindahl-Kiessling and D. Osoba, eds.), pp. 119–125, Academic Press, New York.

Harris, J., and Bagai, R. C., 1972, Immune deficiency states associated with malignant disease in man, *Med. Clin. North Am.* **56**:501–514.

Havemann, K., and Rubin, A. D., 1968, The delayed response of chronic lymphocytic leukemia lymphocytes to PHA *in vitro*, *Proc. Soc. Exp. Biol. Med.* **127**:668–671.

Heath, R. B., Fairley, G. H., and Malpas, J. S., 1964, Production of antibodies against viruses in leukemia and related diseases, *Br. J. Haematol.* **10**:365–370.

Hersh, E. M., and Irvin, W. S., 1969, Blastogenic responses of lymphocytes from patients with untreated lymphomas, *Lymphology* **2**:150–160.

Hersh, E. M., Curtis, J. E., Harris, J. E., McBride, C., Alexanian, R., and Rossen, R., 1970, Host defense mechanisms in lymphoma and leukemia, in: *Leukemia–Lymphoma*, p. 149–167, Year Book Medical Publishers, Chicago.

Hersh, E. M., Guinn, G. A., Rosen, R., Wallace, S., Rose, S., and Freireich, E. S., 1971, Two populations of lymphocytes in chronic lymphocytic leukemia, in: *Proceedings of the 4th Leukocyte Culture Conference* (O. R. McIntyre, ed.), p. 373, Appleton-Century-Crofts, New York.

Hickling, R. A., and Sutliff, W. D., 1928, Pneumonia in a case of chronic lymphatic leukemia, *Am. J. Med. Sci.* **175**:224–228.

Hirschberg, N., 1939, Phagocytic activity in leukemia, *Am. J. Med. Sci.* **197**:706–711.

Holm, G., Perlmann, P., and Johannsson, B., 1967, Impaired phytohaemagglutinin-induced cytotoxicity *in vitro* of lymphocytes from patients with Hodgkin's disease or chronic lymphocytic leukemia, *Clin. Exp. Immunol.* **2**:351–360.

Howell, K. M., 1920, Failure of antibody formation in leukemia, *Arch. Intern. Med.* **26**:706–714.

Huang, A. T., Kremer, W. B., Laszlo, J., and Setlow, R. B., 1972, DNA repair in human leukemic lymphocytes, *Nature (London) New Biol.* **240**:114–116.

Huang, A. T. F., Riddle, M. M., and Koons, L. S., 1975, Some properties of a DNA-unwinding protein unique to lymphocytes from chronic lymphocytic leukemia, *Cancer Res.* **35**:981–986.

Hudson, R., and Wilson, S. J., 1957, Hypogammaglobulinemia and chronic lymphatic leukemia, *J. Lab. Clin. Med.* **50**:829–830.

Insel, R. A., Melewicz, F. M., LaVia, M. F., and Balch, C. M., 1975, Morphology, surface markers, and *in vitro* responses of a human leukemic T cell, *Clin. Immunol. Immunopathol.* **4**:382–391.

Jaffe, E., Shevach, E., and Frank, M., 1974, Nodular lymphoma: Evidence for origin from follicular B lymphocytes, *N. Engl. J. Med.* **290**:813–819.

Jarvis, S. C., Snyderman, R., and Cohen, H. J., 1976, Human lymphocyte motility: Normal characteristics and anomalous behavior of chronic lymphatic leukemia cells, *Blood* **48**:717–729.

Jim, R. T. S., and Reinhard, E. H., 1956, Agammaglobulinemia and chronic lymphocytic leukemia, *Ann. Intern. Med.* **44**:790–796.

Johnson, L. D., and Abell, C. W., 1970, The effects of isoproterenol and cyclic adenosine 3′,5′-phosphate on phytohemagglutinin-stimulated DNA synthesis in lymphocytes obtained from patients with chronic lymphocytic leukemia, *Cancer Res.* **30**:2718–2723.

Kagan, A. R., and Johnson, R. E., 1967, Evaluation of therapy in chronic lymphocytic leukemia using *in vitro* lymphocyte transformation, *Radiology* **88**:352–355.

Kersey, J. H., Spector, B., and Good, R. A., 1973, Immunodeficiency and cancer, *Adv. Cancer Res.* **18**:211–230.

Kersey, J. H., Spector, B., and Good, R. A., 1975, Primary immunodeficiency and malignancy, in: *Immunodeficiency in Man and Animals* (D. Bergsma, ed.), *Birth Defects: Orig. Artic. Ser.* **11**(1):289–298, Sinauer Associates, Sunderland, Massachusetts.

Konig, E., Cohnen, G., Brittinger, G., and Douglas, S. D., 1972, Response to phytohemaglutinin and pokeweed mitogen in chronic lymphocytic leukemia, *Lancet* **1**:795.

Kornfeld, S., 1969, Decreased phytohemagglutinin receptor sites in chronic lymphocytic leukemia, *Biochim. Biophys. Acta* **192**:542–545.

Lamb, D., Pilney, F., Kelly, W. D., and Good, R. A., 1962, A comparative study of the incidence of anergy in patients with carcinoma, leukemia, Hodgkin's disease and other lymphomas, *J. Immunol.* **89**:555–558.

Larson, D. L., and Tomlinson, L. J., 1953, Quantitative antibody studies in man. III. Antibody response in leukemia and other malignant lymphomata, *J. Clin. Invest.* **32**:317–321.

Lawrence, J. H., and Donald, W. G., Jr., 1959, The incidence of cancer in chronic leukemia and in polycythemia vera, *Am. J. Med. Sci.* **237**:488–498.

Leech, J. H., Glick, A. D., Waldron, J. A., Flexner, J. M., Horn, R. G., and Collins, R. D., 1975, Malignant lymphomas of follicular center cell origin in man. I. Immunologic studies, *J. Natl. Cancer Inst.* **54**:11–21.

Leoncini, D., Forni, A., Korngold, L., and Miller, D. G., 1968, A comparison of paper electrophoretic and immunoelectrophoretic studies of serum proteins of patients with lymphomas and leukemias, *Oncology* **22**:81–117.

Libansky, J., 1969, The investigation of the cellular type of immunity in patients with lymphoproliferative and myeloproliferative diseases, *Int. J. Cancer* **4**:288–298.

Lukes, R., and Collins, R., 1974, Immunologic characterization of human malignant lymphoma, *Cancer* **34**:1488–1503.

Mavone, R., and Stramignoni, A., 1974, DNA response of blood and lymph node lymphocytes *in vitro* in malignant lymphomas, *Acta Haematol.* **51**:76–83.

Mellstedt, H., and Pettersson, D., 1974, Lymphocyte subpopulations in chronic lymphocytic leukemia, *Scand. J. Immunol.* **3**:303–310.

Mendes, N. F., Musatti, C. C., and Tolnai, M. E. A., 1974, T and B lymphocyte membrane markers in cells from patients with leukemia and lymphoma, *Int. Arch. Allergy Appl. Immunol.* **46**:695–706.

Milgrom, F., Kano, K., and Fjelde, A., 1973, Studies on heterophil antigen in lymphoma and leukemia spleens by means of absorption of infectious mononucleosis sera, *Int. Arch. Allergy Appl. Immunol.* **45**:631–637.

Miller, D. G., 1965, Immunological disturbances in lymphoma and leukemia, in: *Immunological Diseases* (M. Samter, ed.), pp. 568–570, Little, Brown, Boston.

Miller, D. G., 1962, Patterns of immunological deficiency in lymphomas and leukemias, *Ann. Intern. Med.* **57**:703–716.

Miller, D. G., and Karnofsky, D. A., 1961, Immunologic factors and resistance to infection in chronic lymphatic leukemia, *Am. J. Med.* **3**:748–757.

Miller, D. G., Lizardo, J. G., and Snyderman, R. A., 1961, Homologous and heterologous skin transplantation in patients with lymphomatous disease, *J. Natl. Cancer Inst.* **26**:569–579.

Millian, S. J., Miller, D. G., and Shaefer, N., 1965, Viral complement-fixing antibody in patients with Hodgkin's disease, lymphosarcoma, reticulum cell sarcoma and chronic lymphocytic leukemia, *Cancer* **18**:674–678.

Moayeri, H., Han, T., and Sokal, J. E., 1975, Delayed hypersensitivity responses, palpable disease and survival in chronic lymphocytic leukemia (CLL), *Proc. Am. Assoc. Cancer Res.* **16**:239.

Moertel, C. G., and Hagedorn, A. B., 1957, Leukemia or lymphoma and coexistent primary malignant lesions: A review of the literature and a study of 120 cases, *Blood* **12**:788–803.

Monahan, T. M., Marchand, N. W., Fritz, R. R., and Abell, C. W., 1975, Cyclic adenosine 3'5'-monophosphate levels and activities of related enzymes in normal and leukemic lymphocytes, *Cancer Res.* **35**:2540–2547.

Noguchi, S., Bukowski, R., Deodhar, S., and Hewlitt, J. S., 1976, T and B lymphocytes in non-Hodgkin's lymphoma: A comparison of tumor-derived cells and peripheral blood lymphocytes, *Cancer* **37**:2247–2254.

Norogrodsky, A., Biniaminov, M., Ramot, B., and Katchalski, E., 1972, Binding of concanavalin A to rat, normal human and chronic lymphatic leukemia lymphocytes, *Blood* **40**:311–316.

581

IMMUNO-
DEFICIENCIES
ASSOCIATED WITH
CHRONIC
LYMPHOCYTIC
LEUKEMIA AND
NON-HODGKIN'S
LYMPHOMAS

SUDHIR GUPTA AND
ROBERT A. GOOD

Oppenheim, J. J., Whang, J., and Frei, E., 1963, Immunological and cytogenetic studies of chronic lymphocytic leukemia cells, *Blood* **26**:121–132.

Papac, R. J., 1970, Lymphocyte transformation in malignant lymphoma, *Cancer* **26**:279–286.

Pegorara, L., and Gavosto, F., 1973, Phytohaemagglutinin-responsive lymphocytes in chronic lymphocytic leukaemia, *Lancet* **1**:1508.

Pentycross, C. R., 1974, Chronic lymphocytic leukemia and the mixed lymphocyte reaction, *Lymphology* **7**:7–12.

Perera, D. J. B., and Pegrum, G. D., 1974, The lymphocyte in chronic lymphatic leukemia, *Lancet* **1**:1207–1208.

Peter, C., Mackenzie, M., and Glassy, F., 1974, T and B origin of some non-Hodgkin's lymphomas, *Lancet* **2**:686–688.

Petermann, M. I., Karnofsky, D. A., and Hogness, K. R., 1948, Electrophoretic studies on the plasma proteins of patients with neoplastic disease. III. Lymphomas and leukemia, *Cancer* **1**:109–119.

Pisciotta, A. V., Jermain, L. F., and Hinz, J. E., 1960, Chronic lymphocytic leukemia, hypogammaglobulinemia and autoimmune hemolytic anaemia: An experiment of nature, *Cancer* **1**:109–119.

Polgar, P., Vera, J. C., Kelly, P. R., and Rutenberg, A. M., 1973, Adenylate cyclase activity in normal and leukemic human lymphocytes as determined by a radio-immunoassay for cyclic AMP, *Biochim. Biophys. Acta* **297**:378–383.

Potolsky, A. I., Heath, C. W., Buckley, C. E., and Rowlands, D. T., 1971, Lymphoreticular malignancies and immunologic abnormalities in sibship, *Am. J. Med.* **50**:42–48.

Prasad, A., 1958, The association of hypogammaglobulinemia and chronic lymphatic leukemia, *Am. J. Med. Sci.* **236**:610–613.

Rubin, A. D., 1971, Defective control of ribosomal RNA processing in stimulated leukemic lymphocytes, *J. Clin. Invest.* **50**:2485–2497.

Rubin, A. D., Havemann, K., and Dameshek, W., 1976, Studies in chronic lymphocytic leukemia: Further studies of the proliferative abnormality of the blood lymphocyte, *Blood* **33**:313–328.

Ruhl, H., Vogt, W., Bochert, G., Schmidt, S., Moelle, R., and Schaqua, H., 1976, Mixed lymphocyte culture stimulatory and responding capacity of lymphocytes with lymphoproliferative diseases, *Clin. Exp. Immunol.* **19**:55–65.

Sagone, A., Loguglio, A., and Balcerzak, S. P., 1972, Impaired lymphocytic glucose metabolism in patients with lymphoma, *Clin. Res.* **20**:742.

Saslaw, S., Carlisle, H. O., and Brouncle, B., 1961, Antibody response in hematologic patients, *Proc. Soc. Exp. Biol. Med.* **106**:654–656.

Sbarra, A. J., Shirley, W., Selvaraj, R. J., Ouchie, E., and Rosenbaum, E., 1964, The role of the phagocyte in host–parasite interactions. I. The phagocytic capabilities of leucocytes from lymphoproliferative diseases, *Cancer Res.* **24**:1958–1968.

Scher, N. S., Quagliata, F., Malathi, V. G., Faig, D., Melton, R. A., and Silber, R., 1976, Cyclic adenosine 3′,5′-monophosphate phosphodiesterase activity in normal and chronic lymphocytic leukemia lymphocytes, *Cancer Res.* **36**:3958–3962.

Scholar, E. M., and Calabresi, P., 1973, Identification of the enzymatic pathways of nucleotide metabolism in human lymphocytes and leukemia cells, *Cancer Res.* **33**:94–103.

Schrek, R., 1963, Mobility of normal and leukemia human lymphocytes, *J. Lab. Clin. Med.* **61**:34–43.

Schrek, R., Dolowy, W. C., and Ammeraal, R. N., 1967, L-Asparaginase: Toxicity to normal and leukemic human lymphocytes, *Science* **155**:329–330.

Schultz, E. F., Davis, S., and Rubin, D., 1976, Further characterization of the circulating cells in chronic lymphocytic leukemia, *Blood* **48**:223–234.

Seligmann, M., 1974, B-cell and T-cell markers in lymphoid proliferations (editorial), *N. Engl. J. Med.* **290**:1483–1484.

Selvaraj, R. J., McRipley, R. J., and Sbarra, A. J., 1967, The metabolic activities of leukocytes from lymphoproliferative and myeloproliferative disorders during phagocytosis, *Cancer Res.* **27**:2287–2293.

Shaw, R. K., Szwed, C., Boggs, D. R., Fahey, J. L., Frei, E., III, Morrison, E., and Utz, J. P., 1960, Infection and immunity in chronic lymphocytic leukemia, *Arch. Intern. Med.* **57**:703–716.

Shevach, E., Edelson, R., Frank, M., Lutzner, M., and Green, I., 1974, A human leukemic cell with both T and B cell surface receptors, *Proc. Natl. Acad. Sci. U.S.A.* **71**:863–866.

Smith, M. J., Browne, E., and Slungaard, A., 1973, The impaired responsiveness of chronic lymphatic leukemia (CLL) lymphocytes to allogeneic lymphocytes, *Blood* **41**:505–509.

583

IMMUNO-
DEFICIENCIES
ASSOCIATED WITH
CHRONIC
LYMPHOCYTIC
LEUKEMIA AND
NON-HODGKIN'S
LYMPHOMAS

Sokal, J. E., and Aungst, C. W., 1971, Cellular immune responses and prognosis in malignant lympho-
mas, *Natl. Cancer Inst. Monogr.* **34**:109–112.
Southam, C. M., Goldsmith, Y., and Burchenal, J., 1951, Heterophile antibodies and antigens in
neoplastic diseases, *Cancer* **4**:1036–1042.
Spector, B. D., Good, R. A., and Kersey, J. H., 1978, Immunodeficiency diseases and malignancy, in:
Gastrointestinal Tract Cancer (M. Lipkin and R. A. Good, eds.), pp. 51–70, Plenum Press, New
York.
Spengler, G. A., and Stjernholm, R. L., 1972, A transient lymphotoxic serum factor in a patient with
chronic lymphocytic leukemia, *Am. J. Med. Sci.* **263**:241–251.
Stathopoulos, G., and Elliott, E. V., 1974, Formation of mouse or sheep red blood cell rosettes by
lymphocytes from normal and leukemic individuals, *Lancet* **1**:600–601.
Stryckmans, P. A., Chanana, A. D., Cronkite, E. P., Greenberg, M. L., and Schiff, L. M., 1968, Studies
on lymphocytes. IX. The survival of autotransfused labeled lymphocytes in chronic lymphocytic
leukemia, *Eur. J. Cancer* **4**:241–246.
Sugden, P. J., 1974, Autoinhibition of PHA responses by chronic-lymphocytic leukemia serum, *Lancet*
2:596–597.
Tavadia, H. B., Goudie, R. B., and Nicoll, W. E., 1974, Inhibition of normal lymphocyte transformation
by plasma and lymphocyte factors in chronic lymphatic leukemia, *Clin. Exp. Immunol.* **16**:177–182.
Thomson, A. E. R., and Robinson, M. A., 1967, Cytocidal action of colchicine *in vitro* on lymphocytes in
chronic lymphocytic leukemia, *Lancet* **2**:868–870.
Tung, R., Silber, R., Quagliata, F., Conklyn, M., Gottesman, J., and Hirschhorn, R., 1976, Adenosine
deaminase activity in chronic lymphocytic leukemia, *J. Clin. Invest.* **57**:756–761.
Twomey, J. J., and Douglass, C. C., 1974, An *in vitro* study of lymphocyte and macrophage function with
lymphoproliferative neoplasms, *Cancer* **33**:1034–1038.
Ultmann, J. E., Fisch, W., Osserman, E., and Gellhorn, A., 1959, The clinical implications of hypogam-
maglobulinemia in patients with chronic lymphocytic leukemia and lymphocytic lymphosarcoma,
Ann. Intern. Med. **51**:501–516.
Utsinger, P. D., 1975, Impaired T-cell transformation in chronic lymphocytic leukemia (CLL): Demon-
stration of a blastogenesis inhibitory factor, *Blood* **46**:883–890.
Winter, G. C. B., Osmond, D. G., Yoffey, J. M., and Mahy, D. J., 1964, Leucocyte cultures with
phytohemagglutinin in chronic lymphatic leukemia, *Lancet* **2**:563–565.
Wybran, J., Chantler, S., and Fudenberg, H. H., 1973, Isolation of normal T cells in chronic lymphatic
leukemia, *Lancet* **1**:126–129.
Yadoi, J., Takatsuki, K., and Masuda, T., 1974, Two cases of T-cell chronic lymphocytic leukemia in
Japan, *New Eng. J. Med.* **290**:572–573.

20

Immunological Changes with Hodgkin's Disease

JEREMIAH J. TWOMEY, ROBERT A. GOOD, and
DELVYN C. CASE, JR.

1. Introduction

Hodgkin's disease (HD) is unique among primary tumors of lymphoid tissues. The
histology of Hodgkin's tumors is remarkably pleomorphic. Depletion of lymphoid
cells in blood and tumor tissues occurs with progressive disease. Histological
variability, cellular depletion, and a lack of tissue invasion by a clone of cells are
characteristics of HD that are not typical of a primary neoplastic process.

Improved histological classification, accurate clinical staging, and more effective therapy have dramatically improved prognosis with HD. This progress has
been accomplished largely through a reduction in tumor burden and containment of
residual tumor by the host, rather than complete eradication of the disease (Strum
and Rappaport, 1971). Defense mechanisms that are intrinsic to the host have a
crucial role in maintaining a favorable equilibrium between the patient and residual
HD. The immune system is an essential component of these defense mechanisms.

Patients with lymphocyte-predominant tumors usually have a relatively favorable prognosis (Keller *et al.*, 1968; Neiman *et al.*, 1973). Hodgkin's tumors with an
abundance of lymphocytes probably contain cells that participate in resisting the
disease. Conversely, lymphocyte depletion and immunodeficiency are prognosti-
cally unfavorable findings with HD.

An abundance of information has been collected concerning immunological
changes with HD. This interest reflects the relatively unfavorable prognosis in
patients with reduced immunological competence. The pathophysiology of the
acquired immunodeficiency with HD remains to be explained, but appears to be
related to disease activity. Host defense mechanisms are further compromised by

JEREMIAH J. TWOMEY • Baylor College of Medicine and Veterans Administration Hospital,
Houston, Texas 77211. ROBERT A. GOOD • Memorial Sloan-Kettering Cancer Center, New
York, New York 10021. DELVYN C. CASE, JR. • Portland, Maine.

irradiation and chemotherapy. Progression of the primary disease and infection remain the major threats to life in these immunologically compromised patients. This chapter reviews the complex manifestations of increased and reduced immunological reactivity with HD and their clinical implications.

2. The Importance of Being Immunologically Competent with Hodgkin's Disease

Lymphocyte-depleted Hodgkin's tumors are usually disseminated (Kaplan and Bissinger, 1973). Lymphopenia tends to be most severe in patients with lymphocyte-depleted tumors (Young et al., 1972; Eltringham and Kaplan, 1975). The temporal sequence suggests that HD contributes in some way to the lymphocyte-depleting process. This immunodepletion, in turn, contributes to the immunological deficit that lowers resistance to the disease and to intercurrent infections.

The immune system undergoes involuntary changes with advancing age (see Chapter 3). In particular, the thymus becomes atrophic (Goldstein and Mackay, 1969) and thymic hormone release into the circulation declines after the fourth age decade (Bach et al., 1972; Twomey et al., 1977). Immunological and, in particular, thymic involution may compromise host resistance to HD. This, in fact, appears to be the case. Patients with HD who are over the age of 60 tend to have an atypical distribution of tumor, a greater likelihood of having disseminated lymphocyte-depleted tumors, and a relatively poor clinical prognosis (Kaplan and Bissinger, 1973; Plager and Stutzman, 1971). Conversely, grafts of fetal thymus tissue into patients with lymphocyte-depleted HD have been followed by a degree of immunological reconstitution (Marcolongo and DiPaolo, 1973). Thus, intrinsic immunological reserves determine the capacity of individual patients to resist HD as well as the adverse effect of the disease on immunological capabilities. Age is one factor that affects host resistance.

The high incidence of infections with primary tumors of lymphoid tissues is a reflection of compromised host defense mechanisms. Displacement of normal lymphoid tissues by neoplastic B cells with lymphocytic leukemias or lymphomas (Preud'homme and Seligmann, 1972; Aisenburg and Long, 1975) and by neoplastic T cells with mycosis fungoides (Lutzner et al., 1975) (see Chapter 10) contributes to the high susceptibility to infections among these patients. This contrasts with the lack of cellular invasion of Hodgkin's tumors.

About five times more patients with HD and patients with B- or T-cell lymphoproliferative disorders develop serious infections than do other control patients with coronary artery disease (Casazza et al., 1966; Twomey, 1973) (Table 1). Infections contribute to the death of more than one third of patients with HD or lymphoproliferative disorders. A 60% mortality from infectious complications was reported with disseminated HD (Feld et al., 1974). Even though the literature contains a plethora of reports on uncommon infections due to agents of relatively low virulence, most infectious episodes and deaths are caused by common virulent bacteria. Apart from a slightly higher rate of nonbacterial infections with HD, the overall patterns of infectious complications with this disease and with B- or T-cell neoplasms are remarkably similar.

The incidence of herpes zoster is unusually high among patients with HD. Cutaneous zoster develops in 15–19% of these patients (Casazza et al., 1966; Wilson et al., 1972; Goffinet et al., 1973), as opposed to an incidence of less than

TABLE 1. Frequency and Type of Infections with Hodgkin's Disease and with B- and T-Cell Neoplasms

	Hodgkin's disease		B-cell neoplasms		Mycosis fungoides		Myocardial infarctions	
	N	$\%$	N	$\%$	N	$\%$	N	$\%$
Total number of patients	51		83		36		50	
Patients who developed infections		75		83		74		15
Patients with serious infections at death		35		45		41		0
Total pathogens identified	83		84		54		15	
Bacterial infections		68		77		83		100
Viral infections		20		17		6		0
Fungal infections		12		6		11		0

0.05% in the general population (Weller, 1965). Overall, prognosis tends to be relatively less favorable in patients with HD who develop herpes zoster (Wilson *et al.*, 1972). It is not known why dermatomes exposed to irradiation therapy are most likely to develop zoster in patients with HD but not in other patients with solid tumors who receive irradiation therapy. The incidence of zoster in patients with HD is cumulative after completion of radiation therapy (Schimpff, *et al.*, 1975). A small minority of herpes zoster infections disseminate. The spread of zoster infections has been associated with impaired antibody responses to varicella-zoster antigens (Stevens and Merigan, 1973).

There is an increased incidence of neoplasms among patients with primary immunodeficiencies and also in recipients of renal allografts (see Chapters 7 and 8). About 2.2% of patients with HD, many of whom are immunodeficient, also develop a distinct second neoplasm (Razis *et al.*, 1959). More than 80 cases of coexistent HD and leukemia, which is usually of the myeloid variety, have been reported (Rosner and Grunwald, 1975). In most instances, HD is diagnosed first. Neoplasms develop most often in patients who have received intensive therapy, particularly irradiation therapy (Arceneau *et al.*, 1972). The potential role of HD itself, of its associated immunodeficiencies, and of its therapy in the etiology of subsequent neoplasms in these patients remain to be determined. This becomes an increasingly important issue as survival with HD continues to improve (Kaplan and Bissinger, 1973).

3. Manifestations of Increased Immunological Reactivity

Activation of the immune system initiates a complex series of biological events. These events include cell–cell interactions, DNA, RNA, and protein synthesis, and lymphocyte proliferation. Lymphoid cells may effect immune responses directly or through the release of mediators, immunoglobulins (Ig's), and interferon. Antigenic stimulation also activates macrophages. Activated macrophages ingest and neutralize foreign particulate matter and participate in immune responses. Influenced by mediators released from lymphocytes, macrophages accumulate at sites of immune responses, where they interact with lymphocytes and antigens and become the most populous cell type in delayed hypersensitivity reactions such as in granulomas.

Table 2 lists evidence that the immune system is stimulated in patients with

**TABLE 2. Manifestations of Immunological Activation
with Hodgkin's Disease**

1. Hypertrophy of lymphoid tissues
2. Proliferation of lymphoid cells in tumor tissue
3. High proliferative responses by tissue lymphocytes to T-cell stimuli
4. Elevated percentages of activated T lymphocytes in the circulation
5. Circulating, cell-free macrophage migration inhibitory factor
6. Noncaseating granuloma formation
7. Bone marrow plasmacytosis
8. Hypergammaglobulinemia
9. Increased immunoglobulin synthesis by spleen cells
10. Circulating antigen–antibody complexes

HD. Spleen tissue from patients with HD contains lymphocytes that proliferate briskly when cultured with mitogens (Kaur *et al.*, 1974) and produce elevated amounts of IgG under resting and stimulated conditions (Longmire *et al.*, 1973) except when extensively involved with tumor. Splenomegaly occurs in the absence of detectable tumor involvement (Ultmann, 1970). Conversely, spleens of normal size may contain Hodgkin's tumors. Thus, hypertrophy of immunological tissues in the spleen is not necessarily a local response to the presence of tumor. Instead, splenic hypertrophy is likely to be part of a systemic immunological response in patients with HD.

There is evidence of increased immunological activity in blood from patients with HD. Lymphocytes activated with antigens or mitogens enlarge to a diameter of 15–25 μm and develop basophilic cytoplasm, and DNA synthesis proceeds to cell division. The percentage of activated lymphocytes in normal blood is less than 0.5%, but increases with infections, autoimmune disease, and following immunization (Crowther *et al.*, 1969). An increased density of activated lymphocytes that bear T-cell markers is also present in blood from the majority of patients with HD (Fairley *et al.*, 1973; Huber *et al.*, 1975). Membrane Ig has also been reported on these transformed lymphocytes (Dunbar, 1975). This membrane Ig may be within the cells or adsorbed onto their surfaces.

Various immunobiologically active mediators, such as macrophage migration-inhibition factor (MMIF) are released from activated T and B lymphocytes (Salvin *et al.*, 1973; Rocklin *et al.*, 1974). While mediator function was detected in serum from only 1 of 45 healthy subjects, significant activity was demonstrated in serum from 10 of 13 patients with HD (Cohen *et al.*, 1974). This observation provides additional evidence of systemic immunological activation in patients who have HD.

Plasma cell hyperplasia in the bone marrow (Kass and Votaw, 1975), increased serum IgG levels (Madalinski *et al.*, 1970), and increased IgG synthesis by spleen cells (Kaur *et al.*, 1974) indicate that humoral immunity may be stimulated with HD. Antibodies produced in patients with HD may include responses to disease-related antigens that then participate in formation of antigen–antibody complexes (Amlot *et al.*, 1976). The presence of circulating antigen–antibody complexes with HD tends to coincide with disease activity. Precipitation of these complexes in tissues would explain the presence of γ-globulin and complement deposits in renal glomeruli of some patients (Sutherland *et al.*, 1974). These glomerular deposits may have clinical significance. Coexistent nephrosis, which improves with clinical remission, has been reported in patients with HD (Plager and Stutzman, 1971).

Granulomas develop at sites of cell-mediated immune reactions and occur, for example, with certain intracellular infections or accumulations of lipid. The basis for granuloma formation with an appreciable minority of patients with HD (Kadin *et al.*, 1970) is not known. Most granulomas from patients with HD lack histological evidence of direct tumor involvement (Dorfman, 1970); multinucleated giant cells rather than Reed–Sternberg cells are found in these lesions (Figure 1). Neverthe-

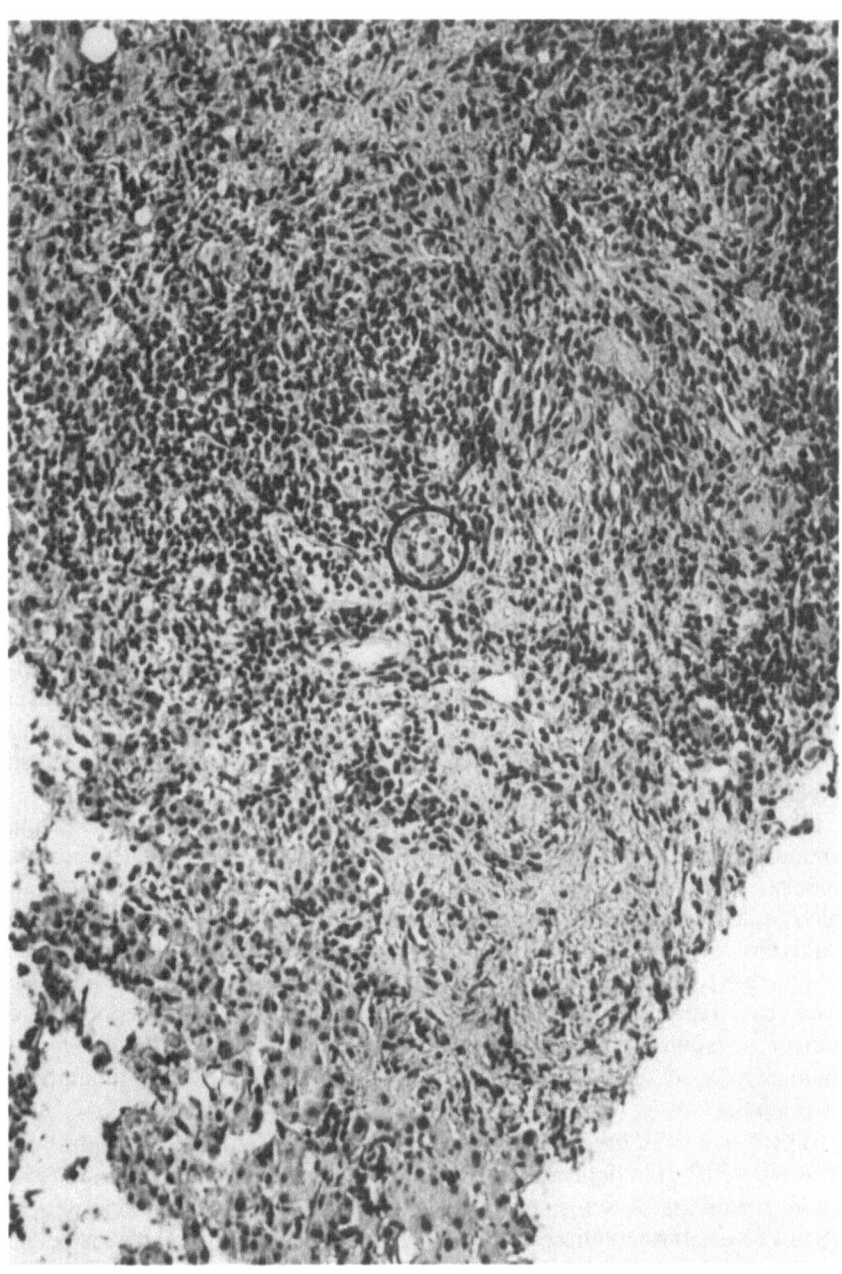

Figure 1. Noncaseating granuloma in a liver biopsy from a patient with Hodgkin's disease. A multinucleated giant cell is circled.

less, these granulomas probably represent intense local responses by the host to the primary disease.

Eosinophilic responses occur with various hypersensitivity reactions. Eosinophilia of blood (Sears, 1932) and bone marrow (Kass and Votaw, 1975) occurs with HD. Histochemical observations suggest that eosinophils that accumulate in Hodgkin's tumors are actively engaged in microendocytosis (Parmley, 1975). The eosinophilic response with HD may also be directed against the disease.

Host defense mechanisms are activated with HD and its infectious complications. These various manifestations of immunological activation do not correlate well with clinical prognosis. One parameter that does correlate with favorable prognosis, however, is the capacity to sustain lymphocyte mass, particularly in tumor tissues (Keller et al., 1968). Lymphocyte depletion occurs with relatively aggressive disease. The coincidence of progressive disease and depletion of immunoreactive cells represents an unfavorable clinical combination. Under these circumstances, the demands placed by the disease itself on host resistance to it are increased while responses by a depleted immune system become less effective. If immunological stimulation and lymphocyte depletion are distinct concurrent events with HD, the severity of lymphocyte depletion may determine the ineffectiveness of host resistance to this disease.

4. Manifestations of Immunodeficiency *in Vivo*

Skin testing is a widely used method for studying cell-mediated immunity (CMI) *in vivo*. These delayed cutaneous responses are determined by a complex series of immunological events: There must be prior sensitization to specific antigens, which must then be retained. An adequate number of the appropriate subpopulations of immune reactive cells must be available to migrate into skin-test sites. These cells must be capable of effecting delayed hypersensitivity reactions. Immunological memory and responsiveness are evaluated by testing with an appropriate battery of recall antigens. The capacity to develop immunity can also be studied by sensitization with new antigens such as keyhole limpet hemocyanin or the chemical allergen dinitrochlorobenzene (DNCB), followed by skin testing for delayed cutaneous responses.

A number of circumstances could be responsible for anergy. Deficits may exist in immunological reactions that precede or occur during delayed hypersensitivity responses. Since responsiveness is determined, in part, by the potency of antigenic challenge, lesser degrees of impairment are not detected when relatively large doses of antigens are used in skin tests (Eltringham and Kaplan, 1975). Negative tests could be due to absence of prior sensitization, which calls for judicious selection of an adequate battery of recall antigens. Interpretation of early reports on delayed cutaneous responsiveness with HD is further complicated by the inclusion of patients who were tested after they had received therapy that had immunosuppressive potential.

There has been considerable interest (Kelley et al., 1960; Good et al., 1962; Lamb et al., 1962) in delayed cutaneous responsiveness with HD since 1954, when Rostenberg and later Schier reported an increased incidence of anergy in patients with this disease (Rostenberg et al., 1954, 1956; Schier, 1954). Inconsistencies in the subsequent literature reflect technical and disease-related variables as well as the complex nature of the responses themselves. Table 3 lists data from three studies

TABLE 3. Anergic Subjects (%) in Three Studies Testing for Delayed Cutaneous Responses with Hodgkin's Disease

	Young *et al.* (1972)[a]	Eltringham and Kaplan (1975)	Case *et al.* (1976)
Total number of patients	103	218	50
Recall antigens			
Hodgkin's disease			
Stages I and II	23	49	12
Stages III and IV	36	64	65
Healthy subjects	12	—	10
DNCB sensitization (dose)	(2000 μg)	(500 μg)	(2000 μg)
Hodgkin's disease			
Stages I and II	24	76	50
Stages III and IV	48	68	45
Healthy subjects	5	17	10

[a]This study used mumps antigens only; the other two studies each used four or more microbial antigens.

that included 371 untreated patients with HD (Young *et al.*, 1972; Eltringham and Kaplan, 1975; Case *et al.*, 1976). These reports document an increased, but variable, incidence of anergy with HD. Eltringham and Kaplan (1975) demonstrated that the frequency of anergy to streptococcal antigens—and, after sensitization, to DNCB—was inversely related to the antigenic potency of the skin-test challenge. This observation probably explains the much higher rate of anergy to DNCB among patients with HD in this survey than in the other two surveys (Young *et al.*, 1972; Case *et al.*, 1977). The high frequency of positive responses to mumps antigen that was evident in the survey of Young *et al.* (1972) may also reflect relatively vigorous skin-test antigenic stimulation. In general, it is possible to demonstrate deficits of CMI *in vivo* in most patients with HD when sensitive skin-testing techniques are employed. Conversely, anergy to vigorous antigenic challenge is usually limited to patients with advanced disease. There is no conclusive evidence that the ability to become sensitized to new antigens is impaired with untreated HD. It is also possible to transfer delayed hypersensitivity with immune RNA to patients who have HD (Han, 1974).

Tests for delayed cutaneous responsiveness have limited practical value with HD. Anergy, with vigorous skin-testing techniques, is associated with a slightly less favorable short-term prognosis than when delayed hypersensitivity responses are elicited under similar conditions (Young *et al.*, 1972). Therapeutic intervention has greatly improved long-term prognosis, however, even in patients with advanced disease (Young *et al.*, 1973). Thus, observations made at diagnosis often become obsolete after patients enter stable remission. Evaluation of delayed hypersensitivity, using sensitive skin-testing techniques, provides useful insight into the adverse effects of HD on immunological competence *in vivo*. These skin-testing techniques have little clinical merit, since the majority of patients with all stages of HD are anergic under these circumstances.

The survival of skin allografts, which is another method for testing cellular immune competence *in vivo*, has been employed on a limited number of patients with HD (Kelly *et al.*, 1960; Miller and Lizardo, 1961; Colombani *et al.*, 1964). It is difficult to assess these studies, since clinical and histological data by modern criteria were not employed and most patients had received prior irradiation therapy.

Nevertheless, the capacity for allograft rejection does appear to be impaired with HD (Miller and Lizardo, 1961). The degree of histocompatibility between donor and recipient appears to be a factor in the duration of skin-graft survival on patients with HD as well as on healthy subjects (Colombani *et al.*, 1964).

5. Lymphocyte Depletion

An absolute count of less than 1500 lymphocytes/mm³ blood constitutes lymphopenia. An appreciable number of patients with HD are lymphopenic (Young *et al.*, 1972; Eltringham and Kaplan, 1975; Aisenberg, 1965a; Swan and Knowelden, 1971; Neiman *et al.*, 1973; Heier and Norman, 1974; Dunbar, 1975). The significance of this lymphopenia with HD has been the subject of extensive studies, the interpretation of which requires careful selection of clinical material. Accurate staging (Rosenberg, 1966) and histological classification (Lukes and Butler, 1966) are essential for comparative analyses. Each clinical stage and histological type of tumor must be represented by an adequate number of cases. Patients with prior therapy that could alter lymphocyte counts must not be included in the clinical material.

The relationship between lymphopenia and clinical stage or tumor histology was analyzed from four adequate series of patients with HD (Young *et al.*, 1972; Eltringham and Kaplan, 1975; Neiman *et al.*, 1973; Heier and Normann, 1974). Overall, lymphopenia was more frequent among patients with disseminated than with localized disease (Figure 2). The most frequent occurrence of lymphopenia with HD was among patients with lymphocyte-depleted tumors, 82% of whom had fewer than 1500 lymphocytes/mm³ blood.

The use of tests that identify T and B subpopulations of lymphocytes has provided additional information on the lymphopenia with HD. These studies should also be limited to untreated patients (Anderson, 1974). Some general conclusions can be drawn from reported data on blood from 113 patients (Case *et al.*, 1976; Anderson, 1974; Bobrove *et al.*, 1975): The number of null lymphocytes in the blood circulation is not altered with HD. Useful information is not likely to be derived from percentage T- and B-cell counts, since these relative values remain within normal limits even with severe lymphopenia. The relative concentrations of

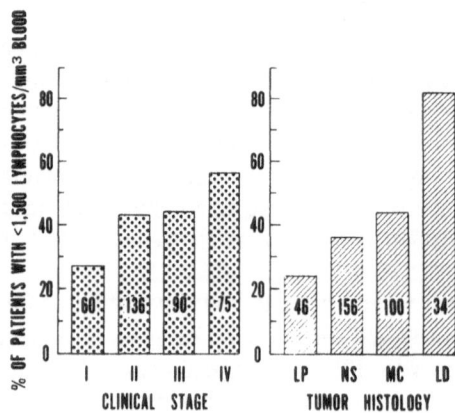

Figure 2. Frequency of lymphopenia with different clinical stages and histological types of Hodgkin's disease. (LP) Lymphocyte predominance; (NS) nodular sclerosis; (MC) mixed cellularity; (LD) lymphocyte depletion. The number on each bar is the number of patients in that group.

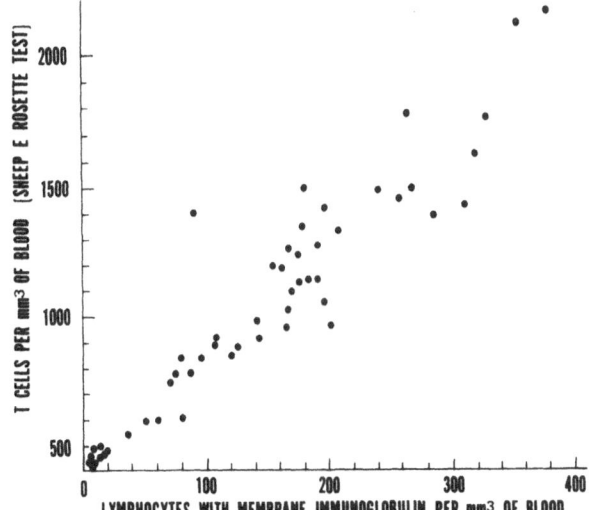

Figure 3. Relationship between absolute SRBC-rosetting lymphocytes and lymphocytes with membrane Ig in the same collections of blood from patients with Hodgkin's disease manifesting different degrees of lymphopenia.

T and B lymphocytes in Hodgkin's tumors are also similar to their concentrations in normal lymphoid tissues (Aisenberg and Long, 1975). Absolute T- and B-cell counts, however, are reduced in lymphopenic blood. A relatively good correlation exists between absolute T- and B-cell counts in the same collections of blood (Figure 3). These values reflect the total lymphocyte content in the same blood specimens. Thus, total lymphocyte counts provide a reasonable estimate of the T- and B-cell contents of blood from patients with HD.

In general, absolute T- and B-cell counts are higher with stage I or II than with stage III or IV HD, and are also higher with lymphocyte-predominant or nodular sclerotic tumors than with mixed-cellularity or lymphocyte-depleted tumors (Case et al., 1976; Anderson, 1974; Bobrove et al., 1975). This relationship follows the general correlation that exists between total lymphocyte counts and the same clinical or histological parameters of the disease (see Figure 2). However, an appreciable minority of patients with apparently localized HD or with tumors that contain an abundance of lymphocytes are lymphopenic (Young et al., 1972; Eltringham and Kaplan, 1975; Heier and Normann, 1974). Lymphocytes from the blood circulation of patients with this disease may also be less responsive than tissue lymphocytes when cultured with mitogens (Kaur et al., 1974; Matchett et al., 1973). These observations suggest that the adverse effects of HD on lymphocytes are more apparent with blood than with tissue lymphocytes. In addition, the distribution of normal lymphocytes throughout the body may be altered in these patients, and this alteration may represent a response on the part of the host against the primary disease (Zatz et al., 1973).

The probability that ecotaxopathy occurs with HD suggests that lymphocyte membranes are concomitantly altered (see Chapter 11). This possibility is supported by experimental data. Normally, a comparable percentage of blood lymphocytes react with antiserum to T-cell membrane antigens and rosette with sheep erythrocytes (SRBC) (Bobrove et al., 1975). With HD, the percentage of blood lymphocytes that rosette with SRBC is appreciably lower than the percentage that react with antiserum to T-cell antigens, unless the lymphocytes under test for rosette formation are preincubated overnight at body temperature. Recent evidence indicates that these rosettes are formed by the attachment of glycopeptides present on the surface of SRBC to receptors for these glycopeptides that are in abundance on the membranes of T lymphocytes (Boldt and Armstrong, 1976). Perhaps a glycopeptide is produced with HD that competitively binds with receptors for SRBC on the membranes of lymphocytes bearing T-cell antigens. The presence of this membrane abnormality correlates with impaired lymphoproliferative responsiveness to mitogens (Bobrove et al., 1975). Studies on membrane cap formation with fluorescein-conjugated concanavalin A (Con A) provide further evidence of lymphocyte membrane change with HD. A reduced percentage of lymphocytes from Hodgkin's tumors and a still lower percentage of blood lymphocytes demonstrate cap formation with Con A (Ben-Bassat and Goldblum, 1975). It therefore seems that changes take place on lymphocyte membranes with HD that may cause ecotaxopathic diversion of lymphocytes from the blood circulation into the tissues.

The lymphopenia with HD cannot be ascribed completely to lymphocyte redistribution. There is evidence that lymphocytes are also damaged with this disease. This evidence includes the presence of an increased percentage of blood lymphocytes with ultrastructural manifestations of injury (Dunbar, 1975), a shortened survival of blood lymphocytes in culture (Hersh and Oppenheim, 1965), and marked lymphocyte depletion of tumor tissue in some severely lymphopenic patients (Neiman et al., 1973). Lymphopoiesis is greatly increased in lymphocyte-depleted tumors (Peckham and Cooper, 1973). This may represent an attempt to compensate for a shortened survival of lymphocytes related to the underlying disease. Additional information is needed on lymphocyte survival and lymphopoiesis with different forms of HD. The potential relationship between the increased incidence of serum lymphocytotoxic antibodies with HD (Arpels and Southam, 1969; Mendius et al., 1976) and lymphocyte injury also remains to be determined.

6. Lymphoproliferative Responses *in Vitro*

The capacity of cultured lymphocytes to proliferate when stimulated with mitogens or antigens has been the subject of extensive investigation. These tests readily detect severe lymphocyte deficits, but are less reliable when used to identify milder degrees of lymphocyte dysfunction. The precision of these tests is limited by a number of technical variables. The artificial standardization of lymphocyte density in most leukocyte culture systems tends to accentuate abnormalities of the concentration of different cell subpopulations (Wybran et al., 1973; Twomey and Douglass, 1974). Most human lymphoproliferative studies have been performed on peripheral blood. Recent evidence suggests that such studies may not reflect immunological capabilities in other tissues (Waddell et al., 1976); indeed, some immune responses occur independently of lymphoproliferation (Rocklin et al., 1974). Thus, the results of lymphoproliferative tests should be interpreted with caution.

The ability of lymphocytes to proliferate *in vitro* is impaired with many immunodeficiency diseases, including HD. Responses to plant mitogens, especially phytohemagglutinin (PHA), have been studied extensively. The sensitivity of the test system is increased by stimulating with suboptimal concentrations of mitogen (Ziegler et al., 1975; Faguet, 1975) and by limiting the culture period to 3 days

(Ippoliti *et al.*, 1974). Responses stimulated by PHA in 3-day cultures are largely effected by T lymphocytes, while both B cells and T cells are stimulated with pokeweed mitogen (PWM) (Chess, *et al.*, 1974). It has been conclusively demonstrated that lymphocytes from the blood circulation of patients with advanced HD are hyporesponsive in culture to PHA (Hersh and Oppenheim, 1965; Aisenberg, 1965b; Papac, 1970; Jackson *et al.*, 1970; Corder *et al.*, 1972). It is also possible to demonstrate hyporesponsiveness to PHA with less extensive disease using sensitive culture techniques (Faguet, 1975). Although HD does not usually impair humoral immunity, lymphoproliferative responses to PWM (which predominantly stimulates B cells) are also reduced (Case *et al.*, 1976; Twomey *et al.*, 1976; Cohnen *et al.*, 1973). Likewise, responses to soluble antigens (Hersh and Oppenheim, 1965) and to alloantigens in the mixed-leukocyte culture reaction (MLR) (Twomey *et al.*, 1976; Lang *et al.*, 1974) are often below normal ranges.

The literature is inconsistent on the frequency of proliferative hyporesponsiveness of blood lymphocytes with different aspects of HD. Responses to PHA are impaired most often with symptomatic (subtype B) disease (Faguet, 1975; Corder *et al.*, 1972). Otherwise, no clear-cut relationship has emerged between responsiveness to PHA and clinical stage (Case *et al.*, 1976; Hersh and Oppenheim, 1965; Papac, 1970; Han and Sokal, 1970; Ziegler *et al.*, 1975; Faguet, 1975; Lang *et al.*, 1974; Corder *et al.*, 1972), tumor histology (Han and Sokal, 1970; Navone and Stramignoni, 1974; Corder *et al.*, 1972), lymphopenia (Han and Sokal, 1970; Ziegler *et al.*, 1975; Faguet, 1975), or cutaneous anergy (Hersh and Oppenheim, 1965; Han and Sokal, 1970; Ziegler *et al.*, 1975; Faguet, 1975; Winkelstein *et al.*, 1974). A disassociation between the ability of patient lymphocytes to proliferate when stimulated with mitogens and with antigens has been reported (Twomey *et al.*, 1976; Lang *et al.*, 1974). The outcome of these extensive studies is to document that the capacity of lymphocytes to proliferate in stimulated cultures is often impaired with HD. The results of these tests on individual patients should not be taken as reliable indicators of various parameters of the disease or of prognosis.

An abundance of lymphocytes in tumor tissue is suggestive of a relatively favorable prognosis with HD (Keller *et al.*, 1968; Neiman *et al.*, 1973). Since these lymphocytes may be actively resisting the primary disease, their functional capacity is of considerable interest. A few studies have been performed on proliferative responses by cultured lymphocytes from Hodgkin's tumors (Twomey *et al.*, 1976; Navone and Stramignoni, 1974; Anderson, 1974). In general, responses by tumor lymphocytes were comparable to those in concomitant cultures by blood lymphocytes from the same patients. However, we have observed higher [^{3}H]thymidine incorporation by stimulated tumor lymphocytes than by blood lymphocytes from patients entering an accelerated phase of disease activity (Twomey *et al.*, 1976). Proliferative responses to mitogens by lymphocytes from tissues without apparent tumor involvement may also be increased (Anderson, 1974). These observations probably reflect disease-related alterations in the distribution of normal lymphocytes.

The proliferative responses by cultured lymphocytes to mitogens and, to a greater degree, to antigens requires the participation of macrophages. Current evidence suggests that macrophages (or at least monocytes) from patients with HD are capable of normal interactions with lymphocytes in lymphoproliferative tests (Blaese *et al.*, 1972; Twomey *et al.*, 1973). Thus, hyporesponsiveness with HD cannot be ascribed to a macrophage deficit. The macrophage series, however, may not be entirely normal with HD. An unusually poor harvest of monocytes using adherence techniques (Blaese *et al.*, 1972) and subnormal phagocytosis of antibody-coated erythrocytes (Urbanitz *et al.*, 1975) were reported with this disease. The relevance of these observations to host defense mechanisms remains to be determined.

7. Abnormalities of Other Immune Responses (Table 4)

Table 4 lists a number of immune responses other than lymphoproliferation that may be impaired with HD.

Activated lymphocytes produce proteins that participate in a variety of immune responses. Normal lymphocytes are stimulated to synthesize protein when cultured with PHA (Rosenberg *et al.*, 1972). Impairment of this response was demonstrated on blood lymphocytes from 19 of 44 untreated patients with HD (Levy and Kaplan, 1974). This abnormality was most apparent with widespread disease, but was also detected with stage IA HD and on treated patients in sustained remission.

At least some mediator responses by lymphocytes involved protein synthesis (Gorski *et al.*, 1975; Rocklin *et al.*, 1972; Rocklin, 1975). Distinct mediator responses inhibit the migration of macrophages (MMIF) and of granulocytes (LMIF) (Rocklin, 1974). These responses may be impaired when protein synthesis is defective. In addition, production of LMIF and MMIF by T cells requires concomitant lymphoproliferation (Rocklin *et al.*, 1974). It is therefore not surprising that these mediator responses may be impaired with HD. Preliminary evidence suggests that MMIF production may be impaired with HD (Churchill *et al.*, 1973). This test, however, may not be a reliable index of CMI competence in these patients (Churchill *et al.*, 1973). It was recently reported that LMIF production was defective in blood lymphocytes from 17 of 19 patients with HD when stimulated in culture with Con A (Gorski *et al.*, 1975). Activated lymphocytes release another mediator that promotes the aggregation of macrophages (MAF) (Lolekha *et al.*, 1970). This response normally correlates well with delayed hypersensitivity and is often impaired with HD (Gotoff *et al.*, 1973).

Normal sensitized T lymphocytes are toxic to appropriate target cells. Lymphocytes that are cultured with PHA become injurious to allogeneic, but not to syngeneic tissue cells (Holm *et al.*, 1964). This *in vitro* test for T-cell function has

TABLE 4.   Immune Responses Other Than Lymphoproliferation That May
Be Impaired with Hodgkin's Disease

Response	Reference
Reduced protein synthesis	Preud'homme and Seligmann (1972)
Impaired release of mediators	
MMIF	Razis *et al.* (1959)
LMIF	Rocklin *et al.* (1972)
MAF	Rocklin (1974)
Lymphocyte-effected cytotoxicity	Rocklin *et al.* (1974)

been applied to the study of HD. Impaired lymphocyte-effected cytotoxicity was demonstrated in 7 of 11 patients (Holm *et al.*, 1967). In general, reduced cytotoxic potential correlated with lymphoproliferative hyporesponsiveness to PHA. While this observation documents an additional deficit of T-cell function with HD, its immunobiological significance is uncertain. The relevance of lymphocyte cytotoxicity to host resistance with this disease therefore remains to be determined. On the other hand, it is possible that abnormal destruction of lymphocytes through immunological mechanisms may contribute to the serious lymphocyte depletion that develops with HD.

8. Suppression of Lymphoproliferative Responses

We recently showed that high concentrations of mononuclear leukocytes from the blood of healthy persons suppress lymphoproliferative responses *in vitro* to mitogens or antigens (Laughter and Twomey, 1977). Suppression in this test system does not require preactivation (e.g., with Con A) and is nonspecific in terms of responding/suppressing cell donor combinations. The suppressor cell adheres to foreign surfaces, resists 2500 rads of X-irradiation, remains functional through at least 5 days in culture, is rich in cytoplasmic nonspecific esterase, and has general morphological characteristics of monocytes. Within the limits of individual collections of blood, inhibition of [^{3}H]thymidine incorporation in the MLR reflects the density of monocytes added to cultures. The cell responsible for this phenomenon must be present in cultures prior to the onset of the proliferative response and must be viable and capable of protein synthesis at the onset of the culture period. There is no evidence that either T cells or B cells participate in this form of lymphoproliferative suppression.

Monocytosis (Maldonado and Hanlon, 1965) and lymphopenia are often present in blood from patients with HD. The altered relative density of these two classes of mononuclear leukocytes is accentuated in cultures in which the number of lymphocytes per unit volume is standardized. The potential of the monocytes to suppress proliferative responses is enhanced by disease-related, lymphocyte hyporesponsiveness with HD. It is therefore not surprising that suppression of proliferative responses *in vitro* occurs with lower concentrations of mononuclear leukocytes from patients with HD than from healthy subjects.

Irradiated mononuclear leukocytes from 16 of 30 patients with HD (at optimal target-cell concentrations for our culture system) stimulated subnormal MLR responses by allogeneic lymphocytes from healthy donors (Twomey *et al.*, 1973, 1975). It can be seen from Table 5 that this abnormality was detected significantly more often with stage III or IV disease than with stage I or II disease, and with lymphocyte-depleted or mixed-cellularity tumors more often than with lymphocyte-predominant or nodular-sclerotic tumors, and was somewhat more prevalent when HD was symptomatic. Conventional chemotherapy or irradiation therapy, *per se*, did not alter results. The abnormality was disease-related, however, in that it became more apparent with clinical progression of the tumor and was no longer demonstrable after patients entered clinical remission. The poor stimulating capacity of patient cells was due to their suppressing the responses under test. Similar observations were made on patients with HD by Kasakura (1975) and on patients

TABLE 5. Frequency of Suppression by Irradiated Mononuclear Leukocytes from Patients with Hodgkin's Disease of MLR Responses by Normal Allogeneic Lymphocytes[a]

Group tested	Number tested	Subnormal MLR stimulation	χ^2 test p value
All Hodgkin's disease patients	30	16	<0.001
Healthy subjects	100	0	
Disease stage			
Stage I or II	8	1	<0.01
Stage III or IV	22	15	
Disease subtype			
Asymptomatic (subtype A)	12	4	>0.05
Symptomatic (subtype B)	18	12	
Tumor type[b]			
LP or NS tumors	10	1	<0.001
LD or MC tumors	20	19	

[a]Cell concentrations were optimal for MLR responses.
[b](LP) Lymphocyte-predominant; (NS) nodular-sclerotic; (LD) lymphocyte-depleted; (MC) mixed-cellularity.

with solid tumors by Berlinger et al., (1976). An excessive level of MLR suppression was not found in tests on blood from 30 patients with non-Hodgkin's lymphomas.

Suppression of MLR responses by relatively low concentrations of mononuclear cells with HD probably involves mechanisms similar to those that we recently identified at much higher cell concentrations with normal mononuclear leukocytes. The phenomenon with HD is also cell-density-dependent and requires the participation of a cell that adheres to glass wool and is ablated by preincubating test cells with inhibitors of protein synthesis (Twomey et al., 1975). Recent evidence suggests that the suppressor effect of monocytes from patients with HD is related to increased release of prostaglandins from adherent leukocytes (Goodwin et al., 1977). When prostaglandin synthesis was inhibited with indomethecin, lymphoproliferative responses by cells from patients with HD approached the normal range. This effect of prostaglandins upon lymphocyte DNA synthesis is probably related to the stimulatory effect of prostaglandins upon cyclic nucleotide generation.

Mononuclear leukocytes from patients with multiple myeloma were recently shown to suppress Ig synthesis by normal allogeneic lymphocytes (Broder et al., 1975). The cell responsible for this suppression also adheres to foreign surfaces and lacks the rosetting property of T cells. Mononuclear leukocytes from patients with multiple myeloma, however, are not abnormally suppressive of MLR responses (Laughter and Twomey, unpublished). Perhaps distinct subpopulations of monocytoid cells suppress MLR proliferative responses and inhibit antibody synthesis. An excess of MLR suppression occurs with HD, and excessive suppression of humoral immunity occurs with multiple myeloma. Further studies are needed to determine whether the pathophysiological mechanism involved is an excessive concentration of normal suppressor cells or the presence of cells with increased suppressor activity, as suggested by Goodwin et al. (1977).

High concentrations of granulocytes inhibit proliferative responses by normal lymphocytes *in vitro* (Bain and Pshyk, 1973). This may have clinical relevance, since delayed cutaneous responses are suppressed during periods of marked polymorphonuclear leukocytosis (Heiss and Palmer, 1974). A variety of circumstances, including lymphopenia, shortened survival, hyporesponsiveness, and suppression by monocytoid cells, all combine to interfere with proliferative responses by cultured lymphocytes from patients with HD. It is therefore not surprising that lymphoproliferative responses by lymphocytes cultured from the blood of patients with HD are interfered with by lower concentrations of granulocytes than are required to interfere with responses by lymphocytes from healthy subjects (Twomey *et al.*, 1975). Indeed, granulocyte concentrations, in the low normal range for peripheral blood, inhibit in cultures that contain mononuclear leukocytes from patients with HD.

Plasma from patients with HD may be inhibitory of lymphoproliferative responses when included in culture medium (Twomey *et al.*, 1976; Gaines *et al.*, 1973). Inhibition is not associated with detectable cytotoxicity in patient plasma. It is also not likely to be due to immune response gene products, since responses by lymphocytes from a number of healthy allogeneic subjects were also inhibited. This phenomenon may be related to the presence of circulating antigen–antibody products (Amlot *et al.*, 1976). Recently, Kaplan and associates (1977) have found that the serum factors inhibitory to normal lymphocyte responses in patients with HD include C-reactive protein coupled with a low-density lipoprotein. The serum lipoprotein appears to be inhibitory to HD lymphocytes even without the C-reactive protein.

The identification of cellular and soluble inhibitors introduces yet another parameter to the immunological deficits with HD. These new data call for reevaluation of mechanisms responsible for subnormal immune responses with this disease that are extensively documented in the literature. The direct relevance of these unusual suppressor phenomena in *in vitro* test systems to immunological competence *in vivo* is still to be determined.

9. Humoral Immunity

Serious infections with HD are usually caused by bacteria similar to those responsible for most infections with lymphoproliferative neoplasms (see Table 1) (Lutzner *et al.*, 1975; Twomey, 1973). Acquired impairment of humoral immunity has been blamed for the high risk from infections with malignancies of the B-cell series (Cone and Uhr, 1964; Fahey *et al.*, 1963). Mechanisms responsible for the high rate of bacterial infections with T-cell neoplasms are not known, although pathological proliferation of suppressor T cells or dysfunction of helper T cells may be postulated. Neoplastic lymphoproliferation is not a primary component of HD. The elucidation of factors that contribute to the high rate of bacterial infections with HD may therefore contribute important information about host defenses against infectious disease. This subject is all the more provocative in light of the fact that the immunodeficiency in these patients primarily involves cell-mediated mechanisms.

About one third of patients with HD are hypergammaglobulinemic (Miller,

1962). Hypogammaglobulinemia is rare, and serum Ig levels are not usually reduced (Fontaine *et al.*, 1974). Most patients have circulating isohemagglutinins and are capable of specific antibody responses (Kelly *et al.*, 1962; Lamb *et al.*, 1962; Aisenberg and Leskowitz, 1963; Chase, 1966; Barr and Fairley, 1961). Primary antibody responses are more likely to be impaired than secondary antibody responses (Barr and Fairley, 1961). In general, humoral immunodeficiency occurs with advanced disease and suggests a poor prognosis (Aisenberg and Leskowitz, 1963; Chase, 1966).

Although there is a proportional decrease in the B- and T-lymphocyte contents of blood with progressive HD, it is cell-mediated and not humoral immunity that usually becomes impaired in these patients. Perhaps extravascular lymphoid tissues of patients with HD contain more B cells than is suggested by studies on peripheral blood. The increased rate of antibody synthesis by stimulated spleen lymphocytes from patients with HD supports this possibility (Longmire *et al.*, 1973), but the reduced percentage of spleen lymphocytes bearing membrane Ig (Kaur *et al.*, 1974) does not. Furthermore, proliferative responses to PHA by tissue T cells exceed responses in paired cultures by T cells from the blood of the same patients (Matchett *et al.*, 1973). Immunological competence is maintained with a much lower concentration in normal blood of B cells than of T cells. The B-cell series may be more efficient than the T-cell series for compensating for lymphocyte depletion with advanced HD. That the humoral immune system may produce enhancing antibodies—perhaps against the primary disease—is suggested by elevated serum IgD levels and the presence of IgD on Reed–Sternberg cells (Madalinski *et al.*, 1970; Rocklin *et al.*, 1974).

There was strong suspicion in the nineteenth century that HD has an infectious etiology. The search for an infectious cause for this disease has recently been directed at viruses and viral genomes (Stevens, 1973). This approach has been encouraged by the convincing evidence that certain experimental tumors of lymphoid tissues and Burkitt's lymphoma in man are due, at least in part, to oncogenic viruses (see Chapters 4 and 13). Since humoral immunity is usually intact with HD, serological surveys for antibodies against specific viral antigens have been employed in these studies.

The recent literature suggests that there is a higher incidence of antibodies against herpes virus type II (Catalano and Goldman, 1972), the Epstein–Barr virus (Langenhuysen *et al.*, 1974; Henle and Henle, 1973), and cytomegalovirus (Langenhuysen *et al.*, 1974) in serum from patients with HD than in serum from healthy populations. There is no apparent correlation between the presence in patient serum of antibodies against any given virus and the presence of HD. The frequency of viral antibodies is highest in patients with advanced disease and in patients with evidence of impaired CMI.

These surveys have so far failed to produce substantial evidence that viruses have a role in the etiology of HD. Perhaps these serological data merely indicate that patients with HD have an increased susceptibility to viral infections, and that infected patients are usually capable of antibody responses to infecting viruses. In studies on experimental Coxsackie B myocarditis, it was shown that antibody suffices to overcome the viral infection and that infected animals do not develop myocarditis when they are incapable of CMI responses (Woodruff and Woodruff, 1974). Perhaps the combination of humoral immune competence and acquired cell-mediated immunodeficiency permits most patients with HD to overcome some viral infections asymptomatically.

10. Therapy of Hodgkin's Disease and Immune Function

Vigorous and prolonged chemotherapy and radiation therapy have greatly improved prognosis with HD. The primary objective of this therapy is to reduce tumor burden and thereby facilitate intrinsic host resistance to the disease. Evidence of residual pockets of tumor in most long-term survivors of HD (Strum and Rappaport, 1971) suggests that reduction of tumor load to a size that permits a symbiotic balance between host and disease is a reasonable therapeutic objective. Prolonged maintainance chemotherapy has been employed to sustain a favorable equilibrium between patient and disease. Intrinsic host defense mechanisms also make important contributions toward maintaining this equilibrium.

The therapeutic agents (Cheema and Hersh, 1971; Weston *et al.*, 1973) and irradiation therapy (Stjernsward *et al.*, 1972) used to treat HD are potent immunosuppressors that have also been used for that purpose in clinical organ transplantation. Prolonged immunosuppression does not follow termination of treatment with chemotherapy or with adrenocorticosteroids. Delayed cutaneous responsiveness to antigens usually recovers within a few months after irradiation therapy (Young *et al.*, 1972; Han and Sokal, 1970; Case *et al.*, 1977). The capacity to become sensitized to DNCB, however, may be impaired for up to 10 years after irradiation therapy (Levy and Kaplan, 1974). Rapid (Han and Sokal, 1970) and delayed (Case *et al.*, 1977) recovery of proliferative responsiveness to mitogens by cultured blood lymphocytes has been reported after patients with HD have received irradiation. Normal absolute and percentage values of T and B blood lymphocytes have been reported after 5 years in clinical remission following irradiation therapy (Case *et al.*, 1977). A reduction of circulating T cells may be an early effect after irradiation therapy for HD (Engeset *et al.*, 1973). Obviously, the results of these studies are influenced by the status of disease activity at the time of testing.

The positive relationship between lymphocyte mass and prognosis with HD suggests that immunological mechanisms contribute significantly to intrinsic host resistance. Lymphocyte depletion and impaired immune function are worrisome complications of HD in terms of host reactivity against the disease. Iatrogenic immunosuppression due to current therapy for HD represents an additional and undesirable acquired deficit of host defense mechanisms. It is therefore not surprising that efforts are being made to enhance immune function with HD. Some success was recently reported with the inclusion of bacillus Calmette Guérin immunotherapy in the treatment of patients with HD (Sokal *et al.*, 1974). More specific T-cell induction in lymphocyte-depleted patients may follow implantation of fetal thymus tissue (Marcolongo and DiPaolo, 1973). Preliminary data suggest that levamisole, which is used primarily to treat intestinal infestations, improves rosette formation between SRBC and lymphocytes from patients with HD (Biniaminov and Ramot, 1975).

This is an era of prognostic optimism for patients with HD. This optimism has encouraged a more vigorous therapeutic attack on the primary disease. Current understanding suggests that careful balance between (1) therapy that reduces tumor mass but causes iatrogenic bone marrow and immunosuppression and (2) efforts to stimulate and maintain the immune system is a desirable approach to the treatment of patients with HD.

11. Commentary

Hodgkin's disease is the most frequently occurring primary tumor of lymphoid tissues. It is traditionally classified with the lymphomas because its most prominent features are enlargement of lymphoid tissues and a progressive clinical course highlighted by acquired immunodeficiency. However, the notable absence of uncontrolled overt proliferation of mononuclear cells, the highly variable histology of Hodgkin's tumors, the usually different anatomical location of disease, and the predominant impairment of CMI distinguish HD from the other lymphomas. In addition, patients with primary immunodeficiencies or allograft recipients are at less risk of developing HD than other lymphoreticular neoplasms (see Chapters 7 and 8). The distinction of HD from non-Hodgkin's lymphomas appears to be valid. It is convenient to consider these nosological entities, collectively, as primary tumors of lymphoid tissues. One can hope that it will later become possible to classify them on an etiological basis.

The exact pathophysiology of HD is not known. Its marked variability raises the possibility of a multifactorial etiology. Alternatively, host responses to this disease may be variable and may, at least in part, determine its clinicopathological immunological expression. It remains to be determined whether immunological activation with HD is primarily a host response to the disease or to concomitant immunological challenge. Alternatively, immunological activation may be intrinsic to HD.

Recent evidence suggests that the monocyte macrophage series may be the primary neoplastic cell with HD. It has proved possible to take cultured cells from HD tumors, implant them in nude athymic mice, and recover a uniform population of cells. These are aneuploid cells of human tumor origin that have a "histiocytic" morphology but lack Fc and complement receptors, but have a cytoplasmic enzyme content suggestive of macrophages (Zamecnik *et al.*, 1977; Long *et al.*, 1977a). Patients with HD who have high serum levels of immune complexes have a serum component which reacts with these cells when tested with antiserum to immunoglobulin or C3 (Long *et al.*, 1977b). Some of these cells are binuclear, with the morphology of Reed–Sternberg cells. Thus, the neoplastic basis for HD seems to have been established. The Reed–Sternberg cell, which is most plentiful in aggressive tumors (Peckham and Cooper, 1973), represents a binucleated or multinucleated form of the primary neoplastic histiocyte. This truly represents a milestone toward our basic understanding of the pathophysiology of HD.

Lymphocyte depletion, which is most apparent in tumor tissue and blood, is an important component of the immunopathology of HD. Both the T-cell and the B-cell series are proportionately depleted. This depletion is due, in part, to maldistribution of lymphocytes throughout the body. However, abnormalities that are intrinsic to lymphocytes also exist with HD. The mechanism or mechanisms responsible for these lymphocyte abnormalities are not known. Lymphocyte survival is probably shortened. Little is known about the status of lymphopoiesis with this disease.

It has been established that immunological reactivity, especially CMI, is increasingly impaired with progressive HD. Various deficits of effector mechanisms are compounded by perturbations of immune regulatory mechanisms. When these complex and variable immunological abnormalities are considered together with disease and host variables, it is not surprising that tests of immune responses have thus far proved unreliable for clinical application. Future efforts should be directed toward identifying mechanisms responsible for lymphocyte depletion and toward devising methods for preventing or reversing this process. Already progress in this direction seems to be in evidence. From recent publications defining HD and its immunologic deficiency, it appears not unreasonable to expect that ongoing analyses will reveal the true nature of the immunodeficiency and thus the increased susceptibility to infection with facultative intracellular bacterial pathogens as well as certain viruses; in fact, these analyses may also elucidate in precise molecular and cellular terms the basis of the decreasing resistance to HD itself. A most provocative recent finding, which suggests that immediate environmental factors play an important role in producing the immunodeficiency and perhaps the disease itself, is the finding of Bjorkholm and Holm (1977) that spouses of patients with HD as well as some family members are immunodeficient and show defective responses to phytomitogens, like PHA.

ACKNOWLEDGMENTS

We wish to thank Ms. Carmen Keltner for her assistance with the preparation of this manuscript.

References

Aisenberg, A. C., 1965a, Lymphocytopenia in Hodgkin's disease, *Blood* **25**:1037–1042.

Aisenberg, A. C., 1965b, Quantitative estimation of reactivity of normal and Hodgkin's disease lymphocytes with thymidine-2¹⁴C, *Nature (London)* **205**:1233–1235.

Aisenberg, A. C., and Leskowitz, S., 1963, Antibody formation in Hodgkin's disease, *N. Engl. J. Med.* **268**:1268–1272.

Aisenberg, A. C., and Long, J. C., 1975, Lymphocyte surface characteristics in malignant lymphoma, *Am. J. Med.* **58**:300–306.

Amlot, P. L., Slaney, J. M., and Williams, B. D., 1976, Circulating immune complexes and symptoms in Hodgkin's disease, *Lancet* **1**:449–451.

Anderson, E., 1974, Depletion of thymus dependent lymphocytes in Hodgkin's disease, *Scand. J. Haematol.* **12**:263–269.

Arceneau, J. C., Sponzo, R. W., Levin, D. L., Schnipper, L. E., Bonner, H., Young, R. C., Canellos, G. P., Johnson, R. E., and DeVita, V. T., 1972, Non-lymphomatous malignant tumors complicating Hodgkin's disease: Possible association with intensive therapy, *N. Engl. J. Med.* **287**:1119–1122.

Arpels, C., and Southam, C. M., 1969, Cytotoxicity of serum from healthy persons and cancer patients, *Int. J. Cancer* **4**:548–559.

Bach, J. F., Paiernik, M., Levasseur, P., Dardenne, M., Barois, A., and LeBrigand, H., 1972, Evidence for a serum factor secreted by the human thymus, *Lancet* **2**:1056–1058.

Bain, B., and Pshyk, K., 1973, Reactivity in mixed cultures of mononuclear leukocytes separated on Ficoll–Hypaque, *Proc. Leukocyte Cult. Conf.* **7**:29–37.

Barr, M., and Fairley, G. H., 1961, Circulating antibodies in reticuloses, *Lancet* **1**:1305–1310.

Ben Bassat, H., and Goldblum, N., 1975, Concanavalin A receptors on the surface membrane of lymphocytes from patients with Hodgkin's and other lymphomas, *Proc. Natl. Acad. Sci. U.S.A.* **72**:1046–1049.

Berlinger, N. T., Lopez, C., and Good, R. A., 1976, Facilitation or attenuation of mixed leukocyte culture responsiveness by adherent cells, *Nature (London)* **260**:145–146.

Biniaminov, M., and Ramot, B., 1975, *In vitro* restoration by levamisole of thymus-derived lymphocyte function in Hodgkin's disease, *Lancet* **1**:464.

Blaese, R. M., Oppenheim, J. J., Seeger, R. C., and Waldmann, T. A., 1972, Lymphocyte–macrophage interaction in antigen-induced *in vitro* lymphocyte transformation in patients with Wiskott–Aldrich syndrome and other diseases with anergy, *Cell. Immunol.* **4**:228–242.

Bobrove, A. M., Fuks, S., Strober, S., and Kaplan, H. S., 1975, Quantitation of T and B lymphocytes and cellular immune function in Hodgkin's disease, *Cancer* **36**:169–179.

Boldt, D., and Armstrong, J. P., 1976, Rosette formation between human lymphocytes and sheep erythrocytes, *J. Clin. Invest.* **57**:1068–1078.

Broder, S., Humphrey, R., Durm, M., Blackman, M., Meade, B., Goldman, G., Strober, W., and Waldmann, T., 1975, Impaired synthesis of polyclonal (nonparaprotein) immunoglobulins by circulating lymphocytes from patients with multiple myeloma, *N. Engl. J. Med.* **293**:887–892.

Casazza, A. R., Duval, C. P., and Carbone, P. P., 1966, Infection in lymphoma, *J. Am. Med. Assoc.* **197**:118–124.

Case, D. C., Hansen, J. A., Corrales, E., Young, C. W., Dupont, B., Pinsky, C. M., and Good, R. A., 1976, Comparison of multiple *in vivo* and *in vitro* parameters in untreated patients with Hodgkin's disease, *Cancer* **38**:1807–1815.

Case, D. C., Hansen, J. A., Corrales, E., Young, C. W., Dupont, B., Pinsky, C. M., and Good, R. A., 1977, Depressed *in vitro* lymphocyte responses to PHA in patients with Hodgkin's disease in continuous long remissions, *Blood* **49**:771–778.

Catalano, L. W., Jr., and Goldman, J. M., 1972, Antibody to herpesvirus hominis types 1 and 2 in patients with Hodgkin's disease and carcinoma of the nasopharynx, *Cancer* **29**:597–602.

Chase, M. W., 1966, Delayed-type hypersensitivity and the immunology of Hodgkin's disease with a parallel examination of sarcoidosis, *Cancer Res.* **26**:1097–1120.

Cheema, A. R., and Hersh, E. M., 1971, Patient survival after chemotherapy and its relationship to *in vitro* lymphocyte blastogenesis, *Cancer* **28**:851–855.

Chess, L., MacDermott, R. P., and Schlossman, S. F., 1974, Immunologic functions of isolated human lymphocyte subpopulations, *J. Immunol.* **113**:1113–1121.

Churchill, W. H., Rocklin, R. R., Maloney, W. C., and David, J. R., 1973, *In vitro* evidence of normal lymphocyte function in some patients with Hodgkin's disease and negative delayed cutaneous hypersensitivity, *Natl. Cancer Inst. Monogr.* **36**:99–106.

Cohen, S., Fisher, B., Yoshida, T., and Bettigole, R. E., 1974, Serum migration-inhibitory activity in patients with lymphoproliferative diseases, *N. Engl. J. Med.* **290**:882–886.

Cohnen, G., Konig, E., Augener, W., and Brittinger, G., 1973, Lymphocyte response to pokeweed mitogen in Hodgkin's disease, *Biomedicine* **19**:239–243.

Colombani, J., Colombani, M., and Dausset, J., 1964, Leukocyte antigens and skin homograft in man, *Ann. N. Y. Acad. Sci.* **120**:307–321.

Cone, L., and Uhr, W., 1964, Immunological deficiency disorders associated with chronic lymphocytic leukemia and multiple myeloma, *J. Clin. Invest.* **12**:2241–2248.

Corder, M. P., Young, R. C., Brown, R. S., and DeVita, V. T., 1972, Phytohemagglutinin-induced lymphocyte transformation: The relationship to prognosis of Hodgkin's disease, *Blood* **39**:595–601.

Crowther, D., Fairley, G. H., and Sewell, R. L., 1969, Significance in the changes in the circulating lymphoid cells in Hodgkin's disease, *Br. Med. J.* **2**:473–477.

Dorfman, R. F., 1970, Granulomas and Hodgkin's disease, *N. Engl. J. Med.* **283**:1410.

Dunbar, J. A., 1975, Injury to large lymphoid cells in Hodgkin's disease, *Lancet* **1**:222–223.

Eltringham, J. R., and Kaplan, H. S., 1975, Immunodeficiency in Hodgkin's disease, *Birth Defects Orig. Artic. Ser.* **11**:278–288.

Engeset, A., Froland, S. S., Bremer, K., and Host, H., 1973, Blood lymphocytes in Hodgkin's disease: Increase of B-lymphocytes following extended field irradiation, *Scand. J. Haematol.* **11**:195–200.

Faguet, G. B., 1975, Quantitation of immunocompetence in Hodgkin's disease, *J. Clin. Invest.* **56**:951–957.

Fahey, J. L., Scoggins, R., Utz, J. P., and Szwed, C. F., 1963, Infection, antibody response and gammaglobulin components in multiple myeloma and macroglobulinemia, *Am. J. Med.* **35**:698–707.

Fairley, G. H., Crowther, D., Prowles, R. L., Sewell, R. L., and Balchin, L. A., 1973, Circulating lymphoid cells in Hodgkin's disease, *Natl. Cancer Inst. Monogr.* **36**:95–98.

Feld, R., Bodye, G. P., Rodriguez, V., and Luna, M., 1974, Causes of death in patients with malignant lymphoma. *Am. J. Med. Sci.* **268**:97–106.

Fontaine, M., Mercier, P., and Mongin, M., 1974, Report of IgA, IgD, IgG and IgM secreting plasma cells in cancerous lymph nodes, *Biomedicine* **21**:168–171.

Gaines, J. D., Gilmer, M. A., and Remington, J. S., 1973, Deficiency of lymphocyte antigen recognition in Hodgkin's disease, *Natl. Cancer Inst. Monogr.* **36**:117–121.

Goffinet, D. R., Goldstein, M. D., and Kaplan, H. S., 1973, Herpes zoster infections in lymphoma patients, *Natl. Cancer Inst. Monogr.* **36**:463–368.

Goldstein, G., and Mackay, I. R., 1969, in: *The Human Thymus*, p. 165, William Heinemann, London.

Goodwin, J. G., Messner, R. P., Bankhurst, A. D., Peake, G. T., Saiki, J. H., and Wilhanes, R. C., 1977, Prostaglandin producing suppressor cells in Hodgkin's disease, *N. Engl. J. Med.* **297**:963–968.

Good, R. A., Kelly, W. D., Rötstein, J., and Varco, R. L., 1962a, Immunological deficiency diseases. Agammaglobulinemia, hypogammaglobulinemia, Hodgkin's disease and sarcoidosis, in: *Progress in Allergy* (P. Kallos and B. H. Waksman, eds.), Vol. 6, pp. 187–319, Karger, Basel, New York.

Good, R. A., Kelly, W. D., and Gabrielsen, A. E., 1962b, Studies of the immunologic deficiency disease: agammaglobulinemia, Hodgkin's disease, and sarcoidosis, in: *Second International Symposium on Immunopathology*, pp. 353–384, Benno Schwabe and Co., Basel, Switzerland.

Gorski, A. J., Dupont, B., Hansen, J. A., and Good, R. A., 1975, Leukocyte migration inhibitory factor induced by concanavalin A: Standardized microassay for production *in vitro, Proc. Natl. Acad. Sci. U.S.A.* **72**:3197–3200.

Gotoff, S. P., Lolekha, S., Lopata, M., Kopp, J., Kopp, R. L., and Malecki, T. J., 1973, The macrophage aggregation assay for cell-mediated immunity in man: Studies of patients with Hodgkin's disease and sarcoidosis, *J. Lab. Clin. Med.* **82**:682–691.

Han, T., 1974, Proceedings: Transfer of cell-mediated skin reactivity with "immune" RNA to Hodgkin's disease and other neoplastic diseases, *Cancer* **33**:497–502.

Han, T., and Sokal, J. E., 1970, Lymphocyte response to phytohemagglutinin in Hodgkin's disease, *Am. J. Med.* **48**:728–734.

Heier, H. E., and Normann, T., 1974, Blood lymphocytes in Hodgkin's disease: Lymphocytopenia related to stages and histologic groups, *Scand. J. Haematol.* **13**:199–202.

Heiss, L. I., and Palmer, D. L., 1974, Anergy in patients with leukocytosis, *Am. J. Med.* **56**:323–332.

Henle, W., and Henle, G., 1973, Epstein–Barr virus-related serology in Hodgkin's disease, *Natl. Cancer Inst. Monogr.* **36**:79–84.

Hersh, E. M., and Oppenheim, J. J., 1965, Impaired *in vitro* lymphocyte transformation in Hodgkin's disease, *N. Engl. J. Med.* **273**:1006–1012.

Holm, G., Perlmann, P., and Werner, B., 1964, Phytohemagglutinin-induced cytotoxic action of normal lymphoid cells on cells in tissue culture, *Nature (London)* **203**:841–843.

Holm, G., Perlmann, P., and Johansson, B., 1967, Impaired phytohemagglutinin-induced cytotoxicity *in vitro* of lymphocytes from patients with Hodgkin's disease or chronic lymphatic leukemia, *Clin. Exp. Immunol.* **2**:351–360.

Huber, C., Michlmayr, G., Falkensamer, M., Fink, U., sur Nedden, G., Braunsteiner, H., and Huber, H., 1975, Increased proliferation of T lymphocytes in the blood of patients with Hodgkin's disease, *Clin. Exp. Immunol.* **21**:47–53.

Ippoliti, G., Marini, G., Ascani, E., and Casirola, G., 1974, The influence of repeated and prolonged stimulation on the PHA-response of lymphocytes in Hodgkin's disease, *Acta Haematol.* **51**:266–269.

Jackson, S. M., Garrett, J. V., and Craig, A. W., 1970, Lymphocyte transformation changes during the clinical course of Hodgkin's disease, *Cancer* **25**:843–850.

Kadin, M. E., Donaldson, S. S., and Dorfman, R. F., 1970, Isolated granulomas in Hodgkin's disease, *N. Engl. J. Med.* **283**:858–861.

Kaplan, H. S., and Bissinger, P. A., 1973, Survival and relapse rates in Hodgkin's disease: Stanford experience 1961–1971, *Natl. Cancer Inst. Monogr.* **36**:487–496.

Kasakura, S., 1975, MLC stimulatory capacity and production of a blastogenic factor in patients with chronic lymphocytic leukemia and Hodgkin's disease, *Blood* **45**:823–832.

Kass, L., and Votaw, M. L., 1975, Esinophilia and plasmacytosis of the bone marrow in Hodgkin's disease, *Am. J. Clin. Pathol.* **64**:248–250.

Kaur, J., Spiers, A. S. D., Catovsky, D., and Galton, D. A. G., 1974, Increase of T lymphocytes in the spleen in Hodgkin's disease, *Lancet* **2**:800–802.

Keller, A. R., Kaplan, H. S., Lukes, R. J., and Rappaport, H., 1968, Correlations of histopathology with other prognostic indicators in Hodgkin's disease, *Cancer* **22**:487–499.

Kelly, W. D., Lamb, D. L., Varco, R. L., and Good, R. A., 1960, An investigation of Hodgkin's disease with respect to the problem of homotransplantation, *Ann. N. Y. Acad. Sci.* **87**:187–202.

Lamb, D., Pilney, F., Kelly, W. D., and Good, R. A., 1962, A comparative study of the incidence of anergy in patients with carcinoma, leukemia, Hodgkin's disease and other lymphomas, *J. Immunol.* **89**:555–558.

Lang, J. M., Oberling, F., Bigel, P., Mayer, S., and Waitz, R., 1974, Lymphocyte reactivity to phytohemagglutinin and allogeneic lymphocytes in 32 untreated patients with Hodgkin's disease, *Biomedicine* **21**:372–377.

Langenhuysen, M. M., Cazemier, T., Houwen, B., Brouwers, T. M., Halie, M. R., The, T. H., and Nieweg, H. O., 1974, Antibodies to Epstein–Barr virus, cytomegalovirus and Australia antigen in Hodgkin's disease, *Cancer* **34**:262–267.

Laughter, A. H., and Twomey, J. J., 1977, Suppression of lymphoproliferation by high concentrations of normal human mononuclear leucocytes, *J. Immunol.* **119**:173–179.

Lee, Y. T., Day, C., and Hori, J. M., 1974, Peripheral lymphocyte counts and prognosis in malignant lymphomas, *Mod. Med. (Minneapolis)* **71**:69–73.

Levy, R., and Kaplan, H. S., 1974, Impaired lymphocyte function in untreated Hodgkin's disease, *N. Engl. J. Med.* **290**:181–186.

Lolekha, S., Dray, S., and Gotoff, S. P., 1970, Macrophage aggregation *in vitro:* A correlate of delayed hypersensitivity, *J. Immunol.* **104**:296–304.

Long, J. C., Zamecnik, P. C., and Aisenberg, A. C., 1977a, Tissue culture studies in Hodgkin's disease: morphologic, cytogenetic cell surface and enzymatic properties of cultures derived from splenic tumors, *J. Exp. Med.* **74**:754–758.

Long, J. C., Hall, C. L., Brown, C. A., Stamatos, C., Weitzman, S. A., and Carey, K., 1977b, Binding of soluble immune complexes in serum of patients with Hodgkin's disease to tissue cultures derived from the tumor, *N. Engl. J. Med.* **297**:295–299.

Longmire, R. L., McMillan, R., Yelenosky, R., Armstrong, S., Lang, J. E., and Craddock, C. G., 1973, *In vitro* splenic Ig synthesis in Hodgkin's disease, *N. Engl. J. Med.* **289**:763–767.

Lukes, R. J., and Butler, J. J., 1966, The pathology and nomenclature of Hodgkin's disease, *Cancer Res.* **26**:1063–1083.

Lutzner, M., Edelson, R., Schein, P., Green, I., Kirkpatrick, C., and Ahmed, A., 1975, Cutaneous T-cell lymphomas: The Sézary syndrome, mycosis fungoides and related disorders, *Ann. Intern. Med.* **83**:534–552.

Madalinski, K., Brzosko, W. S., and Sulawski, M., 1970, Immunoglobulin levels in Hodgkin's disease, *Haematol. Hung.* **4**:333–341.

Maldonado, J. E., and Hanlon, D. G., 1965, Monocytosis: A current appraisal, *Mayo Clin. Proc.* **40**:248–259.

Marcolongo, R., and DiPaolo, N., 1973, Fetal thymic transplant in patients with Hodgkin's disease, *Blood* **41**:625–633.

Matchett, K. M., Huang, A. T., and Kremer, W. B., 1973, Impaired lymphocyte transformation in Hodgkin's disease: Evidence for depletion of circulating T-lymphocytes, *J. Clin. Invest.* **52**:1908–1917.

Mendius, J. R., De Horatius, R. J., Messner, R. P., and Williams, R. C., 1976, Family distribution of lymphocytes in Hodgkin's disease, *Ann. Intern. Med.* **84**:151–156.

Miller, D. G., 1962, Patterns of immunologic deficiency in lymphomas and leukemias, *Ann. Intern. Med.* **57**:703–716.

Miller, D. G., and Lizardo, J. G., 1961, Homologous and heterologous skin transplantation in patients with lymphomatous disease, *J. Natl. Cancer Inst.* **26**:569–583.

Navone, R., and Stramignoni, A., 1974, PHA response of blood and lymph node lymphocytes *in vitro* in malignant lymphomas, *Acta Haematol.* **51**:76–83.

Neiman, R. S., Rosen, P. J., and Lukes, R. J., 1973, Lymphocyte-depleted Hodgkin's disease, *N. Engl. J. Med.* **288**:751–755.

Papac, R. J., 1970, Lymphocyte transformation in malignant lymphomas, *Cancer* **26**:279–286.

Parmley, R. T., 1975, Altered tissue eosinophils in Hodgkin's disease, *Exp. Mol. Pathol.* **23**:70–82.

Peckham, M. J., and Cooper, E. H., 1973, Cell proliferation in Hodgkin's disease, *Natl. Cancer Inst. Monogr.* **36**:179–189.

Plager, J., and Stutzman, L., 1971, Acute nephrotic syndrome as a manifestation of active Hodgkin's disease: Report of four cases and review of the literature, *Am. J. Med.* **50**:56–66.

Preud'homme, J. L., and Seligmann, M., 1972, Surface bound immunoglobulins as a cell marker in human lymphoproliferative diseases, *Blood* **40**:777–794.

Razis, D. V., Diamond, H. D., and Craver, L. F., 1959, Hodgkin's disease associated with other malignant tumors and certain nonneoplastic diseases, *Am. J. Med. Sci.* **238**:327–335.

Rocklin, R. E., 1974, Products of activated lymphocytes: Leukocyte inhibitory factor (LIF) distinct from migration inhibitory factor (MIF), *J. Immunol.* **112**:1461–1466.

Rocklin, R. E., 1975, Partial characterization of leukocyte inhibitory factor by concanavalin A-stimulated human lymphocytes (LIF con A), *J. Immunol.* **114**:1161–1165.

Rocklin, R. E., Remold, H. G., and David, J. R., 1972, Characterization of human migration inhibitory factor (MIF) from antigen-stimulated lymphocytes, *Cell. Immunol.* **5**:436–445.

Rocklin, R. E., MacDermott, R. P., Chess, L., Schlossman, S. F., and David, J. R., 1974, Studies on mediator production by highly purified human T and B lymphocytes, *J. Exp. Med.* **140**:1303–1316.

Rosenberg, S. A., 1966, Report of committee on staging of Hodgkin's disease. *Cancer Res.* **26**:1310.

Rosenberg, S. A., Levy, R., Scheckter, B., Ficker, S., and Terry, W. D., 1972, A rapid microassay of cellular immunity in the guinea pig and mouse, *Transplantation* **13**:541–545.

Rosner, F., and Grunwald, H., 1975, Hodgkin's disease and acute leukemia, *Am. J. Med.* **58**:339–353.

Rostenberg, A., Jr., and Bluefarb, S. M., 1954, Cutaneous reactions in the lymphoblastomas, *Arch. Dermatol.* **69**:195–205.

Rostenberg, A., Jr., McCraney, H. C., and Bluefarb, S. M., 1956, Immunologic studies in the lymphoblastomas. II. The ability to develop an eczematous sensitization to a simple chemical and the ability to accept passive transfer antibody, *J. Invest. Dermatol.* **26**:209–216.

Salvin, S. B., Youngner, J. S., and Lederer, W. H., 1973, Migration inhibitory factor and interferon in the circulation of mice with delayed hypersensitivity, *Infect. Immunol.* **7**:68–75.

Schier, W. W., 1954, Cutaneous anergy and Hodgkin's disease, *N. Engl. J. Med.* **250**:353–361.

Schimpff, S. C., O'Connell, M. H., Greene, W. H., and Wiernik, P. H., 1975, Infections in 92 splenectomized patients with Hodgkin's disease, *Am. J. Med.* **59**:695–701.

Sears, W. G., 1932, The blood in Hodgkin's disease with special reference to eosinophilia, *Guys Hosp. Rep.* **82**:40–54.

Sokal, J. E., Aungst, C. W., and Snyderman, M., 1974, Delay in progression of malignant lymphoma after BCG vaccination, *N. Engl. J. Med.* **291**:1226–1230.

Stevens, D. A., 1973, Oncogenic herpesviruses: A selective review and their possible implications for Hodgkin's disease, *Natl. Cancer Inst. Monogr.*

Stevens, D. A., and Merigan, T. C., 1973, Herpes zoster: Recent studies, *Natl. Cancer Inst. Monogr.* **36**:463–468.

Stjernsward, J., Jondal, M., Vanky, F., Wigzell, H., and Sealy, R., 1972, Lymphopenia and change in distribution of human B and T lymphocytes in peripheral blood induced by irradiation for mammary carcinoma, *Lancet* **1**:1352–1356.

Strum, S. B., and Rappaport, H., 1971, The persistence of Hodgkin's disease in long-term survivors, *Am. J. Med.* **51**:220–240.

Sutherland, J. C., Markham, R. V., Jr., Ramsey, H. E., and Mardiey, M. R., Jr., 1974, Subclinical immune complex nephritis in patients with Hodgkin's disease, *Cancer Res.* **34**:1179–1181.

Swan, H. T., and Knowelden, J., 1971, Prognosis in Hodgkin's disease related to the lymphocyte count, *Br. J. Haematol.* **21**:343–349.

Twomey, J. J., 1973, Infections complicating multiple myeloma and chronic lymphocytic leukemia, *Arch. Intern. Med.* **132**:562–565.

Twomey, J. J., and Douglass, C. C., 1974, An *in vitro* study of lymphocyte and macrophage function with lymphoproliferative neoplasms, *Cancer* **33**:1034–1038.

Twomey, J. J., Douglass, C. C., and Norris, S. M., 1973, Inability of leukocytes to stimulate mixed leukocyte reactions, *J. Natl. Cancer Inst.* **51**:345–351.

Twomey, J. J., Laughter, A. H., Farrow, S., and Douglass, C. C., 1975, Hodgkin's disease: An immunodepleting and immunosuppressive disorder, *J. Clin. Invest.* **56**:467–475.

Twomey, J. J., Laughter, A. H., Lazar, S., and Douglass, C. C., 1976, Reactivity of lymphocytes from primary neoplasms of lymphoid tissues, *Cancer* **38**:740–747.

Twomey, J. J., Lewis, V. M., Bealmear, P., Goldstein, G., and Good, R. A., 1977 (unpublished).

Ultmann, J. E., 1970, Current status: The management of lymphoma, *Semin. Hematol.* **7**:441–460.

Urbanitz, D., Fechner, D., and Gross, R., 1975, Reduced monocyte phagocytosis in patients with advanced Hodgkin's disease and lymphosarcoma. *Klin. Wochenschr.* **53**:437–440.

Waddell, C. C., Taunton, O. D., and Twomey, J. J., 1976, Inhibition of lymphoproliferation of hyperlipoproteinemic plasma, *J. Clin. Invest.* **58**:950–954.

Weller, T. H., 1965, Varicella-herpes zoster virus, in: *Viral and Rickettsial Infections in Man* (F. L. Horsfall and I. Tamm, eds.), 4th Ed., pp. 915–925, Lippincott, Philadelphia.

Weston, W. L., Mandel, M. S., Yeckley, J. A., Krueger, G. G., and Claman, H. N., 1973, Mechanism of cortisol inhibition of adoptive transfer of tuberculin sensitivity, *J. Lab. Clin. Med.* **82**:367–371.

Wilson, J. F., Marsa, W., and Johnson, R. E., 1972, Herpes zoster in Hodgkin's disease: Clinical, histologic and immunologic correlations, *Cancer* **29**:461–465.

Winkelstein, A., Mikulla, J. M., Sartiano, G. P., and Ellis, L. D., 1974, Cellular immunity in Hodgkin's disease: Comparison of cutaneous reactivity and lymphoproliferative responses to phytohemagglutinin, *Cancer* **34**:549–553.

Woodruff, J. F., and Woodruff, J. J., 1974, Involvement of T lymphocytes in the pathogenesis of Coxsackie virus B_3 heart disease, *J. Immunol.* **113**:1726–1734.

Wybran, J., Chandler, S., and Fudenberg, H. H., 1973, Isolation of normal T cells in chronic lymphocytic leukemia, *Lancet* **1**:126–129.

Young, R. C., Corder, M. P., Haynes, H. A., and DeVita, V. T., 1972, Delayed hypersensitivity in Hodgkin's disease, *Am. J. Med.* **52**:63–72.

Young, R. C., Canellos, G. P., Chabner, B. A., Schein, P. S., and DeVita V. T., 1973, Maintenance chemotherapy for advanced Hodgkin's disease in remission, *Lancet* **1**:1339–1343.

Zamecnik, P. C., and Long, J. C., 1977, Growth of cultured cells from patients with Hodgkin's disease and transplantation into nude mice. *Proc. Natl. Acad. Sci. U.S.A.* **74**:754–758.

Zatz, M. M., White, A., and Goldstein, A. L., 1973, Alterations in the lymphocyte populations in tumorgenesis. I. Lymphocyte trapping, *J. Immunol.* **111**:706–711.

Ziegler, J. B., Hausen, P., and Penny, R., 1975, Intrinsic lymphocyte defect in Hodgkin's disease: Analysis of the phytohemagglutinin dose response, *Clin. Immunol. Immunopathol.* **3**:451–460.

21

Non-Hodgkin's Lymphoma in Children: Historical Review, Patterns of Disease, and Future Trends

NORMA WOLLNER

1. Introduction

Non-Hodgkin's lymphoma in children has a different clinical course and survival than its adult counterpart. Although metastatic sites and incidence of recurrence are the same, the length of time for the appearance of recurrence and metastases is much shorter. In patients in the pediatric age group (ages 0–16), a more rapid progression and a fatal outcome are the usual course of this disease (Jones *et al.*, 1972; Levitt *et al.*, 1972; Lemerle *et al.*, 1973; Sullivan, 1973). This chapter discusses the distribution of non-Hodgkin's lymphoma by age, sex, primary site, histology, and stage in a total of 104 patients analyzed from January 1964 to December 1973.

2. Age Distribution

2.1. Total Population

In 104 patients (Figure 1), the only peak observed in occurrence of non-Hodgkin's lymphoma was at age 5, with an almost even distribution among other ages. Figures 2 and 3 show the distribution by age among the 73 males and 31 females.

NORMA WOLLNER • Memorial Sloan-Kettering Cancer Center, New York, New York 10021.

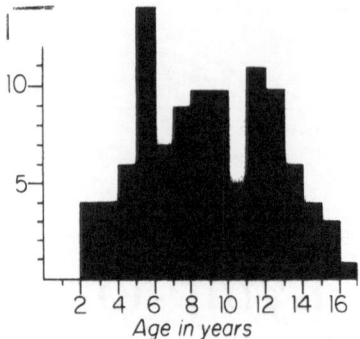

Figure 1. Non-Hodgkin's lymphoma in children: Distribution by age among the 104 patients in the study.

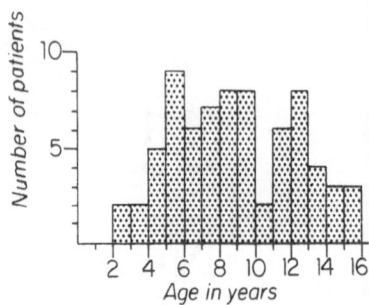

Figure 2. Non-Hodgkin's lymphoma in children: Distribution by age among the 73 male patients in the study.

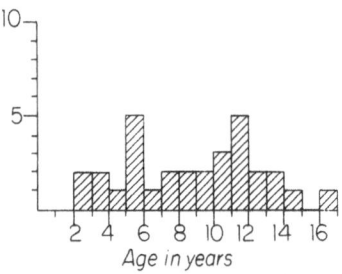

Figure 3. Non-Hodgkin's lymphoma in children: Distribution by age among the 31 female patients in the study.

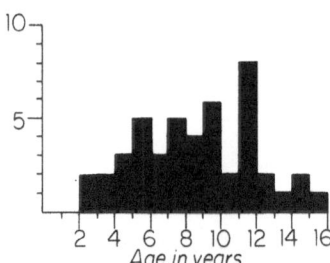

Figure 4. Non-Hodgkin's lymphoma in children: Distribution of primary nodal disease (peripheral nodal and mediastinal) by age among a total of 46 patients.

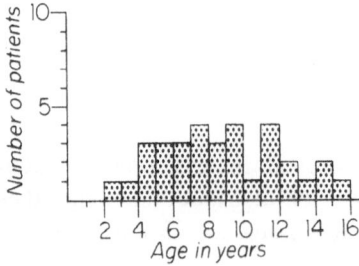

Figure 5. Non-Hodgkin's lymphoma in children: Distribution of primary nodal disease by age among 33 male patients.

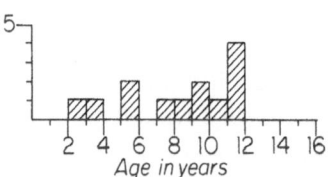

Figure 6. Non-Hodgkin's lymphoma in children: Distribution of primary nodal disease by age among 13 female patients.

2.2. Nodal and Extranodal Disease

611

NON-HODGKIN'S
LYMPHOMA IN
CHILDREN:
HISTORICAL
REVIEW, PATTERNS
OF DISEASE, AND
FUTURE TRENDS

2.2.1. Primary Nodal Disease

The distribution of primary nodal disease, which comprises 46 patients with primary peripheral nodal (25 patients) and mediastinal (21 patients) involvement, shows a slight peak at age 11 (Figure 4). Figures 5 and 6 show the distribution of this type of presentation by age in the male and female population.

2.2.2. Primary Extranodal Disease

In this group, which comprises a total of 58 patients, the distribution of disease by primary site was as follows:

Bowel	21 patients
Skeletal	17
Ovarian	6
Nasopharyngeal	5
Subcutaneous	3
Renal	3
Liver	1
Thyroid	1
CNS	1

In the distribution of primary extranodal disease by age (Figure 7), there were two major peaks—one at age 5, the second at age 12. Figures 8 and 9 show the age distribution by sex.

2.3. Stages

Of the 104 patients in the pediatric age group in the population studied, 26 (25%) presented with local or regional disease. Figure 10 shows the distribution of stages I and II disease in these 26 patients by age, which shows a peak at 5 years. Figures 11 and 12 show the age distribution in this population by sex.

The majority of pediatric patients seen in our institution (75%) presented with far-advanced disease (stages III and IV), as shown in Figure 13. Figures 14 and 15 show the age/sex distribution in patients with stages III and IV disease.

2.4. Pathology

The histological classification of Rappaport (1966) was used in this study. Of the 104 patients, 5 did not have slides available for histological subtyping.

2.4.1. Nodular Histological Pattern

This pattern was observed in 14 (13.5%) of the 104 patients. The distribution of subtyping was as follows:

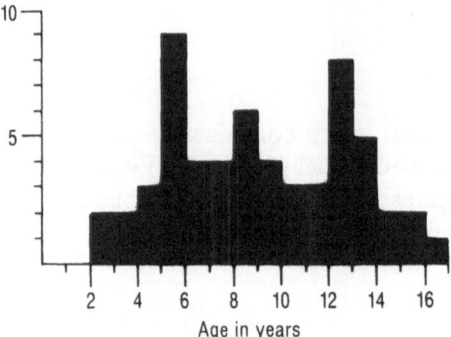

Figure 7. Non-Hodgkin's lymphoma in children: Distribution of primary extranodal disease by age among a total of 58 patients.

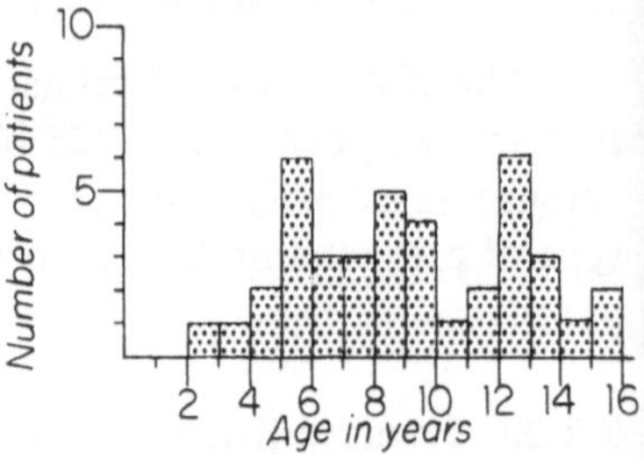

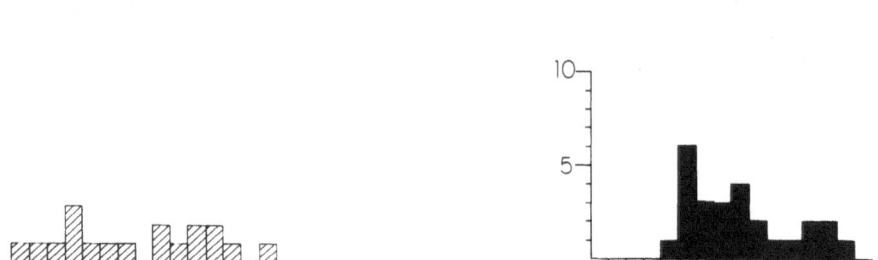

Figure 8. Non-Hodgkin's lymphoma in children: Distribution of primary extranodal disease by age among 40 male patients.

Figure 9. Non-Hodgkin's lymphoma in children: Distribution of primary extranodal disease by age among 18 female patients.

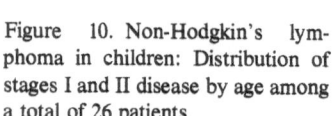

Figure 10. Non-Hodgkin's lymphoma in children: Distribution of stages I and II disease by age among a total of 26 patients.

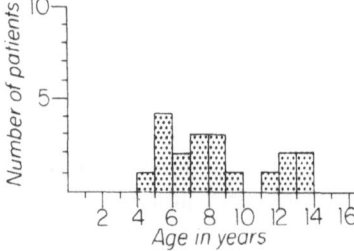

Figure 11. Non-Hodgkin's lymphoma in children: Distribution of stages I and II disease by age among 19 male patients.

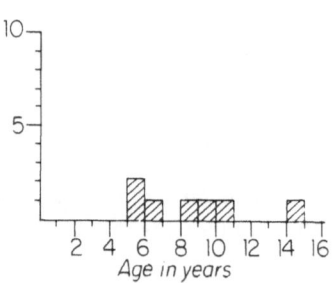

Figure 12. Non-Hodgkin's lymphoma in children: Distribution of Stages I and II disease by age among 7 female patients.

613

NON-HODGKIN'S
LYMPHOMA IN
CHILDREN:
HISTORICAL
REVIEW, PATTERNS
OF DISEASE, AND
FUTURE TRENDS

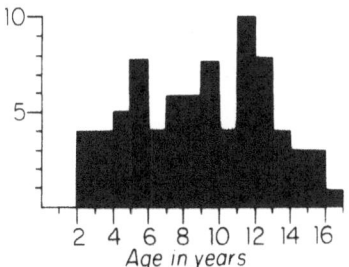

Figure 13. Non-Hodgkin's lymphoma in children: Distribution of stages III and IV disease by age among a total of 78 patients.

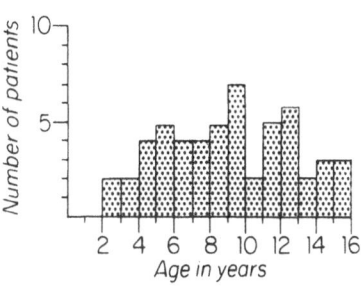

Figure 14. Non-Hodgkin's lymphoma in children: Distribution of stages III and IV disease by age among 54 male patients.

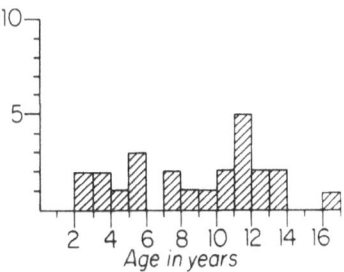

Figure 15. Non-Hodgkin's lymphoma in children: Distribution of stages III and IV disease by age among 24 female patients.

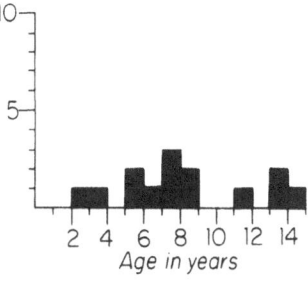

Figure 16. Non-Hodgkin's lymphoma in children: Distribution of nodular pathology by age among a total of 14 patients.

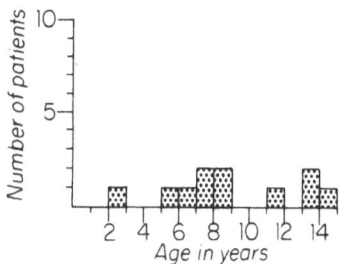

Figure 17. Non-Hodgkin's lymphoma in children: Distribution of nodular pathology by age among 11 male patients.

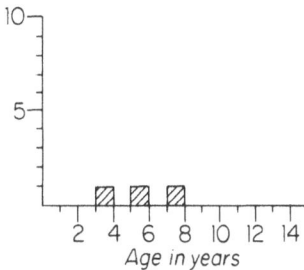

Figure 18. Non-Hodgkin's lymphoma in children: Distribution of nodular pathology by age among 3 female patients.

Nodular lymphocytic, poorly differentiated (NLPD)	8 patients
Nodular lymphocytic, well differentiated (NLWD)	3
Nodular mixed (NM)	2
Nodular undifferentiated (NU)	1

Figure 16 shows the distribution of nodular pathology by age in these 14 patients. Figures 17 and 18 show the age distribution by sex.

2.4.2. Diffuse Histological Pattern

This pattern was observed in 85 (82%) of the 104 patients. The distribution of the different subtypes was as follows:

Diffuse lymphocytic, poorly differentiated (DLPD)	41 patients
Diffuse lymphocytic, well differentiated (DLWD)	5
Diffuse mixed (DM)	1
Diffuse histiocytic (DH)	20
Diffuse undifferentiated (DU)	18

Figure 19 shows the age distribution among the total 85 patients, which has three peaks: one at age 5, another at ages 8 and 9, and a third at ages 11 and 12. Figures 20 and 21 show the breakdown by sex.

2.5. Primary Sites

The distribution by age and sex of the most common primary sites such as peripheral nodal, mediastinal, bowel, and skeletal is shown in Figures 22–25.

3. Natural History with Respect to Primary Sites

3.1. Peripheral Nodal Disease

A total of 25 patients were studied (see Figure 22).

3.1.1. Symptoms

Besides the obvious lymph node enlargement, the following symptoms were encountered: fever, malaise, anorexia, sore throat, cough, weight loss, earache, night sweats, bone pain, and joint pain. These last three are usually found in patients in whom disease has disseminated to bone marrow. All these symptoms are unspecific and at times are responsible for delay in proper diagnosis. Only when no improvement or when progression in lymph node size (despite antibiotic therapy) was seen was the patient referred for biopsy.

3.1.2. Histology

Of the 25 patients, only 1 had no slide review for Rappaport's histological subtyping. In the remaining 24 patients, the histological distribution was as follows: 6 patients had DH disease, 6 had NLPD, 5 had DLPD, 3 had DLWD, 2 had NLWD, 1 had DU, and 1 had NM. Thus, of the 14 patients with nodular histology (see Section 2.4.1), 9 are accounted for in the peripheral nodal disease category.

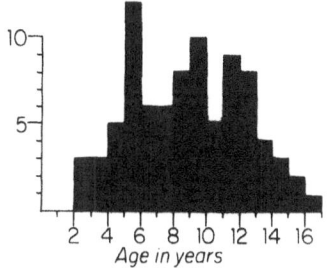

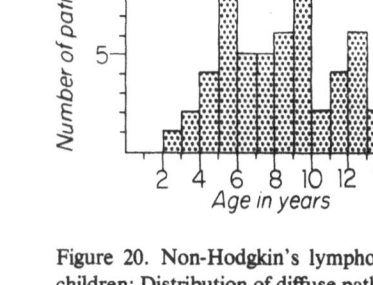

615

NON-HODGKIN'S
LYMPHOMA IN
CHILDREN:
HISTORICAL
REVIEW, PATTERNS
OF DISEASE, AND
FUTURE TRENDS

Figure 19. Non-Hodgkin's lymphoma in children: Distribution of diffuse pathology by age among a total of 85 patients.

Figure 20. Non-Hodgkin's lymphoma in children: Distribution of diffuse pathology by age among 57 male patients.

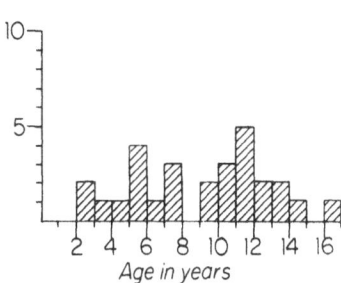

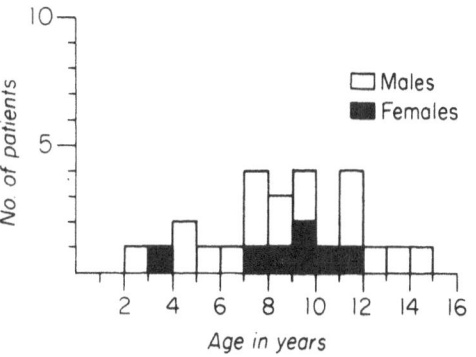

Figure 21. Non-Hodgkin's lymphoma in children: Distribution of diffuse pathology by age among 28 female patients.

Figure 22. Non-Hodgkin's lymphoma in children: Distribution of primary peripheral nodal disease by age and sex among a total of 25 patients (18 males and 7 females).

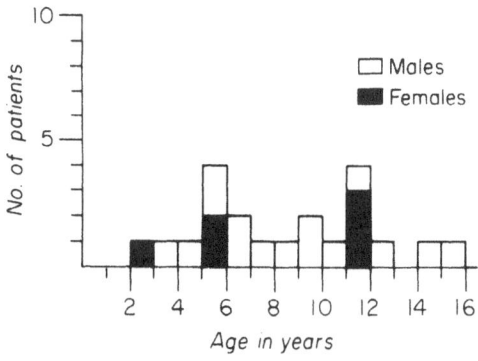

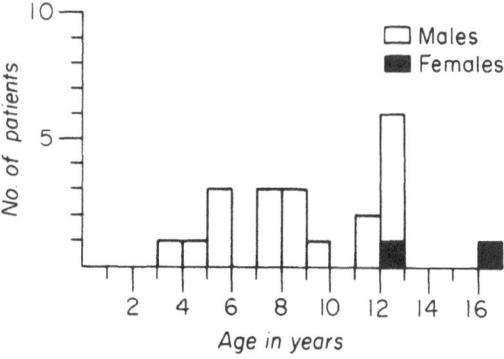

Figure 23. Non-Hodgkin's lymphoma in children: Distribution of primary mediastinal disease by age and sex among a total of 21 patients (15 males and 6 females).

Figure 24. Non-Hodgkin's lymphoma in children: Distribution of primary bowel disease by age and sex among a total of 21 patients (19 males and 2 females).

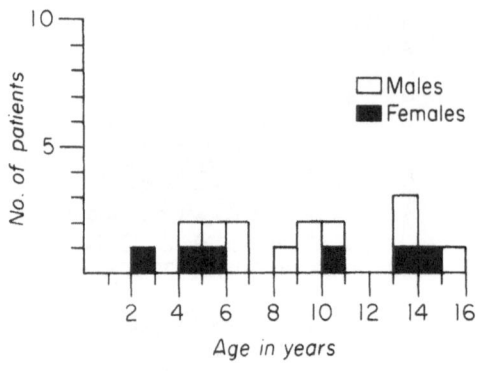

Figure 25. Non-Hodgkin's lymphoma in children: Distribution of primary skeletal disease by age and sex among a total of 17 patients (11 males and 6 females).

3.1.3. Staging

The staging of these 25 patients was as follows: stage I, 5 patients; stage II, 4 patients; stage III, 7 patients; stage IV, 9 patients.

3.1.4. Other Sites of Involvement at the Time of Diagnosis

The presence of a localized lymph node does not preclude disseminated disease, and therefore all patients should be extensively worked up with X rays, scans, and bone marrow aspirations from at least three sites. Of the 25 patients with this type of primary presentation, only 9 had no other site of involvement besides the peripheral nodes.

In the remaining 16 patients, the following additional sites were involved initially:

Bone marrow	9 patients	
Mediastinum	8	
Paraaortic nodes	5	
Bones	4	
Kidneys	3	
Subcutaneous tissue	2	
Nasopharynx	1	(primary superior cervical nodes)
Liver and spleen	1	(initial marrow involvement)
Prostate	1	(primary right upper cervical node)

3.1.5. Recurrence

There was recurrence of primary peripheral nodal disease in 10 of 25 patients as a result of treatment failure, despite adequate therapy. The median time for recurrence was 5 months from diagnosis; the shortest time was 1 month, the longest 22 months.

3.1.6. Metastatic Sites

Besides recurrence, the most common sites for metastatic disease were

Bone marrow   11 patients (in 2 patients it was a recurrence)

617

NON-HODGKIN'S
LYMPHOMA IN
CHILDREN:
HISTORICAL
REVIEW, PATTERNS
OF DISEASE, AND
FUTURE TRENDS

CNS	6 patients
Liver	5
Bowel	4
Spleen	4
Subcutaneous tissues	2
Mediastinum	1
Lung	1
Orbital cavity	1
Kidneys	1
Skeletal	1
Testicles	1

3.2. Primary Mediastinal Disease

A total of 21 patients were studied (see Figure 23).

3.2.1. Symptoms

The most common symptoms in order of decreasing frequency were peripheral adenopathy, fever, cough, dyspnea, fatigue, night sweats, anorexia, vomiting, nausea, subcutaneous nodules, and abdominal mass.

3.2.2. Histology

Of the 21 patients, only 1 slide was not available for retyping. The classification of the 20 patients according to Rappaport's histology was: 12 DLPD, 5 DU, 1 DLWD, 1 DM, and 1 NLPD.

3.2.3. Staging

Of the 21 patients, 14 had stage III and 7 had stage IV disease.

3.2.4. Other Sites of Involvement at the Time of Diagnosis

Other sites of involvement were

Peripheral nodes	18 patients
Pleural effusion	17
Liver	9
Bone marrow	7
Kidney	5
Paraaortic nodes	5
Heart (pericardium)	4
Lungs (by direct extension)	2
Tonsils	2
Bone	2
Subcutaneous tissue	1

The finding of pleural involvement (85%) in patients with mediastinal disease is quite common in non-Hodgkin's lymphoma in children, as opposed to its rare incidence in Hodgkin's disease with mediastinal involvement. Distant metastases at the time of diagnosis are frequent, as seen in the number of patients with involvement of the peripheral and paraaortic nodes, kidney, tonsils, bone marrow, subcutaneous tissue, and bones.

3.2.5. Recurrence

There was recurrence in 13 patients, and in only 3 of these patients was there no mediastinal recurrence. Metastatic sites encountered were

Bone marrow	11 patients
CNS	9
Peripheral nodes	8
Spleen	6
Liver	5
Kidneys	5
Subcutaneous tissue	4
Testicles	4
Bowel	4
Nasopharynx	2
Orbital cavity	1
Pleura	1 (not involved initially)

3.3. Primary Bowel Disease

A total of 21 patients were studied (see Figure 24).

3.3.1. Symptoms

The most common symptoms in order of decreasing frequency were abdominal pain, vomiting, abdominal distension, abdominal mass, fever, diarrhea, anorexia, melena and constipation, intussusception, weight loss, and back pain. Epistaxis occurred in 1 patient in whom there was concomitant nasopharyngeal involvement.

3.3.2. Histology

In 2 patients, slides were not available for subtyping. According to Rappaport's histological classification, there were 11 patients with DLPD, 5 with DH, 2 with DU, and 1 with NLWD.

3.3.3. Staging

The staging of the 21 patients was as follows: stage I, 2 patients; stage II, 3 patients; stage III, 12 patients; stage IV, 4 patients.

3.3.4. Other Sites of Involvement at the Time of Diagnosis

619

NON-HODGKIN'S
LYMPHOMA IN
CHILDREN:
HISTORICAL
REVIEW, PATTERNS
OF DISEASE, AND
FUTURE TRENDS

Only 5 patients had only one site of involvement, the site being bowel in 2 and regional nodes in 3. The remaining 16 patients had the following sites of involvement, excluding the bowel:

Kidneys	11 patients
Peripheral nodes	7
Liver	6
Pleura	5
Paraaortic nodes	5
Bone marrow	4
Testicles	2
Mediastinum	1
Tonsils	1
Ovaries	1
CNS	1

Ascites was present in 5 patients at the time of diagnosis. In all 5, tumor was extensive and unresectable.

3.3.5. Recurrence

Of the total of 21 patients, 12 had recurrence in the primary site and 2 had progressive disease unresponsive to therapy. The median time for recurrence was 3 months from diagnosis; the shortest time was 1 month, the longest 5 months.

3.3.6. Metastatic Sites

Only 6 patients did not have metastases, of which only 1 had local recurrence. Excluding the 2 patients with progressive disease, who died within 1 month of diagnosis, and the 6 patients who did not metastasize, the remaining 13 patients exhibited metastases to the following sites:

Bone marrow	8 patients	
CNS	8	
Pleura	6	(apart from those who presented with it at the time of diagnosis)
Chest wall	4	
Kidney	4	
Peripheral nodes	3	
Liver	3	
Testicles	3	
Paraaortic nodes	2	
Spleen	2	
Bones	2	
Nasopharynx	1	

At the time of recurrence, 6 patients developed ascites. In only 2 of these 6 patients was the ascites recurrent. We feel that the chest wall and pleural involvement is probably due to local recurrent disease and dissemination through the paraaortic gutter to the diaphragm, chest wall, posterior mediastinum, and pleura.

3.4. Primary Skeletal Disease

A total of 17 patients were studied (see Figure 25).

3.4.1. Symptoms

The most common symptoms were bone pain, swelling, lymphadenopathy, anorexia, fever, and weight loss. Abdominal pain, vomiting, and abdominal mass were seen in 1 patient with a jaw mass.

3.4.2. Histology

Of the 17 patients, 6 had DLPD disease, 5 had DU, 5 had DH, and 1 had DLWD.

3.4.3. Staging

There were 3 patients with stage I disease, 1 with stage II, 4 with stage III, and 9 with stage IV.

3.4.4. Other Sites of Involvement at the Time of Diagnosis

Of the 17 patients, 3 had no site other than that of the primary disease involved; 1 had regional node metastases at the time of diagnosis. The remaining 13 patients had the following sites positive at the time of diagnosis:

Peripheral nodes	9 patients
Bone marrow	7
Mediastinum	4
Kidneys	3
Paraaortic nodes	3
CNS	2
Liver and spleen	2
Subcutaneous nodules	2
Pelvic mass	2

3.4.5. Recurrence

Of the 17 patients, 7 had local recurrence despite adequate radiation therapy.

3.4.6. Metastatic Sites

Metastases occurred in the following sites:

Bone marrow	11 patients (6 had no previous involvement)
CNS	7

621

NON-HODGKIN'S
LYMPHOMA IN
CHILDREN:
HISTORICAL
REVIEW, PATTERNS
OF DISEASE, AND
FUTURE TRENDS

Peripheral nodes	3 patients
Other bones	3
Liver	3
Spleen	3
Mediastinum	3
Subcutaneous tissue	2
Bowel	1
Kidneys	1
Tonsils	1
Chest wall	1
Testicles	1

3.5. Primary Ovarian Disease

A total of 6 patients were studied.

3.5.1. Symptoms

The symptoms seen in these patients were abdominal pain, swelling, palpable mass, fever, malaise, weight loss, and constipation.

3.5.2. Histology

Of the 6 patients, 4 had DLPD disease, 1 had DU, and 1 had DH.

3.5.3. Staging

There were no patients with stage I or II disease. Stage III disease was present in 5 patients, stage IV in 1.

3.5.4. Other Sites of Involvement at the Time of Diagnosis

Other sites of involvement were

Paraaortic nodes	3 patients
Kidneys	3
Bowel	2
Mesenteric nodes	2
Liver	2
Mediastinum	2
Peripheral nodes	2
Ascites	2
Bone marrow	1
CNS	1
Tonsils	1
Bones	1
Pleura	1

3.5.5. Recurrence

There was recurrence in 5 of 6 patients within a median time of 3 months.

3.5.6. Metastatic Sites

Metastatic sites encountered were

Bone marrow	4 patients
CNS	4
Peripheral nodes	2
Kidneys	2
Liver	2
Bones	2
Chest wall	1
Mediastinum	1
Pleura	1
Peritoneal cavity with ascites	1

3.6. Primary Nasopharyngeal Disease

A total of 5 patients were studied.

3.6.1. Symptoms

The most common symptoms in order of decreasing frequency were stuffy nose, eye pain and swelling, rhinorrhea, hoarseness, cough, and epistaxis.

3.6.2. Histology

Of the 5 patients, 2 had DU disease, 1 had DH, 1 had NU, and 1 had NLPD.

3.6.3. Staging

In this group, 1 patient had stage I, 3 had stage II, and one had stage IV disease. Regardless of the therapy given (radiation therapy and surgery for 1 patient, high-dose cyclophosphamide and radiation therapy for 1 patient, and the LSA_2-L_2 protocol plus radiation therapy for 3 patients), there were no recurrences or metastases even in the patient with initial paraaortic and bone marrow involvement (stage IV).

3.7. Primary Renal Disease

A total of 3 patients were studied.

3.7.1. Symptoms

The most common symptoms in order of decreasing frequency were abdominal swelling, flank mass, abdominal pain, fever, weight loss, and anorexia.

3.7.2. Histology

Slides were not available in 1 patient for subtyping. The other 2 had DLPD disease.

623

NON-HODGKIN'S
LYMPHOMA IN
CHILDREN:
HISTORICAL
REVIEW, PATTERNS
OF DISEASE, AND
FUTURE TRENDS

3.7.3. Staging

In this group, 1 patient had stage I disease, 1 had stage III, and 1 had stage IV.

3.7.4. Other Sites of Involvement at the Time of Diagnosis

Other sites of involvement were

Peripheral nodes	1 patient
Liver	1
Bowel	1
Bone	1
Bone marrow and CNS	1

3.7.5. Recurrence

There was recurrence in the primary site in only 1 patient.

3.7.6. Metastatic Sites

Sites of metastases were bone marrow and CNS in 1 patient (this was the recurrence of a previous involvement), subcutaneous tissue in 1 patient, bowel in 1 patient, and bone in 1 patient.

3.8. Primary Subcutaneous Tissue Disease

A total of 3 patients were studied.

3.8.1. Symptoms

The following complaints were presented at the time of diagnosis: multiple skin nodules, local inflammatory signs, peripheral node enlargement, cough, fever, and anorexia.

3.8.2. Histology

Histologically, 2 patients had DH disease and 1 had NM.

3.8.3. Staging

Of the 3 patients, 1 had stage II and 2 had stage III disease.

3.8.4. Other Sites of Involvement at the Time of Diagnosis

Other sites of involvement were the peripheral nodes in 3 patients and lung nodules in 1 patient.

3.8.5. Recurrence

Recurrence was seen in 2 of 3 patients—one at 1 year, the second at 25 months, from diagnosis.

3.8.6. Metastatic Sites

No other metastatic sites were encountered, even in those who relapsed.

3.9. Primary Liver Disease

Only 1 patient presented with this type of involvement; he had stage I DU disease. His symptoms were abdominal mass and pain. Recurrence was noted in the primary site within 3 months from diagnosis and metastasized to paraaortic nodes, bone marrow, CNS, kidney, testicles, and subcutaneous tissue.

4. Summary

Even though the majority of symptoms are unspecific, diagnosis in general was not delayed. Diagnosis was within 1–2 months from onset of symptoms in 80% of the patients. Since 75% of the patients had far-advanced disease at the time of diagnosis and about 70% were diagnosed within 1 month from onset of symptoms, one must assume that this disease is very agressive and progresses very rapidly. In those patients in whom diagnosis was not made until several months after onset of symptoms and who had stage I disease at the time of the biopsy and onset of therapy, prognosis was very favorable, indicating in these cases a less agressive tumor, the histological type notwithstanding. Nodular histology does exist in childhood non-Hodgkin's lymphoma and is not associated with good prognosis (40% 5-year survival), as is its counterpart in adults. That stages I and II did not fare so well in the past may have been because only one bone marrow was performed at that time. Further, treatment was not as intensive as it is today.

In the past, the philosophy has been to treat this disease as one treated Hodgkin's disease, i.e., with nitrogen mustard and radiation therapy with or without maintenance therapy (usually one or two drugs). In cases with initial bone marrow involvement, treatment was modeled after the treatment for leukemia at the time, which was also not satisfactory. Non-Hodgkin's lymphoma in children is responsive to most chemotherapeutic agents. The response is rapid, but relapse and resistance are also rapid if treatment is not adequate.

The survival of these patients in the past has ranged from 11% prior to 1968. From 1968 to 1971, with the advent of high-dose cyclophosphamide therapy, the survival improved to 33%. The median time for recurrence and metastases to bone marrow and CNS as well as to other organs did not change much in these two groups of patients.

625

NON-HODGKIN'S
LYMPHOMA IN
CHILDREN:
HISTORICAL
REVIEW, PATTERNS
OF DISEASE, AND
FUTURE TRENDS

5. Present and Future Trends in the Management of Non-Hodgkin's Lymphoma

Beginning April 1971 and continuing until December 1973, 43 patients were included in a treatment protocol called LSA$_2$–L$_2$. The initial work-up, staging, and

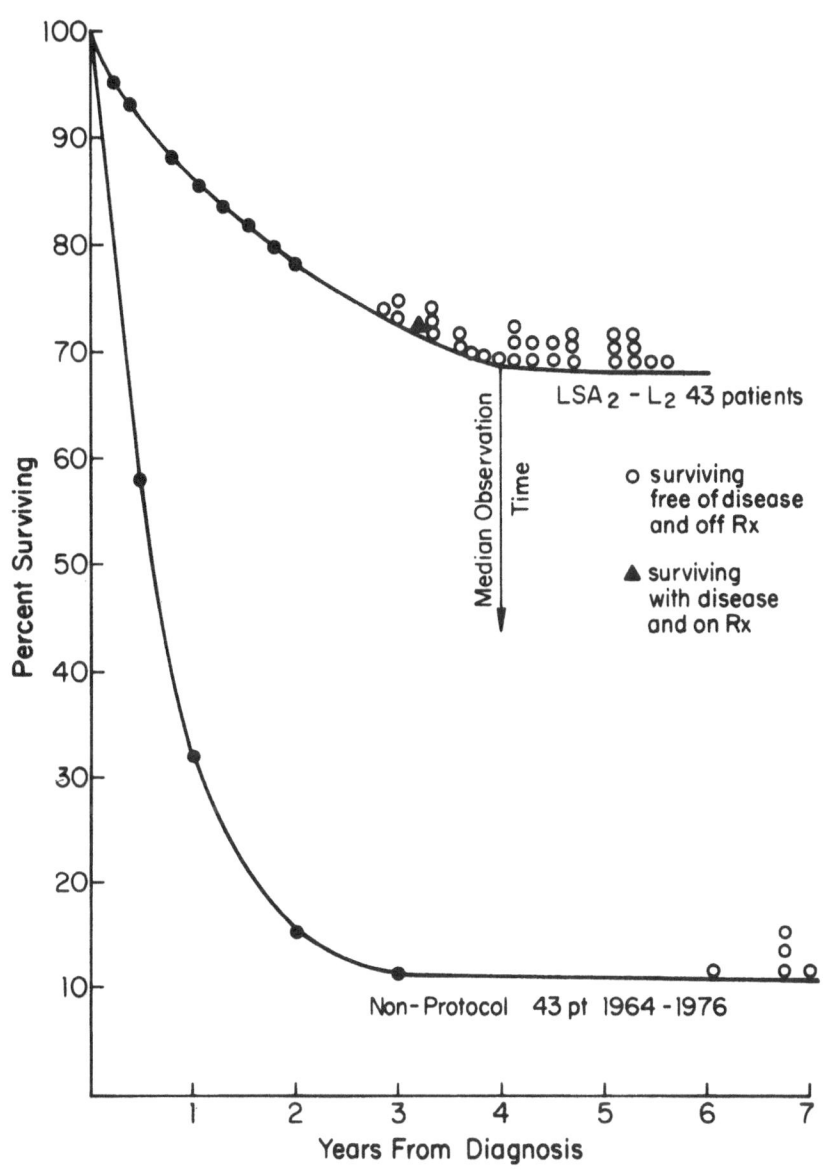

Figure 26. Actuarial survival curves (September 1976) for patients on LSA$_2$–L$_2$ protocol and on nonprotocol treatment.

treatment were detailed elsewhere (Wollner et al., 1974, 1975a,b,c; Wollner, 1976, 1977). The results up until early 1975 were also reported elsewhere (Wollner et al., 1976). After 5½ years of follow-up from the beginning of the study, we will update the information available to us and make future recommendations.

Figure 26 shows the actuarial survival of the 43 patients, previously untreated, on the LSA$_2$–L$_2$ protocol and of a historical group of 43 patients before the advent of high-dose cyclophosphamide. In the latter group, the 5-year survival was only 11%. There were 4 patients with stage I disease and 1 with stage III who at the time of relapse received the LSA$_2$–L$_2$ protocol. The median survival time for this group of patients was 6 months, and 89% were dead at 24 months following multiple relapses. Bone marrow and CNS incidence in this group was high, and occurred within 2–3 months of diagnosis.

In the LSA$_2$–L$_2$ group, the 5-year survival is 69% with all patients off therapy except one, who had a recurrence at 32 months from diagnosis. The median observation time for the group is 48 months, and none of the patients off therapy has active disease.

Table 1 shows the distribution of patients on the LSA$_2$–L$_2$ protocol according to primary site and stage. Of the 43 patients, 21 had nodal and 22 extranodal disease. With regard to staging, 77% had advanced stages (III and IV) and 23% earlier stages, of which only 2% had stage I disease. The median age for the entire group was 8; the youngest was 2 and the oldest 16 years of age.

Table 2 shows the primary sites and the histological types. Of the 43 patients, 15% had a favorable histological type according to the adult criteria. Most of these (4 of 6) had stage IV disease at the time of diagnosis. As to type, 85% had Rappaport's diffuse type of lymphoma. The number of patients with diffuse undifferentiated (DU), a histological type that requires further study, was too small for any definite conclusions, or any comparisons with DLPD and DH.

There are many factors that possibly influence the outcome of a patient with non-Hodgkin's lymphoma, such as clinical and radiological staging, primary sites, histology, and therapy. Figure 26 shows clearly the effect of therapy on survival. We will analyze the remaining factors and determine in general where we failed in

TABLE 1. Non-Hodgkin's Lymphoma in Children: Primary Sites and Staging of 43 Patients on the LSA$_2$–L$_2$ Protocol (September 1976)

Presenting sites	Number of patients	Median age	Stages			
			I	II	III	IV
Peripheral nodal	12	9	1	3	2	6
Mediastinal	9	8	—	—	4	5
Bowel	9	7	—	3	3	3
Skeletal	7	5	—	—	1	6
Nasopharyngeal	3	6	—	3	—	—
Subcutaneous	2	—	—	—	2	—
Ovarian	1	—	—	—	1	—
TOTAL	43		1	9	13	20

627

NON-HODGKIN'S
LYMPHOMA IN
CHILDREN:
HISTORICAL
REVIEW, PATTERNS
OF DISEASE, AND
FUTURE TRENDS

TABLE 2.   Non-Hodgkin's Lymphoma in Children: Primary Sites and Histology of 43 Patients on the LSA$_2$–L$_2$ Protocol (September 1976)

Primary site	Histology							
	NLWD	NM	NLPD	DLWD	DM	DLPD	DH	DU
Peripheral nodal	1	1	2	3	—	3	2	—
Mediastinal	—	—	1	1	1	5	—	1
Bowel	—	—	—	—	—	4	4	1
Skeletal	—	—	—	1	—	4	1	1
Nasopharyngeal	—	—	1	—	—	—	1	1
Subcutaneous	—	—	—	—	—	—	2	—
Ovarian	—	—	—	—	—	1	—	—
TOTAL:	1	1	4	5	1	17	10	4

the 31% that recurred and disseminated and what we may do in the future to improve our results.

5.1.   Stages

Figure 27 shows the actuarial survival of the historical group. There were 10 patients, of which 7 were stage I and 3 were stage II. The 5-year survival rate was 40%. In the LSA$_2$–L$_2$ protocol, there were 9 stage II and one stage I. The 5-year survival rate is 100%.

In the historical group, 6 of 10 patients with adequate staging disseminated and progressed to stage III. We therefore felt that treatment should be as agressive in stage I and II as in stage III disease, knowing we may overtreat 40% of these patients. This is a risk we undertook; we feel that the results of the LSA$_2$–L$_2$ protocol support this concept.

Figure 28 shows the actuarial survival for stage III patients. In the historical control, only 4% survived 5 years free of disease; the 4% represented 1 patient who metastasized early in the course of his treatment and was rescued with the LSA$_2$–L$_2$ protocol. The upper curve shows the actuarial survival of the 13 patients on the LSA$_2$–L$_2$ protocol, with a 61% 5-year survival free of disease. Two patients died without evidence of lymphoma (one from chickenpox and the other from measles and disseminated intravascular coagulation). Thus, only 27% died from lymphoma.

Figure 29 shows the actuarial survival for stage IV patients. The lower curve represents 9 patients of the historical control group, in which there were no survivors. For the 20 patients treated with the LSA$_2$–L$_2$ protocol, the 5-year survival is 58%, with all patients off therapy and a median observation time of 4 years.

Could the survival curve have been improved? The answer is yes. In 1971, the attitude still prevailed among radiation therapists that such far-advanced disease with "leukemic marrow involvement" was beyond hope, and thus radiation therapy

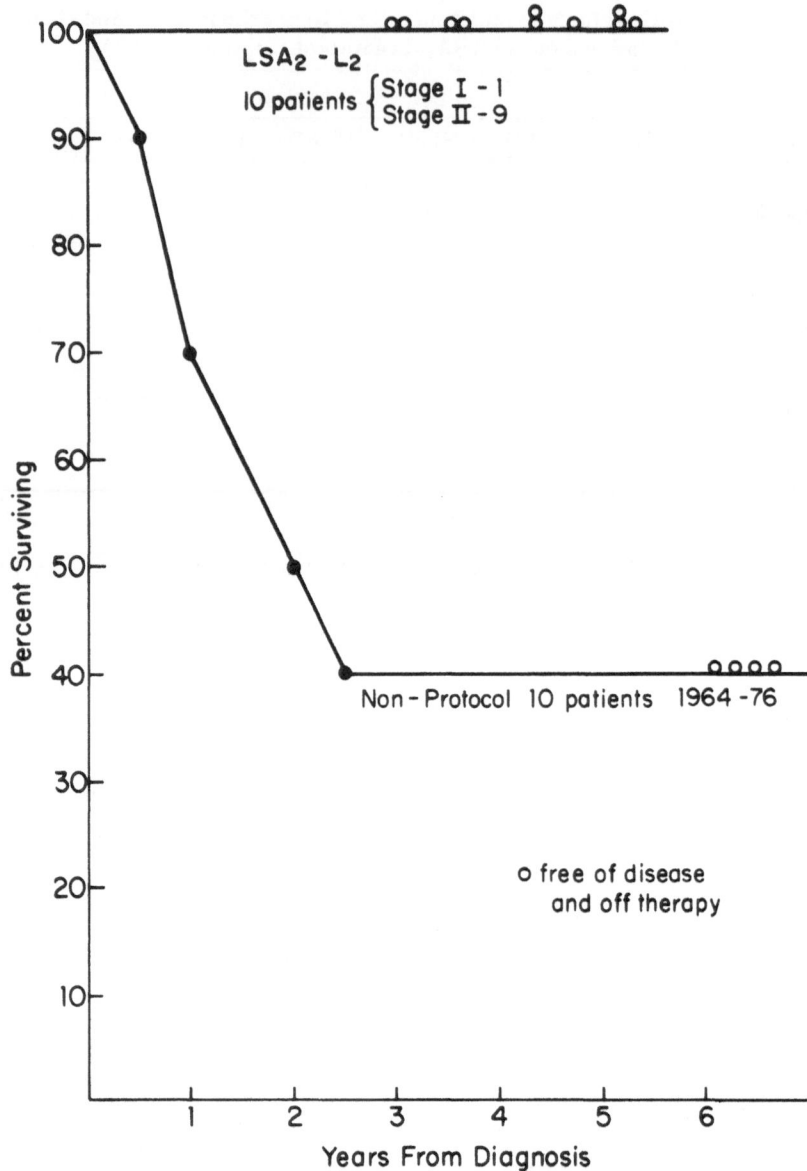

Figure 27. Actuarial survival curve for stages I and II patients (September 1976): LSA$_2$–L$_2$ protocol and nonprotocol.

was given as "palliation" to only a few areas with bulky disease. Also at that time, we were uncertain as to when radiation therapy should be given, and at what dosage, in patients receiving such an intensive chemotherapeutic regimen. Today, we feel we have acquired this knowledge and thus improved the management of these patients on an intensive multidisciplinary approach. Our future results should

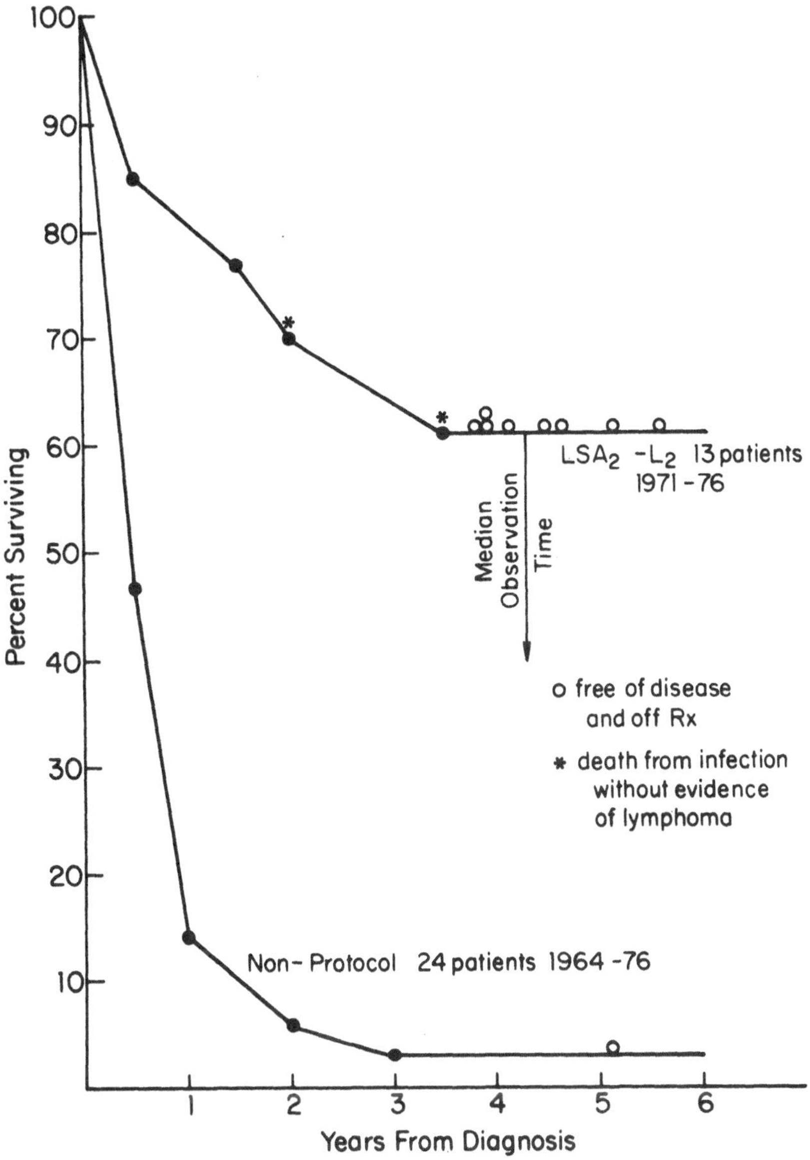

629

NON-HODGKIN'S
LYMPHOMA IN
CHILDREN:
HISTORICAL
REVIEW, PATTERNS
OF DISEASE, AND
FUTURE TRENDS

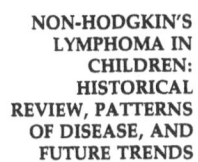

Figure 28. Actuarial survival curve for stage III patients (September 1976): LSA$_2$–L$_2$ protocol and nonprotocol.

reflect this change. We still believe, however, that there will always be patients who are either resistant or are extremely sensitive, with severe and prolonged marrow depression, to this approach, and these patients will fail. Supportive therapy, however, such as white cell, platelet, and red cell transfusions, plus total parenteral nutrition, should prevent some of these failures.

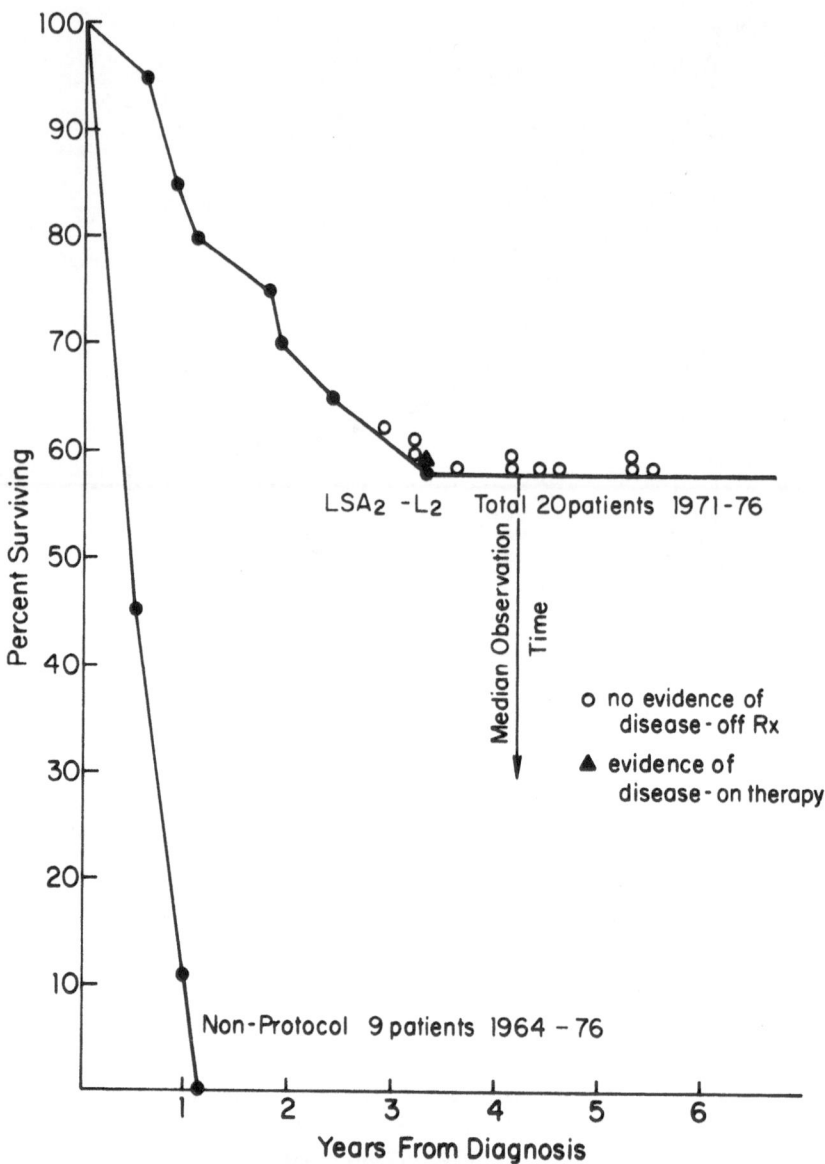

Figure 29. Actuarial survival curve for stage IV patients (September 1976): LSA₂–L₂ protocol and nonprotocol.

5.2. Primary Sites

5.2.1. Peripheral Nodal Disease

Figure 30 shows the actuarial survival of the historical group, with 9 patients and a 5-year survival rate of 34%. Comparison of this rate with the 5-year survival

631

NON-HODGKIN'S
LYMPHOMA IN
CHILDREN:
HISTORICAL
REVIEW, PATTERNS
OF DISEASE, AND
FUTURE TRENDS

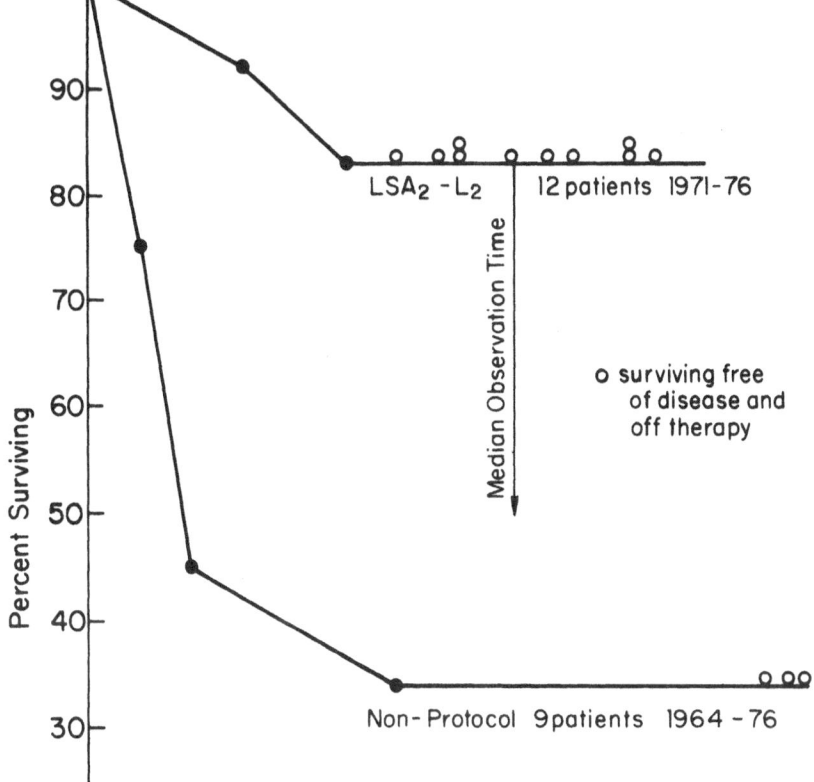

Figure 30. Actuarial survival curves for patients with primary peripheral node disease (September 1976): LSA_2-L_2 protocol and nonprotocol.

rate of 12 patients in the LSA_2-L_2 group of 83% is very encouraging. Again, we feel that some of the patients in this group with stage IV disease (bone marrow, marked nodal involvement) should receive total nodal radiation therapy in addition to the LSA_2-L_2 protocol. We feel that this therapeutic approach will improve these results.

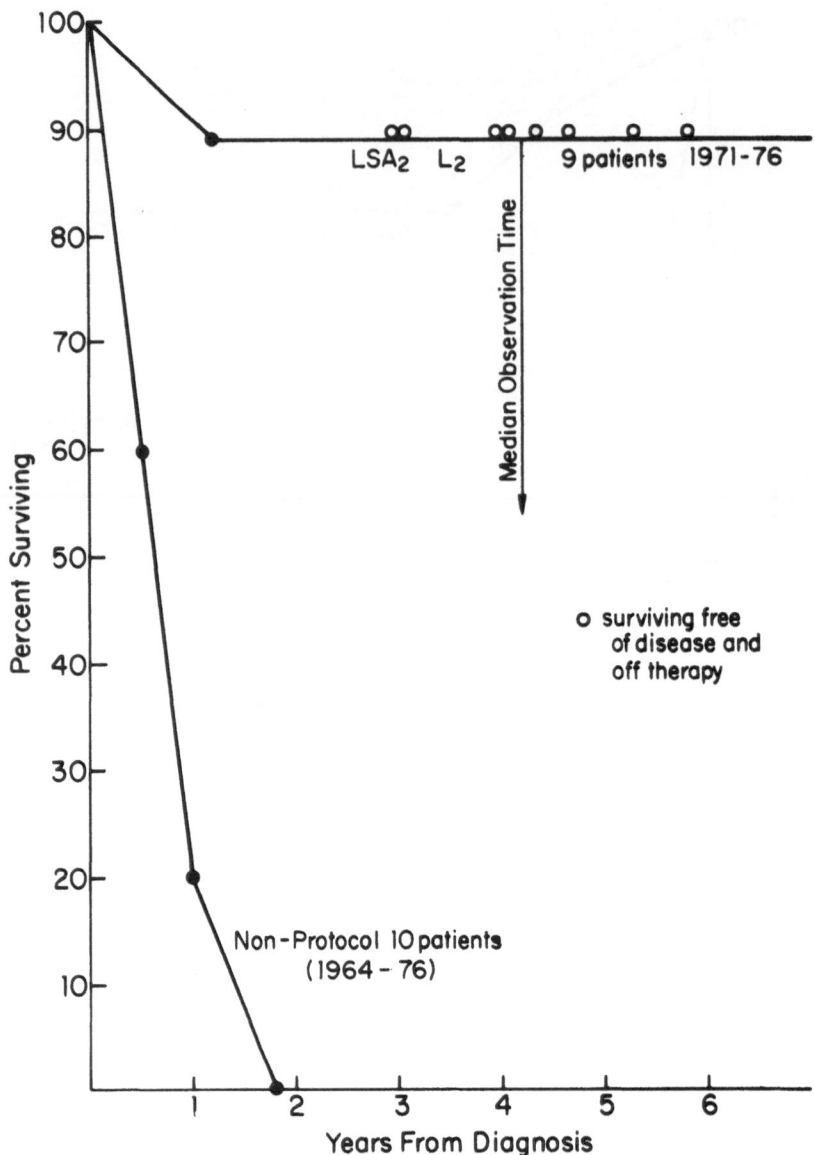

Figure 31. Actuarial survival curves for patients with primary mediastinal disease (September 1976): LSA$_2$–L$_2$ protocol and nonprotocol.

5.2.2. Primary Mediastinal Disease

In this type of primary disease, the difference in survival between the historical control (0%) and the LSA$_2$–L$_2$ group (89%) is striking (Figure 31). The only failure was 1 patient who had mediastinal and pleural disease who did not receive radiation therapy. Since then, the mediastinum and pleura, if involved, are being irradiated, and the results should improve. The timing for radiation therapy to the mediastinum is crucial.

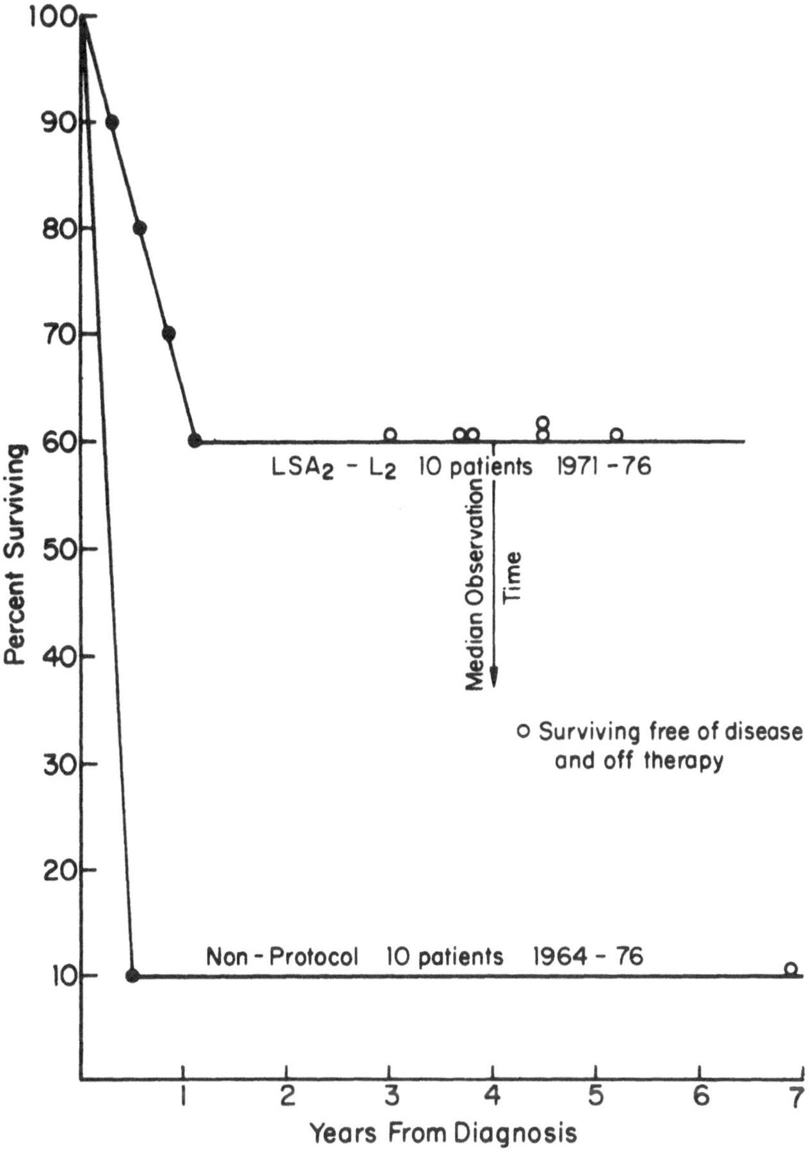

633

NON-HODGKIN'S
LYMPHOMA IN
CHILDREN:
HISTORICAL
REVIEW, PATTERNS
OF DISEASE, AND
FUTURE TRENDS

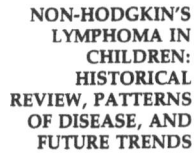

Figure 32. Actuarial survival curves for patients with primary intraabdominal disease (September 1976): LSA$_2$–L$_2$ protocol and nonprotocol.

5.2.3. Primary Intraabdominal Disease

The 5-year actuarial survival for both the LSA$_2$–L$_2$ and the historical control groups are shown in Figure 32. Our major problem has been how to deliver radiation therapy to the entire abdomen in patients with massive disease. To circumvent this difficulty, the following further changes in the management of these patients have been made since 1973:

1. Chemotherapy is started as soon as the patient is staged.
2. At the time of the third injection of vincristine in the induction phase, when the bone marrow has recovered fully, the patient is subjected to a second exploratory laparotomy to determine the feasibility of resecting the previously unresectable tumor, and to delineate other areas of involvement. If the tumor is still unresectable, this area is marked with surgical clips.
3. The area marked with surgical clips is the only area to receive radiation therapy. This amounts to a total dose of 2000 rads in 2 weeks while chemotherapy is continued.

To date, the results with patients treated since 1973 have been encouraging, and the disease-free survival has risen to 75%.

5.2.4. Primary Skeletal Disease

There were no survivors with this primary site in the historical group, as shown in Figure 33. The results of the LSA_2-L_2 protocol were not encouraging (41%), and therefore a change in the protocol was made using high-dose methotrexate (without citrovorum factor rescue). The results so far are encouraging, but more patients are needed and at least 3 years of observation are necessary for any conclusions to be reached.

5.3. Histology

5.3.1. Diffuse and Nodular Lymphocytic, Nodular Lymphocytic, Poorly Differentiated, and Nodular Mixed Well Differentiated

The 5-year actuarial survival for the historical group and the LSA_2-L_2 group show improvement in results (Figure 34). We believe the results of the LSA_2-L_2 patients can be even further improved if adequate radiation therapy is added to the protocol.

5.3.2. Diffuse Lymphocytic Poorly Differentiated

This histological typing, which is considered to signify poor prognosis in adults, does have a good prognosis in children on the LSA_2-L_2 protocol. In this group, 77% have a 5-year survival (Figure 35), and all patients but 1 are off therapy; all are free of disease.

5.3.3. Diffuse Histiocytic

The 5-year survival for the historical group is 13% and for the LSA_2-L_2 group, 53% (Figure 36), with 2 patients dying of other causes, but free of lymphoma. In adults, this histological type has a better prognosis, but in children the survival of the DH, even if corrected for the 2 deaths without lymphoma, does not approach the survival curve of the LSA_2-L_2 patients with DLPD.

635

NON-HODGKIN'S
LYMPHOMA IN
CHILDREN:
HISTORICAL
REVIEW, PATTERNS
OF DISEASE, AND
FUTURE TRENDS

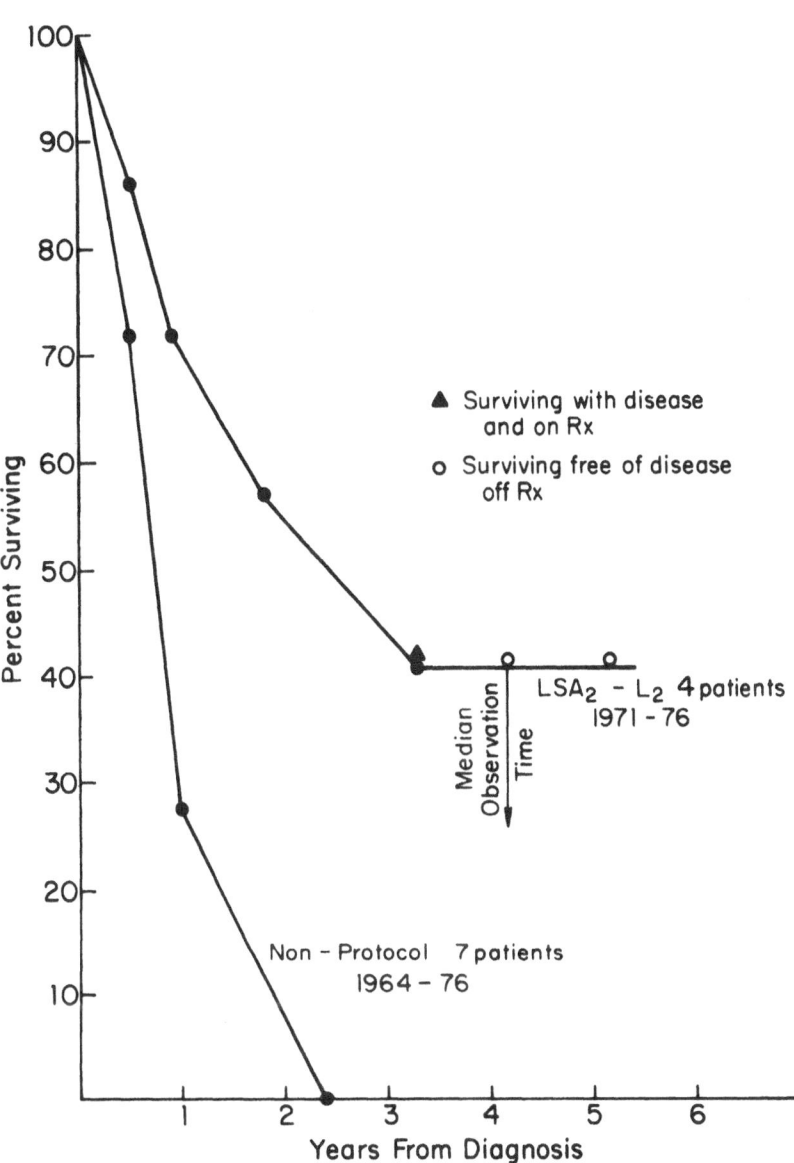

Figure 33. Actuarial survival curves for patients with primary skeletal disease (September 1976): LSA$_2$–L$_2$ protocol and nonprotocol.

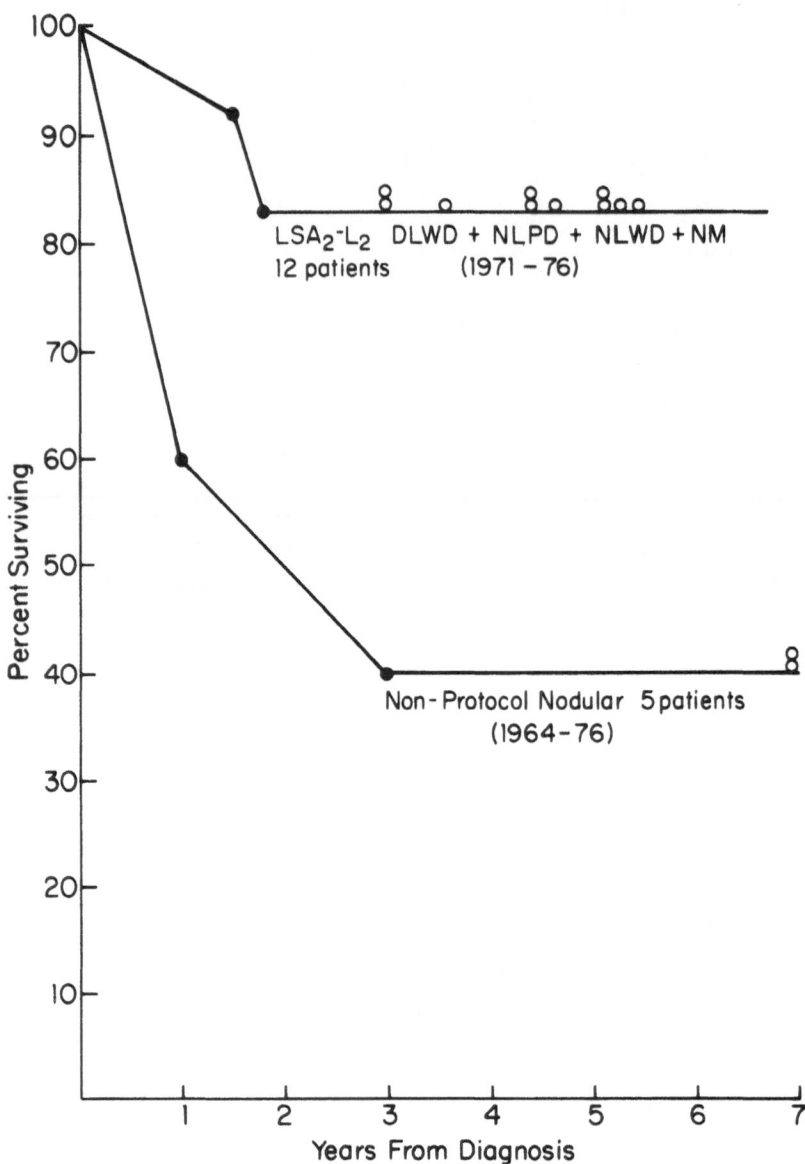

Figure 34. Actuarial survival curves for patients with DLWD, NLWD, NLPD, and NM histology (September 1976): LSA_2-L_2 protocol and nonprotocol.

5.3.4. Diffuse Undifferentiated

The poor results in the LSA_2-L_2 protocol (Figure 37) are due to the following factors:

1. Of the 4 patients, 3 received inadequate radiation or chemotherapy. For this reason, no conclusions can be drawn from this histological type in regard to the poor prognosis.
2. Further, the cases are too few to evaluate for significance.

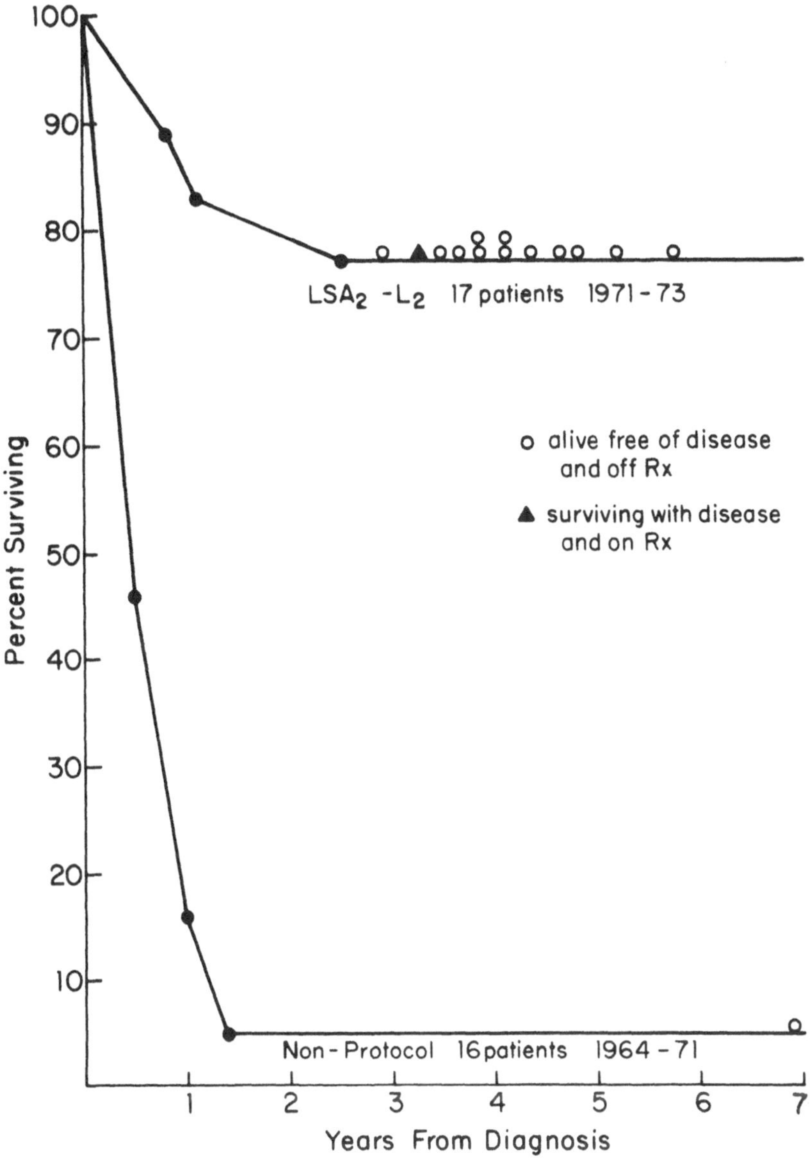

637

NON-HODGKIN'S
LYMPHOMA IN
CHILDREN:
HISTORICAL
REVIEW, PATTERNS
OF DISEASE, AND
FUTURE TRENDS

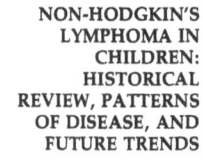

Figure 35. Actuarial survival curves for patients with DLPD histology (September 1976): LSA_2-L_2 protocol and nonprotocol.

6. Conclusions

Further improvement in the survival of children with non-Hodgkin's lymphoma is expected with improved deliverance and timing of radiation and chemotherapy. As we have seen, initial bone marrow involvement, disseminated disease, and histological type have little prognostic implication, if any. The major factors are:

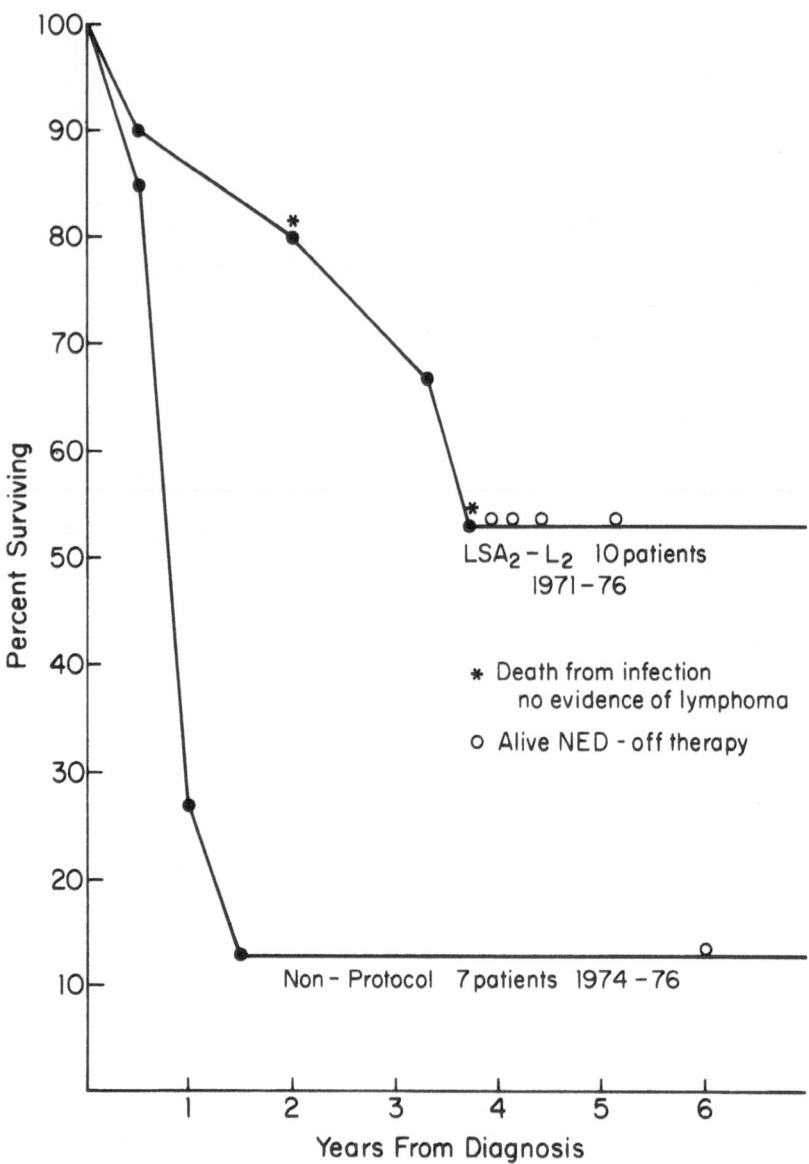

Figure 36. Actuarial survival curves for patients with DH histology (September 1976): LSA$_2$–L$_2$ protocol and nonprotocol.

1. Complete resolution within 1 month of all sites involved at the time of diagnosis (none of the patients who achieved complete remission within 1 month developed CNS involvement).
2. Prevention of bone marrow and CNS disease by an intensive maintenance regimen of intermittent intrathecal injections of methotrexate.

Since non-Hodgkin's lymphoma in children is a disease of rapid progression and the institution of therapy is considered an emergency, few patients have had the chance

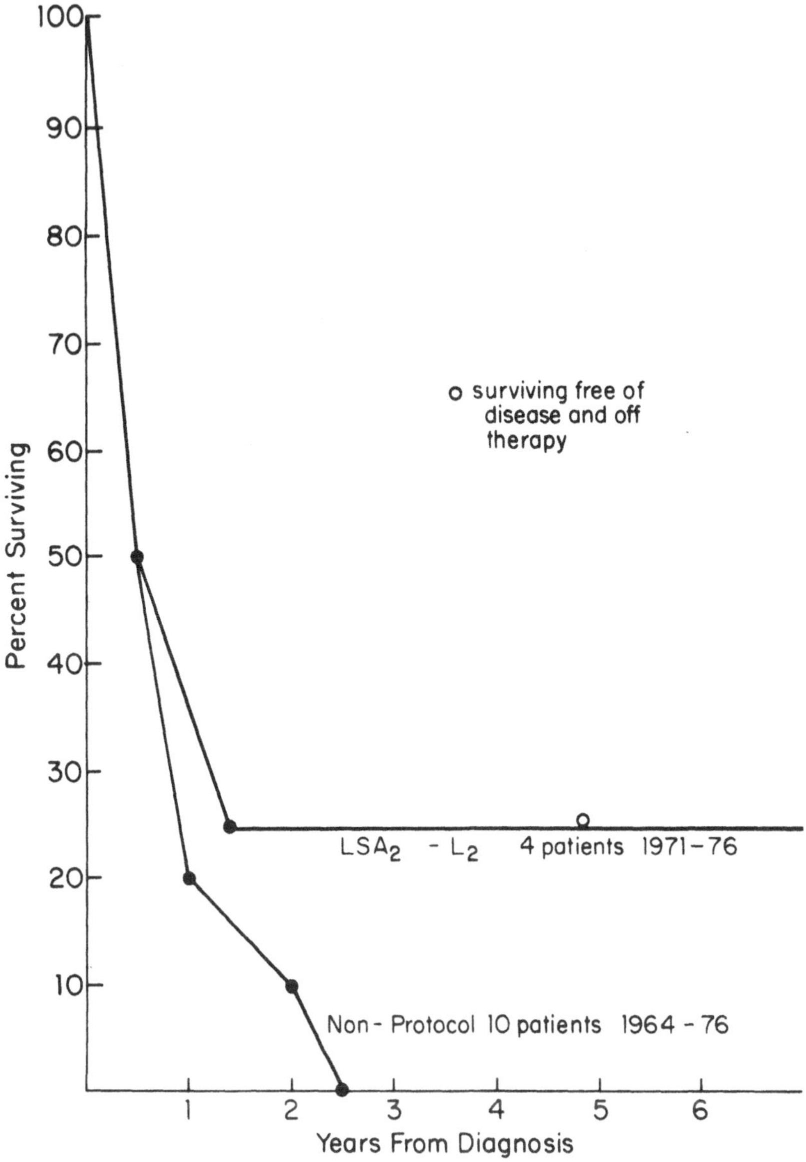

639

NON-HODGKIN'S
LYMPHOMA IN
CHILDREN:
HISTORICAL
REVIEW, PATTERNS
OF DISEASE, AND
FUTURE TRENDS

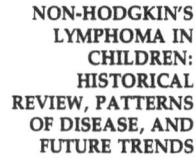

Figure 37. Actuarial survival curves for patients with DU histology (September 1976): LSA$_2$–L$_2$ protocol and nonprotocol.

of a complete work-up for B- and T-cell markers and other immunological parameters. In our patient population, very few cases were studied, and no conclusions can be drawn.

Perhaps appropriate markers would be of prognostic significance in relation to different primary sites and also in cases in which the differential diagnosis between leukemia and non-Hodgkin's lymphoma is difficult (Nathwani *et al.*, 1976; Noguchi *et al.*, 1976).

The question has also arisen many times in our minds whether the poor-prognosis leukemias, such as undifferentiated types and those with high initial white cell count and mediastinal masses, would not eventually be considered a type of non-Hodgkin's lymphoma and therefore benefit from a treatment approach similar to ours.

7. Note Added in Proof

Since this chapter was written another histological review has been carried out to comply with the newer modifications recently made. In this review the number of patients with nodular histology decreased from 14 to 2. In 6 patients there was evidence of surrounding lymphoid tissue with marked nodular hyperplasia. In some of the diffuse lymphocytic poorly differentiated lymphomas the final histology was either maintained or changed to diffuse lymphoblastic convoluted and nonconvoluted. A statistical analysis of these different histological types showed no significant difference in either their responsiveness to therapy or survival. Therefore we feel that histology, while still important for diagnostic purposes, should not be a determinant in prognosis.

References

Jones, E. T., Rosenberg, S. A., Kaplan, H. S., Kadin, M. E., and Dorfman, R. F., 1972, Non-Hodgkin's lymphomas. II. Single agent chemotherapy, *Cancer* **30**:31–38.

Levitt, M., Marsh, J. C., DeConti., R. C., Mitchell, M. S., Skeel, R. T., Farber, L. R., and Bertino, J. R., 1972, Combination sequential chemotherapy in advanced reticulum cell sarcoma, *Cancer* **29**:630–636.

Lemerle, M., Gerard-Marchant, F., Sarrazin, D., Sancho, H., Tchernia, G., Flamant, F., Lemerle, J., and Schweisguth, O., 1973, Lymphosarcoma and reticulum cell sarcoma in children, *Cancer* **32**:1499–1507.

Nathwani, B., Kin, H., and Rappaport, H., 1976, Malignant lymphoblastic lymphoma, *Cancer* **38**:964–983.

Noguchi, S., Bukowski, R., Deodhar, S., and Hewlett, J. S., 1976, T and B lymphocytes in non-Hodgkin's lymphoma: A comparison of tumor derived cells and peripheral blood lymphocytes, *Cancer* **37**:2247–2254.

Rappaport, H., 1966, Tumors of the hematopoietic system, in: *Atlas of Tumor Pathology,* Section III, Fascicle 8, pp. 91–156, Armed Forces Institute of Pathology, Washington, D.C.

Sullivan, M. P., 1973, Non-Hodgkin's lymphoma of childhood, in: *Clinical Pediatric Oncology* (W. W. Sutow, T. J. Vietti, and D. J. Fernbach, eds.), pp. 313–336, C. V. Mosby, St. Louis.

Wollner, N. 1976, Non-Hodgkin's lymphoma in children, *Pediatr. Clin. North Am.* **23** (2):371–378.

Wollner, N., 1977, Central nervous system and bone marrow involvement in childhood non-Hodgkin's lymphoma, in: *Leukemia and Lymphoma in the Nervous System* (C. Pochedly, and A. Mauer, eds.), pp. 152–175, Charles C. Thomas, Springfield.

Wollner, N., Burchenal, J., Lieberman, P., Exelby, P., DiBernardi, B., and Vannucci, R., 1974, Incidence of CNS and bone marrow metastases in non-Hodgkin's lymphoma in children, *Proc. Int. Soc. Pediatr. Oncol.* **6**:51 (abstract).

Wollner, N., Lieberman, P., Exelby, P., D'Angio, G., Burchenal, J., Fang, S., and Murphy, M. L., 1975a, Non-Hodgkin's lymphoma in children: Results of treatment with LSA$_2$–L$_2$ protocol, *Br. J. Cancer Suppl. II* **31**:337–342.

Wollner, N., Burchenal, J. H., Exelby, P., Lieberman, P., D'Angio, G., and Murphy, M. L., 1975b, Non-Hodgkin's lymphoma in children, in: *Proceedings of the Symposium on Conflicts in Childhood Cancer,* Vol. 1, pp. 235–263.

Wollner, N., Burchenal, J., Lieberman, P., Exelby, P., D'Angio, G., and Murphy, M. L., 1975c, Non-Hodgkin's lymphoma in children, *Med. Pediatr. Oncol.* **1**:235–263.

Wollner, N., Burchenal, J. H., Lieberman, P. H., Exelby, P., D'Angio, G., and Murphy, M. L., 1976, Non-Hodgkin's lymphoma in children: A comparative study of two modalities of therapy, *Cancer* **37**:123–134.

22

Biology, Clinical Patterns, and Treatment of Multiple Myeloma and Related Plasma-Cell Dyscrasias

MEHDI FARHANGI and ELLIOTT F. OSSERMAN

1. Plasma-Cell Dyscrasias: Classification, Epidemiology, and Pathogenesis*

The common denominator in all plasma-cell dyscrasias (PCDs) is the inordinate expansion of differentiated B-cell clones (plasma cells) capable of synthesis and secretion of immunoglobulin (Ig) or its subunits. The structurally homogeneous secreted proteins can be demonstrated in the serum and urine of the overwhelming majority of patients. In only rare instances can no secreted product be demonstrated, and infrequently, two or more clones can be shown to occur simultaneously (see Section 4.1.10f).

This functional rather than morphological definition of PCDs includes, by necessity, not only well-differentiated plasma cells but also other cells variously referred to as *lymphoid plasma cells* and *plasmacytoid lymphocytes*. In addition to this definition, PCDs are generally characterized by three cardinal features: (1)

---

*Abbreviations used in this chapter: (CLL) Chronic lymphocytic leukemia; (DNP) dinitrophenyl; (FCR) fractional catabolic rate; (H chain) heavy chain; (HCD) heavy-chain disease; (Ig) immunoglobulin; (L chain) light chain; (MM) multiple myeloma; (PCD) plasma-cell dyscrasia; (PCDUS) plasma-cell dyscrasia(s) of unknown significance; (PHA) phytohemagglutinin; (PV) plasma volume; (RES) reticuloendothelial system; (V region) variable region; (WM) Waldenström's macroglobulinemia; (BMG) benign monoclonal gammopathy; (LM) lichen myxedematosus.

MEHDI FARHANGI • Department of Medicine, University of Missouri–Columbia, Columbia, Missouri 65201.   ELLIOTT F. OSSERMAN • Department of Medicine, College of Physicians and Surgeons, Columbia University, New York, New York.

proliferation of plasma cells, either local or widespread; (2) elaboration of mono-clonal Ig's (MIg's, or M-components) identifiable as IgM, IgG, IgA, IgD, and IgE, or their constituent heavy (H) and light (L) polypeptide chains, albeit structurally defective in some instances; (3) frequently, but not invariably, decreased production of polyclonal Ig's.

The clinical presentations of PCDs are quite variable. Aside from progressive and fatal illnesses such as plasma-cell myeloma (multiple myeloma) (MM), Waldenström's macroglobulinemia (WM), amyloidosis, and the heavy-chain diseases (HCDs), asymptomatic forms are also recognized. Classification of PCDs under two main headings—clinically asymptomatic, or occult, forms (plasma-cell dyscrasias of unknown significance) (PCDUS) and clinically symptomatic, or overt, forms—is presented in Tables 1 and 2.

The knowledge of structure, function, and other biological properties of M-components has contributed to our understanding of mechanisms involved in certain clinical syndromes and laboratory phenomena seen in various PCDs. A group of such clinical syndromes are listed in Table 3 and will be discussed in Section 2.

1.1. Epidemiology and Incidence

The increasing use of serum and urine protein electrophoresis has contributed significantly to the recognition of all forms of PCDs, particularly the asymptomatic forms.

Axelsson *et al.* (1966) used paper electrophoresis to study the serum proteins of 6995 normal Swedish subjects. They found monoclonal proteins in 73 cases, an incidence of about 1.0%. The frequency of serum M components increased significantly with increasing age. For example, the incidence was 0.2% for the 30–39 age group and 5.7% for those 80–89 years of age. Zawadzki and Edwards (1972) used both electrophoresis and immunoelectrophoresis for the detection of M components in the sera of unselected hospitalized male veterans, 70 years or older. Among 748 patients, 55 (7.5%) had monoclonal proteins. In this group, 29 cases were detected by immunoelectrophoresis, and would have been missed by the use of electrophore-

TABLE 1. Plasma-Cell Dyscrasias: Clinically Asymptomatic (Occult) Forms (Plasma-Cell Dyscrasias of Unknown Significance)

   I. Presymptomatic forms evolving into plasma-cell myeloma, Waldenström's macroglobulinemia, and amyloidosis
  II. Asymptomatic forms occurring in old age
 III. Familial forms
  IV. Plasma-cell dyscrasias associated with:
      1. Chronic inflammatory and infectious processes
      2. Autoimmune diseases
      3. Nonreticular neoplasia
      4. Leukemias and myeloproliferative disorders
      5. Gaucher's disease
   V. M components in immune deficiency syndromes
  VI. Plasma-cell dyscrasias associated with malignant lymphoma and chronic lymphocytic leukemia
 VII. Transient plasma-cell dyscrasias

TABLE 2. Plasma-Cell Dyscrasias: Clinically Symptomatic (Overt) Forms

643

BIOLOGY, CLINICAL
PATTERNS, AND
TREATMENT OF
MULTIPLE MYELOMA
AND RELATED
PLASMA-CELL
DYSCRASIAS

TABLE 2. Plasma-Cell Dyscrasias: Clinically Symptomatic (Overt) Forms

Plasma-cell myeloma (multiple myeloma) and the clinical variants:
  Solitary plasmacytoma
  Extraskeletal plasmacytomas
  Plasma-cell leukemia
  Myeloma and acute leukemia, simultaneously occurring
  Osteosclerotic myeloma
  IgD myeloma
  Nonsecretory myeloma
  Biclonal gammopathies
Waldenström's macroglobulinemia
Heavy-chain diseases
  α-Heavy-chain disease
  γ-Heavy-chain disease
  μ-Heavy-chain disease
Deleted heavy- and light-chain disease
Lichen myxedematosus
Amyloidosis

sis alone. The overwhelming majority of patients in both studies had asymptomatic PCDs.

Among symptomatic forms of PCDs, the incidence rate is known for MM. The United States mortality data compiled by the National Institutes of Health (U.S. Cancer Mortality by County: 1950–1969) indicate an incidence of 1.76 per 100,000 white males and 1.24 per 100,000 white females, or approximately 1% of all cancer mortality. The incidence for nonwhite males and females was somewhat higher (2.70 and 1.83, respectively). A study by MacMahon and Clark (1956) also showed a higher incidence and younger onset of MM in the black population in comparison with the Caucasian population of New York City. McPhedran et al. (1972) reported that the diagnosis of MM was made at a rate of 4/100,000 in black and 2.1/100,000 in white residents of metropolitan Atlanta in 1963–1967.

A steady rise in the incidence of MM in the United States is suggested by the mortality data for 1949 and 1963 (0.8 and 1.7 per 100,000, respectively) (Kyle and Bayrd, 1976). In Olmsted County, Minnesota, however, an increase in MM mortality could not be demonstrated for the decade 1955–1964 as compared with 1944–1954 (Kyle et al., 1969).

The data on geographic distribution of cancer mortality in the United States 1950–1969 (Mason et al., 1976) indicate that several areas have a relatively high mortality rate from MM. These areas include several localities in Vermont, Minnesota, North Dakota, Iowa, Montana, Virginia, West Virginia, California, and

TABLE 3. Clinical Syndromes Intimately Related to the M Components

Hyperviscosity syndrome	Xanthomatosis
Cryoglobulinemia	Xanthoderma
Hemostatic abnormalities	Hypercupremia
Cold agglutinin hemolytic anemia	Renal tubular acidosis (Fanconi syndrome)

others. The geographic distribution of the so-called "hot spots" for MM is quite different from that for several other cancers. For example, mortality from cancer of the urinary bladder, which is attributed to industrial carcinogens, is significantly above the United States average in most industrial centers of the Northeast. One might infer, therefore, that if environmental factors are responsible for high incidence of MM in certain areas, these factors are probably different from those responsible for bladder cancer and several other neoplasias.

A cluster of six cases of MM diagnosed in 1 year in one small community in Minnesota was reported by Kyle et al. (1970); there was no detectable rise in the frequency of M-components in others who lived in the same community.

A higher than average incidence of MM has been reported in other areas in the world. For example, Dawson and Ogston (1973) noted an increased rate of MM in Scotland.

1.2. Age

We have already alluded to the increasing chances of discovering a monoclonal Ig in the sera of an aging population. The occurrence of symptomatic PCDs, such as MM and WM, prior to the age of 20 is quite rare. Maeda et al. (1973) reported an unusual case of plasma-cell tumor with an IgA monoclonal protein in a 13-year-old girl. The tumor involved predominantly the breasts, ovaries, and skin. These authors found 10 other previously reported cases in the literature concerning myeloma in children from ages 1½ to 15. Our own youngest patient, a male, was 23 years old at the onset of symptoms (Osserman and Farhangi, 1975); he had documented proteinuria for the preceding 3 years, quite probably the same Bence Jones protein demonstrated when the diagnosis was established. MM in young persons was also reported by Hewell and Alexanian (1976).

The mortality from MM increases progressively from the early 20's (0.01/ 100,000 male and female) until the early 80's (12.41 and 8.37 per 100,000 white males and females, respectively). A modest decline occurs after the age of 85 (Mason et al., 1976). The age and mortality incidence appear to be linearly related, and in this regard, MM resembles many other cancers.

The median age at the time of diagnosis of MM in most series in the United States is reported to be in the late 50's or early 60's (Engle and Wallis, 1969; Isobe and Osserman, 1971; Drivsholm, 1964; Adams et al., 1949; Snapper et al., 1953). In the series of Waldenström (1970) from Malmö, Sweden, the peak incidence was between the ages of 70 and 80.

1.3. Pathogenesis and Suspected Etiological Factors

The etiology of PCDs remains obscure. Studies of plasmacytomas in mice and MM in man, however, have contributed significantly to our current understanding of the pathogenesis of PCDs. There is increasing evidence that chronic stimulation of the lymphoreticular system may play a role in the ultimate development of PCDs. We previously reviewed the supportive data pertinent to this hypothesis (Osserman, 1971). Beginning with animal data, it was noted that old C3H mice (Dunn, 1957; Fahey and Askonas, 1962; Pilgrim, 1965; Potter, 1973a) developed spontaneous plasmacytomas of the ileocecal region. Pilgrim (1965) carried out a compre-

645

BIOLOGY, CLINICAL
PATTERNS, AND
TREATMENT OF
MULTIPLE MYELOMA
AND RELATED
PLASMA-CELL
DYSCRASIAS

hensive histological study of these lesions. Frequently, ulceration of the cecum adjacent to the ileocecal junction was present. He further noted infiltration of mononuclear cells (lymphocytes, plasma cells, histiocytes) surrounding the mucosal ulceration, producing a varied histological picture ranging from an inflammatory reaction to grossly neoplastic lesions. Interestingly, there was a low incidence of plasmacytoma in another group of C3H mice that were raised separately and were found to have infrequent ileocecal ulceration. The spontaneous plasmacytomas in C3H mice, therefore, seem to arise at the site of a chronically sustained inflammatory reaction.

Particularly relevant to the pathogenesis of plasma-cell tumors in mice are the extensive studies by Potter and his associates (Potter, 1962, 1972, 1973a; Potter and Boyce, 1962; Potter and MacCardle, 1964; Potter and Robertson, 1960). These investigators were able to induce plasma-cell tumors in BALB/c mice by intraperitoneal injection or implantation of a variety of substances, including plastics, mineral oil, and branched-chain alkanes, particularly Pristane (2,6,10,14-tetramethyl pentadecane). The sequence of events after the introduction of "irritant" until the development of autonomous transplantable plasmacytomas was carefully studied. Early on, lipogranulomatous lesions on the peritoneum were evident (Potter and MacCardle, 1964). These granulomatous lesions are comprised of lymphocytes, histiocytes, and plasma cells. Concomitantly, diffuse polyclonal hypergammaglobulinemia was demonstrated (Talal et al., 1964). Six to twelve months later, 60–70% of injected mice developed plasmacytomas. These tumors synthesized and secreted M-components and Bence Jones proteins (Potter, 1962; Potter and Robertson, 1960). Furthermore, several cell lines have been established from these tumors (Cohn, 1967; Matsuoka et al., 1967; Namba and Hanaoka, 1969). The susceptibility of BALB/c strain mice to tumor induction is in part related to genetically determined factor(s). This strain of mice has been shown to react strongly to antigenic challenges and this reaction is associated with restricted clonal expansion (Braun et al., 1972; Cerny et al., 1971; Yamada et al., 1969).

An interesting observation by McIntire and Princler (1969) seems to further elucidate the development of plasmacytomas in BALB/c mice. Following intraperitoneal injection of adjuvant in two groups of germ-free and conventional animals, they found an almost equal incidence of neoplasms in both groups. The germ-free animals, however, developed less differentiated tumors that were histologically classified as reticulum-cell sarcomas. Only a few of the animals had plasmacytomas. Most conventional animals, however, developed plasma-cell tumors similar to those in previously mentioned studies. These results suggest that the bacterial flora of the gut may play a role in the development of plasmacytomas.

Other evidence that implicates the role of the gut flora in the induction of plasma-cell tumors in BALB/c mice is derived from studies by Potter and his associates (Potter, 1972, 1973b; Potter and Leon, 1968). These investigators showed that the secreted M components in most plasma-cell tumors were IgA, which is the predominant Ig in the gut. Several mouse M components were also shown to possess antibody activity to antigens of gut flora or constituents of the diet or cage bedding. Some of the antigens corresponding to these monoclonal antibodies are well characterized; these antigens include phosphorylcholine, α1-3 dextran, fructosan, and α-methyl-D-mannose and β1-6 D-galactan. The antibody specificity of these myeloma proteins suggests a close relationship between the neoplastic plasma cell and its normal counterpart (Potter, 1973a). A similar spectrum of antibody activities has been demonstrated for human M components (Seligmann and Brouet, 1973; Nisonoff *et al.*, 1975; Farhangi and Osserman, 1976).

Another experimental model that may provide some insight into the pathogenesis of PCDs is the pattern of immune responses in the New Zealand red rabbit. Krause and his associates (Osterland *et al.*, 1966; Fleischman *et al.*, 1968; Braun and Krause, 1968; Braun *et al.*, 1969) have shown that a small number of these animals, when repeatedly immunized by group A-variant streptococcal vaccine, responded with production of oligoclonal to monoclonal antibodies. These responses were associated with marked plasmacytic proliferation. No plasma-cell tumors were demonstrated, however, and M components subsided after the termination of immunization. This restricted clonal response has been attributed to genetic factors.

Another animal model pertinent to the pathogenesis of PCDs is the Aleutian mink disease (Leader *et al.*, 1963; Porter *et al.*, 1965) caused by a viral agent. In affected animals, there is widespread lymphoreticular hyperplasia and vasculitis. Concomitantly, a diffuse polyclonal hypergammaglobulinemia develops and in 10% of animals, there is transition to monoclonal-type γ-globulin production and Bence Jones proteinuria (Potter, 1962). No plasma-cell tumors were observed, however, although diffuse plasmacytosis occurred in virtually all organs (Leader *et al.*, 1963; Porter *et al.*, 1965). It appears that lymphorecticular hyperplasia and hypergammaglobulinemia in these animals are reactions to tissue injury produced by the virus, rather than against the virus *per se*, since no detectable neutralizing antibody could be demonstrated against the causative agent.

Another animal model that is possibly relevant to human disease is the complex of immunological disorders in inbred New Zealand Black (NZB/B1) mice. These mice develop diffuse lymphoreticular proliferation, vasculitis, and hypergammaglobulinemia (Warner and Wistar, 1968). In addition, Coombs-positive hemolytic anemia, glomerulonephritis, and antinuclear antibodies can be demonstrated with high frequency (Bielschowsky *et al.*, 1959; Helyer and Howie, 1963; Mellors, 1965, 1966). About 20% of these animals ultimately develop lymphoreticular neoplasms, classified histologically as plasmacytoma, reticulum-cell sarcoma, or a pleomorphic Hodgkin's-like lymphoma (Mellors, 1966; Mellors *et al.*, 1969).

In both animal models, the Aleutian mink disease and the disease of NZB/B1 mice, autoimmune mechanisms are operative. True neoplasia, however, develops only in some NZB/B1 mice, with virus particles seen in tumor as well as normal tissues (Mellors *et al.*, 1969; Mellors and Huang, 1966, 1967). It has been hypothesized that the viral agent is transmitted vertically, and causes tissue damage, reticuloendothelial system (RES) proliferation, autoantibody formation, and eventual neoplastic transformation of reactive clones (Mellors, 1966; Mellors *et al.*, 1969, Mellors and Huang, 1966; Staples and Talal, 1969; Warner and Wistar, 1968).

In all of the animal models discussed above, a combination of genetic factors and protracted bacterial, viral, or chemical stimulation of the lymphoreticular system apparently leads to the ultimate development of plasma-cell tumors. Obviously, the relevance of the experimental models to the pathogenesis of PCDs in man is still uncertain. There is, however, circumstantial evidence suggesting that similar mechanisms may be operative in the pathogenesis of human PCDs. This evidence includes the finding of asymptomatic or symptomatic variants of PCD in

647

BIOLOGY, CLINICAL
PATTERNS, AND
TREATMENT OF
MULTIPLE MYELOMA
AND RELATED
PLASMA-CELL
DYSCRASIAS

certain patients with a prolonged history of chronic infection, e.g., chronic osteo-myelitis, pyelonephritis, tuberculosis, and inflammation of the hepatobiliary tracts (Osserman and Takatsuki, 1963a,b, 1964; Isobe and Osserman, 1971; Zawadzki and Edwards, 1972). There are also several case reports of plasma-cell myeloma occurring adjacent to the site of osteomyelitis (Loeper et at., 1947; Heilmann, 1957; Baitz and Kyle, 1964). There are considerable clinical data to relate the occurrence of amyloidosis to preceding chronic infection and inflammatory diseases. This is true not only for "secondary amyloidosis," but also for so-called "primary amyloi-dosis" (Magnus-Levy, 1933, 1952; Osserman et al., 1964; Barth et al., 1968; Isobe and Osserman, 1971).

In many reported patients with γHCD, a background of chronic disorders such as tuberculosis, rheumatoid arthritis, Sjögren's syndrome, myasthenia gravis, systemic lupus erythematosus, hypereosinophilic syndrome, thyroiditis, or nonreticu-lar neoplasia has been documented (Frangione and Franklin, 1973; Loyau et al., 1975; Lyons et al., 1975). Preexisting chronic pyoderma has also been implicated in the pathogenesis of a rare form of PCD, lichen myxedematosus or papular muci-nosis (Perry, H. O., et al., 1960; Osserman and Takatsuki, 1963b; McCarthy et al., 1964; Schneider and Missmahl, 1966).

The association of nonreticular neoplasia with PCDs is also of possible significance (Isobe and Osserman, 1971; see also the review by Zawadzki and Edwards, 1972). A significant rather than a coincidental association is suggested by the observation that the carcinomas in several of these cases were extensively infil-trated with plasma cells, often at the border between normal and cancerous tissue (Bohrod, 1957; Osserman and Takatsuki, 1965). Secondly, there appears to be a particularly high frequency of association of certain cancers with PCD and a low frequency of others. Thus, in 128 cases of asymptomatic PCDs in association with various cancers reported from our clinic (Isobe and Osserman, 1971) 19.6% had adenocarcinoma of the rectosigmoid colon and another 18.8% had adenomatous polyps of the same region. Carcinoma of the prostate and breast were the second and third most frequently encountered tumors (18% and 11%, respectively). Other common tumors, particularly squamous cell carcinoma of the lung, were low on the list.

Finally, the transient occurrence of PCDs has been well documented during the course of acute infections such as viral hepatitis (Seligmann and Basch, 1968), after the insertion of valve prostheses (Young, 1969), and in drug hypersensitivity (Osserman and Takatsuki, 1965). Of particular interest is the case of melanosar-coma reported by Hällén (1966) in which the monoclonal Ig disappeared during the course of treatment. Similarly, in a case of breast carcinoma reported by Bohrod (1957), a monoclonal cryomacroglobulinemia disappeared several weeks after mas-tectomy. Clubb et al. (1964) have described the disappearance of a peak of γ-mobility protein following the removal of parathyroid adenoma. These uncommon but intriguing observations suggest the possibility of an unusual tumor antigenic stimulation leading to a monoclonal expansion of B cells.

1.4. Other Possible Etiological Factors in Plasma-Cell Dyscrasias

We have already indicated the probable importance of genetic factors in both spontaneously occurring and experimentally induced plasmacytomas in mice. In man, there is also some evidence to indicate that the increased frequency of B-cell neoplasias in certain families is more than a chance occurrence (Gunz and Veale, 1969). Several families with multiple cases of asymptomatic PCD have been reported (Spengler et al., 1966–1967; Williams, R. C., et al., 1967; Berlin et al., 1968; Grant et al., 1971; Axelsson and Hällén, 1965; Petite and Cruchaud, 1969–1970). Maldonado and Kyle (1974) have reviewed the literature on the occurrence of MM in two or more first-order relatives. Of this literature, 15 previous reports were considered acceptable, and the authors described eight new families. In the majority, MM was diagnosed in two siblings or in members of two immediate generations. Interestingly, MM developed subsequently in an additional member of two of the families reported by these investigators.

A role for radiation in the causation of certain cases of plasma-cell myeloma is suspected. E. B. Lewis (1963) reported a higher than average incidence of myeloma among radiologists. Also, an increased incidence of malignant lymphoma and MM was documented in survivors of the atomic bomb in Hiroshima (Nishiyama et al., 1973). The risk of developing malignant lymphoma and MM was shown to be higher for people exposed below the age of 25 than for those above this age. Interestingly, a similar increase could not be demonstrated in survivors of the Nagasaki atomic blast. This discrepancy was attributed to the difference in radiation spectrum emitted by the two bombs or biological differences between the two populations of Nagasaki and Hiroshima or both (Nishiyama et al., 1973).

1.5. Carcinogens

No specific carcinogen for MM has yet been described. The occurrence of statistically significant high mortality in certain geographic areas described earlier suggests the possibility of environmental factor(s), although genetic or ethnic differences in population might be operative. Epidemiological and environmental studies of juxtaposed localities with higher and lower than average MM mortality could be informative. Gerber (1970) has reported two cases of MM among 35 cases of proved asbestosis. In one of these cases, an anaplastic carcinoma of the bronchus was also present. Several other hematological dyscrasias were noted in other asbestosis patients. We recently (Perry and Farhangi, 1976) saw a patient with a history of exposure to asbestos and recurrent malignant plasmacytomas, who later developed a mesothelioma in the chest cavity.

1.6. Viral Etiology

Electron-microscopic studies of mouse plasmacytomas have consistently shown viruslike particles and Potter (1973a) has reviewed these observations. Briefly, two kinds of particles, A and C, have been found. A-type particles have been observed in the intracisternal spaces (Dalton and Potter, 1968; Dalton et al., 1961). These particles seem to bud from the rough endoplasmic reticulum and contain small amounts of RNA (Kuff et al., 1972), but lack a dense nucleoid. The structural proteins of these A-type viruses are unrelated to the murine leûkemia virus (MuLV). Two kinds of C-type particles have been demonstrated in mouse plasmacytomas. In one, the structural protein is related to MuLV (Gross) virus, and

649

BIOLOGY, CLINICAL
PATTERNS, AND
TREATMENT OF
MULTIPLE MYELOMA
AND RELATED
PLASMA-CELL
DYSCRASIAS

in the other, called XVEA (Aoki and Takahashi, 1972), no relatedness to MuLV is found.

The significance of the A and C particles in murine plasmacytomas is unknown. Several attempts have been made to transfer a biologically active material from plasma-cell tumor extract into newborn BALB/c mice and all these have failed (Howatson and McCulloch, 1958; Kuff *et al.*, 1968; Parson *et al.*, 1960) except one (Pedio *et al.*, 1968). Viruslike particles were seen in human plasma-cell tumors less frequently than in mouse tumors (Sorenson, 1961, 1965; Tavassoli and Baughan, 1973). In view of the large number of electron microscopic studies of human myeloma cells which have failed to reveal viruslike particles, the significance of these two isolated reports is unclear.

2. Clinical Syndromes Intimately Related to the M Components

Several clinical syndromes (see Table 3) and laboratory phenomena can be directly linked to specific physico-chemical properties of certain M components. The biophysical and functional characteristics of monoclonal proteins appear to be involved in the mechanisms of such manifestations. For example, the intrinsic viscosity of certain proteins, particularly macroglobulins, is the most important factor in the development of the hyperviscosity syndrome. Likewise, the antibody function of other M components may account for hemolysis in some cases of cold agglutinin syndromes. It should be noted, however, that not all of the presently defined biological properties of monoclonal proteins are clinically consequential. For example, M components with binding affinity for streptolysin O, dinitrophenyl (DNP), and phosphorylcholine have thus far not been connected to any specific clinical features. Likewise, the anticomplementary activity occasionally demonstrable in sera with monoclonal proteins appears to be only a "laboratory phenomenon." In this regard, exception should be made for M components with rheumatoid factor and complement-consumption activity (Balazs and Frohlich, 1966; Costanzi *et al.*, 1969; Costanzi and Coltman, 1967). In such cases, a cryoglobulinemia syndrome is frequently present.

The occurrence of M-component-related clinical manifestations can alter the clinical presentation of PCDs and pose diagnostic and therapeutic problems for the clinician. We will discuss these conditions before reviewing the asymptomatic and the clinically-overt forms of PCDs.

2.1. Hyperviscosity Syndrome

Viscosity is defined as internal friction of a fluid which makes it resist a tendency to flow. With respect to blood, the formed elements (red cells, white cells, and platelets) as well as plasma proteins are the principal factors which determine viscosity. Among the formed elements, the contribution of the red cells to blood viscosity is obviously the predominant one, and a linear correlation between blood viscosity and hematocrit was previously demonstrated (McGrath and Penny, 1976). The viscosity of normal plasma falls in a narrow range (McGrath and Penny, 1976). Plasma viscosity may rise significantly, however, when an M component is present. Factors that account for the elevation of viscosity in plasma or serum with M component are (1) the size and shape of the protein molecule; (2) protein concentration; (3) protein–cell interaction; and (4) the properties of the vascular bed (Bloch and Maki, 1973).

The hyperviscosity syndrome in patients with M components occurs most often with IgM monoclonal proteins. In a recent study (MacKenzie and Babcock, 1975), 38% of 34 patients with macroglobulinemia had a serum viscosity, relative to water, of greater than 6.0 (normal: 1.4–1.8). This hyperviscosity was associated with serum IgM levels of greater than 5 g/dl. In another study reported by Fahey *et al.* (1965a,b), most patients with such relative viscosities were symptomatic. IgA M components, due to their tendency to form polymers of varying size (Sugai, 1972), are the second most frequent cause of the hyperviscosity syndrome (Bloch and Maki, 1973). Symptoms of hyperviscosity are uncommon in patients with IgG M components unless the concentration of the monoclonal protein is quite high. In a recent review by Somer (1975), the serum monoclonal IgG in 36 cases with symptomatic hyperviscosity syndrome ranged from 3.6 to 18.0 g/dl, with mean and median values of 9.0 and 8.6 g/dl, respectively. As demonstrated by Capra and Kunkel (1970), IgG3 M components have a particular tendency to form unstable complexes in undiluted serum, thereby raising serum viscosity. It must be understood, however, that the hyperviscosity syndrome can develop with monoclonal IgG's of the other γ-chain subclasses (Benninger and Krebs, 1971; Smith *et al.*, 1965).

The asymmetry of protein molecules contributes significantly to their intrinsic viscosity (MacKenzie *et al.*, 1970; MacKenzie and Babcock, 1975). Thus, the hyperviscosity syndrome may develop with a relatively low concentration of certain monoclonal proteins. Hyperviscosity due to immune complexes, e.g., IgM–IgG, IgG–IgG, and IgA–IgG, has also been well documented in rheumatic diseases (Jasin *et al.*, 1970; Abbruzzo *et al.*, 1970; Bloch and Maki, 1973). It is quite likely that M components with antibody activity for γ chains raise the serum viscosity by virtue of the formation of immune complexes. Such M components are often also associated with cryoglobulinemia (see Section 2.2).

Finally, it should be recognized that the extent and severity of tissue damage due to hyperviscosity is also dependent on the structure of the vascular bed, shear rate, and protein–cell interactions (McGrath and Penny, 1976). A particular case which demonstrated the interplay between an M component and red blood cells was reported by S. Anderson *et al.* (1975). Sickle-cell anemia (S-S hemoglobin) and an IgG M component were diagnosed in the same patient. A marked increase in the viscosity of oxygenated blood at a low shear rate was demonstrated. In a control experiment, the oxygenated S-S hemoglobin, in the absence of the M component, showed a much lower viscosity at a similar shear rate. Thus, the occurrence of symptoms related to blood hyperviscosity depends on several variables. In addition, Fahey and co-workers have stressed the concept of "symptomatic threshold" in the hyperviscosity syndrome (Fahey, 1963; Fahey *et al.*, 1965; Solomon and Fahey, 1963). This threshold viscosity appears to be different from patient to patient, but relatively constant in any given case.

The clinical manifestations of the hyperviscosity syndrome are summarized in Table 4. The anemia is due in part to plasma volume expansion, which occurs predictably in relation to the rise in viscosity (McGrath and Penny, 1976; MacKenzie *et al.*, 1968; Tuddenham and Bradley, 1974). Of particular importance to the

TABLE 4. Signs and Symptoms of the Hyperviscosity Syndrome[a]

Ocular	Distension and tortuosity of retinal veins, "string-of-sausage" appearance, retinal hemorrhage, papilledema
	Disturbance in vision to complete blindness
Hematological	Oozing of blood from oral mucous membranes
	Bleeding from nose and urinary and GI tracts
	Prolonged bleeding at sites of minor surgical procedures
	Anemia
Neurological	Headache, dizziness, vertigo, nystagmus, postural hypotension
	Sommolence, stupor, and coma
	Generalized seizures, EEG changes
Cardiovascular	Congestive heart failure
	Expanded plasma volume
Renal	Glomerular deposits attributable to the hyperviscosity syndrome?
	Diminished concentrating and diluting ability, perhaps attributable to the hyperviscosity syndrome
Subjective	Weakness, fatigue, anorexia

[a]Modified after Fahey *et al.* (1965) by Bloch and Maki (1973) in *Seminars in Hematology* 10:114. Reproduced by permission from Grune & Stratton, Inc., New York, New York.

clinician is the reversibility of most symptoms following adequate plasmapheresis. Cline *et al.* (1963) showed partial reversal of shortened red cell survival following this procedure. Permanent damage such as retinal vein thrombosis (Spalter, 1959) and hearing loss (Afifi and Tawfeek, 1971; Ruben *et al.*, 1969), however, has occurred in some cases.

Plasmapheresis is a relatively simple, safe and effective procedure. Initially, 500 ml of blood is removed, and the red cells are returned to the patient after centrifugation. In severe cases, 3000–4000 ml of blood should be processed in 1–2 days. Maintenance plasmapheresis, weekly to biweekly, may be necessary to maintain the serum viscosity within a tolerable range (Bloch and Maki, 1973).

2.2. Cryoglobulinemia

Although *in vitro* cryoprecipitation can be demonstrated in many sera with M components, clinical manifestations of cryoglobulinemia, i.e., Raynaud's phenomenon, cryosensitivity, skin ulceration, gangrene of the extremities, and progressive renal failure are relatively uncommon. The exceptions are those M components with binding affinity for the γ chain that are frequently associated with purpura in the dependent areas and other clinical manifestations of cryoglobulinemia (Grey and Kohler, 1973; Whitsed and Penny, 1971).

2.3. Hemostatic Abnormalities

Hemostatic abnormalities in PCDs are most often due to factors unrelated to the M components. Thrombocytopenic hemorrhage due to either marrow involvement by the tumor cells or suppression of thrombopoiesis by cytotoxic agents accounts for most bleeding. Autoimmune thrombocytopenia occurs very rarely, and disseminated intravascular coagulation may also develop in patients suffering from PCDs. Hemostatic abnormalities, however, are occasionally related to the M components. We have already alluded to the hemorrhagic manifestation of the hyperviscosity syndrome and purpura associated with some cryoglobulins. M components can also alter platelet function and interfere with the coagulation mechanism. Pachter *et al.* (1959a,b) showed a decrease in the availability of platelet factor 3 in patients with macroglobulinemia. This aberration of platelet function has been confirmed by other investigators [see the review by Lackner (1973)]. The abnormality of platelet aggregation was demonstrated by Doumenc *et al.* (1966). An interesting IgA-myeloma patient with bleeding disorder and normal platelet count was studied by Vigliano and Horowitz (1965, 1967). Collagen exposed to the IgA from this patient was found to lose its platelet-aggregating property. Penny *et al.* (1971) were able to demonstrate evidence for platelet functional abnormalities in seven patients with M components and bleeding manifestations. Bleeding time and platelet adhesiveness were abnormal in six patients. Four patients exhibited a decreased platelet factor 3 release, and in three patients, platelet aggregation was abnormal.

Prolonged thrombin time is a rather common laboratory finding in patients with MM. This laboratory abnormality is attributed to the inhibitory action of the M component on the polymerization of fibrin monomers [see the review by Lackner (1973)]. The severe form of inhibition of fibrin polymerization is associated with the formation of transparent bulky gelatinous clots that fail to retract. The addition of calcium will partially correct the thrombin time abnormality and results in the formation of a less friable clot (Coleman *et al.*, 1972). In one case exhibiting this phenomenon, we were able to extract serum proteins by the addition of 9 volumes of 0.025 M calcium chloride to ACD anticoagulated plasma. The clot thus formed could be readily removed by a wooden applicator (Farhangi and Osserman, 1976). The inhibitory action of the M component on fibrin polymerization has been shown to be related to the Fab portion of the molecule (Coleman *et al.*, 1972). In another study, an IgG-myeloma protein was found to inhibit all three stages of fibrin-clot formation. The M component inhibited the proteolytic action of the thrombin, prevented the polymerization of fibrin monomers, and also interfered with the cross-linking of γ and α chains (Soria *et al.*, 1975).

Factor VIII inhibition by IgM (Castaldi and Penny, 1970) and IgA (Glueck and Hong, 1965) M components has been reported. Abnormal thromboplastin generation was found in a large number of patients in one study (Perkins *et al.*, 1970), without abnormality of the partial thromboplastin time. This lack of correlation between thromboplastin generation time and partial thromboplastin time might have been due to platelet factor 3 unavailability as described above.

Factor X deficiency in amyloidosis is well documented (Howell, 1963; Korsan-Bengsten *et al.*, 1962; Menache and Boivin, 1962; Ottolander and Perret, 1965; Pechet and Kastrul, 1964). No factor X inhibitor, however, has been shown in the sera of the affected patients. The infusion of a large volume of plasma was ineffective in raising the factor X level in the blood (Menache and Boivin, 1962; Bernhardt *et al.*, 1972), thus suggesting either rapid catabolism or the adsorption of factor X by the amyloid tissue. Neither of these two postulated mechanisms has been confirmed experimentally. A recent study by Furie *et al.* (1977) demonstrated rapid clearance of factor X from plasma and its binding to sites probably within the circulatory system.

BIOLOGY, CLINICAL
PATTERNS, AND
TREATMENT OF
MULTIPLE MYELOMA
AND RELATED
PLASMA-CELL
DYSCRASIAS

Cold agglutinins are the earliest examples of M components documented to have antibody activity. Christenson and Dacie (1957) demonstrated a narrow protein band on paper electrophoresis of sera obtained from patients with idiopathic chronic cold hemagglutinin disease. The overwhelming majority of cold agglutinins were later shown to be IgM κ. Harboe *et al.* (1965) studied a large number of cold agglutinins by elution from red cells at 37°C following absorption at 0°C. The isolated antibodies were identified as IgM κ in all cases. Rarely, however, IgM λ (Feizi, 1967) and IgA (Andersen, 1966; Angevine *et al.,* 1966; Williams, R. C., 1971) cold agglutinins have been reported. R. C. Williams *et al.* (1968) demonstrated the sharing of idiotypic specificity among some M components with cold agglutinin activity. The amino acid sequence studies of the amino-terminal end of nine IgM κ cold agglutinins by Capra *et al.* (1972) indicated κ-chain subgroup restriction to κ_3 in most proteins.

The red cell antigens reactive to the cold agglutinins are I and i blood group substances. Rarely, cold agglutinin specific for SP1 (Seligmann and Brouet, 1973), A1 (Rochant *et al.,* 1972), and aged red cells (Ozer and Chaplin, 1963) have been reported. Further insight into the specificity of the anti-I and anti-i antibodies was obtained by the inhibitory activity of glycoproteins extracted from milk (Feizi *et al.,* 1971a,b, 1972).

Chronic cold hemagglutinin disease (Dacie, 1962) is a prototype of clinical syndromes almost totally explainable by the antibody activity and physicochemical property of the corresponding M components. The clinical manifestations of this disease, such as chronic hemolysis, cold sensitivity, and Raynaud's phenomenon, are directly related to the antibody specificity and thermal properties of the monoclonal Ig. Long-term follow-up studies have shown that the concentration of the M component and the cold agglutinin titer generally remain stable for a prolonged period of time (Harboe and Torsvik, 1969). Only exceptionally will a picture of lymphoproliferative disease associated with increasing concentration of IgM ensue.

The M components in WM occasionally exhibit cold agglutinin activity. In such cases, hemolytic anemia, cold sensitivity, and Raynaud's phenomenon may further complicate the clinical manifestations. Transient monoclonal cold agglutinins have also been recognized in association with mycoplasma infection (Feizi and Schumacher, 1968). Most often, however, polyclonal antibodies are responsible for the high cold agglutinin titers in postmycoplasma infection and infectious mononucleosis.

Patients with elevated titers of cold agglutinins, due to either polyclonal or monoclonal antibodies, do not necessarily suffer from hemolytic anemia. The absence of hemolysis is attributed to the difference in the optimal temperature range between the cold agglutinin and the complement activity. It is postulated that hemolysis will develop when these two temperature ranges overlap (Schubothe, 1966).

Protection against exposure to cold often alleviates the hemolysis and reduces other symptoms such as acrocyanosis and gangrene of the extremities. The administration of corticosteroids and splenectomy is generally ineffective (Schubothe, 1966). Cytoxan® and Leukeran®, on the other hand, have been used with some success (Hippe *et al.,* 1970; Olesen, 1964; Dacie and Worlledge, 1969). Blood transfusions should be avoided, if possible, because of the potential hazard of exacerbation of hemolysis (Wintrobe *et al.*, 1974).

2.5. Xanthomatosis and Hyperlipemia Associated with Plasma-Cell Dyscrasias

The mechanisms responsible for xanthomatosis and hyperlipemia in PCDs are complex. A low level of serum cholesterol rather than hypercholesteremia is found in most cases of MM (Seitanichs *et al.*, 1970; Kyle and Bayrd, 1976). Exceptionally, certain cases of MM exhibit xanthomatosis with marked hyperlipemia. Xanthomatosis without hyperlipemia has also been reported (Kint, 1961; Marlen, 1963). The skin lesions are generally described as plane xanthomatous in appearance (Lynch and Winkelmann, 1966). These lesions are yellow to yellowish-brown flat patches distributed over large areas of the body. Tuberous xanthoma and mixed plane and tuberous forms are described in some patients (Potter, 1973b).

Beaumont (1967, 1969) and his associates demonstrated the actual binding of the M component and lipid portion of the lipoprotein, using a red cell agglutination system. These investigators were able to separate the M component from the protein–lipid complex by ultracentrifugation (Beaumont and Lorenzelli, 1967). Both IgA and IgG with lipid-binding properties have been described. Mechanisms other than the affinity of the M component for serum lipid, however, may also be involved in the development of xanthomatosis. For example, Wilson *et al.* (1975) described two cases of lipid abnormalities and cryoglobulinemia associated with IgG κ M components. In one patient, delayed clearance of triglycerides and apolipoprotein was shown; this delay was attributed to the interaction between the M component and heparin. In the second case, the cryoprecipitate contained β and pre-β lipoproteins. Cooper *et al.* (1974) described a monoclonal IgM in a patient with lymphoma and a VDRL titer of 1:4096. Immunochemical studies showed that this monoclonal IgM possessed antibodylike specificity for the phospholipids.

2.6. Xanthoderma

Xanthoderma and xanthotrichia were noted in an elderly patient with otherwise typical MM (Farhangi and Osserman, 1976). The isolated M component, an IgG$_2$ λ (designated IgG^{Gar}), was found to be bound to a bright yellow chromophore that was later identified as riboflavin. IgG^{Gar} exhibited a strong affinity for riboflavin, flavin mononucleotide, and, to a lesser degree, flavin adenine dinucleotide. Other haptens, such as DNP, were also found to bind to IgG^{Gar}. Interestingly, no clinical manifestations of riboflavin deficiency occurred despite the entrapment of large amounts of riboflavin by the M component.

2.7. Hypercupremia

Goodman *et al.* (1967) have reported the presence of a copper-binding IgG κ in a patient with MM. Slit-lamp examination of the eye showed a finely granular discoloration of the corneal endothelium and Descemet's membrane. The posterior surface of the lens was similarly involved. The corneal lesion resembled a Kayser–Fleischer ring, but the deposition of pigment was not confined to the periphery of the cornea. Because of the ocular findings, the concentration of serum copper was

655

BIOLOGY, CLINICAL
PATTERNS, AND
TREATMENT OF
MULTIPLE MYELOMA
AND RELATED
PLASMA-CELL
DYSCRASIAS

determined, and was found to be extremely elevated (3350 $\pm$ 235 μg; normal: < 30μg). The binding of copper to the Ig was shown by electrophoretic separation of serum proteins and the quantitation of copper bound to each fraction. Serum copper was bound almost exclusively to the Ig fraction but the specific binding site for copper was not determined. Short-term treatment of patient with D-penicilla-mine, 1 g/day, resulted in only a very slight increase in the urinary excretion of copper.

In another case of asymptomatic PCD with IgG λ, R. A. Lewis et al. (1975) noted a striking pigment deposition in the Descemet's membrane of the cornea and the lens. Corneal pigmentations were mostly central in distribution and somewhat different from a Kayser–Fleischer ring. Additional studies showed binding of radioactive copper to the M component (Lewis, R. A., et al., 1976).

A large number of monoclonal proteins have been demonstrated to bind streptolysin O, staphylolysin, *Klebsiella, Brucella,* and rubella antigens. Other myeloma proteins have been reported to form complexes with transferrin, serum albumin, and α2 macroglobulin. Binding of haptens such as DNP and phosphoryl-choline has been shown (Seligmann and Brouet, 1973; Potter, 1973b). No discerni-ble clinical features, however, have been linked to these properties of the M components.

2.8. Fanconi Syndrome in Adults

Certain Bence Jones κ proteins appear to exert nephrotoxic effects on the kidney tubules, causing a protracted and long-standing renal tubular acidosis. Maldonado et al. (1975) recently reported three such cases and reviewed 14 previously described patients from the literature. Bence Jones proteinuria was present in all cases, and κ Bence Jones protein was found in all seven patients whose urinary protein was typed. Electron-microscopic examination of the kidneys and bone marrows of several of these cases showed electron-dense inclusion bodies in plasmacytes and the renal tubular cells. Maldonado et al. (1975) pointed out that the clinical picture of Fanconi syndrome and Bence Jones proteinuria in these patients preceded the ultimate development of MM or amyloidosis by several months to several years. MM or amyloidosis eventually occurred in most but not all cases. These clinical features therefore make the Fanconi syndrome in adults with Bence Jones proteinuria a distinct form of PCD.

Bence Jones proteins have been shown to be involved in the pathogenesis of amyloidosis, particularly in cases of myeloma-related and "primary amyloidosis" (see Chapter 12 and Section 4.6 of this chapter).

Bence Jones proteinuria appears to contribute to the development of renal failure in some patients with MM (see Section 4.1.6), although the precise mecha-nisms are not as yet defined.

3. Clinically Asymptomatic (Occult) Forms: Benign Monoclonal Gammopathy; Plasma Cell Dyscrasias of Unknown Significance

At least 32 synonyms have been used to describe various asymptomatic forms of PCD (Ritzmann et al., 1975). A classification based on the clinical features is presented in Table 1. As noted earlier, the more frequent use of serum and urinary protein electrophoresis has been responsible for the increasing recognition of all forms of PCD, particularly the asymptomatic–occult forms. As mentioned earlier the overall incidence of serum M components was about 1.0% in the Swedish adult population (Axelsson *et al.*, 1966). The incidence progressively increased in older groups, particularly after the fifth age decade. In our own experience, the asymptomatic PCDs are diagnosed as frequently as the symptomatic forms. Among 806 cases of PCD previously reported from our laboratory, 367 (45.5%) were asymptomatic, or occult, forms, and 439 (54.5%) were diagnosed as having MM (303 cases), WM (66 cases), or amyloidosis (70 cases) (Isobe and Osserman, 1971). Ritzmann *et al.* (1975) reported 30% asymptomatic PCD among 673 cases. A true incidence of symptomatic vs. asymptomatic forms cannot be ascertained from such data, since these series were gathered selectively from the hospital-referred population. These figures indicate, however, the relatively high frequency with which the physician will face the problem of distinguishing the two groups.

3.1. Differential Diagnosis

Table 5 summarizes some of the more useful criteria for differential diagnosis. Unfortunately, none of the listed criteria is definite and a prolonged period of follow-up is often necessary to determine the true nature of the PCD in a particular case.

The presence of osteolysis (when proved to be due to plasma-cell tumor) or extraskeletal plasmacytomas will, of course, rule out an asymptomatic PCD. Hypercalcemia occurs in approximately 30% of cases of MM (Kyle and Bayrd, 1976), but not in asymptomatic PCD. The stability of the M-component concentration is considered one of the more reliable criteria in favor of asymptomatic PCD or benign monoclonal gammopathy (BMG) (Waldenström, 1973; Hällén, 1969; Axelsson and Hällén, 1968; Seligmann *et al.*, 1971); conversely, in malignant forms of PCD, a progressive rise in M component invariably occurs in untreated cases and in those who do not respond to treatment or are in relapse after clinical remission

TABLE 5. Criteria for the Differentiation of the Clinically Asymptomatic (Occult) Forms (PCDUS) from the Clinically Symptomatic (Overt) Forms of Plasma-Cell Dyscrasia

Criterion	Asymptomatic (occult) (PCDUS)[a]	Symptomatic (overt)[a]
Osteolysis[b]	NO	Yes
Extraskeletal plasma cell tumor	NO	Yes
Hypercalcemia	NO	Yes
Spleen and liver involvement	NO	Yes
Rising M components	NO	YES
Anemia	NO	Yes
Marrow plasmacytosis > 20%[c]	No	Yes
IgG > 2 g/dl, IgA > 1g/dl		
IgM > 1 g/dl, B-J protein > 0.2 g/day	No	Yes
Generalized osteoporosis	No	Yes
Decreased polyclonal Ig's	No	Yes

[a](NO. YES) True in all or the overwhelming majority of patients; (No, Yes) true in some but not all cases.
[b]Osteolysis occurs with other neoplasia; tissue biopsy confirmation is necessary.
[c]Excluding the erythroid elements.

(Waldenström, 1973; Hobbs, 1971; Seligmann *et al.*, 1971; Axelsson and Hällén,

657

BIOLOGY, CLINICAL
PATTERNS, AND
TREATMENT OF
MULTIPLE MYELOMA
AND RELATED
PLASMA-CELL
DYSCRASIAS

1968). Anemia occurs rather frequently in MM and WM, and is generally absent in asymptomatic PCDs. This criterion is useful only if other causes of anemia such as iron deficiency and "anemia of chronic disease" have been clearly ruled out. Bone marrow examination is frequently but not always helpful in establishing the diagnosis. It is true that the majority of patients with MM show a hypercellular marrow with a high percentage of plasma cells but exceptions are common. A marrow plasma cell percentage greater than 20% (excluding erythroid elements) is arbitrarily taken by some investigators to separate the symptomatic from the occult forms (Michaux and Heremans, 1969; Fadem, 1952; Chronic Leukemia–Myeloma Task Force, National Cancer Institute, 1968). The majority of cases of asymptomatic PCD are associated with marrow plasmacytosis of less than 10%. Distinctive ultrastructural features separating malignant myeloma cells from the plasma cells of benign gammopathies have been described (Bernier and Graham, 1976) but the clinical usefulness of these criteria remains to be determined. The concentration of the serum M component is often used to distinguish the malignant from the benign forms of PCD. It should be noted, however, that there is considerable variation in the rate of synthesis of Ig in different cases of MM (Salmon and Durie, 1975), and the catabolic rate of M components is dependent not only on the class and subclasses of the Ig, but also on its serum concentration (see Chapter 12). Despite these reservations it has been suggested that serum concentrations of IgG greater than 2 g/dl, IgA and IgM greater than 1 g/dl (Michaux and Heremans, 1969; Cooke, 1969), and Bence Jones proteinuria greater than 200 mg/day (Osserman, 1971) are consistent with malignant PCD. A serum M component greater than 3 g/dl, regardless of Ig class, has been suggested by others as a more realistic range for separating the two groups (Ritzmann *et al.*, 1975). Most authors agree that the presence of significant amounts of Bence Jones proteinuria is a strong indication of symptomatic and progressive disease (Waldenström, 1970; Hobbs, 1967; Seligmann and Basch, 1968). Exceptional cases of prolonged asymptomatic Bence Jones proteinuria, however, have been reported (Kyle *et al.*, 1973).

It is often difficult to interpret the significance of osteoporosis in patients with PCD whose median age is in the late 50's or early 60's. The high incidence of involutional osteopenia in this age group (Thompson and Frame, 1976) makes the differentiation uncertain. Decreased concentrations of normal Ig's occur more often in symptomatic than in asymptomatic forms of PCD (Hobbs, 1967; Seligmann *et al.*, 1971; Waldenström, 1970; Conklin and Alexanian, 1975).

3.2. Natural History

The natural history of occult PCDs (PCDUS) has been studied in several series (Waldenström, 1973; Zawadzki and Edwards, 1972; Osserman, 1958). It has become evident that the majority of patients remain asymptomatic; exceptionally, however, after several months or years, transition to an overt form of PCD may occur. In a patient described by Salmon (1975), the change from presymptomatic to symptomatic phase occurred progressively. During the 136 days of follow-up, near-doubling of the monoclonal protein and tumor cell number was documented. In other patients, however, after a prolonged stable condition, gradual transition may take place. In a patient whom we have followed for 20 years, an IgG M component associated with carcinoma of the colon was originally documented in 1957. Eleven years later, there was a rise in the concentration of monoclonal protein and development of Bence Jones proteinuria, anemia, and skeletal symptoms, i.e., the full clinical picture of MM. A similar case has been reported by Waldenström (1970).

3.3. Conditions Associated With Asymptomatic Plasma-Cell Dyscrasias

In many patients with asymptomatic PCD's coexistent chronic disease, particularly tuberculosis, syphilis, osteomyelitis, pyelonephritis, and inflammatory diseases of the biliary tract or autoimmune diseases such as rheumatoid arthritis can be documented (Isobe and Osserman, 1971; Hällén, 1966; Zawadzki and Edwards, 1970; Hobbs, 1969a).

The association of asymptomatic as well as symptomatic PCD's with nonreticular neoplasia has been extensively reported (Isobe and Osserman, 1971; Anderson, E. T., and Vye, 1967; Hobbs, 1969a; Osserman and Takatsuki, 1963a; Williams, R. C., et al., 1969; Zawadzki and Edwards, 1972). Other investigators have not found a significant increase in the incidence of PCDs in patients with various cancers (Migliore and Alexanian, 1968). The association of PCDs and nonreticular neoplasia could simply reflect the known increase in second neoplasms in tumor-bearing hosts (Moertel, 1966). However, the histological findings described by us and others (Osserman and Takatsuki, 1965; Williams, R. C., et al., 1969; Bohrod, 1957) indicating heavy infiltration of some nonreticular tumors by plasma cells would suggest an immunological reaction. In a study by R. C. Williams et al. (1969), the antibody produced against the M component was shown to identify clusters of plasma cells infiltrating the carcinoma.

The occurrence of M component in leukemias, particularly monocytic and myelomonocytic leukemias, has been noted by several investigators (DiGuglielmo, 1966; Osserman, 1967, 1969; Poulik et al., 1969; Thijs et al., 1970; Tursz et al., 1974a,b; Law et al., 1976; Bethlenfalvay et al., 1976). An increase in polyclonal Ig's is found rather frequently in patients with monocytic and myelomonocytic leukemia (Brown, R. K., et al., 1948; Ryder, 1966; Osserman and Lawlor, 1966). An increased number of plasmacytes (5.5%) was noted in 11 cases of chronic myelomonocytic leukemia reported by Miescher and Farquet (1974). Lindqvist et al. (1970) reported an interesting case of a child with acute lymphocytic leukemia in whom electrophoresis and Ig quantitation were done serially. The patient developed an IgG M component after several months of chemotherapy. The appearance of the M component was associated with a short-lasting increase in polyclonal Ig's. The M component in this patient, however, could have been the result of immunological stimulation by an infectious agent.

PCDs have been also observed in association with various myeloproliferative syndromes (Zawadzki and Edwards, 1972; Derghazarian and Whittemore, 1974; Isobe and Osserman, 1971). Several cases of Gaucher's disease have been reported to be associated with M components since the first case was described in 1963 (Osserman and Takatsuki, 1963a). The report by Pratt et al. (1968) is particularly interesting in that 4 of 16 cases of Gaucher's disease had an M component, and other patients with splenomegaly and aseptic bone necrosis showed diffuse hypergammaglobulinemia.

659

BIOLOGY, CLINICAL
PATTERNS, AND
TREATMENT OF
MULTIPLE MYELOMA
AND RELATED
PLASMA-CELL
DYSCRASIAS

The occurrence of M components in children with immune deficiency syndromes has been reported (Snapper and Kahn, 1971; Stoop et al., 1962; Cawley and Schenken, 1970; Radl et al., 1967). Since the expected incidence of the M components in young subjects is extremely low, this association is probably significant.

The association of the M component with malignant lymphoma and chronic lymphocytic leukemia (CLL) has been noted by several authors (Azar et al., 1957; Krauss and Sokal, 1966; Michaux and Heremans, 1969). Alexanian (1975) studied 1150 patients with the diagnosis of lymphoma and Hodgkin's disease, in whom serum protein electrophoresis was performed. He found 49 M components: 29 IgM, 15 IgG, and 5 untyped. The incidence of a monoclonal peak, particularly IgM, was significantly higher than expected among patients with diffuse lymphoma (lymphocytic or histiocytic) as well as with CLL. Hodgkin's disease and nodular lymphoma patients did not exhibit an increased frequency of monoclonal peaks. It should be noted, however, that most patients in this series with diffuse lymphoma and monoclonal IgM proteins could be considered as cases of WM. The association of IgM peaks with CLL is quite intriguing. Although the leukemic cells in most CLL patients are B-cell in origin, having 7 S IgM and IgD surface Ig's, the serum component is 19 S macroglobulin. The production of a serum component must therefore be attributed to another clone of B cells that is capable of synthesis and secretion of the pentameric IgM. In an interesting recent study of 29 patients with CLL and lymphosarcoma, Eipe et al. (1975) were able to identify M components in 22 patients by using prolonged cellulose acetate electrophoresis of the serum euglobulin fraction. Antiidiotype antisera prepared against the isolated M components reacted with the autologous but not with the heterologous lymphocytes. These data, if confirmed, would indicate that the incidence of serum M components in lymphoproliferative disease of B-cell origin is much higher than has been previously reported. Furthermore, the M components appear to be the products of a closely related clone of B-cell origin, rather than of an unrelated clone.

The co-occurrence of plasma-cell myeloma with lymphocytic leukemia and lymphosarcoma (Narasimhan et al., 1975) was recently reported. In another account, an IgM monoclonal protein was detected in the serum of a patient with hairy-cell leukemia (Golde et al., 1977).

3.4. Transient Plasma-Cell Dyscrasias

Transient PCDs have been recognized with increasing frequency in recent years. The clinical conditions in which transient PCDs have been described are listed in Table 6. Seligmann et al. (1971) reported transient monoclonal peaks in children with immune deficiency syndromes. It is noteworthy that transient monoclonal proteins were also reported to occur at the time of viral infections in children with acute leukemia who were immunosuppressed by chemotherapy (Stoop et al., 1962; Lindqvist et al., 1970; Vodopick et al., 1974). Infectious diseases that are occasionally noted to be associated with transient PCDs include viral hepatitis (Seligmann et al., 1971; Danon and Seligmann, 1972; Abramson and Shattil, 1973), Mycoplasma pneumonia (Feizi and Schumacher, 1968), and Leptospira pomona infection (Bain et al., 1973). Transient PCDs have also been reported to occur with autoimmune and systemic diseases such as rheumatoid arthritis and periarteritis

**TABLE 6.   Clinical Circumstances Reported to Be Associated with Transient
Plasma-Cell Dyscrasias**

Clinical circumstance	References
Immune deficiencies	Seligmann et al. (1971)
Viral hepatitis	Seligmann et al. (1971), Danon and Seligmann (1972), Abramson and Shattil (1973)
Cytomegalovirus infection	Vodopick et al. (1974), Danon and Seligmann (1972)
Suspected viral infection	Stoop et al. (1968), Lindqvist et al. (1970)
Mycoplasma pneumonia	Feizi and Schumacher (1968)
Leptospira pomona infection	Bain et al. (1973)
Autoimmune and systemic diseases, rheumatoid arthritis, polyarteritis nodosa, cirrhosis	Hällén (1966), Young (1969)
Drug hypersensitivity	Osserman and Takatsuki (1965)
Prosthetic valve surgery	Young (1969)
Parathyroid adenoma	Clubb et al. (1964)
Goiter	Schobel and Wewalka (1965)
Breast carcinoma	Bohrod (1957)
Melanoma	Young (1969), Hällén (1966)
Folic acid deficiency	Roman and Coles (1966)
Methotrexate hepatotoxicity	Abramson and Shattil (1973)
Waldenström's macroglobulinemia	Ferriman and Anderson (1956), Nutter and Kramer (1965)

nodosa (Hällén, 1966; Young, 1969). We observed a patient who, following treatment with sulfonamide (Sulfasoxazole, Gantrisin®) and with a history of recent exposure to penicillin and streptomycin, developed a serum monoclonal peak and Bence-Jones proteinuria (Osserman and Takatsuki, 1965). The follow-up studies of serum and urinary protein 3 months later showed total disappearance of the monoclonal proteins. Transient peaks were also noted following prosthetic heart valve implantation (Young, 1969) and in association with the removal of benign and malignant nonreticular tumors (Clubb et al., 1964; Schobel and Wewalka, 1965; Bohrod, 1957; Young, 1969; Hällén, 1966). Folic acid deficiency and methotrexate-induced hepatotoxicity have been implicated in some cases of transient PCD (Roman and Coles, 1966; Abramson and Shattil, 1973).

Two reported cases of WM who spontaneously remitted (Ferriman and Anderson, 1956; Nutter and Kramer, 1965) are probably examples of an exceptional clinical course in this disease. The serum peaks, together with other organ manifestations of macroglobulinemia, disappeared after a prolonged period of followup. We recently studied an IgA PCD of long-standing (15 years') duration. The monoclonal IgA was shown to have binding affinity for IgG (Farhangi et al., 1977). There was generalized lymphadenopathy, splenomegaly, and marrow plasmacytosis associated with a prominent serum peak (6.0 g/dl). Hemorrhagic episodes and purpura were present, these being attributed to the IgA–IgG complexes demonstrated in the patient's serum. Although the patient was treated with chlorambucil (Leukeran®) early in the course of the disease, several years later, a spontaneous decline in serum peak occurred while the patient was on no chemotherapy.

661

BIOLOGY, CLINICAL
PATTERNS, AND
TREATMENT OF
MULTIPLE MYELOMA
AND RELATED
PLASMA-CELL
DYSCRASIAS

The study of clinical conditions that have been associated with transient PCDs suggests that certain acute inflammatory or immunological reactions such as viral infections, drug hypersensitivity, valve prosthesis surgery or exacerbation of an underlying systemic disease, e.g. rheumatoid arthritis or periarteritis nodosa precedes or coincides with the appearance of the M component. This further suggests that certain unusual antigenic stimulation lead to a restricted clonal proliferation and a monoclonal Ig response.

4. Clinically Symptomatic (Overt) Forms of Plasma-Cell Dyscrasia

Plasma-cell myeloma and Waldenström's macroglobulinemia are the most common symptomatic PCDs (see Table 2). Progress in the elucidation of Ig structure has been responsible in part for the recognition of several newly described entities such as the heavy-chain diseases. Recent studies of amyloid proteins indicate that L-chain fragments are the major constituent of most "primary" and myeloma-related amyloids. This review of the overt forms of PCDs will therefore include a discussion of amyloidosis.

4.1. Plasma-Cell Myeloma (Multiple Myeloma)

In this disease, in addition to the autonomous expansion of a single plasma-cell clone engaged in the production of monoclonal Ig, several characteristics of malignant neoplasia can be recognized. Most clinical manifestations of the disease can be attributed to: (1) the predominant site of tumor-cell distribution, i.e., bone marrow spaces, which results in the destruction of bone and hematopoietic abnormalities; (2) disturbance in immune mechanisms and susceptibility to infection; (3) renal function impairment due to complex mechanisms (see Section 4.1.6); (4) M-component-related clinical manifestations such as the hyperviscosity syndrome, cryoglobulinemia, and hemostatic abnormalities.

4.1.1. The Malignant Plasma Cell

The morphological, ultrastructural, and functional properties of the malignant plasma cell are described elsewhere in this volume. It should be emphasized that the variation in the morphology of plasma cells has been noted frequently both from case to case and within the same case of myeloma (Waldenström, 1970; Snapper and Kahn, 1971; Drivsholm and Clausen, 1964; Maldonado et al., 1965, 1966). A wide range of cellular organelle morphologies has also been described. A rather distinct asynchrony of nuclear and cytoplasmic maturation has been observed to be present in malignant plasma cells and not in asymptomatic PCDs (BMGs) (Smetana et al., 1973; Graham and Bernier, 1975; Turesson, 1975; Bernier and Graham, 1976).

4.1.2. Clinical Manifestations

The clinical features of MM are described in several excellent reviews and monographs (Snapper and Kahn, 1971; Waldenström, 1970; Williams, W. J., et al., 1972; Azar and Potter, 1973; Wintrobe et al., 1974; Kyle and Bayrd, 1976). We will therefore limit our discussion to several major aspects of the disease.

MEHDI FARHANGI
AND ELLIOTT F.
OSSERMAN

4.1.3. Osteolysis and Hypercalcemia

Bone destruction is usually the most prominent clinical feature of MM, and is responsible to a large extent for the patient's symptoms. In the series of cases of MM reported by Kyle (1975), radiological evidence of bony changes in the form of osteolytic lesions, osteoporosis, pathological fractures, or a combination of these changes occurred in 79% of cases, and bone pain as an initial complaint was recorded in 68%. X rays of the vertebrae, pelvis, skull, ribs, and proximal portions of humeri and femurs are generally the most rewarding in delineating the extent of skeletal lesions. Infrequently, the long bones are affected, and may result in pathological fractures. Myelomatous involvement of the mandible and sternum is not uncommon (Kyle and Bayrd, 1976). Bone scan using technetium-99m is less useful than radiography for the detection of myelomatous involvement, evidently due to the paucity of new bone formation at the site of bone resorption. Bone scan may, however, be useful for the survey of ribs, sternum, and long bones (Wahner *et al.*, 1975; Kyle and Bayrd, 1976). Following induction of clinical remission by chemotherapy, the radiographic appearance of preexisting bone lesions often remains unchanged although in some cases osteolytic lesions may recalcify. The disease progression and relapse after the clinical remission are usually associated with the appearance of new lesions and pathological fractures.

The mechanism of osteolysis in MM is thought to be due to tumor growth within the marrow spaces. Recent studies by Mundy *et al.* (1974b) indicate that plasma cells elaborate an osteoclast-activating factor that leads to increased bone resorption. The supernatant from short-term bone marrow cultures from MM patients was found to activate osteoclastic bone resorption similar to the factor elaborated by phytohemagglutinin (PHA)-activated blood leukocytes (Mundy *et al.*, 1974a). Histological evidence for osteoclast activation was demonstrated at the sites where heavy plasma cell infiltration was noted.

Bone destruction in myeloma is associated with increased calcium liberation, and not uncommonly with hypercalcemia. Most frequently, hypercalcemic episodes occur at the time of initial presentation, or at the relapse phase of the disease. In our own series of MM patients treated with melphalan [see Section 4.1.11b(6)], the pretreatment serum calcium value was above 11 mg/dl in 39% of patients and above 13 mg/dl in 24%. In the series of cases reported by Kyle (1975), the initial serum calcium was in an abnormal range in 30% of patients. Hypercalcemia, once developed, causes obligatory diuresis, leading to dehydration and reduced glomerular filtration. Altered renal tubular function then ensues (Epstein, 1968). Phosphate and nitrogen retention are common and usually reversible by appropriate therapeutic measures (see Section 4.1.11a). A condition resembling vasopressin-resistant diabetes insipidus (Zeffren and Heinemann, 1962) and compromised ammonia production and acid excretion has been reported to occur with hypercalcemia (Heinemann, 1963).

4.1.4. Hematopoietic Abnormalities

Hematopoietic abnormalities, particularly anemia, occur frequently in MM. All patients in our own series except one had a pretreatment hemoglobin value of less than 12 g/dl, and 59% of patients had a hemoglobin of less than 10 g/dl. In our series, 32% required repeated blood transfusions to maintain the hemoglobin at 8–9 g/dl

663

BIOLOGY, CLINICAL
PATTERNS, AND
TREATMENT OF
MULTIPLE MYELOMA
AND RELATED
PLASMA-CELL
DYSCRASIAS

(see Table 9). In the series of Kyle (1975), 62% of patients had a pretreatment hemoglobin of less than 12 g/dl. A normocytic, normochromic anemia is the rule. Overt autoimmune hemolytic anemia has been rarely reported in myeloma (Bohrod and Bottcher, 1963; Pirofsky, 1969, Pengelly et al., 1973). Anemia secondary to blood loss due either to thrombocytopenia or to hemostatic abnormalities caused by specific M components may also contribute to the hematological picture. In the presence of hyperviscosity, an increase in plasma volume and proportional decrease in hemoglobin concentration may mimic a "true" anemia (McGrath and Penny, 1976; MacKenzie et al., 1968; Tuddenham and Bradley, 1974).

Pretreatment leukopenia and thrombocytopenia are uncommon. In our series, leukopenia of less than 4000/mm^3 and thrombocytopenia of less than 140,000 per mm^3 occurred in 14 and 25%, respectively, in previously untreated patients. Of the Mayo clinic cases (Kyle, 1975), 16% were also leukopenic (< 4000/mm^3) at the outset, and 12% had thrombocytopenia of less than 100,000/mm^3. Thrombocytosis before treatment or shortly after the onset of treatment with melphalan has been noted (Waldenström, 1970; Zimelman, 1973).

4.1.5. Extraskeletal Tumors

In most cases of MM, extraskeletal tumors are not clinically evident. Occasionally, plasma-cell neoplasia manifests itself primarily in extraskeletal sites (see Section 4.1.10b). In MM, macroscopic and microscopic involvement of the extraskeletal sites at postmortem examination, however, has been reported to be demonstrable in 65–70% of cases (Azar, 1973; Churg and Gordon, 1950). Pasmantier and Azar (1969) autopsied 57 consecutive cases of MM at Francis Delafield Hospital. Organs outside the skeleton were involved in 65% of cases. Spleen, liver, lymph nodes, and kidneys were most frequently affected. The adrenals, thyroid, lungs, pleura, and pancreas were also involved, but to a lesser extent. Gross organ involvement, however, was noted in only one third of cases. Pasmantier and Azar (1969) also reported some correlation between the frequency of involvement of extraskeletal sites and the degree of atypia of plasma cells. During the clinical course of MM, extraskeletal plasma-cell tumors are occasionally recognized. Sporadic case reports dealing with tumors involving practically every organ in the body can be found in the medical literature (McFadzean, 1975; Gupta et al., 1974; Bourreille et al., 1974; Balthazar and Cano, 1975; Mangalik and Gupta, 1974; Higby and Ohnuma, 1975; Kleinholz and Tennebaum, 1973; Yoshimura et al., 1976; Kyle and Bayrd, 1976).

Neurological complications produced by plasma-cell tumors are of particular clinical importance in MM, notably spinal cord compression and involvement of the cauda equina by tumors arising from vertebral bodies or a collapsed vertebral column. Fortunately, the incidence of cord compression and the resultant permanent neurological deficit in the form of paraplegia has declined in recent years (Callis and Sheets, 1974; Farhangi and Osserman, 1973). Early detection of spinal cord compression, decompression surgery followed by radiotherapy, along with more effective chemotherapy have been responsible for this trend. Lumbosacral radiculopathy due to compression or direct tumor involvement is the most common neurological problem, which leads to a vicious cycle of patient immobilization, enhancement of bone resorption, hypercalcemia, and renal failure. Other neurological disorders such as peripheral neuropathies are occasionally seen (Walsh, 1971), particularly in association with osteosclerotic myeloma (see Section 4.1.10e).

Intracranial tumors arising from skull or dura mater, independent of skull lesions, have occasionally been reported (Kyle and Bayrd, 1976). Cases of multifocal leukoencephalopathy have been described (DelDuca and Morningstar, 1967; Gordon *et al.*, 1971; Richardson and Johnson, 1975).

4.1.6. Renal Failure

Renal failure occurs rather frequently with MM. Of patients in our own series, 20% had nonprotein nitrogen levels greater than 50 mg/dl (normal: up to 40 mg/dl) prior to treatment. In the Mayo Clinic series, slightly more than half the patients had elevated initial serum creatinine levels, and in 30% of the patients, the initial serum creatinine was greater than 2.0 mg/dl (Kyle and Bayrd, 1976). Acute renal failure with myeloma often occurs in a clinical setting of hypercalcemia, hyperuricemia, and dehydration at the time of initial presentation or later, when refractoriness to chemotherapy becomes evident.

The causes of renal failure in myeloma are complex and multifactorial. We have already alluded to the renal function impairment associated with hypercalcemia. The hyperuricemia seen in over half of patients (Kyle and Bayrd, 1976) may contribute to renal complications. The role of Bence Jones protein in the causation of the renal failure is not well understood. Some investigators believe that renal failure is more frequent in patients with Bence Jones proteinuria (Hobbs, 1969b) than in those without it. On the basis of data compiled from the medical literature, Jancelewicz *et al.* (1975) noted blood urea nitrogen values above 30 mg/dl in 78% of patients with MM associated with Bence Jones proteinuria alone and in 67% of patients with IgD myeloma known to be associated with a high incidence (92%) of Bence Jones proteinuria. In IgA and IgG myeloma, the incidence was 33 and 14%, respectively (Bence Jones proteinuria was documented in 70 and 60%, correspondingly).

The role of the kidney in the catabolism of Bence Jones proteins has been well established (Solomon *et al.*, 1964; Wochner *et al.*, 1967; Jensen, 1970a,b). In nephrectomized mice given radioiodinated Bence Jones protein, a marked reduction in protein catabolism was noted, as compared with unoperated control animals (Wochner *et al.*, 1967). Interestingly, glomerular filtration and hence tubular reabsorption may not be mandatory for Bence Jones protein catabolism, since the animals with ligated ureters catabolized Bence Jones proteins nearly as well as control animals. The endogenous (primarily kidney) catabolism may account for 50–90% of Bence Jones proteins, and the remainder is excreted in the urine (Solomon *et al.*, 1964). In kidneys with impaired tubular cell function, the L chains are catabolized less efficiently. There is circumstantial evidence for the nephrotoxicity of certain Bence Jones proteins. Ladefoged *et al.* (1970) reported acute renal failure as the presenting manifestation in seven myeloma patients with Bence Jones proteinuria. As mentioned earlier, some cases of Fanconi syndrome in adults have been reported to be associated with Bence Jones κ proteinuria (Maldonado *et al.*, 1975, Engle and Wallis, 1957; Horn *et al.*, 1969; Finkel *et al.*, 1973). Aminoaciduria, renal glycosuria, renal acidosis, hypokalemia, hypophosphatemia, hypouricemia, and elevated alkaline phosphatase were indicative of proximal tubular dysfunction.

665

BIOLOGY, CLINICAL
PATTERNS, AND
TREATMENT OF
MULTIPLE MYELOMA
AND RELATED
PLASMA-CELL
DYSCRASIAS

Moreover, electron-dense crystal-like inclusion bodies were demonstrated in tubular epithelial cells as well as marrow plasma cells (Maldonado *et al.*, 1975). The selective nature of nephrotoxicity due to Bence Jones proteins is suggested by the fact that some patients with a prolonged history of Bence Jones proteinuria remain free of kidney failure (Kyle *et al.*, 1973).

Renal failure associated with defined histological changes in the kidney is often referred to as *myeloma kidney*. Tubular casts, inconsistently marked by eosinophilia, lamellation, and glossy appearance with giant-cell reaction engulfing the casts, are the prominent histological features. The multinucleated giant cells are in continuity with tubular epithelium, and are probably not mononuclear–macrophage in origin. Tubular dilatation and atrophy, interstitial fibrosis, and inflammatory changes are evident in some kidneys. Tubular atrophy is considered more characteristic of myeloma kidney than tubular casts *per se* (Levi *et al.*, 1968). Immunofluorescent studies of kidneys from patients with MM performed by Levi *et al.* (1968) showed tubular casts containing IgG and the L chains of both κ and λ variety, rather than one type of Bence Jones protein.

Most investigators have been unable to demonstrate a consistent correlation between clinical renal failure and the histological findings of "myeloma kidney." Schubert *et al.* (1972) examined the kidneys of 146 patients who died of MM. Premortem clinical data indicative of renal status were available in 65 patients, of whom 56 had renal failure. Myeloma kidney based on histology was diagnosed in 27 cases. Of the remaining 29 patients, 25 had evidence of renal lesions other than myeloma kidney, and 4 had no demonstrable microscopic changes. On the other hand, kidneys with tubular casts may not be associated with discernible functional abnormalities. It is therefore evident that other factors in addition to the precipitation of protein in the kidney tubules, such as hypercalcemia, hypercalciuria, hyperuricemia, and dehydration, play a part in the development of renal failure.

Acute renal failure has been reported following intravenous pyelography (Bartels *et al.*, 1954; Brown, M., and Battle, 1964) and angiographic studies (*New England Journal of Medicine*, 1976). Water deprivation in preparation for the studies was probably responsible for the precipitation of this renal failure (Morgan and Hammack, 1966; Myers and Witten, 1971).

Amyloidosis of the kidney is reported to occur in 7–8% of myeloma patients (Kyle and Bayrd, 1976; Schubert *et al.*, 1972). Renal involvement is often part of a more generalized amyloidosis, which may include the skin, periarticular sites, heart, GI tract, and other tissues, organs, and systems. Nephrotic syndrome and renal insufficiency may supervene as a consequence of renal amyloidosis.

Glomerular nodules resembling diabetic nephrosclerosis were described in nondiabetic myeloma patients (Schubert and Adam, 1974). These investigators noted some ultrastructural features that were distinct from those of diabetic glomerular lesions. Furthermore, a unique collagen was found in the vicinity of the nodules and in the periglomerular interstitium.

The hyperviscosity syndrome associated with the M components is suspected, but not well demonstrated, to cause renal function impairment such as diminished renal concentrating ability (Bloch and Maki, 1973). Cryoglobulinemia, on the other hand, particularly when it is of a mixed type (see Chapter 12), is associated with a high incidence of rapidly progressive renal failure. As mentioned earlier, most cryoglobulins in myeloma remain clinically inconsequential.

Plasma-cell infiltration of the kidney is demonstrated relatively frequently on postmortem examination (Azar, 1973) but it is unlikely to contribute to the impairment of renal function. Plasma cells have also been found in the urine of patients with MM (Rees and Waugh, 1965; Kunwar and Kumar, 1966; Pringle *et al.*, 1974).

As mentioned earlier, a background of chronic or recurrent infection such as urinary tract infection is not unusual in any form of PCD. Renal failure in myeloma patients is not infrequently the result of pyelonephritis (Schubert *et al.*, 1972), obstructive uropathy, stones, or other nephropathy.

4.1.7. M Components in Plasma-Cell Myeloma

Careful examination of the serum and urine of patients with MM by electrophoresis and immunoelectrophoresis will show monoclonal proteins in 99% of cases. Table 7 summarizes our data on 351 cases of plasma-cell myeloma regarding the nature of the M components. Of these patients, 52.1% had an IgG and 21.6% an IgA monoclonal protein. Three patients (0.9%) had an IgD M component, and one patient, a biclonal gammopathy, with IgG and IgA M components. In 25.1% of the patients, Bence Jones protein alone was demonstrated in the urine. Bence Jones proteinuria accompanied the serum M components in another 30% of the cases. We had previously reported 3 cases of so-called "nonsecretory" myeloma (Osserman and Takatsuki, 1963a). Kyle (1975) also observed only 3 such patients among 869 cases of MM. A moderate to marked decrease in polyclonal serum Ig's at the time of diagnosis of MM is the rule rather than the exception. Only rarely is the normal concentration of polyclonal Ig's preserved.

4.1.8. Immune Deficiency and Susceptibility to Infection

The high frequency of pneumococcal and staphylococcal respiratory tract infection and *Escherichia coli* urinary tract infection in MM is well known (Fahey

TABLE 7. Types of Serum M Components and Bence Jones Proteins in 351 Cases of Multiple Myeloma

Serum M component	Urine Bence-Jones protein		Cases	
			Number	%
IgG	—		112	31.9
IgG	+BJ κ		32	9.1
IgG	+BJ λ		39	11.1
		TOTALS:	183	52.1
IgA	—		47	13.4
IgA	+BJ κ		12	3.4
IgA	+BJ λ		17	4.8
		TOTALS:	76	21.6
—	BJ κ only		46	13.1
—	BJ λ only		42	12.0
		TOTALS:	88	25.1
IgD	+BJ λ		3	0.9
IgG κ + IgAλ	+BJ λ		1	0.3

667

BIOLOGY, CLINICAL
PATTERNS, AND
TREATMENT OF
MULTIPLE MYELOMA
AND RELATED
PLASMA-CELL
DYSCRASIAS

et al., 1963; Zinneman and Hall, 1954; Salmon et al., 1967). Meyers et al. (1972) pointed out that infections due to gram-negative microorganisms have been more prevalent in recent years. Among viral illnesses, herpes zoster occurs relatively frequently in MM (Williams, H. M., et al., 1959; Shanbrom et al., 1960; Saidi et al., 1973). As noted above, a moderate to marked decrease in the concentration of polyclonal Ig's can be demonstrated in most cases of MM. An impaired capacity to respond to antigenic stimuli has also been documented (Larson and Tomlinson, 1952; Lawson et al., 1955; Marks, 1953; Dammacco and Clausen, 1966; Harris et al., 1971; Harris and Copeland, 1974). Two mechanisms are implicated to explain the B-cell dysfunction in MM. First, a subpopulation of B cells—"monoclonal lymphocytes"—has been identified in the peripheral blood of MM patients by several investigators using antiidiotype-specific antisera produced against the M components (Lindström et al., 1973; Mellstedt et al., 1974; Abdou and Abdou, 1975; Mellstedt et al., 1976). It has been further shown that those "monoclonal lymphocytes" decrease following chemotherapy (Abdou and Abdou, 1975; Mellstedt et al., 1976). Heller and his associates had earlier shown that following the implantation of plasmacytoma in BALB/c mice there was an increase in the number of receptor-carrying B lymphocytes that shared idiotypic determinants with the M component (Yakulis et al., 1972; Heller et al., 1973). In another study, the recruitment of B cells into "monoclonal lymphocyte" populations by a serum RNA was suggested (Chen et al., 1975), thus making the normal B lymphocytes unavailable to react to various antigens. Broder et al. (1975), on the other hand, identified in the blood of myeloma patients certain phagocytic leukocytes that suppressed polyclonal Ig synthesis by normal peripheral blood lymphocytes stimulated by pokeweed mitogen.

Still other studies indicate that myeloma patients have an impaired ability to develop a delayed hypersensitivity reaction to 2,4-dinitro-1-fluorobenzene (Cone and Uhr, 1964), and depressed function of the RES (Groch et al., 1965), as well as decreased migration of neutrophils to skin windows (Penny et al., 1971). Diminished responses to the nonspecific mitogen PHA have also been reported (Salmon and Fudenberg, 1969; Campbell et al., 1975).

4.1.9. Cell Kinetics in Plasma-Cell Myeloma

Plasma-cell-tumor growth in man, like most spontaneously occurring tumors in animals, is alleged to follow Gompertzian growth kinetics, i.e., an early rapid increase in tumor cell number followed by a decreasing rate of growth that leads to an eventual equilibrium between cell death and cell birth (Laird 1964, 1965; Simpson-Herren and Lloyd, 1970). Salmon and his associates, by sequential quantitation of the tumor cell number and with the aid of a computer program, concluded that the growth of myeloma tumor cells in man likewise follows Gompertzian kinetics (Salmon, 1973). The general approach in quantitating the number of myeloma cells in man is based on the observation made in mouse plasmacytoma, that a linear relationship exists between tumor cell number and the serum concentration of the M component. Nathans et al. (1958) found a good relationship between the estimated total extracellular myeloma protein and the excised tumor weight in C_H3 mice bearing the X5563 plasmacytoma. It is assumed that a similar relationship also exists in human tumors. Total myeloma cell number is determined by using the formula proposed by Salmon and his associates (Salmon and Smith, 1970a; Salmon, 1973):

$$\text{Myeloma cell number} = \frac{\text{Total-body M-component synthesis rate}}{\text{Cellular M-component synthesis rate}}$$

Presuming that a steady state exists at any given time between the synthesis of protein and its catabolism, the total-body M-component synthesis rate is calculated from the fractional catabolic rate (FCR) (Waldmann and Strober, 1969), the plasma volume (PV), and the serum M-component concentration (PPL). Thus, the M-component synthesis rate is equal to FCR × PV × PPL. In this equation, however, the M component distributed outside the vascular system is ignored. In early studies by Salmon and his associates the FCR was determined by measuring the catabolic rate of radioiodinated M component. It was later suggested that this latter step could be bypassed and the appropriate value for FCR obtained from equations and constants developed by Waldmann and Strober (1969). In view of the PV expansion associated with hyperviscosity due to the M component, it would seem necessary to measure the PV directly in such cases. In most studies, however, the PV is calculated from the body surface area and the hematocrit. The cellular M-component synthesis rate is determined *in vitro* by short-term marrow culture (Salmon and Smith, 1970a,b; Salmon, 1973). In this assay, all mononuclear cells (lymphocytes plus plasmacytes) are counted as Ig-synthesizing cells, and the amount of protein synthesized is measured by a sandwich solid-phase radioimmunoassay (Salmon et al., 1969; Salmon and Smith, 1970b). The cellular synthesis rate was found to vary significantly from patient to patient, the range being 2.5–38 pg/cell per day (Salmon and Durie, 1975), with most patients in the range of 10 to 20 pg/cell per day. The synthesis rate for any given patient was found to remain relatively constant (Salmon, 1973, 1975).

Sequential measurement of total myeloma cell mass obtained during the clinical course of myeloma was used to back-track the growth curve of the tumor (Sullivan and Salmon, 1972). Calculation by this method indicated that in most myeloma patients, the preclinical phase would be about 1–3 years (Salmon, 1975). This calculation is in sharp contrast to the earlier estimate made by Hobbs (1969c) on the basis of exponential growth kinetics. Successive measurements of tumor cells were made in several patients who were treated with melphalan alone or in combination with prednisone given continuously or in "pulses." The data obtained indicated that an initial rapid fall in tumor cell number is usually followed by a plateau. This mode of tumor regression is likewise consistent with Gompertzian kinetics (Salmon, 1975; Salmon and Durie, 1975).

The technique of total myeloma cell mass quantitation as detailed above was also tested in mice bearing MOPC 104E plasmacytoma (Ghanta and Hiramoto, 1974) and a good correlation between the actual and calculated cell number was found.

Tritiated-thymidine labeling of marrow cells has been used to measure the fraction of the cell population undergoing mitosis (labeling index, LI) (Salmon, 1975; Alberts and Golde, 1974; Drewinko et al., 1974). Salmon (1975) serially studied one patient in transit from the presymptomatic to the symptomatic phase of myeloma. The initial LI was 6% and the calculated total myeloma cell number was

669

BIOLOGY, CLINICAL
PATTERNS, AND
TREATMENT OF
MULTIPLE MYELOMA
AND RELATED
PLASMA-CELL
DYSCRASIAS

1.7×10^{12}. Five months later, when the total cell number had risen to 3.6×10^{12}, the LI had fallen to 3.1%. In contrast, in a group of eight treated myeloma patients, the LI prior to treatment was 2–7%, and rose to 15–40% after treatment (Salmon, 1975).

Since the determination of tumor cell number is cumbersome and not available in most clinics, Durie and Salmon (1976) have attempted to correlate the clinical and laboratory data with actual measured tumor mass in a series of 85 MM patients. From these studies, they have proposed a staging system for MM (Durie and Salmon 1976). In this system, the clinical and laboratory data are appraised in relation to the actual measured myeloma cell number expressed per square of meter body surface area. The high cell mass ($> 1.2 \times 10^{12}/m^2$) correlated well with the presence of each of the following: hemoglobin, < 8.5 g/dl; serum calcium, > 12 mg/dl; IgG, > 7 g/dl; IgA, > 5 g/dl; urine Bence Jones protein, > 12 g/day; and advanced lytic lesions. The low cell mass ($< 0.6 \times 10^{12}/m^2$) correlated with all the following: hemoglobin, > 10.5 g/dl; serum calcium, normal; IgG, < 5 g/dl; IgA, < 3 g/dl; and urine Bence Jones protein, < 4 g/day. The clinical data that fit neither the high-mass nor the low-mass category correlated with intermediate cell mass (0.6–$1.2 \times 10^{12}/m^2$). A subclassification—A and B—was proposed on the basis of serum creatinine of below or above 2.0 mg/dl.

Although the measured myeloma cell mass appeared to correlate with survival, it had limited predictive value as far as responsiveness to treatment was concerned.

4.1.10. Clinical Variants of Plasma-Cell Myeloma

The clinical variants of plasma-cell myeloma are listed in Table 2. These somewhat atypical forms are distinct from the prototype myeloma cases because of their unusual clinical and laboratory manifestations as well as their course.

a. Solitary Plasmacytoma. An *apparently* solitary plasmacytoma arising from the vertebral column is not uncommon as the initial manifestation of MM. In most cases which present in this way, however, more thorough diagnostic studies reveal the generalized nature of the disease. The recurrence of plasmacytoma in other sites or development into generalized disease in tumors initially diagnosed as solitary is the usual experience. These developments may take place several years after the diagnosis (Yentis, 1956; Kaye *et al.*, 1961; Cohen, D. M., *et al.*, 1964). In some cases, long quiescent intervals were observed between the tumor recurrences (Pankovich and Griem, 1972). In clinical practice, a tentative diagnosis of solitary plasmacytoma should be made after a negative roentgenographic examination of the skeleton and bone marrow biopsy; moreover, the M components should be absent or disappear following treatment of the primary lesion. Supervoltage radiation, 4000–5000 rads, is indicated for curative treatment (Kyle and Bayrd, 1976). Periodic reevaluation still seems to be necessary to recognize late recurrences. True solitary plasmacytomas are occasionally encountered (Lane, 1952; Kaplan and Bennett, 1968; Christopherson and Miller, 1950; Wright, 1961; McLauchlan, 1973).

b. Extraskeletal or Extramedullary Plasmacytomas. We have already described the extramedullary manifestations of MM. Plasma-cell tumors can occur outside the skeleton, however, from the outset. Kyle and Bayrd (1976) recently reviewed the reported cases in the literature. It has become evident that plasmacytoma of the upper airways such as nasal cavities, sinuses, nasopharynx, and larynx are the most common sites of presentation (Dolin and Dewar, 1956). Most of these tumors are probably benign and thus carry a more favorable prognosis than MM (Kotner and Wang, 1972). Plasmacytomas of the GI tract, genital organs, urinary tract, eyes and skin, liver, lymph node, salivary gland, and other sites have been sporadically reported (for references, see Kyle and Bayrd, 1976). In some cases, involvement of the extramedullary sites preceded the eventual development of skeletal manifestation (Webb *et al.*, 1962).

c. **Plasma-Cell Leukemia.** It is not unusual to encounter plasma cells on examination of the blood smear in patients with MM but the percentage and total plasma cell count are generally low. For the diagnosis of plasma-cell leukemia, Kyle *et al.* (1974a) recommended a requirement for an absolute plasma cell count of at least 2000/mm^3 and 20% or more plasma cells on white blood cell differential count. The incidence of plasma-cell leukemia relative to all cases of MM is about 1–2% (Kyle and Bayrd, 1976; Pruzanski *et al.*, 1969). The clinical features of plasma-cell leukemia when diagnosed at the outset (as distinguished from plasma-cell leukemia occurring at the late stage and often the preterminal phase of myeloma) are remarkable in several respects. They include the younger age of the patient at the time of diagnosis in comparison with cases of MM (Kyle *et al.*, 1974a; Moss and Ackerman, 1946), the low incidence of bone pain and bony lesions, the high incidence of hepatosplenomegaly, severe anemia, thrombocytopenia, and renal failure (Kyle *et al.*, 1974a).

The more malignant nature of plasma-cell leukemia is reflected by the short survival in most patients (Pruzanski *et al.*, 1969). In many cases the leukemic plasma cells appear to be poorly differentiated and may create a cytological diagnostic problem. Electron-microscopic features and the documentation of an M component in the serum and urine, as well as immunofluorescent microscopy of leukemic cells, may establish the diagnosis. In their cases of plasma-cell leukemia, Kyle *et al.* (1974a) noted a relatively lower incidence of serum M components detected by electrophoresis (50%) as compared with the incidence in MM (76%). All classes of monoclonal Ig's, Bence Jones proteins, and γH chain (Pruzanski *et al.*, 1969; Keller *et al.*, 1970) have been documented with plasma-cell leukemias. The incidence of plasma-cell leukemia in IgD PCDs is relatively high. Jancelewicz *et al.* (1975) noted that 10 of 81 (12%) previously reported cases of IgD myeloma had plasma-cell leukemia.

The treatment of plasma-cell leukemias is generally unsatisfactory. Melphalan or Cytoxan has produced only short-lived partial remissions. Occasionally, long remissions were obtained using melphalan and prednisone (Kyle and Bayrd, 1976) or a combination of cyclophosphamide, vincristine, cytosine arabinoside, and prednisone followed by a maintenance regimen consisting of melphalan and prednisone (Shaw *et al.*, 1974).

d. **Simultaneously Occurring Myeloma and Acute Leukemia.** The simultaneous occurrence of acute myelomonocytic, monocytic, and myeloblastic leukemias with PCD resembling MM has been observed in several patients who were not previously treated with alkylating agents (Osserman, 1967; Taddeini and Schrader, 1972; Parker, 1973; Tursz *et al.*, 1974a,b; Witwer *et al.*, 1976; Kyle and Bayrd, 1976).

No radiologically discernible osteolytic lesions were detected in reported cases except in one patient (Parker, 1973). The heavy infiltration of marrow by plasma-

cytes indicated a myelomatous process, however, rather than an asymptomatic
PCD. The absence of antecedent chemotherapy distinguishes this group of patients
from cases of leukemia that develop in previously treated myeloma (see Section
4.1.12). The co-occurrence of myeloma and leukemia suggests a common etiological
factor or pathogenic mechanism that is still unclear.

671

BIOLOGY, CLINICAL
PATTERNS, AND
TREATMENT OF
MULTIPLE MYELOMA
AND RELATED
PLASMA-CELL
DYSCRASIAS

e. Osteosclerotic Myeloma. Myeloma associated with osteosclerosis is
rather rare. It has been estimated that 3% of all MM patients present with osteosclerotic lesions (Wiedermann *et al.*, 1966). Lowbeer (1969a,b) reviewed 57 reported
cases, and noted the following distinguishing features: (1) long survival—40% of
patients, most of whom received no alkylating agents, were alive at the end of 30
months; (2) polycythemia, which occurred in several patients; (3) a high incidence
(30–35%) of peripheral neuropathy (*New England Journal of Medicine,* 1972;
Victor *et al.*, 1958; Mangalik and Veliath, 1971; Lowbeer, 1969a,b; Mathews and
Oliver, 1974; Getaz *et al.*, 1974; Rondier *et al.*, 1975). Neuropathy in osteosclerotic
myeloma is often associated with an elevation of spinal fluid protein, and it should
be separated from the radiculopathy caused by vertebral collapse or direct tumor
invasion, that is so common in MM. In osteosclerotic myeloma, the serum and
urinary protein abnormalities are usually similar to cases of typical MM. In several
cases, however, a polyclonal increase in γ-globulins was described, and no M
component was found in the serum or urine (*New England Journal of Medicine,*
1972). Two of the eight cases of IgE myeloma reported so far had diffuse osteosclerosis (Rogers *et al.*, 1977). Osteosclerotic lesions are more often multifocal than
solitary, and not infrequently are associated with osteolytic lesions of the skull or
other skeletal sites. The alkaline phosphatase is rarely elevated, and hypercalcemia
is usually absent.

f. Myeloma Variants Related to the M Components. The clinical manifestations and natural history of the majority of cases of MM are unrelated to the type
of M component produced with the notable exception of those M components with
particular physicochemical or biological properties (See Section 2). However, IgD
myeloma, biclonal gammopathies, and nonsecretory myelomas are sufficiently
distinct in certain respects to warrant further consideration.

Some investigators have suggested that MM cases associated with the production of L chain alone be regarded as a separate category characterized by a more
malignant course (Williams, R. C., *et al.*, 1966; Hobbs, 1971). The association of
Bence-Jones protein and increased "malignancy" is derived in part from the
observations that (1) Bence Jones proteinuria is more common with clinically
symptomatic forms of the PCDs than with clinically asymptomatic forms (Waldenström, 1970; Hobbs, 1967; Seligmann and Basch, 1968) and (2) in some cases of IgG
and IgA myeloma, at the time of terminal relapse, an abrupt and marked increase in
Bence-Jones proteinuria has been noted (Hobbs, 1971). These observations in
human myeloma resemble, to some extent, an experimental mouse myeloma model
(Preud'homme *et al.*, 1973) in which 80% of mutants derived from an IgG-produc-
ing tumor secreted L chain only.

Analysis of survival data in MM by the Cooperative Study by Acute Leukemia
Group B (1975) suggested that patients with Bence Jones proteinuria survived for a
shorter time than those without Bence Jones proteinuria (median: 21 and 34 months,
respectively). Nonazotemic patients with Bence Jones λ did worse than those with
κ (median: 17 and 30 months, respectively), and patients with IgG λ M component

plus λ-type Bence Jones proteinuria did worse than those with IgG λ alone (median: 13 and 47 months, respectively). These data need confirmation, however, since the 270 cases included in the statistical analysis were patients in whom the M components were reliably identified by the reference laboratories and were selected from 774 patients initially randomized for chemotherapy by cooperative institutions.

Shustik *et al.* (1976) noted a significantly shorter survival time in 45 λ-L-chain-disease cases than in 52 patients with κ-L-chain disease (median: 10 and 30 months, respectively). This difference could not be correlated with the response rate to the chemotherapy or the severity of anemia, azotemia, hypercalcemia, hypoalbuminenia, osteolytic lesions, or to the presence of amyloidosis. The marked difference in survival time remained unexplained in this report.

Patients with λ-L-chain disease were shown to excrete more protein than those with κ-L-chain disease (Stone and Frenkel, 1975; Galton and Peto, 1973), which may reflect differing rates of catabolism of these proteins in the kidneys (Wochner *et al.*, 1967). As mentioned earlier, a higher incidence of renal failure has been observed by some investigators in patients with Bence Jones proteinuria than in those without it. Kyle and Bayrd (1976), however, could not confirm this observation from analysis of their own series.

Finally, it appears that the λ L chain is more "amyloidogenic" than the κ L chain (see Section 4.6.1). Aside from the features mentioned above, myeloma associated with the production of the L chain alone does not differ from most other cases.

(1) IgD Myeloma. The frequency of IgD M components is estimated as 0.8% of all M components, and the IgD myelomas comprise 2.1% of all cases of plasma-cell myeloma (Jancelewicz *et al.*, 1975). Following the first report of IgD myeloma by Rowe and Fahey (1965), 133 cases were reported by 1974 (Jancelewicz *et al.*, 1975), and additional reports have appeared since (Isobe *et al.*, 1976; Harisdaugkul *et al.*, 1976). The median age (56 years) in the series gathered by Jancelewicz and colleagues was slightly lower, and the median survival time (9 months) was significantly shorter than has been reported in recent years for non-IgD myeloma patients. The prevalence of lymphadenopathy, hepatomegaly, or splenomegaly, or a combination of these organ involvements (55%), was striking. In some patients, proptosis, subcutaneous plasma cell infiltration, and other soft tissue masses were noted. Plasma-cell leukemia was described in 10 of 81 patients in whom the hematological data were described in detail. Anemia, leukopenia, and thrombocytopenia were common, and renal failure (BUN > 30 mg/dl) occurred in 67% of patients. In 4 patients, overt clinical manifestation of amyloidosis was present. Of patients on whom postmortem examination was performed, 44% were found to have tissue amyloidosis. The concentration IgD M components was generally low and often undetectable by electrophoresis. The high catabolic rate of IgD ($t_{1/2}$ = 2.8 days) may be responsible in part for its relatively low serum concentration. Bence Jones proteinuria occurred in the overwhelming majority of cases (92%), and the λ L chain exceeded the κ by a factor of 9 (Jancelewicz *et al.*, 1975; Hobbs *et al.*, 1966; Fahey *et al.*, 1968; Fine *et al.*, 1974).

(2) Nonsecretory Myeloma. Approximately 1% of patients with MM have no detectable monoclonal protein after careful examination of the serum and urinary proteins by electrophoresis and immunoelectrophoresis (Osserman and Takatsuki,

673

BIOLOGY, CLINICAL
PATTERNS, AND
TREATMENT OF
MULTIPLE MYELOMA
AND RELATED
PLASMA-CELL
DYSCRASIAS

1963a). Diagnosis of nonsecretory myeloma should not be made on the basis of elecrophoresis alone. Some IgA, IgD, and Bence Jones proteins will be missed if the immunoelectrophoretic technique is not employed. In clinical practice, the use of screening devices such as Albustix® and Uristix® may result in the nonrecognition of Bence Jones proteinuria. Although the sulfosalicylic acid test is much superior in this regard, in rare instances, the Bence Jones protein will not precipitate with such acids (Isobe and Osserman, 1974a). Moreover, a negative Bence-Jones heat test alone is also not sufficient to rule out Bence Jones proteinuria. Unfortunately, not all "nonsecretory" myelomas reported in the literature have been examined rigorously. Several well-documented nonsecretory myelomas have been studied in detail, however, with respect to Ig synthesis. By the use of direct or indirect immunofluorescent methods, intracellular Ig chains have been demonstrated in most cases. Thus, the secretion of Ig, rather than the synthesis, appears to be at fault in these clones of plasma cells (Arend and Adamson, 1974; Hurez et al., 1970; Menkes et al., 1972; Stites and Whitehouse, 1975). Occasionally, however, no Ig could be demonstrated in plasma cells (Gach et al., 1971; Indiveri et al., 1974). It is difficult at present to make a clear assessment regarding the prognosis of nonsecretory myelomas. Both favorable (Kim et al., 1972) and unfavorable (Arend and Adamson, 1974; Hobbs, 1969b) prognoses have been described.

(3) Biclonal Gammopathies. Multiple M components comprise about 1% of all serum monoclonal proteins (Bachmann, 1965; Laurell, 1961; Skvaril et al., 1972). Bouvet et al. (1975) recently analyzed 141 reported examples of double paraproteinemias. IgG + IgA were the most common (46 cases), followed by IgM + IgG (34 cases); IgG + IgG (24 cases); IgM + IgA (12 cases); IgM + IgM (11 cases); BJ + BJ proteins (4 cases); IgA + IgA, IgG + BJ, and IgG + IgD (2 cases in each category); and IgA + BJ, IgM + γ chain, IgA + μ chain, and IgG + μ chain (1 case in each category). Among 12 biclonal (IgG + IgG) gammopathies, Skvaril et al. (1972) found IgG_1 M component in all patients. The second M component consisted of IgG_4 in 6, IgG_2 in 4, and IgG_1 in 2 patients. The high incidence of IgG_4 in this group of M components is noteworthy. Multiple M components have been observed in some patients. In one case, IgM, IgG, IgA, and Bence Jones protein were identified (Sanders et al., 1969). Triclonal gammopathies were reported in three cases (Ottó et al., 1972).

Study of Ig's in biclonal gammopathies has been quite rewarding with respect to understanding the genetics of the synthesis of H and L chains. The L chain, in the majority of cases, is the same for both M components. A recent statistical analysis by Bouvet et al. (1975) supported the common cellular origin for both M components. More direct evidence for relatedness of the two seemingly separate clones is obtained by the demonstration of sharing of idiotypic antigenic determinants by the M components (Wang et al., 1970, Penn et al., 1970, Hannestad and Sletten, 1970; Yagi and Pressman, 1973; Rudders et al., 1973; Fair et al., 1974; Wang et al., 1972, 1973; Seon et al., 1973). Extensive studies of a biclonal (IgM κ and IgG κ) gammopathy by Wang et al. (1969) showed near-identical κ chains in both M components. The similarity of L chains was established by peptide mapping and N-terminal sequence analysis of the first 40 amino acids. Study of the variable (V) regions of μ and γ H chains also revealed complete sequence identity for the first 35 residues and for the amino acids from 83 to 103 (Wang et al., 1973). Thus, it was concluded that the genes responsible for the production of the V_L, C_L, and V_H regions were the same for both monoclonal Ig's.

Marrow plasmacytes in biclonal gammopathies have been studied using the immunofluorescent technique. Dittmar *et al.* (1968) noted that marrow plasmacytes in an IgG + IgA biclonal gammopathy stained for either IgG or IgA, but not for both. Bjerrum and Weeks (1968) similarly noted two populations of IgM- and IgG-synthesizing cells in a case of biclonal gammopathy. Costea *et al.* (1967), on the other hand, noted double staining of some plasma cells by anti-IgG and anti-IgA fluorescent antisera. In another case of biclonal gammopathy, Rudders *et al.* (1973) also documented the production of IgA λ and IgG λ in a single plasma cell.

Hopper (1975) studied an interesting biclonal gammopathy (IgM λ + IgG κ). Analyses by antiidiotype antisera indicated that the V_H region of μ and γ chains shared idiotypic antigenic determinants. The antiidiotypic antisera produced against IgM λ and IgG κ each reacted with both IgM Fab and IgG F(ab')$_2$. Amino-terminal sequence studies of patients' μ and γ chains indicated, however, separate subgroup V regions (Hopper *et al.*, 1976). It appears, therefore, that shared idiotypic determinants may occur despite the difference in subgroup V_H regions. Complete sequence studies of V_H regions of the μ and γ chains should reveal the areas of similarity. The sequence of $V_H μ$ has already been reported (Capra and Hopper, 1976), and the study of the sequence of $V_H γ$ is in progress.

The clinical manifestations of biclonal gammopathies resemble those of MM in most patients having IgG and IgA M components. In contrast, patients who have an IgM plus an IgG, IgM, or IgA M component have been reported to have markedly diverse clinical features. Pruzanski *et al.* (1974) reviewed 30 such cases. In 21 patients in whom the clinical data were available, only 1 patient was diagnosed as having MM. The majority of patients were described as having solitary plasmacytomas (3 cases), WM (5 cases), lymphosarcoma (2 cases), and plasma-cell leukemia (1 case). No malignancy was diagnosed in the remaining 9 patients, who were variously affected by polyarthralgia, anemia, thyroiditis, and dermatological disorders.

4.1.11. Treatment of Plasma-Cell Myeloma

Significant progress in the treatment of MM was made in the early 1960's, when the alkylating agents L-phenylalanine nitrogen mustard (Melphalan) and cyclophosphamide (Cytoxan) were introduced into therapeutic regimens. Not only were long clinical remissions free of pain, pathological fracture, renal failure, paraplegia, and other disease manifestations induced in the majority of patients, but also true prolongation of life was accomplished. Whereas prior to the use of these agents the median survival from diagnosis of myeloma was reported as 6–11 months (Osgood, 1960; Midwest Cooperative Chemotherapy Group, 1964; McArthur *et al.*, 1970; Bergsagel *et al.*, 1967; Velez-Garcia and Maldonado, 1971), it rose to 24–34 months after their introduction (Hoogstraten *et al.*, 1967, 1969; Bergsagel *et al.*, 1967; Alexanian *et al.*, 1968, 1969; McArthur *et al.*, 1970; Medical Research Council, 1971; Korst *et al.*, 1964). The median survival from the onset of treatment prolonged to 18–28 months in most large series. Although several cooperative chemotherapy study groups have made efforts in the past decade to refine the dose scheduling and devise combination chemotherapy regimens, no or little additional improvement in survival has been accomplished (Alexanian *et al.*, 1972, 1975b; Costa *et al.*, 1973). The lack of further progress is attributed to (1) the unavailability of new drugs superior to agents now in use; (2) the development of a plateau phase after the initial 1- to 2-log reduction in tumor cell number; and (3) progression of the disease into a more malignant and rapidly evolving terminal phase (Bergsagel, 1976).

675

BIOLOGY, CLINICAL
PATTERNS, AND
TREATMENT OF
MULTIPLE MYELOMA
AND RELATED
PLASMA-CELL
DYSCRASIAS

a. General Management. The principles of general management include the maintenance of maximum ambulation, hydration, the early detection and treatment of infection, adequate analgesics to avoid further immobilization, and close follow-up studies with regular assessment of response, using clinical and laboratory parameters.

The treatment of hypercalcemia warrants special attention. As mentioned previously, the contraction of circulatory volume, azotemia, and hyperuricemia are often present at the time of its recognition. For mild cases (Ca < 12 mg/dl), hydration alone, aimed at 2500–3000 ml urine output, is generally sufficient. In severe forms, (Ca > 12 mg/dl), high doses of glucocorticoids (e.g., prednisone, 60–80 mg/day, or equivalent parenteral preparation) and adequate oral or parenteral hydration to produce 3000–4000 ml urine should be started immediately. Thalassmos and Joplin (1970) reported that the hypercalcemia of myeloma responded to corticosteroids more favorably than did hypercalcemia associated with other neoplasias. Since the calcium excretion increases proportionately with the rate of natriuresis (Suki *et al.*, 1970), it has been recommended that normal saline be used liberally (4–6 liters/day), and that a diuretic agent such as furosemide, 40–120 mg/day, also be administered to force diuresis (Cohen, H. J., and Rundles, 1975). Such a regimen, however, requires meticulous and close monitoring of the cardiovascular system as well as renal status; otherwise, congestive heart failure due to saline load and further aggravation of renal failure due to reduced circulating volume caused by forced diuresis may complicate the picture. Inorganic phosphate (Neutra-Phos®) given orally or via nasogastric tube (150 ml 4 times daily) or a parenteral preparation of sodium and potassium phosphate in doses up to 1 mmol/kg body weight in a 12-hr span should be reserved for the resistant cases of hypercalcemia. Metastatic calcification in kidneys and other organs has occurred with phosphate treatment (Massry *et al.*, 1968). Mithramycin, 25 μg/kg body weight, promptly but transiently reduces the serum calcium (Perlia *et al.*, 1970; Elias *et al.*, 1972). Hyperuricemia can almost always be managed with allopurinol, 300–600 mg/day, and it is seldom necessary to alkalinize the urine with large doses of sodium bicarbonate.

b. Treatment Modalities. *(1) Surgery.* The role of surgery is limited to the biopsy or removal of an extramedullary plasmacytoma for the purpose of tissue diagnosis. Laminectomy and tissue biopsy are frequently carried out in tumors presenting with spinal cord compression. Postoperative radiation therapy is recommended for the treatment of the remaining plasmacytoma. At the same time, the diagnostic evaluation is carried out to assess the extent of the disease. Further treatment with chemotherapy is indicated if the disease is proved to be extensive.

(2) Radiation Therapy. The role of radiation therapy in the treatment of MM has become more clearly defined in recent years. In general, a curative tumoricidal dose of 4000–5000 rads should be delivered to plasma-cell tumors that appear to be solitary lesions. Other indications are for palliative therapy, 1500–2000 rads, to well-circumscribed lesions associated with disabling pain that have failed to respond

to adequate doses of analgesics. The radiation field should be restricted to symptomatic sites to preserve the normal hematopoietic tissue. In patients with adequate marrow reserve, palliative radiotherapy can be administered simultaneously with chemotherapy. It is particularly important to avoid treating one symptomatic area after another with radiation alone. Such a treatment approach almost inevitably results in long delays in the institution of chemotherapy because of marrow suppression. Radiation therapy is also beneficial in preventing pathological fractures of long bones when erosion of the cortex threatens an imminent fracture. Radiation to the site of pathological fracture can hasten pain relief, and will probably improve the chances of bone-healing. Infrequently, MM presents in the form of recurrent plasmacytomas, while the rest of the skeleton is apparently spared. We have chosen to radiate such lesions and at the same time continue with chemotherapy.

(3) Chemotherapeutic Agents.

Melphalan. Melphalan (L-phenylalanine mustard, L-sarcolysin, Alkeran®), an alkylating agent, was introduced for treatment of cancer in the late 1950's (Blokhin *et al.*, 1958). There is a large body of experience in the use of this drug (Bergsagel *et al.*, 1962; Hoogstraten *et al.*, 1967; Alexanian *et al.*, 1968; Farhangi and Osserman, 1973; Waldenström, 1970). In our clinic, we have employed an initial loading dose of melphalan (6–10 mg daily) for 8–10 days, followed by a continuous maintenance dose sufficient to produce an appreciable marrow suppression (WBC 2500–3500/mm^3). We begin the maintenance treatment (usually 2 mg daily) immediately after the completion of the loading dose. We maintain on each case a graphic flow sheet that greatly facilitates the patient's management (Farhangi and Osserman, 1973). Several variables are plotted including the values determined for hemoglobin, WBC, platelet, serum M component, Bence Jones protein, and scores of the severity of pain and performance status.

Bone marrow aspiration and biopsy and X-ray examination of the symptomatic areas can further assess disease progression or relapse. Salmon and his associates have devised a computer program whereby the data on serum M components, cellular synthesis rate, FCRs, and the predicted PV are employed to calculate the total tumor cell number during the course of the treatment (Salmon and Durie, 1975).

Melphalan is given intermittently by other investigators (Alexanian *et al.*, 1969; Kyle and Bayrd, 1976). A 7-day course of 0.15 mg/kg per day by the oral route is repeated every 6 weeks. The subsequent doses are modified upward or downward according to the hematological status (Kyle and Bayrd, 1976). Prednisone, 60 mg daily, is also given for the 7-day duration of each cycle. A favorable response to melphalan can be documented in approximately 70% of patients, and about half the patients will qualify as responders based on the criteria employed by several cooperative chemotherapy groups (for the list of different criteria for responses, see Farhangi and Osserman, 1973). The major side effect of melphalan is bone marrow suppression. Rarely transient thrombocytosis has been observed following the institution of melphalan (Waldenström, 1970, p. 169). The drug has also been implicated in the causation of leukemia occurring in patients after prolonged treatment for myeloma (see Section 4.1.12).

Cyclophosphamide (Cytoxan). Cyclophosphamide is another alkylating agent that is as effective as melphalan in the treatment of MM (Korst *et al.*, 1964; Medical Research Council, 1971; Rivers and Patno, 1969). In our clinic, a continuous oral regimen is started with a daily dose of 200 mg for 5–7 days, and then reduced to 50–

677

BIOLOGY, CLINICAL
PATTERNS, AND
TREATMENT OF
MULTIPLE MYELOMA
AND RELATED
PLASMA-CELL
DYSCRASIAS

100 mg/day, depending on the hematological findings. It has been our intent with both the melphalan and the cyclophosphamide regimen to produce sufficient marrow suppression to cause leukopenia of 2500–3000/mm³. Drug therapy is generally continued unless the leukocyte and platelet counts fall below 2000 and 40,000/mm³, respectively. When therapy is interrupted, we attempt to resume medication as soon as sufficient marrow recovery is documented. Cyclophosphamide may also be given by the intravenous route, 15 mg/kg body weight every 4 weeks (Kyle and Bayrd, 1976), with modification of the subsequent dose according to the hematological status. Besides leukopenia and thrombocytopenia, hemorrhagic cystitis may occur with cyclophosphamide (Korst et al., 1964). Other rare complications are urinary bladder fibrosis (Johnson and Meadows, 1971), carcinoma of the urinary bladder (Wall and Clausen, 1975), and suppression of ovarian and testicular function (Warne et al., 1973; Fairley et al., 1972).

Prednisone. The tumoricidal role of prednisone in human myeloma has remained unclear despite extensive clinical studies. This subject was reviewed by Hoogstraten (1973). The tumoricidal effect of cortisol in plasma-cell tumors of BALB/c mice was demonstrated by Hollander et al. (1968). In another study, however, the administration of prednisone did not prolong the survival of mice with LPC-1 plasma-cell tumor (Abraham et al., 1967). In a cooperative study by the Western Cancer Chemotherapy Group (Mass et al., 1962), prednisone, 40 mg/day, had no therapeutic effect on human myeloma. The administration of high doses of methyl prednisolone to a normal volunteer for 3–5 days caused a pronounced decrease in serum IgG, which was attributed to the suppression of protein synthesis (Butler and Rossen, 1973). Solomon and his associates (Solomon et al., 1975; Solomon, 1976) noted a marked and transient decrease in Bence Jones proteinuria in some patients following the institution of prednisone. Moreover, a protein that was of low molecular weight and Bence-Jones-related, but was not identical to either the V_L or the C_L region of the L chain, was demonstrated in the urine of certain patients. It is concluded, therefore, that the prednisone-induced reduction in serum and urinary monoclonal proteins could be the result of altered protein synthesis, rather than of regression in tumor cell number.

The addition of prednisone to melphalan was reported to augment the response rate, as measured primarily by a 50% decrease in myeloma proteins (Alexanian et al., 1969). In addition, a 3-month prolongation of median survival in a group treated with melphalan plus prednisone, as compared with a group treated with melphalan alone, was reported by Alexanian et al. (1972); the improvement in survival, however, was not significant. In another cooperative study by Acute Leukemia Group B and the Eastern Cooperative Oncology Group, the addition of prednisone or prednisone plus testosterone to melphalan did not improve the median survival time (28, 26, and 27 months, respectively; Cancer and Leukemia Group B, personal communication). Separation of the patients into good- and poor-risk groups,* however, indicated superior, although statistically insignificant, response rate and survival in good-risk patients (Costa et al., 1973). Prednisone apparently had an adverse effect on poor-risk patients. In our opinion, the better survival in prednisone-treated good-risk patients may be attributed to the large percentage of females in this arm of the study protocol.

---

*Good-risk: BUN, ≤ 30 mg/dl; serum calcium, ≤ 12 mg/dl; absence of significant infection; WBC, ≥ 4000/mm³; platelet count, ≥100,000/mm³; estimated survival greater than 2 months. Poor-risk: All other patients.

Although the newer drugs such as the nitrosourea compounds, e.g., 1,3-bis (2-chlorethyl)-1 nitrosourea (BCNU), have been shown by Cancer and Leukemia Group B and others to be effective in myeloma (Salmon, 1976), the survival data have not yet been published. Some chemotherapeutic effects of Adriamycin® in myeloma were shown by O'Bryan et al. (1973). The combination of Adriamycin with other agents such as BCNU (Alberts et al., 1976) and Cytoxan may become an effective regimen, particularly in patients in relapse and in those who fail to respond to melphalan or Cytoxan from the outset.

Among the drugs in use earlier, urethane (ethyl carbamate) was shown to be effective in some patients (Osserman, 1959; Rundles and Coonrad, 1957; Rundles et al., 1950). Because oral urethane causes considerable GI symptoms, the institution of an adequate dose was not possible in most cases. The administration of drugs by suppositories is preferable for the same reason. In a cooperative study, it was considered that the drug was not better than a placebo (Holland et al., 1966). In this study, however, the median dose of drug given was only 145 g for a median duration of 7 weeks. In addition, more azotemic patients were in the urethane-treated group. Urethane toxicity is occasionally severe, and the drug is abandoned in favor of less toxic and more effective agents.

(4) Combination of Chemotherapeutic Agents. Several investigators have recommended a combination drug regimen on the basis of preliminary results. For example, a four-drug combination of melphalan, cyclophosphamide, BCNU, and prednisone was proposed by Harley et al., (1972) and Azam and Delamore, (1974), and this combination plus vincristine was recommended by Lee et al. (1974). The superiority of such drug combinations in comparison with single drugs based on prolongation of survival has yet to be shown. In another study, the addition of procarbazine to melphalan and prednisone did not increase survival (Alexanian et al., 1972). The addition of vincristine, a cell-cycle-specific agent, was shown to further reduce the tumor cell number in a few patients during the plateau phase of melphalan response (Salmon, 1975). In a large cooperative study, however, the addition of vincristine to melphalan, prednisone, and procarbazine did not improve the response rate or survival (Alexanian et al., 1975b).

(5) Drug Regimen for Patient in Relapse. Virtually all MM patients relapse after the initial remission induced by melphalan or cyclophosphamide and there is a great need for a second line of effective agents. Bergsagel et al. (1972) noted good to partial responses in 11 of 19 melphalan-resistant patients using intermittent large doses of cyclophosphamide. Our experience (see the following section) supports his findings. Kyle et al. (1975b), however, found a less favorable result using smaller doses of cyclophosphamide. Adriamycin and BCNU (30 mg/m² of each drug intravenously every 3–4 weeks) were used for the treatment of patients who relapsed after the initial response to alkylating agent or had not responded at all (Alberts et al., 1976). A preliminary report of these studies indicated that 7 of 13 patients were responding.

(6) Single-Agent (Melphalan) Continuous Administration (Our Series). As mentioned earlier, from 1960 to 1971 most patients in our clinic were treated with melphalan and some of the results of these studies were previously reported (Farhangi and Osserman, 1973). It should be recognized that this therapeutic trial was not a randomized and prospective study and the results represent the experience in a single institution. As shown in Table 8, among 76 MM patients referred to us in this period, 41 were treated with an initial loading dose of melphalan followed by a continuous low-dose maintenance regimen. The presenting clinical and labora-

679

BIOLOGY, CLINICAL
PATTERNS, AND
TREATMENT OF
MULTIPLE MYELOMA
AND RELATED
PLASMA-CELL
DYSCRASIAS

TABLE 8. Our Series of Patients with Plasma-Cell Myeloma 1960–1971

Group[a]	Number
Patients treated with a loading dose of melphalan followed by a continuous low-dose daily maintenance	41
Patients treated with cyclophosphamide, melphalan plus prednisone, or interrupted courses of alkylating agents	26
Patients who received no chemotherapy	9
Early death due to sepsis (3)	
Death due to metastatic cervical cancer (1)	
Radiation therapy alone (3)	
Refusal of treatment (1)	
Asymptomatic status in the presence of osteolysis (1)	
TOTAL:	76

[a]Numbers in parentheses indicate number of patients in each category.

tory findings in these 41 cases are summarized in Table 9. The remaining 35 patients were given cylophosphamide (5 cases), melphalan plus prednisone (3 cases), interrupted courses of melphalan or cyclophosphamide (18 cases), and for various reasons no chemotherapy (9 cases). Survival data were available in 71 patients, 5 having been lost to follow-up 12–27 months after the diagnosis.

TABLE 9. Frequency of Clinical and Laboratory Abnormalities at the Onset of Chemotherapy in 41 Melphalan-Treated Patients in Our Series

Abnormality	Patients with the abnormality	
	Number	Percentage of study patients
Pain[a]		
Severe and disabling (3–4)	29	70
Moderate (1–2)	12	30
Performance status[b]		
≤ 40	24	58
50–70	17	42
Hemoglobin		
< 12.0 g/dl	40	97
< 8.5 g/dl	16	39
WBC		
< 4,000/mm³	3	14[c]
Platelets		
< 140,000/mm³	5	23[c]
Serum calcium		
> 12 mg/dl	10	24
Serum uric acid		
≥ 7.0 mg/dl	22	54
Blood nonprotein nitrogen		
> 50 mg/dl	8	20

[a]On a scale of 0–4.
[b]Karnovsky scale (Dollinger et al., 1969).
[c]Of 22 previously untreated patients.

Of 41 melphalan-treated patients, 22 had had no prior treatment of MM; 19 had received urethane (ethyl carbamate), radiotherapy, or short courses of melphalan or cyclophosphamide prior to being referred to our clinic. There were 26 males (63%). The median age was 58 years at the time of diagnosis.

The initial loading dose of melphalan ranged from 6–10 mg daily, according to the patient's size and hematopoietic status, and was continued for 8–10 days. In the first 22 cases, there was a "rest" period of 4–6 weeks (median: 4.6 weeks) between the termination of loading and the onset of daily maintenance treatment. In the remaining 19 patients, daily maintenance therapy was started immediately after the completion of the loading dose. The maintenance dose of melphalan in most cases was 2 mg/daily, but this dosage was adjusted as necessary on the basis of the patient's hematopoietic tolerance. When the WBC dropped below 2500/mm^3, or the platelet count fell below 75,000/mm^3, the melphalan dose was reduced, but not discontinued. It was rarely necessary to interrupt chemotherapy because of excessive marrow toxicity. Calculated as milligrams per kilogram body weight per month of treatment, the actual total loading plus maintenance dose received by 41 patients ranged from 0.39 to 1.31, with a median of 0.90. Concomitant palliative radiotherapy early in the course of treatment in doses of 700–1500 rads was administered to 17 patients.

The response to melphalan was evaluated by the following parameters: hemoglobin, serum M components, Bence Jones protein, skeletal pain, and performance status. The remission duration in responders was calculated from the onset of treatment to the development of relapse. Relapse in most cases was manifested by pain due to new skeletal lesions with radiological confirmation of advancing bony changes, and in some cases by recurrence of hypercalcemia. Relapse was also signalled in several cases by deterioration in hematological status, not accounted for by marrow toxicity. Increasing concentrations of serum M components and/or Bence-Jones proteinemia preceded the other signs of relapse in several cases.

Results. Pain disappeared completely in 85% of patients. The interval from the onset of treatment to pain-free status ranged from 1 to 16 months, with a median of 5.7 months. In 75% of patients, the performance status improved significantly. The median pretreatment performance score on the Karnofsky scale (Dollinger *et al.,* 1969) was 40, and rose to 80 during remission. Most patients in this group returned to normal activities. The interval between the onset of treatment and achievement of best performance ranged from 2 to 18 months, with a median of 9 months. In the remaining patients, there was no or a modest improvement in performance. The hemoglobin continued to decline early in the course of treatment, reaching a nadir 3–4 weeks after the initiation of therapy. Later on, however, it rose 2–7.5 g above the pretreatment value in 66% of patients. There was a period of 6–27 months between the onset of treatment and the achievement of best hemoglobin value. A 50% or greater decrease in serum M components and a 75% or greater decrease in Bence Jones proteinuria occurred in 23 (67.5%) of 34 patients in whom serial quantitations could be made. Among these patients, in 3 cases the serum M component became undetectable by electrophoresis and in 4 cases there was no residual Bence Jones proteinuria. Of the remaining 7 patients, 2 died within the first month of treatment due to sepsis, and the effect of melphalan with respect to the M components could not be evaluated. One patient had nonsecretory myeloma and did not respond to melphalan. This patient, 12 years prior to the diagnosis of plasma-cell myeloma, had been successfully treated with radiation therapy for

681

BIOLOGY, CLINICAL
PATTERNS, AND
TREATMENT OF
MULTIPLE MYELOMA
AND RELATED
PLASMA-CELL
DYSCRASIAS

localized Hodgkin's disease. In 4 patients, the concentrations of monoclonal proteins were low and not suitable for serial assessment (IgA, 2 cases; Bence Jones proteinemia, 1 case; Bence Jones proteinuria, 1 case). All 4 patients, however, showed marked improvements in other parameters of response.

Remission Duration and Survival Data. Of the 41 patients treated with melphalan, 2 died within the first month of chemotherapy due to sepsis. In 30 patients (73%), marked improvement in all or the majority of abnormal parameters was noted, and the patients were considered to have gone into remission; the remission duration in this group ranged from 7 to 120 months (mean: 38 months; median: 29 months). Survival data were calculated according to the life-table method (Cutler and Ederer, 1958). The median survival from diagnosis in all 76 myeloma patients was 40 months; in the 41 melphalan-treated patients, including the 2 early deaths and 9 nonresponding patients, it was 49 months. The median survival from diagnosis in 15 female patients (53 months) was 10 months longer than in male patients. This difference, however, was not significant ($p = 0.25$). The median survival from the onset of treatment in the 41 melphalan-treated patients was 40 months.

Effect of Interruption of Chemotherapy During Remission Induction. As previously mentioned, an interval ("rest period") of 4–6 weeks (median: 4.6 weeks) was interposed between the loading period and the institution of maintenance therapy in the first 22 patients. In most cases, following administration of the loading dose, there was a decrease in Bence Jones proteinuria. At the end of the "rest period" or shortly after the onset of maintenance treatment, however, there was a rebound, with a rapid rise in urinary Bence Jones proteins. Figure 1 illustrates the effect of the "rest period" on urinary excretion of Bence Jones (λ) and serum IgA M component in one of our patients. In Figure 2, the effect of "rest periods" on Bence Jones proteinuria and serum M components of 7 such patients is shown. A rebound phenomenon was observed in most patients with Bence Jones proteinuria. The effect of rest periods on serum M components was less obvious due to the slower turnover rate of complete Ig's.

It appears, therefore, that in some tumors a quick recovery can occur during the short period of chemotherapy interruption. For this reason, in the subsequent 19 patients, the daily maintenance dose was started immediately after the loading dose. No rebound phenomenon was observed in this group.

M-Component Response Rate and Duration of Remission. No correlation was found between the magnitude of reduction in the M components and the duration of remission. It was noted, however, that "fast responders," i.e. cases in which a 50% reduction in the serum M components was observed in the first 2 months of chemotherapy, remained in remission for a shorter time than did those who responded at a slower pace. Table 10 demonstrates the rank correlation between remission duration and the slope of change in serum M components during the first year of treatment. A significant correlation ($p < 0.01$) was found in the group of 19 responding patients in whom the final remission duration was known (patients still in remission were not included). Although a similar trend was observed with regard to Bence Jones protein response, the rank correlation was not statistically significant ($p > 0.25$).

Response to Cyclophosphamide after the Development of Resistance to Melphalan. A second course of chemotherapy was generally given to patients who demonstrated signs of relapse after the first remission and to those patients who did not respond to melphalan. Cyclophosphamide was given in a daily oral dose of 50–

MEHDI FARHANGI
AND ELLIOTT F.
OSSERMAN

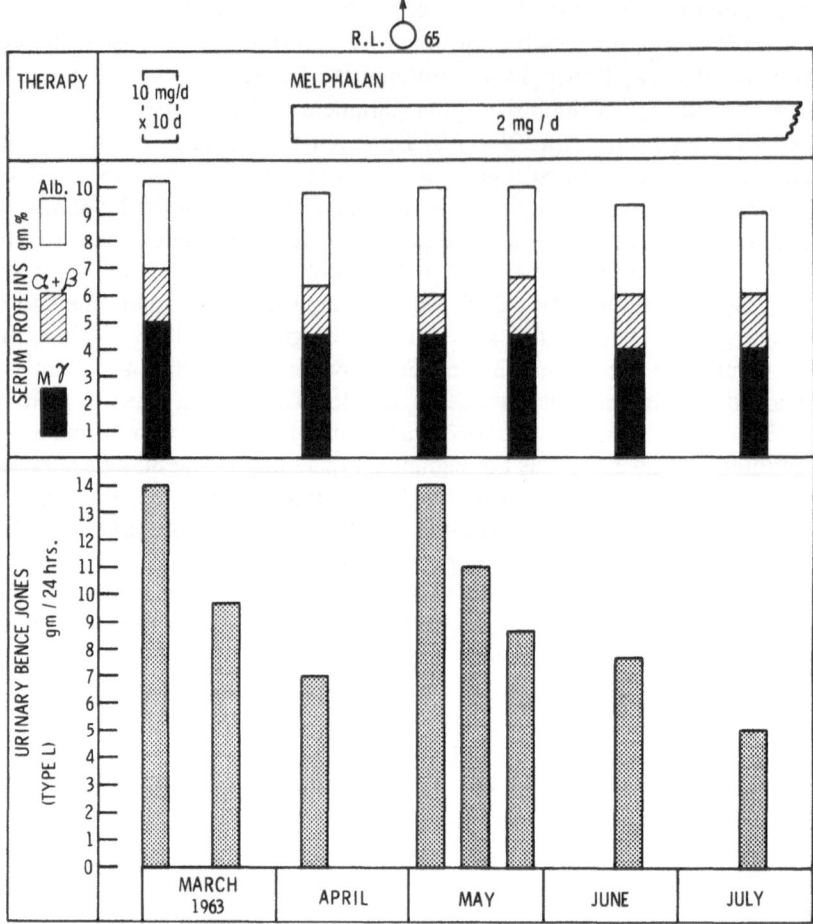

Figure 1. Effect of interruption of chemotherapy—"rest period"—following the loading dose on serum IgA, M component (Mγ), and urinary Bence Jones λ protein in patient R.L. A rebound in Bence Jones proteinuria occurred following the cessation of treatment.

100 mg. Retreatment was attempted in 16 such patients, of whom 5 received less than 8 weeks of therapy and died of infections or renal complications. Of the remaining 11 patients, 5 responded with remissions lasting from 15 to 39+ months (mean: 28 months); in 6 patients, although improvement in some parameters was noted, a status quo was generally maintained for 3–30 months (mean: 12.5 months).

Terminal Events. Table 11 summarizes the terminal events in the 41 melphalan-treated patients. Six patients were alive and still in remission. The majority of the patients died while myeloma was active, due either to lack of response or to relapse of the disease following one or two clinical remissions. The terminal relapse was generally characterized by a more malignant pattern of disease. For example, three patients relapsed with the clinical and hematological features of plasma-cell leukemia. Two patients terminated with monomyelocytic leukemia at a time when little or no clinical and laboratory evidence of myeloma activity was present. Four patients died of unrelated causes while in clinical remission.

BIOLOGY, CLINICAL
PATTERNS, AND
TREATMENT OF
MULTIPLE MYELOMA
AND RELATED
PLASMA-CELL
DYSCRASIAS

In 1964, the discovery of an extremely cationic homogeneous protein in the urine of a patient with MM and Bence Jones κ proteinuria led to the identification of this protein as lysozyme (Osserman and Lawlor, 1966). The patient, a 41-year-old male, was diagnosed in 1960 as having MM with osteolysis and marrow plasmacytosis (55%). He was treated with urethane, prednisone, and radiotherapy. In 1962, macroglossia and other manifestations of amyloidosis were noted. Later in 1963–1964, a course of melphalan and prednisone was instituted, which resulted in symptomatic improvement and marked reduction in Bence Jones proteinuria. In

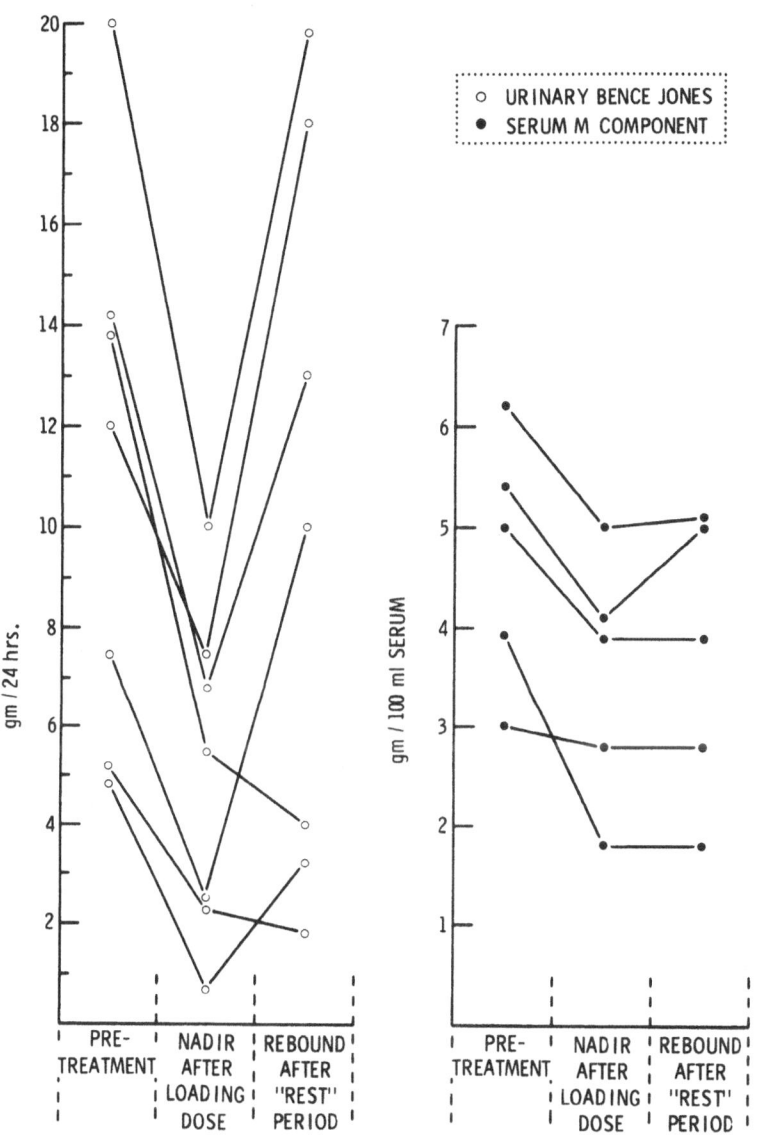

Figure 2. Changes in urinary Bence Jones protein and serum M components following the "rest period."

TABLE 10. Rank Correlation Between Remission Duration and Slope of Change in Serum M Components During the First Year of Treatment in Our Series

Patient	Slope[a]	Rank[b]	Remission (months)	Rank[b]
1	−18.76	7	15	1.4
2	−26.26	4	15	1.5
3	−27.06	3	16	3
4	−20.04	6	17	4
5	−11.82	14	21	5
6	−32.96	2	25	6.5
7	− 9.33	15	25	6.5
8	−25.33	5	27	8.5
9	−14.80	12	27	8.5
10	−15.12	11	28	10
11	−16.38	8	30	11
12	−15.16	10	33	12
13	−33.70	1	40	13
14	− 0.30	18	45	14
15	− 2.01	17	55	15
16	− 7.36	16	61	16
17	+11.09	19	66	17
18	−15.45	9	75	18
19	−12.29	13	95	19

[a] Slope of percentage change of initial value with log time in weeks. Slope is estimated by least squares for the data of the first year.
[b] Rank correlation: $z = 0.53$; standard deviation; $z = 2.58$; $p < 0.01$.

TABLE 11. Terminal Events in 41 Melphalan-Treated Patients in Our Series

Group[a]	Number
Alive and in clinical remission	6
Died while myeloma was active	29
Early death due to sepsis (2)	
Unresponsive to treatment (7)	
Relapsed following clinical remission (17)	
Relapsed into plasma-cell leukemia following clinical remission (3)	
Died of monomyelocytic leukemia while myeloma was inactive	2
Died of unrelated causes while myeloma was inactive	4
Renal failure due to chronic pyelonephritis (2)	
Myocardial infarction (1)	
Suicide (1)	
TOTAL:	41

[a] Numbers in parentheses indicate number of patients in each category.

685

BIOLOGY, CLINICAL
PATTERNS, AND
TREATMENT OF
MULTIPLE MYELOMA
AND RELATED
PLASMA-CELL
DYSCRASIAS

October 1964, profound pancytopenia preceded the development of an acute mono-myelocytic leukemia associated with marked elevation of serum and urine lysozyme (Osserman, 1969). This patient and two additional cases from our clinic were subsequently reported (Farhangi and Osserman, 1970). The diagnosis of MM was made 4, 6, and 7 years prior to the development of leukemia and lysozymuria, and all 3 patients were treated with alkylating agents for prolonged periods of time. We recently observed two additional cases, one treated with melphalan (for 10 years) and one with Cytoxan (for 30 months). Of these 5 leukemias, 4 occurred in the 76 patients listed in Table 8—an incidence of 5%.

The common features among these cases were: (1) lengthy clinical remissions prior to the development of leukemia; (2) absence of myelomatous activity at the time of leukemic manifestations; (3) profound cytopenia antecedent to the leukemic manifestation that could not be attributed to the marrow toxicity or relapse of myeloma; and (4) marked elevation of serum and urinary lysozyme in 4 of the 5 cases. Similar features have been described by other investigators (Kyle *et al.*, 1970, 1975a; Rosner and Grünwald, 1974). Ring sideroblasts and displastic changes of erythropoiesis were noted by Khaleeli *et al.* (1973). Erythroleukemia following melphalan therapy for MM was reported by Fishman and Ritz (1975). In one study, marked aneuploidy was noted in six patients in whom cytogenetic studies were performed (Hossfeld *et al.*, 1975). The incidence of aneuploidy appeared to be much higher in these patients than in cases of spontaneously occurring leukemia (Gonzales *et al.*, 1977).

The treatment of the leukemia supervening in cases of MM has been uniformly disappointing. The etiological role of alkylating agents in the genesis of these leukemias has been emphasized (Kyle *et al.*, 1975a). This hypothesis is supported by the fact that patients with other diseases treated with alkylating agents have also developed acute leukemia (Kyle and Bayrd, 1976, p. 179). As noted previously, however, leukemias have also been reported to occur simultaneously with PCDs without antecedent chemotherapy. It is therefore possible that some as yet poorly understood etiological or pathogenic relationship exists between the two neoplasias.

4.1.13. Prognostic Factors in Plasma-Cell Myeloma

We have already noted that certain clinical variants of MM have distinctly different natural courses. For example, survival in IgD myeloma and plasma-cell leukemias is far worse than in average cases of myelomas. In contrast, some extramedullary plasmacytomas and rare osteosclerotic forms of myeloma are char-acterized by prolonged survival. There is lack of agreement as to whether myelomas associated with Bence Jones proteinuria alone comprise a somewhat more malig-nant form of the disease (see Section 4.1.10f).

Several factors have been recognized as influencing survival in MM. Carbone *et al.* (1967) noted that pretreatment hemoglobin levels of less than 9 g/dl, blood urea concentration above 30 mg/dl, serum calcium above 12 mg/dl, and poor performance status all negatively influenced survival. Low serum albumin was also reported to have an adverse prognostic significance (Medical Research Council, 1973). The detrimental consequence of renal failure on survival was noted in several series (Hoogstraten *et al.*, 1967; Costa *et al.*, 1969; Dawson and Ogston, 1971; Kyle and Bayrd, 1976, p. 162). It should be emphasized, however, that pretreatment renal failure in the majority of patients occurred in a setting of hypercalcemia, dehydration, and hyperuricemia, with or without Bence Jones proteinuria. The reversibility of renal failure depends greatly on early recognition and treatment of hypercalcemia, hyperuricemia, and dehydration. In our opinion, survival in MM can be materially improved if early deaths due to renal failure are avoided by early diagnosis and appropriate treatment.

Kiang *et al.* (1974) analyzed survival in 138 cases of MM. The factors that were found to influence survival were, in descending order of importance: hemoglobin, age, serum calcium, sex, plasma-cell morphology, Bence Jones protein, serum albumin, blood urea nitrogen, and the presence of osteolytic lesions. Salmon and Durie (1975) evaluated several clinical and laboratory variables in 85 cases of MM in relation to measured tumor cell number. Each of the following factors correlated with high ($> 1.2 \times 10^{12}/m^2$) myeloma cell mass: hemoglobin, < 8.5 g/dl; serum calcium, > 12 mg/dl; advanced lytic bone lesions; and high concentration of M components (IgG, > 7 g/dl; IgA, > 5 g/dl; Bence Jones protein, > 12 g/24 hr). Patients with low myeloma cell mass ($< 0.6 \times 10^{12}/m^2$) had all the following features: hemoglobin, > 10.5 g/dl; serum calcium, normal; low levels of M components (IgG, < 5.0 g/dl; IgA, < 3.0 g/dl; Bence Jones protein, < 4 g/day); and no lytic lesions on skeletal survey. Patients with intermediate myeloma cell mass ($0.6–1.2 \times 10^{12}/m^2$) had intermediate levels of these parameters.

In this study, the myeloma cell mass correlated with survival; it had limited predictive value, however, as far as responsiveness to treatment was concerned. Alexanian *et al.* (1975a) noted a significant difference in survival and remission duration in 482 patients treated with melphalan and prednisone when comparison was made between hemoglobin (< 8.5 vs. > 10.5 g/dl), serum calcium (> 12.5 vs. < 11.5 mg/dl), and serum M component (> 7.0 vs. < 5.0 g/dl).

One of the more paradoxical factors that may influence survival of patients with MM and is recognized only retrospectively is the adverse effect of a rapid response of M-component levels on survival. Waldenström (1970, p. 179) noted a shorter survival in patients in whom a 50% reduction in M component was achieved during the first year of treatment. Hansen *et al.* (1973) also reported that a rapid decline in serum M components during the first 2 months of treatment (≥ 0.6 g/dl) was associated with short survivals (median: 13 months), whereas the slow responder lived much longer (median: 62 months). Our data [see section 4.1.11b (6)] based on rank correlation between the remission duration and the slope of change in the serum M components during the first year of treatment support these observations. It is not known which biological properties of the tumor are responsible for this phenomenon. The adverse contribution of rapid responders to overall survival has not been analyzed in most previously reported series but this factor may account for some of the variation in the results of a given chemotherapeutic regimen when administered by the same group of investigators.

4.2. Waldenström's Macroglobulinemia

The study of hypergammaglobulinemic sera by electrophoresis and ultra-centrifugation led to the discovery of the macroglobulins and the description of a new syndrome i.e., WM (Waldenström, 1944). The serum paraprotein of these patients was later identified as IgM. Waldenström's earlier patients were mostly elderly men. Anemia, high sedimentation rate, adenopathy, and splenomegaly, in the absence of skeletal manifestations, were features that distinguished WM from MM (Waldenström, 1965). It was later demonstrated that the serum M component was the secretory product of a differentiated B-cell clone having surface Ig that shared idiotypic antigenic determinants with the circulating protein (Preud'homme and Seligmann, 1972).

687

BIOLOGY, CLINICAL
PATTERNS, AND
TREATMENT OF
MULTIPLE MYELOMA
AND RELATED
PLASMA-CELL
DYSCRASIAS

4.2.1. Protein Abnormality

The serum of all patients with WM contains high levels of 19 S (pentameric) IgM that often migrates in the fast γ or β region on electrophoresis. In many cases of WM, in addition to the 19 S IgM, the serum also contains low-molecular-weight 7 S IgM that may comprise as much as 40% of the total serum macroglobulin (McDougal *et al.*, 1975; Solomon and Kunkel, 1967; Bush *et al.*, 1969). The presence of low-molecular-weight IgM results in the overestimation of IgM by immune quantitation methods. The ratio of κ:λ L chains on IgM components is of the order of 2.4:1 and significantly higher than IgG or IgA components (Oberdorfer *et al.*, 1973). Bence-Jones proteinuria is variously reported as occurring in one third (McCallister *et al.*, 1967) to almost all cases (Carter and Hobbs, 1971; Dammacco and Waldenström, 1968). In a recent report by Krajny and Pruzanski (1976), Bence-Jones proteinuria was documented in 71% of 45 patients, but the daily urinary excretion was usually low. Bence Jones proteinuria exceeded 200 mg/24 hr in only 9 cases. The concentrations of IgG and IgA are often depressed; normal values do occur, however, in a significant number of patients (Stein *et al.*, 1975). An IgA PCD with clinical manifestations resembling those of WM was recently reported (Hijmans, 1975). The intrinsic physicochemical and functional properties of the macroglobulins are frequently responsible for the hyperviscosity syndrome, cryoglobulinemia, hemostatic abnormalities, and other aberrations that are discussed earlier in this chapter.

4.2.2. Cellular and Histological Features

In the bone marrow, lymph nodes and spleen of patients with WM, there characteristically are increased numbers of mononuclear cells that are described as lymphocytes, plasmacystoid-lymphocytes, or plasmacytes. Not infrequently, increased numbers of both plasma cells and lymphocytes are found. Periodic acid–Schiff-positive droplets, due to carbohydrate-rich IgM, are seen in the cytoplasm of such lymphoid cells (Dutcher and Fahey, 1969). Well-developed rough endoplasmic reticulum was demonstrated on electron microscopy (Brecher *et al.*, 1964). The bone marrow biopsy frequently demonstrates hypercellular marrow, diffusely infiltrated by lymphoplasmacytic elements. In addition, an increased number of mast cells is noted. Diffuse nodular lesions and malignant lymph nodules have also been described (Rywlin *et al.*, 1975).

The histology of the lymph node in WM resembles that in lymphosarcoma or CLL although certain distinguishing morphological features may be recognized (Harrison, 1972).

MEHDI FARHANGI
AND ELLIOTT F.
OSSERMAN

4.2.3. Clinical Features

A median age of about 60 and a predilection for men have been reported in most series. Weakness, fatigue, and bleeding from oral and nasal mucosal membranes are the most frequent complaints. Symptoms related to hyperviscosity, cryoglobulinemia, and cold agglutinin hemolytic anemia occasionally dominate the clinical picture. Pallor, peripheral adenopathy, and hepatosplenomegaly are the most common physical findings (McCallister *et al.*, 1967; MacKenzie and Fudenberg, 1972; Krajny and Pruzanski, 1976). Anemia occurs in the majority of patients MacKenzie and Fudenberg, 1972). Expansion of the PV due to hyperviscosity contributes significantly to the apparent anemia.

Infiltration of the bone marrow by the monoclonal B cells, shortened red cell survival, hypersplenism, and blood loss all participate in the pathogenesis of anemia in WM (Cline *et al.*, 1963). Hemolysis due to IgM cold agglutinins is discussed in Section 2.4. Autoimmune hemolytic anemia associated with a positive direct Coombs test due to IgG antibody has been reported (MacCallister *et al.*, 1967). Rouleau formation is regularly seen on blood smear; the WBC is usually normal, low, or slightly elevated with a relatively mild lymphocytosis. Monocytosis is occasionally noted and serum lysozyme levels are normal or slightly elevated, in contradistinction to the low levels of serum lysozyme usually found in cases of CLL.

Neurological manifestations associated with the hyperviscosity syndrome, such as vertigo, ataxia, dizziness, and altered sensorium, are common in WM. Peripheral neuropathy occurs rather frequently and myelin degeneration, not associated with tumor cell infiltration, is found on histological examination (Darnley, 1962; Dayan and Lewis, 1966). Neuropathy associated with amyloidosis has also been observed in WM.

An increased incidence of infection (Fahey *et al.*, 1963) can be attributed to impaired immunological mechanisms (see Chapter 18). Renal failure is much less common in WM than in MM. Passive deposition of IgM on the endothelial side of the glomerular basement membrane may account for some of the renal functional abnormalities. Progressive renal failure can occur with cryoglobulinemia (see Chapter 12). Renal amyloidosis may also complicate WM. The nephrotic syndrome was reported in case of biclonal gammopathy with serum IgM κ, IgG κ, free γ chain, and urinary γ and κ chains (Martelo *et al.*, 1975). Immunofluorescence studies of the kidney showed glomerular deposits of IgM, IgG, and C3.

Pleural and pulmonary involvement in cases of WM has been increasingly appreciated in recent years (Winterbauer *et al.*, 1974). Gastrointestinal manifestations, particularly diarrhea, steatorrhea, and malabsorption have been associated in some cases with the deposition of amorphous material in the lamina propria and the lymphatics of the bowel (Beker *et al.*, 1971; Bedine *et al.*, 1973). Immunofluorescence studies of these deposits in one patient with an IgM λ M-component showed reactivity with anti-μ and anti-λ antisera (Pruzanski et al., 1973). Portal hypertension was reported in a 60-year-old man with WM (Brooks, 1976). Blood flow measurements and catheterization data were consistent with a presinusoidal cause for the portal hypertension due to tumor-cell infiltration.

Osteolysis of the bone is rarely observed, although osteoporosis is relatively common. Single or scattered osteolytic lesions have been occasionally described in the course of the disease (Vermess *et al.*, 1972). In a recent report by Stein *et al.* (1975), 2 patients among 34 subjects who had IgM M components were classified as having plasma-cell myeloma because of multiple lytic lesions and greater than 25% plasma cells in the bone marrow.

4.2.4. Diagnosis

The demonstration of a monoclonal IgM is not sufficient to establish the diagnosis of WM. Monoclonal IgM components may be found in the serum of apparently healthy subjects without anemia, lymphadenopathy, splenomegaly, or other manifestations of disease. In these cases, the concentration of serum M component is usually < 1.0 g/dl. Low-molecular-weight IgM is also generally not present in the serum of these patients (Carter and Hobbs, 1971). Some of these apparently benign IgM PCDs however, may terminate in clinically overt and symptomatic disease (Martin, 1960; Kyle and Bayrd, 1976, p. 211). Cases of chronic cold hemagglutinin disease are generally considered examples of benign gammopathy since these patients would remain asymptomatic if it were not for the antibody activity of their M component. As mentioned earlier, the concentration of monoclonal IgM in these patients characteristically remains constant for a prolonged period of time although a terminal lymphoproliferative condition may supervene. At the other end of the spectrum, some patients with IgM M components initially present with the clinical and hematological features of CLL or lymphosarcoma (Stein *et al.*, 1975). Thus, it must be understood that the distinction between lymphosarcoma CLL associated with an IgM M component and WM is often arbitrary.

4.2.5. Prognosis

The natural course of WM is extremely variable. The mean survival from diagnosis was 49.5 months in a recently reported series (Krajny and Pruzanski, 1976). MacKenzie and Fudenberg (1972) reported a mean survival from diagnosis of 49.2 months in responders and 24.1 months in nonresponders. WM occasionally evolves into a rapidly progressive malignancy with the histological features of reticulum-cell sarcoma (Wanebo and Clarkson, 1956) or lymphoblastic lymphosarcoma (Wood and Frenkel, 1967). We recently observed a terminal diffuse histiocytic lymphoma in a patient who was previously reported by Essig *et al.* (1974) to have plasma-cell interstitial pneumonia and macroglobulinemia.

4.2.6. Treatment

We have already discussed the usefulness of adequate plasmapheresis in patients with the neurological, hematological, and cardiovascular manifestations of hyperviscosity. Chlorambucil (Leukeran) given daily for a prolonged period of time has been shown to be quite useful in the control of WM (Bayrd, 1961; Clatanoff and Meyer, 1963; McCallister *et al.*, 1967; Waldenström, 1961). A daily dose of 6–8 mg is instituted, and should subsequently be adjusted according to the white cell and platelet counts. It is desirable to maintain the WBC above 3000/mm³ and the platelet count above 100,000/mm³. Daily continuous doses of cyclophosphamide are also employed successfully (Bouroncle *et al.*, 1964). We have noted some success using a combination of cyclophosphamide, vincristine, and prednisone in patients refractory to chlorambucil.

4.3. Heavy-Chain Diseases

Since the recognition and first description of γ, α, and μHCD, approximately 35 cases of γ, 80 cases of α, and 11 cases of μHCD have been reported (Franklin and Frangione, 1975; Seligmann, 1975; Mihaesco *et al.*, 1976; Faguet *et al.*, 1977; Jonsson *et al.*, 1976). No δ or ϵHCD has been described. The structural features of the corresponding monoclonal proteins are discussed in Chapter 12. αHCD is described in Chapter 14. In this section, we will limit our consideration to the clinical features of γ and μHCD.

4.3.1. γ-Heavy-Chain Disease

Franklin *et al.* (1964) described the first case of PCD associated with the production of a fragment of Ig closely related to γ chain. The patient, a 44-year-old black male, presented with a marked cervical adenopathy—"bull neck"—that became massive 6 months later. Fever and considerable palatal edema were noted to be present. His spleen became palpable and then massive in dimensions at a later date. Rapidly evolving disease ensued with the development of ascites, pleural effusion, edema, anemia, leukopenia, thrombocytopenia, and susceptibility to pneumococcal infection (eight bouts were treated with penicillin). Histological studies of the cervical nodes showed dense lymphocytic infiltration and focal collections of large mononuclear ("reticulum") cells with pale eosinophilic granular cytoplasm. The bone marrow contained a small number of plasma cells (2%), which increased subsequently to 25%

Following this discovery, four additional cases were described by Osserman and Takatsuki (1964). The predominant clinical features in these cases were again lymphadenopathy, splenomegaly, fever, palatal erythema and marked susceptibility to bacterial infection. In one case, a skin nodule was present on the right cheek 6 months before the development of these systemic manifestations. Biopsy of this lesion showed an atypical granulomalike process with central "epitheloid" cells surrounded by lymphocytes and plasma cells. Subsequent lymph node biopsy showed abnormal nodal architecture with immature plasma cells, lymphocytes, reticulum cells, and eosinophiles as the predominant cellular elements.

Frangione and Franklin (1973) reviewed all 30 cases of γHCD reported prior to August 1972. There were 19 males and 11 females. Their ages ranged between 18 and 76 years. Slightly more than half the patients had an insidious onset of disease; in the others, the manifestations developed rather rapidly. Lymphadenopathy, fever, splenomegaly, hepatomegaly, and anemia were the most common features. An unusual waxing and waning of adenopathy was observed during the early course of some patients. Palatal erythema and edema were described in 8 patients, and appeared to be related to involvement of Waldeyer's ring with the disease process. Moderate anemia, leukopenia, and thrombocytopenia primarily ascribed to hypersplenism were the major hematological manifestations. Eosinophilia was present in

691

BIOLOGY, CLINICAL
PATTERNS, AND
TREATMENT OF
MULTIPLE MYELOMA
AND RELATED
PLASMA-CELL
DYSCRASIAS

several cases, and plasma cell leukemia was diagnosed in 2 cases. No skeletal findings were described in any of 20 patients who had bone X rays. The duration of the disease was from 5 weeks to 5 years, and most patients died of sepsis or malignancy.

In almost half the patients, the serum M component was greater than 2 g/dl. The serum peaks appeared broad-based and polydispersed on electrophoresis, and were invariably associated with a marked decrease in polyclonal Ig's. Proteinuria occurred in all patients, with a range of 0.5–20 g/day in half the patients, and only trace amounts of protein in the other half. The M components were confirmed by appropriate immunological and chromatographic analyses to be incomplete γ chains lacking L chains. Bence-Jones protein was absent in all except 1 atypical case who was also shown to have an IgM M component in the serum (Keller *et al.*, 1970). More recently, another patient has been reported with rheumatoid arthritis, γHCD, Bence-Jones proteinuria, and cryoglobulinemia (Kretschmer *et al.*, 1974).

In patients with γHCD, a background of chronic disorders has been reported in several cases. These conditions include tuberculosis, rheumatoid arthritis, Sjögren's syndrome, myasthenia gravis, systemic lupus erythematosus, discoid lupus, hemolytic anemia, hypereosinophilic syndrome, thyroiditis, vasculitis, hypocomplementemia, and nonreticular neoplasia (Frangione and Franklin, 1973; Loyau *et al.*, 1975; Lyons *et al.*, 1975).

Treatment. Review of the reported cases of γHCD suggests that to arrive at a therapeutic decision, a clinical assessment of each case is necessary. This evaluation should be focused on the rapidity of disease processes since it appears that more aggressive chemotherapy is indicated in patients with rapidly progressive disease. A regimen of intravenous cyclophosphamide (500 mg) and prednisone (100 mg/day for 4 days) every 4 to 6 weeks was reported to have controlled the disease for over 2 years in one patient (Lyons *et al.*, 1975). The necessity for prompt antibiotic therapy of intercurrent infection cannot be overemphasized. The usefulness of γ-globulin supplementation for prevention of infection has not been systematically studied but is probably indicated.

4.3.2. μ-Heavy-Chain Disease

Since the first descriptions of μHCD in a patient with CLL and amyloidosis (Forte *et al.*, 1970; Ballard *et al.*, 1970), 10 other cases have been reported (for the references, see Jonsson *et al.*, 1976). The clinical manifestations in the majority of reported cases have been quite similar to those in the first patient. Antecedent CLL was documented in 9 patients. All subjects were older than 39, their ages ranging from 39 to 79 years. Vacuolated plasma cells were noted in the bone marrow of most patients. Serum protein electrophoresis showed no distinct peak in 9 patients, although a monoclonal μ-chain protein was demonstrated by immunochemical methods. Bence-Jones κ protein was present in the urine of most patients (Franklin, 1975; Jonsson *et al.*, 1976). The absence of the μ-chain-related protein in the urine is attributed to the large size of the pentameric structure, which lacks L chains, has deletions in the V regions, and has an approximate molecular weight of 520,000 daltons. A recent study by Mihaesco *et al.* (1976) provides further insight into the structural and immunochemical aspects of μHCD proteins.

Two cases of μHCD reported from Africa (Bonhomme *et al.*, 1974; Danon *et al.*, 1975) differ from the other reported cases in several respects. No history of antecedent CLL was present in either case. Serum electrophoresis of both patients showed a detectable β mobility peak, and no Bence Jones protein was excreted in the urine. Massive hepatosplenomegaly occurred in the case reported by Bonhomme and co-workers, and cirrhosis of the liver was present in the patient described by Danon and co-workers (1975). μ-Chain-related protein was demonstrated in the urine of the first African case. Thus, two distinct sets of clinical and laboratory manifestations of μHCD have so far been described. Moreover, in the non-African cases associated with an antecedent history of CLL, the abnormality of the structure of the deleted μ chain seems to be responsible for its lack of pairing with the L chain, while in the African form of the disease, the L chain is apparently not synthesized. In both situations, partially deleted pentameric molecule $(Fc\mu)_5$ is found in the sera of the affected patients.

4.4. Deleted Heavy- and Light-Chain Disease

In 1974, we described a case of PCD in a 51-year-old male with an insidious onset of fatigue, weakness, adenopathy, and hepatosplenomegaly associated with anemia, leukopenia, thrombocytopenia, and no skeletal disease (Isobe and Osserman, 1974a). The lymph node biopsy and bone marrow aspirate showed marked plasma-cell infiltration. The serum showed a broad-based "peak" extending from the γ_1 to the β region, and the urine contained a polydispersed protein traversing the fast γ to the α region on electrophoresis. Immunochemical studies of serum and urinary proteins showed: (1) IgG1 λ serum globulin with deletions in both H and L chains and an estimated molecular weight of 110,000; (2) free γ (Fc fragment) in the serum and urine; and (3) deleted Bence Jones λ protein in the urine with an approximate molecular weight of 15,000. Subsequent determination of the complete sequence of the λ L chain demonstrated that 80 residues in the V region (from position 30 to the V-C "switch") were missing. The C region was intact (Garver *et al.*, 1975). The γ chains in this case were deleted to a comparable extent, but detailed sequence studies have not been completed.

Another patient, described by A. F. Lewis *et al.* (1968), was found to have an IgG1 M component with apparently similar deletions in the L and H chains (Connel *et al.*, 1970; Parr *et al.*, 1972; Smithies *et al.*, 1971). This patient was a 53-year-old female with a prolonged history of a sclerodermalike condition. The clinical manifestations at the time of recognition of PCD were anemia, leukopenia, thrombocytopenia, splenomegaly, and marrow plasmacytosis.

Several other PCDs with structurally defective proteins, such as half IgG and IgA, have been studied (see Chapter 12). It is not evident, however, that particular clinical features can be ascribed to these cases.

4.5. Lichen Myxedematosus (Papular Mucinosis, Scleromyxedema, Lichen Amyloidosis)

Lichen myxedematosus (LM) is a rare skin disease characterized by dermal lesions consisting of papules, macules, and plaques, mostly involving the upper half of the body. The lesions may progress to the point of limiting body movements.

693

BIOLOGY, CLINICAL
PATTERNS, AND
TREATMENT OF
MULTIPLE MYELOMA
AND RELATED
PLASMA-CELL
DYSCRASIAS

This condition appears to be a specific form of tissue proteinosis associated with an underlying PCD. Although the disease involves mostly the skin and remains relatively benign in the majority of cases, some evidence for generalized disease is obtained from the autopsy findings. Mucicarmine-positive materials are seen in the media and adventitia of the vessels of the heart, kidney, adrenal, and pancreas (McCuistion and Schoch, 1956), as well as in the renal papillae, bronchial epithelium, and ductal epithelium of the pancreas (Perry, H. O., et al., 1960).

Osserman and Takatsuki (1963b) first noted an extremely cationic IgG M component in the serum of a patient with lichen myxedematosus. They isolated this protein and demonstrated that it had strong binding affinity for normal skin, suggesting an auto-antibody-like activity. Subsequent studies by other investigators have confirmed the presence of a PCD with cationic IgG λ M components in the majority of cases of LM. (James et al., 1967). Danby et al. (1976) reported a case of LM associated with an IgG κ M component and reviewed 27 other previously reported cases. The majority of the M components were IgG λ although 3 were IgG κ (Lai A Fat et al., 1973; Epstein, W. L., 1974; Bridgen, 1974). Moreover, both IgA (Fowlkes et al., 1967; Pambor and Höfs, 1968) and IgM (Bohnstedt and Ehlors, 1967; Huth et al., 1972) monoclonal protein have been described with this disease.

The progression of the underlying PCD into frank MM was reported in one case of LM (Perry, H. O., et al., 1960). Treatment of LM patients with melphalan has been shown to reduce the concentration of the serum M component concomitant with a significant regression of the skin lesions (Feldman et al., 1969; Kyle and Bayrd, 1976, p. 293).

4.6. Amyloidosis

Tissue amyloidosis is perhaps best defined by ultrastructural features as determined by electron microscopy. In all variants of amyloidosis, a fibrillar structure has been observed to be deposited in the extracellular spaces (Cohen, A. S., and Calkins, 1959; Spiro, 1959; Gueft et al., 1968). Amyloid fibrils are linear and nonbranching and measure 75–100 Å in width and 300–10,000 Å in length (Glenner and Page, 1976). They consist of two or several parallel filaments. X-ray diffraction studies of amyloid fibrils indicated a "cross-β" pleated sheet conformation (Eanes and Glenner, 1968; Glenner et al., 1972b). Congo red staining of the amyloid tissue, which was introduced by Bennhold (1922), has greatly facilitated the histological diagnosis of the amyloidosis. This dye augments the double refractile property of the amyloid deposits. Thus, by the use of an appropriate optical system, a characteristic yellow-green dichroism, typical of amyloid, can be demonstrated (Missmahl and Hartwig, 1953). Several other staining methods with varying degrees of sensitivity associated with false-negative and false-positive reactions have also been employed (Glenner and Page, 1976).

Significant progress in understanding the nature of amyloid proteins was accomplished with the demonstration that isolated amyloid fibril concentrates could be solubilized in the presence of 6 M guanidine HCl (Glenner et al., 1969, 1972a,b). Extensive immunological and immunochemical studies of solubilized proteins obtained from amyloid cases, particularly from patients diagnosed as having "primary amyloidosis," demonstrated the presence of an L-chain fragment (Glenner et al., 1969, 1970, 1971a, 1973). The amino acid sequence analysis of several amyloid proteins confirmed areas of structural homology between these proteins and the amino-terminal portions of κ or λ L chains (Glenner *et al.*, 1971a). In one case, a complete L chain was demonstrated to be present in the amyloid protein, and the amino acid sequence of the amyloid protein was identical to the sequence of the patient's urinary Bence Jones protein (Terry *et al.*, 1973).

Concomitant with these observations, studies of the amyloid protein solubilized from some cases of "secondary amyloidosis" revealed a protein with 79 amino acids and no apparent homology with immunoglobulins (Benditt *et al.*, 1971; Ein *et al.*, 1972a,b; Levin *et al.*, 1972). This protein was designated as AA or *amyloid of unknown origin* (AUO). The complete amino acid sequence of a varient of AA consisting of 64 residues was recently reported (Sletten *et al.*, 1976a).

It should be pointed out that proteins homologous to Ig L chain structure have been isolated from cases of so-called "secondary" amyloidosis. Protein AA has been found in some cases of so-called "primary" amyloidosis (Glenner and Page, 1976). It is suggested that protein AA is derived from the pentagonal structures that are seen by electron microscopy in all cases of amyloidosis (Benditt and Eriksen, 1966). It is not clear, however, whether Ig fragment and protein AA are present simultaneously in all amyloid cases (Glenner and Page, 1976). A serum protein related to protein AA (SAA) was discovered by Franklin and co-workers (Levin *et al.*, 1973). This protein was characterized as 12,000 daltons in molecular size, somewhat larger than its tissue counterpart (8500 daltons), both having the identical first 11 amino acids from the amino-terminal end. Thus, protein AA appears to be an amino-terminal fragment of SAA protein (Rosenthal *et al.*, 1976). This group subsequently reported that 85,000 SAA (Franklin *et al.*, 1975) is apparently a complex form that contains 12,000-dalton subunits.

Further evidence of the diverse nature of amyloid proteins is the recent demonstration of a calciotonin-related structure in the amyloid fibril protein obtained from medullary carcinoma of the thyroid (Sletten *et al.*, 1976b). Furthermore, an insulin-related amyloid protein is suggested to be present in cases of insulinoma (Pearse *et al.*, 1972).

4.6.1. Association of Amyloidosis and Plasma-Cell Dyscrasias

The frequent association of Bence Jones proteinuria in patients with so-called "primary" amyloidosis was first appreciated by Magnus-Levy (1931). Apitz (1940) subsequently noted the bone marrow plasmacytosis in cases with this pattern of distribution of amyloidosis. Subsequent clinical studies provided further evidence of the association of "primary"-type amyloidosis, Bence Jones proteins and PCD (Osserman, 1959, 1961; Osserman *et al.*, 1961, 1964; Kyle and Bayrd, 1967, 1975; Hällen and Rudin, 1966; Pruzanski and Katz, 1976).

On the basis of analyses of 100 cases of amyloidosis studied in our clinic, we (Isobe and Osserman, 1974b), have suggested the following classification based on the predominant clinical pattern of amyloid distribution:

Pattern I: Principal involvement of the tongue (macroglossia), carpal ligaments (carpal tunnel syndrome), skin, nerves (peripheral neuropathy), skeletal and smooth muscles, heart and GI tract. This pattern of amyloid distribution encompasses most cases of "primary" and MM-related amyloidosis.

695

BIOLOGY, CLINICAL
PATTERNS, AND
TREATMENT OF
MULTIPLE MYELOMA
AND RELATED
PLASMA-CELL
DYSCRASIAS

Pattern II: Principal involvement of the spleen, liver, kidneys, and adrenals. This type of amyloid distribution is most commonly observed in "secondary" amyloidosis occurring in patients with osteomyelitis, rheumatoid arthritis, Hodgkin's disease, and Familial Mediterranean fever.

Mixed Pattern I and II: Amyloid distribution includes Pattern I and II sites.

Of our 100 cases of amyloidosis, 50 cases exhibited the Pattern I distribution, 17 had Pattern II, and 30 had Mixed Pattern I and II distribution. The amyloidosis in 3 patients was localized.

Monoclonal proteins were demonstrated in *all* Pattern I, in 87% of Mixed Pattern I and II, and in 53% of Pattern II cases. Bence Jones proteins, predominantly the λ type, were present in 92% of Pattern I cases, and monoclonal IgG, IgA, IgD, and IgM were more frequently associated with Pattern II and Mixed Pattern I and II cases. Thus, this classification of amyloidosis based solely on the tissue distribution of deposits may have some pathogenic significance.

The clinical manifestations, natural history and pathophysiology of the various forms of amyloidosis have been reviewed in detail by Kyle and Bayrd (1975, 1976) and will not be considered here.

4.6.2. Possible Mechanisms to Explain the Role of Bence Jones Proteins in Amyloidosis

Although the precise role of Bence Jones proteins in the pathogenesis of amyloidosis is still not defined, our investigations (Osserman *et al.*, 1964) provided evidence that amyloid-related Bence Jones proteins had a greater binding affinity for normal tissues than Bence Jones proteins from patients without amyloidosis. We therefore postulated that amyloid-related Bence Jones proteins might represent L chains of autoantibodies. More recently, from analyses of the amino acid sequences of 2 amyloid-related Bence Jones proteins, BJ_κ^{TEW} (Putnam *et al.*, 1973) and BJ_λ^{MCG} (Fett and Deutsch, 1974), we have suggested that a specific residue at position 30 in the first hypervariable region may have particular relevance to the "amyloidogenicity" of certain Bence Jones proteins (Osserman, 1976). Further sequence data are needed to confirm or refute this hypothesis.

To explain the finding of incomplete L chains in amyloid, it has been postulated that these may either be synthesized *de novo* by abnormal plasma cells or may be formed *in situ* by partial proteolytic cleavage by the proteases of macrophages or leukocytes (Glenner *et al.*, 1971b; Glenner and Page, 1976).

4.6.3. Treatment of Amyloidosis

No generally efficacious treatment for amyloidosis is available at present but the fact that certain forms of amyloid are potentially reversible is well-documented. Prior to the availability of antibiotics, H. Waldenström* (1928) observed the regression of hepatic enlargement and the nephrotic syndrome due to amyloidosis in cases of osteomyelitis treated with drainage and curettage. Fitchen (1975) reported a case of granulomatous ileocolitis and extensive amyloidosis of the liver and kidneys in

---

*H. Waldenström was the father of Jan Waldenström.

whom resection of the involved bowel resulted in a striking decrease in liver amyloid deposits and disappearance of proteinuria. Paraf *et al.* (1970) have reported the regression of hepatic amyloidosis in a patient with an hypernephroma following its surgical removal.

In patients with amyloidosis related to an underlying PCD, therapy with melphalan or cyclophosphamide has been sporadically effective particularly in those cases with overt MM in whom a major remission with marked reduction in Bence Jones proteinuria is concomitantly achieved (Osserman *et al.*, 1964; Jones *et al.*, 1972; Lessin *et al.*, 1972; Cohen, H. J., *et al.*, 1975; Kyle *et al.*, 1974a,b; Kyle and Bayrd, 1975). Unfortunately, however, the majority of cases are unresponsive to alkylating agents, either alone or in combination with corticosteroids.

Because of the evidence that noncovalent (hydrogen) bonds are primarily involved in the polymerization of the protein subunits of amyloid fibrils, we have investigated the possible therapeutic usefulness of dimethyl sulfoxide (DMSO), an agent which is known to dissociate these types of bonds. DMSO was found (Isobe and Osserman, 1976) to block the characteristic heat-precipitation reaction of Bence Jones proteins, which is probably dependent on similar physicochemical mechanisms. DMSO was also shown to effect the solubility of amyloid fibrils and to reduce the extent of casein-induced amyloidosis in C3H mice (Isobe and Osserman, 1976). These latter results have recently been confirmed by Kedar *et al.*, (1977). On the basis of these findings, a clinical trial of DMSO was considered warranted and six patients were treated for periods ranging from 1 to 12 months with daily doses of 5–15 grams orally. In 2 of the 6 cases, there was clinical evidence of amyloid regression, most notably a decrease in macroglossia, increase in EKG voltage and increase in blood pressure. In the other 4 cases there were no demonstrable effects. Although these limited trials of DMSO were not particularly encouraging, further studies including cases of other clinical forms of amyloidosis are probably warranted. Along these lines, Ravid *et al.* (1977) have recently reported an increased excretion of amyloid fibrils in the urine of patients with renal amyloidosis secondary to Familial Mediterranean Fever following the intravenous administration of DMSO. Recognizing the differences in the chemical composition of different amyloids, we would expect different solubility properties, rates of deposition and turnover. These factors will almost certainly influence responsiveness to DMSO or to any other therapy.

ACKNOWLEDGMENT

The authors would like to thank Dr. Andre O. Varma, School of Public Health, Columbia University, for the analysis of the data in Table 10.

References

Abbruzzo, J. L., Heimer, R., Guiliano, V., and Marting, J., 1970, The hyperviscosity syndrome, polysynovitis, polymyositis and an unusual 13 S serum IgG component, *Am. J. Med.* **49**:258.

Abdou, N. I., and Abdou, N. L., 1975, The monoclonal nature of lymphocytes in multiple myeloma, *Ann. Intern. Med.* **83**:42–45.

Abraham, D., Carbone, P. P., Venditti, J. M., Kline, I., and Goldin, A., 1967, Evaluation of chemical agents against the plasma cell tumor LPC-1 in mice, *Biochem. Pharmacol.* **16**:665.

Abramson, N., and Shattil, S. J., 1973, M-components, *J. Am. Med. Assoc.* **223**:156.

697

BIOLOGY, CLINICAL
PATTERNS, AND
TREATMENT OF
MULTIPLE MYELOMA
AND RELATED
PLASMA-CELL
DYSCRASIAS

Adams, W. S., Alling, E. L., and Lawrence, J. S., 1949, Multiple myeloma: Its clinical and laboratory diagnosis with emphasis on electrophoretic abnormalities, *Am. J. Med.* **6**:141.

Afifi, A. M., and Tawfeek, S., 1971, Deafness due to Waldenström's macroglobulinemia, *J. Laryngol. Otol.* **85**:275.

Alberts, D. S., and Golde, D. W., 1974, DNA synthesis in multiple myeloma cells following cell cycle-nonspecific chemotherapy, *Cancer Res.* **34**:2911–2914.

Alberts, D. S., Durie, B. G., and Salmon, S. E., 1976, Doxorubicin/B.C.N.U. chemotherapy for multiple myeloma in relapse, *Lancet* **1**:926–928.

Alexanian, R., 1975, Monoclonal gammopathy in lymphoma, *Arch. Intern. Med.* **135**:62–66.

Alexanian, R., Bergsagel, D. E., Migliore, P. J., Vaughn, W. K., and Howe, C. D., 1968, Melphalan therapy for plasma cell myeloma, *Blood* **31**:1.

Alexanian, R., Haut, A., Khan, A. U., Lane, M., McKelvey, E. M., Migliore, P. J., Stuckey, W. J., Jr., and Wilson, H. E., 1969, Treatment for multiple myeloma, *J. Am. Med. Assoc.* **208**:1680.

Alexanian, R., Bonnet, J., Gehan, E., Haut, A., Hewlett, J., Lane, M., Monto, R., and Wilson, H., 1972, Combination chemotherapy for multiple myeloma, *Cancer* **30**:382–389.

Alexanian, R., Balcerzak, S., Bonnet, J. D., Gehan, E. A., Haut, A., Hewlett, J. S., and Monto, R. W., 1975a, Prognostic factor in multiple myeloma, *Cancer* **36**:1192–1201.

Alexanian, R., Balcerzak, S., Haut, A., Hewitt, J., and Gehan, E. (for the Southwest Oncology Group), 1975b, Remission maintenance therapy for multiple myeloma, *Arch. Intern. Med.* **135**:147.

Andersen, B. R., 1966, Gamma A-cold agglutinin: Importance of disulfide bonds in activity and structure, *Science* **154**:281–283.

Anderson, E. T., and Vye, M. V., 1967, Dysproteinemia of the myeloma type associated with a thymoma, *Ann. Intern. Med.* **66**:141.

Anderson, S., Yeung, K., Hillman, D., and Lessin, L., 1975, Multiple myeloma in a patient with sickle cell anemia: Interesting effects on blood viscosity, *Am. J. Med.* **59**:568–574.

Angevine, C. D., Andersen, B. R., and Barnett, E. V., 1966, A cold agglutinin of IgA class, *J. Immunol.* **96**:578.

Aoki, T., and Takahashi, T., 1972, Viral and cellular surface antigens of murine leukemias and myelomas, *J. Exp. Med.* **135**:433.

Apitz, K., 1940, Die Paraproteinosen (über die Störung des Eiweisstoffwechsels bei Plasmacytom), *Virchows Arch. Pathol. Anat.* **306**:631.

Arend, W. P., and Adamson, J. W., 1974, Nonsecretory myeloma: Immunofluorescent demonstration of paraprotein within bone marrow plasma cells, *Cancer* **33**:721–728.

Axelsson, U., and Hällén, J., 1965, Familial occurrence of pathological serum-proteins of different γ-globulin groups, *Lancet* **2**:369.

Axelsson, U., and Hällén, J., 1968, Review of 54 subjects with monoclonal gammopathy, *Br. J. Haematol.* **15**:417–420.

Axelsson, U., Bachmann, R., and Hällén, J., 1966, Frequency of pathological proteins (M components) in 6,995 sera from an adult population, *Acta Med. Scand.* **179**:235–247.

Azam, L., and Delamore, I. W., 1974, Combination therapy for myelomatosis, *Br. Med. J.* **4**:560–564.

Azar, H. A., 1973, Pathology of multiple myeloma and related growths, in: *Multiple Myeloma and Related Disorders*, Vol. I (H. A. Azar and M. Potter, eds.), pp. 1–85, Harper and Row, New York.

Azar, H. A., and Potter, M. (eds.), 1973, *Multiple Myeloma and Related Disorders*, Vol. I, Harper and Row, New York.

Azar, H. A., Hill, W. T., and Osserman, E. F., 1957, Malignant lymphoma and lymphocytic leukemia associated with myeloma type serum proteins, *Am. J. Med.* **23**:239–249.

Bachmann, R., 1965, Simultaneous occurrence of two immunologically different M components in serum, *Acta Med. Scand.* **177**:593.

Bain, B. J., Ribush, N. T., McPath, P. N., Whitesed, H. M., and Morgan, T. D., 1973, Renal failure and transient paraproteinemia due to *Leptospira pomoma*, *Arch. Intern. Med.* **131**:740–745.

Baitz, T., and Kyle, R. A., 1964, Solitary myeloma in chronic osteomyelitis, *Arch. Intern. Med.* **113**:872–876.

Balazs, V., and Frohlich, M. M., 1966, Anti-complementary effect of cryoglobulinemic sera and isolated cryoglobulins, *Am. J. Med. Sci.* **251**:51–56.

Ballard, H. S., Hamilton, L. M., Marcus, A. J., and Illes, C. H., 1970, A new variant of heavy-chain disease (μ-chain disease), *N. Engl. J. Med.* **282**:1060–1062.

Balthazar, E. J., and Cano, R., 1975, The radiology corner: Gastric myeloma, *Am. J. Gastroenterol.* **63**(4):340–344.

Bartels, E. D., Brun, G. C., Gammeltoft, A., and Gjørup, P. A., 1954, Acute anuria following intravenous pyelography in a patient with myelomatosis, *Acta Med. Scand.* **150**:297–302.

Barth, W. F., Glenner, G. G., Waldmann, T. A., and Zelis, R. F., 1968, Primary amyloidosis, *Ann. Intern. Med.* **69**:787–805.

Bayrd, E. D., 1961, Continuous chlorambucil therapy in primary macroglobulinemia of Waldenström: Report of four cases, *Proc. Staff Meet. Mayo Clin.* **36**:135–147.

Beaumont, J. L., 1967, Une specificité commune aux α- et β-lipoproteines du serum revelée par un auto-anticorps de myelome, *C. R. Acad. Sci. Ser. D* **264**:183–188.

Beaumont, J. L., 1969, Gamma-globulines et hyperlipidémie par auto-anticorps, *Ann. Biol. Clin. (Paris)* **27**:611–635.

Beaumont, J. L., and Lorenzelli, L., 1967, L'auto-anticorps antilipoproteins (anti-Pg) du γ-A-myelome avec hyperlipidemie: Methode d'isolement et de purification a partir des complexes circulant, *Ann. Biol. Clin. (Paris)* **25**:655–675.

Bedine, M. S., Yardley, J. H., Elliott, H. I., Banwell, J. G., and Hendrix, T. R., 1973, Intestinal involvement in Waldenström's macroglobulinemia, *Gastroenterology* **65**:308–315.

Beker, S. G., Grases, P. J., Merino, F., Arends, T., and Guevara, J., 1971, Intestinal malabsorption in macroglobulinemia, *Am. J. Dig. Dis. New Ser.* **16**:648–656.

Benditt, E. P., and Eriksen, N., 1966, Amyloid. III. A protein related to the subunit structure of human amyloid fibrils, *Proc. Natl. Acad. Sci. U.S.A.* **55**:308.

Benditt, E. P., Eriksen, N., Hermodson, M. A., and Ericsson, L. H., 1971, The major proteins of human and monkey amyloid substance: Common properties including unusual *N*-terminal amino acid sequences, *FEBS Lett.* **19**:169.

Benhold, H., 1922, Eine spezifische Amyloid färbung mit Kongorot, *Muench. Med. Wochenschr.* **2**:1537.

Benninger, G. W., and Kreps, S. I., 1971, Aggregation phenomenon in an IgG multiple myeloma resulting in the hyperviscosity syndrome, *Am. J. Med.* **51**:287.

Bergsagel, D. E., 1976, The treatment of plasma cell myeloma, *Br. J. Haematol.* **33**(4):443–449.

Bergsagel, D. E., Sprague, C. C., Austin, C., and Griffith, K. M., 1962, Evaluation of new chemotherapeutic agents in the treatment of multiple myeloma. IV. 1-Phenylalanine mustard (NSC-8806), *Cancer Chemother. Rep.* **21**:87–99.

Bergsagel, D. E., Griffith, K. M., Haut, A., and Stuckey, W. J., Jr., 1967, The treatment of multiple myeloma, *Adv. Cancer Res.* **10**:311.

Bergsagel, D. E., Cowan, D. H., and Hasselback, R., 1972, Plasma cell myeloma: Response of melphalan-resistant patients to high-dose intermittent cyclophosphamide, *Can. Med. Assoc. J.* **107**:851–855.

Berlin, S.-O., Odeberg, H., and Weingart, L., 1968, Familial occurrence of M-components, *Acta Med. Scand.* **183**:347.

Bernhardt, B., Valbetta, M., Brook, J., and Lejnieks, I., 1972, Case report, amyloidosis with factor X deficiency, *Am. J. Med. Sci.* **264**:411–414.

Bernier, G. M., and Graham, R. C., Jr., 1976, Plasma cell asynchrony in myeloma: Correlation of light and electron microscopy, *Semin. Hematol.* **13**:239–245.

Bethlenfalvay, N. C., Henley, L. E., Rupp, T. D., and Phyliky, R. L., 1976, Nonsecretory plasma cell dyscrasia followed by acute granulocytic leukemia 25 years after thorotrast administration, *Cancer* **37**(3):1449–1453.

Bielschowsky, M., Helyer, B. J., and Howie, J. B., 1959, Spontaneous haemolytic anaemia in mice of the NZB/B1 strain, *Proc. Univ. Otago Med. Sch.* **37**:9.

Bjerrum, O. J., and Weeks, B., 1968, Two M-components, γGK, γML, in different cells in the same patients, *Scand. J. Haematol.* **5**:215.

Bloch, K. J., and Maki, D. G., 1973, Hyperviscosity syndromes associated with immunoglobulin abnormalities, *Semin. Hematol.* **10**:113–124.

Blokhin, N., Larionov, L., Perevodchikova, N., Chebotareva, L., and Merkulova, N., 1958, Clinical experiences with sarcolysin in neoplastic diseases, *Ann. N.Y. Acad. Sci.* **68**:1128–1132.

Bohnstedt, R. M., and Ehlers, G., 1967, Mucinosis Papulosa (Myxomatosis cutis Papulosa, Lichen Myxoedematosus) beim Macroglobulinämie Waldenström, *Proc. 13th Int. Congr. Dermatol. Munich* **3**:142.

Bohrod, M. G., 1957, Plasmacytosis and cryoglobulinemia in cancer, *J. Am. Med. Assoc.* **164**:18.

Bohrod, M. G., and Bottcher, E. J., 1963, Multiple myeloma, hemolytic anemia and protein phagocytosis, *Arch. Pathol.* **76**:700–707.

Bonhomme, J., Seligmann, M., Mihaesco, C., Clauvel, J. P., Danon, F., Brouet, J. C., Bouvry, P., Martine, J., and Clerc, M., 1974, Mu-chain disease in an African patient, *Blood* **43**:485–492.

699

BIOLOGY, CLINICAL
PATTERNS, AND
TREATMENT OF
MULTIPLE MYELOMA
AND RELATED
PLASMA-CELL
DYSCRASIAS

Bouroncle, B. A., Datta, P., and Frajola, W. J., 1964, Waldenström's macroglobulinemia: Report of three patients treated with cyclophosphamide, *J. Am. Med. Assoc.* **189**:729–732.

Bourreille, J., Hemet, J., Tayot, J., and Maitre, A.-M., 1974, Gastric localization of multiple myeloma, *Sem. Hop.* **50**(25):1737–1742.

Bouvet, J. P., Feingold, J., Oriol, R., and Liacopoulos, P., 1975, Statistical study on double paraprotein-emias: Evidence for a common cellular origin of both myeloma globulins, *Biomedicine* **22**:517–523.

Braun, D. G., and Krause, R. M., 1968, The individual antigenic specificity of antibodies to streptococcal carbohydrates, *J. Exp. Med.* **128**:969.

Braun, D. G., Eichmann, K., and Krause, R. M., 1969, Rabbit antibodies to streptococcal carbohydrates, *J. Exp. Med.* **129**:809.

Braun, D. G., Kindred, B., and Jacobson, E. B., 1972, Streptococcal group A carbohydrate antibodies in mice: Evidence for strain differences in magnitude and restriction of the response and for thymus dependence, *Eur. J. Immunol.* **2**:138.

Brecher, G., Tanaka, Y., Malmgren, R. A., and Fahey, J. L., 1964, Morphology and protein synthesis in multiple myeloma and macroglobulinemia, *Ann. N.Y. Acad. Sci.* **113**:642–653.

Bridgen, W. D., 1974, Papular mucinosis (scleromyxoedema of Arndt–Gottron) associated with parapro-tein IgG kappa type, *Proc. R. Soc. Med.* **67**:200.

Broder, S., Humphrey, R., Durm, M., Blackman, M., Meade, B., Goldman, C., Strober, W., and Waldmann, T., 1975, Impaired synthesis of polyclonal (non-paraprotein) immunoglobulins by circulating lymphocytes from patients with multiple myeloma: Role of suppressor cells, *N. Engl. J. Med.* **293**:887–892.

Brooks, A. P., 1976, Portal hypertension in Waldenström's macroglobulinemia, *Br. Med. J.* **1**(6011):689–690.

Brown, M., and Battle, J. D., Jr., 1964, The effect of urography on renal function in patients with multiple myeloma, *Can. Med. Assoc. J.* **91**:786–790.

Brown, R. K., Read, J. T., Wiseman, B. K., and France, W. G., 1948, The electrophoretic analysis of serum proteins of the blood dyscrasias, *J. Lab. Clin. Med.* **33**:1523.

Bush, S. T., Swedlund, H. A., and Gleich, G. J., 1969, Low molecular weight IgM in human sera, *J. Lab. Clin. Med.* **73**:194–201.

Butler, W. T., and Rossen, R. D., 1973, Effect of corticosteroids on immunity in man. I. Decreased serum IgG concentration caused by 3 or 5 days of high doses of methylprednisolone, *J. Clin. Invest.* **52**:2629–2640.

Callis, M. N., and Sheets, R. F., 1974, Multiple myeloma in Iowa, *J. Iowa Med. Soc.* **64**:429–433.

Campbell, A. E., De Vine, J., Azam, L., Hamid, J., Delamore, I. W., and McFarlane, H., 1975, Lymphocyte transformation in patients with paraproteinaemia, *Br. J. Haematol.* **29**:179–188.

Capra, J. D., and Hopper, J. E., 1976, Comparative studies on monotypic IgM λ and IgG κ from an individual patient. III. The complete aminoacid sequence of the V_H region of the IgM paraprotein, *Immunochemistry* **13**:995–999.

Capra, J. D., and Kunkel, H. G., 1970, Aggregation of γG3 proteins: Relevance to the hyperviscosity syndrome, *J. Clin. Invest.* **49**:610.

Capra, J. D., Kehoe, J. M., Williams, R. C., Jr., Feizi, T., and Kunkel, H. G., 1972, Light chain sequences of human IgM cold agglutinins, *Proc. Natl. Acad. Sci. U.S.A.* **69**:40–43.

Carbone, P. P., Kellerhouse, I. E., and Gehan, E. A., 1967, Plasmacytic myeloma: A study of the relationship of survival to various clinical manifestations and anomalous protein type in 112 patients, *Am. J. Med.* **12**:937–948.

Carter, P. M., and Hobbs, J. R., 1971, Clinical significance of 7 S IgM in monoclonal IgM diseases, *Br. Med. J.* **2**:260.

Castaldi, P. A., and Penny, R., 1970, A macroglobulin with antibody activity against coagulation factor VIII, *Blood* **35**:370.

Cawley, L. P., and Schenken, J. R., 1970, Monoclonal hypergammaglobulinemia of the γM type in a nine-year-old girl with ataxia–telangiectasia, *Am. J. Clin. Pathol.* **54**:790.

Cerny, J., McAlack, R. F., Sajid, M. A. and Friedman, H., 1971, Genetic differences in the immunocytic response of mice to separate determinants on one bacterial antigen, *Nature (London) New Biol.* **230**:247.

Chen, Y., Bhoopalam, N., Yakulis, V., and Heller, P., 1975, Changes in lymphocytes surface immuno-globulins in myeloma and the effect of a RNA-containing plasma factor, *Ann. Intern. Med.* **83**:625.

Christenson, W. N., and Dacie, J. V., 1957, Serum proteins in acquired hemolytic anemia (auto-antibody type), *Br. J. Haematol.* **3**:153–163.

Christopherson, W. M., and Miller, A. J., 1950, A re-evaluation of solitary plasma cell myeloma of bone, *Cancer* 3:240–252.

Chronic Leukemia–Myeloma Task Force, National Cancer Institute, 1968, Proposed guidelines for protocol studies. II. Plasma cell myeloma, *Cancer Chemother. Rep.* 1:17.

Churg, J., and Gordon, A. J., 1950, Myltiple myeloma: Lesions of the extra-osseous hematopoietic system, *Am. J. Clin. Pathol.* 20:934–945.

Clatanoff, D. V., and Meyer, O. O., 1963, Response to chlorambucil in macroglobulinemia, *J. Am. Med. Assoc.* 183:40–44.

Cline, M. J., Solomon, A., Berlin, N. I., and Fahey, J. L., 1963, Anemia in macroglobulinemia, *Am. J. Med.* 34:213–220.

Clubb, J. S., Posen, S., and Neale, F. C., 1964, Disappearance of a serum paraprotein after parathyroidectomy, *Arch. Intern. Med.* 114:616.

Cohen, A. S., and Calkins, E., 1959, Electron microscopic observations on a fibrous component in amyloid of diverse origins (letter to the editor), *Nature (London)* 183:1202–1203.

Cohen, D. M., Svien, H. J., and Dahlin, D. C., 1964, Long-term survival of patients with myeloma of the vertebral column, *J. Am. Med. Assoc.* 187:914–917.

Cohen, H. J., and Rundles, R. W., 1975, Managing the complications of plasma cell myeloma, *Arch. Intern. Med.* 135:177–184.

Cohen, H. J., Lessin, L. S., Hallal, J., and Burkholder, P., 1975, Resolution of primary amyloidosis during chemotherapy: Studies in a patient with nephrotic syndrome, *Ann. Intern. Med.* 82:466–473.

Cohn, M., 1967, Natural history of the myeloma, *Cold Spring Harbor Symp. Quant. Biol.* 32:211.

Coleman, M., Vigliano, E. M., Weksler, M. E., and Nachman, R. L., 1972, Inhibition of fibrin monomer polymorization by lambda myeloma globulins, *Blood* 39:210–223.

Cone, L., and Uhr, J. W., 1964, Immunological deficiency disorders associated with chronic lymphocytic leukemia and multiple myeloma, *J. Clin. Invest.* 43:2241–2248.

Conklin, R., and Alexanian, R., 1975, Clinical classification of plasma cell myeloma, *Arch. Intern. Med.* 135:139–143.

Connell, G. E., Dorrington, K. J., Lewis, A. F., and Parr, D. M., 1970, The confirmation of an atypical IgG myeloma protein and its pepsin fragments, *Can. J. Biochem.* 48:784.

Cooke, K. B., 1969, Essential paraproteinaemia, *Proc. R. Soc. Med.* 62:777–778.

Cooperative Study by Acute Leukemia Group B, 1975, Correlation of abnormal immunoglobulin with clinical features of myeloma, *Arch. Intern. Med.* 135:46–52.

Cooper, M. R., Cohen, H. J., Huntley, C. C., Waite, B. M., Spees, L., and Spurr, C. L., 1974, A monoclonal IgM with antibody-like specificity for phospholipids in a patient with lymphoma, *Blood* 43:493–504.

Costa, G., Engle, R. L., and Taliente, P., 1969, Criteria for defining risk groups and response to chemotherapy in multiple myeloma, *Proc. Am. Assoc. Cancer Res.* 10:15 (abstract).

Costa, G., Engle, R. L., Jr., Schilling, A., Carbone, P., Kochwa, S., Nachman, R. I., and Glidewell, O., 1973, Melphalan and prednisone: An effective combination for the treatment of multiple myeloma, *Am. J. Med.* 51:589–599.

Costanzi, J. J., and Coltman, C. A., Jr., 1967, Kappa chain cold precipitable immunoglobulin G (IgG) associated with cold urticaria, *Clin. Exp. Immunol.* 2:167–178.

Costanzi, J. J., Coltman, C. A., Jr., and Donaldson, V. H., 1969, Activation of complement by a monoclonal cryoglobulin associated with cold urticaria, *J. Lab. Clin. Med.* 74:902–910.

Costea, N., Yakulis, V. J., Libnoch, J. A., Pilz, C. G., and Heller, P., 1967, Two myeloma globulins (IgG and IgA) in one subject and one cell line, *Am. J. Med.* 42:630.

Cutler, S. J., and Ederer, F., 1958, Maximum utilization of the life table method in analyzing survival, *J. Chronic Dis.* 8:699.

Dacie, J. V., 1962, *The Hemolytic Anemias: Congenital and Acquired,* Part II, 2nd Ed., Churchill, London.

Dacie, J. V., and Worlledge, S. M., 1969, Autoimmune hemolytic anemias, *Prog. Hematol.* 6:82.

Dalton, A. J., and Potter, M., 1968, Electron microscopic study of the mammary tumor agent in plasma cell tumors, *J. Natl. Cancer Inst.* 40:1375.

Dalton, A. J., Potter, M., and Merwin, R. M., 1961, Some ultrastructural characteristics of a series of primary and transplanted plasma cell tumors of the mouse, *J. Natl. Cancer Inst.* 26:1221.

Dammacco, F., and Clausen, J., 1966, Antibody deficiency in paraproteinemia, *Acta Med. Scand.* 179:755–768.

Dammacco, F., and Waldenström, J., 1968, Serum and urine light chain levels in benign monoclonal

BIOLOGY, CLINICAL
PATTERNS, AND
TREATMENT OF
MULTIPLE MYELOMA
AND RELATED
PLASMA-CELL
DYSCRASIAS

gammapathies, multiple myeloma and Waldenström's macroglobulinemia, *Clin. Exp. Immunol.* **3**:911.

Danby, F. W., Danby, C. W. D., and Pruzanski, W., 1976, Papular mucinosis with IgG(κ) M component, *Can. Med. Assoc. J.* **114**:920–922.

Danon, F., and Seligmann, M., 1972, Transient human monoclonal immunoglobulins, *Scand. J. Immunol.* **1**:323.

Danon, F., Michaesco, E., Bouvry, M., Clere, M., and Seligmann, M., 1975, A new case of heavy μ-chain disease, *Scand. J. Haematol.* **15**(1):5–9.

Darnley, J. D., 1962, Polyneuropathy in Waldenström's macroglobulinemia: Case report and discussion, *Neurology* **12**:617–623.

Dawson, A. A., and Ogston, D., 1971, Factors influencing the prognosis in myelomatosis, *Postgrad. Med. J.* **47**:635–638.

Dawson, A. A., and Ogston, D., 1973, High incidence of myelomatosis in north-east Scotland, *Scott. Med. J.* **18**:75–77.

Dayan, A. D., and Lewis, P. D., 1966, Demyelinating neuropathy in macrocryoglobulinemia, *Neurology* **16**:1141–1144.

DelDuca, V., Jr., and Morningstar, W. A., 1967, Multiple myeloma associated with progressive multifocal leukoencephalopathy, *J. Am. Med. Assoc.* **199**:671–673.

Derghazarian, C., and Whittemore, N. B., 1974, Multiple myeloma superimposed on chronic myelocytic leukemia, *Can. Med. Assoc. J.* **110**:1047–1050.

DiGuglielmo, R., 1966, Unusual morphologic and humoral conditions in the field of plasmocytoms and M-dysproteinemia, *Acta Med. Scand.* **179**(Suppl. 445):206.

Dittmar, K., Kochwa, S., Zucker-Franklin D., Gralnick, H., and Wasserman, L. R., 1968, Coexistence of polycythemia and biclonal gammapathy (gamma GK and gamma AL) with two Bence-Jones proteins (BJK and BJL), *Blood* **31**:881.

Dolin, S., and Dewar, J. P., 1956, Extramedullary plasmacytoma, *Am. J. Pathol.* **32**:83–103.

Dollinger, M. R., Golby, R. B., and Karnofky, D. A., 1969, Cancer chemotherapy, *Dis. Mon.* April, p. 11.

Doumenc, J., Prost, R. J., Samama, M., and Bousser, J., 1966, Anomalie de l'agrégation plaquettaire au cours de la maladie de Waldenström (à propos de 3 cas), *Nouv. Rev. Fr. Hematol.* **6**:734.

Drewinko, B., Brown, B. W., Humphrey, R., and Alexanian, R., 1974, Effect of chemotherapy on the labeling index of myeloma cells, *Cancer* **34**:526.

Drivsholm, A., 1964, Myelomatosis, *Acta Med. Scand.* **176**:509.

Drivsholm, A., and Clausen, J., 1964, The relationship between the cytology and the immunoelectrophoretic pattern in 105 cases of myelomatosis, *Acta Med. Scand.* **175**:609.

Dunn, T. B., 1957, Plasma-cell neoplasms beginning in the ileocecal area in strain C_3H mice, *J. Natl. Cancer Inst.* **19**:371.

Durie, B. G., and Salmon, S. E., 1976, A clinical staging system for multiple myeloma: Correlation of measured myeloma cell mass with presenting clinical features, response to treatment and survival, *Cancer* **36**:842–854.

Dutcher, T. F., and Fahey, J. L., 1959, The histopathology of the macroglobulinemia of Waldenström, *J. Natl. Cancer Inst.* **22**:887–917.

Eanes, E. D., and Glenner, G. G., 1968, X-ray diffraction studies on amyloid filaments, *J. Histochem. Cytochem.* **16**:673.

Ein, D., Kimura, S., and Glenner, G. G., 1972a, An amyloid fibril protein of unknown origin: Partial amino acid sequence analysis, *Biochem. Biophys. Res. Commun.* **46**:498.

Ein, D., Kimura, S., Terry, W. D., Magnotta, J., and Glenner, G. G., 1972b, Amino acid sequence of an amyloid fibril protein of unknown origin, *J. Biol. Chem.* **247**:5653.

Eipe, J., Yakulis, V., and Costea, N., 1975, Idiotypic specificity of lymphocyte surface Ig (S Ig) and serum monoclonal IgM in patients with malignant lymphoproliferative disorders, Abstract 107, American Society of Hematology (Eighteenth Annual Meeting), Dallas, Texas.

Elias, E. G., Reynoso, G., and Mittlemann, A., 1972, Control of hypercalcemia with mithramycin, *Ann. Surg.* **175**:431–435.

Engle, R. I., Jr., and Wallis, I. A., 1957, Multiple myeloma and the adult Fanconi syndrome. 1. Report of a case with crystal-like deposits in the tumor cells and in the epithelial cells of the kidney, *Am. J. Med.* **22**:5–12.

Engle, R. L., Jr., and Wallis, L. A., 1969, *Immunoglobulinopathies,* Charles C. Thomas, Springfield, Illinois.

Epstein, F. H., 1968, Calcium and the kidney, *Am. J. Med.* **45**:700.

Epstein, W. L., 1974, Connective tissue diseases, in: *Year Book of Dermatology* (F. D. Malkinson and R. W. Pearson, eds.), p. 271, Year Book Medical Publishers, Chicago.

Essig, L. J., Timms, E. S., Hancock, D. E., and Sharp, G. C., 1974, Plasma cell interstitial pneumonia and macroglobulinemia: A response to corticosteroid and cyclophosphamide therapy, *Am. J. Med.* **56**:398.

Fadem, R. S., 1952, Differentiation of plasmacytic responses from myelomatous diseases on the basis of bone marrow findings, *Cancer* **5**:128–137.

Faguet, G. B., Barton, B. P., Smith, L. L. and Garver, F. A., 1977, Gamma heavy chain disease: Clinical aspects and characterization of a deleted, moncovalently linked γ1 heavy chain dimer (BAZ), *Blood* **49**:495–505.

Fahey, J. L., 1963, Serum protein disorders causing clinical symptoms in malignant neoplastic disease, *J. Chronic Dis.* **16**:703–712.

Fahey, J. L., and Askonas, B. A., 1962, Enzymatically produced sub-units of proteins formed by plasma cells in mice. I. γ-Globulin and γ-myeloma proteins, *J. Exp. Med.* **115**:623.

Fahey, J. L., Scoggins, R., Utz, J. P., and Szwed, C. F., 1963, Infection, antibody response and gamma globulin components in multiple myeloma and macroglobulinemia, *Am. J. Med.* **35**:698–707.

Fahey, J. L., Barth, W. F., and Solomon, A., 1965, Serum hyperviscosity syndrome, *J. Am. Med. Assoc.* **192**:464–467.

Fahey, J. L., Carbone, P. P., Rowe, D. S., and Bachmann, R., 1968, Plasma cell myeloma with D-myeloma protein (IgD myeloma), *Am. J. Med.* **45**:373–380.

Fair, D. S., Krueger, R. G., Gleich, G. J. and Kyle, R., 1974, Studies on IgA and IgG monoclonal proteins derived from a single patient. 1. Evidence for shared individually specific antigenic determinants, *J. Immunol.* **1974**:112–201.

Fairley, K. F., Barrie, J. U., and Johnson, W., 1972, Sterility and testicular atrophy related to cyclophosphamide therapy, *Lancet* **1**:568–569.

Farhangi, M., and Osserman, E. F., 1970, Monocytic and monomyelocytic leukemia with lysozymuria as a late complication in plasma cell leukemia, in: *Proceedings of the 13th International Congress on Hematology*, p. 192, J. F. Lehmanns Verlag, Munich.

Farhangi, M., and Osserman, E. F., 1973, The treatment of multiple myeloma, *Semin. Hematol.* **10**:149–161.

Farhangi, M., and Osserman, E. F., 1976, Myeloma with xanthoderma due to an IgG λ monoclonal anti-flavin antibody, *N. Engl. J. Med.* **294**:177.

Farhangi, M., Bukstein, D., Lay, D. E., and Morris, A. D., 1977, Hyperviscosity syndrome and purpura associated with a transient IgA(κ) monoclonal anti-Ig G in a patient with rheumatoid arthritis, *Clin. Res.* **25**:52A.

Feizi, T., 1967, Lambda chain in cold agglutinins, *Science* **156**:1111–1112.

Feizi, T., and Schumacher, M., 1968, Light chain homogeneity of postinfective cold agglutinins, *Clin. Exp. Immunol.* **3**:923–929.

Feizi, T., Kabat, E. A., Vicari, G., Anderson, B., and Marsh, W. L., 1971a, Immunochemical studies on blood groups. XLVII. The I antigen complex-precursors in the A, B, H, Le[a] and Le[b] blood group system—Hemagglutination–inhibition studies, *J. Exp. Med.* **133**:39.

Feizi, T., Kabat, E. A., Vicari, G., Anderson, B., and Marsh, W. L., 1971b, Immunochemical studies on blood groups. XLIX. The I antigen complex: Specificity differences among anti-I sera revealed by quantitative precipitin studies: Partial structure of the I determinant specific for one anti I serum, *J. Immunol.* **106**:1578.

Feizi, T., Kabat, E. A., Vicari, G., Anderson, B., and Marsh, W. L., 1972, Immunochemical studies on blood groups. LIV. Classification of anti-I and anti-i sera into groups based on reactivity patterns with various antigens related to the blood group A, B, H, Le[a], Le[b] and precursor substances, *J. Exp. Med.* **135**:1247.

Feldman, P., Shapiro, L., Pick, A., and Slatkin, M., 1969, Scleromyxedema: A dramatic response to melphalan, *Arch. Dermatol.* **99**:51.

Ferriman, D. G., and Anderson, A. B., 1956, Macroglobulinemia of Waldenström, *Br. Med. J.* **2**:402–403.

Fett, J. W., and Deutsch, H. F., 1974, The primary structure of the Mcg λ-chain, *Biochemistry* **13**(20):4102–4114.

Fine, J. M., Rivat, C., Lambin, P., and Ropartz, C., 1974, Monoclonal IgD: A comparative study of 60 sera with IgD "M" component, *Biomedicine Express (Paris)* **21**:119–125.

703

BIOLOGY, CLINICAL
PATTERNS, AND
TREATMENT OF
MULTIPLE MYELOMA
AND RELATED
PLASMA-CELL
DYSCRASIAS

Finkel, P. N., Kronenberg, K., Pesce, A. J., Pollak, V. E., and Pirani, C. L., 1973, Adult Fanconi syndrome, amyloidosis and marked κ-light chain proteinuria, *Nephron* **10**:1–24.

Fishman, S. A., and Ritz, N. D., 1975, Erythroleukemia following melphalan therapy for multiple myeloma, *N.Y. State J. Med.* **75**(13):2402–2404.

Fitchen, J. H., 1975, Amyloidosis and granulomatous ileocolitis: Regression after surgical removal of the involved bowel, *N. Engl. J. Med.* **292**:352–353.

Fleischman, J. B., Braun, D. G., and Krause, R. M., 1968, Streptococcal group-specific antibodies: Occurrence of a restricted population following secondary immunization, *Proc. Natl. Acad. Sci. U.S.A.* **60**:134.

Forte, F. A., Prelli, F., Yount, W. J., Jerry, L. M., Kochwa, S., Franklin, E. C., and Kunkel, H. G., 1970, Heavy chain disease of the μ (γ M) type: Report of the first case, *Blood* **36**:137–144.

Fowlkes, R. W., Blaylock, W. K., and Mullinax, F., 1967, Immunologic studies in lichen myxedematosus, *Arch. Dermatol.* **95**:370.

Frangione, B., and Franklin, E. C., 1973, Heavy chain diseases: Clinical features and molecular significance of the disordered immunoglobulin structure, *Semin. Hematol.* **10**:53–64.

Franklin, E. C., 1975, μ-Chain disease, *Arch. Intern. Med.* **135**:71–72.

Franklin, E. C., and Frangione, B., 1975, Structural variants of human and murine immunoglobulins, in: *Contemporary Topics in Molecular Immunology*, Vol. 4 (F. P. Inman and W. J. Mandy, eds.), p. 89, Plenum Press, New York.

Franklin, E. C., Lowenstein, J., Bigelow, B., and Meltzer, M., 1964, Heavy chain disease—a new disorder of serum γ-globulins: Report of the first case, *Am. J. Med.* **37**:332–350.

Franklin, E. C., Rosenthal, C. J., and Pras, M., 1975, Studies on the amyloid A protein (AA protein) and a related serum component: Purification, partial characterization and tissue origin and distribution in different types of amyloidosis, *Adv. Nephrol.* **5**:89.

Fudenberg, J. K., Epstein, H., Shuster, W. L., and Shuster, J., 1967, Studies on a unique diagnostic serum globulin in papular mucinosis (lichen myxedematosus), *Clin. Exp. Immunol.* **2**:153–166.

Furie, B., Green, E., and Furie, B. C., 1977, Syndrome of acquired factor X deficiency and systemic amyloidosis. *In vivo* studies of the metabolic fate of factor X, *N. Engl. J. Med.* **297**:81–85.

Gach, J., Simar, I., and Salmon, J., 1971, Multiple myeloma without M-type proteinemia: Report of a case with immunologic and ultrastructure studies, *Am. J. Med.* **50**:835–844.

Galton, D. A. G., and Peto, R., 1973, Report on first myelomatosis trial. I. Analysis of presenting features of prognostic importance, *Br. J. Haematol.* **24**:123.

Garver, F. A., Chang, L., Mendicino, J., Isobe, T., and Osserman, E. F., 1975, Primary structure of a deleted human lambda type immunoglobulin light chain containing carbohydrate protein Sm λ, *Proc. Natl. Acad. Sci. U.S.A.* **72**:4559–4563.

Gerber, M. A., 1970, Asbestosis and neoplastic disorders of the hematopoietic system, *Am. J. Clin. Pathol.* **53**:204–208.

Getaz, P., Handler, L., and Tunley, P. J. I., 1974, Osteosclerotic myeloma with peripheral neuropathy, *S. Afr. Med. J.* **48**(29):1246–1250.

Ghanta, V. K., and Hiramoto, R. N., 1974, Quantitation of total-body tumor cells (MOPC 104E), 1. Subcutaneous tumor model, *J. Natl. Cancer Inst.* **52**:1199–1202.

Glenner, G. G., and Page, D. L., 1976, Amyloid, amyloidosis, and amyloidogenesis, *Int. Rev. Exp. Pathol.* **15**:1–92.

Glenner, G. G., Cuatrecasas, P., Isersky, C., Bladen, H. A., and Eanes, E. D., 1969, Physical and chemical properties of amyloid fibers. II. Isolation of a unique protein constituting the major component from human splenic amyloid fibril concentrates, *J. Histochem. Cytochem.* **17**:769.

Glenner, G. G., Harbaugh, J., Ohms, J. L., Harada, M., and Cuatrecasas, P., 1970, An amyloid protein: The amino-terminal variable fragment of an immunoglobulin light chain, *Biochem. Biophys. Res. Commun.* **41**:1287.

Glenner, G. G., Terry, W., Harada, M., Isersky, C., and Page, D., 1971a, Amyloid fibril proteins: Proof of homology with immunoglobulin light chains by sequence analysis, *Science* **172**:1150.

Glenner, G. G., Ein, D., Eanes, E. D., Bladen, H. A., Terry, W., and Page, D., 1971b, The creation of "amyloid" fibrils from Bence Jones proteins *in vitro*, *Science* **174**:712.

Glenner, G. G., Harada, M., and Isersky, C., 1972a, The purification of amyloid fibril proteins, *Prep. Biochem.* **2**:39.

Glenner, G. G., Eanes, E. D., and Page, D. L., 1972b, The relation of Congo red staining of amyloid fibrils to the β-conformation, *J. Histochem. Cytochem.* **20**:821.

Glenner, G. G., Terry, W. D., and Isersky, C., 1973, Amyloidosis: Its nature and pathogenesis, *Semin. Hematol.* **10**:65.

Glueck, H. I., and Hong, R., 1965, A circulating anticoagulant in γl-A multiple myeloma: Its modification by penicillin, *J. Clin. Invest.* **44**:1866.

Golde, D. W., Saxon, A., and Stevens, R. H., 1977, Macroglobulinemia and hairy-cell leukemia, *N. Engl. J. Med.* **296**:92–93.

Gonzales, F., Trujilio, J. M., and Alexanian, R., 1977, Acute leukemia in multiple myeloma, *Ann. Intern. Med.* **86**:440–443.

Goodman, S. I., Rodgerson, D. O., and Kauffman, J., 1967, Hypercupremia in a patient with multiple myeloma, *J. Lab. Clin. Med.* **70**:57–62.

Gordon, H., Bandmann, M., and Sandbank, U., 1971, Multiple myeloma associated with progressive multifocal leukoencephalopathy and *Pneumocystis carinii* pneumonia, *Isr. J. Med. Sci.* **7**:581–588.

Graham, R. C., Jr., and Bernier, G. M., 1975, The bone marrow in multiple myeloma: Correlation of plasma cell ultrastructure and clinical state, *Medicine (Baltimore)* **54**:225–243.

Grant, J. A., Blumenschein, G. R., and Buckley, C. E., III, 1971, Familial paraproteinemia, *Arch. Intern. Med.* **128**:427.

Grey, H. M., and Kohler, P. F., 1973, Cryoimmunoglobulins, *Semin. Hematol.* **10**:87–112.

Groch, G. S., Perillie, P. E., and Finch, S. C., 1965, Reticuloendothelial phagocytic function in patients with leukemia, lymphoma and multiple myeloma, *Blood* **26**:489–499.

Gueft, B., Kikkawa, Y., and Hirschel, S., 1968, An electron-microscopic study of amyloidosis from different species, in: *Amyloidosis* (E. Mandema, L. Ruinen, J. H. Scholten, and A. S. Cohen, eds.), pp. 172–183, Excerpta Medica, Amsterdam.

Gunz, F. W., and Veale, A. M. O., 1969, Leukemia in close relatives—accident or predisposition?, *J. Natl. Cancer Inst.* **42**:517.

Gupta, N. M., Datta, B. N., and Talwar, B. L., 1974, Plasmacytoma of stomach—A case report and review of literature, *Indian J. Cancer* **11**(3):355–359.

Hällén, J., 1966, Discrete gammoglobulin (M-) components in serum, *Acta Med. Scand.* **179**(Suppl. 462).

Hällén, J., 1969, Differentialdiagnostik vid monoclonal gammapati, *Nord. Med.* **82**:885–890.

Hïlén, J., and Rudin, R., 1966, Peri-collagenous amyloidosis, a study of 51 cases, *Acta Med. Scand.* **179**:483.

Hannestad, K., and Sletten, K., 1971, Multiple M-components in a single individual. III. Heterogeneity of M-components in two macroglobulinemia sera with anti-polysaccharide activity, *J. Biol. Chem.* **246**(22):6982–6990.

Hansen, O. P., Jessen, B., and Videback, A., 1973, Prognosis of myelomatosis on treatment with prednisone and cytostatics, *Scand. J. Haematol.* **10**:282–290.

Harboe, M., and Torsvik, H., 1969, Protein abnormalities in the cold hemagglutination syndrome, *Scand. J. Haematol.* **6**:416–426.

Harboe, M., Van Furth, R., Schubothe, H., Lind, K., and Evans, R. S., 1965, Exchange occurrence of κ-chains in isolated cold hemagglutinins, *Scand. J. Haematol.* **2**:259–266.

Harisdaugkul, V., and Srichaikul, T., 1976, A case of IgD myeloma with clinical manifestation resembling malignant lymphoma, *J. Med. Assoc. Thailand* **59**:331–337.

Harley, J. B., Ramanan, S. V., Kim, I., Thiagarajan, P. V., Chen, J. H., Gomez, R., Koppel, D., Hyde, F., Gustke, S., and Krall, J., 1972, The cyclic use of multiple alkylating agents in multiple myeloma, *W. V. Med. J.* **68**:1–3.

Harris, J., and Copeland, D., 1974, Impaired immunoresponsiveness in tumor patients, *Ann. N.Y. Acad Sci.* **230**:56–85.

Harris, J., Alexanian, R., Hersh, E., and Migliore, P., 1971, Immune function in multiple myeloma: Impaired responsiveness to keyhole limpet hemocyanin, *Can. Med. Assoc. J.* **104**:389–392.

Harrison, C. V., 1972, The morphology of the lymph node in the macroglobulinaemia of Waldenström, *J. Clin. Pathol.* **25**:12–16.

Heilmann, D., 1957, Plasmocytom auf dem Boden einer chronischen Osteomyelitis bei gleichzeitiger Osteitis deformans, *Muench. Med. Wochenschr.* **99**:1586.

Heinemann, H. O., 1963, Reversible defect in renal ammonia excretion in patients with hypercalcemia, *Metabolism* **12**:792.

Heller, P., *et al.*, 1973, The role of RNA in the immunological deficiency of plasmacytoma, *Ann. N.Y. Acad. Sci.* **207**:468–480.

Helyer, B. J., and Howie, J. B., 1963, Spontaneous autoimmune disease in NZB/B1 mice, *Br. J. Haematol.* **9**:119.

Howell, G. M., and Alexanian, R., 1976, Multiple myeloma in young persons, *Ann. Intern. Med.* **84**:441–443.

Higby, D. J., and Ohnuma, T., 1975, Plasmacytoma cell ascites, *N.Y. State J. Med.* **75**(7):1074–1076.

Hijmans, W., 1975, Waldenström's disease with an IgA paraprotein, *Acta Med. Scand.* **198**(6):519–523.

Hippe, E., Jensen, K. B., Olesen, H., Lind, K., and Thornsen, P. E. B., 1970, Chlorambucil treatment of patients with cold agglutinin syndrome, *Blood* **35**:68.

Hobbs, J. R., 1967, Paraproteins, benign or malignant?, *Br. Med. J.* **3**:699–704.

Hobbs, J. R., 1969a, Paraproteinemia, *Proc. R. Soc. Med.* **62**:773.

Hobbs, J. R., 1969b, Immunochemical classes of myelomatosis: Including data from a therapeutic trial concluded by a Medical Research Council working party, *Br. J. Haematol.* **16**:599–606.

Hobbs, J. R., 1969c, Growth rate and responses to treatment in human myelomatosis, *Br. J. Haematol.* **16**:607–617.

Hobbs, J. R., 1971, Immunocytoma o'mice an' man, *Br. Med. J.* **2**:67–72.

Hobbs, J. R., Slot, G. M. J., Campbell, C. H., Clein, G. P., Scott, J. T., Crowther, D., and Swan, H. T., 1966, Six cases of gamma-D myelomatosis, *Lancet* **2**:614–618.

Holland, J. F., Hosley, H., Scharlau, C., Carbone, P. P., Frei, E., III, Brindley, C. O., Hall, T. C., Shnider, B. I., Gold, G. L., Lasagna, L., Owens, A. H., Jr., and Miller, S. P., 1966, A control trial of urethane treatment in multiple myeloma, *Blood* **27**:328.

Hollander, V. P., Takakura, K., and Yamada, H., 1968, Endocrine factors in the pathogenesis of plasma cell tumors, *Recent Prog. Horm. Res.* **24**:81–137.

Hoogstraten, B., 1973, Steroid therapy of multiple myeloma and macroglobulinemia, *Med. Clin. North Am.* **57**:1321–1330.

Hoogstraten, B., Sheehe, P. R., Cuttner, J., Cooper, T., Kyle, R. A., Oberfield, R. A., Townsend, S. R., Harley, J. B., Hayes, D. M., Costa, G., and Holland, J. F., 1967, Melphalan in multiple myeloma, *Blood* **30**:74.

Hoogstraten, B., Costa, J., Cuttner, J., Forcier, J., Leone, L. A., Harley, J. R., and Glidewell, O. J., 1969, Intermittent melphalan therapy in multiple myeloma, *J. Am. Med. Assoc.* **209**:251.

Hopper, J. E., 1975, Comparative studies on monotypic IgM λ and IgG κ from an individual patient. I. Evidence for shared V_H idiotypic determinants, *J. Immunol.* **115**:1101–1107.

Hopper, J. E., Noyes, C., Heinrikson, R., and Kessel, J. W., 1976, Comparative studies on monotypic IgMλ and IgGκ from an individual patient. II. Amino-terminal sequence analyses, *J. Immunol.* **116**:743.

Horn, M. F., Knapp, M. S., Page, F. T., and Walker, W. H. C., 1969, Adult Fanconi syndrome and multiple myelomatosis, *J. Clin. Pathol.* **22**:414–416.

Hossfeld, D. K., Holland, J. F., Cooper, R. G., and Ellison, R. R., 1975, Chromosome studies in acute leukemias developing in patients with multiple myeloma, *Cancer Res.* **35**(10):2808–2813.

Howatson, A. F., and McCulloch, E. A., 1958, Viruslike bodies in a transplantable mouse plasma cell tumor, *Nature (London)* **181**:1213–1214.

Howell, M., 1963, Acquired factor X deficiency associated with systematized amyloidosis: Report of a case, *Blood* **21**:739–744.

Hurez, D., Preud'homme, J. L., and Seligmann, M., 1970, Intracellular "monoclonal" immunoglobulin in nonsecretory human myeloma, *J. Immunol.* **101**:263–264.

Huth, K., Ehlers, G., Knoth, W., Kunze, K., Löffler, H., Mähr, G., and Petzoldt, 1972, Lichen myxoedematosus bei Makroglobulinämie Waldenström mit Polyneuropathie und Carpal-tunnel-syndrome, *Dtsch. Med. Wochenschr.* **97**:152.

Indiveri, F., Barabino, A., Santolini, M. E., and Santolini, B., 1974, "Nonsecretory" multiple myeloma: Report of a case, *Acta Haematol (Basel)* **51**:302–309.

Isobe, T. and Osserman, E. F., 1971, Pathologic conditions associated with plasma cell dyscrasias: A study of 806 cases, *Ann. N.Y. Acad. Sci.* **190**:507–518.

Isobe, T., and Osserman, E. F., 1974a, Plasma cell dyscrasia associated wih the production of incomplete (?deleted) IgG λ molecules, gamma heavy chains, and free lambda chains containing carbohydrate: Description of the first case, *Blood* **43**:505–526.

Isobe, T., and Osserman, E. F., 1974b, Patterns of amyloidosis and their association with plasma cell dyscrasia, monoclonal immunoglobulins and Bence-Jones proteins, *N. Engl. J. Med.* **290**:473–477.

BIOLOGY, CLINICAL
PATTERNS, AND
TREATMENT OF
MULTIPLE MYELOMA
AND RELATED
PLASMA-CELL
DYSCRASIAS

Isobe, T., and Osserman, E. F., 1976, Effect of dimethyl sulfoxide (DMSO) on Bence-Jones proteins, amyloid fibrils and casein-induced amyloidosis, in: *Amyloidosis* (O. Vegelius and A. Pasternack, eds.), p. 247, Academic Press, London.

Isobe, T., Ikeda, Y., Ohta, H., and Sinura, H., 1976, IgD myeloma, a clinical study of 9 cases, *Acta Haematol. Jpn.* **39**:343–344.

James, K., Fudenberg, H., Epstein, W. L., and Shuster, J., 1967, Studies on a unique diagnostic serum globulin in papular mucinosis (lichen myxedematosus), *Clin. Exp. Immunol.* **2**:153–166.

Jancelewicz, Z., Takatsuki, K., Sugai, S., and Pruzanski, W., 1975, IgD multiple myeloma: Review of 133 cases, *Arch. Intern. Med.* **135**:87–93.

Jasin, J. E., LoSpalluto, J., and Ziff, M., 1970, Rheumatoid hyperviscosity syndrome, *Am. J. Med.* **49**:484.

Jensen, K., 1970a, Metabolism of Bence Jones proteins in non-myeloma patients with normal renal function, *Scand. J. Clin. Lab. Invest.* **25**:281–289.

Jensen, K., 1970b, Metabolism of Bence Jones proteins in multiple myeloma patients and in patients with renal disease, *Scand. J. Clin. Lab. Invest.* **26**:13–21.

Johnson, W. W., and Meadows, D. C., 1971, Urinary-bladder fibrosis and telangiectasia associated with long-term cyclophosphamide therapy, *N. Engl. J. Med.* **284**:290–294.

Jones, N. F., Hilton, P. J., Tighe, J. R., and Hobbs, J. R., 1972, Treatment of "primary" renal amyloidosis with melphalan, *Lancet* **2**:616–619.

Jonsson, V., Videbek, A., Axelsen, N. H., and Harhoe, M., 1976, μ-Chain disease in a case of chronic lymphocytic leukemia and malignant histiocytoma. I. Clinical aspects, *Scand. J. Haematol.* **16**(3):209–217.

Kaplan, G. A., and Bennett, J., 1968, Solitary myeloma of the lumbar spine successfully treated with radiation: Report of a case, *Radiology* **91**:1017–1018, 1032.

Kaye, R. L., Martin, W. J., Campbell, D. C., and Lipscomb, P. R., 1961, Long survival in disseminated myeloma with onset as solitary lesion: Two cases, *Ann. Intern. Med.* **54**:535–544.

Kedar (Keizman), I., Greenwald, M., and Ravid, M., 1977, Treatment of experimental murine amyloidosis with dimethyl sulfoxide, *Eur. J. Clin. Invest.* **7**:149.

Keller, H., Spengler, G. A., Skvaril, F., Flury, W., Noseda, G., and Riva, G., 1970, Zur Frage der Heavy chain disease: Ein Fall von IgG-heavy-chain-Fragment-und IgM-Typ K-Para-proteinämie mit Plasmazellenleukämie, *Schweiz. Med. Wochenschr.* **100**:1012–1022.

Khaleeli, M., Keane, W. M., and Lee, G. R., 1973, Sideroblastic anemia in multiple myeloma: A preleukemic change, *Blood* **41**:17–25.

Kiang, D. T., Sundberg, R. D., Fortuny, I. E., Brunning, R. D., Theologides, A., Goldman, A., and Kennedy, B. J., 1974, Multiple myeloma: Clinical evolution, *Minn. Med.* **57**:542–548.

Kim, L., Harley, J. B., and Weksler, B., 1972, Multiple myeloma without initial paraproteins, *Am. J. Med. Sci.* **264**:267–275.

Kint, A., 1961, Les manifestations cutanées de la maladie de Kahler, *Arch. Belg. Dermatol. Syphiligr.* **17**:148.

Kleinholz, E. J., Jr., and Tennebaum, M. J., 1973, Pleural plasmacytoma presenting as pleural effusion, *V. Med. Mon.* **100**:1035–1040.

Korsan-Bengsten, K., Hjort, P. F., and Ygge, J., 1962, Acquired factor X deficiency in a patient with amyloidosis, *Thromb. Diath. Haemorrh.* **7**:558–566.

Korst, D. R., Clifford, G. O., Fowler, W. M., Louis, J., Will, J., and Wilson, H. E., 1964, Multiple myeloma. II. Analysis of cyclophosphamide therapy in 165 patients, *J. Am. Med. Assoc.* **189**:758.

Kotner, L. M., and Wang, C. G., 1972, Plasmacytoma of the upper air and food passages, *Cancer* **30**:414–418.

Krajny, M., and Pruzanski, W., 1976, Waldenström's macroglobulinemia: Review of 45 cases, *Can. Med. Assoc. J.* **114**(10):899–905.

Krauss, S., and Sokal, J. E., 1966, Paraproteinemias in the lymphomas, *Am. J. Med.* **40**:400–413.

Kretschmer, R. R., Pizzuto, J., González, J., and López, M., 1974, Heavy chain disease, rheumatoid arthritis and cryoglobulinemia, *Clin. Immunol. Immunopathol.* **2**:195–215.

Kuff, E. L., Wivel, N. A., and Lueders, K. R., 1968, The extraction of intracisternal A particles from a mouse plasma-cell tumor, *Cancer Res.* **28**:2137–2148.

Kuff, E. L., Lueders, K. K., Ozer, H. L., and Wivel, N., 1972, Some structural and antigenic properties of intracisternal A particles occurring in mouse tumors, *Proc. Natl. Acad. Sci. U.S.A.* **69**:218.

707

BIOLOGY, CLINICAL
PATTERNS, AND
TREATMENT OF
MULTIPLE MYELOMA
AND RELATED
PLASMA-CELL
DYSCRASIAS

Kunwar, K. B., and Kumar, S., 1966, Multiple myeloma with myeloma cells in the urine: Case report, *Indian J. Med. Sci.* **20**:641–643.

Kyle, R. A., 1975, Multiple myeloma: Review of 869 cases, *Mayo Clin. Proc.* **50**:29–40.

Kyle, R. A., and Bayrd, E. D., 1961, "Primary" systemic amyloidosis and myeloma: Discussion of relationship and review of 81 cases, *Arch. Intern. Med.* **107**:344–353.

Kyle, R. A. and Bayrd E. D. 1975: Amyloidosis: review of 236 cases. *Med.* (Baltimore) **54**:271–299.

Kyle, R. A., and Bayrd, E. D., 1976, *The Monoclonal Gammopathies, Multiple Myeloma and Related Plasma-cell Disorders,* Charles C. Thomas, Springfield, Illinois.

Kyle, R. A., Nobrega, F. T., and Kurland, L. T., 1969, Multiple myeloma in Olmsted County, Minnesota, 1945–1964, *Blood* **33**:739–745.

Kyle, R. A., Pierre, R. V., and Bayrd, E. D., 1970, Multiple myeloma and acute myclononocytic leukemia: Report of four cases possibly related to melphalan, *N. Engl. J Med.* **283**:1121–1125.

Kyle, R. A., Maldonado, J. E., and Bayrd, E. D., 1973, Idiopathic Bence Jones proteinuria: A distinct entity?, *Am. J. Med.* **55**:222–226.

Kyle, R. A., Maldonado, J. E., and Bayrd, E. D., 1974a, Plasma cell leukemia: Report on 17 cases, *Arch. Intern. Med.* **133**:813–818.

Kyle, R. A., Pierre, R. V., and Bayrd, E. D., 1974b, Primary amyloidosis and acute leukemia associated with melphalan therapy, *Blood* **44**:333–337.

Kyle, R. A., Pierre, R. V., and Bayrd, E. D., 1975a, Multiple myeloma and acute leukemia associated with alkylating agents, *Arch. Intern. Med.* **135**:185–192.

Kyle, R. A., Seligman, B. R., Wallace, H. J., Jr., Silver, R. T., Glidewell, O., and Holland, J. F., 1975b, Multiple myeloma resistant to melphalan (NSC-8806) treated with cyclophosphamide (NSC-26271), prednisone (NSC-10023), and chloroquine (NSC-187208), *Cancer Chemother. Rep.* **59**:557–562.

Lackner, H., 1973, Hemostatic abnormalities associated with dysproteinemias, *Semin. Hematol.* **10**:125–133.

Ladefoged, A. J., Nielsen, B., and Pedersen, K., 1970, Akut nyreinsufficiens ved myelomatose, *Ugeskr. Laeg.* **132**:641–646.

Lai A Fat, R. F. M., Suurmond, D., Rádl, J., and van Furth, R., 1973, Scleromyxoedema (lichen myxoedematosus) associated with a paraprotein, IgG$_1$ of type kappa, *Br. J. Dermatol.* **88**:107–116.

Laird, A. K., 1964, Dynamics of tumor growth, *Br. J. Cancer* **18**:490.

Laird, A. K., 1965, Dynamics of tumor growth: Comparison of growth rates and extrapolation of growth curve to one cell, *Br. J. Cancer* **19**:278.

Lane, S. L., 1952, Plasmacytoma of the mandible, *Oral Surg.* **5**:134–142.

Larson, D. L., and Tomlinson, L. J., 1952, Quantitative antibody studies on man. II. Relation of serum proteins to antibody production, *J. Lab. Clin. Med.* **39**:129.

Laurell, C. B., 1961, Studies on abnormal serum globulins, *Acta Med. Scand.,* Suppl. 367, p. 17.

Law, I. P., Koch, F. J., Cannon, G. B., Herberman, R. B., and Oldham, R. K., 1976, Acute myelomonocytic leukemia associated with paraproteinemia, *Cancer* **37**(3):1359–1364.

Lawson, H. A., Stuart, C. A., Paull, A. M., Phillips, A. M., and Phillips, R. W., 1955, Observations on antibody content of blood in patients with multiple myeloma, *N. Engl. J. Med.* **252**:13.

Leader, R. W., Wagner, B. M., Henson, J. B., and Gorham, J. R., 1963, Structural and histochemical observations of liver and kidney in Aleutian disease of mink, *Am. J. Pathol.* **43**:33.

Lee, B. J., Sahakian, G., Clarkson, B. D., and Krakoff, I. H., 1974, Combination chemotherapy of multiple myeloma with Alkeran, Cytoxan, vincristine, prednisone, and BCNU, *Cancer* **33**:533–538.

Lessin, L. S., Hallal, J., Burkholder, P., and Cohen, H., 1972, Ultrastructural studies of the role of the reticuloendothelial (RE) cell in clinical resolution of amyloidosis, *Clin. Res.* **20**:512.

Levi, D. F., Williams, R. C., Jr., and Lindström, F. D., 1968, Immunofluorescent studies on the myeloma kidney with special reference to light chain disease, *Am. J. Med.* **44**:922–933.

Levin, M., Franklin, E. C., Frangione, B., and Pras, M., 1972, The amino acid sequence of a major nonimmunoglobulin component of some amyloid fibrils, *J. Clin. Invest.* **51**:2773–2776.

Levin, M., Pras, M., and Franklin, E. C., 1973, Immunologic studies of the major nonimmunoglobulin protein of amyloid. I. Identification and partial characterization of a related serum component, *J. Exp. Med.* **138**:373.

Lewis, A. F., Bergsagel, D. E., Bruce-Robertson, A., Schachter, R. K., and Connell, G. E., 1968, An atypical immunoglobulin, *Blood* **32**:189.

Lewis, E. B., 1963, Leukemia, multiple myeloma, and aplastic anemia in American radiologists, *Science* **142**:1492–1494.

Lewis, R. A., Falls, H. F., and Troyer, D. O., 1975, Ocular manifestations of hypercupremia associated with multiple myeloma, *Arch. Ophthalmol.* **93**:1050–1053.

Lewis, R. A., Hultquist, D. E., Baker, B. L., Falls, H. F., Gershowitz, H., and Penner, J. A., 1976, Hypercupremia associated with a monoclonal immunoglobulin, *J. Lab. Clin. Med.* **88**(3):375–388.

Lindqvist, K. J., Ragale, A. H., and Osterland, C. K., 1970, Paraproteinemia in a child with leukemia, *Blood* **35**:213–221.

Lindström, F. D., Hardy, W. R., Eberle, B. J. and Williams, R. C., Jr., 1973, Multiple myeloma and benign monoclonal gammopathy: Differentiation by immunofluorescence of lymphocytes, *Ann. Intern. Med.* **78**:837–844.

Loeper, M., Vignalou, J., and Borreau, T., 1947, Le myclome suite de traumatisme osseux et d'osteomyelite, *Prog. Med. (Paris)* **75**:51.

Lowbeer, L., 1969a, Occurrence of osteosclerosis in multiple myeloma, *Lab. Med. Bull. Pathol.*, pp. 396–397.

Lowbeer, L., 1969b, Osteosclerosis in multiple myeloma, *Am. J. Clin. Pathol.* **52**:757.

Loyau, G., Barre, J. P., L'Hirondel, J. L., Laniece, M., and Preud'homme, J. L., 1975, Maladie des chaines lourdes gamma: A propos d'une nouvelle observation, *Nouv. Presse Med.* **4**(13):957–959.

Lynch, P. J., and Winkelmann, R. K., 1966, Generalized plane xanthoma and systemic disease, *Arch. Dermatol.* **93**:639.

Lyons, R. M., Chaplin, H., Tillack, T. W., and Majerus, P. W., 1975, Gamma heavy chain disease: Rapid sustained response to cyclophosphamide and prednisone, *Blood* **46**:1–19.

MacKenzie, M. R., and Babcock, J., 1975, Studies of the hyperviscosity syndrome. II. Macroglobulinemia, *J. Lab. Clin. Med.* **85**:227–234.

MacKenzie, M. R., and Fudenberg, H. H., 1972, Macroglobulinemia: An analysis for forty patients, *Blood* **39**:874–889.

MacKenzie, M. R., Brown, E., and Fudenberg, H. H., 1968, Hypervolemia in the hyperviscosity syndrome of macroglobulinemia, *J. Clin. Invest.* **47**:64a.

MacKenzie, M. R., Fudenberg, H. H., and O'Reilly, R. A., 1970, The hyperviscosity syndrome. I. In IgG myeloma: The role of protein concentration and molecular shape, *J. Clin. Invest.* **49**:15.

MacMahon, B., and Clark, D. W., 1956, The incidence of multiple myeloma, *J. Chronic Dis.* **4**:508.

Maeda, K., Abesamis, C. M., Kuhn, L. M., and Hyun, B. H., 1973, Multiple myeloma in childhood: Report of a case with breast tumors as a presenting manifestation, *Am. J. Clin. Pathol.* **60**:552–558.

Magnus-Levy, A., 1931, Bence-Jones-Eiweiss und Amyloid, *Z. Klin. Med.* **116**:510–531.

Magnus-Levy, A., 1933, Multiple myeloma. VII. Euglobulinämie zur Klinik und Pathologie; Amyloidosis, *Z. Klin. Med.* **126**:62.

Magnus-Levy, A., 1952, Amyloidosis in multiple myeloma: Progress noted in 50 years of personal observation, *J. Mt. Sinai Hosp. N.Y.* **19**:8.

Maldonado, J. E., and Kyle, R. A., 1974, Familial myeloma: Report of eight families and a study of serum proteins in their relatives, *Am. J. Med.* **57**:875–884.

Maldonado, J., Bayrd, E. D., and Brown, A. L., 1965, The flaming cell in multiple myeloma: A light and electron microscopy study, *Am. J. Clin. Pathol.* **44**:605.

Maldonado, J., Kyle, R. A., Brown, A. L., and Bayrd, E. D., 1966, "Intermediate" cell types and mixed cell proliferations in multiple myeloma: Electron microscopic observations, *Blood* **27**:212.

Maldonado, J. E., Velosa, J. A., Kyle, R. A., Wagoner, R. D., Holly, K. E., and Salassa, R. M., 1975, Fanconi syndrome in adults: A manifestation of a latent form of myeloma, *Am. J. Med.* **58**:354–364.

Mangalik, A., and Veliath, A. J., 1971, Osteosclerotic myeloma and peripheral neuropathy: A case report, *Cancer* **28**:1040–1045.

Mangalik, A., and Gupta, P. K., 1974, Soft tissue involvement in plasmacytoma and multiple myeloma: A report of seven cases, *Indian J. Pathol. Bacteriol.* **17**(1):45–53.

Marks, J., 1953, Antibody formation in myelomatosis, *J. Clin. Pathol.* **6**:62–63.

Marlen, R. H., 1963, Xanthomatosis and myelomatosis, *Proc. R. Soc. Med.* **55**:318.

Martelo, O. J., Schultz, D. R., Pardo, V., and Perez-Stable, E., 1975, Immunologically-mediated renal disease in Waldenström's macroglobulinemia, *Am. J. Med.* **58**(4):567–575.

Martin, N. H., 1960, Macroglobulinemia: A clinical and pathological study, *Q. J. Med.* **29**:179.

Mason, T. J., McKay, F. W., Hoover, R., Blot, W. J., and Fraumeni, J. F., Jr., 1976, Atlas of cancer mortality for U.S. Counties: 1950–1969, Publication No. (NIH) 75-780, Department of Health, Education and Welfare, Washington, D.C.

Mass, R. E., 1962, A comparison of the effect of prednisone and a placebo in the treatment of multiple myeloma, *Cancer Chemother. Rep.* **16**:257.

Massry, S. G., Mueller, E., Silverman, A. G., and Kleeman, C. R., 1968, Inorganic phosphate treatment of hypercalcemia, *Arch. Intern. Med.* **121**:307–312.

Mathews, J. W., Jr., and Oliver, C. A., 1974, Osteoblastic multiple myeloma, *South. Med. J.* **67**:318.

Matsuoka, Y., Moore, G. E., Yagi, Y., and Pressman, D., 1967, Production of free light chains of immunoglobulins by a mematopoietic cell line derived from a patient with multiple myeloma, *Proc. Soc. Exp. Biol. Med.* **125**:1246.

McArthur, J. R., Athens, J. W., Wintrobe, M. M., and Cartwright, G. E., 1970, Melphalan and myeloma: Experience with a low-dose continuous regimen, *Ann. Intern. Med.* **72**:665.

McCallister, B. D., Bayrd, E. D., Harrison, E. G., Jr., and McGuckin, W. F., 1967, Primary macroglobulinemia: Review with a report of thirty-one cases and notes on the value of continuous chlorambucil therapy, *Am. J. Med.* **43**:394–434.

McCarthy, J. T., Osserman, E. F., Lombardo, P. C., and Takatsuki, K., 1964, An abnormal serum globulin in lichen myxedematosus, *Arch. Dermatol.* **89**:446.

McCuistion, C. H., and Schoch, E. P., Jr., 1956, Autopsy findings in lichen myxedematosus, *Arch. Dermatol.* **74**:259.

McDougal, J. S., Hardisdangkul, V., and Christian, C. L., 1975, Naturally occurring low molecular weight IgM in patients with rheumatoid arthritis, systemic lupus erythematosus, and macroglobulinemia. II. Structural studies and comparison of some physiochemical properties of reduced and alkylated IgM, and low molecular weight IgM, *J. Immunol.* **115**:223–229.

McFadzean, R. M., 1975, Orbital plasma cell myeloma, *Br. J. Ophthalmol.* **59**(3):164–165.

McGrath, M. A., and Penny, R., 1976, Blood hyperviscosity and clinical manifestations, *J. Clin. Invest.* **58**:1155–1162.

McIntire, K. R., and Princler, G. L., 1969, Prolonged adjuvant stimulation in germ free BALB/c mice: Development of plasma cell neoplasia, *Immunology* **17**:181.

McLauchlan, J., 1973, Solitary myeloma of the clavicle with long survival after total excision: Report of a case, *J. Bone Joint Surg. Br. Vol.* **55**:357–358.

McPhedran, P., Heath, C. W., Jr., and Garcia, J., 1972, Multiple myeloma incidence in metropolitan Atlanta, Georgia: Racial and seasonal variations, *Blood* **39**:866.

Medical Research Council, 1971, Myelomatosis: Comparison of melphalan and cyclophosphamide therapy, *Br. Med. J.* **1**:640.

Medical Research Council, 1973, Working Party for Therapeutic Trials in Leukaemia, Report on the first myelomatosis trial. I. Analysis of presenting features of prognostic importance, *Br. J. Haematol.* **21**:123–139.

Mellors, R. C., 1965, Autoimmune disease in NZB/B1 mice. I. Pathology and pathogenesis of a model system of spontaneous glomerulonephritis, *J. Exp. Med.* **122**:25.

Mellors, R. C., 1966, Autoimmune disease in NZB/B1 mice. II. Autoimmunity and malignant lymphoma, *Blood* **27**:435.

Mellors, R. C., and Huang, C. Y., 1966, Immunopathology of NZB/B1 mice. V. Virus-like (filterable) agent separable from lymphoma cells and identifiable by electron microscopy, *J. Exp. Med.* **124**:1031.

Mellors, R. C., and Huang, C. Y., 1967, Immunopathology of NZB/B1 mice. VI. Virus separable from spleen and pathogenic for Swiss mice, *J. Exp. Med.* **126**:53.

Mellors, R. C., Aoki, T., and Huebner, R. J., 1969, Further implications of murine leukemia-like virus in the disorders of NZB mice, *J. Exp. Med.* **129**:1045.

Mellstedt, H., Hammarström, S., and Holm, G., 1974, Monoclonal lymphocyte population in human plasma cell myeloma, *Clin. Exp. Immunol.* **17**:371–384.

Mellstedt, H., Pettersson, D., and Holm, G., 1976, Monoclonal B-lymphocytes in peripheral blood of patients with plasma cell myeloma: Relation to activity of the disease, *Scand. J. Haematol.* **16**:112–120.

Menache, D., and Boivin, P., 1962, Deficit acquis en facteur X chez un malade atteint d'amylose primitive: Injection d'une fraction C.S.B., *Nouv. Rev. Fr. Hematol.* **2**:868–887.

709

BIOLOGY, CLINICAL
PATTERNS, AND
TREATMENT OF
MULTIPLE MYELOMA
AND RELATED
PLASMA-CELL
DYSCRASIAS

Menkes, C. J., Herreman, G., Preud'homme, J. L., Godeau, P., and Delbarre, F., 1972, Myélome à plasmocytes non excrétants (à propos de deux nouvelles observations), *Nouv. Presse Med.* 1:309–312.

Meyers, B. R., Hirschman, S. Z., and Axelrod, J. A., 1972, Current patterns of infection in multiple myeloma, *Am. J. Med.* **52**:87–92.

Michaux, J. L., and Heremans, J. F., 1969, Thirty cases of monoclonal immunoglobulin disorders other than myeloma or macroglobulinemia: A classification of diseases associated with the production of monoclonal-type immunoglobulins, *Am. J. Med.* **46**:562–579.

Midwest Cooperative Chemotherapy Group, 1964, Multiple myeloma, *J. Am. Med. Assoc.* **188**:741.

Miescher, P. A., and Farquet, J. J., 1974, Chronic myelomonocytic leukemia in adults, *Semin. Hematol.* **11**:129–139.

Migliore, P. J., and Alexanian, R., 1968, Monoclonal gammopathy in human neoplasia, *Cancer* **21**:1127.

Mihaesco, C., Mihaesco, E., Miglierina, R., Lamaziere, J., Roy, J. P., and Seligmann, M., 1976, Physiochemical and immunological properties of a mu chain disease protein, *Immunochemistry* **13**(1):39–45.

Missmahl, H. P., and Hartwig, M., 1953, *Virchows Arch. Pathol. Anat. Physiol.* **324**:480.

Moertel, C. G., 1966, Multiple primary malignant neoplasms, their incidence and significance, *Recent Results Cancer Res.* **7**:1–108.

Morgan, C., Jr., and Hammack, W. J., 1966, Intravenous urography in multiple myeloma, *N. Engl. J. Med.* **275**:77–79.

Moss, W. T., and Ackerman, L. V., 1946, Plasma cell leukemia, *Blood* **1**:396.

Mundy, G. R., Lulien, R. A., Raisz, L. G., Oppenheim, J. J., and Buell, D. N., 1974a, Bone resolving activity in supernatants from lymphoid cell lines, *N. Engl. J. Med.* **290**:867–871.

Mundy, G. R., Raisz, L. G., Cooper, R. A., Schechter, G. P., and Salmon, S. E., 1974b, Evidence for the secretion of an osteoclast stimulating factor in myeloma, *N. Engl. J. Med.* **291**:1041–1046.

Myers, G. H., Jr., and Witten, D. M., 1971, Acute renal failure after excretory urography in multiple myeloma (editorial), *Am. J. Roentgenol. Radium Ther. Nucl. Med.* **113**:583–588.

Namba, Y., and Hanaoka, M., 1969, Immunoglobulin synthesis by cultured mouse myeloma cells, *J. Immunol.* **102**:1486.

Narasimhan, P., Jagathambal, K., Elizalde, A. M., and Rosner, F., 1975, Chronic lymphocytic leukemia and lymphosarcoma associated with multiple myeloma: Report of three cases, *Arch. Intern. Med.* **135**(5):729–732.

Nathans, D., Fahey, J. L., and Potter, M., 1958, The formation of myeloma protein by a mouse plasma cell tumor, *J. Exp. Med.* **108**:121–129.

New England Journal of Medicine, 1972, Case records of the Massachusetts General Hospital, Case 29-1972, **287**:138–143.

New England Journal of Medicine, 1976, Case records of the Massachusetts General Hospital, Case 18-1976, **294**:998–1002.

Nishiyama, H., Anderson, R. E., Ishimaru, T., Ishida, K., Ii, Y., and Okabe, N., 1973, The incidence of malignant lymphoma and multiple myeloma in Hiroshima and Nagasaki atomic bomb survivors, *Cancer* **32**:1301–1309.

Nosonoff, A., Hopper, J. E., and Spring, S. B., 1975, *The Antibody Molecule*, Academic Press, New York.

Nutter, D. O., and Kramer, N. C., 1965, Macrocryogelglobulinemia: Report of a case, with unusual spontaneous recovery, *Am. J. Med.* **38**:462.

von Oberdorfer, A., Schnauffer, K., Lange, H.-J., und Neiss, A., 1973, Zur Verteilung von Paraproteinamien nach Geschlecht und Alter der Patienten, Paraprotein-Klassen, -Subklassen und Leichtketten-Typen. *Z. Klin. Chem. Klin. Biochem.* **11**:51–64.

O'Bryan, R. M., Luce, J. K., Talley, R. W., Gottlieb, J. A., Baker, L. H., and Bonadonna, G., 1973, Phase II evaluation of adriamycin in human neoplasia, *Cancer* **32**:1–8.

Olesen, H., 1964, Chlorambucil treatment in the cold agglutinin syndrome, *Scand. J. Haematol.* **1**:116.

Osgood, E. E., 1960, Survival time of patients with plasmacytic myeloma, *Cancer Chemother. Rep.* **9**:1.

Osserman, E. F., 1958, Natural history of multiple myeloma before radiological evidence of disease, *Radiology* **71**:157.

Osserman, E. F., 1959, Plasma-cell myeloma. II. Clinical aspects, *N. Engl. J. Med.* **261**:952 and 1006.

Osserman, E. F., 1961, The plasmacytic dyscrasias, *Am. J. Med.* **31**:671.

711

BIOLOGY, CLINICAL
PATTERNS, AND
TREATMENT OF
MULTIPLE MYELOMA
AND RELATED
PLASMA-CELL
DYSCRASIAS

Osserman, E. F., 1967, The association between plasmacytic and monocytic discrasias in man: Clinical and biochemical studies, in: *Nobel Symposium 3: Gamma Globulins: Structure and Control of Biosynthesis* (J. Killander, ed.), p. 573, Almquist and Wiksell, Stockholm.

Osserman, E. F., 1969, Clinical and biochemical studies of plasmacytic and monocytic dyscrasias and their interrelationships, *Trans. Coll. Physicians Philadelphia* **36**:134.

Osserman, E. F., 1971, Multiple myeloma and related plasma cell dyscrasias, in: *Immunological Diseases*, 3rd Ed. (M. Samter, ed.), pp. 520–547, Little, Brown and Company, Boston.

Osserman, E. F., 1976, Analysis of amyloid-related Bence-Jones proteins (TEW BJκ and MCG BJλ) and the "non-immunoglobulin" amyloid protein (AUO); hypervariable region homologies and their possible significance, in: *Amyloidosis* (O. Vegelius and A. Pasternack, eds.), p. 223, Academic Press, London.

Osserman, E. F., and Farhangi, M., 1972, Plasma cell myeloma, in: *Hematology* (Williams, Beutler, Erslev, and Rundles, eds.), pp. 956–968, McGraw-Hill, New York.

Osserman, E. F., and Farhangi, M., 1975, Plasma cell and monocyte (mono-myelocyte) dyscrasias and their specific protein markers—monoclonal immunoglobulins and lysozyme, in: *Excerpta Medica Int. Congr. Ser.*, No. 349, Vol. 1, *Cell Biology and Tumor Immunology: Proceedings of the 12th International Cancer Congress*, Florence 1974 (P. Buculossi, U. Verones', and N. Cascinelli, eds.), pp. 142–148, Excerpta Medica, Amsterdam.

Osserman, E. F., and Lawlor, D. P., 1966, Serum and urinary lysozyme (muramidase) in monocytic and monomyelocytic leukemia, *J. Exp. Med.* **124**:921.

Osserman, E. F., and Takatsuki, K., 1963a, Plasma cell myeloma: Gamma globulin synthesis and structure, *Medicine (Baltimore)* **42**:357.

Osserman, E. F., and Takatsuki, K., 1963b, Role of an abnormal, myeloma-type serum gamma globulin in the pathogenesis of the skin lesions of papular mucinosis (lichen myxedematosus), *J. Clin. Invest.* **42**:962.

Osserman, E. F., and Takatsuki, K., 1964, Clinical and immunochemical studies of four cases of heavy (H γ-²) chain disease, *Am. J. Med.* **37**:351–373.

Osserman, E. F., and Takatsuki, K., 1965, Considerations regarding the pathogenesis of the plasmacytic dyscrasias, *Scand. J. Haematol.* **4**(Suppl.):28.

Osserman, E. F., Talal, N., and Takatsuki, K., 1961, Amyloidosis: Tissue proteinosis: Gammaloidosis (editorial), *Ann. Intern. Med.* **55**:1033.

Osserman, E. F., Takatsuki, K., and Talal, N., 1964, The pathogenesis of "amyloidosis": Studies on the role of abnormal gammaglobulins and gammaglobulin fragments of the Bence-Jones (L-polypeptide) types in the pathogenesis of "primary" and "secondary" amyloidosis associated with plasma cell myeloma, *Semin. Hematol.* **1**:3.

Osserman, E. F., Isobe, T., and Farhangi, M., 1976, Effect of dimethyl sulfoxide (DMSO) in the treatment of amyloidosis, in: *Amyloidosis* (O. Vegelius and A. Pasternack, eds.), p. 553, Academic Press, London.

Osterland, C. K., Miller, E. J., Karakawa, W. W., and Krause, R. M., 1966, Characteristics of streptococcal group-specific antibody isolated from hyperimmune rabbits, *J. Exp. Med.* **123**: 599.

Ottó, S., Puskás, É., Medgyeski, G. A., and Gergely, J., 1972, Diclonal and multiple gammopathies, *Haematologia (Budapest)* **6**:471–487.

Ottolander, G. J. H. Den, and Perret, L. J., 1965, Verworven hemorragische idathese ten gevolge van geisoleerde factor X-deficientie, *Med. Tijdschr. Geneeskd.* **109**:852–854.

Ozer, F. L., and Chaplin, H., 1963, Agglutination of stored erythrocytes by a human serum, characterization of the serum factor and erythocyte changes, *J. Clin. Invest.* **42**:1735.

Pachter, M. R., Johnson, S. A., Neblett, T. R., and Truant, J. P., 1959a, Bleeding, platelets, and macroglobulinemia, *Am. J. Clin. Pathol.* **31**:467.

Pachter, M. R., Johnson, S. A., and Basinski, D. H., 1959b, The effect of macroglobulins and their dissociation units on release of platelet factor 3, *Thromb. Diath. Haemorrh.* **3**:501.

Pambor, M., and Höfs, W., 1968, Lichen myxoedematosus mit konsekutivem Skleromyxödem Arndt Gottron bei Paraproteinämie, seroaktiver Toxoplasmose und Myokardhypoxie, *Arch. Klin. Exp. Dermatol.* **232**:127.

Pankovich, A. M., and Griem, M. L., 1972, Plasma-cell myeloma: A thirty-year follow-up, *Radiology* **104**:521–522.

Paraf, A., Coste, T., Rautureau, J., and Texier, J., 1970, La régression de l'amylose: Disparition d'une amylose hépatique massive après nephrectomie pour cancer, *Presse Med.* **78**:547–548.

Parker, A. C., 1973, A case of acute myelomonocytic leukaemia associated with myelomatosis, *Scand. J. Haematol.* **11**:257–260.

Parr, D. M., Percy, M. E., and Connell, G. E., 1972, A human immunoglobulin G with deletions in both heavy and light polypeptide chains, *Immunochemistry* **9**:51–63.

Parson, D. F., Darden, E. B., Jr., Lindsley, D. L., Pratt, G. T., and Edwards, M. P., 1960, Electron microscopy of plasma-cell tumors of the mouse. I. MPC-1 and X5563 tumors, *J. Biophys. Biochem. Cytol.* **9**:353–368.

Pasmantier, M. W., and Azar, H. A., 1969, Extraskeletal spread in multiple plasma cell myeloma: A review of 57 autopsied cases, *Cancer* **23**:167–174.

Pearse, A. G. E., Ewen, S. W. B., and Polak, J. M., 1972, The genesis apudamyloid in endocrine polypeptide tumors: Histochemical distinction from immunoamyloid, *Virchows Arch. Pathol. Anat.* **B10**:93.

Pechet, L., and Kastrul, J. J., 1964, Amyloidosis associated with factor X (Stuart) deficiency, *Ann. Intern. Med.* **61**:315–318.

Pedio, G., Grieshaber, E., and Ruttner, J. R., 1968, On plasmacytoma-oncogenesis of mice. II. Differential ultracentrifugate which contains RNA virus-like particles from HIPA tumor, inducing a plasmacytoid neoplasia in BALB/c mice, *Pathol. Microbiol.* **32**:241.

Pengelly, C. D., Mondal, B. K., and Barua, A. R., 1973, Hemolytic anemia in myelomatosis, *Postgrad. Med. J.* **49**:279–281.

Penn, G. M., Kunkel, H. G., and Grey, H. M., 1970, Sharing of individual antigenic determinants between a gamma G and a gamma M protein in a myeloma serum, *Proc. Soc. Exp. Biol. Med.* **135**:660.

Penny, R., Castaldi, P. A., and Whitsed, H. M., 1971, Inflammation and haemostasis in paraproteinaemias, *Br. J. Haematol.* **20**:35–44.

Perkins, H. A., MacKenzie, M. R., and Fudenberg, H. H., 1970, Hemostatic defects in dysproteinemias, *Blood* **35**:695.

Perlia, C. P., Gubisch, N. J., Wolter, J., Edelberg, D., Dederick, M. M., and Taylor, S. G., 1970, Mithramycin treatment of hypercalcemia, *Cancer* **25**:389–394.

Perry, H. O., Montgomery, H., and Stickney, J. M., 1960, Further observations on lichen myxedematosus, *Ann. Intern. Med.* **53**: 955.

Perry, M. C., and Farhangi, M., 1976 (unpublished case).

Petite, J., and Cruchaud, A., 1969–1970, Qualitative and quantitative abnormalities of immunoglobulins in relatives of patients with idiopathic paraproteinemia: A study of 12 families, *Helv. Med. Acta* **35**:248.

Pilgrim, H. I., 1965, The relationship of chronic ulceration of the ileocecal junction to the development of reticuloendothelial tumors in C_3H mice, *Cancer Res.* **25**:53.

Pirofsky, B., 1969, *Autoimmunization and Autoimmune Hemolytic Anemias,* pp. 127–131, Williams and Wilkins Co., Baltimore.

Porter, D. D., Dixon, F. J., and Larsen, A. E., 1965, The development of a myeloma-like condition in mink with Aleutian disease, *Blood* **25**:736.

Potter, M., 1962, Plasma cell neoplasia in a single host: A mosaic of different protein-producing cell types, *J. Exp. Med.* **115**:339.

Potter, M., 1972, Immunoglobulin-producing tumors and myeloma proteins of mice, *Physiol. Res.* **52**:631.

Potter, M., 1973a, The developmental history of the neoplastic plasma cell in mice: A brief review of recent developments, *Semin. Hematol.* **10**:19.

Potter, M., 1973b, Antigen binding M-components in man and mouse, in: *Multiple Myeloma and Related Disorders* (H. A. Azar and M. Potter, eds.), pp. 195–246, Harper and Row, New York.

Potter, M., and Boyce, C. R., 1962, Induction of plasma-cell neoplasms in strain BALB/c mice with mineral oil and mineral-oil adjuvants, *Nature (London)* **193**:1086.

Potter, M., and Leon, M. A., 1968, Three IgA myeloma immunoglobulins from the BALB/c mouse: Precipitation with pneumococcal C polysaccharide, *Science* **162**:369.

Potter, M., and MacCardle, R. C., 1964, Histology of developing plasma cell neoplasia induced by mineral oil in BALB/c mice, *J. Natl. Cancer Inst.* **33**:497.

713

BIOLOGY, CLINICAL
PATTERNS, AND
TREATMENT OF
MULTIPLE MYELOMA
AND RELATED
PLASMA-CELL
DYSCRASIAS

Potter, M., and Robertson, C. L., 1960, Development of plasma-cell neoplasms in BALB/c mice after intraperitoneal injection of paraffin-oil adjuvant, heat killed *Staphylococcus* mixtures, *J. Natl. Cancer Inst.* **25**:847.

Potter, M., Fahey, J. L., and Pilgrim, H. I., 1957, Abnormal serum protein and bone destruction in transmissible mouse plasma-cell neoplasm, *Proc. Soc. Exp. Biol. Med.* **94**:327.

Poulik, D., Berman, L., and Prasad, A. S., 1969, "Myeloma protein" in a patient with monocytic leukemia, *Blood* **33**:746.

Pratt, P. W., Estren, S., and Kochwa, S., 1968, Immunoglobulin abnormalities in Gaucher's disease: Report of 16 cases, *Blood* **31**:633–640.

Preud'homme, J. L., and Seligmann, M., 1972, Immunoglobulins on the surface of lymphoid cells in Waldenström's macroglobulinemia, *J. Clin. Invest.* **51**:701–705.

Preud'homme, J. L., Buxbaum, J., and Scharff, M. O., 1973, Mutagenesis of mouse myeloma cells with "melphalan," *Nature (London)* **245**:320.

Pringle, J. P., Graham, R. C., and Bernier, G. M., 1974, Detection of myeloma cells in the urine sediment, *Blood* **43**:137–143.

Pruzanski, W., and Katz, A., 1976, Clinical and laboratory findings in primary generalized and multiple-myeloma-related amyloidosis, *Can. Med. Assoc. J.* **114**:906–909.

Pruzanski, W., Platts, M. E., and Ogryzlo, M. A., 1969, Leukemic form of immunocytic dyscrasia (plasma cell leukemia): A study of ten cases and a review of the literature, *Am. J. Med.* **47**:60–74.

Pruzanski, W., Warren, R. F., Goldie, J. H. and Katz, A., 1973, Malabsorption syndrome with infiltration of the intestinal wall by extracellular monoclonal macroglobulin, *Am. J. Med.* **54**:811–818.

Pruzanski, W., Underdown, B., Silver, E. H., and Katz, A., 1974, Macroglobulinemia–myeloma double gammopathy: A study of four cases and a review of the literature, *Am. J. Med.* **57**:259–266.

Putnam, F. W., Whitley, E. J., Jr., Paul, C., and Davidson, J. N., 1973, Amino acid sequence of a Bence Jones protein from a case of primary amyloidosis, *Biochemistry* **12**:3763.

Radl, J., Masopust, J., Houstek, J., and Hrodek, O., 1967, Paraproteinaemia and unusual dys-γ-globulinaemia in a case of Wiskott–Aldrich syndrome. *Arch. Dis. Child.* **42**:608.

Ravid, M., Kedar (Keizman), I., and Sohar, E., 1977, Effect of a single dose of dimethyl sulfoxide on renal amyloidosis, *Lancet* **1**(8014):730–731.

Rees, E. D., and Waugh, W. H., 1965, Factors in the renal failure of multiple myeloma, *Arch. Intern. Med.* **116**:400–405.

Richardson, E. P., Jr., and Johnson, P. C., 1975, Atypical progressive multifocal leukoencephalopathy with plasma-cell infiltrates, *Acta Neuropathol. Suppl.* **6/247-250**:2784.

Ritzmann, S. E., Loukas, D., Sakai, H., Daniels, J. C., and Levin, W. C., 1975, Idiopathic (asymptomatic) monoclonal gammopathies, *Arch. Intern. Med.* **135**:95–106.

Rivers, S. L., and Patno, M. E., 1969, Cyclophosphamide vs. melphalan in treatment of plasma cell myeloma, *J. Am. Med. Assoc.* **207**:1328.

Rochant, H., Tonthat, H., Etrevenant, M. F., Intrator, L., Sylvestre, R., and Dryfus, B., 1972, Lambda cold agglutinin with anti-A1 specificity in a patient with a reticulo-sarcoma, *Vox Sang.* **1**:45.

Rogers, J. S., II., Spahr, J., Judge, D. M., Varano, L. A., and Eyster, M. E., 1977, IgE myeloma with osteoblastic lesions, *Blood* **49**:295–299.

Roman, W., and Coles, M., 1966, Paraproteins in folic-acid deficiency, *Lancet* **1**:211–212.

Rondier, J., Simon, F., Cayla, J., Diebold, J., Bontoux, D., and Delbarre, F., 1975, Myeloma and osteocondensation (apropos of 2 cases), *Sem. Hop.* **51**(3):157–167 (English abstract).

Rosenthal, C. J., Franklin, E. C., Frangione, B., and Greenspan, J., 1976, Isolation and partial characterization of SAA—an amyloid-related protein from human serum, *J. Immunol.* **116**:1415–1418.

Rosner, F., and Grünwald, H., 1974 (for Acute Leukemia Group B), Multiple myeloma terminating in acute leukemia: Report of 12 cases and review of the literature, *Am. J. Med.* **57**:927–939.

Rowe, D. S., and Fahey, J. L., 1965, A new class of human immunoglobulins. I. A unique myeloma protein, *J. Exp. Med.* **121**:171–184.

Ruben, R. J., Distenfeld, A., Berg, P., and Carr, R., 1969, Sudden sequential deafness as the presenting symptom of macroglobulinemia, *J. Am. Med. Assoc.* **209**:1364.

Rudders, R. A., Yakulis, V., and Heller, P., 1973, Double myeloma: Production of both IgG type lambda and IgA type lambda myeloma proteins by a single plasma cell line, *Am. J. Med.* **55**:215.

Rundles, R. W., and Coonrad, E. F., 1957, The treatment of multiple myeloma, in: *Proceedings of the Third National Cancer Conference*, p. 389, J. B. Lippincott, Philadelphia.

Rundles, R. W., Dillon, M. L., and Dillon, E. S., 1950, Multiple myeloma. III. Effect of urethane therapy on plasma cell growth, abnormal serum protein components and Bence Jones proteinuria, *J. Clin. Invest.* **29**:1243.

Ryder, R. J. W., 1966, Chronic monocytic leukemia, *Blut* **14**:47.

Rywlin, A. M., Civantos, F., Ortega, R. S., and Ocminguez, C. J., 1975, Bone marrow histology in monoclonal macroglobulinemia, *Am. J. Clin. Pathol.* **63**(6):769–778.

Saidi, P., Uhlman, W. E., and Goldberg, I., 1973, Herpes zoster and multiple myeloma, *J. Med. Soc. N.J.* **70**:836–838.

Salmon, S. E., 1973, Immunoglobulin synthesis and tumor kinetics of multiple myeloma, *Semin. Hematol.* **10**:135–147.

Salmon, S. E., 1975, Expansion of the growth fraction in multiple myeloma with alkylating agents, *Blood* **45**:119–129.

Salmon, S. E., 1976, Nitrosoureas in multiple myeloma, *Cancer Treatment Rep.* **60**:789–794.

Salmon, S. E., and Durie, B. G. M., 1975, Cellular kinetics in multiple myeloma: A new approach to staging and treatment, *Arch. Intern. Med.* **135**:131–138.

Salmon, S. E., and Fudenberg, H. H., 1969, Abnormal nucleic acid metabolism of lymphocytes in plasma cell myeloma and macroglobulinemia, *Blood* **33**:300–312.

Salmon, S. E., and Smith, B. A., 1970a, Immunoglobulin synthesis and total body tumor cell number in IgG multiple myeloma, *J. Clin. Invest.* **49**:1114–1121.

Salmon, S. E., and Smith, B. A., 1970b, Sandwich solid phase radioimmunoassays for the characterization of human immunoglobulins synthesized *in vitro, J. Immunol.* **104**:665.

Salmon, S. E., Samal, B. A., Hayes, D. M., Hosley, H., Miller, S. P., and Schilling, A., 1967, Role of gamma globulin for immunoprophylaxis in multiple myeloma, *N. Engl. J. Med.* **277**:1336.

Salmon, S. E., Mackey, G., and Fudenberg, H. H., 1969, "Sandwich" solid phase radioimmunoassay for the quantitative determination of human immunoglobulins, *J. Immunol.* **103**:129.

Sanders, J. H., Fahey, J. L., Finegold, L., Ein, D., Reisfeld, R., and Berard, C., 1969, Multiple anomalous immunoglobulins, clinical structural and cellular studies in three patients, *Am. J. Med.* **47**:43.

Schneider, W., and Missmahl, H. P., 1966, Leichen amyloidosis als Beispiel der perikollagenen, primären, hautbeschränkten und vorweigend umschriebenen Amyloidose, *Arch. Klin. Exp. Dermatol.* **224**:235.

Schobel, B., and Wewalka, F., 1965, Temporäre "kryptogenetische" Paraproteinämie, *Schweiz. Med. Wochenschr.* **95**:1301–1304.

Schubert, G. E., and Adam, A., 1974, Glomerular nodules and long-spacing collagen in kidneys of patients with multiple myeloma, *J. Clin. Pathol.* **27**:800–805.

Schubert, G. E., Veigel, J., and Lennert, K., 1972, Structure and function of the kidney in multiple myeloma, *Virchows Arch. A* **355**:135–157.

Schubothe, H., 1966, The cold hemagglutinin disease, *Semin. Hematol.* **3**:27.

Seitanichs, B. A., Shulman, G., and Hobbs, J. R., 1970, Low serum cholesterol with IgA-myelomatosis, *Clin. Chim. Acta* **29**:93.

Seligmann, M., 1975, Immunochemical, clinical and pathological features of α-chain disease, *Arch. Intern. Med.* **135**:78–82.

Seligmann, M., and Basch, A., 1968, The clinical significance of pathological immunoglobulins, plenary session papers, in: *Twelfth Congress of the International Society of Hematology* (E. R. Jaffé, ed.), p. 21–31, Grune & Stratton, New York.

Seligmann, M., and Brouet, J. C., 1973, Antibody activities of human myeloma globulin, *Semin. Hematol.* **10**:163.

Seligmann, M., Danon, F., and Clauvel, J. P., 1971, Natural history of monoclonal immunoglobulins (Myeloma Workshop), *Br. Med. J.* **2**:321.

Seon, B. K., Yagi, Y., and Pressman, D. J., 1973, Comparative chemical study of α-μ chains from a single patient (SC), *J. Immunol.* **111**:1285.

Shanbrom, E., Miller, S., and Haar, H., 1960, Herpes zoster in hematologic neoplasias: Some unusual manifestations. *Ann. Intern. Med.* **53**:523–533.

Shaw, M. T., Twele, T. W., and Nordquist, R. E., 1974, Plasma cell leukemia: Detailed studies and response to therapy. *Cancer* **33**:619–625.

715

BIOLOGY, CLINICAL
PATTERNS, AND
TREATMENT OF
MULTIPLE MYELOMA
AND RELATED
PLASMA-CELL
DYSCRASIAS

Shustik, C., Bergsagel, D. E., and Pruzanski, W., 1976, κ and λ light chain disease: Survival rates and clinical manifestations, *Blood* **48**:41–51.

Simpson-Harren, L., and Lloyd, H. H., 1970, Kinetic parameter and growth curves for experimental tumor systems, *Cancer Chemother. Rep.* **54**:143–150.

Skvaril, F., Morell, A., and Barandun, S., 1972, The IgG subclass distribution in 659 myeloma sera, *Vox Sang.* **23**:546.

Sletten, K., Husby, G., and Natvig, J. B., 1976a, The complete amino acid sequence of an amyloid fibril protein AAl of unusual size (64 residues), *Biochem. Biophys. Res. Commun.* **69**:19–25.

Sletten, K., Westermark, P., and Natvig, J. B., 1976b, Characterization of amyloid fibril proteins from medullary carcinoma of the thyroid, *J. Exp. Med.* **143**:993–998.

Smetana, K., Gyorkey, F., Gyorkey, P., and Busch, H., 1973, Ultrastructural studies on human myeloma plasmacytes, *Cancer Res.* **33**:2300–2309.

Smith, E., Kochwa, S., and Wasserman, L. R., 1965, Aggregation of IgG globulin *in vivo*. I. The hyperviscosity syndrome in multiple myeloma, *Am. J. Med.* **39**:35.

Smithies, O., Gibson, D., Fanning, E. M., Goodfliesh, R. M., Gilman, J. G., and Ballantyne, D. L., 1971, Quantitative procedures for use with the Edman-Begg sequenator. Partial sequences of two unusual immunoglobulin light chains, Rzf and Sac. *Biochemistry* **10**:4912.

Snapper, I., and Kahn, A., 1971, *Myelomatosis. Fundamentals and Clinical Features,* University Park Press, Baltimore.

Snapper, I., Turner, L. B., and Moscovitz, H. L., 1953, *Multiple Myeloma,* Grune & Stratton, New York.

Solomon, A., 1976, Bence-Jones proteins and light chains of immunoglobulins, *N. Engl. J. Med.* **294**:91–98.

Solomon, A., and Fahey, J. L., 1963, Plasmapheresis therapy in macroglobulinemia, *Ann. Intern. Med.* **58**:789–800.

Solomon, A., and Kunkel, H. G., 1967, A "monoclonal" type low molecular weight protein related to γM-macroglobulins, *Am. J. Med.* **42**:958–967.

Solomon, A., Waldmann, T. A., Fahey, J. L., and McFarlane, A. S., 1964. Metabolism of Bence Jones proteins, *J. Clin. Invest.* **43**:103–117.

Solomon, A., McLaughlin, C. L., and Capra, J. D., 1975, Bence proteins and light chains of immunoglobulins. XI. A transient Bence Jones-related protein associated with corticosteroid therapy, *J. Clin. Invest.* **55**:579–585.

Somer, T., 1975, Hyperviscosity syndrome in plasma cell dyscrasias, *Adv. Microcirc.* **6**:1–55.

Sorenson, G. D., 1961, Electron microscopic observations of viral particles within myeloma cells of man, *Exp. Cell Res.* **25**:219.

Sorenson, G. D., 1965, Virus-like particles in myeloma cells of man, *Proc. Soc. Exp. Biol. Med.* **118**:250.

Soria, J., Soria, C., Samama, M., Fine, J. M., and Bousser, J., 1975, Analysis of fibrin abnormality in case of multiple myeloma, *Scand. J. Haematol.* **15**:207–218.

Spalter, H. F., 1959, Abnormal serum proteins, and retinal vein thrombosis, *Arch. Ophthalmol.* **62**:868.

Spengler, G. A., Bütler, R., Fischer, C., Ryssel, H. J., Schmid, E., and Siebner, H., 1966–1967, On the question of familial occurrence of paraproteinemia, *Helv. Med. Acta* **33**:208.

Spiro, D., 1959, The structural basis of proteinuria in man: Electron microscopic studies of renal biopsy specimens from patients with lipid nephrosis, amyloidosis, and subacute and chronic glomerulonephritis, *Am. J. Pathol.* **35**:47.

Staples, P. J., and Talal, N., 1969, Relative inability to induce tolerance in adult NZB and NZB/NZW F_1 mice, *J. Exp. Med.* **129**:123.

Stein, R. S., Ellman, L., and Bloch, K. J., 1975, The clinical correlates of IgM M-components: An analysis of thirty-four patients, *Am. J. Med. Sci.* **269**:209–216.

Stites, D. P., and Whitehouse, M. J., 1975, Evolution of multiple myeloma with nonsecreted paraproteins, *Clin. Res.* **23**:283A (abstract).

Stone, M. J., and Frenkel, E. P., 1975, The clinical spectrum of light chain myeloma: A study of 35 patients with special reference to the occurrence of amyloidosis, *Am. J. Med.* **58**:601–619.

Stoop, J. W., Ballieux, R. E., and Weyers, H. A., 1962, Paraproteinemia with secondary immuneglobulin deficiency in an infant, *Pediatrics* **29**:97.

Stoop, J. W., Zegers, J. M., Van Heiden, C., and Ballieux, R. E., 1968, Monoclonal gammapathy in a child with leukemia, *Blood* **32**:774.

Sugai, S., 1972, IgA pyroglobulin, hyperviscosity syndrome and coagulation abnormality in a patient with multiple myeloma, *Blood* **39**:224.

Suki, W. N., Yium, J. J., Von Minden, M., Saller-Herbert, C., Eknoyan, G. and Martinez-Maldonado, M., 1970, Acute treatment of hypercalcemia with furosemide, *N. Engl. J. Med.* **283**:836–841.

Sullivan, P. W., and Salmon, S. E., 1972, Kinetics of growth and regression in IgG multiple myeloma, *J. Clin. Invest.* **51**:1697–1708.

Taddeini, L., and Schrader, W., 1972, Concomitant myelomonocytic leukemia and multiple myeloma, *Minn. Med.* **55**:446–448.

Talal, N., Hermann, G., de Vaux St. Cyr, C., and Grabar, P., 1964, Immunoelectrophoretic changes in mouse γ-globulin after intraperitoneal injection of Bayol F, *J. Immunol.* **92**:747.

Tavassoli, M., and Baughan, M., 1973, Virus like particle in human myeloma without paraproteinemia, *Arch. Pathol.* **96**:347–349.

Terry, W. D., Page, D. L., Kimura, S., Isobe, T., Osserman, E. F., and Glenner, G. G., 1973, Structural identity of Bence Jones and amyloid fibril proteins in a patient with plasma cell dyscrasia and amyloidosis, *J. Clin. Invest.* **52**:1276–1281.

Thalassmos, N. C., and Joplin, G. F., 1970, Failure of corticosteroid therapy to correct the hypercalcemia of malignant disease, *Lancet* **2**:537–539.

Thijs, L. G., Hijmans, W., Leene, W., Muntinghe, O. G., Pietersz, R. N. I., and Ploem, J. E., 1970, Blast cell leukaemia associated with IgA paraproteinaemia and Bence Jones protein, *Br. J. Haematol.* **19**:485.

Thompson, D. L., and Frame, B., 1976, Involutional osteopenia: Current concepts, *Ann. Intern. Med.* **85**:789–803.

Tuddenham, E. G. C., and Bradley, J., 1974, Plasma volume expansion and increased serum viscosity in myeloma and macroglobulinemia, *Clin. Exp. Immunol.* **16**:169–176.

Turesson, I., 1975, Nuclear size in benign and malignant plasma cell proliferation, *Acta Med. Scand.* **197**:7–14.

Tursz, T., Flandrin, G., Brouet, J. C., Briere, J., and Seligmann, M., 1974a, Simultaneous occurrence of acute myeloblastic leukaemia and multiple myeloma without previous chemotherapy, *Br. Med. J.* **2**:642–643.

Tursz, T., Flandrin, G., Brouet, J. C., and Seligmann, M., 1974b, Coexistence of a myeloma and a granulocytic leukemia in the absence of any treatment: Study of 4 cases, *Nouv. Rev. Fr. Hematol.* **14**:693–704.

U.S. Cancer Mortality by County: 1950–1969, U.S. Department of Health, Education and Welfare, Public Health Service, National Institutes of Health, DHEW Publication No. (NIH) 74-615.

Velez-Garcia, E., and Maldonado, N., 1971, Long term follow-up and therapy in multiple myeloma, *Cancer* **27**:44.

Vermess, M., Pearson, K. D., Einstein, A. B., and Fahey, J. L., 1972, Osseous manifestations of Waldenström's macroglobulinemia, *Radiology* **102**:497–504.

Victor, M., Banker, B. Q., and Adams, R. D., 1958, The neuropathy of multiple myeloma, *J. Neurol. Neurosurg. Psychiatry* **21**:73–88.

Vigliano, E. M., and Horowitz, H. I., 1965, Bleeding syndrome caused by interaction of IgA myeloma protein and connective tissue, *Blood* **26**:880.

Vigliano, E. M., and Horowitz, H. I., 1967, Bleeding syndrome in a patient with IgA myeloma: Interaction of protein and connective tissue, *Blood* **29**:823.

Vodopick, H., Chaskes, S. J., Solomon, A., and Stewart, J. A., 1974, Transient monoclonal gammopathy associated with cytomegalovirus infection, *Blood* **44**:189–195.

Wahner, H. W., Kyle, R. A., and Beabow, J. W., 1975, Imaging of multiple myeloma with Tc-99m labeled dyphosphonate, *J. Nucl. Med.* **16**:579 (abstract).

Waldenström, H. J., 1928, On the formation and disappearance of amyloid in man, *Acta Chir. Scand.* **63**:479.

Waldenström, J., 1944, Incipient myelomatosis or "essential" hyperglobulinemia with fibrogenopenia: A new syndrome?, *Acta Med. Scand.* **117**:216–247.

Waldenström, J., 1961, Studies on conditions associated with disturbed gamma globulin formation (gammopathies), *Harvey Lect.* **56**:211.

Waldenström, J., 1965, Macroglobulinemia, in: *Immunological Diseases* (M. Samter, ed.), Little, Brown and Company, Boston.

Waldenström, J., 1970, *Diagnosis and Treatment of Multiple Myeloma*, Grune & Stratton, New York.

717

BIOLOGY, CLINICAL
PATTERNS, AND
TREATMENT OF
MULTIPLE MYELOMA
AND RELATED
PLASMA-CELL
DYSCRASIAS

Waldenström, J., 1973, Benign monoclonal gammopathies, in: *Multiple Myeloma and Related Disorders* (H. A. Azar and M. Potter, Eds.), pp. Harper & Row, New York.

Waldmann, T. A., and Strober, W., 1969, Metabolism of immunoglobulins, *Prog. Allergy* **13**:1.

Wall, R. L., and Clausen, K. P., 1975, Carcinoma of the urinary bladder in patients receiving cyclophosphamide, *N. Engl. J. Med.* **293**:271–273.

Walsh, J. C., 1971, The neuropathy of multiple myeloma: An electrophysiological and histological study, *Arch Neurol.* **25**:404–414.

Wanebo, H. J., and Clarkson, B. D., 1965, Essential macroglobulinemia: Report of a case including immunofluorescent and electron microscopic studies, *Ann. Intern. Med.* **62**:1025–1045.

Wang, A. C., Wang, I. Y. F., McCormick, J. N., and Fudenberg, H. H., 1969, The identity of light chains of monoclonal IgG and monoclonal IgM in one patient, *Immunochemistry* **6**:451.

Wang, A. C., Wilson, S. K., Hopper, J. E., Fudenberg, H. H., and Nisonoff, A., 1970, Evidence for control of synthesis of the variable regions of the heavy chains of immunoglobulins G and M by the same gene, *Proc. Natl. Acad. Sci. USA* **66**:337.

Wang, A. C., Fudenberg, H. H., Goldrosen, M. H., and Freedman, M. H., 1972, Chemical studies of heavy chains of two IgG-λ myeloma proteins from a single patient, *Immunochemistry* **9**:473.

Wang, A. C., Gergely, J., and Fudenberg, H. H., 1973, Aminoacid sequences at constant and variable regions of heavy chains of monotypic immunoglobulins G and M of a single patient, *Biochemistry* **12**:528.

Warne, G. L., Fairley, K. F., Hobbs, J. B., and Martin, F. I. R., 1973, Cyclophosphamide-induced ovarian failure, *N. Engl. J. Med.* **289**:1159–1162.

Warner, N. L., and Wistar, R., 1968, Immunoglobulins in NZB/B1 mice: I. Serum immunoglobulin levels and immunoglobulin class of erythrocyte antibody, *J. Exp. Med.* **127**:169.

Webb, H. E., Harrison, E. G., Jr., Masson, J. K., and ReMine, W. H., 1962, Solitary extramedullary myeloma (plasmacytoma) of the upper part of the respiratory tract and oropharynx, *Cancer* **15**:1142–1155.

Whitsed, H. M., and Penny, R., 1971, IgA-IgG, cryoglobulinemia with vasculitis, *Clin. Exp. Immunol.* **9**:183.

Wiedermann, B., Krc, C., Soyka, O., and Vykydal, J., 1966, Plasmozytome mit generalisieter Osteosklerose, *Folia Haematol. (Leipzig)* **86**:47–69.

Williams, H. M., Diamond, H. D., Graver, L. F., and Parsons, H., 1959, *Neurological Complications of Lymphomas and Leukemias*, Charles C. Thomas, Springfield, Illinois.

Williams, R. C., Jr., 1971, Cold agglutinins: Studies of primary structure, serologic activity and antigenic uniqueness, *Ann. N.Y. Acad. Sci.* **190**:330–341.

Williams, R. C., Brunning, R. D., and Wollheim, F. A., 1966, Light chain disease: An abortive variant of multiple myeloma, *Ann. Intern. Med.* **65**:471.

Williams, R. C., Jr., Erickson, J. L., Polesky, H. F., and Swaim, W. R., 1967, Studies of monoclonal immunoglobulins (M-components) in various kindreds, *Ann. Intern. Med.* **67**:309.

Williams, R. C., Jr., Kunkel, H. G., and Capra, J. D., 1968, Antigenic specifities related to the cold agglutinin activity of gamma M globulins, *Science* **161**:379–381.

Williams, R. C., Bailly, R. C., and Howe, R. B., 1969, Studies of "benign" serum M-components, *Am. J. Med. Sci.* **257**:275.

Williams, W. J., Beutler, E., Erslev, A. J., and Rundles, R. W., 1972, *Hematology*, McGraw-Hill, New York.

Wilson, D. E., Flowers, C. M., Hershgold, E. J., and Eaton, R. P., 1975, Multiple myeloma, cryoglobulinemia and xanthomatosis: Distinct clinical biochemical syndromes in two patients, *Amer. J. Med.* **59**:721–729.

Winterbauer, R. H., Riggins, R. C. K., Griesman, F. A., and Bauermeister, D. E., 1974, Pleuropulmonary manifestations of Waldenström's macroglobulinemia, *Chest* **66**:368–375.

Wintrobe, M. M., Lee, R. G., Buggs, D. R., Bithell, T. C., Athens, J. W., and Foerster, J., 1974, *Clinical Hematology*, 7th Ed., Lea and Febiger, Philadelphia.

Witwer, M. W., Schmid, F. R., and Tesar, J. T., 1976, Acute myelomonocytic leukaemia and multiple myeloma after sulphinpyrazone and colchicine treatment of gout, *Br. Med. J.* **2**(6027):89.

Wochner, R. D., Strober, W., and Waldmann, T. A., 1967, The role of the kidney in the catabolism of Bence Jones proteins and immunoglobulin fragments, *J. Exp. Med.* **126**:207–221.

Wood, T. A., and Frenkel, E. P., 1967, An unusual case of macroglobulinemia, *Arch. Intern. Med.* **119**:631–637.

Wright, C. J. E., 1961, Long survival in solitary plasmacytoma of bone, *J Bone Joint Surg. Br. Vol.* **43**:767–771.

Yagi, Y., and Pressman, D., 1973, Monoclonal IgA and IgM in the serum of a single patient. I. Sharing of individually specific determinants between IgA and IgM, *J. Immunol.* **110**:335.

Yakulis, V., Bhoopalam, N., Schade, S., and Heller, P., 1972, Surface immunoglobulins of circulating lymphocytes in mouse plasmacytoma. I. Characteristics of lymphocyte surface immunoglobulins, *Blood* **39**:453–464.

Yamada, H., Washburn, L. T., Takakura, K., and Hollander, V. P., 1969, The correlation between plasma cell tumor development and antibody response in inbred strains of mice, *Proc. Soc. Exp. Biol. Med.* **131**:947.

Yentis, L., 1956, The so-called solitary plasmocytoma of bone, *J. Fac. Radiol. London* **8**:132–144.

Yoshimura, Y., Takada, K., Kawai, N., Hasegawa, K., and Ishikawa, T., 1976, Two cases of plasmacytoma in the oral cavity, *Int. J. Oral Surg.* **5**(2):82–91.

Young, V. H., 1969, Transient paraproteins, *Proc. R. Soc. Med.* **62**:778.

Zawadzki, Z. A., and Edwards, G. A., 1970, Dysimmunoglobulinemia associated with hepatobiliary disorders, *Am. J. Med.* **48**:196.

Zawadzki, Z. A., and Edwards, G. A., 1972, Non-myelomatous monoclonal immunoglobulinemia, in: *Progress in Clinical Immunology*, Vol. 1 (R. S. Schwartz, ed.), pp. 105–156, Grune & Stratton, New York.

Zeffren, J. L., and Heinemann, H. O., 1962, Reversible defect in renal concentrating mechanism in patients with hypercalcemia, *Am. J. Med.* **33**:54.

Zimelman, A. P., 1973, Thrombocytosis in multiple myeloma (letter to the editor), *Ann. Intern. Med.* **78**:970–971.

Zinneman, H. H., and Hall, W. H., 1954, Recurrent pneumonia in multiple myeloma and some observations on immunologic response, *Ann. Intern. Med.* **41**:1152.

23

Treatment of Primary Neoplasms of Lymphoid Tissues

SAUL A. ROSENBERG

1. Introduction

A discussion of the management of adult patients with primary neoplasms of lymphoid tissues cannot be separated from a recognition of problems and controversies in nomenclature and classification. Clinicians are faced with the challenge of understanding and judging numerous histopathological proposals and new immunological and lymphoid physiological concepts at the same time as rapidly changing diagnostic and therapeutic programs are being developed and proposed. The experienced clinician is constantly aware, by observing patients with these diseases, that current and proposed understanding of the nature of lymphoid neoplasms is still imprecise and inadequate. Yet, despite the apparent confusion and complexity of this field to the student or the inexperienced, the situation is improving. Advances are being made in predicting clinical behavior and treatment responses based on good clinicopathological correlative studies and insights. As a result, the management of patients with neoplasms of lymphoid tissues is among the most rewarding and satisfying in the difficult area of clinical oncology.

This chapter will present the clinical and therapeutic aspects of primary lymphoid neoplasms of adults. Of necessity, the material is not comprehensive and represents the opinions and judgment of the author, based primarily on the extensive clinical experience of the author and his colleagues at Stanford University. Specific clinicopathological disease entities presented in earlier chapters (Chapters 13, 14, 16, 17, and 20) will not be described in detail.

SAUL A. ROSENBERG • Division of Oncology, Stanford University School of Medicine, Stanford, California 94305.

2. Histopathological Classifications

SAUL A. ROSENBERG

Patients with lymphoid neoplasms often referred to as malignant lymphomas present with a wide spectrum of clinical problems. The disease processes may be among the most aggressive and rapidly fatal known, despite all available therapy, or among the most indolent and well tolerated, requiring no therapy at all. During the past one hundred years, pathologists have been able to gradually clarify and recognize histopathological appearances that correlate with clinical behavior.

On the basis of classic histological methods of light microscopy, numerous classifications and separations have been proposed. In the extremes, these schemes have been so complex and with so many subgroups as to be of little utility to other than the proposer (Robb-Smith, 1938) or so oversimplified (Warthin, 1931) as to lose all correlative value. The overlap of leukemias of lymphoid origin with the lymphomas has always presented a problem in nomenclature and classification. Nonetheless, the studies and efforts of numerous pathologists have provided clinicians with a reasonably useful and reproducible classification. It is recommended that the nomenclature and system described by Rappaport (1966) in the United States Armed Forces fascicle be used by practicing pathologists and clinicians. That this system contains errors and deficiencies is readily acknowledged and is evidenced by this book. Changes in our standard nomenclature should be gradual, however, and by agreement among the most experienced investigators and clinicians in this field. New classifications should always include parallel reference to the standardized classification of Rappaport, whenever possible.

Table 1, adapted from Rappaport, lists the major clinicopathological groups of adult lymphoid neoplasms. It is widely accepted and useful to separate Hodgkin's disease from other lymphomas that do not contain the characteristic multinucleated giant cells diagnostic of that disorder. The unfortunate but widely used term *non-*

TABLE 1. Recommended Histopathological Classifications of the Malignant Lymphomas[a]

Hodgkin's disease[b]	Non-Hodgkin's lymphomas[c]		
	Nodular		Diffuse
Lymphocyte predominance		Lymphocytic, well differentiated	
10–15 years	NLWD		DLWD
	10+ years		10 years
Nodular sclerosis		Lymphocytic, poorly differentiated	
5–10 years	NLPD		DLPD
	7–8 years		2 years
Mixed cellularity		Mixed, lymphocytic and histiocytic	
2–3 years	NM		DM
	7–8 years		1–2 years
Lymphocyte depletion		Histiocytic	
1 year	NH		DH
	3 years		1 year
		Undifferentiated	
			DU
			1 year

[a]The survival figures are estimated median survival from retrospective studies not utilizing currently available management programs.
[b]As agreed on at the Rye Conference in 1965 (see Lukes *et al.*, 1966b).
[c]From Rappaport (1966).

Hodgkin's lymphomas is applied to all other primary lymphoid neoplasms. This group contains a wide spectrum of clinical disorders.

Some 30 years ago, Jackson and Parker (1947) put forward their classic histopathological classification, which divided Hodgkin's disease into three categories: paragranuloma, granuloma, and sarcoma. Unfortunately, this classification proved of little value in clinical practice, since nearly 90% of all cases were found to fall in the granuloma category. More recently, principally as a result of the work of Lukes *et al.* (1966a), an important subgroup of the former granuloma category, designated nodular sclerosis, has been delineated. This refinement and other refinements have permitted the development of a new histopathological classification (Lukes *et al.*, 1966b), the essential features of which were agreed on at the Rye and Paris Conferences in 1965 (Lukes *et al.*, 1966b; Bernard *et al.*, 1966). Four histopathological groups were identified, each of which has a different prognosis and predicts to a moderate degree certain clinical features of the disease. The *lymphocyte predominance* group has the best overall prognosis and the *lymphocyte depletion* group the worst. The *nodular sclerosis* group in general has a very good natural history and prognosis, though individual patients with this histopathological type may have a very aggressive short course. The *mixed cellularity* picture identifies a relatively unfavorable group of patients. The prognostic variables of the histopathological classification are not totally independent of other important variables such as the sites and extent of involvement, age, sex, and the presence or absence of systemic symptoms (Kaplan, 1972). Moreover, the results of current highly successful treatment programs are reducing the differences in survival formerly observed among the various histopathological types of Hodgkin's disease (Rosenberg and Kaplan, 1975a).

The studies and proposals of Rappaport and his colleagues have considerably improved the clinicopathological understanding of the non-Hodgkin's lymphomas. Former groups called lymphosarcoma, reticulum-cell sarcoma, and giant follicle lymphoma did not convey adequate clinical or even morphological meaning to those who had to utilize these terms. The major value of the so-called Rappaport classification was the identification and development of criteria for two major groups, those with *nodular* and those with *diffuse* histological patterns. Within these major subdivisions, the major cell type or types are identified, creating a classification of nine subtypes (see Table 1).

It is now well established that patients who present with lymph node patterns that are nodular have a significantly more favorable prognosis and natural history for the same cell type(s) than do those who present with diffuse patterns (Jones *et al.*, 1973a). In general, those who present with neoplasms of well-differentiated lymphocytes have a better prognosis than those with poorly differentiated lymphocytes. Patients with neoplasms composed of so-called histiocytes have poorer prognoses than those with lymphocytes, and patients with undifferentiated cytologies have the worst prognoses. Patients with nodular architecutre and well-differentiated small lymphocytes are rare, and nodular architecture with undifferentiated cells has not been described. Patients with a mixture of poorly differentiated lymphocytes and histiocytes are often seen and acknowledged in the Rappaport classification. Their prognoses are similar to those of patients with predominantly poorly differentiated lymphocytes, though they do present several unique clinical characteristics.

The newer concepts of lymphoid physiology reviewed by Lukes (Chapter 9) and Siegal (Chapter 10) and others have challenged the validity and usefulness of the Rappaport classification (Berard and Dorfman, 1974). Concepts of T- and B-cell origin, surface immunoglobulin markers, and the probable rarity of "true" histiocytic cell neoplasms raise serious problems for the Rappaport terminology and classification. It can be anticipated that these new concepts will result in a classification of greater value than the Rappaport system in the years ahead. This is not yet the case, however, and for clinical purposes, the Rappaport system is recommended for general clinical and clinical investigative usage.

In most textbooks and classifications, chronic lymphocytic leukemia (CLL) is not discussed with the malignant lymphomas. Yet if a lymph node from a patient with CLL were examined, it would be indistinguishable from lymph nodes from patients with a diffuse lymphoma composed of well-differentiated or small lymphocytes (DLWD). The distinction between CLL and DLWD is an arbitrary one based on clinical rather than morphological features, primarily on the presence and extent of bone marrow infiltration. Patients with CLL do not ordinarily present findings or problems that relate to acute lymphocytic leukemia (ALL) either at the outset of their illness or later in the course of the disease. Neither does the disease CLL have similarities in clinical problems or management approaches to chronic myelocytic leukemia (CML). Yet in most textbooks, CLL is discussed in the same context as the other leukemias, ALL and CML.

Clinically and immunologically, CLL is a primary neoplasm of the lymphoid tissues and bears many similarities to other lymphocytic lymphomas. Given the present state of our knowledge, therefore, a discussion of CLL relating it to the other primary lymphoid neoplasms is presented. Using the Rappaport terminology, CLL would be included in the category of diffuse lymphoma, well-differentiated lymphocytic type (DLWD).

3. Diagnostic Methods

The diagnosis of a lymphoid neoplasm must be made by examination of satisfactory tissue by an experienced pathologist. A patient may present with clinical problems strongly suggestive of a malignant lymphoma, even of a particular subtype, but the clinical similarities between infectious diseases and lymphoid neoplasms on the one hand and nonlymphoid neoplasms on the other make tissue confirmation essential for the diagnosis. Moreover, the various subtypes within the malignant lymphoma groups overlap clinically, but have very different natural histories and indications for management, depending on expert pathological interpretations.

Once the diagnosis is established, it is very important that patients be carefully evaluated diagnostically to determine the extent of their disease prior to embarking on a therapeutic program. The progress that has been made in the treatment of these diseases, especially of Hodgkin's disease, has paralleled the improvement of techniques for identifying the extent of the disease in the untreated patient and carefully documenting the response to therapy (Rosenberg, 1971; Kaplan, 1972).

Table 2 lists the diagnostic procedures that should be utilized in these patients unless there are specific contraindications. Each patient situation must be individualized, however, in terms of age, coexistent medical and other problems, and therapeutic options. The diagnostic routine is therefore prescribed as an important guideline, and should not be followed without regard for the context of each patient situation.

TABLE 2. Recommended Diagnostic Procedures for Previously Untreated Patients
with Primary Lymphoid Neoplasms

1. Careful history and physical examination
2. Routine chest roentgenogram
3. Whole-lung tomography if routine roentgenogram is abnormal
4. Complete blood count, including differential count, platelet count, and erythrocyte sedimentation rate
5. Urinalysis, serum creatinine or BUN
6. Stool examination for occult blood
7. Serum alkaline phosphatase
8. Bilateral lower-extremity lymphogram
9. Needle bone marrow biopsy
10. Exploratory laparotomy and splenectomy for selected patients depending on clinical stage and histological group
11. Intravenous pyelogram if lymphogram is abnormal

Optional procedures of limited value in selected patients

12. Skeletal and gastrointestinal roentgenograms
13. Radioisotopic scans of liver, spleen, bones, and brain
14. Gallium scans
15. Percutaneous liver biopsy
16. Laparoscopy, especially for patients with non-Hodgkin's lymphomas
17. Serum protein immunoelectrophoresis

A careful history and physical examination are essential to uncover characteristic systemic symptoms and to describe all the lymph node areas of the body. Not all palpable lymph nodes are pathological in the sense that they contain disease. However, if there are suspicious lymph nodes that, if involved, would change the therapeutic approach, biopsy should be done for confirmation. The lymphoid tissues in the oropharynx and nasopharynx should be evaluated by a skilled examiner. The size of the liver and spleen must be determined as carefully as possible. The bones should be examined for areas of tenderness.

Radiological examinations should include routine chest films and whole-lung tomography to identify mediastinal and hilar lymphadenopathy and pulmonary involvement (Davidson and Clarke, 1968). Lower-extremity lymphography is essential in all patients, unless pulmonary function is seriously limited or bone marrow or other disseminated extralymphatic involvement has been documented. A skeletal survey complemented by bone scans is desirable to detect osseous lesions in selected patients. Routine blood cell counts and determination of sedimentation rate, serum alkaline phosphatase, urinalysis, and evaluation of renal function are the minimal laboratory studies required for evaluation. Bone marrow biopsy is especially important for all patients with non-Hodgkin's lymphomas of the lymphocytic types and in all other patients with advanced lymph node involvement (Rosenberg, 1975).

In recent years, exploratory laparotomy and splenectomy have been employed to identify and confirm the presence of Hodgkin's disease in the abdomen and pelvis (Glatstein *et al.,* 1969; Ultmann, 1970; Rosenberg, 1972). Studies have demonstrated that approximately half of patients with clinical enlargement of the spleen do not have histological involvement of that organ; conversely, in approximately 1 patient in 4, spleens of normal size have demonstrable foci of Hodgkin's disease. The identification of involvement of the liver by Hodgkin's disease is especially difficult. It is unusual for marked and obvious liver involvement to occur early in the course of the disease. Abnormalities of liver function tests, including the bromsulphthalein excretion, serum alkaline phosphatase, and other enzymes, modest hepatomegaly, and nonspecific hepatic scan abnormalities may all be misleading. These abnormalities may occur nonspecifically, especially in patients with systemic symptoms, and histological verification of hepatic involvement should be sought. Conversely, liver involvement can be demonstrated, although rarely, at laparotomy, with no laboratory abnormalities thought to be characteristic of that condition.

The indications for exploratory laparotomy and splenectomy for patients with non-Hodgkin's lymphoma remain to be determined. Studies demonstrate that considerable information is obtained by the surgical procedure. Mesenteric involvement is much more frequent than suspected or found in Hodgkin's disease, occurring in approximately half the patients explored. The morbidity of the procedure is greater, however, in the older age population of these patients, whose disease may be indolent in some or very aggressive in others. It has not yet been determined to what extent, if any, therapeutic results will be improved by employing diagnostic laparotomy. The procedure should therefore be reserved for selected patients or for groups involved in careful clinical investigations (Goffinet *et al.*, 1973; Rosenberg *et al.*, 1975).

4. Staging of Lymphomas

There have been several attempts to classify the extent of disease in previously untreated patients with primary neoplasms of lymphoid tissues (Peters, 1950; Hoster *et al.*, 1948). The most utilized staging system for Hodgkin's disease, which is based on good prognostic data, has evolved at several international meetings (Rosenberg, 1966; Carbone *et al.*, 1971). The definitions of stages and important prognostic symptoms formulated at a conference in Ann Arbor in 1971 are shown in Table 3 (Carbone *et al.*, 1971). This system acknowledges the poor prognostic significance of widespread disease, certain systemic symptoms, and the involvement of multiple extralymphatic sites or tissues.

TABLE 3. Ann Arbor Staging Classification of the Lymphomas[a]

Stage	Definition
I	Involvement of a single lymph node region (I) or of a single extralymphatic organ or site (I_E)
II	Involvement of two or more lymph node regions on the same side of the diaphragm alone (II) or with involvement of limited, contiguous extralymphatic organ or tissue (II_E)
III	Involvement of lymph node regions on both sides of the diaphragm (III), which may include the spleen (III_S), or limited contiguous extralymphatic organ or site (III_E), or both (III_{ES})
IV	Multiple or disseminated foci of involvement of one or more extralymphatic organs or tissues, with or without lymphatic involvement

[a] All cases are subclassified to indicate the absence (A) or presence (B) of the systemic symptoms of significant fever, night sweats, or unexplained weight loss of greater than 10% of normal body weight. The clinical stage (CS) denotes the stage as determined by all diagnostic examinations and a single diagnostic biopsy only. If a second biopsy of any kind has been obtained, whether negative or positive, the term *pathological stage* (PS) will be used and the results of the additional biopsies shown by an agreed on designation. See Carbone *et al.* (1971).

TABLE 4. Proposed Staging System for Chronic Lymphocytic Leukemia[a]

Stage	0	Bone marrow and blood lymphocytosis only
Stage	I	Lymphocytosis and lymphadenopathy
Stage	II	Lymphocytosis and enlargement of the spleen or liver or both
Stage	III	Lymphocytosis with anemia
Stage	IV	Lymphocytosis with thrombocytopenia

[a]From Rai et al. (1975).

The Ann Arbor staging system also acknowledges the importance of defining the diagnostic studies employed in arriving at a staging designation. Since different centers and physicians employ different diagnostic procedures, the Ann Arbor system defines a clinical stage (CS) to indicate the extent of disease utilizing only the initial diagnostic biopsy and all clinical, laboratory, radiological, and scintographic procedures. The pathological stage (PS) is used to indicate the extent of disease determined by further biopsy or operative procedures such as bone marrow biopsy, second lymph node biopsy, and/or exploratory laparotomy with splenectomy. A system of subscripts to indicate the type and results of extensive pathological staging procedures is included in the Ann Arbor system (Carbone et al., 1971).

The Ann Arbor staging system was developed from data and is most useful for patients with Hodgkin's disease. It is also used for patients with the non-Hodgkin's lymphomas. For the various subtypes of the non-Hodgkin's lymphomas, the system has good descriptive value, but only limited prognostic value (Jones et al., 1973a). The prognostic importance of systemic symptoms for these groups of patients has not been well documented. For some subgroups, such as those with lymphocytic cell types, the great majority of patients have widespread disease, with very few in the stage I or II categories after complete evaluation. In some of the subtypes, there are minimal prognostic differences, depending on the extent of disease.

It will be necessary to develop new staging systems for the various non-Hodgkin's lymphomas. Until these are agreed on, however, the Ann Arbor system is a useful and standardized descriptive staging system that should be employed, despite its limitations.

A recent proposal attempts to classify patients with CLL into a five-group staging classification (Rai et al., 1975) (Table 4). This appears to be a useful prognostic system based on clinical variables that experienced clinicians have utilized for some time. There has not yet been general or international agreement on this proposal as there has been for Hodgkin's disease. Review of the data presented for the CLL staging system suggests that stages I and II may be combined in one stage and stages III and IV in another, simplifying the proposal to a three-stage system for prognostic purposes.

The importance of accepted staging classifications is to give an estimate of prognosis, to facilitate the selection of appropriate treatment programs, and to permit valid comparisons among medical centers for evaluation of therapeutic results and investigative programs. It can be predicted that as more successful treatment programs are developed for these responsive diseases, previous prognostic differences of staging designations will be obscured. This is already occurring for Hodgkin's disease (Rosenberg et al., 1977).

SAUL A. ROSENBERG

5. Clinical Manifestations

Though there are some similarities in the clinical picture of patients with primary neoplasms of lymphoid tissues, such as enlargement of the lymph nodes and involvement of the spleen and often the bone marrow, there is a considerable spectrum in the clinical manifestations of the various subgroups. Typical clinical presentations and courses will be presented for several of the major subtypes.

5.1. Hodgkin's Disease

A typical onset is in the observation, usually by the patient, of a painless, enlarging mass, most commonly in the neck, but occasionally in the axillary or inguinal–femoral region. On examination, this is found to be a discrete, rubbery, painless lymphadenopathy, frequently surrounded by enlarged lymph nodes. In other instances, a routine chest roentgenogram demonstrates mediastinal node enlargement; examination may then disclose lower cervical lymphadenopathy, which had not been noticed by the patient. Although these typical presentations occur at any age and with any histopathological type, the patients are usually between 15 and 35 years of age and have the histological variety of nodular sclerosis.

As the typical asymptomatic patient is evaluated more thoroughly, the anatomical extent of disease is usually more widespread than was apparent on physical examination. In significant numbers of such patients, mediastinal enlargement is found on routine or detailed radiological examination, paraaortic involvement is noted on lower extremity lymphography, or splenic involvement is found at exploratory laparotomy.

Occasionally, the lymphadenopathy makes itself known to the patient or his physician by producing local symptoms of pain, lymphatic or venous obstruction in an extremity, vena-caval obstruction, or airway narrowing. The duration of lymphadenopathy prior to diagnosis is extremely variable. Some patients report that a mass has been present for several years, even waxing and waning in size. Typically, several weeks to several months elapse between the time of the patient's first observation and the diagnostic biopsy.

In another group of patients with Hodgkin's disease, unexplained and persistent fever or night sweats or both are the initial symptoms. Fatigue and weight loss may be associated complaints as these symptoms become more severe and prolonged. These patients tend to be in the older age groups, are more often male than female, and when evaluated, are found to have more widespread disease than the typical patient presenting without symptoms. Occasionally in older patients, usually past the age of 40, the systemic symptoms are severe and often associated with anemia, but the lymphadenopathy is minimal. Extensive diagnostic efforts may be required to uncover the cause of the symptoms, including lymphography, bone marrow and liver biopsies, or even exploratory laparotomy. In rare cases, the diagnosis is not made before a postmortem examination. These older patients, with predominant systemic symptoms at the onset, usually show histological varieties of mixed cellularity or lymphocyte depletion (Nieman *et al.*, 1973).

Some patients with Hodgkin's disease have intermittent evening fever lasting several days, alternating with afebrile periods lasting days or weeks. Usually, the fever gradually becomes more severe and more continuous. This cyclic fever has been labeled the Pel–Ebstein or Murchison type, and is rarely a presenting manifestation of the disease.

Pruritus, usually generalized and severe, is another characteristic systemic symptom of Hodgkin's disease. It may appear in a mild, localized form, but if caused by Hodgkin's disease, it usually progresses and becomes generalized. The pruritus may be the only systemic symptom in the otherwise typical presentation of a young person, especially in women. Generalized severe pruritus may occur in patients with lymphoma other than Hodgkin's disease and in other systemic and dermatological conditions, but its presence should always suggest Hodgkin's disease. Its cause is unknown.

Occasionally, patients complain of pain in the region of enlarged lymph nodes within a few minutes after drinking alcoholic beverages. Although this is suggestive of Hodgkin's disease, it is not diagnostic. Its mechanism is also not known.

A wide variety of other symptoms may initially call the attention of the patient and his physician to the disease. These same problems occur with increasing frequency as the disease progresses.

The clinical course of the disease can be extremely variable. In addition, almost all patients receive treatment that may profoundly affect the course of the disease, sometimes resulting in apparent cure, and in many instances also resulting in complications that become difficult to separate from the disease itself.

In the typical young patient, Hodgkin's disease progresses at a variable rate, over a period of months or years, to involve adjacent lymph nodes. In time, if the disease is not controlled, extensions beyond the lymph nodes occur. There may be intrathoracic problems with compression of the airway or great veins, involvement of the pleura or pericardium or both with resultant effusions, increasing pulmonary parenchymal involvement, or local osseous involvement of the sternum, clavicle, ribs, or vertebrae.

Often, patients with early disease, apparently localized in the neck, develop disease of the lymph nodes in the upper paraaortic region or spleen or both. Later, as though there has been a loss of defense mechanisms, even the young patient with an initially favorable prognosis may develop widespread problems. At this stage, the bone marrow may become focally or diffusely involved. Multiple osseous lesions may occur, usually of an osteoblastic or mixed osteoblastic and osteolytic radiological appearance. These lesions may produce pain, but rarely result in fractures. The liver may become progressively involved with diffuse infiltration of the portal spaces. Laboratory tests confirm intrahepatic biliary obstruction. Hepatic failure may appear and result in death. Liver involvement in Hodgkin's disease has been noted to be closely, if not uniformly, associated with involvement of the spleen. Peripheral neuropathies and epidural cord compression may occur as a direct result of tumor growth as the disease progresses.

In time, virtually all patients with untreated or uncontrollable Hodgkin's disease develop increasingly severe systemic symptoms as their disease progresses. High continuous fever, drenching night sweats, malaise, fatigue, anorexia, and weight loss are all characteristic of the terminal picture. Selected aspects of some of the clinical problems of patients with Hodgkin's disease require further discussion.

Hematological Abnormalities. It is difficult to separate the effects of therapy for Hodgkin's disease from the effects of the disease itself on hematological parameters. Anemia of a moderate degree may be found in patients who have widespread Hodgkin's disease, often associated with systemic symptoms. The red blood cell indices are usually normal, the reticulocyte count normal or low, and the Coombs test negative. There may be shortened red blood cell survival with inadequate marrow response, as is also seen in patients with advanced cancer or chronic infection. Some patients develop profound anemia at the onset, but more commonly during the course of the disease. This may be due to extensive bone marrow involvement with the disease, hypersplenism, or rarely, a Coombs-positive hemolytic process. Often, combinations of these factors are responsible for the most severe anemias. The toxic effects of therapy may aggravate all the hematological abnormalities.

Bone marrow involvement with Hodgkin's disease can only rarely be demonstrated by the usual marrow aspirate technique and examination of marrow smears, the reason being that the marrow involvement is focal and often associated with fibrosis. It can therefore be discovered more readily by a marrow biopsy performed with a large-bore needle or open surgery (Grann et al., 1966; Rosenberg, 1972).

The sedimentation rate is commonly elevated in patients with active disease, and sometimes it may be the only evidence that the disease has been inadequately treated or that clinical recurrence is imminent. Numerous other laboratory abnormalities have been reported to be correlated with disease activity. These include elevations of plasma fibrinogen, serum α_2-globulin, haptoglobin, copper, zinc, and ceruloplasmin; depression of serum iron and iron-binding capacity; elevation of leukocyte alkaline phosphatase; and increase in urinary hydroxproline and muramidase (Teillet et al., 1971).

In the untreated or minimally treated patient, moderate to marked neutrophilic leukocytosis and thrombocytosis characterize active, symptomatic Hodgkin's disease. Occasionally, the granulocytosis may be so marked as to suggest chronic granulocytic leukemia. More careful study, however, usually demonstrates that this is a "leukemoid" reaction. Eosinophilia of a mild degree may be present, and occasionally is moderate or marked, often in patients with severe and long-standing pruritus. Absolute lymphopenia, even in untreated patients, is seen in a small percentage of cases and, when present, is a grave prognostic sign (Aisenberg, 1965). Absolute lymphocytosis is seen rarely if ever in Hodgkin's disease, and should always suggest an error in diagnosis. Reed–Sternberg cells have been described in the peripheral blood in studies employing special techniques (Bouroncle, 1966), but they are seldom recognized with usual hematological techniques. Rarely, leukemia of the acute myelomonocytic type occurs in patients with long-standing Hodgkin's disease (Ezdinli et al., 1969; Arseneau et al., 1972).

5.2. Nodular Lymphoma, Poorly Differentiated Lymphocytic Type

Nodular lymphoma of the poorly differentiated lymphocytic type (NLPD) is the most common type of nodular lymphoma and presents a more uniform clinical picture than the other nodular types.

The disease occurs in adults, usually over the age of 40, with a median age of about 55. It is very rare in young adults or children, although instances below the age of 15 are known.

It is almost always an asymptomatic illness at onset, characterized by painless adenopathy in the cervical, axillary, and inguinal–femoral regions. In some patients, large abdominal masses of retroperitoneal or mesenteric lymph nodes cause symptoms that bring the patient to a physician. Even though the patient may be aware of only one or several enlarged lymph nodes, examination and study with lymphography and laparotomy may reveal widespread, often symmetrical, lymph-adenopathy. In contrast to other lymphomas, especially Hodgkin's disease, anterior mediastinal adenopathy is not common, but symmetrical hilar adenopathy can occur. The lymph node enlargement may have been present for several, even many, years, but so gradual or fluctuating in its appearance that patients have not been concerned enough to seek medical attention. Occasionally, an enlarged lymph node removed years earlier and thought to be "hyperplastic" or "atypical" will on review, be diagnostic of nodular lymphoma.

The spleen is often enlarged, but rarely symptomatic, at the onset of the disease. Subsequently, it may become considerably enlarged, producing local symptoms and significant hypersplenism.

Involvement of the lymphoid tissue in Waldeyer's ring is uncommon.

Other than the bone marrow, nodular lymphomas of this type or other types do not often symptomatically involve nonlymphatic organs and tissues such as the lung, liver, bones, and skin. Paravertebral lymphoid masses may result in chylous pleural effusions or ascites or both, presumably because of lymphatic obstruction. It is extremely rare for the CNS to become involved, although peripheral nerve compression and epidural tumor masses may develop.

The peripheral blood picture is usually normal at the onset of the disease, although careful examination of the blood smear may reveal notched or cleft so-called "buttock" cells thought to be characteristic, but not diagnostic, of nodular lymphomas. Ordinary bone marrow aspirations are usually normal. Study of the bone marrow by the needle or open biopsy technique, however, will reveal focal bone marrow involvement in up to 75% of patients with NLPD even at the onset of the disease (Ribas-Mundo and Rosenberg, 1977).

Histological examination will reveal nodular lymphoma in some patients who present an otherwise typical clinical picture of chronic lymphocytic leukemia, with white blood cell counts as high as 100,000 or more. In a small proportion of patients, such an extreme lymphocytosis may appear during the course of the disease. It remains to be determined whether these patients differ significantly from those with typical chronic lymphocytic leukemia, in whom the histological picture of the lymph nodes is that of a diffuse lymphoma of the well-differentiated lymphocytic type.

The clinical course of this type of nodular lymphoma is usually an indolent one. Lymphadenopathy may have been present for years prior to establishment of the diagnosis and be well tolerated for 5–10 years or more after the diagnosis. This is a malignant disease, however, and though there may be spontaneous regression of lymphadenopathy, clinical problems gradually appear. In a rare patient, the tempo of the disease accelerates, and the patient may experience difficulties within months of the diagnosis.

After years of being well tolerated, the disease may become much more aggressive. Lymph node masses may grow rapidly, often in localized or asymmetrical locations. They cause serious local problems and are less responsive to previously effective treatment. Systemic symptoms of fever, night sweats, and weight loss may appear. Nonlymphoid organs and tissues become involved, and the prognosis grows very poor. If biopsy is repeated at this time, change in histological appearance is usually seen, characterized by a diffuse pattern, and often a larger cell type corresponding to the diffuse histiocytic lymphoma of Rappaport. It seems probable that currently available immunological techniques will clarify the relationship of the original nodular lymphoma and the later diffuse type of apparently different cytology (Lukes and Collins, 1975).

The other nodular lymphomas are: (1) nodular lymphocytic, well differentiated (NLWD); (2) nodular mixed (NM); and (3) nodular histiocytic (NH). These types differ somewhat in overall prognosis, frequency of initial bone marrow involvement, and type and location of lymph node enlargement (Jones *et al.*, 1973a; Rosenberg, 1975). The NH group has the poorest prognosis of the nodular group, and the rare NLWD probably the best. The NM type is similar to the NLPD group in many respects, though bone marrow involvement at onset is less common, and large abdominal masses may be seen more often.

In general, the nodular lymphomas should be considered systemic malignancies, since the actual or potential involvement of the B-cell distribution of lymphocytes is very high. Therapeutic programs should be based on this consideration, as well as on the variable but favorable natural history in older patients.

5.3. Diffuse Non-Hodgkin's Lymphomas

This group of lymphomas is extremely variable in its clinical expression. The diffuse histiocytic (DH) type is the most common, and will be presented in detail. Each of the other varieties has a unique clinical course, the diffuse lymphomas ranging from some of the most rapidly progressive malignant diseases to some of the most indolent.

The category of DH lymphoma is often equated with the term "reticulum-cell sarcoma" of the older literature, but the groups and criteria for diagnosis are not identical. Undoubtedly, the occasional indolent course of patients with reticulum-cell sarcoma seen in the past is explained by some degree of nodular architecture, which under current criteria would place the patient in a nodular subgroup. Other tumors that have been called reticulum-cell sarcoma are now categorized on the basis of their content of large relatively undifferentiated lymphoid cells, or convoluted nuclear cell types, which are not included in the DH subgroup. Much remains to be done to clarify the clinicopathological understanding of these diffuse lymphomas of large cell types.

In general, patients with DH lymphomas present with relatively localized but rapidly progressing tumor masses. These masses are often in lymph nodes, almost anywhere in the body. More often than any other lymphoma, this disease presents in nonlymphatic sites. Presentation in the GI tract, bone, thyroid, testes, and the lymphoid tissue of Waldeyer's ring all occur. In approximately half the patients, extensive diagnostic efforts demonstrate that the disease is relatively localized, involving contiguous lymphoid regions, of stage I or II extent. The bone marrow is affected initially in less than 10% of patients, and involvement even late in the course of the disease is uncommon (Ribas-Mundo and Rosenberg, 1977). Invasion by tumor masses is more common, causing peripheral nerve compression and venacaval and airway compression. Epidural tumors and destructive osseous lesions also occur during the course of the disease. The skin, liver, lung, and even the brain may become involved. Bone marrow involvement can, but rarely does, cause the appearance in the peripheral blood of large monocytoid or very undifferentiated cells.

5.4. Chronic Lymphocytic Leukemia

Chronic lymphocytic leukemia (CLL) is a disease that in its typical form is easily distinguished from the other primary neoplasms of lymphoid tissues. Typically, it affects an older age group, with a median age of 60 years. There is small- to moderate-sized generalized, symmetrical lymphadenopathy, modest splenomegaly, little or no mediastinal adenopathy, and easily demonstrated diffuse involvement of the bone marrow with a peripheral blood picture with a preponderance of numerous, relatively mature small lymphocytes. Patients are often asymptomatic at the onset of their illness, with lymphadenopathy or splenomegaly or both discovered by themselves or on a routine physical examination, or their illness is discovered at the time of routine peripheral blood examination obtained for an unrelated purpose.

Signs, symptoms, and problems with CLL are related to the progressive infiltration of the bone marrow, lymph nodes, and spleen, and less commonly other tissues and viscera, such as the liver, skin, GI tract, and lungs. Symptoms of fatigue, night sweats, fever, and weight loss become more prominent as the disease progresses beyond control.

The white blood count is high, almost by definition of the disorder, but may vary, with an absolute lymphocyte count of 5000 to over 200,000 cells/mm^3. Patients with advancing disease, and occasionally at onset, have difficulty with anemia, granulocytopenia, and thrombocytopenia. About 1 patient in 5 develops a positive Coomb's test with symptomatic autoimmune hemolytic anemia. Some degree of hypersplenism is common. Abnormalities of γ-globulin production are common in patients with CLL, and they are particularly sensitive to certain infections (see Chapters 18 and 19).

The proposed clinical staging system described in Table 4 acknowledges the variable prognosis of patients with CLL (Rai *et al.*, 1975). Those presenting with lymphocytosis only (stage 0) have a very good prognosis and may survive for many years, often without requiring therapy. Those who present with lymphadenopathy, with or without hepatosplenomegaly but no anemia or thrombocytopenia (stages I and II), have a median survival of 5–8 years, and those with anemia or thrombocytopenia or both at onset (stages III and IV) have the poorest prognoses, with a median of approximately 2 years.

There is difficulty in distinguishing some lymphocytic non-Hodgkin's lymphomas that involve the bone marrow from CLL. In general, patients with CLL have (1) diffuse, rather than focal, involvement of the bone marrow; (2) lymph nodes of a diffuse, well-differentiated lymphocytic morphological appearance, rather than a nodular pattern or less differentiated cytology; and (3) a greater number of more mature-appearing peripheral blood lymphocytes than patients with non-Hodgkin's lymphomas. It may well be, however, that the clinical picture of CLL represents merely one end of a spectrum of advanced disease, which in its more localized presentation cannot be distinguished from the better-differentiated lymphocytic non-Hodgkin's lymphomas.

Fortunately, management decisions, given our present state of knowledge, do not depend on the separation of CLL patients from those with lymphocytic non-Hodgkin's lymphoma. Rather, therapeutic decisions are based on the extent and sites of disease.

6. Treatment

The discussion of treatment of the primary neoplasms of lymphoid tissue must separate Hodgkin's disease from the non-Hodgkin's lymphomas. Considerable progress and understanding of treatment indications have been made for Hodgkin's disease. These same concepts and approaches are often erroneously applied to the non-Hodgkin's lymphomas as well. Clinical studies designed to improve the therapeutic results for the non-Hodgkin's lymphomas have been frustrated by inadequate pathological and clinical staging classifications. Only since 1970 has there been enough clarification of the natural history of these lymphomas to design meaningful therapeutic programs and trials. In some instances, it is premature to be certain about indicated treatment methods.

6.1. Hodgkin's Disease

The treatment of Hodgkin's disease has undergone radical changes since 1940. These changes have resulted from advances in the availability and techniques of supervoltage radiotherapy, effectiveness of chemotherapeutic agents, especially when used in combination, and the realization that patients can be cured (Easson and Russell, 1963; Kaplan, 1962, 1972).

The advances and enthusiasm for aggressive treatment since 1960 have appeared and evolved rapidly. It is not yet possible to make an accurate assessment of the true curative potential of modern treatment. Nonethless, there can be no doubt that considerable improvement in overall survival rates is being observed, and a significant number of patients are being cured by appropriate evaluation and staging and the application of concepts of tolerable aggressive therapy.

6.1.1. Radiotherapy

The basic concepts of modern radiotherapy for Hodgkin's disease were proposed by the Swiss radiotherapist René Gilbert (1939), and were effectively put into practice by Peters, Kaplan, Johnson, and others (Peters, 1950; Rosenberg et al., 1978; Johnson, 1969; Kaplan, 1962, 1972).

The major considerations that determine the success of radiation therapy are the radiation dose employed, the extent of the fields, and the energy of the radiation source. It is inappropriate to employ kilovoltage X rays in a curative attempt for a patient with Hodgkin's disease. Doses of 3500–4500 rads to relatively large fields are required to effect permanent eradication of any given site (Kaplan, 1966). Because of the limitations of present diagnostic methods in determining the true extent of the disease, lymphoid regions adjacent to known disease or contiguous via lymphatic channels are usually treated to full dose to achieve the best results. Modern equipment and methods permit the treatment of most of the commonly involved lymphoid tissues in two or three large single fields, the "mantle" or supradiaphragmatic field and the "inverted-Y" below the diaphragm (Page et al., 1970).

Data are accumulating that support this philosophy of therapy for all carefully studied patients with stage I, II, and IIIA disease in providing relapse-free survival and probably increased cure rates as well.

6.1.2. Chemotherapy

Drugs that can result in significant regression of Hodgkin's disease have been available since nitrogen mustard was tested during World War II. There are effective agents representing a number of different classes of compounds and mechanisms of action. These drugs include the alkylating agents (nitrogen mustard, chlorambucil, cyclophosphamide, melphalan), the vinca alkaloids (vinblastine, vincristine), procarbazine, the nitrosoureas, bleomycin, doxorubicin, and to a limited extent the corticosterioids.

Though effective palliation for patients with Hodgkin's disease can be obtained with single-agent chemotherapy, the potential for prolonged disease-free results by using aggressive combination chemotherapy relegates the use of single-agent treatment programs to late-stage patients who no longer have the reserve or tolerance for potential curative combination chemotherapy programs.

There are several effective combination chemotherapy programs for Hodgkin's disease, but the most successful and widely used is the MOPP program, developed at the National Cancer Institute (DeVita *et al.*, 1970). This program consists of at least six 2-week cycles of therapy employing nitrogen mustard, vincristine, procarbazine, and prednisone. Since 2-week rest periods intervene between successive cycles, the entire course requires approximately 6 months.

The chemotherapy program is indicated at present for patients who have stage IV disease that is beyond the extent that can be treated with radiotherapy and for those patients who have developed recurrent disease after initial radiation therapy programs. Some 70–80% of such patients can be expected to have a complete regression of their disease. Approximately half of such patients have remained free of evidence of disease, in some cases as long as 10 years.

Combination chemotherapy is being evaluated as an adjuvant to radiation therapy in certain settings and stages of the disease, and is proving to be a superior primary therapy for patients with stage IIIB disease. Rarely, the drug program has been used for even more limited extent of the disease, which can be controlled with irradiation in 60–90% of cases (DeVita *et al.*, 1976; Olweny *et al.*, 1974). In some of these settings, the use of chemotherapy (along with or in place of radiation therapy) is still in a developmental state that will require 5–10 years to evaluate adequately. Table 5 lists the recommended therapy for each stage of Hodgkin's disease, as well as treatment programs being studied.

6.2. Non-Hodgkin's Lymphomas

The precise roles of radiation therapy, chemotherapy, and combined modality therapy, and which drug combinations are the most effective for the treatment of non-Hodgkin's lymphomas, remain to be determined by careful clinical investigations. Only general and tentative recommendations can be made at this time.

The principles of effective radiation therapy described for Hodgkin's disease are much the same for the non-Hodgkin's lymphomas when irradiation is selected for the primary potentially curative treatment approach. In general, such an approach should be used for the more aggressive lymphomas in the younger patients, with the most localized disease extent. When radiation fields are planned, the radiotherapist must take into consideration the more frequent or potential involvement of Waldeyer's ring, the mesenteric lymph nodes, and the lower incidence of mediastinal disease than occurs in Hodgkin's disease.

Patients, usually over the age of 50, who have the more indolent lymphomas of the nodular or well-differentiated lymphocytic types with clinical or pathologic stage III or IV disease should be approached conservatively with palliative radiotherapy or chemotherapy programs. In many instances, the disease can remain

SAUL A. ROSENBERG

TABLE 5.   Therapeutic Recommendations and Estimated Prognoses for the Lymphomas (September 1976)[a]

Subgroup	Pathological stage	Recommended therapy	5-Year disease-free survival	Experimental therapy programs
Hodgkin's disease	IA and IIA	Subtotal lymphoid irradiation	90%	Limited-field irradiation ± combination chemotherapy
	IB, IIB, II$_E$A, II$_E$B	Total lymphoid irradiation	75%	Total lymphoid irradiation + combination chemotherapy
	IIIA, III$_S$A, II$_{ES}$A	Total lymphoid irradiation	60%	Combination chemotherapy ± total lymphoid irradiation
	IIIB, III$_S$B, III$_{ES}$B	Combination chemotherapy	50%	Combination chemotherapy + total lymphoid irradiation
	IVA, IVB	Combination chemotherapy	25–40%	Combination chemotherapy + limited-field or total lymphoid irradiation
Non-Hodgkin's lymphomas				
NLWD, NLPD, NM, DLWD	I and II	Limited-field irradiation	75%	Total lymphoid irradiation ± combination chemotherapy
NH, DLPD, DM, DH, DU	I and II	Total lymphoid irradiation	60%	Total lymphoid irradiation + combination chemotherapy
NLWD, NLPD, NM, DLWD	III and IV	Palliative chemotherapy	?None[b]	Total-body irradiation or Total lymphoid irradiation ± combination chemotherapy or combination chemotherapy alone
NH, DLPD, DM, DH, DU	III and IV	Combination chemotherapy	10–50%	Combination chemotherapy + limited-field or total lymphoid irradiation

[a]These recommendations are for adults only. Childhood lymphomas of the Burkitt's, mediastinal, and other types require different approaches. Childhood Hodgkin's disease requires lower irradiation doses supplemented by combination chemotherapy.
[b]The 5-year survival will be approximately 75%.

untreated until the tempo of activity of the disease is gauged to be rapid, or until local or general symptoms require treatment. Since the risk of recurrent disease in these patients continues for many years (despite apparent complete regression with aggressive treatment programs), it has not yet been established that such potentially curative approaches are successful or justified.

The natural history of the diffuse lymphomas of poor prognosis, however, justifies aggressive staging, radiation, and chemotherapy programs despite uncertainties in this field that remain to be resolved.

The chemotherapeutic agents available and employed for the non-Hodgkin's lymphomas are much the same as those effective for Hodgkin's disease. Many combinations are being developed and evaluated, and only certain general recommendations can be made at this time.

Combinations that include cyclophosphamide, vincristine, and prednisone are effective for all the nodular and diffuse lymphocytic lymphomas (Schein *et al.*, 1974; Portlock and Rosenberg, 1976). A variation of the MOPP program substituting cyclophosphamide for nitrogen mustard has been reported to produce 30–40% long-term remissions for the diffuse lymphomas of poor prognosis (DeVita *et al.*, 1975). Adriamycin is an effective drug for the DH group of patients, and combinations employing that drug appear to have the highest response rate available (Bonadonna *et al.*, 1975). Agents that are cycle-specific are being included in combinations for the rapidly proliferating tumors of this group. Such combinations include cytosine arabinoside, 6-thioguanine, and methotrexate with or without leucovorin "rescue" (Levitt *et al.*, 1972; Rosenberg and Kaplan, 1975b). Bleomycin is useful as a single agent and in combinations because of its minimal marrow-suppressing effect.

When palliation or minimal treatment programs are decided on for the nodular and diffuse lymphocytic lymphomas and CLL, the oral alkylating agents, chlorambucil, or cyclophosphamide in continuous daily or intermittent oral schedules can be very effective and well tolerated (Portlock *et al.*, 1976).

Radiation therapy should always be considered for serious local problems in which rapid and prolonged control is required and for most histological varieties no matter what the stage of disease. Such serious problems as spinal cord compression, vena-caval obstruction, ureteral obstruction, localized neuropathies, and fluid accumulation should be considered for irradiation within the limitations of field size, marrow tolerance, and other sites of active disease. These decisions require the close collaboration of medical oncologists, radiation therapists, and diagnostic radiologists.

6.3. Chronic Lymphocytic Leukemia

The therapy of CLL has proceeded along different lines than regimens that have developed for the other primary neoplasms of lymphoid tissues. Hematologists have generally acknowledged the systemic nature and incurability of CLL. It remains to be tested whether or not early aggressive treatment programs that have been utilized so successfully for widespread Hodgkin's disease and some of the non-Hodgkin's lymphomas might be of value in treating CLL.

Usually patients who are asymptomatic, with stable normal or near-normal blood counts, are not treated no matter what the peripheral lymphocyte count and the appearance of the bone marrow. Localized cosmetic or mechanical problems caused by lymphadenopathy can be satisfactorily treated with modest doses of irradiation. Prominent splenomegaly can also be treated with irradiation, often with an improvement in systemic symptoms and peripheral blood counts.

When systemic therapy is required because of important symptoms, oral alkylating agents are very effective. If the platelet count is low, corticosteroids may be successful as a lymphocytolytic agent without direct bone marrow suppression. Alkylating agents or corticosteroids or both may be given continuously or on intermittent oral schedules. After improvement, the drugs are either discontinued or given on a maintenance schedule with the lowest possible dose to achieve the palliative effect.

Whole-body low-dose irradiation was recently revived as an effective palliative therapy for patients requiring treatment for CLL (Johnson, 1975). It should not be employed routinely because of the need for special treatment techniques or when the platelet count is low.

6.4. Complications of Therapy

The current and recommended management approach to the majority of patients with these neoplasms is optimistic, aggressive, and demanding. Invasive diagnostic techniques are required to intelligently select the most successful therapeutic programs. Though the diseases are usually quite responsive to treatment programs, maximal treatment is usually required to achieve the highest probabilities of cure (Rosenberg and Kaplan, 1975b). The complications and cost of these management programs are acceptable but nonetheless considerable (Glicksman and Nickson, 1973; Kaplan, 1972; Arseneau et al., 1972).

The full treatment programs, including staging and irradiation or chemotherapy or both, may require many months and sometimes more than a year. Radiation doses are maximal in terms of normal adjacent tissue tolerance, especially of the lungs, heart, liver, kidneys, thyroid, spinal cord, and bone marrow. Potentially curative chemotherapy results in serious bone marrow suppression and depending on the drugs employed may seriously injure the gonads, heart, lungs, bladder, and other sites. Though reversible, the acute toxicities of radiation and chemotherapy of the type required for cure are very considerable (Glicksman and Nickson, 1973). In particular, GI side effects, hair loss, skin changes, impotence, weight loss, fatigue, and emotional disturbances require very skillful management and the best motivation of the patient, the patient's family, and the treatment team, which must include skilled oncology nurses.

It remains to be completely known what the late complications of curative irradiation or chemotherapy programs may be. Radiation-induced neoplasms are well known and can be expected in a small percentage of patients 5–10 years or more after treatment. Chemotherapeutic agents are also potent mutagens and carcinogens, and acute leukemias of the myelomonocytic type have been described after the long-term use of alkylating agents. The use of multiple drugs with or without irradiation can be expected to result in an increased frequency of late nonlymphomatous neoplasms, but the precise risk is still unknown (Arseneau et al., 1972; Rosenberg and Kaplan, 1975a). From available data, it can be estimated that the overall risk of these neoplastic late complications will be less than 5% and probably less than 2%. As unfortunate and tragic as these occurrences are, they are part of the cost paid for the considerable improvement in overall cure and survival rates now possible.

Earlier chapters present in detail the major problems of these patients. Bacterial, viral, fungal, and so-called "opportunistic" infections are serious problems that assume major proportions in patients being treated with curative intent, but also in the natural history of their disease. The appearance in patients on prolonged immunosuppressive therapy of peculiar neoplasms, such as the "immunoblastic sarcoma" of Lukes (Lukes and Collins, 1975), can be expected in patients treated for primary neoplasms of the lymphoid tissues. These clinical situations will be especially complex and require careful documentation and clinicopathological study to understand.

7. Concept of Cure

It had long been thought that primary neoplasms of lymphoid tissues were qualitatively different from other neoplasms. They were thought to be systemic diseases and incurable by methods utilized for other neoplasms. In part, this philosophy seems to have been justified by the widespread distribution of these diseases throughout the lymphoid system, often extending to extralymphatic tissues, especially late in the course of the diseases and at postmortem examination. This concept was certainly supported, in the past, by treatment approaches that were relatively ineffective, at least in terms of cure.

These concepts have gradually come under challenge, primarily by radiotherapists. Easson and Russell (1963) and others were able to demonstrate that very long-term control—in fact, cure—of patients with localized Hodgkin's disease and some of the other lymphomas was possible when they were treated with adequate doses of irradiation. As improved diagnostic methods became available, especially lower-extremity lymphography, patterns of disease in untreated patients could be shown to be compatible with the concept that lymphomas arose and spread much like other neoplasms, along lymphatic channels (Rosenberg and Kaplan, 1966; Kaplan, 1972). Again, this has been more clearly demonstrated for patients with Hodgkin's disease than for those with other lymphoid neoplasms, but may well be true for several of the subtypes other than Hodgkin's disease, in particular the diffuse lymphomas of large cell types (Jones et al., 1973b).

During this same period of improved diagnostic technology, therapeutic programs were improving and investigators were demonstrating progressively improved treatment results. An increasing number of patients with both Hodgkin's disease and the non-Hodgkin's lymphomas were obtaining initial complete control of their disease with no subsequent recurrence for many years (Rosenberg and Kaplan, 1975b; O'Connell et al., 1975; DeVita et al., 1975).

Analysis of recurrence rates after initial therapy in carefully followed large patient series has demonstrated a progressively reduced risk of recurrence of disease with time. This is clearly the case for Hodgkin's disease, whether treated with irradiation or chemotherapy, when the subsequent risk of recurrence falls to an almost insignificant probability 5 years after induction of a complete remission of the disease (Kaplan, 1972). This also appears to be true for non-Hodgkin's lymphomas of the DH type of the Rappaport system (DeVita *et al.,* 1975). Despite the overall poor prognosis of this group of patients, recurrence of the disease after a sustained disease-free period of 2 years is distinctly uncommon.

In contrast, those patients with the better-tolerated, more indolent non-Hodgkin's lymphomas, in particular the nodular subtypes, appear to have a continuous risk of recurrence after complete remission induction for as long as they have been followed (Schein *et al.,* 1975; Jones *et al.,* 1973b). There continues to be a significant proportion of patients whose disease activity reappears 5–10 years after an apparent complete remission induced by initial aggressive treatment programs.

It remains to be determined what the curative possibilities of modern treatment programs may be for all the different subtypes of these neoplasms, but there is no longer any question that permanent eradication of these diseases is possible and is being achieved in an increasing proportion of patients. This is true both for patients with Hodgkin's disease and with the non-Hodgkin's lymphomas, and for both localized and widespread disease. Though many years are required to establish the curative potential of new treatment programs for some of these diseases, the previous notion that these diseases are incurable is no longer tenable.

Table 5 provides an estimate of the probability of cure utilizing the recommended treatment programs listed for the various groups and stages of patients with primary neoplasms of lymphoid tissues. In some cases, these probabilities are well established on the basis of reported clinical studies with adequate follow-up. In others, they are the best estimates available to the author from actual studies and reports from responsible investigators and medical centers.

Potentially curative treatment programs have not been applied systematically to patients with CLL. The reason is primarily that this disease affecting an elderly population may be tolerated for many years and often is not the direct cause of death of the patient. Much the same is true for patients with nodular lymphoma in the elderly. These are progressive neoplasms in the majority of patients, however, and may affect younger patients, whose longevity will be significantly reduced by the disease. Potentially curative programs should be developed and carefully evaluated for all these patients and selectively applied on the basis of the results of such studies.

8. Summary

The management of patients with primary neoplasms of lymphoid tissue, the so-called "malignant lymphomas," is a dynamic and rewarding endeavor that has undergone remarkable change during the past 20 years. These changes have resulted from improved histopathological classifications, technical advances in radiotherapy, more successful use of potent chemotherapeutic agents, and an optimistic, aggressive philosophy of therapy. Continued improvement in treatment results can be expected following these same concepts not only to develop more curative treatment programs, but also to minimize treatment morbidity. The more significant clinical advances in this field will come, however, when there is a better understanding of the etiology and pathogenesis of lymphoid neoplasms. It may then be possible to prevent or reverse the disease process, rather than having to identify and eradicate all sites of the disease with nonspecific destructive therapies.

References

Aisenberg, A. C., 1965, Lymphocytopenia in Hodgkin's disease, *Blood* **25**:1037–1042.

Arseneau, J. C., Sponzo, R. W., Levin, D. L., Schnipper, L. E., Bonner, H., Young, R. C., Canellos, G. P., Johnson, R. E., and DeVita, V. T., 1972, Nonlymphomatous malignant tumors complicating Hodgkin's disease, *N. Engl. J. Med.* **287**:1119–1122.

Berard, C. W., and Dorfman, R. F., 1974, Histopathology of malignant lymphomas, in: *Clinics in Haematology* (S. Rosenberg, guest ed.), **3**:39–76.

Bernard, J., Chiappa, S., Denoix, P., Kaplan, H. S., Laugier, A., Lukes, R. J., Mathe, G., Nezeloff, G., Peters, V., Ratti, A., and Tubiana, M., 1966, Proposition d'une classification des différentes formes cliniques de la maladie de Hodgkin, *Nouv. Rev. Franc. Hemat.* **6**:175–176.

Bonadonna, F., DeLena, M., Lattuada, A., Milani, F., Monfardini, S., and Baretta, G., 1975, Combination chemotherapy and radiotherapy in non-Hodgkin's lymphomata, *Br. J. Cancer* **31**(Suppl. II):481–488.

Bouroncle, B. A., 1966, Sternberg–Reed cells in the peripheral blood of patients with Hodgkin's disease, *Blood* **27**:544–556.

Carbone, P. P., Kaplan, H. S., Musshoff, K., Smithers, D. W., and Tubiana, M., 1971, Report of the committee on Hodgkin's disease staging classification, *Cancer Res.* **31**:1860–1861.

Davidson, J. W., and Clarke, E. A., 1968, Influence of modern radiological techniques on clinical staging of malignant lymphomas, *Can. Med. Assoc. J.* **99**:1196–1204.

DeVita, V. T., Serpick, A., and Carbone, P. P., 1970, Combination chemotherapy in the treatment of advanced Hodgkin's disease, *Ann. Intern. Med.* **73**:881–895.

DeVita, V. T., Jr., Canellos, G. P., Chabner, B., Schein, P., Hubbard, S. P., and Young, R. C., 1975, Advanced diffuse histiocytic lymphoma, a potentially curable disease, *Lancet* **1**:248–250.

DeVita, V. T., Canellos, G., Hubbard, S., Chabner, B., and Young, R., 1976, Chemotherapy of Hodgkin's disease (HD) with MOPP: A ten year progress report, *Proc. Am. Assoc. Cancer Res., Am. Soc. Clin. Oncol.* **17**:269 (Abs. C-131).

Easson, E. C., and Russell, M. H., 1963, The cure of Hodgkin's disease, *Br. Med. J.* **1**:1704–1707.

Ezdinli, E. Z., Sokal, J. E., Aungst, C. W., Kim, U., and Sandberg, A. A., 1969, Myeloid leukemia in Hodgkin's disease: Chromosomal abnormalities, *Ann. Intern. Med.* **71**:1097–1104.

Gilbert, R., 1939, Radiotherapy in Hodgkin's disease (malignant granulomatosis), *Am. J. Roentgenol. Radium Ther.* **41**:198–241.

Glatstein, E., Guernsey, J. M., Rosenberg, S. A., and Kaplan, H. S., 1969, The value of laparotomy and splenectomy in the staging of Hodgkin's disease, *Cancer* **24**:709–718.

Glicksman, A. S., and Nickson, J. J., 1973, Acute and late reactions to irradiation in the treatment of Hodgkin's disease, *Arch. Intern. Med.* **131**:369–373.

Goffinet, D. R., Castellino, R. A., Kim, H., Dorfman, R. F., Fuks, Z., Rosenberg, S. A., Nelsen, T., and Kaplan, H. S., 1973, Staging laparotomies in unselected previously untreated patients with non-Hodgkin's lymphomas, *Cancer* **32**:672–681.

Grann, V., Pool, J. L., and Mayer, K., 1966, Comparative study of bone marrow aspiration and biopsy in patients with neoplastic disease, *Cancer* **19**:1898–1900.

Hoster, H. A., Dratman, M. B., Craver, L. F., and Rolnick, H. A., 1948, Hodgkin's disease, (Part 1) 1832–1947, *Cancer Res.* **8**:1–78.

Jackson, H., Jr., and Parker, F., Jr., 1947, *Hodgkin's Disease and Allied Disorders,* Oxford University Press, New York.

Johnson, R. E., 1969, Modern approaches to the radiotherapy of lymphoma, *Semin. Hematol.* **6**:357–375.

Johnson, R. E., 1975, Management of generalized malignant lymphomata with "systemic" radiotherapy, *Br. J. Cancer* **31**(Suppl. II):450–455.

Jones, S. E., Fuks, Z., Bull, M., Kadin, M. D., Dorfman, R. F., Kaplan, H. S., Rosenberg, S. A., and Kim, H., 1973a, Non-Hodgkin's lymphomas. IV. Clinicopathologic correlation in 405 cases, *Cancer* **31**:806–823.

Jones, S. E., Fuks, Z., Kaplan, H. S., and Rosenberg, S. A., 1973b, Non-Hodgkin's lymphomas. V. Results of radiotherapy, *Cancer* **32**:682–691.

Kaplan, H. S., 1962, The radical radiotherapy of regionally localized Hodgkin's disease, *Radiology* **78**:553–561.

Kaplan, H. S., 1966, Evidence for a tumoricidal dose level in the radiotherapy of Hodgkin's disease, *Cancer Res.* **26**:1221–1224.

Kaplan, H. S., 1972, *Hodgkin's Disease,* Harvard University Press, Cambridge.

Levitt, M., Marsh, J. C., DeConti, R. C., Mitchell, M. S., Skeel, R. T., Farber, L. R., and Bertino, J. R., 1972, Combination sequential chemotherapy in advanced reticulum cell sarcoma, *Cancer* **29**:630–636.

Lukes, R. J., and Collins, R. D., 1975, New approaches to the classification of the lymphomata, *Br. J. Cancer* **31**(Suppl. II):1–28.

Lukes, R. J., and Butler, J. J., and Hicks, E. B., 1966a, Natural history of Hodgkin's disease as related to its pathologic picture, *Cancer* **19**:317–344.

Lukes, R. J., Craver, L. F., Hall, T. C., Rappaport, H., and Rubin, P., 1966b, Report of the Nomenclature Committee, *Cancer Res.* **26**:1311.

Neiman, R. S., Rosen, P. J., and Lukes, R. J., 1973, Lymphocyte-depletion Hodgkin's disease: A clinicopathological entity, *N. Engl. J. Med.* **288**:751–755.

O'Connell, M. J., Wiernik, P. H., Brace, K. C., Byhardt, R. W., and Greene, W. H., 1975, A combined modality approach to the treatment of Hodgkin's disease: Preliminary results of a prospectively randomized clinical trial, *Cancer* **35**:1055–1065.

Olweny, C. L. M., Mbidde, E. K., Nkwocha, J., Magrath, I., and Ziegler, J. L., 1974, Chemotherapy of Hodgkin's disease, *Lancet* **2**:1397.

Page, V., Gardner, A., and Karzmark, C. J., 1970, Physical and dosimetric aspects of the radiotherapy of malignant lymphomas, I. The mantle technique. II. The inverted Y technique. *Radiology* **96**:609–626.

Peters, M. V., 1950, A study of survivals in Hodgkin's disease treated radiologically, *Am. J. Roentgenol.* **63**:299–311.

Portlock, C. S., and Rosenberg, S. A., 1976, Combination chemotherapy with cyclophosphamide, vincristine and prednisone in advanced non-Hodgkin's lymphomas, *Cancer* **37**:1275–1282.

Portlock, C. S., Rosenberg, S. A., Glatstein, E., and Kaplan, H. S., 1976, Treatment of advanced non-Hodgkin's lymphomas with favorable histologies: Preliminary results of a prospective trial, *Blood* **47**:747–756.

Rai, K. R., Sawitsky, A., Cronkite, E. P., Chanana, A. D., Levy, R. N., and Pasternack, B. S., 1975, Clinical staging of chronic lymphocytic leukemia, *Blood* **46**:219–234.

Rappaport, H., 1966, Tumors of the hematopoietic system, in: *Atlas of Tumor Pathology,* Section III, Fascicle 8, pp. 91–156, Armed Forces Institute of Pathology, Washington, D.C.

Ribas-Mundo, M., and Rosenberg, S. A., 1977 (unpublished).

Robb-Smith, A. H. T., 1938, Reticulosis and reticulosarcoma: A histologic classification, *J. Pathol. Bacteriol.* **47**:457–480.

Rosenberg, S. A., 1966, Report of the committee on the staging of Hodgkin's disease, *Cancer Res.* **26**:1310.

Rosenberg, S. A., 1971, Hodgkin's disease of the bone marrow, *Cancer Res.* **31**:1733–1736.

Rosenberg, S. A., 1972, Splenectomy in the management of Hodgkin's disease, *Br. J. Haematol.* **23**:271–276.

Rosenberg, S. A., 1975, Bone marrow involvement in the non-Hodgkin's lymphomata, *Br. J. Cancer* **31**(Suppl. II):261–264.

Rosenberg, S. A., and Kaplan, H. S., 1966, Evidence for an orderly progression in the spread of Hodgkin's disease, *Cancer Res.* **26**:1225–1231.

Rosenberg, S. A., and Kaplan, H. S., 1975a, The management of stages I, II, and III Hodgkin's disease with combined radiotherapy and chemotherapy, *Cancer* **35**:55–63.

Rosenberg, S. A., and Kaplan, H. S., 1975b, Clinical trials in the non-Hodgkin's lymphomata at Stanford University: Experimental design and preliminary results, *Br. J. Cancer* **31**(Suppl. II):456–464.

Rosenberg, S. A., Dorfman, R. F., and Kaplan, H. S., 1975, The value of sequential bone marrow biopsy and laparotomy and splenectomy in a series of 127 consecutive untreated patients with non-Hodgkin's lymphoma, *Br. J. Cancer* **31**(Suppl. II):221–227.

Rosenberg, S. A., Kaplan, H. S., Glatstein, E. J., and Portlock, C. S., 1978, Combined modality therapy of Hodgkin's disease: A report on the Stanford trials, *Cancer* (in press).

Schein, P. S., Chabner, B. A., Canellos, G. P., Young, R. C., Berard, C., and DeVita, V. T., Jr., 1974, Potential for prolonged disease-free survival following combination chemotherapy of non-Hodgkin's lymphomas, *Blood* **43**:181–189.

Schein, P. S., Chabner, B. A., Canellos, G. P., Young, R. C., and DeVita, V. T., 1975, Non-Hodgkin's lymphoma: Patterns of relapse from complete remission after combination chemotherapy, *Cancer* **35**:354–357.

Teillet, F., Boiron, M., and Bernard, J., 1971, A reappraisal of clinical and biological signs in staging of Hodgkin's disease, *Cancer Res.* **31**:1723–1729.

Ultmann, J. E., 1970, Current status: The management of lymphoma, *Semin. Hematol.* **7**:441–460.

Warthin, A. S., 1931, The genetic neoplastic relationships of Hodgkin's disease, aleukemic and leukemic lymphoblastoma and mycosis fungoides, *Ann. Surg.* **93**:153–161.

Index